DAVIS'S

DISEASES DISORDERS

A Nursing Therapeutics Manual

Seventh Edition

Marilyn Sawyer Sommers, PhD, RN, FAAN

Professor Emerita
University of Pennsylvania School of Nursing
Philadelphia, Pennsylvania

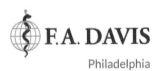

F.A. DAVIS

Philadelphia

F. A. Davis Company
1915 Arch Street
Philadelphia, PA 19103
www.fadavis.com

Printed in the United States

Last digit indicates print number: 10 9 8 7 6 5 4 3 2 1

Publisher, Nursing: Terri W. Allen
Senior Content Project Manager: Amy M. Romano
Illustration and Design Manager: Carolyn O'Brien

As new scientific information becomes available through basic and clinical research, recommended treatments and drug therapies undergo changes. The authors and publisher have done everything possible to make this book accurate, up to date, and in accord with accepted standards at the time of publication. The authors, editors, and publisher are not responsible for errors or omissions or for consequences from application of the book, and make no warranty, expressed or implied, in regard to the contents of the book. Any practice described in this book should be applied by the reader in accordance with professional standards of care used in regard to the unique circumstances that may apply in each situation. The reader is advised always to check product information (package inserts) for changes and new information regarding dose and contraindications before administering any drug. Caution is especially urged when using new or infrequently ordered drugs.

Library of Congress Cataloging-in-Publication Data

Names: Sommers, Marilyn Sawyer, author.
Title: Davis's diseases and disorders : a nursing therapeutic manual / Marilyn Sawyer
      Sommers.
Other titles: Diseases and disorders
Description: Seventh edition. | Philadelphia : F.A. Davis Company, 2022. | Includes
      bibliographical references and index.
Identifiers: LCCN 2022004787 (print) | LCCN 2022004788 (ebook) | ISBN 9781719645492
      (paperback) | ISBN 9781719648394 (ebook)
Subjects: MESH: Nursing Care--methods | Nursing Process | Handbook
Classification: LCC RT51 (print) | LCC RT51 (ebook) | NLM WY 49 | DDC
      610.73--dc23/eng/20220207
LC record available at https://lccn.loc.gov/2022004787
LC ebook record available at https://lccn.loc.gov/2022004788

Dedication

With a loving eye on the future: To Abigail, Sophia, Joshua, Jonah, and Ari

With a grateful eye on the past: To Mother and Dad

MSS

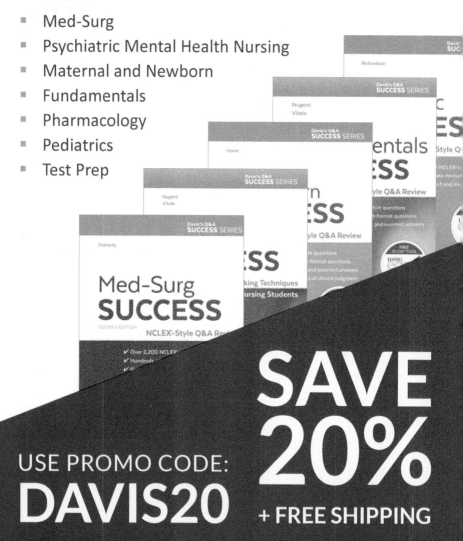

Preface

The seventh edition of *Davis's Diseases and Disorders* was revised during the year of an outbreak of the severe acute respiratory syndrome coronavirus 2 (SARS-CoV-2), more commonly known as COVID-19. The World Health Organization declared a global pandemic on March 11, 2020 (Majumder & Minko, 2021), and the revision of the book was completed during 2021 as infections waxed and waned across the world. Just as COVID-19 affected all of us with respect to our individual, family, and work lives, it also affected the revision of the book. First, it highlighted the fact that emerging infectious diseases may be our future way of life. They are outbreaks of previously unknown diseases that persist in an uncontrolled manner and respect no national boundaries. They threaten the health and safety of all people because prevention strategies, control recommendations, and care guidelines may not be immediately available when the disease appears (National Institute of Allergy and Infectious Diseases, 2018). Second, COVID-19 also brought to the forefront inequities and disparities in the risk of disease and healthcare delivery that people experience (see **Emerging Infectious Diseases**).

Health disparities are preventable differences in the burden of disease, injury, and violence, or in opportunities to achieve optimal health experienced by socially disadvantaged racial, ethnic, income, and other population groups and communities (CDC, 2017; Healthy People, 2021). While health disparities have been an issue of concern for many years, COVID-19 brought these differences into high relief over a short period of time. The most persistent disparities in the incidence of COVID-19 occurred in Native Hawaiian and Pacific Islander, American Indian, Alaska Native, Hispanic, and Black persons as compared to non-Hispanic White persons (Van Dyke et al., 2021). The reasons for these discrepancies may include inequities in COVID-19 testing and the fact that Hispanic and Black persons are overrepresented in the essential workforce leading to higher risk for exposure. The U.S. Commission on Civil Rights (2021) reported that COVID-19 has had a disproportionate toll on Native American communities as well. They note that the Navajo Nation experienced one of the highest infection rates in the United States. Additionally, discrimination in healthcare and living in urban areas may increase risk for exposure. In contrast, people living in rural areas may have longer distances to travel to receive healthcare from COVID-19 specialists and are less likely to receive medical care guided by standard guidelines than those at large medical centers. Because sexual and gender minority persons have been historically affected disproportionately by lack of health insurance, poverty, discrimination, mental health disorders, and substance use disorders as compared to nongender and sexual minority persons, COVID-19 presents additional burdens for them (O'Neill, 2020).

While these issues are specific to COVID-19, investigation into the healthcare literature demonstrates the particular need to highlight health disparities in multiple conditions such as Heart Failure and Cerebral Concussion. For this reason, a new section titled **Health Disparities and Sexual/Gender Minority Health** has been added in all entries to reflect the importance of differences in health risks and outcomes across populations. The term sexual/gender minority health describes the unique healthcare needs of persons including but not limited to those who identify as lesbian, gay, bisexual, transgender, or queer, all of whom face unique stigma and discrimination in the healthcare setting. The section titled **Global Health Considerations** has been updated to reflect a global society where many families migrate to, travel to, and live on multiple continents. This section acknowledges that the health of world populations becomes as important as the health of a neighborhood. Human papillomavirus and *Trichomonas vaginalis* infections are threatening the health of a generation of young people. In addition to infectious diseases, cardiovascular disease, lung disease, poor nutrition, violence, and injury cause death and disability around the world. By cultivating a global perspective, students and practicing nurses can prepare themselves for the next decades of healthcare. In the section titled **Evidence-Based Practice and Health Policy**, specific research studies or policy briefs have been chosen that relate to each entry and provide current information to guide nursing practice. The cited studies were selected because of their timeliness, relationship to nursing practice, and introduction of innovative therapies to improve health. I am indebted to Kaitlyn Shen, a geneticist at the University of Pennsylvania, who worked with me to update and expand the **Genetic Considerations** sections. As the volume of material about the genetic basis of disease proliferates, and as our understanding increases about how genetic and environmental factors relate to health and disease, this content has become essential to nursing practice.

Each entry begins with the Diagnosis Related Group (DRG) category. DRGs were initiated by the Health Care Financing Administration to serve as an organizing framework to group related conditions and to stabilize reimbursements. Because they provide a convenient standard to evaluate hospital care, DRGs are used by institutions and disciplines to measure utilization and to allocate resources. DRGs are included to indicate the expected norms in average length of hospital stay for each entry (Mean LOS). In addition, entries begin with the background information on epidemiology and physiology, causation, and considerations including genetics, gender, race/ethnicity, life span, health disparities, gender/minority health, and global health. I recognize that race, ethnicity, and gender are social and political constructs. Just as there are many races, there are also many genders, and categorizing people into groups, including a gender binary of male and female, does not represent the individuals for whom we provide care. I have tried to consider issues of race, ethnicity, and gender without stereotyping, but rather to inform nursing care. I will continue to work toward a goal of health equity in coming editions. Each entry follows the nursing process, with assessment information incorporated in the **History** and **Physical Assessment** sections, **Psychosocial Assessment**, and **Diagnostic Highlights**. These detailed, specific sections provide the foundation needed to perform a comprehensive assessment of the patient's condition so that a **Primary Nursing Diagnosis** can be formulated that is appropriate to the patient's specific needs (Butcher et al., 2018; Herdman et al., 2021; Moorhead et al., 2018). The **Planning and Implementation** section is divided into **Collaborative** and **Independent** interventions. The intent of the Collaborative section is to detail the goals of a multidisciplinary plan of care to manage the condition or disease. As in the first six editions, there is an expanded section on **Pharmacologic Highlights** that explores commonly used drugs, along with their doses, mechanisms of action, and rationales for use. The **Independent** section focuses on independent nursing interventions that demonstrate the core of the art and science of nursing. Each entry then finishes with **Evidence-Based Practice and Health Policy, Documentation Guidelines,** and **Discharge and Home Healthcare Guidelines** to help nurses evaluate the outcomes of care and to prepare hospitalized patients for discharge.

As with each preceding edition, the team at F. A. Davis has made the revision of the book much easier, and I am grateful to Rob Allen, Terri Allen, and Amy Romano for their patience, support, and assistance. I am also particularly grateful to Gloria Coats, Taralyn McMullan, and Karyn Morgan, who made important contributions to the revision of the seventh edition. The entire reason to revise this book is to provide practicing nurses a concise yet current and scientifically sound text to guide the professional practice of nursing. The provision of nursing care in the 21st century presents us with overwhelming challenges, and yet nursing is the discipline of choice for millions of practitioners. I hope this book honors the science of nursing and makes it easier to practice the art of nursing.

MARILYN (LYNN) S. SOMMERS

REFERENCES

Butcher, H., Bulechek, G., Dochterman, J., & Wagner, C. (2018). *Nursing interventions classification* (7th ed.). Elsevier.

Centers for Disease Control and Prevention. (2017). *Health disparities.* https://www.cdc.gov/aging/disparities/index.htm

Healthy People. (2021). *Disparities.* https://www.healthypeople.gov/2020/about/foundation-health-measures/Disparities

Herdman, T., Kamitsuru, S., & Lopes, C. (2021). *NANDA International, Inc. nursing diagnoses: Definitions and classification, 2021–2023.* Thieme.

Majumder, J., & Minko, T. (2021). Recent developments on therapeutic and diagnostic approaches for COVID-19. *AAPS Journal, 23*(14). https://doi.org/10.1208/s12248-020-00532-2

Moorhead, S., Swanson, E., Johnson, M., & Maas, M. (2018). *Nursing Outcomes Classification: Measurement of health outcomes* (6th ed.). Elsevier.

National Institute of Allergy and Infectious Diseases. (2018). *NIAID emerging infectious diseases/pathogens.* https://www.niaid.nih.gov/research/emerging-infectious-diseases-pathogens

O'Neill, K. (2020). *Economic vulnerabilities to COVID-19 among LGBT adults in California.* https://escholarship.org/uc/item/1zh0q62v

U.S. Commission on Civil Rights. (2021). *The COVID-19 and Native American community.* https://www.usccr.gov/files/2021/05-19-AZ-Memo-COVID-19-Native-Americans.pdf

Van Dyke, M., Mendoza, M., Li, W., Parker, E., Belay, B., Davis, E., Quint, J., Penman-Aguilar, A., & Clarke, K. (2021). Racial and ethnic disparities in COVID-19 incidence by age, sex, and period among persons aged < 25 years—16 US jurisdictions, January 1–December 31, 2020. *Morbidity and Mortality Weekly Reports, 70*(11), 382–388.

Consultants for 7th Edition

Kaitlyn M. Shen, BS, PhDc
University of Pennsylvania
Philadelphia, Pennsylvania

Gloria Haile Coats, MSN, RN, FNP
Professor Emerta
Modesto Junior College, Modesto,
  California
Assistant Clinical Professor
California State University, Stanislaus,
  California

Taralyn McMullan, DNP, RN, CNS-BC
Associate Professor
University of South Alabama
Mobile, Alabama

Karyn I. Morgan, MSN, APRN-CNS
Professor Emerita
University of Akron
Akron, Ohio

Reviewers

Dr. Victoria Haynes, DNP, APRN, FNP-C
Tenured Professor of Nursing
Coordinator of Diversity & Cultural
  Competency
MidAmerica Nazarene University
Olathe, Kansas

**Hiba Wehbe-Alamah, PhD, RN,
FNP-BC, CTN-A, FAAN**
Professor, School of Nursing
Michigan Distinguished Professor
University of Michigan-Flint
Flint, Michigan

Contents

Nursing Diagnoses Accepted for Use and Research*

Activity Intolerance
Activity Intolerance, risk for
Airway Clearance, ineffective
Allergy Response, latex
Allergy Response, risk for latex
Anxiety [mild, moderate, severe, panic]
Anxiety, death
Aspiration, risk for
Attachment, risk for impaired
  parent/child
Autonomic Dysreflexia
Autonomic Dysreflexia, risk for

Behavior, risk-prone health
Body Image, disturbed
Body Temperature, risk for imbalanced
Bowel Incontinence
Breastfeeding, effective
Breastfeeding, ineffective
Breastfeeding, interrupted
Breathing Pattern, ineffective

Cardiac Output, decreased
Caregiver Role Strain
Caregiver Role Strain, risk for
Comfort, readiness for enhanced
Communication, impaired verbal
Communication, readiness for enhanced
Conflict, decisional (specify)
Conflict, parental role
Confusion, acute
Confusion, chronic
Constipation
Constipation, perceived
Constipation, risk for
Contamination
Contamination, risk for
Coping, compromised family
Coping, defensive
Coping, disabled family
Coping, ineffective
Coping, ineffective community
Coping, readiness for enhanced
Coping, readiness for enhanced
  community
Coping, readiness for enhanced family

Death Syndrome, risk for sudden infant
Decision Making, readiness for enhanced
Denial, ineffective
Dentition, impaired
Development, risk for delayed
Diarrhea
Disuse Syndrome, risk for
Diversional Activity, deficient

Energy Field, disturbed
Environmental Interpretation Syndrome,
  impaired
Failure to Thrive, adult
Falls, risk for
Family Processes: alcoholism,
  dysfunctional
Family Processes, interrupted
Family Processes, readiness for enhanced
Fear [specify focus]
Fluid Balance, readiness for enhanced
Fluid Volume, deficient (hyper/hypotonic)
Fluid Volume, deficient (isotonic)
Fluid Volume, excess
Fluid Volume, risk for deficient
Fluid Volume, risk for imbalanced

Gas Exchange, impaired
Glucose, risk for unstable blood
Grieving
Grieving, complicated
Grieving, risk for complicated
Growth, risk for disproportionate
Growth and Development, delayed

Health Maintenance, ineffective
Health-Seeking Behaviors (specify)
Home Maintenance, impaired
Hope, readiness for enhanced
Hopelessness
Hyperthermia
Hypothermia

Identity, disturbed personal
Immunization Status, readiness for
  enhanced
Infant Behavior, disorganized

Infant Behavior, readiness for enhanced organized
Infant Behavior, risk for disorganized
Infant Feeding Pattern, ineffective
Infection, risk for
Injury, risk for
Injury, risk for perioperative positioning
Insomnia
Intracranial Adaptive Capacity, decreased

Knowledge (specify), readiness for enhanced

Lifestyle, sedentary
Liver Function, risk for impaired
Loneliness, risk for

Memory, impaired
Mobility, impaired bed
Mobility, impaired physical [specify level]
Moral Distress

Neglect, unilateral
Noncompliance [Adherence, ineffective] (specify)
Nutrition: less than body requirements, imbalanced
Nutrition: more than body requirements, imbalanced
Nutrition, readiness for enhanced
Nutrition: risk for more than body requirements, imbalanced

Oral Mucous Membrane, impaired

Pain, acute
Pain, chronic
Parenting, impaired
Parenting, readiness for enhanced
Parenting, risk for impaired
Peripheral Neurovascular Dysfunction, risk for
Poisoning, risk for
Post-Trauma Syndrome [specify stage]
Post-Trauma Syndrome, risk for
Power, readiness for enhanced
Powerlessness [specify level]
Powerlessness, risk for
Protection, ineffective

Rape-Trauma Syndrome
Rape-Trauma Syndrome: compound reaction

Rape-Trauma Syndrome: silent reaction
Religiosity, impaired
Religiosity, readiness for enhanced
Religiosity, risk for impaired
Relocation Stress Syndrome, risk for
Role Performance, ineffective

Self-Care, readiness for enhanced
Self-Care Deficit [specify level]: feeding, bathing/hygiene, dressing/grooming, toileting
Self-Concept, readiness for enhanced
Self-Esteem, chronic low
Self-Esteem, situational low
Self-Esteem, risk for situational low
Self-Mutilation
Self-Mutilation, risk for
Sensory Perception, disturbed (specify: visual, auditory, kinesthetic, gustatory, tactile, olfactory)
Sexuality Dysfunction
Sexuality Patterns, ineffective
Skin Integrity, impaired
Skin Integrity, risk for impaired
Sleep, readiness for enhanced
Social Interaction, impaired
Social Isolation
Sorrow, chronic
Spiritual Distress
Spiritual Distress, risk for
Spiritual Well-Being, readiness for enhanced
Stress Overload
Suffocation, risk for
Suicide, risk for
Surgical Recovery, delayed
Swallowing, impaired

Therapeutic Regimen Management, effective
Therapeutic Regimen Management, ineffective
Therapeutic Regimen Management, ineffective community
Therapeutic Regimen Management, ineffective family
Therapeutic Regimen Management, readiness for enhanced
Thermoregulation, ineffective
Thought Processes, disturbed
Tissue Integrity, impaired

Tissue Perfusion, ineffective (specify):
  renal, cerebral, cardiopulmonary,
  gastrointestinal, peripheral
Transfer Ability, impaired
Trauma, risk for

Urinary Elimination, impaired
Urinary Elimination, readiness for enhanced
Urinary Incontinence, functional
Urinary Incontinence, overflow
Urinary Incontinence, reflex
Urinary Incontinence, risk for urge
Urinary Incontinence, stress
Urinary Incontinence, total
Urinary Incontinence, urge
Urinary Retention [acute/chronic]

Ventilation, impaired spontaneous
Ventilatory Weaning Response, dysfunctional

Violence, [actual]/risk for other-directed
Violence, [actual]/risk for self-directed

Walking, impaired
Wandering [specify sporadic or continual]

T. Heather Herdman/Shigemi Kamitsuru
  (Eds.), NANDA International, Inc.
  Nursing Diagnoses: Definitions and
  Classification 2018–2020, Eleventh
  Edition © 2017 NANDA International,
  ISBN 978-1-6262-3929-6. Used by
  arrangement with the Thieme Group,
  Stuttgart/New York.
Information that appears in brackets has
  been added by the authors to clarify
  and enhance the use of these nursing
  diagnoses.

---

*In order to make safe and effective judgments using NANDA-I nursing diagnoses, it is essential that nurses refer to the definitions and defining characteristics of the diagnoses listed in this work.

Abdominal Aortic Aneurysm

DRG Category:	270
Mean LOS:	9.4 days
Description:	SURGICAL: Other Major Cardiovascular Procedures With Major Complication or Comorbidity
DRG Category:	300
Mean LOS:	4.0 days
Description:	MEDICAL: Peripheral Vascular Disorder With Complication or Comorbidity

An abdominal aortic aneurysm (AAA) is a localized outpouching or dilation of the arterial wall in the latter portion of the descending segment of the aorta. It is most commonly located in the infrarenal aorta (below the kidneys). The dilation increases the diameter of the vessel by at least 50% from baseline, with the aortic diameter reaching at least 3 cm. AAAs are the most common type of arterial aneurysms, occurring in 3% to 10% of people older than 50 years of age in the United States. AAAs may be fusiform (spindle-shaped) or saccular (pouchlike) in shape. A fusiform aneurysm in which the dilated area encircles the entire aorta is most common. A saccular aneurysm has a dilated area on only one side of the vessel.

The outpouching of the wall of the aorta occurs when the musculoelastic middle layer or media of the artery becomes weak. Degradation of structural proteins (elastin and collagen), inflammation and immune responses, stress and stretching of the inner and outer layers of the arterial wall, and genetic changes are all important mechanisms in the development of aneurysms. AAAs often occur in people with advanced atherosclerosis, which may lead to weakening of the aortic wall and degenerative changes. While the two conditions (AAA and atherosclerosis) are associated with each other, most experts suggest that the development of AAAs occurs because of multiple factors. People who experience a ruptured AAA are gravely ill, and more than half do not survive if the rupture occurs outside the hospital. Early detection and elective rather than emergent repair are therefore the goals of care. More than half of people with untreated aneurysms die of aneurysm rupture within 2 years.

CAUSES

Ninety percent of AAAs are believed to be degenerative in origin; 5% are inflammatory. Other causes include high blood pressure, heredity, connective tissue disorders, trauma, and infections (syphilis, tuberculosis, and endocarditis). Chronic obstructive pulmonary disease is a risk factor as are increased height and weight (increased body surface areas), and smoking is a contributing cause.

GENETIC CONSIDERATIONS

It is increasingly clear that there are genetic factors that make one susceptible to an AAA, with an estimated heritability of 70%. There have been observations of both autosomal dominant and recessive inheritance patterns. Recent work has provided evidence for genetic heterogeneity and the presence of susceptibility loci for AAAs on chromosomes 1q32.3, 4q31, 9p21, 12q13.3, 13q12.11, 19q13, and 21q22.2. Family clustering of AAAs has been noted in 15% to 25% of patients undergoing surgery for AAAs. In addition, AAAs are seen in rare genetic diseases such as Ehlers-Danlos syndrome or Marfan syndrome.

SEX AND LIFE SPAN CONSIDERATIONS

Abdominal aneurysms are more common in hypertensive men than women; from four to five times as many men as women develop AAAs. Estimates are that they are found in 1% to 2% of all men over age 55 years. The incidence of AAA increases with age and peaks in the eighth decade of life. The occurrence is rare before age 50 years, common between the ages of 60 and 80 years, and more pronounced in men who have a smoking history. Aneurysms in women are known to rupture at a smaller size than in men.

HEALTH DISPARITIES AND SEXUAL/GENDER MINORITY HEALTH

AAAs are 3.5 times more common in White men than men of other races and ethnicities. AAAs are uncommon in Black, Asian, and Hispanic people. In a large study of more than 100,000 people living in five states in the United States who underwent AAA repair, uninsured and Medicaid patients had a higher mortality rate when compared to insured patients (Rozental et al., 2020). This study demonstrated that lower income and lack of insurance contributed to health disparities. Experts have found that gay men report higher rates of smoking, a contributing cause of AAA, than heterosexual men, placing gay men at risk. Sexual minority women report a higher number of risk factors for AAA as compared to heterosexual women, including mental distress, current smoking, and obesity (Caceres et al., 2019).

GLOBAL HEALTH CONSIDERATIONS

The incidence of AAAs is 4% to 9% in men and 1% in women who live in Asia and Europe.

▒ ASSESSMENT

HISTORY. Seventy-five percent of AAAs are **asymptomatic** and are found by screening or incidentally during radiological procedures such as computed tomography (CT). When the aorta enlarges and compresses the surrounding structures, patients may describe back, flank, abdominal, or groin **pain**; epigastric discomfort; or altered bowel or urinary elimination. The pain may be deep and steady with no change if the patient shifts position. If the patient reports severe back and abdominal pain, rupture of the AAA may be imminent.

PHYSICAL EXAMINATION. Symptoms of an AAA may be vague, and misdiagnosis is fairly common. Inspect the patient's abdomen for a pulsating abdominal mass in the periumbilical area, slightly to the left of midline. Auscultate over the pulsating area for an audible bruit. Gently palpate the area to determine the size of the mass and whether tenderness is present.

Watch for signs that may indicate impending aneurysm rupture, such as **syncope** (transient loss of consciousness and postural tone). Note subtle changes, such as a change in the characteristics and quality of peripheral pulses, changes in neurological status, and changes in vital signs such as a drop in blood pressure, increased pulse, and increased respirations. An abdominal aneurysm can impair flow to the lower extremities and cause what are known as the five Ps of ischemia: pain, pallor, pulselessness, paresthesias, and paralysis.

Because emergency surgery is indicated for both a rupture and a threatened rupture, serial and thorough assessments are important. When the aneurysm ruptures into the retroperitoneal space, hemorrhage is confined by surrounding structures, preventing immediate death by loss of blood. Examine the patient for signs of shock, including decreased capillary refill, increased pulse and respirations, a drop in urine output, weak peripheral pulses, and cool and clammy skin. When the rupture occurs anteriorly into the peritoneal cavity, rapid hemorrhage generally occurs. The patient's vital signs and vital functions diminish rapidly, and the patient may exhibit frank shock (cyanosis, mottling, loss of consciousness, cardiovascular collapse). The shorter the time to surgery, the better is the outcome.

PSYCHOSOCIAL. In most cases, the patient with an AAA faces hospitalization, a surgical procedure, a possible stay in an intensive care unit, and a substantial recovery period. Therefore, assess the patient's coping mechanisms and existing support systems. Assess the patient's and significant others' anxiety levels regarding surgery and the recovery process.

Diagnostic Highlights

General Comments: Because this condition often causes no symptoms, it may be diagnosed through routine physical examinations or abdominal x-rays.

Test	Normal Result	Abnormality With Condition	Explanation
Standard test: Abdominal ultrasonography for initial diagnosis	Normal aortic diameter (2-cm diameter)	Widened aorta > 3 cm in diameter	Determines presence of dilation of the infrarenal aorta
CT scan	Normal aortic diameter (2-cm diameter)	Locates outpouching within the aortic wall; widened aorta > 3 cm	Reliable assessment of size and location of aneurysm; aortic diameter exceeds 3 cm but usually will not rupture until > 5 cm; contrast-enhanced CT shows arterial anatomy; intra-aortic computed tomography angiography (IA-CTA) allows for visualization of the Adamkiewicz artery, which is important for spinal cord perfusion
Abdominal x-ray	Negative study	May show location of aneurysm with an "eggshell" appearance; AAA is evident by curvilinear calcification in the anterior wall of the aorta, displaced significantly anterior from the vertebrae	Assesses size and location of aneurysm; aortic wall calcification is seen only 50% of the time (low sensitivity); should not be used for sole purpose of evaluating a suspected AAA because of low diagnostic value

Other Tests: Magnetic resonance, aortography, complete blood count.

PRIMARY NURSING DIAGNOSIS

DIAGNOSIS. Risk for bleeding as evidenced by active fluid volume loss from hemorrhage

OUTCOMES. Fluid balance; Blood loss severity; Circulation status; Cardiac pump effectiveness; Cardiopulmonary status

INTERVENTIONS. Shock management: Volume; Fluid resuscitation; Blood product administration; IV therapy; Bleeding reduction; Fluid management

⬛ PLANNING AND IMPLEMENTATION

Collaborative

PREOPERATIVE. Over time, most patients without symptoms eventually require surgery because long-term mortality approaches 100% without intervention. The choice of surgical repair depends on careful decision making about risk and benefit by the patient, family, and healthcare team. The treatment for AAAs 5.5 cm or greater in size is generally surgical repair, although some experts recommend following patients with ultrasound imaging regularly without surgery. If the AAA is 3 to 4.5 cm, the patient usually will have regular monitoring with ultrasound imaging, with surgical intervention only if the aneurysm expands. Generally, patients with AAAs greater than 4.5 cm are referred to a vascular surgeon. There is increasing evidence suggesting that a beta blocker, particularly propranolol, may decrease the rate of AAA expansion, and blood pressure control and smoking cessation are important. Other experts suggest elective surgical repair regardless of aneurysm size. If the aneurysm is leaking or about to rupture, immediate surgical intervention is required to improve survival rates. Approximately 80% of people with an aortic rupture do not survive.

SURGICAL. Endovascular aneurysm repair (EVAR) is the most common approach to repair an AAA, although open surgical repair is also used. EVAR is a minimally invasive method that involves the placement of an expandable stent graft within the aorta through a small incision in the groin. EVAR is associated with lower perioperative and long-term mortality than is open surgical repair, as well as with more graft-related complications, higher cost, and generally a shorter hospital stay. With the open approach, typically, an abdominal or retroperitoneal incision is made, the aneurysm is opened, clots and debris are removed, and a synthetic graft is inserted within the natural arterial wall and then sutured. During this procedure, the aorta is cross-clamped proximally and distally to the aneurysm to allow the graft to take hold. The patient is treated with heparin during the procedure to decrease the clotting of pooled blood in the lower extremities.

POSTOPERATIVE. Patients with EVAR are usually sent to a floor care area for several days. Endoleaks (blood leaking back into the aneurysm) are the most common complication with EVAR. Other complications that may occur following EVAR include bleeding or infection at the groin site, loss of circulation in the legs and bowels, deep vein thrombosis, graft infection, and nerve damage that may affect sexual functioning in males. Following the open procedure, patients typically spend 2 to 3 days in the intensive care setting until their condition stabilizes. Monitor their cardiac and circulatory status closely, and pay particular attention to the presence or absence of peripheral pulses and the temperature and color of the feet. Immediately report to the physician any absent or diminished pulse or cool, pale, mottled, or painful extremity. These signs could indicate an obstructed or leaking graft. Ventricular dysrhythmias are common in the postoperative period because of hypoxemia (deficient oxygen in the blood), hypothermia (temperature drop), and electrolyte imbalances. An endotracheal tube may be inserted to support ventilation. An arterial line, central venous pressure line, and peripheral IV lines are all typically ordered to maintain and monitor fluid balance. Adequate blood volume is supported to ensure patency of the graft and to prevent clotting of the graft as a result of low blood flow. Foley catheters are also used to assist with urinary drainage as well as with accurate intake and output measurements. Monitor for signs of infection; watch for temperature and white blood cell count elevations. Observe the abdominal wound closely, noting poor wound approximation, redness, swelling, drainage, or odor. Also report pain, tenderness, and redness in the calf of the patient's leg. These symptoms may indicate thrombophlebitis from clot formation. If the patient develops severe postoperative back pain, notify the surgeon immediately; pain may indicate that a graft is tearing.

Pharmacologic Highlights

Medication or Drug Class	Dosage	Description	Rationale
Morphine	1–10 mg IV	Opioid analgesic	Relieves surgical pain
Fentanyl	50–100 mcg IV	Opioid analgesic	Relieves surgical pain
Antihypertensives and/or diuretics	Varies by drug	Varies by drug	Rising blood pressure may stress graft suture lines

Ultrashort-acting beta1 blocker, esmolol, may be used for elevated arterial pressure and is often used in conjunction with nitroprusside. If surgical treatment is contraindicated or not required, evidence exists that the following drugs may decrease the risk of AAA expansion or reduce the potential for complications: statins, antiplatelet therapy, angiotensin-converting enzyme inhibitors, roxithromycin, and doxycycline.

Independent

PREOPERATIVE. Teach the patient about the disease process, breathing and leg exercises, the surgical procedure, and postoperative routines. Support the patient by encouraging them to share fears, questions, and concerns. When appropriate, include support persons in the discussions. Note that the surgical procedure may be performed on an emergency basis, which limits the time available for preoperative instruction. If the patient is admitted in shock, support airway, breathing, and circulation, and expedite the surgical procedure. If the patient is to have ongoing surveillance rather than surgery, provide information on follow-up annual diagnostic testing.

POSTOPERATIVE. Keep the incision clean and dry. Inspect the dressing every hour to check for bleeding. Use sterile techniques for all dressing changes. If the open procedure is warranted, assist the patient with coughing and deep breathing after extubation. Splint the incision with pillows, provide adequate pain relief prior to coughing sessions, and position the patient with the head of the bed elevated to facilitate coughing. Turn the patient side to side every 2 hours to promote good ventilation and to limit skin breakdown.

Remember that emergency surgery is a time of extreme anxiety for both the patient and the significant others. Answer all questions, provide emotional support, and explain all procedures carefully. If the patient or family is not able to cope effectively, you may need to refer them for counseling.

Evidence-Based Practice and Health Policy

Antoniou, G. A., Antoniou, S. A., & Torella, F. (2020). Endovascular vs. open repair for abdominal aortic aneurysm: Systemic review and meta-analysis of updated peri-operative and long term data of randomized controlled trials. *European Journal of Vascular Surgery, 59*(3), 385–397.

- The authors studied data from seven randomized controlled trials reporting on the outcomes of EVAR as compared to open repair in patients with nonruptured AAA. The trials included 2,938 patients.
- They found significantly lower odds of 30-day and in-hospital mortality with EVAR as compared to open repair. Long-term outcomes (over 8 years), however, demonstrated lower risk of aneurysm-related mortality and aneurysm rupture in patients with the open repair as compared to EVAR. In the short term, EVAR was related to lower risk, but in the long term, open repair was related to lower risk.

DOCUMENTATION GUIDELINES

- Location, intensity, and frequency of pain and the factors that relieve pain
- Appearance of groin or abdominal wound (color, temperature, intactness, drainage)
- Evidence of stability of vital signs, hydration status, bowel sounds, electrolytes
- Presence of complications: EVAR: Endoleaks, male sexual dysfunction, infection, bleeding, thrombophlebitis. Open procedure: Hypotension, graft occlusion, hypertension, cardiac dysrhythmias, infection, low urine output, thrombophlebitis, changes in consciousness, aneurysm rupture, excessive anxiety, poor wound healing

DISCHARGE AND HOME HEALTHCARE GUIDELINES

WOUND CARE. Explain the need to keep the surgical wound clean and dry. Teach the patient to observe the wound and report to the physician/practitioner any increased swelling, redness, drainage, odor, or separation of the wound edges. Also instruct the patient to notify the physician if a fever develops.

ACTIVITY RESTRICTIONS. Following EVAR, patients can walk several times a day but should limit climbing stairs to two times a day for the first few days after the procedure. They should avoid yard work, driving, and playing sports for 2 to 3 days and avoid lifting more than 10 pounds for 2 weeks. Following open repair, the activity restriction is more severe. Instruct the patient to lift nothing heavier than 5 pounds for about 6 to 12 weeks and to avoid driving until her or his physician/practitioner permits. Braking while driving may increase intra-abdominal pressure and disrupt the suture line. Most surgeons temporarily discourage activities that require pulling, pushing, or stretching, such as vacuuming, changing sheets, playing tennis and golf, mowing grass, and chopping wood.

SMOKING CESSATION. Encourage the patient to stop smoking and to attend smoking-cessation classes. Smoking-cessation materials are available through the Agency for Healthcare Research and Quality (https://www.ahrq.gov) or the National Institute on Drug Abuse (https://www.nida.nih.gov).

COMPLICATIONS FOLLOWING SURGERY. Discuss with the patient the possibility of clot formation or graft blockage. Symptoms of a clot may include pain or tenderness in the calf, and these symptoms may be accompanied by redness and warmth in the calf. Signs of graft blockage include a diminished or absent pulse and a cool, pale extremity. Tell patients to report such signs to the physician immediately. Endoleaks following EVAR generally do not cause symptoms and are usually found on follow-up visits with the physician through CT or ultrasound studies.

COMPLICATIONS FOR PATIENTS NOT REQUIRING SURGERY. Compliance with the regime of monitoring the size of the aneurysm by CT or ultrasound over time is essential. The patient needs to understand the prescribed medication to control hypertension. Advise the patient to report abdominal fullness or back pain, which may indicate a pending rupture.

Abdominal Trauma

DRG Category: 326
Mean LOS: 13.2 days
Description: SURGICAL: Stomach, Esophageal, and Duodenal Procedures With Major Complication or Comorbidity

DRG Category: 394
Mean LOS: 3.8 days
Description: MEDICAL: Other Digestive System Diagnoses With Complication or Comorbidity

Abdominal trauma accounts for approximately 15% to 20% of all trauma-related deaths. Intra-abdominal trauma is usually not a single organ system injury; as more organs are injured, the risks of organ dysfunction and death climb. The abdominal cavity contains solid, gas-filled, fluid-filled, and encapsulated organs. These organs are at greater risk for injury than other organs of the body because they have few bony structures to protect them. Although the last five ribs serve as some protection, if they are fractured, the sharp-edged bony fragments can cause further organ damage from lacerations or organ penetration (Table 1).

• **TABLE 1** Injuries to the Abdomen

ORGAN OR TISSUE	COMMON INJURIES	SYMPTOMS
Diaphragm	• Partially protected by bony structures, the diaphragm is most commonly injured by penetrating trauma (particularly gunshot wounds to the lower chest) • Automobile deceleration may lead to rapid rise in intra-abdominal pressure and a burst injury • Diaphragmatic tear usually indicates multi-organ involvement	• Decreased breath sounds • Abdominal peristalsis heard in thorax • Acute chest pain and shortness of breath may indicate diaphragmatic tear • May be hard to diagnose because of multisystem trauma, or the liver may "plug" the defect and mask it
Esophagus	• Penetrating injury is more common than blunt injury • May be caused by knives, bullets, foreign body obstruction, usually in the upper esophagus • May be caused by iatrogenic perforation • May be associated with cervical spine injury	• Pain at site of perforation • Fever • Difficulty swallowing • Cervical tenderness • Peritoneal irritation

(table continues on page 8)

• TABLE 1 Injuries to the Abdomen (continued)

ORGAN OR TISSUE	COMMON INJURIES	SYMPTOMS
Stomach	• Penetrating injury is more common than blunt injury; in one-third of patients, both the anterior and the posterior walls are penetrated • May occur as a complication from cardiopulmonary resuscitation or from gastric dilation	• Epigastric pain • Epigastric tenderness • Signs of peritonitis • Bloody gastric drainage
Liver	• Most commonly injured organ (both blunt and penetrating injuries); blunt injuries (70% of total) usually occur from motor vehicle crashes and steering wheel trauma • Highest mortality from blunt injury (more common in suburban areas) and gunshot wound (more common in urban areas) • Hemorrhage is most common cause of death from liver injury; overall mortality 10%–15%	• Persistent hypotension despite adequate fluid resuscitation • Guarding over right upper or lower quadrant; rebound abdominal tenderness • Dullness to percussion • Abdominal distention and peritoneal irritation • Persistent thoracic bleeding
Spleen	• Commonly injured organ with blunt abdominal trauma, often in motor vehicle crashes; most common organ injured during sports • Injured in penetrating trauma of the left upper quadrant	• Hypotension, tachycardia, shortness of breath • Peritoneal irritation • Abdominal wall tenderness • Left upper quadrant pain; pain may radiate to left shoulder • Fixed dullness to percussion in left flank; dullness to percussion in right flank that disappears with change of position
Pancreas	• Most often penetrating injury (gunshot wounds at close range) • Blunt injury from deceleration; injury from steering wheel • Often associated (40%) with other organ damage (liver, spleen, vessels)	• Pain over pancreas • Paralytic ileus • Symptoms may occur late (after 24 hr); epigastric pain radiating to back; nausea, vomiting • Tenderness to deep palpation
Small intestines	• Duodenum, ileum, and jejunum; hollow viscous structure most often injured by penetrating trauma • Gunshot wounds account for 70% of cases • Incidence of injury is third only to liver and spleen injury • When small bowel ruptures from blunt injury, rupture occurs most often at proximal jejunum and terminal ileum	• Testicular pain • Referred pain to shoulders, chest, back • Mild abdominal pain • Peritoneal irritation • Fever, jaundice, intestinal obstruction

• TABLE 1 Injuries to the Abdomen (continued)

ORGAN OR TISSUE	COMMON INJURIES	SYMPTOMS
Large intestines	• One of the more lethal injuries because of fecal contamination; occurs in 5% of abdominal injuries • More than 90% of incidences are penetrating injuries • Blunt injuries are often from safety restraints in motor vehicle crashes	• Pain, muscle rigidity • Guarding, rebound tenderness • Blood on rectal examination • Fever

Abdominal trauma can be blunt or penetrating. *Blunt injuries* occur when there is no break in the skin; they often occur as multiple injuries. In blunt injuries, the spleen and liver are the most commonly injured organs. Injury occurs from concussive and compressive forces that cause tears and hematomas to the solid organs, such as the liver, and from deceleration forces. These forces can also cause hollow organs such as the small intestines to deform; if the intraluminal pressure of hollow organs increases as they deform, the organ may rupture. Deceleration forces, such as those that occur from a sudden stop in a car or truck, may also cause stretching and tears along ligaments that support or connect organs, resulting in bleeding and organ damage. Examples of deceleration injuries include hepatic tears along the ligamentum teres (round ligament that is the fibrous remnant of the left umbilical vein of the fetus, originates at the umbilicus, and may attach to the inferior margin of the liver), damage to the renal artery intima, and mesenteric tears of the bowel.

Penetrating injuries are those associated with foreign bodies (knives, bullets) set into motion. The foreign object penetrates the abdominal cavity and dissipates energy into the organ(s) and surrounding areas. The abdominal organs and structures most commonly involved with penetrating trauma include the small bowel, colon, liver, diaphragm, and abdominal vascular structures. The most common cause of mortality in the first 24 hours is hemorrhagic shock. Complications following abdominal trauma include profuse bleeding from aortic dissection or other vascular structures, hemorrhagic shock, peritonitis, abscess formation, septic shock, paralytic ileus, ischemic bowel syndrome, acute renal failure, liver failure, adult respiratory distress syndrome, disseminated intravascular coagulation, and death.

CAUSES

More than half of the cases of blunt abdominal trauma are caused by motor vehicle crashes (MVCs) and auto-pedestrian collisions. These injuries are often associated with head and chest injuries as well. Other causes of blunt injury include falls, aggravated assaults, and contact sports. Penetrating injuries can occur from gunshot wounds (64% of total), stab wounds (31% of total), shotgun wounds (5% of total), and impalements (< 1% of total).

GENETIC CONSIDERATIONS

No clear genetic contributions to susceptibility have been defined.

SEX AND LIFE SPAN CONSIDERATIONS

Traumatic injuries, which are usually preventable, are the leading cause of death in the first four decades of life. Most blunt abdominal trauma is associated with MVCs, which are two to three times more common in males than in females in the 15- to 24-year-old age group. Penetrating injuries from gunshot wounds and stab wounds, which are on the increase in U.S. preteens, teens, and young adults, are more common in males than females. Men have different patterns of injury than women and a higher injury severity. Analysis of trauma outcomes indicates that, following traumatic injury, males have higher rates of multiple organ failure, pneumonia, and sepsis than females, creating health disparities for men (Marcolini, 2019). Trauma is the third leading cause of death in people 45 to 65 years old and the seventh leading cause of death in people older than 65 years.

HEALTH DISPARITIES AND SEXUAL/GENDER MINORITY HEALTH

In recent years, Black persons have been killed in traffic crashes at a rate almost 25% higher than White persons (National Highway Traffic Safety Administration [NHTSA, 2021]). Native American persons have the highest rate of MVC injury in the United States, more than twice the rate of Black persons (NHTSA, 2021). Experts have noted that Black and Native American communities tend to be crisscrossed by more dangerous roads than other locations, placing people from those communities at risk for injury. Penetrating injuries from gunshot wounds and stab wounds are more common in non-Hispanic Black persons than in non-Hispanic White persons. Non-Hispanic Black males have adjusted firearm death rates from two to seven times higher than males of other groups. Healthy People 2020 reports that non-Hispanic Black persons have the highest injury death rate in the United States (79.9 injury deaths per 100,000 persons), followed by non-Hispanic White persons (79.2), Native American persons (78.2), Hispanic persons (45.5), and Asian/Pacific Islander persons (25.6). Recent work has shown evidence that rural populations have injury mortality rates that are more than twice as high as urban rates. Many factors contribute to these health disparities, including the risk of traffic injury on narrow rural roads, the lack of graded curves and lighted traffic signals on rural highways, and the distance from major trauma centers. Many of the most dangerous occupations, such as mining and agriculture, are found in rural areas and can result in injury, disability, and death. Sexual and gender minority persons have high risk for dating and interpersonal violence, violence related to bullying, and intentional and unintentional injury (National Center for Health Statistics, 2021).

GLOBAL HEALTH CONSIDERATIONS

According to the World Health Organization (WHO), falls from heights of less than 5 meters are the leading cause of injury globally, but estimates are that only 6% of those are related to abdominal trauma. WHO estimates that 1.35 million people die each year from MVCs and cost most countries 3% of their gross domestic product. Globally, more than half of all traffic injuries are among vulnerable road users such as pedestrians, cyclists, and motorcyclists. More than 90% of the world's fatalities in traffic injuries occur in low- and middle-income countries. Even in high-income countries, people from lower socioeconomic backgrounds are more likely to be involved in road traffic crashes than other groups. Sub-Saharan Africa has the highest death rate from traumatic injuries in the world. Rates of firearm injury vary widely around the world, with low rates in Japan and high rates in the United States. Penetrating injury rates depend on industrialization, weapon availability, and the degree of military conflict.

ASSESSMENT

HISTORY. For patients who have experienced abdominal trauma, establish a history of the mechanism of injury by including a detailed report from the prehospital professionals, witnesses, or significant others. SAMPLE is a useful mnemonic in trauma assessment: **S**igns and symptoms, **A**llergies, **M**edications, **P**ast medical history, **L**ast meal, and **E**vents or environment leading to presentation. Information regarding the type of trauma (blunt or penetrating) is helpful. If the patient was in an MVC, determine the speed and type of the vehicle, whether the patient was restrained, the patient's position in the vehicle, and whether the patient was thrown from the vehicle on impact. If the patient was injured in a motorcycle crash, determine whether the patient was wearing a helmet. In cases of traumatic injuries from falls, determine the point of impact, the distance of the fall, and the type of landing surface. If the patient has been shot, ask the paramedics or police for ballistics information, including the caliber of the weapon and the range at which the person was shot.

PHYSICAL EXAMINATION. The patient's appearance may range from anxious but stable to critically injured with full cardiopulmonary arrest. If the patient is hemorrhaging from a critical abdominal injury, they may be profoundly hypotensive with the symptoms of hypovolemic shock (see **Hypovolemic/Hemorrhagic Shock,** p. 653). The initial evaluation or primary survey of the trauma patient is centered on assessing the Airway, Breathing, Circulation, Disability (neurological status), and Exposure (by completely undressing the patient to check all body surfaces for wounds), known as the *ABCDEs* of trauma care. The primary survey provides an initial general impression to determine the seriousness of the patient's condition. Life-saving interventions may accompany assessments made during the primary survey in the presence of life- and limb-threatening injuries. The primary survey is followed by a secondary survey, a thorough head-to-toe assessment of all organ systems with a focused history and physical examination. The assessment of the injured patient should be systematic, constant, and include reevaluation. Serial assessments are critical because large amounts of blood can accumulate in the peritoneal or pelvic cavities without early changes in the physical examination. Once the patient is stable, a tertiary survey (complete repetition of the primary and secondary surveys) is completed to determine any injuries that might have been missed during the primary and secondary surveys.

The most common signs and symptoms are **pain, abdominal tenderness,** and **gastrointestinal hemorrhage** in the alert patient. When you inspect the patient's abdomen, note any disruption from the normal appearance, such as distention, lacerations, ecchymoses, and penetrating wounds. Inspect for any signs of obvious bleeding, such as ecchymoses around the umbilicus (Cullen sign) or over the left upper quadrant, which may occur with a ruptured spleen (although these signs usually take several hours to develop). Note that Grey Turner sign, bruising of the flank area, may indicate retroperitoneal bleeding. Inspect the perineum for accompanying urinary tract injuries that may lead to bleeding from the urinary meatus, vagina, and rectum. If the patient is obviously pregnant, determine the fetal age, and monitor the patient for premature labor.

Auscultate all four abdominal quadrants for 2 minutes per quadrant to determine the presence of bowel sounds. Although the absence of bowel sounds can indicate underlying bleeding, their absence does not always indicate injury. Bowel sounds heard in the chest cavity may indicate a tear in the diaphragm. Trauma to the large abdominal blood vessels may lead to a friction rub or bruit. Bradycardia may indicate the presence of free intraperitoneal blood. Percussion of the abdomen identifies air, fluid, or tissue intra-abdominally. Air-filled spaces produce tympanic sounds as heard over the stomach. Abnormal hyperresonance can indicate free air; abnormal dullness may indicate bleeding. When you palpate the abdomen and flanks, note any increase in tenderness, which can be indicative of an underlying injury. Note any masses, rigidity, pain, and guarding. Kehr sign—radiating pain to the left shoulder when you palpate the left upper quadrant—is associated with injury to the spleen. Palpate the pelvis for injury.

PSYCHOSOCIAL. Changes in lifestyle may be required depending on the type of injury. Large incisions and scars may be present. If injury to the colon has occurred, a colostomy, whether temporary or permanent, alters the patient's body image and lifestyle. The sudden alteration in comfort, potential body image changes, and possible impaired functioning of vital organ systems can often be overwhelming and lead to maladaptive coping. Physical injury can lead to long-standing psychological trauma, posttraumatic stress disorder, and depression. Injuries that occur in the home, particularly in children, pregnant women, or older patients, may be the result of neglect, abuse, or violence. Providers are responsible for inquiring about possible neglect, abuse, or violence, which may have mandatory reporting requirements. If alcohol or other drugs of abuse were involved in the injury, determine if assessment and follow-up are needed.

Diagnostic Highlights

Test	Normal Result	Abnormality With Condition	Explanation
Contrast-enhanced computed tomography (CT) scan	Normal and intact abdominal structures	Injured or ruptured organs; accumulation of blood or air in the peritoneum, in the retroperitoneum, or above the diaphragm	Provides detailed pictures of the intra-abdominal and retroperitoneal structures, the presence of bleeding, hematoma formation, abdominal fluid accumulation, and the grade of injury
Focused abdominal sonogram for trauma (FAST); four acoustic windows (pericardiac, perihepatic, perisplenic, pelvic)	No fluid seen in four acoustic windows	Positive scan shows accumulation of blood or free fluid in the peritoneum	Provides rapid evaluation of hemoperitoneum; experts consider FAST's accuracy equal to that of diagnostic peritoneal lavage (DPL) (see below) (high specificity) to identify fluid accumulation, but negative FAST results cannot be relied on to rule out intraperitoneal injury (low sensitivity)
DPL; indicated in spinal cord injury, multiple injuries with unexplained shock, intoxicated or unresponsive patients with possible abdominal injury; in many institutions, DPL has been replaced by FAST and/or CT	Negative lavage without presence of excessive bleeding or bilious or fecal material	Direct aspiration of 15–20 mL of blood, bile, or fecal material from a peritoneal catheter; following lavage with 1 L of normal saline, the presence of 100,000/mm^3 red cells or 100–500/mm^3 white cells is a positive lavage; this is 90% sensitive for detecting intra-abdominal hemorrhage	Determines presence of intra-abdominal hemorrhage or rupture of hollow organs; contraindicated when there are existing indications for laparotomy

Other Tests: Complete blood count; coagulation profile; blood type, screen, and crossmatch; serum drug and alcohol screens; serum chemistries; serum glucose; serum amylase; serum lipase; abdominal, chest, and cervical spine radiographs; urinalysis and excretory urograms; arteriography; magnetic resonance cholangiopancreatography (MRCP) for the diagnosis of bile duct injuries.

PRIMARY NURSING DIAGNOSIS

DIAGNOSIS. Ineffective breathing pattern related to pain and abdominal distension as evidenced by tachypnea, altered chest excursion, decreased vital capacity, hypoxemia, and/or hypoventilation

OUTCOMES. Respiratory status: Gas exchange; Respiratory status: Ventilation; Symptom control; Treatment behavior: Illness or injury; Pain control; Comfort status: Physical

INTERVENTIONS. Airway management; Anxiety reduction; Oxygen therapy; Airway insertion and stabilization; Pain management: Acute; Mechanical ventilation: Pneumonia prevention; Positioning; Respiratory monitoring

PLANNING AND IMPLEMENTATION

Collaborative

The initial care of the patient with abdominal trauma follows the ABCDEs of trauma care. Measures to ensure adequate oxygenation and tissue perfusion include the establishment of an effective airway and a supplemental oxygen source, support of breathing, control of the source of blood loss, and replacement of intravascular volume. Titrate IV fluids to maintain a systolic blood pressure of 100 mm Hg; overaggressive fluid replacement may lead to recurrent or increased hemorrhage and should be avoided prior to surgical intervention to repair damage. As with any traumatic injury, treatment and stabilization of any life-threatening injuries are completed immediately.

SURGICAL. The focus is on four broad components of care: control of bleeding, identification of injuries, control of contamination, and reconstruction of the injured area. Generally, a laparotomy is performed for signs of peritonitis, rapid clinical deterioration, uncontrolled shock or hemorrhage, or positive findings on the FAST or DPL. Damage control surgery, or damage control laparotomy, is an abbreviated laparotomy that occurs after control of bleeding or hemorrhage. Techniques include intra-abdominal packing or leaving the abdominal fascia open after the surgery. Definitive surgical repair with reconstruction of the abdomen occurs 24 to 48 hours after injury. Some patients may have their intra-abdominal pressure monitored after surgery to prevent abdominal compartment syndrome.

Diaphragmatic tears are repaired surgically to prevent visceral herniation in later years. Esophageal and gastric injury are often managed with gastric decompression with a nasogastric tube, antibiotic therapy, and surgical repair of the esophageal tear. Liver injury may be managed nonoperatively or operatively, depending on the degree of injury and the amount of bleeding. Patients with liver injury are apt to experience problems with albumin formation, serum glucose levels (hypoglycemia in particular), blood coagulation, resistance to infection, and nutritional balance. Management of injuries to the spleen depends on the patient's age, stability, associated injuries, and type of splenic injury. Because removal of the spleen places the patient at risk for immune compromise, splenectomy is the treatment of choice only when the spleen is totally separated from the blood supply, when the patient is markedly hemodynamically unstable, or when the spleen is totally macerated. Treatment of pancreatic injury depends on the degree of pancreatic damage, but drainage of the area is usually necessary to prevent pancreatic fistula formation and surrounding tissue damage from pancreatic enzymes. Small and large bowel perforation or lacerations are managed by surgical exploration and repair. Preoperative and postoperative antibiotics are administered to prevent sepsis, and the patient may need to be rewarmed if hypothermia occurs.

NUTRITIONAL. Nutritional requirements may be met with the use of a small-bore feeding tube placed in the duodenum during the initial surgical procedure or at the bedside under fluoroscopy. It may be necessary to eliminate gastrointestinal feedings for extended periods of time depending on the injury and the surgical intervention required. Total parenteral nutrition may be used to provide nutritional requirements.

Pharmacologic Highlights

Medication or Drug Class	Dosage	Description	Rationale
Histamine-2 blockers	Varies with drug	Ranitidine (Zantac), cimetidine (Tagamet), famotidine (Pepcid), nizatidine (Axid)	Block gastric secretion and maintain pH of gastric contents above 4, thereby decreasing inflammation
Antibiotics	Varies with drug	Cefotetan (Cefotan) or combined therapy, often an aminoglycoside (gentamicin, tobramycin) and clindamycin (Cleocin) or metronidazole (Flagyl)	Prophylaxis to prevent infection after penetrating trauma; treatment of bacterial infection

Other Therapies: Narcotic analgesia to manage pain and limit atelectasis and pneumonia; morphine sulfate and fentanyl are the drugs of choice; axiolytics such as lorazepam reduce anxiety; generally a tetanus toxoid booster is administered.

Independent

The most important priority is the maintenance of an adequate airway, oxygen supply, breathing patterns, and circulatory status. Be prepared to assist with endotracheal intubation and mechanical ventilation by maintaining an intubation tray within immediate reach at all times. Maintain a working endotracheal suction at the bedside as well. If the patient is hemodynamically stable, position the patient for full lung expansion, usually in the semi-Fowler position with the arms elevated on pillows. If the cervical spine is at risk after an injury, maintain the body alignment and prevent flexion and extension by using a cervical collar or other strategy as dictated by trauma service protocol.

The nurse is the key to providing adequate pain control. Encourage the patient to describe and rate the pain on a scale of 1 through 10 to help you evaluate whether the pain is being controlled successfully. Consider using nonpharmacologic strategies, such as diversionary activities or massage, to manage pain as an adjunct to analgesia.

Emotional support of the patient and family is also a key nursing intervention. Patients and their families are often frightened and anxious. If the patient is awake as you implement strategies to manage the ABCs, provide a running explanation of the procedures to reassure the patient. Explain to the family the treatment alternatives and keep them updated as to the patient's response to therapy. Notify the physician if the family needs to speak to the physician about the patient's progress. If blood component therapy is essential to manage bleeding, answer the patient's and family's questions about the risks of hepatitis and HIV transmission.

Evidence-Based Practice and Health Policy

Hanna, K., Asmar, S., Ditillo, M., Chehab, M., Khurrum, M., Bible, L., Douglas, M., & Joseph, B. (2021). Readmission with major abdominal complications after penetrating abdominal trauma. *Journal of Surgical Research, 257*, 69–78.

- Major abdominal complications are a frequent occurrence following surgical treatment for penetrating abdominal trauma. The authors proposed to study all patients who had an exploratory laparotomy and were readmitted within 6 months of the injury to determine complication rates.
- They studied 4,473 patients with a mean age of 32 years. The rate of major abdominal complications within 6 months was 22%. Further analysis predicted that complications were most often associated with firearm injuries, damage control laparotomy, large bowel perforation, biliary-pancreatic injury, hepatic injury, and blood transfusion.

• Firearm injuries have a higher potential than other injuries to lead to major abdominal complications, particularly after damage control laparotomy.

DOCUMENTATION GUIDELINES

• Abdominal assessment: Description of wounds or surgical incisions, wound healing, presence of bowel sounds, location of bowel sounds, number and quality of bowel movements, patency of drainage tubes, color of urine, presence of bloody urine or clots, amount of urine, appearance of catheter insertion site, fluid balance (intake and output, patency of IV catheters, speed of fluid resuscitation)
• Comfort: Location, duration, precipitating factors of pain; response to medications; degree of pain control
• Presence of complications: Pulmonary infection, peritonitis, hemorrhage, wound infection, alcohol withdrawal
• Assessment of level of anxiety or depression, degree of understanding, adjustment, family's or partner's response, coping skills
• Understanding of and interest in patient teaching

DISCHARGE AND HOME HEALTHCARE GUIDELINES

Provide a complete explanation of all emergency treatments, and answer the patient's and family's questions. Explain the possibility of complications to recovery, such as poor wound healing, infection, and bleeding. Explain the risks of blood transfusions and answer any questions about exposure to blood-borne infections. If needed, provide information about any follow-up laboratory procedures that might be required after discharge. Provide the dates and times that the patient is to receive follow-up care with the primary healthcare provider or the trauma clinic. Give the patient a phone number to call with questions or concerns. Work with the trauma team to assess the need for home health assistance following discharge. Provide demonstration and information on how to manage any drainage systems, colostomy, IV therapies, or surgical wounds.

Abnormal Uterine Bleeding

DRG Category:	744
Mean LOS:	5.8 days
Description:	SURGICAL: Dilation and Curettage, Conization, Laparoscopy and Tubal Interruption With Complication or Comorbidity or Major Complication or Comorbidity
DRG Category:	760
Mean LOS:	3.4 days
Description:	MEDICAL: Menstrual and Other Female Reproductive System Disorders With Complication or Comorbidity or Major Complication or Comorbidity

Abnormal uterine bleeding (AUB), also known as *dysfunctional uterine bleeding*, is menorrhagia with no discernible organic cause. It is a leading cause of outpatient visits in the healthcare system in the United States. As many as 10% of women with normal ovulatory cycles experience AUB, and one in every 20 women ages 30 to 49 years consults a practitioner for the condition. The normal menstrual cycle is dependent on the influence of four hormones: estrogen, which predominates during the proliferative phase (generally days 1 to 14); progesterone, which predominates during the secretory phase (generally days 15 to 28); and follicle-stimulating hormone (FSH) and luteinizing hormone (LH), both of which stimulate the ovarian follicle to mature. Disrupting the balance of these four hormones usually results in anovulation and AUB, which is an abnormal amount, duration, or timing of bleeding.

During an anovulatory cycle, the corpus luteum does not form; thus, progesterone is not secreted. Failure of progesterone secretion allows continuous unopposed production of estradiol, which stimulates the overgrowth of the endometrium. This results in an overproduction of the uterine blood flow. Complications of AUB include anemia, infection from prolonged use of tampons, and in rare situations, hemorrhagic shock.

CAUSES

The cause of AUB is unknown. Dysfunctional bleeding indicates that it is occurring without an organic cause; thus, it is a diagnosis of exclusion. It is associated with polycystic ovarian disease and obesity; in both conditions, the endometrium is chronically stimulated by estrogen. Other possible associated factors are cancer of the vagina, cervix, ovaries, and uterus; fibroids, polyps, ectopic pregnancy, or molar pregnancy; and excessive weight gain, stress, and increased exercise performance. AUB may also occur from the use of progestin-only compounds for birth control or from contraceptive intrauterine devices (IUDs), which can cause variable vaginal bleeding for the first few cycles after placement.

GENETIC CONSIDERATIONS

Excessive menstrual bleeding is a common clinical problem in women of reproductive age. Multiple hereditary bleeding disorders, such as von Willebrand disease, factor X deficiency, or factor VII deficiency, are among the genetic causes of menorrhagia.

SEX AND LIFE SPAN CONSIDERATIONS

AUB can occur from menarche to postmenopause. AUB occurs in teenagers as the result of anovulatory cycles that are related to the immaturity of the hypothalamic-pituitary-gonadal axis. AUB is most common in the perimenopausal person as the result of changing hormonal levels. Older people approaching menopause possibly suffer from AUB because of a decreased sensitivity of the ovary to FSH and LH. Adolescent girls who suffer from AUB have significantly larger uterine volume than healthy girls, a finding that does not depend on endometrial thickness.

HEALTH DISPARITIES AND SEXUAL/GENDER MINORITY HEALTH

While AUB has no predilection for race, Black women have a higher incidence of leiomyomas and higher levels of estrogen and, as a result, are prone to experiencing more episodes of abnormal vaginal bleeding. Transgender is a term used to describe persons whose gender identity is different from their sex assigned at birth. Approximately 1% of the U.S. population identify themselves as transgender. Gender-affirming hormone therapy is the use of hormone therapy for gender transition or gender affirmation and can be masculinizing for transgender men. Typically, transgender men on testosterone can expect the end of menses within 6 months, but if they have previously had frequent cycles or heavy irregular bleeding, they may experience complications as they wait for cessation of menses. Transgender men not on testosterone and who have chosen not to undergo hysterectomy or gender-affirming genital procedures may experience AUB (Cacerese, Jackman, et al., 2020; Connelly et al., 2019; Obedin-Maliver, 2016).

GLOBAL HEALTH CONSIDERATIONS

Countries that have a large population of female athletes have a higher prevalence of AUB. Global prevalence data are not available.

☀ ASSESSMENT

HISTORY. Determine the duration of the present bleeding, the amount of blood loss, and the presence of associated symptoms such as cramping, nausea and vomiting, fever, abdominal pain, or passing of blood clots. Ask the patient to compare the number of pads or tampons used in a normal period with the amount they are presently using. Obtain a menstrual and obstetric history. Recent episodes of easy bruising or prolonged, heavy bleeding may indicate abnormal clotting times. Take a birth control history to determine if the patient is using contraceptives or an IUD. Other possible causative factors, such as pregnancy, pelvic inflammatory disease, or other medical conditions, can be ruled out through a complete history.

PHYSICAL EXAMINATION. The most common symptom is unpredictable heavy or light **irregular vaginal bleeding**. A complete examination is essential to eliminate organic causes of bleeding. A pelvic speculum and bimanual examination should be done, with particular attention paid to the presence of cervical erosion, polyps, presumptive signs of pregnancy, masses, tenderness or guarding, or other signs of pathology that may cause abnormal uterine bleeding. Assess for petechiae, purpura, and mucosal bleeding (gums) to rule out hematological pathology. Check for pallor and absence of conjunctival vessels to gauge anemia.

PSYCHOSOCIAL. For many women, AUB results in distress related to the uncertainty of the timing, duration, and amount of bleeding. Pain is a common symptom of AUB. Patients may feel that their usual activities need to be curtailed, a situation that may contribute to feelings of loss of control. Assess the severity of the symptoms as well as concerns and coping patterns to establish a framework for determining appropriate interventions.

Diagnostic Highlights

General Comments: Diagnosis of AUB is made by ruling out organic causes.

Test	Normal Result	Abnormality With Condition	Explanation
Pelvic ultrasonography or transvaginal ultrasonography	Normal uterine and ovarian structures	Abnormal structures such as ovarian cysts, fibroids, pregnancy, structural lesions	Identifies structure of uterus and ovaries
Endometrial biopsy	Presence of a "secretory-type" endometrium 3–5 days before normal menses; no pathological conditions	Hyperplastic proliferative polyps are found with AUB (polyps stimulate estrogen); with anovulation, no secretory changes are noted; adenocarcinoma indicates uterine cancer	Other organic conditions must be ruled out before a diagnosis of AUB is made
Hysteroscopy	No pathology visualized	Polyps indicate AUB; other tumors or structural variations may be seen with other conditions	Direct visualization of the uterus with biopsy

Other Tests: Pelvic examination, Pap smear, uterine ultrasound, complete blood count, cultures for sexually transmitted infections; prothrombin time, activated partial thromboplastin time, human chorionic gonadotropin (to rule out pregnancy), thyroid tests

PRIMARY NURSING DIAGNOSIS

DIAGNOSIS. Risk for bleeding as evidenced by active hemorrhage, tachycardia, hypotension, and/or pallor

OUTCOMES. Blood loss severity; Fluid balance; Hydration; Circulation status

INTERVENTIONS. Bleeding reduction; Blood product administration; Fluid monitoring; IV therapy; Shock prevention; Shock management: Volume

PLANNING AND IMPLEMENTATION

Collaborative

The patient may be confronted with a prolonged evaluation and a variety of treatments before uterine bleeding resumes a more normal pattern or stops completely. Activities are not restricted and can be continued as the patient tolerates them. If infection or anemia is identified, appropriate pharmacologic therapy is initiated. Hormonal manipulation may be indicated, requiring careful dosing and attention to compliance with the treatment plan. Surgical management, a last resort, typically begins with dilation and curettage to remove excessive endometrial buildup, but may include intrauterine cryosurgery; laser ablation of the endometrium; or, as a last resort, a hysterectomy. Hysteroscopic tubal sterilization can be performed along with the endometrial ablation if the patient desires permanent contraception.

Pharmacologic Highlights

Medication or Drug Class	Dosage	Description	Rationale
Levonorgestrel intrauterine system	Release of 20 mcg/day; system lasts for 5 yr	Intrauterine contraceptive with synthetic female hormone, levonorgestrel, which is released slowly into the uterus	Progesterone agonist
Oral contraceptives	Varies with drug	Combination (estrogen and progestin) oral contraceptives	Suppresses endometrial development, reestablishes predictable menstrual patterns and decreases flow, and lowers the risk of anemia
Naproxen	500 mg q 12 hr PO as needed	Anti-inflammatory	To reduce pain from cramping
Medroxyprogesterone acetate (Provera)	10 mg PO daily, for 10 days (days 16–25 of the menstrual cycle)	Synthetic progestin	Transforms proliferative endometrium into secretory endometrium
Conjugated estrogen (Premarin)	25 mg IV q 4 hr for three doses or until bleeding stops	Natural estrogen	Emergency treatment for severe bleeding, follow with progestins
Desmopressin	0.05 mg q 12 hr intranasally	Vasopressin-related analog	Last-resort medication for heavy bleeding

Independent

Important interventions include strategies to assist the patient in maintaining normal activities during the evaluation. Instruct the patient about the signs and symptoms of toxic shock syndrome (fever, joint and muscle aches, malaise, weakness) if they continue to use tampons; more frequent than normal changes of the tampon may be indicated. The use of incontinence pads may be more beneficial than the standard sanitary napkin in the presence of heavy bleeding.

Issues related to sexuality, especially if hysterectomy is indicated, require an accepting, open attitude of the nurse. A woman may feel her femininity is threatened but may have difficulty expressing these feelings. You may need to initiate discussions regarding the impact of evaluation and treatment on the patient. If appropriate, consider the effect on the patient's partner, and include the partner in all discussions.

Evidence-Based Practice and Health Policy

Henry, C., Jefferies, R., Ekeroma, A., & Filoche, S. (2020). Beyond the numbers—Understanding women's experiences of accessing care for abnormal uterine bleeding (AUB): A qualitative study. *British Medical Journal Open Access, 10*, Advance online publication. https://doi.org/10.1136/bmjopen-2020-041853

- The purpose of this qualitative study was to gain a deeper understanding of women's experiences of accessing care for abnormal uterine bleeding. They conducted semistructured interviews with 15 women receiving a gynecological consultation for AUB. For all women, AUB had a traumatic impact on their quality of life including relationships, education, and work.
- All women in the study sought treatment from their primary care providers. Many reported negative experiences and inadequate care. Many women were frustrated that treatment was given without investigating the cause of the abnormal bleeding. The authors note that with endometrial cancer rates rising, access and appropriate care for AUB should not be overlooked. Healthcare providers need better practice guidelines, and women need to be better educated about abnormal uterine bleeding through public health campaigns.

DOCUMENTATION GUIDELINES

- Findings on history and physical examination; complete blood count
- Records of the bleeding patterns kept by the patient
- Presence of symptoms from complications such as anemia

DISCHARGE AND HOME HEALTHCARE GUIDELINES

Provide a list of prescribed medications, if any, that includes the name, dosage, route, and side effects and the signs and symptoms of potential complications, including hypotensive episodes. Explain the need for careful monitoring and follow-up of the bleeding. Encourage the patient to keep a menstrual calendar and record daily bleeding patterns. Teach the patient to have appropriate laboratory follow-up of the complete blood count if indicated.

Abortion, Spontaneous

DRG Category:	770
Mean LOS:	2.1 days
Description:	SURGICAL: Abortion With Dilation and Curettage, Aspiration, Curettage, or Hysterectomy
DRG Category:	779
Mean LOS:	2.9 days
Description:	MEDICAL: Abortion Without Dilation and Curettage

Spontaneous abortion (SAB) is the termination of pregnancy from natural causes before the fetus is viable. Other terms include *miscarriage* and *spontaneous early pregnancy loss*. Viability is defined as 20 to 24 weeks' gestation or a fetal weight of more than 500 grams. SABs are a common occurrence in human reproduction, occurring in approximately 15% to 22% of all pregnancies. If the abortion occurs very early in the gestational period, the ovum detaches and stimulates uterine contractions that result in its expulsion. Hemorrhage into the decidua basalis followed by necrosis of tissue adjacent to the bleeding usually accompany the abortion. If the abortion occurs later in the gestation, maceration of the fetus occurs; the skull bones collapse, the abdomen distends with blood-stained fluid, and the internal organs degenerate. In addition, if the amniotic fluid is absorbed, the fetus becomes compressed and desiccated.

There are four types of SABs, classified according to symptoms (Table 1), as well as a threatened abortion. The four types of actual abortion are inevitable, incomplete, complete, and missed. A threatened abortion occurs when there is slight bleeding and cramping very early in the pregnancy; about 50% of pregnant people in this category abort. An inevitable abortion occurs when the membranes rupture, the cervix dilates, and bleeding increases. An incomplete abortion occurs when the uterus retains parts of the products of conception and the placenta. Sometimes the fetus and placenta are expelled, but part of the placenta may adhere to the wall of the uterus and lead to continued bleeding. A complete abortion occurs when all the products of conception are passed through the cervix. A missed abortion occurs when the products of conception are retained for 2 months or more after the death of the fetus. Complications include infection, bleeding, and shock. Signs and symptoms of these five types of abortion involve varying degrees of vaginal bleeding, cervical dilatation, and uterine cramping.

• TABLE 1 Types of SABs

TYPE OF ABORTION	BLEEDING	PAIN	CERVICAL DILATION	TISSUE PASSAGE
Threatened	Slight	Mild cramping	No	No
Inevitable	Moderate	Moderate cramping	Yes	No
Incomplete	Heavy	Severe cramping	Yes	Yes
Complete	Decreased; slight	Mild cramping	No	Yes
Missed	None; slight	None	No	No

CAUSES

The majority of SABs are caused by chromosomal abnormalities that are incompatible with life; the majority also have autosomal trisomies. Infections in the pregnant person, such as *Mycoplasma hominis*, *Ureaplasma urealyticum*, syphilis, HIV, group B streptococci, and second-trimester bacterial vaginosis, increase the risk for an SAB. Inherited disorders or abnormal embryonic development resulting from environmental factors (teratogens) may also play a role. A pregnant person's occupation, such as a hairstylist, may also be a factor in SAB if they are exposed to teratogens. Unfavorable environmental factors also include interpersonal violence, as pregnant people who are in abusive relationships have a 50% higher chance of pregnancy loss. Alcohol is a significant risk factor. Each additional week of alcohol exposure during the first trimester increases the risk of SAB, even at low levels of consumption.

Patients who are classified as habitual aborters (three or more consecutive SABs) usually have an incompetent cervix—that is, a situation in which the cervix is weak and does not stay closed to maintain the pregnancy. Another reason for habitual abortions may be antiphospholipid antibodies and polycystic ovarian disease. Risk factors include advanced age of pregnant person, young age of pregnant person, previous miscarriages, infections, chronic conditions such as diabetes and hypertension, exposure to chemicals, incompetent cervix, tobacco use, recent term delivery, underweight or overweight, and prenatal tests such as villus sampling and amniocentesis.

GENETIC CONSIDERATIONS

Approximately 15% of clinically recognized pregnancies end in spontaneous abortion during the first trimester. It is estimated that 50% to 70% of these fetuses have significant chromosomal abnormalities; 60% are trisomies, 20% are monosomy X, and 20% are polyploidies (multiples of a complete set of chromosomes). About 9% of aborted fetuses and 2.5% of stillbirths are due to trisomy 13, 18, or 21. Infants with trisomy 13 or 18 rarely survive the perinatal period. These abnormalities result from chromosomal nondisjunction during meiosis, a phenomenon that itself appears to have some genetic influences. Monogenetic factors include mutations in pregnancy-specific glycoproteins (PSGs), cytochrome c oxidase (*SCO2*), *NALP7*, methylenetetrahydrofolate reductase (*MTHFR*), prothrombin (F2), coagulation factor V gene (F5), and skewed X-chromosome inactivation, which can all cause spontaneous abortions. Deficiencies of *A4GALT* or *B3GALT3* can also cause hemolytic disease of the newborn and spontaneous abortion via anti-P/P(k) antibodies. Additionally, there are likely to be complex genetic contributions such as multifactorial inheritance, methylation status, and mitochondrial function contributing to pregnancy loss.

SEX AND LIFE SPAN CONSIDERATIONS

More than 80% of abortions occur in the first 12 weeks of pregnancy. SABs are more common in teens (12%), elderly primigravidas (26%), and those pregnant people who engage in high-risk behaviors, such as drug and alcohol use or multiple sex partners. The incidence of abortion increases if a pregnant person conceives within 3 months of term delivery. Advanced paternal age is associated with increased risk of SAB, and poor preconception paternal health is also associated with a higher risk of pregnancy loss (Fosse et al., 2020).

HEALTH DISPARITIES AND SEXUAL/GENDER MINORITY HEALTH

Surveillance data for pregnancy indicate that Black women have a higher risk of SAB than White and Asian women. Women in vulnerable situations, such as immigrants, women with a low socioeconomic status, or childless women, are particularly vulnerable to mental health problems after a SAB. The risk of SAB in rural areas is greater than in urban areas, and agricultural workers have a higher risk of SAB compared to factory and professional workers, possibly due to exposure to chemicals. Women with low income have an increased risk of SAB as do women with low educational attainment for unknown reasons. Sexual and gender minority status has no known effect on the risk for SAB.

GLOBAL HEALTH CONSIDERATIONS

International rates of SAB vary, likely dependent on how data are collected. In an English study, researchers found that ultrasound screening at 10 to 13 weeks of gestation revealed a 2.8% rate of pregnancy failure. Approximately 13% of all pregnancy-related deaths are due to abortion worldwide, whereas in the United States, about 4% of pregnancy-associated deaths are related to induced and spontaneous abortions.

ASSESSMENT

HISTORY. Obtain a complete obstetric history. Determine the date of the last menstrual period to calculate the fetus's gestational age. Vaginal bleeding is usually the first symptom that signals the onset of a spontaneous abortion. Question the patient as to the onset and amount of bleeding. Saturating a pad or more per hour would be an alarming amount of blood, and the patient should receive immediate care from a healthcare provider if that occurs. Inquire further about a small gush of fluid, which indicates a rupture of membranes, although at this early point in gestation, there is only a small amount of amniotic fluid expelled. Ask the patient to describe the duration, location, and intensity of any pain. Although it is a sensitive topic, ask the patient about the passage of fetal tissue. If possible, the patient should bring the tissue passed at home into the hospital because sometimes laboratory pathological analysis can reveal the cause of the abortion. With a missed abortion, early signs of pregnancy cease; thus, inquire about nausea, vomiting, breast tenderness, urinary frequency, and leukorrhea (white or yellow mucous discharge from the vagina).

PHYSICAL EXAMINATION. Begin the examination by taking vital signs and making an abdominal assessment to determine the presence of distention, suprapubic tenderness, and rebound tenderness. The pulse and blood pressure will indicate if the patient is hemodynamically stable. In addition, pallor, cool and clammy skin, and changes in the level of consciousness are symptoms of shock. **Pain** varies from mild cramping to severe abdominal pain, depending on the type of abortion; pain can also occur as a backache or pelvic pressure. Examine the patient's peripad for **vaginal blood loss**, and determine if any tissue has been expelled. Sometimes tissue can be observed at the introitus, but do not perform a vaginal examination if that situation occurs. A pelvic examination may show blood on the perineum or vagina and no cervical motion tenderness. A closed cervical canal will be seen with complete or threatened abortion. An open os and a uterus smaller than one would expect given the gestational age will be seen with inevitable or incomplete abortion.

PSYCHOSOCIAL. Assess the patient's emotional status, as well as that of the baby's other parent and other family members. Often this hospital admission is the first one for the patient, and it may cause anxiety and fear. The other parent may withhold expressing their **grief**, feeling that they need to "be strong" for the pregnant person.

Diagnostic Highlights

General Comments: Most of the time, diagnosis of SAB is made on the basis of patient symptoms and the documentation of a positive pregnancy test.

Test	Normal Result	Abnormality With Condition	Explanation
Human chorionic gonadotropin (hCG)	Negative < 5 mIU/mL	> 5 mIU/mL, increases as the gestation progresses	hCG normally is not present in nonpregnant people
Ultrasound (transvaginal, transabdominal)	Positive fetal heartbeat; growth within normal limits	Heartbeat absent; gestational sac appears shriveled or shrinking	Used to diagnose a missed abortion
Red blood cells; hemoglobin; hematocrit	4.2–5.4 mL/mm^3; 12–16 g/dL; 37%–47%	These three values will decrease several hours after significant blood loss has occurred	With active bleeding, red blood cells are lost

Other Tests: Blood type and crossmatch, white blood cells; habitual aborters should also undergo additional testing to rule out causes other than an incompetent cervix (thyroid-stimulating hormone, mid-luteal phase serum progesterone measurement, hysterosalpingogram, and screening for lupus anticoagulant).

IU = International unit.

PRIMARY NURSING DIAGNOSIS

DIAGNOSIS. Risk for maladaptive grieving as evidenced by blaming, despair, guilt, distress, psychological distress, and/or personal growth

OUTCOMES. Grief resolution; Guilt resolution

INTERVENTIONS. Grief work facilitation: Perinatal death; Guilt work facilitation; Active listening; Presence; Truth telling; Support group

PLANNING AND IMPLEMENTATION

Collaborative

MEDICAL. Threatened abortions are treated conservatively with bedrest at home, although there is no evidence to support bedrest as altering the course of a threatened abortion. Acetaminophen is prescribed for mild pain. Patients are instructed to abstain from intercourse for at least 2 weeks following the cessation of bleeding. Approximately 50% of patients who are diagnosed with a threatened abortion carry their pregnancies to term. Inevitable and incomplete abortions are considered obstetric emergencies. IV fluids are started immediately for fluid replacement, and narcotic analgesics are administered to decrease the pain. Oxytocics, when given IV, help decrease the bleeding. With any type of abortion, it is critical to determine the patient's blood Rh status. Any patient who is Rh-negative is given an injection of an $Rh_o(D)$ immune globulin (RhoGAM) to prevent Rh isoimmunization in future pregnancies, but there is little evidence that RhoGAM administration is necessary for first-trimester losses. To determine the patient's response to treatment, monitor the patient's vital signs, color, level of consciousness, and response to fluid replacement.

SURGICAL. A dilation and curettage (D&C) is usually indicated. This procedure involves dilating the cervix and scraping the products of conception out of the uterus with a curette. The nurse's role in this procedure is to explain the procedure to the patient and family, assist the patient to the lithotomy position in the operating room, perform the surgical prep, and support the patient during the procedure.

A D&C is not indicated in the case of a complete abortion because the patient has passed all tissue. Bleeding and cramping are minimal. Monitor the patient for complications, such as excessive bleeding and infection. With a missed abortion, the physician can wait for up to 1 month for the products of conception to pass independently; however, disseminated intravascular coagulation (DIC) or sepsis may occur during the wait. Clotting factors and white blood cell counts should be monitored during this waiting time. The physician can remove the products of conception if an SAB does not occur.

Pharmacologic Highlights

Medication or Drug Class	Dosage	Description	Rationale
Oxytocin (Pitocin)	10–20 U IV after passage of tissue	Oxytocic	Stimulates uterine contractions to decrease postpartum bleeding
Misoprostol	600 mcg sublingually single dose	Prostaglandin	Treatment for missed abortion, inevitable abortion, or incomplete abortion; increases uterine contractions and softens cervix to allow passage of products of conception
RhoGAM	1500 IU (300 mcg) IM within 2 hr; if SAB is within 13 weeks, give 250 IU (50 mcg) IM (minidose)	Immune serum	Prevents Rh isoimmunizations in future pregnancies; given if pregnant person is Rh negative and infant is Rh positive

(highlight box continues on page 24)

Pharmacologic Highlights (continued)

Medication or Drug Class	Dosage	Description	Rationale
Methotrexate	50 mg/m² IM or 50 mg PO	Antineoplastic	Inhibits embryonic cell reproduction; used for missed abortion
Methergine	0.2 mg IM or IV	Oxytocic	Acts on uterine muscle, causing uterine contraction to reduce bleeding

Independent

PREOPERATIVE. Monitor for shock in patients who are bleeding. Nursing interventions are complex because of the profound physiological and psychological changes that a pregnant person experiences with a spontaneous abortion. Monitor emotional status. Emotional support of this patient is very important. In cases of a threatened abortion, avoid offering false reassurance because the patient may lose the pregnancy despite taking precautions. Phrases such as "I'm sorry" and "Is there anything I can do?" are helpful. It is not helpful to say, "If the baby had lived, the baby would probably be disabled" or "You are young; you can get pregnant again." Inform the patient of perinatal grief support groups.

POSTOPERATIVE. Expect the patient to experience very mild uterine cramping and minimal vaginal bleeding. Patients become very drowsy from the anesthesia; ensure that a call light is within easy reach and side rails are up for safety. Assist the patient to the bathroom; syncope is possible because of anesthesia and blood loss. Continue to support the patient emotionally. Patients should be offered the opportunity to see the products of conception.

Evidence-Based Practice and Health Policy

Boryri, T., Navidian, A., & Hashem Zehi, F. (2020). Assessing the effect of self-care education on anxiety and depression among pregnant women with a history of spontaneous abortion. *Journal of Education and Health Promotion, 9,* 347–350.

• Increased anxiety and stress can lead to premature birth, increased complications, and increased medical interventions for the pregnant mother and fetus. The purpose of this study was to determine the effects of a self-care educational intervention on anxiety and depression among pregnant women ($N = 90$) with a past medical history of SAB. Between 6 and 12 weeks of gestation, the control group received usual prenatal care education. The intervention group received usual care along with more self-care education about strategies to reduce anxiety.
• The authors found that there was no significant difference between the two groups in terms of anxiety and depression at baseline. At 4 weeks, the mean scores of anxiety and depression in the intervention group were significantly lower than the scores in the control group and were also significantly lower than at baseline. The authors concluded that self-care training was a useful intervention after SAB to reduce anxiety and depression.

DOCUMENTATION GUIDELINES

• Amount and characteristics of blood loss, passage of fetal tissue, severity and location of pain, vital signs
• Signs of hypovolemic shock (pallor; cold, clammy skin; change in level of consciousness)
• Patient's (and other parent's) emotional response to losing the pregnancy

DISCHARGE AND HOME HEALTHCARE GUIDELINES

PREVENTION. Use extreme caution not to make the patient feel guilty about the cause of the SAB; however, it is important that the patient be made aware of factors that might contribute to the occurrence of an SAB (such as cigarette smoking, alcohol and drug use, exposure to x-rays or environmental teratogens). Preconception care should be encouraged should the patient decide to become pregnant again.

COMPLICATIONS. Teach the patient to notify the physician of an increase in bleeding, return of painful uterine cramping, malodorous vaginal discharge, temperature greater than 100.4°F (38°C), or persistent feelings of depression.

HOME CARE. Teach the patient to avoid strenuous activities for a few days. Encourage the patient to use peripads instead of tampons for light vaginal discharge to decrease the likelihood of an infection. Explain that the patient should avoid intercourse for at least 1 week and then use some method of birth control until a future pregnancy can be discussed with the physician. Follow-up is suggested. A phone call to the patient on their due date will demonstrate support and provide an outlet for the patient to express their grief. Provide contact information for a support group. Explain that help is available because pregnant people who experience spontaneous abortions are at high risk for depression.

Abruptio Placentae

DRG Category:	806
Mean LOS:	2.7 days
Description:	MEDICAL: Vaginal Delivery Without Sterilization or Dilation & Curettage With Complication or Comorbidity

Abruptio placentae is the premature separation of a normally implanted placenta before the delivery of the baby. It is characterized by a triad of symptoms: vaginal bleeding, uterine hypertonus, and fetal distress. It can occur during the prenatal or intrapartum period. In a marginal abruption, separation begins at the periphery, and bleeding accumulates between the membranes and the uterus and eventually passes through the cervix, becoming an external hemorrhage. In a central abruption, the separation occurs in the middle, and bleeding is trapped between the detached placenta and the uterus, concealing the hemorrhage. Frank vaginal bleeding also does not occur if the fetal head is tightly engaged. Since bleeding can be concealed, note that the apparent bleeding does not always indicate actual blood loss. If the placenta completely detaches, massive vaginal bleeding is seen. Abruptions are graded according to the percentage of the placental surface that detaches (see Table 1). Visual inspection of an abrupted placenta reveals circumscribed depressions on its parental surface, and it is covered by dark, clotted blood. Destruction and loss of function of the placenta result in fetal distress, neurological deficits such as cerebral palsy, or fetal death. Complications for the pregnant person include shock, disseminated intravascular coagulation, and/or renal failure, and for the baby, premature birth or stillbirth.

● **TABLE 1** Classification System for Abruptions

Class 0	Less than 10% of the total placental surface has detached; the patient has no symptoms; however, a small retroplacental clot is noted at birth
Class I	Approximately 10%–20% of the total placental surface has detached; no vaginal bleeding to mild vaginal bleeding and slightly tender uterus are noted; however, the pregnant person and fetus are in no distress
Class II	Approximately 20%–50% of the total placental surface has detached; the patient has moderate to severe uterine tenderness and tetanic contractions; bleeding can be concealed or is obvious; signs of fetal distress are noted; the patient is not in hypovolemic shock, but orthostatic changes in blood pressure may occur
Class III	More than 50% of the placental surface has detached; uterine tetany is severe; bleeding can be concealed or is obvious; the patient is in shock and often experiencing coagulopathy; fetal death occurs

CAUSES

The cause of abruptio placentae is unknown; however, any condition that causes vascular changes at the placental level may contribute to premature separation of the placenta. Hypertension, preterm premature rupture of membranes, smoking, heavy alcohol consumption, pregnant person trauma, trauma related to intimate partner violence, motor vehicle crashes, and crack/cocaine abuse are the most common risk factors. A short umbilical cord, fibroids (especially those located behind the placental implantation site), severe diabetes or renal disease, advanced age of pregnant person, and vena caval compression are other predisposing factors. Chronic upper respiratory infections and chronic bronchitis also increase the incidence of abruptio placentae.

GENETIC CONSIDERATIONS

Multiple studies have shown possible genetic loci linked to placental abruption (PA), including *ABCC8*, *KCNJ11*, *ZNF28*, *CTNND2*, and *ADAM12*. Several SNPs in these genes have been mapped to trophoblast-like cell chromatin interactions, suggesting a potential role in pregnancy-specific regulatory activity. Additionally, several genes involved in coagulation have been associated with PA, including the factor V Leiden SNP.

SEX AND LIFE SPAN CONSIDERATIONS

Increased incidence of abruption is noted in those with multiparity, in pregnant people over age 40 years, and for those with a history of past abruptio placentae. Abruptions occur in 1 of 200 deliveries and are responsible for 10% of third-trimester stillbirths. Severe abruptions are associated with a 25% to 35% perinatal mortality rate.

HEALTH DISPARITIES AND SEXUAL/GENDER MINORITY HEALTH

While abruptio placentae is more common in Black pregnant people than in White or Latina pregnant people, experts are unsure of the cause of these differences. However, lower gestational age at delivery is the most important risk factor for poor neonatal outcomes in Black pregnant people with abruptio placentae. A nationwide population-based study showed that nurses had a higher risk for abruptio placentae than nonmedical working pregnant people (Huang et al., 2016). White-collar workers had a significantly higher risk of placental abruption than physicians. Sexual and gender minority status has no known effect on the risk for abruptio placentae.

GLOBAL HEALTH CONSIDERATIONS

Experts estimate that abruptio placentae occurs in 1% of all pregnancies regardless of country or origin.

☀ ASSESSMENT

HISTORY. Obtain an obstetric history. Determine the date of the last menstrual period to calculate the estimated day of delivery and gestational age of the infant. Inquire about alcohol, tobacco, and drug usage and any trauma or abuse situations during pregnancy. Ask the patient to describe the onset of bleeding (the circumstances, amount, and presence of pain). When obtaining a history from a patient with an abruption, recognize that it is possible for the patient to be disoriented from blood loss and/or cocaine or other drug usage. Generally, patients have one of the risk factors, but sometimes no clear precursor is identifiable.

PHYSICAL EXAMINATION. The most common symptoms include **vaginal bleeding, abdominal or back pain and tenderness, fetal distress,** and **abnormal uterine contractions.** Assess the amount and character of vaginal bleeding; blood is often dark red in color, and the amount may vary depending on the location of abruption. Palpate the uterus; patients complain of uterine tenderness and abdominal and back pain. The fundal height may be increased due to an expanding uterine hematoma. The fundus is extremely firm, with a poor resting tone between contractions. With a mild placental separation, contractions are usually of normal frequency, intensity, and duration. If the abruption is more severe, strong and erratic contractions occur. Assess for signs of concealed hemorrhage: slight or absent vaginal bleeding; an increase in fundal height; a rigid, board-like abdomen; poor resting tone; constant abdominal pain; and late decelerations or decreased variability of the fetal heart rate. A vaginal examination should not be done until an ultrasound is performed to rule out placenta previa.

Using electronic fetal monitoring, determine the baseline fetal heart rate and presence or absence of accelerations, decelerations, and variability. At times, persistent uterine hypertonus is noted with an elevated baseline resting tone of 20 to 25 mm Hg. Ask the patient if they feel the fetal movement. Fetal position and presentation can be assessed by Leopold maneuvers. Assess the contraction status, and view the fetal monitor strip to note the frequency and duration of contractions. Throughout labor, monitor the patient's bleeding, vital signs, color, urine output, level of consciousness, uterine resting tone and contractions, and cervical dilation. If placenta previa has been ruled out, perform sterile vaginal examinations to determine the progress of labor. Assess the patient's abdominal girth hourly by placing a tape measure at the level of the umbilicus. Maintain continuous fetal monitoring.

PSYCHOSOCIAL. Assess the patient's understanding of the situation and the significant other's degree of anxiety, coping ability, and willingness to support the patient. Assess the patient for intimate partner violence or other violence in the home.

Diagnostic Highlights

General Comments: Abruptio placentae is diagnosed based on the clinical symptoms, and the diagnosis is confirmed after delivery by examining the placenta.

Test	Normal Result	Abnormality With Condition	Explanation
Pelvic ultrasound	Placenta is visualized in the fundus of the uterus	None; ultrasound is used to rule out a previa	If the placenta is in the lower uterine segment, a previa (not an abruption) exists; while ultrasonography helps to determine the location of the placenta, it is not always useful in diagnosing abruptio placentae. A normal sonogram does not exclude the condition.

Other Tests: Complete blood count; coagulation studies including fibrinogen, prothrombin time, and activated partial thromboplastin time; type and crossmatch; magnetic resonance imaging; a nonstress test and biophysical profile are done to assess fetal well-being.

PRIMARY NURSING DIAGNOSIS

DIAGNOSIS. Risk for bleeding as evidenced by pregnancy complications and/or vaginal bloody discharge

OUTCOMES. Blood loss severity; Fluid balance; Hydration; Fetal status: Antepartum; Fetal status: Intrapartum; Circulation status; Shock severity: Hypovolemic

INTERVENTIONS. Bleeding reduction: Antepartum uterus; Labor suppression; IV insertion; Blood products administration; IV therapy; Shock management: Volume

PLANNING AND IMPLEMENTATION

Collaborative

If the fetus is immature (< 37 weeks) and the abruption is mild, conservative treatment may be indicated. However, conservative treatment is rare because the benefits of aggressive treatment far outweigh the risk of the rapid deterioration that can result from an abruption. Conservative treatment includes bedrest, tocolytic (inhibition of uterine contractions) therapy, oxygen, and constant patient and fetal surveillance. Generally, an IV line should be started, and a type and crossmatch completed in case of the need for administration of IV fluids and/or blood. $Rh_o(D)$ immune globulin (RhoGAM) is given if the patient is Rh-negative due to the increased chance of fetal cells entering the patient's circulation.

If the patient's condition is more severe, aggressive, expedient, and frequent assessments of blood loss, vital signs, and fetal heart rate pattern and variability are performed. Give a lactated Ringer solution IV via a large-gauge peripheral catheter. At times, two IV catheters are needed, especially if a blood transfusion is anticipated and the fluid loss has been great. If there has been excessive blood loss, blood transfusions and central venous pressure (CVP) monitoring may be ordered.

If the pregnant person or fetus is in distress, an emergency cesarean section is indicated. If any signs of fetal distress are noted (flat variability, late decelerations, bradycardia, tachycardia), turn the patient to their left side, increase the rate of their IV infusion, administer oxygen via face mask, and notify the physician. If a cesarean section is planned, see that informed consent is obtained in accordance with unit policy, prepare the patient's abdomen for surgery, insert a Foley catheter, administer preoperative medications as ordered, and notify the necessary personnel to attend the operation.

After delivery, monitor the degree of bleeding and perform fundal checks frequently. The fundus should be firm, midline, and at or below the level of the umbilicus. Determine the Rh status of the patient; if the patient is Rh-negative and the fetus is Rh-positive with a negative Coombs test, administer RhoGAM.

Pharmacologic Highlights

Medication or Drug Class	Dosage	Description	Rationale
Magnesium sulfate	4–5 g IV loading dose, 1–2 g/hr IV maintenance	Anticonvulsant	Effective tocolytic; relaxes the uterus, slowing the abruption
Oxytocin (Pitocin)	10–40 U in 500–1,000 mL of IV fluid	Oxytocic	Assists the uterus to contract after delivery to prevent hemorrhage

Independent

During prenatal visits, explain the risk factors and the relationship of alcohol and substance abuse to the condition. Teach the patient to report any signs of abruption, such as cramping and bleeding. If the patient develops abruptio placentae and a vaginal delivery is chosen as the treatment option, the patient should not receive analgesics because of the fetus's prematurity; regional anesthesia may be considered. The labor, therefore, may be more painful than most patients experience; provide support during labor. Keep the patient and the significant others informed of the progress of labor as well as the condition of the patient and fetus. Monitor the fetal heart rate for repetitive late decelerations, decreased variability, and bradycardia. If noted, turn the patient on their left side, apply oxygen, increase the rate of the IV, and notify the physician immediately.

Offer as many choices as possible to increase the patient's sense of control. Reassure the significant others that both the fetus and the patient are being monitored for complications and that surgical intervention may be indicated. Provide the patient and family with an honest commentary about the risks. Discuss the possibility of an emergency cesarean section or the delivery of a premature infant. Answer the patient's questions honestly about the risk of a neonatal death. If the fetus does not survive, support the patient and listen to the family's feelings about the loss.

Evidence-Based Practice and Health Policy
Odendaal, H., Wright, C., Schubert, P., Boyd, T., Roberts, D., Brink, L., Nel, D., & Groenewald, C. (2020). Associations of maternal smoking and drinking with fetal growth and placental abruption. *European Journal of Obstetrics & Gynecology and Reproductive Biology, 253,* 95–102.

• The authors aimed to determine if the individual and combined effects of smoking and drinking alcohol during pregnancy increased the risk of placental abruption. They analyzed data from 7,000 maternal-neonatal dyads in the United States and South Africa (Safe Passage Study). High smoking constituted 10 or more cigarettes per day, and high drinking was considered four or more binge drinking episodes or 32 or more standard drinks during pregnancy.
• When compared to the no drinking and no smoking participants, the high drinking and high smoking participants were older, had a higher gravidity, had lower household income, and fewer were employed. The low drinking and low smoking participants had a higher prevalence rate of placental abruption than the no smoking and no drinking group. In addition, the study did not demonstrate an association with increased risk of placental abruption with smoking alone but did determine a significant risk of placenta abruption related to the combined effect of smoking and alcohol consumption.

DOCUMENTATION GUIDELINES
• Amount and character of bleeding: Uterine resting tone; intensity, frequency, and duration of contractions and uterine irritability
• Response to treatment: IV fluids, blood transfusion, medications, surgical interventions
• Fetal heart rate baseline, variability, absence or presence of accelerations or decelerations, bradycardia, tachycardia

DISCHARGE AND HOME HEALTHCARE GUIDELINES
Discharge before delivery (if the fetus is very immature and the patient and infant are stable).

MEDICATIONS. Instruct the patient not to miss a dose of the tocolytic medication; usually the medication is prescribed for every 4 hours and is to be taken throughout the day and night. Tell the patient to expect side effects of palpitations, fast heart rate, and restlessness. Teach the patient to notify the doctor and come to the hospital immediately if they experience any bleeding or contractions. Note that being on tocolytic therapy may mask contractions. Therefore, if the patient feels any uterine contractions, they may be developing abruptio placentae.

POSTPARTUM. Give the usual postpartum instructions for avoiding complications. Inform the patient that they are at much higher risk of developing abruptio placentae in subsequent pregnancies. Instruct the patient on how to provide safe care of the infant. If the fetus has not survived, provide a list of referrals to the patient and significant others to help them manage their loss.

Acid-Base Imbalances: Metabolic Acidosis and Alkalosis; Respiratory Acidosis and Alkalosis

DRG Category: 640
Mean LOS: 4.5 days
Description: MEDICAL: Miscellaneous Disorders of Nutrition, Metabolism, Fluids, and Electrolytes With Major Complication or Comorbidity

The hydrogen ion concentration ($[H^+]$) of the body, described as the pH or negative log of the $[H^+]$, is maintained in a narrow range to promote health and homeostasis. The body has many regulatory mechanisms that counteract even a slight deviation from normal pH. An acid-base imbalance can alter many physiological processes and lead to serious problems or, if left untreated, to coma and death. A pH below 7.35 is considered acidosis and above 7.45 is alkalosis. Alterations in hydrogen ion concentration can be metabolic or respiratory in origin or they may have a mixed origin.

Metabolic acidosis results from any nonpulmonary condition that leads to an excess of acids as compared to bases and can have long-term consequences. For example, damaged kidneys in patients with renal failure lead to decreased acid excretion and chronic acidemia. Skeletal problems then occur as calcium and phosphate are released from bone to help with the buffering of acids. Loss of bicarbonate in patients with severe diarrhea or with gastrointestinal fistulae can also lead to metabolic acidosis. Metabolic alkalosis results from any nonpulmonary condition that leads to an excess of bases over acids. Metabolic alkalosis results from one of two mechanisms: loss of acids or excess of bases. Prolonged vomiting, hyperaldosteronism, and diuretic therapy lead to loss of acids. Patients with a history of heart failure and hypertension who are on sodium-restricted diets and diuretics may develop metabolic alkalosis from increased urinary acid secretion. Ingestion or infusion of bases such as sodium bicarbonate can also lead to metabolic alkalosis.

Respiratory acidosis is a pH imbalance that results from alveolar hypoventilation and an accumulation of carbon dioxide. It can be classified as either acute or chronic. Acute respiratory acidosis is associated with a sudden failure in ventilation, such as conditions like obstructive sleep apnea and pneumothorax. Chronic respiratory acidosis is seen in patients with chronic pulmonary disease in whom long-term hypoventilation results in a chronic elevation (> 45 mm Hg) of $Paco_2$ levels (hypercapnia), which renders the primary mechanism of inspiration, an elevated $Paco_2$, unreliable. The major drive for respiration in patients with chronic pulmonary disease then becomes a low oxygen level (hypoxemia). Respiratory alkalosis is a pH imbalance that results from the excessive loss of carbon dioxide through hyperventilation ($Paco_2 < 35$ mm Hg). Respiratory alkalosis is the most frequently occurring acid-base imbalance of hospitalized patients. When the central respiratory center is stimulated by anxiety, pain, or fever, respiratory alkalosis may occur. Improper use of mechanical ventilators with a rapid respiratory rate per minute can cause iatrogenic respiratory alkalosis, whereas secondary respiratory alkalosis may develop from hyperventilation stimulated by metabolic or respiratory acidosis. Patients with respiratory alkalosis are at risk for hypokalemia, hypocalcemia, and hypophosphatemia.

CAUSES

See Table 1.

• TABLE 1 Common Causes of Acid-Base Disorders

ACID-BASE DISORDER	COMMON CAUSES
Metabolic acidosis	Decreased acid excretion: chronic renal disease results in decreased acid excretion and is the most common cause of chronic metabolic acidosis Excessive acid production: oxygen tissue deprivation with shock and cardio-pulmonary arrest, vigorous exercise (transient), prolonged periods of fever, ketoacidosis in insulin-dependent diabetics, alcoholic ketoacidosis, and ingestion of drugs and chemicals (methanol, ethylene glycol, aspirin) Underproduction of bicarbonate: pancreatitis Excessive loss of bicarbonate: severe diarrhea; intestinal obstruction; small bowel, pancreatic, ileostomy, or biliary fistula drainage Hyperchloremic acidosis, an increase in the extracellular concentration of chloride, also promotes bicarbonate loss
Metabolic alkalosis	Most common: vomiting and nasogastric (NG) suction Other: ingestion of bicarbonates, carbonates, acetates, citrates, and lactates found in total parenteral nutrition solutions, Ringer lactate, and sodium bicarbonate administration; rapid administration of stored blood and volume expanders with high citrate and acetate levels; excessive intake of antacids, which are composed of sodium bicarbonate or calcium carbonate; loss of acids (gastric fluid loss, diuretic therapy, excessive mineralocorticoid release); hypercalcemia; diuretic therapy; aldosterone excess
Respiratory acidosis	Depression of respiratory center in the medulla: head injury, drug ingestion (anesthetics, opiates, barbiturates, ethanol) Decreased amount of functioning lung tissue: bronchial asthma, chronic bronchitis, emphysema, pneumonia, hemothorax, pneumothorax, pulmonary edema Airway obstruction: foreign body aspiration, obstructive sleep apnea, bronchospasm, laryngospasm Disorders of the chest wall: flail chest, impaired diaphragm movement (pain, splinting, chest burns, tight chest or abdominal dressings) Abdominal distention: obesity, ascites, bowel obstruction Disorders of respiratory muscles: severe hypokalemia, amyotrophic lateral sclerosis, Guillain-Barré syndrome, poliomyelitis, myasthenia gravis, drugs (curare, succinylcholine)
Respiratory alkalosis	Hyperventilation due to hypoxemia (a decrease in the oxygen content of blood) or improper ventilator settings: anemia; hypotension; high altitudes; and pulmonary disease, such as pneumonia, interstitial lung disease, pulmonary vascular disease, and acute asthma Direct stimulation of the central respiratory center: anxiety, pain, fever, sepsis, salicylate ingestion, head trauma, central nervous system (CNS) disease (inflammation, lesions)
Examples of mixed disorders	Respiratory acidosis and metabolic alkalosis: chronic obstructive pulmonary disease (COPD) produces chronically elevated $PaCO_2$ levels and high HCO_3 levels as a compensatory mechanism. If the chronically elevated $PaCO_2$ is rapidly decreased, as it would be with aggressive mechanical ventilation, HCO_3 levels remain elevated, causing metabolic alkalosis. Respiratory alkalosis and metabolic acidosis: salicylate ingestion directly stimulates the respiratory center, resulting in an increased rate and depth of breathing; ingestion of large amounts of salicylates can also produce metabolic acidosis; respiratory alkalosis results from the "blowing off" of CO_2

GENETIC CONSIDERATIONS

A number of inherited disorders can result in acid-base imbalances. Bartter syndrome (a group of several disorders of impaired salt reabsorption in the thick ascending loop of Henle) results in metabolic alkalosis along with hypokalemia and hyperaldosteronism. Bartter syndrome is inherited in an autosomal recessive pattern. Liddle syndrome is inherited in an autosomal dominant pattern and results in metabolic alkalosis due to dysregulation of the epithelial sodium channel. Metabolic acidosis is often seen with inborn errors of metabolism, such as Gaucher disease (autosomal recessive transmission) or from mutations in the pyruvate dehydrogenase complex genes (autosomal recessive or X-linked inheritance).

SEX AND LIFE SPAN CONSIDERATIONS

Metabolic acidosis occurs primarily in patients with insulin-dependent diabetes mellitus (IDDM) and chronic renal failure regardless of age. Metabolic acidosis from severe diarrhea can occur at any age, but children and older adults are at greater risk because of associated fluid imbalances. Young people are at an increased risk of metabolic acidosis because of popular fad diets that lead to starvation.

Metabolic alkalosis is a common disorder of adult hospitalized patients. Older patients are at risk for metabolic alkalosis because of their delicate fluid and electrolyte status. Young people who practice self-induced vomiting to lose weight are also at risk for developing metabolic alkalosis. Finally, middle-aged people with chronic hypercapnia respiratory failure are at risk for metabolic alkalosis if their $Paco_2$ levels are rapidly decreased with mechanical ventilation, corticosteroids, or antacids.

Patients of all ages are at risk for acute respiratory acidosis when an injury or illness results in alveolar hypoventilation. Older adults are at high risk for electrolyte and fluid imbalances, which can lead to respiratory depression. Patients with COPD are at highest risk for chronic respiratory acidosis. The typical COPD patient is a middle-aged man with a history of smoking. Older children and adults are at risk for respiratory alkalosis with large-dose salicylate ingestion. Older adults are at an increased risk for respiratory alkalosis because of the high incidence of pulmonary disorders, specifically pneumonia, in their population. Identification of respiratory alkalosis may be more difficult in older patients because the early symptoms of increased respirations and altered neurological status may be attributed to other disease processes.

HEALTH DISPARITIES AND SEXUAL/GENDER MINORITY HEALTH

Ethnicity, race, and sexual/gender minority status have no known effect on the risk for acid-base imbalance.

GLOBAL HEALTH CONSIDERATIONS

No data are available.

☀ ASSESSMENT

HISTORY
Metabolic Acidosis. Establish a history of renal disease, IDDM, or hepatic or pancreatic disease. Determine if the patient has experienced seizure activity, starvation, shock, acid ingestion, diarrhea, nausea, vomiting, anorexia, or abdominal pain or dehydration. Ask if the patient has experienced dyspnea with activity or at rest, as well as weakness, fatigue, headache, or confusion.

Metabolic Alkalosis. Establish a history of prolonged vomiting, NG suctioning, hypercalcemia, hypokalemia, or hyperaldosteronism. Determine if the patient has been taking thiazide diuretics, has been receiving potassium-free IV infusions, eats large quantities of licorice, or regularly uses nasal sprays. Elicit a history of lightheadedness; agitation; muscle weakness, cramping, and twitching or tingling; or circumoral (around the mouth) paresthesia. Ask the patient if they have experienced anorexia, nausea, or vomiting.

Respiratory Acidosis. Establish a history of impaired ventilation or breathlessness. The initial manifestations of respiratory acidosis involve changes in a patient's behavior. Investigate early signs of confusion, impaired judgment, lack of motor coordination, and restlessness. Determine if the patient has experienced headache, lethargy, blurred vision, confusion, or nausea.

Respiratory Alkalosis. Establish a history of hyperventilation from anxiety or mechanical over-ventilation. Early manifestations involve changes in neurological and neuromuscular status due to decreased $Paco_2$ levels (hypocapnia), which may lead to decreased cerebral perfusion. Determine if the patient has experienced lightheadedness, anxiety, inability to concentrate, or confusion. Elicit a patient history of muscle cramps, spasms, tingling (paresthesia) of the extremities, and circumoral numbness. Other possible symptoms are nausea and vomiting, caused by a low potassium level.

PHYSICAL EXAMINATION

Metabolic Acidosis. Inspect the patient's skin, noting if it feels warm. Note a **flushed appearance**. Assess the patient's breathing pattern for **Kussmaul breathing**, a compensatory mechanism that the body uses to attempt to balance the pH by blowing off carbon dioxide. Check for an **increased heart rate** caused by stimulation of the sympathetic nervous system. To detect changes in cardiac performance, use a cardiac monitor for patients with a pH less than 7 and a potassium level greater than 5 mEq/L. Assess for changes in heart rate, ventricular ectopics, T-wave configuration, QRS, and PR intervals. Include neurological status checks at least every 4 hours or more frequently if the patient is confused or lethargic.

Metabolic Alkalosis. The patient with metabolic alkalosis demonstrates signs associated with the accompanying electrolyte imbalances. If hypocalcemia is present, the patient may demonstrate **positive Chvosteks and Trousseau signs** (see **Hypocalcemia**, p. 614). Hypocalcemia and hypokalemia affect muscle strength and irritability. Assess the strength of the patient's hand grasps. Observe the patient's gait for unsteadiness, and note the presence of any hyperactive reflexes, such as spasms and seizures. Observe the patient's breathing patterns for a compensatory decrease in the rate and depth of breathing. Use continuous cardiac monitoring, and check for an increased heart rate or ventricular dysrhythmias. Assess the patient for atrial tachycardias, ventricular dysrhythmias, and a prolonged QT interval.

Respiratory Acidosis. Assess the patient for an **increased heart rate**. As Pao_2 decreases and $Paco_2$ increases, the sympathetic nervous system is stimulated, resulting in a release of catecholamines, epinephrine, and norepinephrine, which causes an increase in heart rate and cardiac output. Note cardiovascular abnormalities, such as tachycardia, hypertension, and atrial and ventricular dysrhythmias. During periods of acute respiratory acidosis, monitor the cardiac rhythm continuously. Take the patient's pulse, noting a bounding quality that may occur with hypercapnia. If the cause of the respiratory acidosis is respiratory center depression or respiratory muscle paralysis, **respirations are slow and shallow**. As respiratory acidosis worsens and respiratory muscles fail, the rate of respirations decreases.

Respiratory Alkalosis. The hallmark sign of respiratory alkalosis is **hyperventilation**; the patient may be taking 40 or more respirations per minute and may manifest a breathing pattern that is reminiscent of Kussmaul breathing caused by diabetic acidosis. Check the patient for an increased heart rate caused by hypoxemia. Test the patient's hand grasps for signs of weakness. Observe the patient's gait for unsteadiness, and note any indications of hyperactive reflexes such as spasms, tetany, and seizures. The presence of a positive Chvostek or Trousseau sign may indicate hypocalcemia (see **Hypocalcemia**, p. 614), which may occur from lower amounts of ionized calcium during periods of alkalosis.

PSYCHOSOCIAL. Acid-base imbalances frequently affect patients with both acute and chronic illnesses. Their response to yet another problem is at best unpredictable. Neurological changes such as confusion, agitation, or psychosis are upsetting if they occur, as are electrolyte disturbances. Anticipate the patient feeling powerless and plan care to support all psychological needs.

Diagnostic Highlights

Test	Normal Result	Abnormality With Condition	Explanation
Arterial blood gases (ABGs)	pH 7.35–7.45; PaO_2 80–100 mm Hg; $PaCO_2$ 35–45 mm Hg; SaO_2 > 95%; HCO_3 22–26 mEq/L	Metabolic acidosis: pH < 7.35; HCO_3 < 22 mEq/L; metabolic alkalosis: pH > 7.45; HCO_3 > 26 mEq/L; respiratory acidosis: pH < 7.35; $PaCO_2$ > 45 mm Hg; respiratory alkalosis: pH > 7.45; $PaCO_2$ < 35 mm Hg	Hydrogen ion concentration varies based on condition

Other Tests: Electrocardiogram; serum electrolyte levels (sodium, chloride, calcium, potassium, magnesium); glucose; lactate; total protein; blood urea nitrogen; creatinine; urine pH

PRIMARY NURSING DIAGNOSIS

DIAGNOSIS. Risk for electrolyte imbalance as evidenced by compromised pulmonary and/or renal function

OUTCOMES. Metabolic acidosis severity; Metabolic alkalosis severity; Metabolic function; Acute respiratory acidosis severity; Acute respiratory alkalosis severity; Respiratory status; Electrolyte & acid/base balance; Electrolyte balance

INTERVENTIONS. Acid-base management: Metabolic acidosis, Metabolic alkalosis, Respiratory acidosis, Respiratory alkalosis; Acid-base monitoring; Electrolyte monitoring

PLANNING AND IMPLEMENTATION

Collaborative

GENERAL. The highest priority for all patients with acid-base imbalances is to maintain the adequacy of airway, breathing, and circulation. An important focus for collaborative treatment is to deliver oxygen, remove carbon dioxide, and monitor gas exchange. Treatment is focused on correcting the cause and restoring fluids and electrolytes to a normal range. Provide constant cardiac monitoring for patients with hypokalemia, hypocalcemia, and hypomagnesemia. Consult with a dietitian to provide foods that can help restore electrolyte balance and increase oral intake. If a patient demonstrates impaired physical mobility, consult a physical therapist to evaluate the patient's abilities and to recommend needed strengthening exercises and assist devices.

Metabolic Acidosis. Sodium bicarbonate may be administered to treat normal anion gap metabolic acidosis, but it is controversial in treating increased anion gap metabolic acidosis. Research has shown that administering sodium bicarbonate may inhibit hemoglobin release of oxygen to the tissues, thus increasing the acidosis. Sodium bicarbonate is recommended if the pH is greatly reduced (< 7.1). Sodium bicarbonate may be administered by IV drip or by IV push. Overmedication of sodium bicarbonate may cause metabolic alkalosis, fluid volume overload, hypokalemia, and worsened acidosis. Potassium-sparing diuretics, amphotericin B, and large quantities of isotonic saline solutions should not be administered to patients with suspected renal failure. These drugs may contribute to the development of metabolic acidosis.

Metabolic Alkalosis. Pharmacologic therapy may include IV saline solutions, potassium supplements, histamine antagonists, and carbonic anhydrase inhibitors. IV saline solutions (0.9% or 0.45%) may be used to replace lost volume and chloride ions. Causes of metabolic alkalosis that respond favorably to saline therapy include vomiting, NG suctioning, postchronic hypercapnia, and diuretic therapy. The causes of metabolic alkalosis that do not respond favorably to the administration of saline include hypokalemia and mineralocorticoid excess. Potassium chloride is used to treat hypokalemia in a patient with metabolic alkalosis. Dietary supplements of potassium are not effective unless chloride levels are stabilized.

Histamine H_2 receptor antagonists, particularly cimetidine and ranitidine, reduce the production of hydrochloric acid in the stomach and may prevent the occurrence of metabolic alkalosis in patients with NG suctioning and vomiting. In severe cases of metabolic alkalosis (pH > 7.55), IV hydrochloric acid may be indicated.

The carbonic anhydrase inhibitor acetazolamide (Diamox) is useful for correcting metabolic alkalosis in patients with congestive heart failure who cannot tolerate fluid volume administration. Acetazolamide promotes the renal excretion of bicarbonate. Severe metabolic alkalosis may require the administration of weak acid solutions. Because acetazolamide promotes the excretion of potassium, it is not given until serum potassium levels are evaluated as safe.

Potassium-sparing diuretics, such as spironolactone, may be used if diuretics are needed. Anticonvulsants are usually not needed because the risk for seizures decreases as fluid and electrolyte imbalances are corrected.

Respiratory Acidosis. Although oxygen therapy is required to treat the hypoxemia that accompanies respiratory acidosis, a fraction of inspired air (FIO_2) of less than 0.40 is desirable. Oxygen concentrations greater than 0.80 are toxic to the lung over a 5- to 6-day time period. Caution: The use of oxygen for patients with COPD and hypercapnia may remove the stimulus for respiration and result in respiratory depression. If the $PaCO_2$ is greater than 60 mm Hg or the PaO_2 is less than 50 mm Hg with high levels of supplemental oxygen, intubation and mechanical ventilation are required. Pharmacologic therapy for respiratory acidosis depends on the cause and severity of acidosis. The administration of sodium bicarbonate is controversial for a pH greater than 7.0. If the pH is below 7.0, sodium bicarbonate administration is recommended. Bronchodilators may be used to decrease bronchospasms. Antibiotics are prescribed for respiratory infections, but sedatives that depress respirations are limited.

Respiratory Alkalosis. Because the most common cause of respiratory alkalosis is anxiety, reassurance and sedation may be all that are needed. Pharmacologic therapy most likely includes the administration of antianxiety medications and potassium supplements. Benzodiazepines, commonly used to control acute anxiety attacks, are administered intramuscularly or intravenously. If the anxiety is more severe and the respiratory alkalosis is pronounced, rebreathing small amounts of exhaled air with a paper bag or a rebreather mask helps increase arterial $PaCO_2$ levels and decrease arterial pH. If the cause of the hyperventilation is hypoxemia, oxygen therapy is needed. Overventilation by mechanical ventilation can be easily remedied by decreasing the respiratory rate or tidal volume. If ventilator changes do not decrease the pH, dead space can be added to the ventilator tubing. Dead space provides a smaller volume of air so that less CO_2 can be expired.

Independent

For patients who are acutely ill, the priority is to maintain a patent airway, which can be managed through positioning or the use of an oral airway or endotracheal tube. Position the patient in a semi-Fowler position to allow for optimal chest wall expansion, patient comfort, and adequate gas exchange. Aggressive pulmonary hygiene techniques are used to mobilize secretions and increase alveolar ventilation. These measures should include turning, coughing, and deep breathing every 2 hours; postural drainage and percussion every 4 hours; and sitting up in a chair twice per day.

Orient a confused patient to person, time, and place. Use clocks, calendars, family photos, and scheduled rest periods to help maintain orientation. Assist the patient in using hearing aids and glasses to ensure an accurate interpretation of surroundings. Consider using restraints according to hospital policy if the risk for injury is high. Remove the restraints every 2 hours to allow for range-of-motion exercises. Incorporate the patient's normal sleep routines into the care plan. Schedule collaborative activities to allow at least two 1-hour rest periods during the day and one 4-hour rest period at night.

Provide assistance as needed in feeding, bathing, toileting, and dressing. Provide frequent mouth care (every 2 hr) to ensure patient comfort. If the patient is able to swallow, offer sips of water or ice chips every hour. Avoid lemon glycerine swabs, which may cause dryness. The patient is not discharged until the cause of the acid-base alteration has been resolved; in many patients, however, underlying organ diseases may not be resolved.

Evidence-Based Practice and Health Policy

Lo, K., Garvia, V., Stempel, J., Ram, P., & Rangaswami, J. (2020). Bicarbonate use and mortality outcome among critically ill patients with metabolic acidosis: A meta analysis. *Heart & Lung, 49*, 167–174.

• The authors studied the role of sodium bicarbonate in the treatment of severe acidosis in the intensive care unit (ICU) setting.
• They studied all available articles in several healthcare databases and located 202 articles addressing bicarbonate use in ICUs. Five studies evaluated mortality.
• Following advanced analysis, the authors found that mortality was not improved by the use of bicarbonate in severe acidosis unless actual bicarbonate loss is the primary mechanism for acidosis.

DOCUMENTATION GUIDELINES

• Physical findings: Flushed, dry, warm skin; mental status (presence of disorientation or confusion); respiratory rate and pattern, breath sounds; cardiac rhythm and rate, blood pressure, quality of pulses, urine output; level of consciousness, orientation, ability to concentrate, motor strength, and seizure activity (if seizures are present, the following information should be charted: time the seizure began, parts of the body involved in the seizure, progression of the seizure, type of body movements, pupil size and reaction, eye movements, vital signs during seizure, and postictal state)
• Response to therapy: Medications, activity, interventions
• Laboratory values: ABGs and serum potassium, calcium, sodium, chloride, and magnesium

DISCHARGE AND HOME HEALTHCARE GUIDELINES

The patients at highest risk for a recurrence of acid-base imbalances are those who consume large quantities of thiazide diuretics, antacids, and licorice, as well as those who have chronic renal, pulmonary, cardiac, and neurological disorders and IDDM. Make sure these patients understand the importance of maintaining the prescribed treatment regimen. Teach patients on diuretic therapy the signs and symptoms of the associated fluid and electrolyte disturbances of hypovolemia and hypokalemia. Teach patients the action, dose, and side effects of all medications. Teach the patient with mild to moderate anxiety progressive muscle relaxation, therapeutic breathing, and visualization techniques to control anxiety.

Acromegaly

DRG Category: 644
Mean LOS: 4.3 days
Description: MEDICAL: Endocrine Disorders With Complication or Comorbidity

Acromegaly is a rare, chronic, and disabling disorder of body growth and endocrine dysfunction in adults (after closure of the epiphyses) that is caused by excessive levels of insulinlike growth factor (IGF-1). It occurs in approximately 60 out of 1 million individuals. When it occurs while the epiphyseal growth plates are open during childhood (up until a child is 15 to 17 years of age), the disorder is considered giantism. Growth hormone (GH) and IGF-1 are related. GH is secreted from the anterior pituitary gland and is responsible for linear growth. GH stimulates the formation of IGF-1 (also known as *somatomedin C*), which is produced primarily by the liver and is the primary mediator of the growth-promoting effects of GH. In adults, acromegaly is almost always due to a GH-secreting pituitary adenoma. The excess production of GH causes enlargement of tissues and an altered production of glucocorticoids, mineralocorticoids, and gonadotropins. Left untreated, acromegaly causes gross physical deformities, crippling neuromuscular alterations, major organ dysfunctions, and decreased visual acuity. Arthritis or carpal tunnel syndrome may also develop. Acromegaly increases an individual's risk for heart disease, diabetes mellitus, stroke, and gallstones. The resultant cardiac disease reduces life expectancy.

CAUSES

The overproduction of GH and IGF-1 is a result of hyperpituitarism. More than 90% of patients have a GH-secreting pituitary adenoma. The etiology of adenomas is unknown, and less than 1% of the tumors are malignant. Hyperpituitarism can also occur with lung, gastric, breast, and ovarian cancers and may have a genetic cause.

GENETIC CONSIDERATIONS

While most cases of acromegaly are not inherited, there are now 10 known mutations that contribute to acromegaly. Many of these mutations are inherited in an autosomal dominant fashion and also contribute to gigantism. The most frequent genetic causes of acromegaly are mutations in the *AIP* gene (aryl hydrocarbon receptor-interacting protein), which causes the disorder familial isolated pituitary adenoma (*FIPA*), and newly identified microduplications of the *GPR101* gene on the X chromosome, which causes X-linked acrogigantism. In addition, mutations in the *GNAS1* gene can cause GH-secreting pituitary adenomas (somatotropinomas), which are transmitted in an autosomal dominant pattern. Familial acromegaly may also be a feature of multiple endocrine neoplasia type I (MEN I), an autosomal dominant disorder that includes peptic ulcer disease and pituitary, parathyroid, and pancreas endocrine abnormalities.

SEX AND LIFE SPAN CONSIDERATIONS

The average onset of acromegaly is in the third decade of life, but diagnosis usually occurs after the age of 40 years in men and 45 years in women. It occurs more frequently in women than in men.

HEALTH DISPARITIES AND SEXUAL/GENDER MINORITY HEALTH

Ethnicity, race, and sexual/gender minority status have no known effect on the risk for acromegaly.

GLOBAL HEALTH CONSIDERATIONS

No global data are available.

☀ ASSESSMENT

HISTORY. The course of acromegaly is slow, with very gradual changes over 7 to 10 years. Reviewing a patient's old photographs may reveal the progressive **changes in facial features.** Determine if the patient has had a change in hat, glove, ring, or shoe size because of an overgrowth of the hands and feet. Ask the patient if they have had **headaches** or **visual disturbances** (primarily bitemporal hemianopsia, partial blindness where vision is missing in outer half of both visual fields), which in acromegaly are caused by the growth of the adenoma, which exerts pressure on brain tissue and cranial nerves III, IV, and VI. Establish a history of altered sexual function, which may be an indicator of decreased gonadotropin production. Ask about the presence of pain in the hands, feet, and spine, which is probably caused by bone growth; also ask about problems with chewing, swallowing, or talking, which may be caused by tongue, jaw, and teeth enlargement. Note the presence of a deepening of the voice, recurrent bronchitis, excessive sweating, heat intolerance, fatigue, and muscle weakness. Check for a family history of pituitary tumors.

PHYSICAL EXAMINATION. Patients often have tall stature and mild to moderate obesity (giantism). The initial physical changes that occur with acromegaly result from an enlargement of the bones in the head, hands, and feet. The parts of the head that may be enlarged by acromegaly include the jaw, forehead, nose, tongue, and teeth. Observe the patient's facial appearance, noting an enlarged supraorbital ridge, thickened ears and nose, or jutting of the jaw (prognathism). The patient may have increased skin pigmentation. If the patient has an enlarged tongue, note any respiratory alterations. High blood pressure and cardiac hypertrophy often occur in people with acromegaly.

Examine the patient's fingers for signs of thickening. Inspect the patient's torso, noting a barrel chest or kyphosis. Note any signs of bowed legs. Assess the patient's skin for signs of oiliness or excessive sweating (diaphoresis). Assess the patient's hand strength. A soft, "doughy," damp handshake is characteristics of the disorder. Test the patient's vision for bitemporal hemianopsia and loss of visual acuity. Note a deep, hollow-sounding voice.

PSYCHOSOCIAL. Patients with acromegaly undergo some dramatic physical changes that can lead to permanent dysfunctions. These changes affect the patient's self-concept and ability to perform expected roles. Note any irritability, hostility, or depression.

Diagnostic Highlights

Test	Normal Result	Abnormality With Condition	Explanation
Magnetic resonance imaging	No visual evidence of tumors; normal brain structure	Provides visual evidence of pituitary adenoma	Standard imaging test to identify pituitary tumors; can identify macroadenomas and microadenomas larger than 3 mm; can locate small abnormalities in pituitary gland unrelated to symptoms

Diagnostic Highlights (continued)

Test	Normal Result	Abnormality With Condition	Explanation
GH level by radioimmunoassay	Men: < 5 ng/mL; women: < 10 ng/mL; child: 0–20 ng/mL; newborn: 10–40 ng/mL	Levels are measured after 100 mg of glucose orally, and GH measurements are made at 30, 60, 90, and 120 minutes; failure to suppress GH to < 10 ng/mL confirms diagnosis of acromegaly	Overproduction of GH
Plasma insulin like growth factor (IGF-1) (plasma somatomedin C)	Varies by age; adults 21–25 years of age: 116–341 ng/mL	Increased to over five times normal. If levels are only moderately elevated, diagnosis is confirmed by giving 75 mg of glucose orally and measuring serum GH at 1 hr; failure to suppress GH to < 12 ng/mL confirms diagnosis of acromegaly.	Small polypeptide produced in the liver; mediates most effects of GH; directly stimulates growth and proliferation of normal cells and predicts overproduction of GH

Other Tests: Computed tomography; x-rays of skull, hands, feet; serum glucose levels, serum sodium levels

PRIMARY NURSING DIAGNOSIS

DIAGNOSIS. Disturbed body image related to anxiety about changes in body structures as evidenced by distress, fear, and/or apprehension

OUTCOMES. Self-esteem; Body image; Anxiety level

INTERVENTIONS. Body image enhancement; Coping enhancement; Emotional support; Self-esteem enhancement; Support group; Anxiety reduction

PLANNING AND IMPLEMENTATION

Collaborative

SURGICAL. The goal of treatment is to normalize pituitary function. Pituitary adenomas are frequently removed by endoscopic, transnasal, transsphenoidal pituitary microsurgery. Surgery cures approximately 60% of people with acromegaly. Although the surgeon removes the adenoma, the procedure usually preserves anterior pituitary function. A transfrontal craniotomy may be used if the tumor is large or if a transsphenoidal approach is contraindicated. Because many patients have macroadenomas, complete tumor resection with a cure of acromegaly may be impossible, and radiotherapy may be used to prevent regrowth and control symptoms.

POSTOPERATIVE. After surgery, assess the patient's neurological status and report significant changes. Also check for the presence of pain. Antibiotics, antipyretics, and analgesics may be used to control infection and pain. Check any nasal drainage for the presence of glucose, which indicates cerebrospinal fluid drainage. Monitor blood glucose and serum sodium levels. GH levels generally fall rapidly after surgery, thus removing an insulin-antagonist effect and possibly causing hypoglycemia. Hyponatremia may occur 4 to 13 days after surgery. Pituitary dysfunction occurs in about one-fifth of patients after surgery and requires glucocorticoids, gonadotropins, and thyroid replacement hormone therapy. If a complete remission has not occurred following surgery or medical therapy, the patient may be treated with stereotactic radiosurgery via gamma knife, heavy particle radiation, or adapted linear accelerator. Medical therapy is prescribed to patients with continuing postoperative disease or for people who cannot tolerate surgery.

Pharmacologic Highlights

Medication or Drug Class	Dosage	Description	Rationale
Octreotide and lanreotide	Octreotide (maintenance dose): 100 mcg SC tid; or in a long-acting depot form, 10–30 mg IM per month; lanreotide: 60–120 mg per month	Somatostatin analog	Suppresses GH secretion while the effect of radiation is being awaited after surgery or if radiation is used to prevent regrowth
Pegvisomant	10–30 mg SC qd	GH antagonist	Lowers IGF-1 to normal levels

Patients who do not have remission after surgery may be treated with cabergoline, somatostatin analogs, pegvisomant, or a combination of drugs.

Independent

PREOPERATIVE. At the time of diagnosis, the patient requires education and emotional support. Focus education on the cause of the disease, the prescribed medical regime, and preparation for surgery. Encourage the patient to interact with family and significant others. Reassure the patient that treatment reverses some of the physical deformities. If you note disabling behavior, refer the patient to psychiatric resources.

Prepare the patient and family for surgery. Explain the preoperative diagnostic tests and examinations.

POSTOPERATIVE. Elevate the patient's head to facilitate breathing and fluid drainage. Do not encourage the patient to cough, as this interferes with the healing of the operative site. Provide frequent mouth care and keep the skin dry. To promote maximum joint mobility, perform or assist with range-of-motion exercises. Encourage the patient to ambulate within 1 to 2 days of the surgery. To ensure healing of the incision site, explain the need to avoid activities that increase intracranial pressure, such as toothbrushing, coughing, sneezing, nose blowing, and bending.

Evidence-Based Practice and Health Policy

Parolin, M., Dassie, F., Alessio, L., Wennberg, A., Rossato, M., Vettor, R., Maffei, L., & Pagano, C. (2020). Obstructive sleep apnea in acromegaly and the effect of treatment: A systemic review and meta-analyses. *Journal of Clinical Endocrinology & Metabolism, 105,* e24–e32.

- The authors conducted a study to determine the risk for obstructive sleep apnea in acromegaly, with particular focus on the role of the disease activity and the effect of treatment. They retrieved 21 articles including 24 studies with a total sample of 734 patients.
- Obstructive sleep apnea occurred with similar prevalence rates in patients with both active and inactive disease. After treatment for acromegaly, the apnea-hypopnea index improved, showing improvement in obstructive sleep apnea outcomes.

DOCUMENTATION GUIDELINES

- Physical findings: Respiratory rate and pattern; nasal drainage: color, amount, and presence of glucose
- Neurological status: Level of consciousness, motor strength, sensation, and vision

- Presence of postoperative complications: Diabetes insipidus, hypopituitarism, meningitis, hypoglycemia, and hyponatremia
- Psychosocial assessment: Self-esteem, coping, interpersonal relationships, and sexual dysfunction

DISCHARGE AND HOME HEALTHCARE GUIDELINES

REFERRALS. Refer to a physical therapist patients with advanced acromegaly who experience arthritic changes and require assist devices for ambulation and activities of daily living.

ACTIVITY RESTRICTIONS. Instruct the patient to avoid activities that increase intracranial pressure for up to 2 months after surgery. Toothbrushing can be resumed in 2 weeks. Instruct the patient to report increased nasal drainage. Incisional numbness and altered olfaction may occur for 4 months after surgery.

MEDICATIONS. If octreotide or lanreotide are prescribed, the patient must be able to demonstrate how to administer a subcutaneous or intramuscular injection.

FOLLOW-UP. Patients need to be monitored for development of cardiac disease, diabetes mellitus, and gallstones and a recurrence of symptoms. Advise the patient to wear a medical identification bracelet.

Adrenal Crisis, Acute

DRG Category:	644
Mean LOS:	4.3 days
Description:	MEDICAL: Endocrine Disorders With Complication or Comorbidity

Acute adrenal crisis is a life-threatening endocrine emergency caused by a deficit of glucocorticoids (primarily cortisol) or mineralocorticoids (primarily aldosterone). The anterior pituitary gland produces adrenocorticotropic hormone (ACTH), which causes the adrenal cortex to produce more than 50 steroid hormones. Cortisol and aldosterone are the most physiologically active of these hormones. In primary adrenocortical insufficiency, the impairment occurs within the adrenal gland, which does not produce adequate levels of glucocorticoids and mineralocorticoids to sustain normal function. Secondary adrenal insufficiency is caused by impairment of the pituitary gland or hypothalamus. Acute adrenocortical insufficiency is a difficult diagnosis to make. Acute adrenal crisis rarely occurs without an accompanying serious injury or illness. The diagnosis is difficult because many of the signs and symptoms are nonspecific. However, when left untreated, a person with acute adrenal insufficiency has a very poor prognosis for survival.

Glucocorticoids are cardiac stimulants that activate release of essential vasoactive substances. Without cortisol, stress results in hypotension, shock, and death. A deficiency of cortisol produces many metabolic abnormalities, such as decreases in glucose production, protein and fat metabolism, appetite, and digestion. Serious systemic effects include a decrease in vascular tone and a diminished effect of catecholamines, such as epinephrine and norepinephrine. Normally, a body under stress releases cortisol and other corticosteroids. Both the decrease in the vascular tone of the blood vessels and the decreased effect of catecholamines in an individual in an adrenal crisis can cause shock. The deficiency of aldosterone results in profound fluid and electrolyte imbalances: a decrease in sodium and water retention, a decrease in circulating blood volume, and an increase in both potassium and hydrogen ion reabsorption.

CAUSES

Acute adrenal insufficiency is most commonly caused by acute withdrawal of chronic corticosteroid therapy (secondary insufficiency). It can also occur from immune destruction of the adrenal cortex, adrenal hemorrhage, or from infiltration by metastatic carcinoma (primary insufficiency). Before signs and symptoms appear, at least 90% or more of the adrenal cortex has been damaged by the disorder, resulting in deficient glucocorticoid and mineralocorticoid hormones. Some medications (ketoconazole, phenytoin, rifampin, mitotane) are also associated with the condition. Other causes include physiological stress, including surgery, infection, sepsis, septic shock, burns, anesthesia, fluid volume loss, trauma, asthma, hypothermia, alcohol abuse, myocardial infarction, fever, hypoglycemia, pain, and depression. Critically ill patients without a baseline deficit of glucocorticoids or mineralocorticoids before the critical illness have an incidence of acute adrenal crisis of approximately 20% to 50%.

GENETIC CONSIDERATIONS

Addison disease, which can lead to acute adrenal crisis, has a strong genetic component, with a recent twin study estimating a heritability of 97%. The most well-established risk factors include variants in the human leukocyte antigen (HLA) genes, which follow a recessive pattern of inheritance. There is also a rare form of X-linked congenital adrenal insufficiency that is associated with mutations in the *NR0B1* gene that produce the DAX1 protein. Congenital adrenal hyperplasia is characterized by autosomal recessive mutations in one of the enzymes required for cortisol synthesis, impairing cortisol production. Adrenal insufficiency is often seen in families in association with other autoimmune disorders, most commonly with autoimmune polyendocrine syndrome (APS).

SEX AND LIFE SPAN CONSIDERATIONS

Males and females are affected by adrenocortical insufficiency at the same rate, but women develop the idiopathic autoimmune form of adrenal insufficiency more often than men. Idiopathic autoimmune adrenal insufficiency generally occurs in young and middle adulthood, but adrenal crisis may occur at any age, without regard to gender, and may be associated with developmental or genetic abnormalities. In children, the most common cause of acute adrenal crisis is an overwhelming infection with *Pseudomonas* or meningococcal meningitis (also known as Waterhouse-Friderichsen syndrome). In adults, acute adrenal crisis is more commonly associated with hemorrhagic destruction because of anticoagulant therapy or aggravation of adrenal hypofunction during periods of major stress but also occurs during critical illnesses such as septic shock. Mortality rates are highest for people older than 60 years and in people with comorbidities such as diabetes mellitus.

HEALTH DISPARITIES AND SEXUAL/GENDER MINORITY HEALTH

Ethnicity and race have no known effect on the risk for acute adrenal crisis. Sexual and gender minority persons have higher rates of multiple chronic conditions, poor quality of life, mental distress (stigma, social stress, victimization), and more cardiovascular disease compared to other groups (Caceres et al., 2019; Downing & Przedworski, 2018). These conditions place them at risk for acute adrenal crisis.

GLOBAL HEALTH CONSIDERATIONS

In developed countries, the incidence of primary adrenocortical insufficiency is approximately 50 cases per 1 million persons. No data are available on Eastern countries or many developing countries.

ASSESSMENT

HISTORY. Elicit a medication history, with particular attention to such medications as corticosteroids, phenytoin, barbiturates, anticoagulants, and rifampin. People with a history of corticosteroid use who are most at risk have taken at least 20 mg per day for at least 5 days during the past year. Note a history of cancer, autoimmune diseases requiring treatment with corticosteroids, critical illness, or radiation to the head or abdomen. A family history of either Addison disease or an autoimmune disease may be important.

Inquire about a recent decrease in appetite, abdominal pain, weight loss, or salt craving. Often, in crisis, the patient or family may describe fever, nausea, and vomiting. Determine if the patient has experienced signs and symptoms such as generalized fatigue, apathy, dizziness, weakness, headache, flank pain, hypothermia, hyperthermia, or changes in skin pigmentation. Some patients describe central nervous system effects such as confusion, irritability, psychoses, emotional lability, or even seizures. Women may describe a decreased libido and amenorrhea.

PHYSICAL EXAMINATION. The patient appears to be critically ill with **unexplained shock** and weakness. Because of decreased fluid volume caused by a decrease in water reabsorption, the patient may arrive at the hospital with severe hypotension; tachycardia; decreased cardiac output; weak and rapid pulses; and cool, pale skin. Peripheral pulses may be weak and irregular. Urine output is usually quite low. The blood pressure may be very hard to maintain because a decrease in the catecholamines can result in decreased vascular tone. Other symptoms include **nausea**, **vomiting**, **flank pain**, and **hypothermia**. Some patients have signs of an acute abdomen (distention, pain, abdominal rigidity) or high fever.

An increase in skin pigmentation (bronze color) is noticeable in people with pale skin tones. Areas most often affected include the mucous membranes and areas over joints and scars. A loss of pubic hair may also occur from a decreased level of adrenal androgens.

PSYCHOSOCIAL. Assess the patient's and significant others' ability to cope with a critical illness and the presence of a social network for support during a serious illness.

Diagnostic Highlights

Test	Normal Result	Abnormality With Condition	Explanation
Serum cortisol level (adult)	6 to 8 a.m., 5–25 mcg/dL	Decreased	Determines the ability of the adrenal gland to produce glucocorticoids
Serum electrolytes and chemistries (adult)	Sodium 135–145 mEq/L; potassium 3.5–5.3 mEq/L; blood urea nitrogen 8–21 mg/dL; glucose 70–100 mg/dL; anion gap 8–16 mEq/L	Hyponatremia; hyperkalemia; metabolic acidosis; azotemia; hypoglycemia	Values reflect sodium loss from a deficit in mineralocorticoids with loss of fluids and poor glucose control because of decreased gluconeogenesis; shock leads to acidosis (elevated anion gap); some patients may not have abnormalities
ACTH stimulation test; determine baseline serum cortisol, then administer 250 mcg ACTH intravenously and draw serum cortisol level 30–60 min later	Normal serum cortisol level (see above)	Less than 20 mcg after ACTH stimulation; increase of less than 9 mcg/dL determines the diagnosis of adrenal insufficiency	Normal adrenal gland greatly increases production of cortisol when stimulated by ACTH

(highlight box continues on page 44)

Diagnostic Highlights (continued)

Other Tests: Blood and other cultures and sensitivities; computed tomography (CT) of the abdomen; complete blood count; serum calcium; skull x-rays; thyroid-stimulating hormone; thyroid hormone levels; pituitary and adrenal imaging

PRIMARY NURSING DIAGNOSIS

DIAGNOSIS. Deficient fluid volume related to electrolyte imbalance as evidenced by decrease in blood pressure and/or increase in heart rate

OUTCOMES. Fluid balance; Electrolyte & acid base balance; Hypoglycemia severity; Hyponatremia severity; Hyperkalemia severity; Circulation status; Cardiac pump effectiveness; Hydration; Nutritional status

INTERVENTIONS. Fluid/electrolyte management; Hypoglycemia management; IV therapy; Fluid monitoring; Medication administration: IV; Electrolyte management: Hyponatremia, hyperkalemia

☀ PLANNING AND IMPLEMENTATION

Collaborative

Patients with acute adrenal crisis are critically ill and have a potentially fatal condition. Rapid intervention is necessary, and the highest priority is to maintain airway, breathing, and circulation. If the patient is unresponsive, providers may initiate a coma protocol and administer glucose in case of diabetic shock, thiamine in case of thiamine deficiency, and/or naloxone in case of drug overdose. Pharmacologic treatment centers on fluid and electrolyte replacement and hormonal supplements (see Pharmacologic Highlights box). Fluid replacement with dextrose- and sodium-containing solutions allows for correction of hypovolemia and hypoglycemia. As much as 5 L or more of fluid may be needed to maintain an adequate blood pressure, circulation, and urine output and to replace the fluid deficit. Correct sodium, potassium, calcium, and glucose abnormalities. Always treat the underlying problem that precipitated adrenal crisis.

Pharmacologic Highlights

Medication or Drug Class	Dosage	Description	Rationale
Dexamethasone	4 mg IV	Corticosteroid	Substitution therapy in deficiency state; drug does not interfere with serum cortisol assay; dangerous to delay glucocorticoid replacement while awaiting ACTH stimulation test results; drug does not have mineralocorticoid activity and therefore needs to be accompanied by fluid and electrolyte replacement
Hydrocortisone sodium succinate	100 mg IV q 6–8 hr	Corticosteroid	Substitution therapy in deficiency state

Other Therapies: Cortisone acetate (Cortone); fludrocortisone acetate (Florinef) for primary insufficiency

Independent

During the initial hours of managing a patient with acute adrenal crisis, the first priority is to maintain airway, breathing, and circulation. Patients who receive large amounts of room-temperature fluids are at risk for hypothermia. Keep the temperature of the room warm and the bed linens dry. If possible, keep the patient fully covered. During massive fluid replacement, administer warmed (body-temperature) fluids if possible.

Teach the patient on corticosteroids about the medication and the need to continue to take it until the physician tapers the dose and then finally discontinues it. Explain the symptoms of adrenal crisis to any patient who is undergoing anticoagulant therapy. Explain the effects of stress on the disease and the need for adjustment of medications during times of stress.

Patients with altered tissue perfusion require frequent skin care. If the patient is immobile, perform active and passive range-of-motion exercises at least every 8 hours. Encourage coughing and deep breathing to limit the complications from immobility. Provide small, frequent meals and make referrals to the dietitian early in the hospitalization.

Evidence-Based Practice and Health Policy

Martin-Grace, J., Dineen, R., Sherlock, M., & Thompson, C. (2020). Adrenal insufficiency: Physiology, clinical presentation and diagnostic challenges. *Clinica Chimica Acta*, *505*, 78–91.

- The authors described the normal physiology of the hypothalamic-pituitary-adrenal axis and how it relates to the signs and symptoms of adrenal crisis.
- Adrenal insufficiency is associated with increased morbidity and mortality and reduction of quality of life. The most common cause is autoimmune adrenalitis and is also associated with other autoimmune conditions such as thyroid disease, celiac disease, pernicious anemia, and type 1 diabetes mellitus. People with untreated acute adrenal insufficiency often have chronic fatigue, weight loss, and vulnerability to infection.
- While vague specific symptoms can make early diagnosis challenging, rapid treatment is important to reverse the patient's acute illness.

DOCUMENTATION GUIDELINES

- Physical findings: Vital signs and pulse oximetry; mental status, pulmonary artery/central venous catheter pressure readings; monitoring of airway, breathing, circulation; urine output; mental status
- Important changes in laboratory values: Plasma cortisol, serum glucose, serum sodium and potassium, pH, oxygen saturation
- Presence of complications: Infection, cardiac dysrhythmias, hypotension/shock, fluid and electrolyte imbalance, weight loss
- Response to therapy: Daily weights, appetite, level of hydration

DISCHARGE AND HOME HEALTHCARE GUIDELINES

PATIENT TEACHING. Teach the patient and significant others about the disease and the factors that aggravate it. Provide suggestions about rest and activity and stress reduction. Explain the signs and symptoms that may lead to crisis.

PREVENTION. Identify the stressors and the need to increase medication during times of stress. Teach the patient and family when the physician needs to be notified.

MEDICATIONS. Teach the patient the name, dosage, action, and side effects of drugs and the need to continue using them for life. Provide written instruction about medications and follow-up physician's appointments.

Adrenal Insufficiency (Addison Disease)

DRG Category: 644
Mean LOS: 4.3 days
Description: MEDICAL: Endocrine Disorders With Complication or Comorbidity

Adrenal insufficiency occurs when the adrenal glands do not produce adequate amounts of hormones to support the body's function. The medulla, the inner portion of the adrenal gland, is responsible for the secretion of the catecholamines epinephrine and norepinephrine; the cortex, or outer portion, is responsible for the secretion of glucocorticoids, mineralocorticoids, and androgen. The principal glucocorticoid, cortisol, helps regulate blood pressure, metabolism, anti-inflammatory response, and emotional behavior. The principal mineralocorticoid, aldosterone, is important for regulating sodium levels. Adrenal insufficiency is characterized by the decreased production of cortisol, aldosterone, and androgen. Cortisol deficiency causes altered metabolism, decreased stress tolerance, and emotional lability. Aldosterone deficiency causes urinary loss of sodium, chloride, and water, resulting in dehydration and electrolyte imbalances. Androgen deficiency leads to the loss of secondary sex characteristics. The major cause of illness or death for people with adrenal insufficiency is a delay in making the diagnosis, or failure to begin appropriate therapy with glucocorticoids and/or mineralocorticoids. Complications include bone loss, hypothyroidism, ischemic heart disease, acute adrenal insufficiency, and shock.

CAUSES

Adrenal insufficiency can be primary or secondary. Addison disease, or primary adrenal insufficiency, occurs rarely, but when it occurs, there is loss of at least 90% of the adrenal cortex. Idiopathic adrenal atrophy is the most common cause of primary adrenal insufficiency. It is not known exactly why this occurs, but it is believed to be related to an autoimmune response that results in the slow destruction of adrenal tissue. Tuberculosis, histoplasmosis, AIDS, malignancies, and hemorrhage into the adrenal glands have all been associated with destruction of the adrenal glands. Secondary insufficiency occurs from disorders of the pituitary gland, which produces hormones to regulate the adrenal gland. It results from hypopituitarism due to hypothalamic-pituitary disease or suppression of the hypothalamic-pituitary axis by corticosteroid therapy. Secondary adrenal failure can also occur with adrenocorticotropic hormone (ACTH) deficiency caused by disorders of the pituitary. Other causes include physiological stress, including surgery, anesthesia, fluid volume loss, trauma, asthma, hypothermia, alcohol abuse, myocardial infarction, fever, hypoglycemia, pain, and depression. Approximately 8% of people with adrenal insufficiency require hospital treatment each year for adrenal crisis (see **Adrenal Crisis, Acute**).

GENETIC CONSIDERATIONS

Addison disease has a strong genetic component, with a recent twin study estimating a heritability of 97%. The most well-established risk factors include variants in the human leukocyte antigen (HLA) genes, which follow a recessive pattern of inheritance. There is also a rare form of X-linked congenital adrenal insufficiency that is associated with mutations in the *NR0B1* gene that produce the DAX1 protein. Congenital adrenal hyperplasia is characterized by autosomal recessive mutations in one of the enzymes required for cortisol synthesis, impairing cortisol production. Adrenal insufficiency is often seen in families in association with other autoimmune disorders, most commonly with autoimmune polyendocrine syndrome (APS).

SEX AND LIFE SPAN CONSIDERATIONS

Addison disease, particularly idiopathic autoimmune Addison disease, occurs most often in adults from ages 30 to 50 years and affects females more than males. Children may develop the condition if they have genetic susceptibility.

HEALTH DISPARITIES AND SEXUAL/GENDER MINORITY HEALTH

Ethnicity, race, and sexual/gender minority status have no known effect on the risk for Addison disease.

GLOBAL HEALTH CONSIDERATIONS

In developed countries, the incidence in Western countries is 50 cases per 1 million persons. No data are available on Eastern countries or many developing countries.

ASSESSMENT

HISTORY. Determine if the patient has a history of recent infection, use of corticosteroids such as prednisone, or adrenal or pituitary surgery. Patients may describe vague symptoms such as weakness, fatigue, dizziness, and weight loss. They may experience **hyperpigmentation** of the skin (particularly on the knuckles, elbows, knees, palmar creases), nailbeds, and mucous membranes because of melanin overproduction. Hyperpigmentation may have lasted for months or even years. Establish a history of poor tolerance for stress, weakness, fatigue, and activity intolerance. Ask if the patient has experienced **anorexia, nausea, vomiting,** or **diarrhea** as a result of altered metabolism. Some patients have **dizziness with orthostasis** due to hypotension. Elicit a history of craving for salt or intolerance to cold. Determine presence of altered menses in females and impotence in males.

PHYSICAL EXAMINATION. Assess the patient for signs of dehydration such as tachycardia, altered level of consciousness, dry skin with poor turgor, dry mucous membranes, weight loss, and weak peripheral pulses. Check for postural hypotension—that is, a drop in systolic blood pressure greater than 15 mm Hg when the patient is moved from a lying position to a sitting or standing position.

Inspect the skin for pigmentation changes caused by an altered regulation of melanin, noting if surgical scars, skin folds, and genitalia show a characteristic bronze color. Inspect the patient's gums and oral mucous membranes to see if they are bluish-black. Take the patient's temperature to see if it is subnormal. Note any loss of axillary and pubic hair that could be caused by decreased androgen levels.

PSYCHOSOCIAL. Because an acute adrenal crisis may be precipitated by emotional stress, periodic psychosocial assessments are necessary for patients with adrenal insufficiency. Patients with an adrenal insufficiency frequently complain of weakness and fatigue, which are also characteristic of an emotional problem. However, weakness and fatigue of an emotional origin seem to have a pattern of being worse in the morning and lessening throughout the day, whereas the weakness and fatigue of adrenal insufficiency seem to be precipitated by activity and lessen with rest. Patients with adrenal insufficiency may show signs of depression and irritability from decreased cortisol levels.

Diagnostic Highlights

General Comments: To determine if a cortisol deficit exists, a plasma cortisol level is drawn in the morning; less than 10 mcg/dL suggests adrenal insufficiency; further testing may be needed to determine if the adrenal glands have a primary deficiency or if the pituitary cannot produce enough ACTH (secondary adrenal failure).

(highlight box continues on page 48)

Diagnostic Highlights (continued)

Test	Normal Result	Abnormality With Condition	Explanation
Serum cortisol level (adult)	6–8 a.m. levels should be 5–25 mcg/dL	Decreased	Determines the ability of the adrenal gland to produce glucocorticoids
Serum electrolytes and chemistries (adult)	Sodium 135–145 mEq/L; potassium 3.5–5.3 mEq/L; blood urea nitrogen 8–21 mg/dL; glucose 70–100 mg/dL	Hyponatremia; hyperkalemia; azotemia; hypoglycemia	Values reflect sodium loss from a deficit in mineralocorticoids with loss of fluids and poor glucose control because of decreased gluconeogenesis; most consistent finding is elevated blood urea nitrogen due to hypovolemia, decreased glomerular filtration rate, and decreased renal plasma flow
ACTH stimulation test	15–30 minutes after infusion of ACTH, the adrenal cortex releases two to five times its normal plasma cortisol level; the cortisol value should be above 20 mcg/dL and have increased at least 7 mcg/dL above baseline readings	Level ≤ 20 mcg/dL in 30 or 60 min	Adrenal glands cannot respond to the stimulation from ACTH and demonstrate that they are not functioning normally

Other Tests: Computed tomography of the abdomen; chest x-ray to determine heart size or presence of tuberculosis or fungal infections; metyrapone suppression test; urine 17-hydroxycorticosteroids (17-OHCS) and 17-ketosteroids (17-KS); thyroid-stimulating hormone; serum calcium; and electrocardiogram (ECG)

PRIMARY NURSING DIAGNOSIS

DIAGNOSIS. Imbalanced nutrition: less than body requirements related to insufficient dietary intake as evidenced by anorexia, nausea, vomiting, and/or diarrhea

OUTCOMES. Fluid balance; Hydration; Nutritional status: Food and fluid intake; Nutritional status: Energy; Electrolyte & acid-base balance; Hypoglycemia severity; Hyponatremia severity; Hyperkalemia severity

INTERVENTIONS. Fluid/electrolyte management: Hyponatremia, hyperkalemia; Hypoglycemia management; Nutritional management; Nutritional counseling

☀ PLANNING AND IMPLEMENTATION

Collaborative

Collaborative treatment of adrenal insufficiency focuses on restoring fluid, electrolyte, and hormone balances. The fluid used for adrenal insufficiency will most likely be 5% dextrose in 0.9% sodium chloride to replace fluid volume, glucose, and serum sodium. Correct sodium, potassium, calcium, and glucose abnormalities. Patients with adrenal insufficiency will require lifelong replacement glucocorticoid and mineralocorticoid therapy, which needs careful monitoring for signs of inadequate replacement. Patients on an appropriate maintenance dose should not experience morning weakness, dizziness, and headaches. Patients with diabetes mellitus will require insulin adjustments for elevated serum glucose levels.

Pharmacologic Highlights

General Comments: Fludrocortisone promotes kidney reabsorption of sodium and the excretion of potassium. Overtreatment can result in fluid retention and possibly congestive heart failure; therefore, monitor serum potassium and sodium levels frequently during fludrocortisone administration.

Medication or Drug Class	Dosage	Description	Rationale
Glucocorticoids such as hydrocortisone, dexamethasone, and prednisone	Varies by drug	Corticosteroid	Replacement therapy in deficiency state
Fludrocortisone	0.1 mg PO daily	Mineralocorticoid	Replacement therapy in deficiency state

Independent

Because of the negative effect of physical and emotional stress on the patient with adrenal insufficiency, promote strategies that reduce stress. If the patient develops an infection or heavy cold, or has a procedure such as a minor surgery or tooth extraction, teach the patient to double or triple their corticosteroid dose or to check with the provider about increasing the dose. Teach the patient to rest between activities to conserve energy and to wear warm clothing to increase comfort and limit heat loss. To limit the risk of infection, encourage the patient to use good hand-washing techniques and to limit exposure to people with infections. To prevent complications, teach the patient to avoid using lotions that contain alcohol to prevent skin dryness and breakdown and to eat a nutritious diet that has adequate proteins, fats, and carbohydrates to maintain sodium and potassium balance.

Finally, the prospect of a chronic disease and the need to avoid stress may lead patients to impaired social interaction and ineffective coping. Discuss with the patient the presence of support systems and coping patterns. Provide emotional support by encouraging the patient to verbalize feelings about an altered body image and anxieties about the disease process. Incorporate the patient's unique positive characteristics and strengths into the care plan. Encourage the patient to interact with family and significant others. Before discharge, refer patients who exhibit disabling behaviors to therapists, self-help groups, or crisis intervention centers.

Evidence-Based Practice and Health Policy

Margulies, S., Corrigan, K., Bathgate, S., & Macri, C. (2020). Addison's disease in pregnancy: Case report, management, and review of literature. *Journal of Neonatal-Prenatal Medicine, 13,* 275–278.

- While adrenal insufficiency is an unusual complication of pregnancy, pregnant patients are at risk for multiple complications. The authors reviewed symptoms that can occur and provided a case study.
- Complications that occurred in a healthy, 34-year-old woman included lethargy, skin hyperpigmentation, frequent urination, and salt craving. Her laboratory results showed hyperkalemia, hyponatremia, elevated adrenocorticotropic hormone, and low cortisol.
- She was treated with hydrocortisone and fludrocortisone, which resolved her symptoms. The authors suggested that during pregnancy, patients with adrenal insufficiency have their medications increased due to the stress of pregnancy.

DOCUMENTATION GUIDELINES

- Physical findings: Cardiovascular status, including blood pressure and heart rate; tissue perfusion status, including level of consciousness, skin temperature, peripheral pulses, and

urine output; fluid volume status, including neck vein assessment, daily weights, and fluid input and output
• Laboratory findings: Blood levels of potassium, sodium, hematocrit, and blood urea nitrogen (BUN)

DISCHARGE AND HOME HEALTHCARE GUIDELINES

PREVENTION. To prevent acute adrenal crisis, teach patients how to avoid stress. Emphasize the need to take medications as prescribed and to contact the physician if the patient becomes stressed or unable to take medications. Make sure the patient knows to alert the surgeon about adrenal insufficiency prior to all surgical procedures. Parenteral corticosteroids will likely be prescribed during any major procedure or times of major stress or trauma.

MEDICATIONS. Be sure the patient understands the reason for steroids that are prescribed. (See Box 1 for a full explanation.) Some patients will be taught to give themselves an IM injection of steroids to be administered if they are unable to take their medication orally.

RESOURCES. Referrals may be necessary to identify potential physical and emotional problems. Notify the hospital's social service department before patient discharge if you have identified obvious environmental stressors. Initiate home health nursing to ensure compliance with medical therapy and early detection of complications. If you identify emotional problems, refer the patient to therapists or self-help groups.

• BOX 1 Patient Teaching for Corticosteroids

• Emphasize the lifetime nature of taking corticosteroids.
• Provide name, dosage, and action of the prescribed medication.
• Explain the common side effects of weight gain, swelling around the face and eyes, insomnia, bruising, gastric distress, gastric bleeding, and petechiae.
• Advise the patient to take the medication with meals to avoid gastric irritation and to take the medication at the time of day prescribed, usually in the morning.
• Suggest the patient weigh self daily, at the same time each day, and call the healthcare provider if weight changes by 5 pounds.
• Emphasize that the patient should always take the medication. Not taking it can cause life-threatening complications. Tell the patient to call the healthcare provider if they are unable to take medication for more than 24 hours.
• Explain that periods of stress require more medication. Tell the patient to call the healthcare provider for changes in dose if they experience extra physical or emotional stress. Illness and temperature extremes are considered stressors.
• Explain preventative measures. Tell the patient that to prevent getting ill, they should avoid being in groups with people who are ill and environments where temperatures change from very hot to very cold.
• Teach the patient to recognize signs of undermedication: weakness, fatigue, and dizziness. Emphasize the need to report underdosing to the healthcare provider.
• Teach the patient to avoid dizziness by moving from a sitting to a standing position slowly.
• Urge the patient to always wear a medical alert necklace or bracelet to inform healthcare professionals of the diagnosis.

Air Embolism

DRG Category:	175
Mean LOS:	5.1 days
Description:	MEDICAL: Pulmonary Embolism With Major Complication or Comorbidity or Acute Cor Pulmonale

An air embolism is an obstruction in a vein or artery caused by a bubble of atmospheric gas. Air enters the circulatory system when the pressure gradient favors movement of air or gas from the environment into the blood. A venous air embolism is the most common form of air embolism. It occurs when air enters the venous circulation. It can then pass through the right side of the heart and proceed to the lungs. A small volume of air is broken up in the capillaries, or the lungs can filter the air and absorb it without complications. When large amounts of air (80–100 mL) are introduced into the body, however, the lungs no longer have the capacity to filter the air, and the patient has serious or even lethal complications. Complications occur if a large air bubble blocks the outflow of blood from the right ventricle into the lungs, preventing the blood from moving forward. The patient develops cardiogenic shock because of insufficient cardiac output. Experts have found that the risk from air embolism increases as both the volume and the speed of air injection increase.

An arterial embolism occurs when air gains entry into the pulmonary venous circulation and then passes through the heart and into the systemic arterial circulation. An arterial embolism can also form in the patient who has a venous embolism and a right-to-left shunt (often caused by a septal defect in the heart) so that the air bubble moves into the left ventricle without passing through the lungs. Pulmonary capillary shunts can produce the same effect. The arterial embolism may cause serious or even lethal complications in the brain and heart. Scientists have found that as little as 0.5 mL of air in the coronary arteries can cause ventricular fibrillation or death.

CAUSES

The two major causes of air embolism are iatrogenic and environmental. Iatrogenic complications are those that occur as a result of a diagnostic or therapeutic procedure. One common situation in which iatrogenic injury may occur is during insertion, maintenance, or removal of a central line. The risk is highest during catheter insertion because the large-bore needle, which is in the vein, is at the hub while the catheter is threaded into the vein. The frequency of clinically recognized venous air embolism following central line insertion is less than 2%, but in that setting, it has a mortality rate as high as 30%. In addition, air can be pulled into the circulation whenever the catheter is disconnected for a tubing change or the catheter tubing system is accidentally disconnected or broken. When the catheter is removed, air can also enter the fibrin tract that was caused by the catheter during the brief period between removal and sealing of the tract. Other procedures that can lead to air embolism are cardiac catheterization, coronary arteriography, transcutaneous angioplasty, embolectomy, high-pressure mechanical ventilation, epidural anesthesia, and hemodialysis. Both blunt and penetrating trauma to the head and face, neck, thorax, or abdomen can lead to air embolism. Some surgical procedures also place the patient at particular risk, including orthopedic, urological, gynecological, open heart, cervical spine, and brain surgery, particularly when the procedure is performed with the patient in an upright position. Conditions such as multiple trauma, placenta previa, and pneumoperitoneum have also been associated with air embolism.

Environmental causes occur when a person is exposed to atmospheric pressures that are markedly different from atmospheric pressure at sea level. Two such examples are deep-sea diving (scuba diving) and high-altitude flying. Excessive pressures force nitrogen, which is not absorbable, into body tissues and the circulation. Nitrogen accumulates in the extracellular spaces, forms bubbles, and enters into the bloodstream as emboli.

GENETIC CONSIDERATIONS

No clear genetic contributions to susceptibility have been defined.

SEX AND LIFE SPAN CONSIDERATIONS

An air embolism can occur at any age if individuals are in a situation that places them at risk for either an iatrogenic or an environmental cause.

HEALTH DISPARITIES AND SEXUAL/GENDER MINORITY HEALTH

Ethnicity, race, and sexual/gender minority status have no known effect on the risk for air embolism.

GLOBAL HEALTH CONSIDERATIONS

No data are available.

ASSESSMENT

HISTORY. The patient may have been scuba diving or flying at the onset of symptoms. Usually patients who develop an iatrogenic air embolism are under the care of the healthcare team, who assesses the signs and symptoms of air embolism as a complication of treatment. Some patients have a **gasp or cough** when the initial infusion of air moves into the pulmonary circulation. Suspect an air embolism immediately when a patient becomes symptomatic following insertion, maintenance, or removal of a central access catheter. Patients suddenly become **dyspneic, dizzy, nauseated, confused,** and **anxious,** and they may complain of **substernal chest pain.** Some patients describe the feeling of "impending doom." Other symptoms may include headaches, slurred speech, blurred vision, syncope, or seizures.

PHYSICAL EXAMINATION. On inspection, the patient may appear in acute distress with cyanosis, jugular neck vein distension, or even seizures and unresponsiveness. Some reports explain that more than 40% of patients with an air embolism have central nervous system effects, such as altered mental status or coma. When auscultating the patient's heart, listen for a "mill-wheel murmur" produced by air bubbles in the right ventricle and heard throughout the cardiac cycle. The murmur may be loud enough to be heard without a stethoscope but is only temporarily audible and is usually a late sign. More common than the mill-wheel murmur is a harsh systolic murmur or normal heart sounds. Most patients have a rapid apical pulse and low blood pressure. You may also hear wheezing from acute bronchospasm. The patient may have increased central venous pressure, pulmonary artery pressure, increased systemic vascular resistance, and decreased cardiac output.

PSYCHOSOCIAL. Most patients respond with fear, confusion, and anxiety. Usually patients are immediately transported to a setting for diagnostic testing or emergency/critical care and undergo a variety of emergency measures. Evaluate the patient's and family's ability to cope with the crisis, and provide the appropriate support. If the cause is iatrogenic, use honesty in discussing the situation.

Diagnostic Highlights

Test	Normal Result	Abnormality With Condition	Explanation
Arterial blood gases	Pao₂ 80–95 mm Hg; Paco₂ 35–45 mm Hg; SaO₂ > 95%	Pao₂ < 80 mm Hg; Paco₂ varies; SaO₂ < 95%	Poor gas exchange leads to hypoxemia and hypercapnea from dead-space ventilation

Other Tests: Supporting tests include electrocardiogram, chest x-ray, transthoracic or transesophageal echocardiography, precordial Doppler ultrasound, computed tomography, and magnetic resonance imaging.

PRIMARY NURSING DIAGNOSIS

DIAGNOSIS. Decreased cardiac output related to blocked right ventricular filling as evidenced by decreased preload, decreased stroke volume, and/or tachycardia

OUTCOMES. Cardiac pump effectiveness; Circulation status; Tissue perfusion: Cerebral, Cardiac, Respiratory, Peripheral

INTERVENTIONS. Oxygen therapy; Positioning; Cardiac care: Acute; Shock management: Cardiac; Hemodynamic regulation

PLANNING AND IMPLEMENTATION

Collaborative

PREVENTION. Several strategies can help prevent development of air embolism. First, maintain the patient's level of hydration because dehydration predisposes the patient to decreased venous pressures. Second, some clinicians recommend that you position the patient in the supine position with the head lowered (Trendelenburg position) during central line insertion and removal because the position increases central venous pressure. Third, instruct patients to hold their breath or perform the Valsalva maneuver on exhalation during central line insertion or removal to increase intrathoracic pressure and thereby increase central venous pressure.

Prime all tubings with IV fluid prior to connecting the system to the catheter. Immediately apply an occlusive pressure dressing after catheter removal and maintain the site with an occlusive dressing for at least 24 hours. To prevent air embolism during surgical procedures, the surgeon floods the surgical field with liquid in some situations so that liquid rather than air enters the circulation.

TREATMENT. If an air embolus occurs, the first efforts are focused on preventing more air from entering the circulation. Any central line procedure that is in progress should be immediately terminated with the line clamped. The catheter should not be removed unless it cannot be clamped. Place the patient on 100% oxygen immediately to facilitate the washout of nitrogen from the bubble of atmospheric gas. Place the patient in the left lateral decubitus position. This position allows the obstructing air bubble in the pulmonary outflow tract to float toward the apex of the right ventricle, which relieves the obstruction. Use the Trendelenburg position to relieve the obstruction caused by air bubbles. Other suggested strategies are to aspirate the air from the right atrium, to use closed-chest cardiac compressions, and to administer fluids to maintain vascular volume. Hyperbaric oxygen therapy may improve the patient's condition as well. This therapy increases nitrogen washout in the air bubble, thereby reducing the bubble's size and the absorption of air. Note that if the patient has to be transferred to a hyperbaric facility, the decrease in atmospheric pressure that occurs at high altitudes during fixed-wing or helicopter transport may worsen the patient's condition because of bubble enlargement or "bubble explosion." Ground transport or transport in a low-flying helicopter is recommended, along with administering 100% oxygen and adequate hydration during transport.

Independent

If the patient suddenly develops the symptoms of an air embolism, place the patient on the left side with the head of the bed down to allow the air to float out of the outflow track. Notify the physician immediately and position the resuscitation cart in close proximity. Initiate 100% oxygen via a nonrebreather mask immediately before the physician arrives according to unit policy. Be prepared for a sudden deterioration in cardiopulmonary status and potential for cardiac arrest.

The patient and family need a great deal of support. Remain in the patient's room at all times, and if the patient finds touch reassuring, hold the patient's hand. Provide an ongoing summary of the patient's condition to the family. Expect the patient to be extremely frightened and the family to be anxious or even angry. Ask the chaplain, clinical nurse specialist, nursing supervisor, or social worker to remain with the family during the period of crisis.

Evidence-Based Practice and Health Policy

Capron, T., Guinde, J., Laroumagne, S., Dutau, H., & Astoul, P. (2020). Cerebral air embolism after pleural lavage for empyema. *Annals of Thoracic Surgery*, *110*, e289–e291.

- The authors reported on a case of cerebral embolism during a pleural lavage for the management of an empyema (collection of pus in the cavity between the lung and the membrane that surrounds the lung). The risk of an air embolus during this procedure is approximately 5%.
- Immediately after the procedure, the patient developed hypoxemia, bradycardia, and loss of consciousness. Her neurological examination included right hemiplegia, facial paralysis, and seizure activity. Following hyperbaric oxygen therapy, her condition improved rapidly, and she had no long-term consequences of the air embolus.

DOCUMENTATION GUIDELINES

- Physical findings: Changes in vital signs, cardiopulmonary assessment, skin color, capillary blanch, level of activity, changes in level of consciousness
- Pain: Location, duration, precipitating factors, response to interventions
- Responses to interventions: Positioning, oxygen, hyperbaric oxygen, evacuation of air, cardiopulmonary resuscitation
- Development of complications: Seizures, cardiac arrest, severe anxiety, ineffective patient or family coping

DISCHARGE AND HOME HEALTHCARE GUIDELINES

PREVENTION. Instruct the patient to report any signs of complications. Make sure that the patient and family are aware of the next follow-up visit with the healthcare provider. If the patient is being discharged with central IV access, make sure that the caregiver understands the risk of air embolism and can describe all preventive strategies to limit the risk of air embolism.

Alcohol Intoxication, Acute

DRG Category: 895
Mean LOS: 12.4 days
Description: MEDICAL: Alcohol, Drug Abuse or Dependence With Rehabilitation Therapy

In the United States, an estimated 95,000 people die each year from alcohol-related causes, making alcohol the third-leading preventable cause of death. Acute alcohol intoxication occurs when a person consumes large quantities of alcohol. In most states, legal intoxication occurs at a blood alcohol level of 80 mg/dL (0.08 g/dL or 0.08%) or more. Acute alcohol intoxication leads to complex physiological interactions that can affect the central nervous system (CNS), lungs, heart, and the gastrointestinal (GI) system. Because alcohol is a primary and continuous depressant of the CNS, patients may seem stimulated initially because alcohol depresses inhibitory control mechanisms. Other effects on the CNS include loss of memory, concentration, insight, and motor control, and advanced intoxication can produce coma and general anesthesia, hypoglycemia, and hypothermia. Chronic intoxication may lead to brain damage, memory loss, sleep disturbances, and psychoses. Respiratory effects also include apnea, decreased diaphragmatic excursion, diminished respiratory drive, impaired glottal reflexes, and vascular shunts in lung tissue. The risk of aspiration and pulmonary infection increases while respiratory depression and apnea occur.

The cardiovascular system becomes depressed, leading to depression of the vasomotor center in the brain and to hypotension. Conversely, in some individuals, intoxication causes the release of catecholamines from adrenal glands, which leads to hypertension. Intoxication also depresses leukocyte movement into areas of inflammation, depresses platelet function, and leads to fibrinogen and clotting factor deficiency, thrombocytopenia, and decreased platelet function.

The effects on the GI system include stimulation of gastric secretions, mucosal irritation, cessation of motor function of the gut, and delayed absorption. Pylorospasm and vomiting may occur. Complications include pulmonary aspiration, impaired judgment and impaired motor coordination leading to injury or violence, interpersonal violence, disorderly conduct, GI disturbances such as nausea and vomiting, hypothermia, apnea, and death.

CAUSES

Alcohol is metabolized at a rate of approximately 15 to 25 g/hour in people who are not heavy drinkers; thus alcohol intoxication occurs when persons ingest alcohol at a rate faster than their body can metabolize it. One standard drink (12 ounces of beer, 5 ounces of wine, or 1.5 ounces of whiskey) provides about 14 g of alcohol. When people drink faster than the body metabolizes alcohol, they become intoxicated when blood alcohol levels reach 100 mg/dL, although the physiological effects occur at levels as low as 40 mg/dL.

GENETIC CONSIDERATIONS

Susceptibility to alcohol misuse appears to be both genetic and environmental, with an estimated heritability of 50%. Genetic differences in alcohol metabolism may result in increased levels of a metabolite that produces pleasure for those with a predisposition toward alcohol misuse. Associations between alcoholism and certain alleles of alcohol dehydrogenase (*ADH2*, *ADH3*, and *ADH7*) are the most well documented. A recent Genome Wide Association Study (GWAS) found five loci (*ADH1B*, *ADH1C*, *FTO*, *GCKR*, and *SLC39A8*) significantly associated with high alcohol consumption and alcohol use disorder (AUD, chronic relapsing brain disorder characterized by an impaired ability to stop or control alcohol use despite adverse social, occupational, or health consequences; National Institute on Alcohol Abuse and Alcoholism, 2021), eight loci (*VRK2, DCLK2, ISL1, IGF2BP1, PPR1R3B, BRAP, BAHCC1,* and *RBX1*) significantly associated with only high consumption, and four loci (*ADH4, DRD2, SIX3,* and chr10q25.1) significantly associated with only AUD.

SEX AND LIFE SPAN CONSIDERATIONS

Acute alcohol intoxication can affect people of any age, gender, race, or socioeconomic background. Alcohol use should be considered when a patient is seen for trauma, acute abdominal pain, cardiac dysrhythmias, cardiomyopathy, encephalopathy, coma, seizures, pancreatitis, sepsis, anxiety, delirium, depression, or suicide attempt. Males drink more alcohol than females.

TEENAGERS AND YOUNG ADULTS. The use of alcohol is seen as a part of growing up for many individuals. Binge drinking (four or more drinks in 2 hours for females, five or more drinks in 2 hours for males) is common and dangerous. The combination of alcohol and potentially risky activities, such as driving or sex, is a source of high morbidity and mortality for teens. An emerging trend, high-intensity drinking, is defined as consuming alcohol at levels that are two or more times the sex-specific binge drinking thresholds (NIAAA, 2021). Experts note people who engage in high-intensity drinking are 70 to 90 times more likely to have an alcohol-related emergency department visit than those who do not binge drink. Female teens and young women are drinking more as sex differences are shrinking in drinking patterns, AUD, hospitalizations, and emergency department visits.

PREGNANT PEOPLE. Alcohol is a potent teratogen. Binge drinking and moderate to heavy drinking have been associated with many fetal abnormalities. There is no currently known safe drinking level during pregnancy.

OLDER ADULTS. Loss of friends and family, loss of income, decreased mobility, and chronic illness or pain may increase isolation and loneliness and lead to an increased use of alcohol.

HEALTH DISPARITIES AND SEXUAL/GENDER MINORITY HEALTH

Data from 2021 show that in teenagers and young adults 12 to 20 years of age, approximately 21% of White youths drink alcohol, as compared to 16% of Hispanic and 10% of Black youths. Across all ages, alcohol consumption is most prevalent among White persons, followed by Native American, Hispanic, and Black people (NIAAA, 2021). The National Survey on Drug Use and Health (SAMHSA, 2021) has reported that sexual minority persons are more likely to engage in binge drinking and heavy alcohol use as compared to their heterosexual counterparts. Sexual minority persons are also more likely to continue heavy drinking into later life. The Centers for Disease Control and Prevention (CDC) note that alcohol use may be a reaction to homophobia, violence, or discrimination for sexual minorities (CDC, 2021). Transgender is a term used to describe persons whose gender identity is different from their sex assigned at birth. Approximately 1% of the U.S. population identify themselves as transgender. Male to female transgender persons have higher rates of heavy, episodic drinking when compared to cisgender females (Downing & Przedworski, 2018). Cisgender persons have gender identity and gender expression that are aligned with the assigned sex listed on their birth certificate. There are no specific data known that explain the prevalence of alcohol withdrawal in sexual and gender minority persons.

GLOBAL HEALTH CONSIDERATIONS

Three million deaths every year around the globe result from harmful use of alcohol, representing 5.3% of all deaths (World Health Organization [WHO], 2018). WHO reports that alcohol contributed to more than 200 diseases and injury-related health conditions, ranging from liver diseases, road traffic injuries and violence, to cancers, cardiovascular diseases, suicides, tuberculosis, and HIV. Globally, alcohol misuse has been identified as the seventh leading risk factor for premature death and disability, and, among people aged 15 to 49 years of age, it has been identified as the first leading risk factor. The WHO (2021) reports that in high income countries, about 20% of fatally injured drivers have excess alcohol in their blood, while in low and middle income countries, these figures may be up to 69%. Alcohol consumption has increased greatly in developing countries and is a health concern because, first, it is occurring in countries without a tradition of alcohol use, and second, these countries have few strategies for prevention or treatment.

ASSESSMENT

HISTORY. Ask the patient how much alcohol they consumed and over what period of time. Elicit a history of past patterns of alcohol consumption. You may need to consult other sources, such as family or friends, to obtain accurate information when the patient is acutely intoxicated upon admission.

PHYSICAL EXAMINATION. The intoxicated individual needs to have a careful respiratory, cardiovascular, and neurological evaluation. In life-threatening situations, conduct a brief survey to identify serious problems and begin stabilization. Begin with assessment of the airway, breathing, and circulation (ABCs).

Respiratory. Assess the patency of the patient's airway. Check the patient's respiratory rate and rhythm and listen to the breath sounds. Monitor the patient carefully for **apnea and respiratory depression** throughout the period of intoxication. Determine the adequacy of the patient's breathing.

Cardiovascular. Check the strength and regularity of the patient's peripheral pulses. Take the patient's blood pressure to ascertain if there are any orthostatic changes, **hypotension**, or **tachycardia**. Note that early intoxication may be associated with tachycardia and hypertension, whereas later intoxication may be associated with hypotension. Check the patient's heart rate, rhythm, and heart sounds. Inspect for jugular distension and assess the patient's skin color, temperature, and capillary refill.

Neurological. Assess the patient's level of consciousness. The brief mental status examination includes general appearance and behavior, levels of consciousness and orientation, emotional status, attention level, language and speech, and memory. Conduct an examination of the cranial nerves. Assess the patient's deep tendon and stretch reflexes. Perform a sensory examination by assessing the patient's response to painful stimuli, and check for autonomic evidence of sympathetic stimulation. Check the adequacy of the gag reflex. Alcohol intoxication is associated with CNS depression including **unresponsiveness, hypothermia**, and **loss of gross motor control (ataxia, slurred speech)**.

Gastrointestinal/Genitourinary. The patient may experience nausea, vomiting, and diuresis. Depression of the gag reflex from alcohol leads to the risk for aspiration of stomach contents.

PSYCHOSOCIAL. Individuals admitted to the hospital during episodes of acute alcohol intoxication need both a thorough investigation of the physiological responses and a careful assessment of their lifestyle, attitudes, and stressors. People with binge drinking and AUD have complex psychosocial needs. Identify the patient's support systems (family and friends) and assess the effect of those systems on the patient's health maintenance. Alcohol intoxication is identified as a risk factor for suicide. Screening for suicide lethality risk is an essential part of the assessment process.

Diagnostic Highlights

Test	Normal Result	Abnormality With Condition	Explanation
Blood alcohol concentration	Negative (< 10 mg/dL or 0.01 g/dL)	Positive (> 10 mg/dL or 0.01 g/dL); intoxication (inebriation) 80–150 mg/dL; loss of muscle coordination 150–200 mg/dL; decreased level of consciousness 200–300 mg/dL; death 300–500 mg/dL	Legal intoxication in most states is 80–100 mg/dL
Serum glucose	Fasting: < 100 mg/dL	Hyperglycemia > 110 mg/dL; hypoglycemia < 50 mg/dL	Calories in alcohol may increase glucose levels, particularly in diabetics; at high doses of alcohol, the depressant effects may lead to low glucose levels. Elevated or low blood glucose levels without a family history of diabetes mellitus indicate chronic alcohol use.
Carbohydrate deficient transferrin (CDT)	0–26 units/L for women; 0–20 units/L for men; results may be calculated as proportion of the CDT in relation to total transferrin; normal values are < 3%	> 20 units/L or > 3%; if daily consumption is over 60 g/day for at least 3 weeks, the CDT is likely to be 18%	Demonstrates excessive alcohol consumption for 1–4 weeks
Gammaglutamyl transferase (GGT)	0–24 units/L (females); 0–30 units/L (males)	Elevated above normal	Evidence of liver disease or alcoholism
Aspartate aminotransferase (AST)	10–35 units/L	Elevated above normal	Evidence of liver disease or alcoholism
Alanine aminotransferase (ALT)	10–40 units/L	Elevated above normal	Evidence of liver disease or alcoholism

PRIMARY NURSING DIAGNOSIS

DIAGNOSIS. Risk-prone health behavior related to stressors, social anxiety, or low self-efficacy as evidenced by substance (alcohol) misuse

OUTCOMES. Alcohol abuse cessation behavior; Substance withdrawal severity; Electrolyte & acid/base balance; Fluid balance; Neurological status; Anxiety self-control

INTERVENTIONS. Substance use treatment: Alcohol withdrawal; Airway management; Aspiration precautions; Delirium management; Environmental management: Safety; Surveillance

PLANNING AND IMPLEMENTATION

Collaborative

MEDICAL. Provide supportive care during the acute phase by maintaining ABCs. Mechanical ventilation may be necessary. Ensure that the patient maintains a normal body temperature;

initiate body warming procedures for hypothermia. Electrolyte replacement, especially magnesium and potassium, may be necessary. Dehydration is a common problem, and adequate fluid replacement is important. IV fluids may be necessary. Assess the patient for hypoglycemia. During periods of acute intoxication, use care in administering medications that potentiate the effects of alcohol, such as sedatives and analgesics. Calculate when the alcohol will be fully metabolized and out of the patient's system by dividing the blood alcohol level on admission by 20 mg/dL. The result is the number of hours the patient needs to metabolize the alcohol fully.

Anticipate withdrawal syndrome with any intoxicated patient. Formal withdrawal assessment instruments, such as the Clinical Institute Withdrawal Assessment of Alcohol (revised) scale (CIWA-Ar), are available to help guide early intervention and the need for medication such as benzodiazepines to prevent more serious consequences of alcohol withdrawal. If the patient has an AUD, an alcohol referral to social service, psychiatric consultation service, or a clinical nurse specialist is important. Brief interventions (short counseling sessions that focus on helping people cut back on drinking) are appropriate for people who drink in ways that are harmful or abusive, and such interventions can be delivered by clinicians who are trained in the technique.

Pharmacologic Highlights

Medication or Drug Class	Dosage	Description	Rationale
Thiamine	100 mg IV	Vitamin supplement	Counters effects of nutritional deficiencies
Benzodiazepines	Varies by drug	Antianxiety	Manage alcohol withdrawal

Independent

Create a safe environment to reduce the risk of injury. Make sure the patient's airway is patent and the patient has adequate breathing, circulation, and body temperature. Reorient the patient frequently to people and the environment as the level of intoxication changes. Create a calm, nonjudgmental atmosphere to reduce anxiety and agitation.

Symptoms of alcoholic withdrawal can occur as early as 4 to 12 hours after the last drink in individuals with heavy and prolonged use. Usually withdrawal symptoms improve within 3 to 5 days, but in some individuals, it may last for weeks. Monitor for early signs such as tremors, agitation, restlessness, increased or decreased blood pressure, increased pulse, and confusion. Delirium tremens (DTs), a serious medical condition associated with alcohol withdrawal, may include dehydration, rapid heartbeat, hallucinations, and seizures. While it only occurs in about 5% of individuals going through alcohol withdrawal, it can be fatal. Medications such as benzodiazepines are often used in tapering doses to reduce the risks associated with alcohol withdrawal. Keep the room dark and decrease environmental stimulation. Avoid using the intercom. Remain with the patient as much as possible. Encourage the patient to take fluids to diminish the effects of dehydration. Avoid using restraints unless patients are at risk for injuring themselves or others.

As the patient recovers, perform a complete nutritional assessment with a dietary consultation if appropriate.

Evidence-Based Practice and Health Policy

Davies, E., Cooke, R., Maier, L., Winstock, A., & Ferris, J. (2020). Drinking to excess and the tipping point: An international study of alcohol intoxication in 61,000 people. *International Journal of Drug Policy, 83*. Advance online publication. https://doi.org/10.1016/j.drugpo.2020.102867

• The authors aimed to explore three stages of intoxication: the feeling effects, being as drunk as you would like to be, and reaching the tipping point (feeling more drunk than you want to be). They drew data from 61,043 participants in an international study, the Global Drug Survey. The investigators assessed the prevalence of alcohol use disorder, substance use, mental health, and social status in 631 young adults 18 to 30 years of age at 7 years following an emergency department admission for alcohol intoxication.

- Males consumed 87.55 grams of alcohol to be as drunk as they would want to be, and females consumed 70.16 grams. Twenty percent of the sample reached their tipping point on a monthly basis. The tipping point was reached at 138.65 grams for males and 106.54 grams for females. The authors concluded that the amount of alcohol being consumed to reach a desired point of intoxication is much higher than the maximum daily, and sometimes weekly, amount. The authors concluded that an effective intervention based on encouraging people to avoid reaching their tipping point may be a useful strategy during alcohol counseling.

DOCUMENTATION GUIDELINES

- Physical findings: Initial neurological, respiratory, and cardiovascular function and ongoing monitoring of these systems
- Alcohol history, assessment, and interventions (note that history is confidential)
- Response to referral to substance abuse screening and diagnosis if appropriate
- Symptoms of withdrawal and response to treatment
- Response to nutrition counseling
- Federal regulations, as outlined in the *Federal Register* (Title 42 Code of Federal Regulations Part 2; https://www.govinfo.gov/content/pkg/FR-2017-01-18/pdf/2017-00719.pdf), were established to add a layer of protection for confidentiality of medical records addressing substance use disorders. These regulations are intended to make sure that persons receiving treatment in a drug program do not face adverse consequences, such as in criminal proceedings or domestic proceedings (divorce, child custody) or during their employment. Documentation should contain only information essential to the care and management of people under treatment and should be factual and free of bias or opinion.

DISCHARGE AND HOME HEALTHCARE GUIDELINES

PREVENTION. Focus teaching on the problems associated with intoxication and strategies to avoid further intoxication. Encourage the patient to adapt proper nutrition.

REFERRALS. Refer the patient to appropriate outpatient rehabilitation programs and substance abuse support groups such as Alcoholics Anonymous (AA).

Alcohol Withdrawal

DRG Category:	895
Mean LOS:	12.4 days
Description:	MEDICAL: Alcohol, Drug Abuse or Dependence With Rehabilitation Therapy

Withdrawal is a pattern of physiological responses to the discontinuation of a drug or substance such as alcohol. Tolerance occurs when consistent and long-term use of a substance leads to cellular adaptation so that increasing amounts of the substance are needed to produce the substance effect. Most central nervous system (CNS) depressants produce similar responses, but alcohol is the primary substance with which withdrawal is life-threatening. Withdrawal symptoms should be anticipated with any patient who has been drinking the alcohol equivalent of a six-pack of beer on a daily basis for a period of 6 months; patients with smaller body sizes who have drunk less may exhibit the same symptoms. Alcohol withdrawal involves CNS excitation, respiratory alkalosis, and low serum magnesium levels, leading to an increase in neurological excitement (Table 1). The primary pathophysiologic mechanism is exposure to and then withdrawal of alcohol to neuroreceptors in the brain, which changes receptor interaction with neuroreceptors, such as gamma-aminobutyric acid, glutamate, and opiates.

• TABLE 1 Pathophysiology of Alcohol Withdrawal

MECHANISM	EXPLANATION
Respiratory alkalosis	Alcohol produces a depressant effect on the respiratory center, depressing a person's respirations and increasing the level of CO_2. Once the person ceases the intake of alcohol, the respiratory center depressions cease, leaving an increased sensitivity to CO_2. This increase in sensitivity produces an increase in the rate and depth of the person's respirations (hyperventilation) and lowered levels of CO_2 (respiratory alkalosis).
Low magnesium levels	Many people with alcohol use disorder (AUD) have low magnesium intake because of inadequate nutrition. Compounding the problem is the loss of magnesium from the gastrointestinal tract caused by alcohol-related diarrhea and the loss of magnesium in the urine caused by alcohol-related diuresis. Maintaining magnesium levels in the normal range of 1.8–2.5 mEq/L decreases neuromuscular irritability during withdrawal.
CNS excitation	Chronic alcohol use alters cell membrane proteins that normally open and close ion channels to allow electrolytes to enter and exit the cell. With the cessation of alcohol intake, the altered proteins produce an increase in neurological excitement.

Withdrawal occurs within 4 to 12 hours of the last drink and is associated with tremors, anxiety, nausea, vomiting, increase or decrease in blood pressure, rapid pulse, and restlessness. Within 24 to 48 hours of the last drink, hallucinations, tremors, vomiting, seizures, and hypertension may occur. Delirium tremens (DTs) are the most severe form of alcohol withdrawal. Symptoms include profound confusion, sympathetic nervous system activation (hypertension, tachycardia, and diaphoresis), visual and auditory hallucinations, and even cardiovascular collapse. DT typically appear 3 to 5 days after the last drink, but in some individuals, symptoms may last for weeks. Approximately 5% of people who are admitted to the hospital for alcohol-related issues may develop DTs. The mortality rate of DTs is 20% if it is left untreated.

The National Institute on Alcohol Abuse and Alcoholism (NIAAA, 2021) defines alcohol misuse as drinking in a manner, situation, amount, or frequency that could cause harm to the person engaging in drinking or those around them. When alcohol misuse is identified as a problem by a healthcare provider, the diagnosis is described as AUD. Alcohol withdrawal is a potentially dangerous complication of AUD, a chronic relapsing brain disorder characterized by an impaired ability to stop or control alcohol use despite adverse social, occupational, or health consequences (NIAAA, 2021). An estimated 15 million people in the United States have AUD (NIAAA, 2021) on a continuum of alcohol misuse ranging from mild to severe. Approximately 8% of hospitalized patients with AUD will experience alcohol withdrawal. While many hospitalized patients have AUD, only 2% of them have an admitting primary or secondary diagnosis of AUD. The other 28% have been admitted for a variety of reasons. Illnesses such as esophagitis, gastritis, ulcers, hypoglycemia, pancreatitis, and some anemias can be attributed directly to alcohol usage. AUD is the most common cause of cardiomyopathy, and it is also related to injuries, falls, and hip fractures related to high blood alcohol levels.

CAUSES

When a heavy drinker takes a drink, it has a calming effect, and the person experiences a sense of tranquility. As alcohol consumption continues, the CNS is increasingly depressed, leading to a sleep state. The brain (reticular activating system) attempts to counteract sleepiness and the depression with a "wake-up" mechanism. The reticular activating system works through chemical stimulation to keep the body and mind alert. The individual who drinks on a daily basis builds up a tolerance to the alcohol, requiring increasing amounts to maintain the calming effect. If no alcohol is consumed for 24 hours, the reticular activating system nonetheless continues to produce the stimulants to maintain alertness, which leads the individual to experience an over-stimulated state and the development of alcohol withdrawal symptoms.

GENETIC CONSIDERATIONS

Susceptibility to alcohol withdrawal shares many genetic components with tendency toward alcohol abuse (see Alcohol Intoxication, Acute). However, recent studies implicate the genes *FKBP5* and *SORCS2* in the severity of alcohol withdrawal.

SEX AND LIFE SPAN CONSIDERATIONS

Alcohol misuse and AUD are seen in all age groups over 12 years of age and in females and males, although the prevalence is higher in males. Increasing numbers of teens are identified as having AUD and should have their alcohol usage assessed on admission to the hospital or clinic. Binge drinking (more than five drinks at one time for males and four for females) is a persistent problem among college students. An emerging trend in teenagers and young adults, high-intensity drinking is defined as consuming alcohol at levels that are two or more times the sex-specific binge drinking thresholds (NIAAA, 2021). Experts note people who engage in high-intensity drinking are 70 to 90 times more likely to have an alcohol-related emergency department visit than those who do not binge drink. Female teens and young women are drinking more as sex differences are shrinking in drinking patterns, AUD, hospitalizations, and emergency department visits. Approximately 60% of people with AUD are males, but women are more likely to hide their problem. Of growing concern is the number of older adults who are misusing alcohol as a way to deal with their grief, loneliness, and depression.

HEALTH DISPARITIES AND SEXUAL/GENDER MINORITY HEALTH

AUD is more prevalent in White and Native American persons, as well as younger adults, as compared to other groups. There is some evidence to suggest that Black and Hispanic men report more symptoms of AUD than White men, and experience more functional impairment and social consequences than White men. Data from 2021 show that in teenagers and young adults 12 to 20 years of age, approximately 21% of White youths drink alcohol, as compared to 16% of Hispanic and 10% of Black youths. Across all ages, alcohol consumption is most prevalent among White persons, followed by Native American, Hispanic, and Black persons (NIAAA, 2021). In hospitals, White patients seem to have a higher risk of alcohol withdrawal than do Black patients. Experts note that Black patients may receive less adequate care than other patients. One of the monitoring instruments for alcohol withdrawal, the Clinical Institute Withdrawal Assessment for Alcohol, Revised (CIWA-Ar), is used less often for Black patients than other patients (Steel et al., 2021). The National Survey on Drug Use and Health (SAMHSA, 2021) has reported that sexual minority persons are more likely to engage in binge drinking and heavy alcohol use as compared to their heterosexual counterparts. Sexual minority persons are also more likely to continue heavy drinking into later life. The Centers for Disease Control and Prevention (CDC) note that alcohol use may be a reaction to homophobia, violence, or discrimination for sexual minority persons (CDC, 2021). Transgender is a term used to describe persons whose gender identity is different from their sex assigned at birth. Approximately 1% of the U.S. population identify themselves as transgender. Male to female transgender people have higher rates of heavy, episodic drinking when compared to cisgender females (Downing & Predworski, 2018). Cisgender persons have gender identity and gender expression that are aligned with the assigned sex listed on their birth certificate.

GLOBAL HEALTH CONSIDERATIONS

Three million deaths every year around the globe result from harmful use of alcohol, representing 5.3% of all deaths (World Health Organization [WHO], 2018). The WHO reports that alcohol contributed to more than 200 diseases and injury-related health conditions, ranging from liver diseases, road traffic injuries and violence, to cancers, cardiovascular diseases, suicides, tuberculosis, and HIV. Globally, alcohol misuse has been identified as the seventh leading risk factor for premature death and disability, and among people aged 15 to 49 years of age, it has been identified as the first leading risk factor. The WHO (2021) reports that in high income countries, about 20% of fatally injured drivers have excess alcohol in their blood, while in low and middle income countries, these figures may be up to 69%. Alcohol consumption has increased greatly in developing countries and is a health concern because, first, it is occurring in countries without a tradition of alcohol use, and second, these countries have few strategies for prevention or treatment.

ASSESSMENT

HISTORY. Determine when the patient had their last drink to assess the risk of alcohol withdrawal. Do not ask, "Do you drink?" but rather, "When did you have your last drink?" Asking the patient's significant others about their alcohol use may be another way to establish a history of alcohol abuse; however, significant others may also be unwilling to answer potentially embarrassing questions honestly.

PHYSICAL EXAMINATION. Use the CAGE questionnaire, an alcoholism screening instrument. CAGE is an acronym for key words in the questions that follow. Affirmative answers to two or more of the CAGE screening questions identify individuals who require more intensive evaluation:

- Have you ever felt the need to CUT down on drinking?
- Have you ever felt ANNOYED by criticisms of your drinking?
- Have you ever had GUILTY feelings about drinking?
- Have you ever taken a morning EYE opener?

To predict whether alcohol withdrawal will occur, use the Prediction of Alcohol Withdrawal Severity Scale. To assess the severity of alcohol withdrawal, the CIWA-Ar is the gold standard assessment instrument. It takes 5 minutes to administer and is freely available in the public domain. It includes questions such as, Do you feel sick to your stomach?, Have you vomited?, and Do you feel nervous? Determine if the patient has a history of poor nutrition or an illness or infection that has responded poorly to treatment; these are possible signs of AUD. Ask the patient if they have experienced any **agitation, restlessness, anxiety, disorientation**, or **tremors** in the past few hours, which are signs of the onset of early stage alcohol withdrawal. Determine if the patient has been **sweating** excessively; feeling weak in the muscles; or experiencing **rapid breathing, vomiting**, or **diarrhea**.

Although many people with AUD appear normal, look for clues of alcohol use, particularly if the patient has not been forthcoming during the history taking. Note the odor of alcohol on the breath or clothing. Inspect arms and legs for bruising or burns that may have been caused by injury. Inspect for edema around the eyes or tibia and a flushed face from small vessel vaso-dilation. Observe general appearance, noting if the patient appears haggard or older than the stated age.

The first symptoms of alcohol withdrawal can appear as soon as 4 hours after the last drink. Note any comments made by the patient about drinking, even in jest. Observe any defensiveness or guarded responses to questions about drinking patterns. Note if the patient requests sedation. If you suspect that a patient may have been abusing alcohol, assess the vital signs every 2 hours for the first 12 hours. If the patient remains stable, vital signs can be assessed less frequently; however, monitor the patient carefully for signs of mild anxiety or nervousness that could indicate alcohol withdrawal. Temperature, blood pressure, and heart rate begin to elevate. Hyper-alertness and irritability increase. The patient may remark that they feel "trembly" or nervous on the "inside" (internal tremors). Temperature, blood pressure, and heart rate continue to elevate. Mild disorientation and diaphoresis are present. External tremors are visible. If the brain is still not sedated, the patient can have seizures, cardiac failure, and death unless medication protocols are instituted.

PSYCHOSOCIAL. Patients who have previously experienced active withdrawal may have little trust or confidence that they will receive adequate amounts of medication to help them manage their withdrawal. Patients need to feel secure that you will be there to keep them safe and that all symptoms will be managed. Individuals who are alcohol dependent may be in denial or very embarrassed at having their drinking exposed. Maintain a nonjudgmental, supportive approach. Assess the patient's coping mechanisms and support system.

Diagnostic Highlights

Test	Normal Result	Abnormality With Condition	Explanation
Blood alcohol concentration	Negative (< 10 mg/dL or 0.01 g/dL)	Positive (> 10 mg/dL or 0.01 g/dL)	Legal intoxication in most states is 80 mg/dL
Gamma-glutamyl transpeptidase	0–24 units/L (females); 0–30 units/L (males)	Elevated above normal	Evidence of liver disease or alcoholism
Aspartate aminotransferase	10–35 units/L	Elevated above normal	Evidence of liver disease or alcoholism
Alanine aminotransferase	10–40 units/L	Elevated above normal	Evidence of liver disease or alcoholism

Other Tests: Blood glucose levels: Elevated or low blood glucose levels without a family history of diabetes mellitus indicate chronic alcohol use. Chest x-ray: Approximately 50% of patients with DT who have fever will also have an infection and, in particular, pneumonia.

PRIMARY NURSING DIAGNOSIS

DIAGNOSIS. Deficient fluid volume related to active water loss as evidenced by thirst, alter-nations in mental status, and/or increase in body temperature

OUTCOMES. Fluid balance; Circulation status; Cardiac pump effectiveness; Hydration; Vital signs; Electrolyte balance

INTERVENTIONS. Fluid/electrolyte management; Fluid monitoring; Shock prevention; Shock management: Volume; Medication administration; Fluid resuscitation

☀ PLANNING AND IMPLEMENTATION

Collaborative

Upon assessment of a pattern of heavy drinking, the patient is often placed on prophylactic benzodiazepines. These medications are particularly important if the patient develops early signs of withdrawal, such as irritability, anxiety, tremors, restlessness, confusion, mild hypertension (blood pressure > 140/90), tachycardia (heart rate > 100), and a low-grade fever (temperature > 100°F [37.8°C]). Keeping the patient safe during the withdrawal process depends on managing the physiological changes, the signs and symptoms, and the appropriate drug protocols. The goal is to keep the patient mildly sedated or in a calm and tranquil state while still allowing for easy arousal.

Although sedation should prevent withdrawal, if withdrawal occurs, patients will often require IV hydration, with fluid requirements ranging from 4 to 10 L in the first 24 hours. Hypoglycemia is common, and often a 5% dextrose solution in 0.90% or 0.45% saline will be used. Monitoring the patient's airway and maintaining airway patency are important strategies for people with altered mental status. Because patients with AUD often have low calcium, magnesium, phosphorous, and potassium levels, they may need electrolyte replacement.

Once the patient's nausea and vomiting have been controlled, encourage a well-balanced diet. Monitor the patient continually for signs of dehydration, such as poor skin turgor, dry mucous membranes, weight loss, concentrated urine, and hypotension. Record intake and output. If the patient's blood pressure drops below 90 mm Hg, a significant fluid volume loss has occurred; notify the physician immediately.

Pharmacologic Highlights

Medication or Drug Class	Dosage	Description	Rationale
Thiamine; multivitamin supplements	100 mg IV; 1 amp multivitamin	Vitamin supplement	Counters effects of nutritional deficiencies
Benzodiazepines	Varies by drug	Antianxiety	Manages alcohol withdrawal; prescribed for their sedating effect and to control the tremors or seizures, which can be life-threatening

Other Drugs: Electrolyte replacement, phenobarbital, carbamazepine, gabapentin, and midazolam; clonidine and beta blockers may be administered to suppress the cardiovascular signs of withdrawal. It is not appropriate to administer alcohol in any form to manage DT or withdrawal.

Independent

Managing the potential for airway compromise and managing fluid volume deficit are the top priorities in nursing care. If the patient is able to maintain the airway and swallow, encourage the patient to drink fluids, particularly citrus juices, to help replace needed electrolytes. Caution the patient to avoid caffeine, which stimulates the CNS. Maintain a quiet environment to assist in limiting sensory or perceptual alterations and sleep pattern disturbance.

An appropriately sedated patient should not undergo acute withdrawal. If symptoms occur, however, stay at the bedside during episodes of extreme agitation to reassure the patient and to maintain patient safety. Avoid using restraints.

When patients are awake, alert, and appropriately oriented, discuss their drinking and the effect of drinking on the illness. Encourage the patient to seek help from Alcoholics Anonymous (AA) or to see a counselor or attend a support group. Refer the patient to a clinical nurse specialist if appropriate.

Evidence-Based Practice and Health Policy

Sherk, A., Thomas, G., Churchill, S., & Stockwell, T. (2020). Does drinking within low-risk guidelines prevent harm? Implications for high-income countries using the international model of alcohol harms and policies. *Journal of Studies on Alcohol and Drugs, 81*, 352–361.

• The authors note that low-risk drinking is not without harm, even though many countries have low-risk guidelines. They applied the International Model of Alcohol Harms and Policies to quantify the alcohol-caused harms experienced by people drinking within those guidelines. They used medical record data and applied the model to estimate alcohol-attributable deaths and hospital stays for people drinking.

• More men (18%) than women (7%) drank above the low-risk amount and for all consumption levels, men had a higher relative risk than women. Those drinking within the guidelines had 140 more deaths and 3,663 more hospital stays than the group who abstained. Among those drinking within the low-risk drinking guidelines, the lowest risk was associated with a consumption level of 10 grams per day. The authors conclude that low-risk drinking guidelines should reflect a consumption level of no more than 10 grams of alcohol per day (or roughly one drink).

DOCUMENTATION GUIDELINES

• Physical findings: Airway status, vital signs, fluid intake and output, skin turgor, presence of tremors or seizures
• Mental status: Anxiety level, auditory-visual hallucinations, confusion, violent behavior
• Reactions to the alcohol withdrawal experience
• Federal regulations, as outlined in the *Federal Register* (Title 42 Code of Federal Regulations Part 2; https://www.govinfo.gov/content/pkg/FR-2017-01-18/pdf/2017-00719.pdf), were established to add a layer of protection for confidentiality of medical records addressing substance use disorders. These regulations are intended to make sure that persons receiving treatment in a drug program do not face adverse consequences, such as in criminal proceedings or domestic proceedings (divorce, child custody) or during their employment. Documentation should contain only information essential to the care and management of people under treatment and should be factual and free of bias or opinion.

DISCHARGE AND HOME HEALTHCARE GUIDELINES

TEACHING. Teach the patient to eat a well-balanced diet with sufficient fluids. Emphasize the value of exercise and adequate rest. Encourage the patient to develop adequate coping strategies.

FOLLOW-UP. Following an alcohol withdrawal experience, the patient may be able to accept that they have a problem with alcohol misuse. Discharge plans may include behavior modification programs, sometimes in conjunction with disulfiram (Antabuse) or participation in Alcoholics Anonymous. Families and significant others must also be involved in the treatment planning to gain an understanding of the part that family dynamics play in people with AUD.

Allergic Purpura

DRG Category:	813
Mean LOS:	4.9 days
Description:	MEDICAL: Coagulation Disorders

Allergic purpura (AP) is an allergic reaction mediated by immunoglobulin A (IgA) that leads to acute or chronic inflammation of the vessels of the skin, joints, gastrointestinal (GI) tract, and genitourinary (GU) tract, primarily in children. It is also called *Henoch-Schönlein purpura*, named after the two physicians who first identified the disease, and is the most common acute vasculitis among children. AP occurs as an acquired, abnormal immune response to a variety of agents that normally do not cause allergy. It is manifested by a purple spotted skin rash, bleeding into the tissues, organs, and joints, which leads to organ dysfunction, pain, and immobility. An acute attack of AP can last for several weeks, but usually episodes of the disease subside without treatment within 1 to 6 weeks. Patients with chronic AP can have a persistent and debilitating disease. The most severe complications are acute glomerulonephritis and renal failure. Hypertension often complicates the course. If bleeding into tissues and organs is excessive, the patient can develop a fluid volume deficit. On rare occasions, patients may be at risk for airway compromise from laryngeal edema.

CAUSES

While the cause of AP has not been clearly defined, experts suggest that it occurs as an allergic response to antigens such as bacteria, viruses, drugs (particularly antibiotics or vaccines), food (wheat, eggs, chocolate, milk), or bee stings. The allergic reaction is probably an autoimmune response directed against the vessel walls. Most patients have experienced an upper respiratory or GI infection 1 to 3 weeks prior to the development of allergic purpura.

GENETIC CONSIDERATIONS

Over 20 genes have been associated with the development of allergy, and heritability has been estimated at 60% to 80%. Implicated genes include those that code for IL-4, the IL-4 receptor, interferon gamma, β-adrenergic receptor, 5 lipoxygenase, PHF1, TARC, and leukotriene C4 synthetase. Some alleles of the *MEFV* and *ACE* genes, along with various HLA alleles, are also associated with allergic purpura.

SEX AND LIFE SPAN CONSIDERATIONS

AP can occur at any age, but it is most common in children between 2 and 11 years old with the peak prevalence at age 5 years. Children tend to have a less serious course of the disease than adults, who are more apt to have involvement of the kidneys. The condition is more common in males than in females. In North America, the disease occurs mostly from November to January. In one-half to two-thirds of children, an upper respiratory or GI tract infection precedes the clinical onset by 1 to 3 weeks, and children are mildly ill with a fever.

HEALTH DISPARITIES AND SEXUAL/GENDER MINORITY HEALTH

White persons are more affected than Black persons. Sexual and gender minority status has no known effect on the risk for AP.

GLOBAL HEALTH CONSIDERATIONS

Studies of children with AP have been completed in Thailand, China, Korea, Taiwan, and Turkey, and the authors report similar epidemiology to U.S. findings.

☀ ASSESSMENT

HISTORY. Patients with AP typically have headache, anorexia, and fever, with a rash most commonly on the legs. Approximately half have GU symptoms such as **dysuria** and **hematuria**. Other symptoms include peripheral edema and joint pain of the knees and ankles. Young children may refuse to walk because of joint pain. The **skin lesions are accompanied by pruritus, paresthesia, and angioedema** (swelling of the skin, mucous membranes, or organs). Other patients describe severe GI symptoms such as spasm, colic, constipation, bloody vomitus, and bloody stools. In unusual situations, the GI symptoms from AP can resemble an abdominal emergency and result in small bowel infarction and perforation.

PHYSICAL EXAMINATION. Inspect the patient's skin for the typical skin lesions— patches of purple macular lesions of various sizes that result from vascular leakage into the skin and mucous membranes. The skin lesions are most common on the legs, buttocks, and abdomen. Note that in children, the lesions more commonly start as urticarial areas that then expand into hemorrhagic lesions. Determine if the patient has any peripheral swelling, particularly in the hands and face. Perform gentle range of motion of the extremities to determine the presence and location of joint pain. Assess the color of the patient's urine and stool, and note any bleeding.

PSYCHOSOCIAL. The patient may experience a disturbance in body image because of the disfigurement caused by the rash and swelling. The discomforts involved with AP are distressing to children and parents, who need to participate in their management. Determine the patient's response to their appearance, and identify whether the changes interfere with implementing various roles, such as parenting or work.

Diagnostic Highlights

No single laboratory test identifies AP. The diagnosis is based on clinical presentation rather than laboratory tests. Supporting tests include complete blood count, erythrocyte sedimentation rate, urinalysis, blood urea nitrogen, creatinine, and coagulation profile. A biopsy may be taken from the skin, kidneys, or other tissues and may show high levels of IgA. If abdominal pain is severe, bowel imaging may be necessary.

PRIMARY NURSING DIAGNOSIS

DIAGNOSIS. Impaired skin integrity related to damage and inflammation of vessels as evidenced by localized red-purple rash and/or swelling

OUTCOMES. Tissue integrity: Skin and mucous membranes; Wound healing: Primary intention; Body image

INTERVENTIONS. Skin surveillance; Wound care; Body image enhancement

☀ PLANNING AND IMPLEMENTATION

Collaborative

Treatment is based on the acuity and severity of the symptoms. To date, no treatment has been found to shorten the duration of AP. Some patients are treated pharmacologically with corticosteroids to relieve edema, but few studies support their effectiveness. Analgesics, particularly ibuprofen, are used to manage joint discomfort. Allergy testing to identify the provocative allergen is usually performed, and the allergen is immediately discontinued. If the allergen is a food or medication, the patient needs to avoid ingesting the allergen for the rest of the patient's life. Patients who are placed on corticosteroids or immunosuppressive therapy need an environment that protects them as much as possible from secondary infection. If the patient is on corticosteroids, monitor the patient for signs of Cushing syndrome and the complications of corticosteroids, such as labile emotions, fluid retention, hyperglycemia, and osteoporosis. Patients should be monitored for kidney disease and referred to a nephrologist as needed for increased blood pressure or creatinine levels, or hematuria and proteinurea.

Pharmacologic Highlights

Medication or Drug Class	Dosage	Description	Rationale
Glucocorticoids	Varies by drug	Corticosteroid	Relieves edema; analgesics may be needed to manage joint and GI discomfort
Cyclosporine	Varies by age and whether it is initial or maintenance dose	Immunosuppressant	Suppresses cell-mediated hypersensitivity

Independent
If the patient has alterations in coagulation, create a safe environment to prevent bleeding from falls or other injuries. Protect open or irritated skin lesions from further tissue trauma and infection. Apply unguents and soothing creams, if appropriate, to manage discomfort. Assist the patient with colloidal baths and activities of daily living if joint pain and the lesions give the patient limited activity tolerance. Reassure the patient that the lesions are of short duration prior to healing. Explore possible sources of the allergy. Allow the patient time to discuss concerns about the disease. If the patient or significant other appears to be coping ineffectively, provide a referral to a clinical nurse specialist or counselor.

Evidence-Based Practice and Health Policy
Zheng, X., Chen, Q., & Chen, L. (2019). Obesity is associated with Henoch-Schönlein Purpura Nephritis (HSP) and development of end-stage renal disease in children. *Renal Failure, 41,* 1016–1020.

• The authors proposed a retrospective study of patients diagnosed with HSP to determine the association of obesity, the occurrence of HSP nephritis, and the development of end-stage renal disease (ESRD) in children. Variables included obesity as defined by body mass index (BMI), laboratory data, and clinical features such as angioedema. The results indicated that 35.2% of the children had HSP nephritis.
• Additional findings demonstrated that obesity, age over 6 years at onset, and the occurrence of angioedema are linked to an increased risk of HSP nephritis. At 52 months' follow-up, 5.2% of the children developed ESRD. The authors conclude that obesity is associated with an increased risk of renal involvement in these children.

DOCUMENTATION GUIDELINES
• Extent, location, and description of rash; degree of discomfort; signs of wound infection; presence and description of edema
• Response to allergy testing and withdrawal of the provocative agent if identified
• Response to treatments: Medications, creams, and colloidal baths
• Emotional response to the condition; problems coping; body image disturbance

DISCHARGE AND HOME HEALTHCARE GUIDELINES

PREVENTION. Teach the patient about the disease and its cause. If the allergen is identified, assist the patient in eliminating the allergen, if possible. Teach the patient to protect lesions from additional trauma by wearing long-sleeved blouses or shirts. Teach the patient to pay particular attention to edematous areas where skin breaks down easily if injured. Encourage the patient to prevent secondary infections by avoiding contact with others and by using good hand-washing techniques. Encourage the patient to report recurrent signs and symptoms, which are most likely to occur 6 weeks after the initial onset of symptoms.

MEDICATIONS. Provide the patient with information about the medications, including dosage, route, action, and side effects. Provide the patient with written information so that the patient can refer to it for questions at home.

Alzheimer Disease

DRG Category:	57
Mean LOS:	5.6 days
Description:	MEDICAL: Degenerative Nervous System Disorders Without Major Complication or Comorbidity

Alzheimer disease (AD) is an incurable, degenerative disorder of the brain that is manifested by dementia and progressive physiological impairment. AD, the most common cause of dementia in older adults, although not a normal part of aging, affects 5.8 million Americans. An even larger number of people have mild cognitive impairment, which often evolves into dementia. The prevalence of dementia doubles every 5 years in people older than 65 years, with 80% of all cases among those aged 75 years and older. It involves progressive decline in two or more of the following areas of cognition: memory, language, calculation, visuospatial perception, judgment, abstraction, and behavior. Dementia is classified in the *Diagnostic and Statistical Manual of Mental Disorders* (5th ed., *DSM-5*; American Psychiatric Association [APA], 2013) as one type of major neurocognitive disorder (NCD), and AD accounts for 60% to 80% of all NCD cases. The pathophysiological changes are complex. In the brain, the microtubules that form a support structure in neurons disintegrate into tangled structures (neurofibrillary tangles [NFT]), leading to problems with neuronal communication. Senile plaques (SP), also known as beta-amyloid plaques, accumulate outside and around neurons and develop in the hippocampus (where memories are encoded) and in the cerebral cortex (responsible for perceiving, thinking, and understanding language). Other changes that occur, causing neuronal damage to the brain, include activation of the inflammatory response, cholinergic and estrogen deficiency, and oxidative stress.

The life expectancy of a patient with NCD due to AD is reduced 30% to 60%. The average time from onset of symptoms to death is 4 to 8 years. Complications include difficulty concentrating, sleep disturbance, falls, wandering, bowel and bladder incontinence, depression, unstable mood, pneumonia, malnutrition, and dehydration.

CAUSES

The cause of AD is unknown, but knowledge about the hereditary links is growing (see Genetic Considerations). Individuals with Down syndrome have an increased risk of early onset AD, and many people with Down syndrome develop AD in older adulthood. Risk factors for AD include advancing age, family history, and genetic predisposition (apolipoprotein E [*APOE*] genotype), depression, brain injury, Down syndrome, hypertension, obesity, and insulin resistance.

GENETIC CONSIDERATIONS

AD is a complex disorder with a significant genetic component (heritability between 60% and 80%). There are two basic types of AD from a genetic standpoint: familial and sporadic (associated with late-onset disease). Familial AD (FAD) is a rare form of AD that has an early onset before age 65 years and affects less than 10% of patients with AD. FAD is caused by gene mutations on chromosomes 1, 14, and 21 (definitively, within the *PSEN2*, *PSEN1*, and *APP* genes, respectively) and has an autosomal dominant inheritance pattern. Therefore, if one of these mutated genes is inherited from a parent, the person will almost always develop early onset AD.

The majority of AD cases are late onset (developing after age 65 years), and while there have been over 20 genes recently identified to play a role in AD, there is still no clear inheritance pattern. The greatest genetic risk factor for late-onset AD is linked with the *APOE* gene on chromosome 19. It is involved with making APOE, a substance that transports cholesterol in the bloodstream. The *APOE* gene comes in several different alleles, and individuals have different combinations of the e2, e3, and e4 alleles. The most common allele is e3 (~79% of individuals have at least one copy). However, those with two copies of the e4 allele have an increased risk of AD (approximately ninefold), whereas those with the e2 allele have a decreased risk (approximately threefold). Specific polymorphisms that are associated with AD have been identified in recent genome-wide association studies. Notable findings include *CLU*, which encodes clusterin/apolipoprotein J, *SORL1*, which is involved in amyloid processing, and the genes *PLCG2*, *AB13*, and *TREM2*, which are components of microglial innate immunity pathways.

SEX AND LIFE SPAN CONSIDERATIONS

The onset of AD may occur at any age but is rare before age 50 years; the average onset occurs after age 65 years. The prevalence of AD increases dramatically with age, affecting about 3% of individuals between 65 and 74 years, 17% of individuals between 75 and 84 years, and 32% of individuals 85 years and older. More women than men have the disease, although the higher proportion may be related to women having a longer life expectancy.

HEALTH DISPARITIES AND SEXUAL/GENDER MINORITY HEALTH

AD is disproportionately more common in Black and Hispanic persons as compared to White persons. Native American and Alaskan Native persons in the United States may be more prone to AD due to long-standing inequities in access to healthcare and the physical, emotional, and psychological stresses associated with their history. Experts note that these groups have socioeconomic disadvantages, exposure to poor housing conditions, poverty, and geographical isolation, which may contribute to the risks for AD. Rural patients with AD have more difficulty locating resources to manage the disease and rely more heavily on emergency departments for preventive healthcare as compared to their urban counterparts. Sexual and gender minority persons with AD face a heightened risk for unmet needs due to cognitive impairment because of discrimination, barriers to healthcare access, limited availability of caregivers, and higher rates of some chronic diseases (Fredriksen-Goldsen et al., 2018).

GLOBAL HEALTH CONSIDERATIONS

The World Health Organization reports that worldwide, about 50 million people have dementia, and about 60% are living in low- and middle-income countries. The majority (60%–70%) of cases are attributed to AD. The estimated proportion of the general population aged 60 years and over with dementia at a given time is between 5% and 8%, and every year there are almost 10 million new cases.

ASSESSMENT

HISTORY. AD is a disease process that begins years before the onset of symptoms and when symptoms do appear, the course is slow, progressive, and deteriorating. Depending on the degree of cognitive impairment, secondary sources may be needed to obtain a history and make a diagnosis because the patient is often unaware of their difficulty with thought processing. Because many patients lack insight into their own impairments, consider the patient's responses carefully. Some patients may deny deficits. It is important to determine the time and nature of the onset of symptoms so that other conditions can be considered for a differential diagnosis. Past medical history should be evaluated for previous head injury, surgery, recent falls, headache, and family history of AD.

PHYSICAL EXAMINATION. The history will help determine which stage the disease process has reached at the time of patient assessment. The following four-stage scale reflects the progressive symptoms of AD:

- Stage 1 (preclinical) is characterized by recent **memory loss**, increased **irritability, impaired judgment, loss of interest in life, decline of problem-solving ability**, and reduction in abstract thinking. Remote memory and neurological examination remain unchanged from baseline.
- Stage 2 (mild) lasts 2 to 4 years. Patients may get lost when traveling to familiar places, and daily tasks may take longer than previously. They may have problems managing finances and have compromised judgment. There is a decline in the patient's ability to manage personal and business affairs, an inability to remember shapes of objects, continued repetition of a meaningless word or phrase (perseveration), wandering or circular speech patterns (circumlocution dysphasia), wandering at night, restlessness, depression, anxiety, and intensification of the cognitive and emotional changes of stage 1.
- Stage 3 (moderate) is associated with significant changes in the cerebral cortex location responsible for thinking, language, and reasoning. It is characterized by impaired ability to speak (aphasia), inability to recognize familiar objects (agnosia), inability to use objects properly (apraxia), inattention, distractibility, involuntary emotional outbursts, urinary or fecal incontinence, lint-picking motion, and chewing movements. Patients may have loss of impulse control and use vulgar language. Progression through stages 2 and 3 varies from 2 to 12 years.
- Stage 4 (severe), which may last approximately 1 year, reveals a patient with a masklike facial expression, no communication, apathy, withdrawal, eventual immobility, assumed fetal position, no appetite, and emaciation.

The neurological examination remains almost normal except for increased deep tendon reflexes and the presence of snout, root, and grasp reflexes that appear in stage 3. In stage 4, there may be generalized seizures and immobility, which precipitate flexion contractures.

Appearance may range from manifesting normal patient hygiene in the early stage to a total lack of interest in hygiene in the later stages. Some patients also demonstrate abusive language, inappropriate sexual behaviors, and paranoia. The Folstein Mini Mental State Exam is a quick evaluation tool that can assist in diagnosis and monitoring of the disease's progression.

PSYCHOSOCIAL. The nurse needs to assess the family for its ability to cope with this progressive disease, to provide physical and emotional care for the patient, and to meet financial responsibilities. A multidisciplinary team assessment approach is recommended for the patient and family.

Diagnostic Highlights

Diagnostic tests generally are completed to rule out a treatable condition that could be causing dementia, such as thyroid disease, stroke, vitamin deficiency, brain tumor, drug and medication effects, infection, anemia, and depression. Imaging studies such as computed tomography (CT) and magnetic resonance imaging (MRI) help exclude other possible causes for dementia, but clinical criteria rather than biological testing are used to make the diagnosis of AD.

Test	Normal Result	Abnormality With Condition	Explanation
Brain biopsy upon autopsy	Negative	Positive for cellular changes that are associated with the disease	No diagnostic tests have been definitive for AD. Clinical criteria for diagnosis of AD: (1) presence of at least two cognitive deficits, (2) onset occurring between ages 40 and 90 years, (3) progressive deterioration, (4) all other causes ruled out

Other Tests: Most patients will receive neuroimaging (CT, MRI) as part of the diagnostic work-up to rule out other conditions, such as subdural hematoma, brain tumors, and stroke. Supporting tests include CT scan, MRI, and positron emission tomography (PET). During the early stages of dementia, CT and MRI may be normal, but in later stages, an MRI may show a decrease in the size of the cerebral cortex or of the area of the brain responsible for memory, particularly the hippocampus. Genetic testing for the *APOE* gene is available, and the presence of the gene is a risk factor for AD. Genetic tests may be helpful in diagnosis, but further studies are needed to confirm their reliability. A number of studies have sought to identify biomarkers of AD before the onset of symptoms. They report evidence that a blood test for amyloid levels, especially when considered along with age and the presence of the apolipoprotein E4 (*APOE4*) gene variant, is 94% accurate in identifying people with early brain changes indicative of AD. This blood test is not yet available for clinical use, but it is hoped that such a test will pave the way for research and avenues for early diagnosis and treatment.

PRIMARY NURSING DIAGNOSIS

DIAGNOSIS. Disturbed personal identity related to organic brain disorder as evidenced by inconsistent behaviors, ineffective relationships, and/or ineffective role performance

OUTCOMES. Self-care: Activities of daily living (Bathing, Hygiene, Eating, Toileting); Cognitive orientation; Comfort status; Role performance; Social interaction skills; Hope

INTERVENTIONS. Self-care assistance: Bathing/hygiene/dressing/grooming; Oral health maintenance; Behavior management; Body image enhancement; Emotional support; Mutual goal setting; Exercise therapy: Ambulation and balance; Discharge planning

PLANNING AND IMPLEMENTATION

Collaborative

The initial management of the patient begins with education of the family and caregivers regarding the disease, the prognosis, and changes in lifestyle that are necessary as the disease progresses. Basic collaborative principles include:

- Keep requests for the patient simple
- Avoid confrontation and requests that might lead to frustration
- Remain calm and supportive if the patient becomes upset

- Maintain a consistent environment
- Provide frequent cues and reminders to reorient the patient
- Adjust expectations for the patient as they decline in capacity

Pharmacologic Highlights

Generally, therapy is focused on symptoms with an attempt to maintain cognition.

Medication or Drug Class	Dosage	Description	Rationale
Donepezil	5–10 mg PO qd	Cholinesterase inhibitor; elevates acetylcholine concentration in cerebral cortex by slowing degradation of acetylcholine released by intact neurons; other drugs in this class include galantamine and rivastigmine	Improves cognitive symptoms; improves cognitive function in the early stages of the disease only; drug effects diminish as the disease progresses
Memantine	5–20 mg PO qd	N-methyl-D-aspartate (NMDA) receptor antagonist	Delays progression of cognitive impairment symptoms
Antidepressants	Varies with drug	Selective serotonin reuptake inhibitors; increase activity of serotonin in the brain	Treat depression, anxiety, and irritability
Atypical antipsychotics	Varies with drug	Risperidone, olanzapine, quetiapine, aripiprazole, clozapine, ziprasidone	Treat psychosis but should be avoided in people with the risk of stroke and weight gain; drugs are expensive and may increase mortality but might be better tolerated; use must be weighed carefully
Anxiolytics	Varies with drug	Lorazepam, oxazepam	Short-term use to manage episodes of anxiety

Other Therapies: Some evidence supports the benefit of vitamin E in delaying the progression of mild to moderate disease, and omega-3s may lower the risk of developing dementia. Other herbs that have been studied, including Ginkgo biloba and curcumin, have not demonstrated benefits in clinical trials. Secondary treatments are aimed at treating depression, psychosis, and agitation. To control night wandering and behavioral outbursts, physicians prescribe mild sedatives such as diphenhydramine. Barbiturates are avoided because they can precipitate confusion. Depression is treated with antidepressants (trazodone). Psychotic behaviors may be treated with antipsychotics (chlorpromazine or haloperidol), but the risks and benefits must be carefully assessed since all antipsychotics carry a black box warning about increased risk of death in older patients with NCD. Consider hospitalization for any unstable medical condition, such as an infectious or metabolic process, that may complicate the patient's treatment. If the patient becomes a danger to themselves or a danger to others, a short hospitalization may be indicated to adjust psychotropic medications.

Independent

For patients with mild impairment, some experts recommend providing mentally challenging activities to slow disease progression. Although the long-term benefits of activities such as word games and puzzles are not known, these activities are appropriate for some patients.

Promote patient activities of daily living to the fullest, considering the patient's functional ability. Give the patient variable assistance or simple directions to perform those activities. Anticipate and assess the patient's needs mainly through nonverbal communication because of the patient's inability to communicate meaningfully through speech. Emotional outbursts or changes in behavior often are a signal of the patient's toileting needs, discomfort, hunger, or infection.

To maximize orientation and memory, provide a calendar and clock for the patient. Encourage the patient to reminisce, since loss of short-term memory triggers anxiety in the patient. Emotional outbursts usually occur when the patient is fatigued, so it is best to plan for frequent rest periods throughout the day.

Maintain physical safety of the patient by securing loose rugs, supervising electrical devices, and locking doors and windows. Lock up toxic substances and medications. Supervise cooking, bathing, and outdoor recreation. Be sure that the patient wears appropriate identification in case they get lost. Terminate driving by removing the car keys or the car. Provide a safe area for wandering. Encourage and anticipate toileting at 2- to 3-hour intervals. Change incontinence pads as needed, but use them only as a last resort. Bowel and bladder programs can be beneficial in the early stage of the disease.

Provide structured activity during the day to prevent night wandering. If confusion and agitated wandering occur at night, provide toileting, fluids, orientation, night lights, and familiar objects within a patient's view. Some patients respond calmly when given the security of a stuffed animal or a familiar blanket.

Families should be referred to the Alzheimer's Association Web site (https://www.alz.org) and the many pamphlets and books available to provide information on this disease. Encourage family members to verbalize their emotional concerns, coping strategies, and other aspects of caregiver role strain. Discuss appropriate referrals to local support groups, clergy, social workers, respite care, day care, and attorneys. Provide information about advanced directives (living wills and durable power of attorney for healthcare).

Evidence-Based Practice and Health Policy

Wang, F., Tang, Q., Zhang, L., Yang, J., Li, Y., Peng, H., & Wang, S. (2020). Effects of mindfulness-based interventions on dementia patients: A meta-analysis. *Western Journal of Nursing Research, 42*, 1163–1173.

- Mindfulness-based interventions are directed toward guiding a patient to focus on the present moment and are often a facet of meditation for relaxation and developing awareness of "the here and now." This meta-analysis of nine studies sought to determine the efficacy of mindfulness-based interventions in improving mental health and quality of life for people with dementia.
- The meta-analysis found a statistically significant decrease in depressive symptoms among people with dementia who were treated with mindfulness-based interventions. The findings suggest that the intervention may be a beneficial alternative treatment for people with dementia who have depression. However, there were no noted improvements in anxiety, stress, or overall quality of life.

DOCUMENTATION GUIDELINES

- Any changes in cognitive function: Confused orientation (time, place, person), emotional outbursts, forgetfulness, paranoia, decreased short-term memory, impaired judgment, loss of speech, disturbed affect, decline of problem-solving ability, and reduction in abstract thinking
- Response to medications (anxiolytics, antipsychotics, cholinesterase inhibitors, antidepressants, sedatives)
- Verbal and nonverbal methods that effectively meet or communicate the patient's needs
- Caregiver response to patient behaviors and information about AD
- Ability to perform the activities of daily living

DISCHARGE AND HOME HEALTHCARE GUIDELINES

MEDICATIONS. Be sure the caregiver understands all medications, including the dosage, route, action, and adverse effects.

SAFETY. Explain the need to supervise outdoor activity, cooking, and bathing. Lock doors and windows, and lock up medications and toxic chemicals. Make sure the patient wears identification to provide a safe return if the patient becomes lost. Commercially made products are available that trigger an alarm if the patient wanders out of safe territory.

Amputation

DRG Category:	239
Mean LOS:	12.8 days
Description:	SURGICAL: Amputation for Circulatory System Disorders Except Upper Limb and Toe With Major Complication or Comorbidity
DRG Category:	908
Mean LOS:	5.3 days
Description:	SURGICAL: Other Operating Room Procedures for Injuries With Complication or Comorbidity

Amputation is the surgical severing of any body part. Amputations can be surgical (therapeutic) or traumatic (emergencies resulting from injury). The type of amputation performed in the Civil War era by a surgeon called a "sawbones" was straight across the leg, with all bone and soft tissue severed at the same level. That procedure, known as a guillotine (or open) amputation, is still seen today.

In the United States, 30,000 to 40,000 amputations are performed annually. Most amputations are performed for ischemic diseases of the lower extremities, such as peripheral arterial disease (PAD) in people with diabetes mellitus. A traumatic amputation is usually the result of an industrial or home-based accident, in which blades of heavy machinery sever part of a limb. A healthy young person who suffers a traumatic amputation without other injuries is often a good candidate for limb salvage. Reattachment of a limb will take place as soon as possible following the injury. The chief problems are hemorrhage and nerve damage. A closed amputation is the most common surgical procedure today. The bone is severed somewhat higher than the surrounding tissue, with a skin flap pulled over the bone end, usually from the posterior surface. This procedure provides more even pressure for a weight-bearing surface, promoting healing and more successful use of a prosthesis. Patients may experience postoperative edema near the surgical site, wound breakdown, swelling, pain, joint contractures, and phantom limb sensation. Serious complications include hemorrhage, shock, and infection. (See Table 1 for levels of amputations.)

• TABLE 1 Levels of Amputation

TYPE	DESCRIPTION
Transfemoral amputation (above-the-knee)	Performed to remove the lower limb above the knee joint when the limb has been severely damaged or the blood flow is so severely compromised that lower leg surgery is prohibited
Transtibial (below-the-knee)	Most common surgical site, performed rather than above-the-knee amputation whenever possible because the higher the amputation performed, the greater the energy required for mobility
Syme procedure (foot amputation)	Partial amputation with salvage of the ankle; has advantages over loss of the limb higher up because it does not require a prosthesis and produces less weight-bearing pain
Transmetatarsal (forefoot amputation)	Involves removal of the front part of the foot with an attempt to retain as much function as possible; requires little rehabilitation but may create problems with balance or gait
Hip disarticulation/extensive hemipelvectomy (full leg)	Usually performed for malignancies; because of the surgery involved and the extremely bulky prosthesis required for ambulation, these procedures are used either as life-saving measures in young patients or as a surgery of last resort for pain control
Upper extremity	Performed with salvage of as much normal tissue as possible. Function of the upper extremity is vital to normal activities of daily living. Much research is being conducted at the current time to manufacture and refine prostheses that can substitute for the patient's arm and hand, providing both gross and fine movement. Cosmetic considerations are extremely important in the loss of the upper extremity for many patients.

Note: The terms *below-the-knee amputation* (BKA) and *above-the-knee amputation* (AKA) are also commonly used.

CAUSES

Diabetes with PAD is a more frequent cause of amputation than are traumatic injuries. Diabetic patients having an amputation related to PAD have a 50% to 75% five-year mortality rate due to cardiovascular complications. Poor foot care, impaired circulation, and peripheral neuropathy lead to serious ulcerations, which may be undetected until it is too late to salvage the foot or even the entire limb. Congenital deformity, severe burns, and crushing injuries that render a limb permanently unsightly, painful, or nonfunctional may be treated with surgical amputation. Tumors (usually malignant) and chronic osteomyelitis that does not respond to other treatment may also necessitate amputation.

GENETIC CONSIDERATIONS

No clear genetic contributions to susceptibility have been defined.

SEX AND LIFE SPAN CONSIDERATIONS

Amputations are seen in people of all ages. Children who have an amputation very early in life and are fitted with new and appropriate prostheses as they outgrow the old ones have the best physical and psychological adjustment to amputation. The greatest number of amputations are performed in older adults. In young adulthood, more men than women suffer traumatic amputations brought about by hazardous conditions in both the workplace and recreation. The greatest number of amputations are performed in men over 60 years old.

HEALTH DISPARITIES AND SEXUAL/GENDER MINORITY HEALTH

Black, Native American, and low-income persons have the highest rates of amputation in patients with diabetes and peripheral artery disease compared to their White counterparts (Barnes et al., 2020). Experts suggest that Black and Hispanic persons are less likely to receive a second opinion or having additional diagnostic testing to determine if other options exist, creating health disparities. In a series of studies of Veterans Administration patient treatment files, Black and Hispanic veterans with diabetes or peripheral arterial occlusive disease had higher odds of a lower extremity amputation than White patients. Sexual and gender minority status has no known effect on the risk for amputation.

GLOBAL HEALTH CONSIDERATIONS

No empirical data are available. Countries with high levels of civil strife or at war will have a higher prevalence of amputations because of injury from land mines, bullet wounds, and knife wounds. Areas with social deprivation and high rates of diabetes will have comparatively high rates of amputation.

☼ ASSESSMENT

HISTORY. Seek information in such areas as the control of diabetes and hypertension, diet, smoking, and any other activities that may affect the condition and rehabilitation of the patient.

PHYSICAL EXAMINATION. Inspection of the limb prior to surgery should focus on the area close to the expected site of amputation. If peripheral vascular disease is present, because of limited circulation, the limb often feels **cool to the touch**. Any **lacerations, abrasions**, or **contusions** may indicate additional problems with healing and should be made known to the surgeon. For patients with a severe traumatic injury, **hemorrhage, limb transection**, or a severe open fracture with irreparable neurovascular injury may occur. If the limb is so severely injured that a reconstructed limb will be less functional than an amputated limb, the amputation is performed.

PSYCHOSOCIAL. The loss of a limb creates stigma as society may view the person as incomplete or damaged. The young patient with a traumatic amputation may be in the denial phase of grief. The older patient with a long history of peripheral vascular problems, culminating in loss of a limb, may fear the loss of independence. Patients may show hostility or make demands of the nurse that seem unreasonable. Incomplete grieving, along with depression and false cheerfulness, can indicate psychological problems that predispose to phantom limb pain and prolonged rehabilitation.

Those patients who are reluctant to have visitors while they are hospitalized following an amputation may have problems with depression later. Psychological support is essential throughout the surgical and rehabilitation phases.

Diagnostic Highlights

Test	Normal Result	Abnormality With Condition	Explanation
Ankle-brachial index (ABI)	ABI > 1	ABI < 0.6	Ratio of the blood pressure in the leg to that in the arm; identifies people with severe aortoiliac occlusive disease

Other Tests: C-reactive protein (indicates infection), complete blood count, limb blood pressure, extremity x-rays, Doppler ultrasonography, ultrasonic duplex scanning, technetium-99m pyrophosphate bone scan, plethysmography, computed tomography

PRIMARY NURSING DIAGNOSIS

DIAGNOSIS. Impaired physical mobility related to loss of lower extremity as evidenced by alterations in gait

OUTCOMES. Balance; Body positioning: Self-initiated; Ambulation; Bone healing; Comfort status; Joint movement; Mobility; Muscloskeletal rehabilitation participation; Pain level; Wound healing: Primary intention; Fall prevention behavior

INTERVENTIONS. Positioning; Body image enhancement; Fall prevention; Exercise promotion; Exercise therapy: Ambulation and balance; Pain management: Acute and chronic; Positioning; Skin surveillance; Wound care

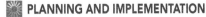 PLANNING AND IMPLEMENTATION

Collaborative

MANAGEMENT OF TRAUMATIC AMPUTATION. Lower extremity amputation has been performed since the time of Hippocrates, with improvements since then in control of bleeding, relief of pain, and sterile operative conditions. If complete amputation of a body part occurs in the field, flush the wound with sterile normal saline, apply a sterile pressure dressing, and elevate the limb. Do not apply a tourniquet to the extremity. Wrap the amputated body part in a wet sterile dressing that has been soaked with sterile normal saline solution, and place a towel around the body part. Place the body part in a clean, dry plastic bag; label the bag; and seal it. Place the bag in ice, and transport it with the trauma patient. If possible, cool the amputated part to 39°F (4°C). Do not store the amputated part on dry ice or in normal saline. Estimate the blood lost at the scene. Following reimplantation surgery, assess the color, temperature, peripheral pulses, and capillary refill of the reimplanted body part every 15 minutes. If the skin temperature declines below the recommended temperature or if perfusion decreases, notify the surgeon immediately.

POSTOPERATIVE MANAGEMENT. Many interventions can help improve the patient's mobility—for example, care of the surgical wound, control of pain, and prevention of further injury. If any excessive bleeding occurs, notify the surgeon immediately and place direct pressure on the area of hemorrhage. Patients may return from surgery with a soft dressing with pressure wrap, semirigid dressings including plaster splints, or rigid dressings, which are used with care because they reduce access to the surgical wound. They may return with an immediate postsurgical fitted prosthesis already in place. Explain that the device is intended to aid ambulation and prevent the complications of immobility.

A particular danger to mobility for the patient with a lower limb amputation is contracture of the nearest joint. Elevate the stump on a pillow for the first 24 hours following surgery to control edema. However, after 24 hours, do not elevate the stump any longer, or the patient may develop contractures. To prevent contractures, turn the patient prone for 15 to 30 minutes twice a day with the limb extended if the patient can tolerate it. If not, keep the joints extended rather than flexed.

Pharmacologic Highlights

Medication or Drug Class	Dosage	Description	Rationale
Analgesia	Varies by drug	The amputation procedure is painful and generally requires narcotic analgesia	Relieves pain and allows for increasing mobility to limit surgical complications

(highlight box continues on page 80)

Pharmacologic Highlights (continued)

Other Therapies: Intense burning, crushing, or knifelike pain responds to anticonvulsants such as gabapentin (Neurontin), pregabalin (Lyrica), and carbamazepine (Tegretol). The severe muscle cramps or spasmodic sensations that other patients experience respond better to a central-acting skeletal muscle relaxant such as baclofen (Lioresal). Narcotics such as tramadol (ConZip) may be used to relieve nerve pain, and beta blockers, such as propranolol, may be used to manage constant, dull, burning ache.

Independent

The discomfort that patients experience varies over time. Postoperative pain located specifically in the stump can be severe and is not usually aided by positioning, distraction, or other nonpharmacologic measures. True stump pain should be short term and should decrease as healing begins. If severe stump pain continues after healing progresses, it may indicate infection and should be investigated. Phantom limb pain, very real physical discomfort, usually begins about 2 weeks after surgery. It may be triggered by multiple factors, including neuroma formation, ischemia, scar tissue, urination, defecation, and even a cold temperature of the limb.

Grieving over loss of a body part is a normal experience and a necessary condition for successful rehabilitation. It becomes excessive when it dominates the person's life and interferes seriously with other functions. Explore concerns and help the patient and family determine which are real and which are feared.

Looking at the stump when the dressing is first changed is usually difficult for the patient. It triggers a body image disturbance that may take weeks or months to overcome. The nurse's calm manner in observing and caring for the stump encourages the patient to move toward accepting the changes in the patient's body.

Regardless of the type of dressing, stump sock, or temporary prosthesis, inspect the surgical area of an amputation every 8 hours for healing. The goal of bandaging is to reduce edema and shrink the stump into shape for a future prosthesis. Keep the wound clean and free of infection.

Many problems of safety or potential for injury exist for the patient who reestablishes their center of balance and relearns ambulation. Urge caution, especially with the young patient who denies having any disability. Safety concerns play a prominent role in planning for discharge. The nurse or physical therapist assesses the home situation.

Evidence-Based Practice and Health Policy

Minc, S., Hendricks, B., Misra, R., Ren, Y., Thibault, D., Marone, L., & Smith, G. (2020). Geographic variation in amputation rates among patients with diabetes and/or peripheral arterial disease in the rural state of West Virginia identifies areas for improved care. *Journal of Vascular Surgery, 71*, 1708–1717.

- The authors note that amputation is a devastating but preventable complication of diabetes and PAD. They proposed to identify the prevalence of major and minor amputation among patients with diabetes and PAD in rural West Virginia to establish high-risk geographical areas.
- They initiated a medical records review over 6 years of data to describe patients with diabetes and PAD with and without amputation. They found a prevalence of amputation that equals 4.9 per 1,000, with the highest risk in the central and northeastern counties of West Virginia. They suggest that these results should be used for public policy and public health initiatives.

DOCUMENTATION GUIDELINES

• Condition of the surgical site, including signs of irritation, infection, edema, and shrinkage of tissue
• Control of initial postoperative pain by pain medication
• Measures, both effective and ineffective, in control of phantom limb pain
• Ability to look at the stump and take part in its care
• Participation in physical therapy, including reluctance to try new skills
• Presence of any complication: Bleeding, thrombophlebitis, contractures, infection, return of pain after initial postoperative period

DISCHARGE AND HOME HEALTHCARE GUIDELINES

PREVENTION OF COMPLICATIONS. Teach the patient to wash the stump daily with plain soap and water, inspecting for signs of irritation, infection, edema, or pressure. Remind the patient not to elevate the stump on pillows, as a contracture may still occur in the nearest joint.

PHANTOM LIMB PAIN. Teach the patient to apply gentle pressure to the stump with the hands to control occasional phantom limb pain and to report frequent phantom limb pain to the physician.

PHYSICAL THERAPY. Give the patient the physical therapy or exercise schedule the patient is to follow, and make sure the patient understands it. If the patient needs to return to the hospital for physical therapy, check on the availability of transportation.

SUPPLIES AND EQUIPMENT. Make sure that the patient is provided with needed supplies and equipment, such as stump socks and a well-fitting prosthesis.

ENVIRONMENT. Instruct the patient to avoid environmental hazards, such as throw rugs and steps without banisters.

SUPPORT SERVICES. Many communities have support services for amputees and for patients who have suffered a loss (including a body part). Help the patient locate the appropriate service or refer the patient to the social service department for future support.

Amyloidosis

DRG Category:	546
Mean LOS:	4.4 days
Description:	MEDICAL: Connective Tissue Disorders With Complication or Comorbidity

Amyloidosis is a rare, chronic metabolic disorder characterized by the extracellular deposition of amyloid, a fibrous protein, in one or more locations of the body. Technically, amyloidosis is a constellation of disorders. Primary amyloidosis is a monoclonal plasma cell disorder, and the abnormal protein is an immunoglobulin; it is not associated with other clinical conditions and is considered idiopathic because it arises spontaneously. Secondary amyloidosis occurs as a result of chronic infection, inflammation, or malignancy and is caused by the degradation of the acute-phase reactant serum amyloid; familial amyloidosis results from accumulation of a mutated version of a plasma protein. Because normally soluble proteins are folded or pleated, they become deposited as insoluble fibrils that progressively disrupt tissue structure and function. The modern classification of amyloidosis is based on the chemistry of the protein. The disease is referred to with an *A* followed by an abbreviation of the fibril protein. Most people with primary amyloidosis have a fibril protein that is a light chain, abbreviated *L*. Therefore, most people with primary amyloidosis have light chain amyloidosis (AL). Eight out of 1 million people develop amyloidosis, and the average age of diagnosis is 65 years. The Amyloidosis Foundation estimates that approximately 4,500 people are diagnosed with AL each year in the United States. AL is caused by a disorder of the bone marrow, which produces plasma cells that make an abnormal immunoglobin (antibody) that is deposited in organs and other tissues. Organ dysfunction results from accumulation and infiltration of amyloid into tissues, which ultimately puts pressure on surrounding tissues and causes atrophy of cells. Some forms of amyloidosis cause reticuloendothelial cell dysfunction and abnormal immunoglobulin synthesis.

The associated disease states may be inflammatory, hereditary, or neoplastic; deposition can be localized or systemic. Secondary amyloidosis is associated with such chronic diseases as tuberculosis, syphilis, HIV, Hodgkin disease, and rheumatoid arthritis and with extensive tissue destruction. Amyloidosis occurs in about 5% to 10% of patients who have multiple myeloma, the second-most common malignant tumor of bone. The spleen, liver, kidneys, and adrenal cortex are the organs most frequently involved. For a patient with generalized amyloidosis, the average survival rate is 1 to 4 years. Some patients have lived longer, but amyloidosis can result in permanent or life-threatening organ damage. The major causes of death are renal failure and cardiac failure. When heart failure is associated with amyloidosis, the average survival rate is less than a year.

CAUSES

The precise causes of amyloidosis are unknown, although some experts suspect an immunobiological basis for the disease. The disease has complex causes, with both immune and genetic factors involved. It may be due to an enzyme defect or an altered immune response. Some forms of amyloidosis appear to have a genetic cause. Another form of amyloidosis appears to be related to Alzheimer disease.

GENETIC CONSIDERATIONS

While not specifically a genetic disease, several genes have been associated with amyloidosis. These include the apolipoprotein A1 gene (*APOA1*), the fibrinogen alpha-chain gene (*FGA*), and the lysozyme gene (*LYZ*). Amyloidosis can also occur as a feature of heritable diseases, such as familial Mediterranean fever (FMF), which is an autosomal recessive disease more common among persons of Mediterranean origin; autosomal dominant cases have also been reported. FMF causes fever and pain in the joints, chest, and abdomen. Amyloid aggregation has also been linked to familial amyloid neuropathies, which are usually caused by mutations in transthyretin (*TTR*), apolipoprotein A1 (*APOA1*), or gelsolin (*GSN*).

SEX AND LIFE SPAN CONSIDERATIONS

Amyloidosis is seen more in adult populations than in children and adolescents. Older individuals, especially those with Alzheimer disease and rheumatoid arthritis, are at risk. In the United States, because of higher rates of rheumatoid arthritis in women, inflammatory (secondary) amyloidosis is more common in women than in men. Considering all forms of amyloidosis, the male-to-female ratio is 2:1 because males have higher incidence of primary amyloidosis than females.

HEALTH DISPARITIES AND SEXUAL/GENDER MINORITY HEALTH

Some studies show that Black persons have a higher risk for cardiac-related amyloidosis leading to cardiomyopathy and a more aggressive form of the disease than do other groups. Sexual and gender minority status has no known effect on the risk for amyloidosis.

GLOBAL HEALTH CONSIDERATIONS

Amyloidosis occurs around the world, but no prevalence data are available. International rates depend on the prevalence of associated diseases in the country of origin. Patients whose origins are Portuguese, Japanese, Swedish, Greek, and Italian may be more susceptible.

◼ ASSESSMENT

HISTORY. Establish a history of **weakness, weight loss, lightheadedness,** or **fainting** (syncope). Ask the patient if they have experienced **difficulty breathing.** Determine if the patient has experienced difficulty in swallowing, diarrhea, or constipation, which are signs of gastrointestinal (GI) involvement. Determine if the patient has experienced **joint pain,** which is a sign of amyloid arthritis. Elicit a history of potential risk factors.

PHYSICAL EXAMINATION. Assess for kidney involvement by inspecting the patient's feet for signs of pedal edema and the patient's face for signs of periorbital edema. Take the patient's pulse, noting changes in rhythm and regularity. Note any changes in the patient's blood pressure. Auscultate the patient's heart sounds for the presence of dysrhythmias, murmurs, or adventitious sounds. Auscultate the breath sounds and observe for dyspnea.

Observe the patient's tongue for swelling and stiffness, and assess the patient's ability to speak and swallow. Auscultate bowel sounds, noting hypoactivity. Palpate the patient's abdomen, noting any enlargement of the liver. Observe the patient for signs of abdominal pain, and check the patient's stool for blood.

Assess the patient's skin turgor and color, noting any evidence of jaundice. The patient may have petechiae and bruising. Malabsorption occurs with GI involvement, leading to malnourishment. Observe the patient's skin for the presence of lesions that may indicate nutrient or vitamin deficiencies. Palpate the axillary, inguinal, and anal regions for the presence of plaques or elevated papules. Inspect the patient's neck and mucosal areas, such as the ear or tongue, for lesions. Observe the patient's eyes, noting any periorbital ecchymoses ("black-eye syndrome"). Neurological testing may reveal decreased pain sensation and muscle strength in the extremities.

PSYCHOSOCIAL. Because the patient with amyloidosis may be asymptomatic, the suddenness of the revelation of the disease can be traumatic. Patients with facial lesions may be upset at the change in their appearance. Depending on the type and progression of amyloidosis, the patient's life expectancy may be shortened, and counseling may be helpful. The need for long-term health planning, palliative care, and support for caregiving are important components to consider.

Diagnostic Highlights

Test	Normal Result	Abnormality With Condition	Explanation
Serum protein electrophoresis, urine protein electrophoresis, serum and urine protein immunoelectrophoresis	Negative	Identification of abnormal immunoglobulins; serum free light chains can be measured	To determine the immune response
Biopsy, usually taken from the rectal mucosa or subcutaneous abdominal fat pads; other sites include skin and gums	Negative	Positive for amyloid usually with Congo red staining techniques	Identifies the presence of amyloid with appropriate stains

Other Tests: Electrocardiogram, echocardiogram, cardiac magnetic resonance, troponin T, troponin I, brain natriuretic peptide, serum alkaline phosphatase, urinalysis, blood urea nitrogen and creatinine

PRIMARY NURSING DIAGNOSIS

DIAGNOSIS. Decreased cardiac output related to an ineffective ventricular pump as evidenced by dyspnea, tachycardia, and/or peripheral edema

OUTCOMES. Cardiac pump: Effectiveness; Circulation status; Tissue perfusion: Abdominal organs and peripheral; Vital signs; Electrolyte & acid base balance; Endurance; Energy conservation; Fluid balance

INTERVENTIONS. Cardiac care; Fluid/electrolyte management; Medication administration; Medication management; Oxygen therapy; Vital signs monitoring

PLANNING AND IMPLEMENTATION

Collaborative

Therapy is targeted to support care that manages symptoms of the underlying organ dysfunction through pharmacologic therapy, but there is no known cure. Autologous blood stem cell transplant is a treatment option for people whose disease is not advanced with good cardiac function, but only a minority of patients with AL are eligible for this procedure. Chemotherapy and immunomodulator therapy may also be administered. Surgical procedures may be used to treat severe symptoms. The patient may develop a complication of the tongue called macroglossia. If this occurs, a tracheotomy may be necessary to maintain oxygenation. Patients with severe renal amyloidosis and azotemia may undergo bilateral nephrectomy and renal transplantation followed by immune therapy, although the donor kidney may be susceptible to amyloidosis as well. Strict control of blood glucose levels and treatment of hypertension are important for people with renal amyloidosis.

OTHER MANAGEMENT. A dietary consultation can provide the patient with a plan to supplement needed nutrients and bulk-forming foods based on the patient's symptoms. Unless the patient requires fluid restriction, they need to drink at least 2 L of fluid per day. A referral to a speech therapist may be necessary if the patient's tongue prevents clear communication.

Pharmacologic Highlights

Medication or Drug Class	Dosage	Description	Rationale
Melphalan and prednisone combined therapy	Varies with drug protocol	Antineoplastic alkylating agent and corticosteroid	Interrupts the growth of the abnormal cells that produce amyloid protein; decreases amyloid deposits; no known effective therapy to reverse amyloidosis

Other Therapies: Drug combinations are tailored to individual patients to enable the best course of treatment. New and experimental combinations include cyclophosphamide, proteasome inhibitors, and immunomodulators such as thalidomide. Dimethylsulfoxide (DMSO) and colchicine have been used at times to decrease amyloid deposits. Doxycycline may be used to reduce joint pain and increase range of motion. To prevent serious cardiac complications in patients with cardiac amyloidosis, antidysrhythmic agents are prescribed. Digitalis is avoided because patients are susceptible to toxicity. Vitamin K is used to treat coagulation problems, and analgesics are prescribed for pain. As the disease progresses and malabsorption develops secondary to GI involvement, parenteral nutrition is used to meet nutritional needs.

Independent

Maintain a patent airway when the patient's tongue is involved. Prevent respiratory tract complications by gentle and adequate suctioning when necessary. Keep a tracheotomy tray at the patient's bedside in case of airway obstruction. When the patient is placed on bedrest, institute measures to prevent atrophy of the muscles, development of contractures, and formation of pressure ulcers.

Provide a pleasant environment to stimulate the patient's appetite. Give oral hygiene before and after meals and assist the patient as needed with feeding. Note that the disease puts tremendous stressors on the family and patient as they cope with a chronic disease without hope of recovery. Encourage the patient to verbalize their feelings. Involve loved ones in the care of the patient, and involve the patient in all discussions surrounding their care. Present a realistic picture of the prognosis of the illness, but do not remove the patient's hope. This illness tends to be progressive and debilitating with significant dysfunction of the involved organs. Long-term health planning is essential. Refer the patient and family to the chaplain or a clinical nurse specialist for counseling if appropriate.

Evidence-Based Practice and Health Policy

Rubin, J., & Maurer, M. (2020). Cardiac amyloidosis: Overlooked, underappreciated, and treatable. *Annual Review of Medicine, 71*, 203–219.

• The authors proposed to review the literature that explains cardiac amyloidosis, a disease that leads to infiltrative and restrictive cardiomyopathy and ultimately to heart failure. Cardiac amyloidosis is often underdiagnosed. Diagnostic testing such as nuclear scintigraphy has reduced the need for patients to undergo a biopsy to make the diagnosis. In nuclear scintigraphy, radioisotopes are attached to drugs that are injected, travel to the heart, and allow for capture of two-dimensional images.

• In addition to sodium restrictions and diuretic use, advanced chemotherapies are being targeted to different stages of the disease process depending on the pathophysiology of the disease.

DOCUMENTATION GUIDELINES

• Physical findings: Adequacy of airway, degree of hydration or dehydration, presence of lesions, macroglossia, edema
• Ability to use extremities: Range of motion, weakness, gait, activity tolerance
• Nutritional status
• Changes in heart and lung sounds, presence of dysrhythmias
• Response to medications, speech therapy, counseling, surgery
• Emotional responses to disease: Degree of hope, resiliency, family support, ability to cope
• Understanding of and interest in patient teaching

DISCHARGE AND HOME HEALTHCARE GUIDELINES

MEDICATIONS. Teach the patient the purpose, dosage, schedule, precautions and potential side effects, interactions, and adverse reactions of all prescribed medications.

COMPLICATIONS. Teach the patient to examine their legs daily for signs of swelling. Instruct the patient to monitor urinary output for a decrease in quantity. Teach the patient to test the stool for bleeding. Advise the patient to report breathing difficulties or irregular heartbeats.

FOLLOW-UP. Explain to the patient and significant others that a variety of counseling and social supports are available to help as the disease progresses. Give the patient a phone number to call if some health assistance is needed. Provide the patient and family with information about the Amyloidosis Foundation (https://amyloidosis.org).

Amyotrophic Lateral Sclerosis

DRG Category: 57
Mean LOS: 5.6 days
Description: MEDICAL: Degenerative Nervous System Disorders Without Major Complication or Comorbidity

Amyotrophic lateral sclerosis (ALS) is a degenerative, progressive disease that causes atrophy (wasting) of muscle fibers that control voluntary muscle movement. ALS is a fatal disease with an average life expectancy after diagnosis of approximately 3 years, although some persons live as long as 10 or 15 years with a benign form of the disease. There are approximately 18,000 Americans living with the disease at any one time, and each year in the United States, there are 5,600 new cases. ALS is often referred to as Lou Gehrig disease after the baseball player who died from it. ALS is characterized by a progressive loss of motor neurons (in both the cerebral cortex and the spinal cord). The muscular atrophy is called *amyotrophy*. As motor neurons are destroyed in the cerebral cortex, the long axons and the myelin sheaths that make up the corticospinal nerve tracts disappear. The loss of fibers in the nerve tracts and development of a firmness in the tissues lead to the designation *lateral sclerosis*. One important feature of the disease is the selective nature of neuronal cell death. The sensory networks and the portions of the brain needed for control and regulation of movement, intellect, and thinking are not affected, while motor function deteriorates. The most common complications of ALS are respiratory dysfunction, and death may occur because of pneumonia or respiratory failure.

CAUSES

The precise cause of ALS is unknown. Only 5% to 10% of patients have the inherited form. These people have a closely related family member with ALS, and the disease is referred to as *familial* ALS (FALS). Most people with adult-onset ALS have no family history of ALS. This isolated situation is referred to as *sporadic* ALS (SALS), and although there is likely a genetic predisposition involved, it is not inherited.

Theories of disease development center on an interaction between genetics, environment, and age-related risk factors; experts suggest that a biochemical transformation occurs (such as a viral infection), which creates a metabolic disturbance in motor neurons or an autoimmune response directed against motor neurons. Most scientists agree that smoking is an environmental risk factor. Other possible risk factors are serving in the military, head trauma, and living in the Western Pacific islands (most commonly Guam), as well as physical exhaustion, severe stress, viral infections, and conditions such as myocardial infarction and malnutrition. Data from recent studies raise concerns that athletes in the sports of American football, European football, soccer, and boxing may be at risk.

GENETIC CONSIDERATIONS

Like Alzheimer disease, ALS has both familial and sporadic forms. Approximately 10% of ALS is familial and follows an autosomal dominant pattern of inheritance. A recently identified mutation in the gene *C9orf72* is responsible for approximately 50% of FALS and for 5% to 10% of SALS. Another 15% to 20% of FALS cases have been linked with mutations in the superoxide dismutase-1 gene (*SOD1*). Juvenile-onset forms of ALS are more likely to be familial and have been associated with mutations in the alsin (*ALS2*), senataxin (*SETX*), and Spatacsin (*SPG11*) genes, among others. Other rarer mutations in *FUS, VAPB, ANG, TARDBP,* and *FIG4* cause adult-onset ALS, whereas modifying mutations in *NEFH, PRPH, ATXN2,* and *DCTN1* appear to affect susceptibility to SALS.

SEX AND LIFE SPAN CONSIDERATIONS

There is a higher incidence of ALS in men than in women, although after menopause, the male-to-female ratio equalizes. Women have more problems with speech dysfunction than men. The onset of the disease usually occurs in middle age, predominantly in the fifth or sixth decade. Mean age of onset is 65 years. If the symptoms develop during the teenage years, the patient probably has FALS.

HEALTH DISPARITIES AND SEXUAL/GENDER MINORITY HEALTH

In the United States, ALS affects White persons more than other racial/ethnic groups or persons with mixed races/ethnicities. In contrast, Black persons live longer with ALS than White persons. Recent work suggests that this may occur because Black persons opt for tracheostomy and invasive ventilation use more than other groups. Data suggest that persons with Pacific Islander ancestry may have a higher prevalence of the disease than other populations. Sexual and gender minority status has no known effect on the risk for ALS.

GLOBAL HEALTH CONSIDERATIONS

ALS occurs in people around the world. The frequency of ALS in European countries is similar to that among the U.S. population: 2 per 100,000 persons per year. Finland and Japan have a higher incidence than most other populations, as do Guam, New Guinea, and the Marianas Island. There are no data available for the disease in developing countries.

✴ ASSESSMENT

HISTORY. The first evidence of the disease is often gradually developing **asymmetrical painless weakness in one limb** without accompanying loss in sensation. Establish a recent history of muscle weakness or **involuntary contractions** (fasciculations) of the muscles, especially in the tongue, feet, and hands. The dominant arm is more commonly affected than the nondominant arm. People with upper extremity onset may complain of finger cramping, stiffness, or weakness, whereas people with lower extremity onset may experience tripping or a stumbling, awkward gait. Ask whether the patient has lost weight, experienced **problems with speech**, has had difficulty in chewing or swallowing, or has been drooling. Elicit a history of breathing difficulties or choking. Ask if the patient has experienced any speech dysfunction, crying spells, or periods of inappropriate laughter, which can be caused by progressive bulbar palsy (degeneration of upper motor neurons in the medulla oblongata).

PHYSICAL EXAMINATION. Determine how the disease is affecting the patient's functioning and ability to carry out the activities of daily living. Assess for the characteristic atrophic changes such as weakness or fasciculation in the muscles of the forearms, hands, and legs. The muscles may lose their bulk because of atrophy. One side of the body may have more muscle involvement than the other. Assess the patient's respiratory status, noting rate and pattern and the patient's breath sounds.

As the disease progresses, muscle weakness that began asymmetrically becomes symmetrical. The patient may develop foot drop. Muscles of chewing, swallowing, and tongue movement are affected. Note facial symmetry, the presence or absence of a gag reflex, slurred speech, and the ability to swallow. Note any tendency to drool or any tongue tremors. Over time, speech becomes difficult with a strained quality. Standardized assessment for people with ALS can be accomplished with the ALS Functional Rating Scale Revised, a questionnaire that can provide important information as the disease progresses (Cedarbaum et al., 1999).

PSYCHOSOCIAL. The patient with ALS is confronted with a progressive fatal illness. Because mental capacity is not affected by this disease, the patient remains alert even in the late stages of the disease. Living with this disease presents extraordinary challenges to patients and families. Patients with ALS usually experience depression and need a great deal of emotional support, as do their families and significant others.

Diagnostic Highlights

General Comments: Because ALS is currently untreatable, it is essential that other potential causes of motor neuron dysfunction be excluded by diagnostic testing.

Test	Normal Result	Abnormality With Condition	Explanation
Needle electromyography and nerve conduction studies at three levels of the paraspinal muscles (cervical, thoracic, lumbar) and of the bulbar muscles	Normal conduction velocity 40–80 m/sec after a nerve is stimulated with normal muscle action potentials	Diffuse denervation signs, decreased amplitude of compound muscle action potentials, and normal conduction velocities	Rules out other muscle diseases; often reflects a decrease in motor units of the affected muscles

Other Tests: Muscle biopsy, cerebrospinal fluid analysis, pulmonary function tests, computed tomography scan, magnetic resonance imaging, other conduction studies; genetic testing and genetic counseling; serum protein immunoelectrophoresis, HIV testing, and Lyme disease serology to rule out other disorders

PRIMARY NURSING DIAGNOSIS

DIAGNOSIS. Ineffective airway clearance related to ineffective cough as evidenced by dyspnea, absence of cough, restlessness, altered respiratory rhythm

OUTCOMES. Respiratory status: Airway patency; Respiratory status: Gas exchange; Respiratory status: Ventilation; Oral health

INTERVENTIONS. Airway insertion and stabilization; Airway management; Airway suctioning; Oral health promotion; Oxygen therapy; Respiratory monitoring; Ventilation assistance

☀ PLANNING AND IMPLEMENTATION

Collaborative

Management of ALS is focused on the treatment of symptoms, maintaining quality of life, and rehabilitation measures. No specific treatment for the disease exists that will influence the underlying pathophysiology.

REHABILITATION. Rehabilitation aids are available to overcome the effects of muscular disability and to support weakened muscles. A planned program of exercise helps patients function for a longer period of time.

AIRWAY MANAGEMENT. Supporting the patient's airway and breathing becomes essential as the disease progresses. Noninvasive ventilation (NIV) is the use of breathing support under positive pressure using a face mask, nasal mask, or helmet. Oxygen can be added to the air, and generally the amount of pressure is alternated depending on the phase of breathing (inspiration or expiration). Experts suggest that NIV is the most effective treatment for prolonging life in people with ALS. The patient's deteriorating respiratory status may eventually require mechanical ventilation in certain situations. If a ventilator is being used at home, the patient and significant others will need instructions on ventilatory management.

NUTRITION. When the patient can no longer maintain nutrition, enteral or parenteral feedings may be initiated. Experts suggest percutaneous endoscopic gastrostomy for long-term nutritional management as the patient's appetite declines and as swallowing becomes impaired.

Pharmacologic Highlights

Medication or Drug Class	Dosage	Description	Rationale
Riluzole	50 mg PO q 12 hr	Central nervous system agent	Inhibits presynaptic release of glutamic acid in the central nervous system; prolongs tracheostomy-free survival by decreasing injury of neurons by glutamic acid
Baclofen	5–10 mg PO tid	Skeletal muscle relaxant	Manages muscle spasticity
Tizanidine	4–8 mg PO qid	Skeletal muscle relaxant	Manages muscle spasticity

Other Therapy: NSAIDs, tramadol, detorolac for pain; benzodiazepines or anticonvulsants for cramps.

Independent

MANAGING THE DISEASE. A variety of mobile chairs are available to help maintain the patient's quality of life and independence. Teach the patient breathing exercises, methods to change positions, chest physical therapy techniques, and incentive spirometry. Explore measures to reduce the risk of aspiration. Encourage rest periods prior to meals to decrease muscle fatigue. Have the patient sit in an upright position with the neck slightly flexed during meals, use a neck support such as a cervical collar, and serve foods with a soft consistency. Encourage the patient to remain in an upright position for at least 30 minutes after a meal. If the patient is having problems handling oral secretions, teach them how to use oral suction.

As the disease worsens, the patient may lose the ability to speak. Work with the patient and family to develop alternate methods of communication, such as tablet computers, picture or word charts, or computers with artificial speech or synthesizers. When the patient's immobility increases, teach the family to provide skin care to all pressure points. The patient needs to be turned and positioned frequently. The use of a pressure-reducing mattress will also help maintain skin integrity.

ACTIVITIES OF DAILY LIVING. To achieve maximum mobility and independence, institute an exercise regimen with active or passive range-of-motion (ROM) exercises. Use supportive devices for mobility and transfer, and instruct the patient on the use of splints. Establish regular bowel and bladder routines. Work with the patient and significant others to develop a pattern for activities of daily living that allows the patient to participate but not to become overly fatigued. As mobility decreases, help the patient obtain equipment such as a walker, a wheelchair, or a lift. Ask the patient or family to describe the living environment (or perform a home assessment) to identify areas that may cause potential injury or to recommend modifications to the environment.

EMOTIONAL SUPPORT. Early in the disease process, expect the patient and family to be angry, deny the probable disease outcome (death), or show extreme anxiety. The patient and family will most likely experience periods of depression and may need a referral to a counselor or support group. Recognize that the disease is a catastrophic event in the family's life and will change the family forever. Most communities have local chapters of the Amyotrophic

Lateral Sclerosis Association, and its Web site is very helpful for patients and families: https://www.alsa.org.

END-OF-LIFE PLANNING. Planning with a palliative care specialist is critical to ensure that wishes of the patient and family are incorporated into a palliative plan of care. In addition to supporting the patient as symptoms worsen, disabilities increase, and death approaches, end-of-life care will support the patient's and caregivers' quality of life, spiritual needs, and mental health needs.

Evidence-Based Practice and Health Policy

Kim, G., Gautier, O., Tassoni-Tsuchida, E., Ma, X., & Gitler, A. (2020). ALS genetics: Gains, losses, and implications for future therapies. *Neuron, 108*, 822–842.

- The authors reviewed background information about ALS, a fatal neurodegenerative disorder caused by the loss of motor neurons from the brain and spinal cord. The patient experiences progressive loss of motor function and ultimately the loss of respiratory function that leads to death. The authors note that the genetic changes that occur with ALS are similar to those that occur with some types of dementia, which is helpful as the focus on both conditions is to find therapies related to genetic function.
- Loss of function mutations of genes may modify the severity of or susceptibility to ALS and are targets for therapeutic strategies. Current efforts focus on personalized therapies for individual patients with specific targets for medications.

DOCUMENTATION GUIDELINES

- Physical findings related to the patient's respiratory status, including respiratory rate, depth, rhythm, breathing pattern, respiratory excursion, breath sounds, and cough effort
- Responses to the nursing interventions taken to support the patient's respiratory function, such as coughing, deep breathing, frequent position changes, and incentive spirometry
- Nutritional status: Patient's weight, measure to maintain nutrition (feeding patient, soft or pureed food, tube feeding)
- Patient's ability to perform activities of daily living and maintain mobility
- Responses to all ROM exercises or active exercises
- Responses to equipment or assistive devices such as splints necessary in patient care
- Response to managing a debilitative disease and to end-of-life planning

DISCHARGE AND HOME HEALTHCARE GUIDELINES

PREVENTION OF ASPIRATION. Teach the family or caregivers how to protect the patient's airway and dislodge food if the patient aspirates. Teach the patient or family how to suction the patient.

TREATMENT. Provide information regarding home healthcare products that are available and explain how to get them. Explain to the patient and family treatment options such as NIV, mechanical ventilation, and tracheostomy.

EMOTIONAL. Explore coping strategies. Recommend communication strategies such as tablet computers. Support groups for ALS patients are available in many cities. Refer the patient or family to respite care or the Amyotrophic Lateral Sclerosis Association.

Anaphylaxis

DRG Category:	916
Mean LOS:	2.2 days
Description:	MEDICAL: Allergic Reactions Without Major Complication or Comorbidity

Anaphylactic shock, or anaphylaxis, is an immediate, life-threatening, multiple organ (skin, respiratory tract, cardiovascular system, gastrointestinal system) allergic reaction caused by a systemic antigen-antibody immune response to a substance (antigen) introduced into the body. The classic form of anaphylaxis results from prior sensitization to the antigen, with later reexposure producing symptoms of shock through an immunological mechanism. The term was first coined in 1902 when a second dose of a vaccination caused the death of an animal; the animal's death was described as the opposite of prophylaxis and was therefore called *anaphylaxis*, which means "without protection." In the United States, experts estimate that from 20,000 to 50,000 people have anaphylactic shock each year; fatalities are infrequent, but as many as 1,000 people may die in the United States each year. Experts suggest that up to 15% of the North American population is at risk of experiencing anaphylaxis.

Traditionally, most experts have considered that classic anaphylaxis is caused by a type I, immunoglobulin E (IgE)–mediated hypersensitivity reaction only. The antigen combines with IgE on the surface of the mast cells and precipitates a release of histamine and other chemical mediators, such as serotonin and slow-reacting substance of anaphylaxis (SRS-A). The resulting increased capillary permeability, smooth muscle contraction, and vasodilation account for the cardiovascular collapse. More recently, the World Allergy Organization has broadened the definition of anaphylaxis to include not only IgE-mediated but also non-IgE-mediated and nonimmunological anaphylaxis events. Non-IgE anaphylaxis results from IgG- and complement-mediated activation, whereas nonimmunological anaphylaxis results from mast cell and basophil degranulation without the presence of immunoglobulins.

Bronchoconstriction, bronchospasm, and relative hypovolemia result in impaired airway, breathing, and circulation; vasodilation, increased vascular permeability, and nerve stimulation occurs, and death may follow if anaphylaxis is not promptly reversed. Although a delayed reaction may occur 24 hours after the exposure to an antigen, most reactions occur within minutes after exposure, and a recurrence of symptoms may occur after 4 to 8 hours. The most common causes of death from anaphylaxis are airway obstruction and hypotension.

CAUSES

Anaphylaxis can result from a variety of causes, but it most commonly occurs in response to food, medications, and insect bites. Severe reactions to penicillin occur with a frequency of 1 to 5 patients per 10,000 courses of medication, and deaths from penicillin occur in 1 case per 50,000 to 100,000 courses of medication. Insect stings cause 25 to 50 deaths per year in the United States. In population-based studies in the United States, ingestion of a specific food was responsible for 33% of cases, insect stings for 18.5% of cases, and medications for 13.7% of cases. Twenty-five percent of cases had no identifiable cause. Common sources are iodine-based contrast materials and medications that are derived from biological protein sources. These medications can include those derived from horse sera, vaccines, enzymes, and hormones. Foods such as fish, eggs, peanuts, milk products, and chocolate can cause allergic reactions and anaphylaxis. Rarely, anaphylaxis can also be caused by vigorous exercise such as jogging, tennis, soccer, and bicycling.

GENETIC CONSIDERATIONS

While susceptibility to anaphylaxis is increased among those who have inherited sensitivity to antigens, the genetic component has not been well defined. Several genes have been implicated specifically in development of anaphylaxis (*IL4R*, *IL10*, *IL13*) and in modulating the severity of anaphylaxis (PAF-AH, cKIT). More broadly, over 20 genes have been associated with the development of allergy, and of these, many are passed on in families. Family studies indicate that if both parents suffer from allergies, the allergy risk in their offspring is 80%. In addition to the genes involved in anaphylaxis, it is thought that interferon gamma (*IFNG*), β-adrenergic receptor (*ADRB2*), 5 lipoxygenase (*ALOX5*), *PHF1*, *TARC*, and the leukotriene C4 synthetase (*LTC4S*) genes play a role in allergy risk. Animal studies indicate that mutations in the transient receptor potential cation channel (*TRPM4*), which controls calcium influx, particularly in T cells and mast cells, can augment anaphylaxis.

SEX AND LIFE SPAN CONSIDERATIONS

Anaphylactic shock can occur at any age and in both men and women, but women seem a little more susceptible than men. Individuals with food allergies (particularly shellfish, peanuts, and tree nuts) and asthma may be at increased risk for having a life-threatening anaphylactic reaction. People near the end of the life span are most at risk. To prevent infants and children from experiencing severe allergic reactions, pediatricians carefully plan vaccines and diet to limit the risk of allergic reaction until a child's immune system is more mature. Severe food allergy is more common in children than in adults, but diagnostic contrast, insect stings, and anesthetics are more common in adults than in children. Teenagers with food allergies and asthma may be at high risk for an allergic reaction because they are more likely to eat outside the home and less likely to carry their medications. Some experts suggest that latex, aspirin, and muscle relaxant reactions are more common in women and insect sting anaphylaxes are more common in men. Older adults also have a great risk of anaphylaxis, and their risk of death is high owing to the presence of preexisting diseases.

HEALTH DISPARITIES AND SEXUAL/GENDER MINORITY HEALTH

Allergy rates in children seem to vary by race and ethnicity. Black children have more allergies to wheat, soy, corn, fish, and shellfish than White children. Hispanic children have more allergies to corn, fish, and shellfish than White children. This same study suggested that Black and Hispanic children are at higher risk of adverse outcomes, a shorter duration of follow-up with an allergy specialist, and higher rates of anaphylaxis as compared to White children (Mahdavinia et al., 2017). Sexual and gender minority status has no known effect on the risk for anaphylaxis.

GLOBAL HEALTH CONSIDERATIONS

The global incidence of anaphylaxis is unknown, but fatal anaphylaxis is relatively rare, whereas milder forms occur more frequently. Internationally, the frequency of anaphylaxis is increasing due to an increase in exposure to allergens. Allergic reactions to insects, venomous plants, and venomous animals are more prevalent in tropical areas.

✵ ASSESSMENT

HISTORY. Obtain information about any recent food intake, medication ingestion, outdoor activities, exercise, exposure to insects, or known allergies. Symptoms usually begin within 5 to 30 minutes, and the earlier the signs and symptoms begin, the more severe the reaction. Often the signs and symptoms begin with skin and respiratory involvement and include those listed in Box 1.

• BOX 1 Signs and Symptoms of Anaphylaxis

Skin	**Urticaria (rash), flushing, angioedema, sneezing, conjunctival pruritus, swelling, diaphoresis**
Respiratory	Nasal congestion, rhinorrhea, **throat tightness, shortness of breath**, cough, hoarseness, nasal congestion, bronchospasm, **swelling of lips and tongue**
Gastrointestinal	Nausea, vomiting, diarrhea, pain, cramping
Cardiovascular	**Tachycardia**, syncope, dizziness, chest pain
Neurological (rare)	Headache, seizure, hypoxemia may lead to confusion
General	Weakness, lightheadedness, sense of impending doom

Ask family members about a family history of drug allergies or a history of previous reactions.

PHYSICAL EXAMINATION. Note any hives, which appear as well-defined areas of redness with raised borders and blanched centers. Generalized symptoms include flushing, tingling, pruritus, and angioedema around the mouth, tongue, eyes, and hands. Wheezing, stridor, loss of the voice, and difficulty breathing indicate laryngeal edema and bronchospasm and may indicate the need for emergency intubation. Auscultate the patient's blood pressure with a high suspicion for hypotension. Auscultate the patient's heart to identify cardiac dysrhythmias, which may precipitate vascular collapse. Palpate the patient's extremities for signs of cardiovascular compromise, such as weak peripheral pulses and delayed capillary refill.

PSYCHOSOCIAL. The patient who is experiencing an anaphylactic reaction is often panicky and fearful. Although alert, the patient may express a feeling of helplessness, loss of control, and impending doom. In addition, the family, parents, or significant others are likely to be fearful and severely anxious.

Diagnostic Highlights

No specific laboratory tests are required to make the diagnosis of anaphylactic shock, although diagnostic tests may be performed to rule out other causes of the symptoms, such as congestive heart failure, myocardial infarction, or status asthmaticus. If a patient is seen soon after the event, the following diagnostic tests may be helpful in confirming the diagnosis: plasma histamine, urinary histamine metabolites, or serum tryptase.

PRIMARY NURSING DIAGNOSIS

DIAGNOSIS. Ineffective airway clearance related to laryngeal edema and bronchospasm as evidenced by hoarseness, shortness of breath, and/or apnea

OUTCOMES. Allergic response: Systemic; Respiratory status: Airway patency; Respiratory status: Gas exchange; Respiratory status: Ventilation; Anxiety level; Risk control

INTERVENTIONS. Airway insertion and stabilization; Airway management; Oxygen therapy; Respiratory monitoring; Ventilation assistance; Allergy management; Anaphylaxis management; Anxiety reduction

☀ PLANNING AND IMPLEMENTATION

Collaborative

The plan of care depends on the severity of the reaction, but airway management is the first priority. Discontinue the administration of any possible allergen immediately. Consider applying a tourniquet to the extremity with the antigen source; this procedure can retard antigen exposure to the systemic circulation, but the tourniquet needs to be released every 5 minutes, and it should not be left in place longer than 30 minutes. Complete an assessment of the patient's airway to ensure patency, adequate breathing, and oxygenation. If the patient has airway compromise, endotracheal intubation and noninvasive ventilation or mechanical ventilation with oxygenation may be necessary. More severe or prolonged cases of anaphylactic shock are aggressively treated with the establishment of IV access and infusion of normal saline or lactated Ringer solution as well as supplemental oxygen therapy. The patient may require urinary catheterization to monitor urinary output during periods of instability.

Pharmacologic Highlights

Medication or Drug Class	Dosage	Description	Rationale
Epinephrine	Preparation and dose vary by route, which can be IV, subcutaneous, intramuscular, sublingually, or down the endotracheal tube; subcutaneous dose is 0.3–0.5 mg of a 1:1,000 solution and repeated at 20-min intervals; an IV drip may be used for protracted cases; prefilled syringe is often used	Catecholamine	Decreases inflammation and allergic response
Diphenhydramine (Benadryl; H$_1$ blocker) may be given to inhibit further histamine release; ranitidine (H$_2$ blocker) may be given at the same time	25–50 mg IV with 50 mg of ranitidine IV	Antihistamine	Inhibits histamine release and relieves skin symptoms but has no immediate effect on the systemic reaction; combination of H$_1$ and H$_2$ blockers together have been found to be effective

Other Medications: Corticosteroids (methylprednisolone) and aminophylline for swelling and bronchospasm; inhaled beta-adrenergic agonists such as albuterol; severe hypotension can be treated with vasopressor agents such as dopamine. Glucagon may be useful in treating cardiovascular effects for patients taking beta blockers.

Independent

The most important priority for nurses is to ensure adequacy of the airway, breathing, and circulation. Keep intubation equipment available for immediate use. Insert an oral or nasal airway if the patient is at risk for airway occlusion but has adequate breathing. Use an oral airway for unresponsive patients and a nasal airway for patients who are responsive. If endotracheal intubation is necessary, secure the tube firmly and suction the patient as needed to maintain the airway. If the patient has a compromised circulation that does not respond to pharmacologic intervention, begin cardiopulmonary resuscitation with chest compressions.

Teach the patient and family how to prevent future allergic reactions. Explain the nature of the allergy, the signs and symptoms to expect, and measures to perform if the patient is exposed to the allergen. Teach the patient that if shortness of breath, difficulty swallowing, or the formation of the "lump in the throat" occurs, they should go to an emergency department immediately. If the allergen is a medication, make sure the patient and family understand that they must avoid the various sources of the medication in both prescription drugs and over-the-counter preparations for the rest of their lives. Encourage the patient to notify all healthcare providers of the allergy prior to treatment.

Evidence-Based Practice and Health Policy

Turner, P., Campbell, D., Motosue, M., & Campbell, R. (2020). Global trends in anaphylaxis epidemiology and clinical implications. *Journal of Allergy and Clinical Immunology: In Practice, 8*, 1169–1176.

- Anaphylaxis is an emergency situation that occurs with an acute systemic allergic reaction that can be fatal. The true global incidence of anaphylaxis is difficult to determine because many times it occurs in community and not hospital settings. In spite of difficulties quantifying the incidence, the authors suggest that a global increase is occurring because of allergies to medication and food. Anaphylaxis accounts for less than 1% of hospital admissions, with most of the Western developed countries with increasing rates and Taiwan with decreasing rates.
- In spite of this increase, mortality rates have not increased. The authors suggest that older age, delayed administration of epinephrine, and keeping a patient in an upright position with a dependent lower body are risk factors for fatal anaphylaxis.

DOCUMENTATION GUIDELINES

- Adequacy of airway: Patency of airway, ease of respirations, chest expansion, respiratory rate, presence of stridor or wheezes
- Skin assessment: Swelling, rash, itching
- Cardiovascular assessment: Changes in vital signs (particularly blood pressure and heart rate), skin color, cardiac rhythm
- Assessment of level of anxiety, degree of understanding, adjustment, and coping skills

DISCHARGE AND HOME HEALTHCARE GUIDELINES

FOLLOW-UP. Provide a complete explanation of all allergic responses and how to avoid future reactions. If the patient has a reaction to a food or medication, instruct the patient and family about the substance itself and all potential sources. If the patient has a food allergy, you may need to include a dietitian in the patient teaching. Encourage the patient to carry an anaphylaxis kit with epinephrine. Teach the patient and family to administer subcutaneous epinephrine in case of emergencies. Encourage the patient to wear an identification bracelet at all times that specifies the allergy.

Angina Pectoris

DRG Category: 287
Mean LOS: 3.0 days
Description: MEDICAL: Circulatory Disorders Except Acute Myocardial Infarction, With Cardiac Catheterization Without Major Complication or Comorbidity
DRG Category: 311
Mean LOS: 2.4 days
Description: MEDICAL: Angina Pectoris

Angina pectoris is a symptom of ischemic heart disease characterized by paroxysmal and usually recurring substernal or precordial chest pain or discomfort. The term comes from the Latin words meaning "choking of the chest." About 10 million Americans experience angina each year, and approximately 500,000 new cases of angina occur every year. Angina pectoris is caused by varying combinations of increased myocardial demand, decreased myocardial perfusion, and reduced oxygen-carrrying capacity of the blood. Blood flow through the coronary arteries is partially or completely obstructed because of coronary artery spasm, fixed stenosing plaques, disrupted plaques, thrombosis, platelet aggregation, and/or embolization. Pain or discomfort results from chemical and mechanical stimulation of nerve endings in the coronary circulation and heart muscle as myocardial cells switch from aerobic to anaerobic metabolism.

Angina can be classified as chronic exertional (stable, typical) angina, variant angina (Prinzmetal), unstable or crescendo angina, or silent ischemia (Table 1). Chronic exertional angina is usually caused by obstructive coronary artery disease that causes the heart to be vulnerable to further ischemia whenever there is increased demand or workload. Variant angina may occur in people with normal coronary arteries who have cyclically recurring angina at rest, unrelated to effort. Unstable angina is diagnosed in patients who report a changing character, duration, and intensity of their pain. Experts are also recognizing that not all ischemic events are perceived by patients, even though such events, called silent ischemia, may have adverse implications for the patient.

• TABLE 1 Classification of Angina Pectoris

TYPE	CAUSE	DESCRIPTION	DURATION	CESSATION
Stable (typical)	Reduction of coronary perfusion by chronic stenosing coronary atherosclerosis; relieved by rest; related to activities that increase myocardial demand	Chest discomfort is produced by exertion; pain may occur after meals or be brought on by emotional tension or exertion; reproducible pattern of symptoms	3–15 min	Relieved by rest and/or nitroglycerin (NTG)

• TABLE 1 Classification of Angina Pectoris (continued)

TYPE	CAUSE	DESCRIPTION	DURATION	CESSATION
Prinzmetal variant angina	Coronary artery spasm without increased myocardial oxygen demand; coronary arteries are normal with angiogram	Occurs at rest, often during sleep in early morning hours or with exertion; associated with elevation of the ST segment of the electrocardiogram, which indicates transmural ischemia	Tends to last longer than other forms of angina	May subside with exercise
Unstable angina	Disruption of an atherosclerotic plaque or vasospasm or both; myocardial ischemia without detectable biomarkers of myocardial necrosis	Pattern of pain with progressively increasing frequency and precipitated with progressively less effort; may occur at rest	Prolonged duration longer than that of stable angina	May not be relieved by NTG or rest; 10%–20% of untreated patients may progress to myocardial infarction (MI)
Microvascular angina or cardiac syndrome X	Normal (or near normal) coronary arteries and without a known cause; may be due to inadequate flow reserve in the microvascular circulation of the heart	Chest pain, chest heaviness, squeezing chest pressure, triggered by exertion, travels to back, neck, jaw, shoulder, arm	Lasts longer than 10 min	Usually relieved with rest and/or nitrates
Silent ischemia	Exact mechanism is unknown, but possible explanations include autonomic dysfunction, high threshold, and production of excessive quantities of endorphins	Angina without pain; as many as 90% of attacks of angina may be silent; most happen in the early morning hours; may result in problems with contractility	Transient ST depression persisting for at least 1 min	Usually unrecognized by patients

CAUSES

Most recurrent angina pectoris is caused by atherosclerosis, which is the most common cause of coronary artery disease (CAD) and continues to be the leading cause of death for both women and men in the United States. Atherosclerotic lesions lead to decreased myocardial blood supply. However, angina may occur in patients with normal coronary arteries as well. Approximately 90% of patients with recurrent angina pectoris have hemodynamically significant stenosis or occlusion of a major coronary artery. Other causes include severe myocardial hypertrophy, severe aortic stenosis or regurgitation, cardiac dysrhythmias, increased metabolic demand, marked anemia, or inadequate flow reserve in the microcirculation. Risk factors include tobacco use, diabetes mellitus, hypertension, sedentary lifestyle, alcohol abuse, obesity, elevated cholesterol, older age, and stress.

GENETIC CONSIDERATIONS

Combination of genetics and environment appear to account for the vast majority of cases of coronary heart disease (CHD) and angina. First-degree relatives of patients with CHD are at higher risk of developing the disease and developing it earlier than the general population. Over 250 genes have been implicated in the onset of CHD, making it a prime example of the combination of multiple genes and environment seen in complex disease. Defects in genes involved with low-density lipoprotein (LDL) metabolism, homocysteine metabolism, muscle development, and blood pressure regulation have been associated with CAD development. Other associated genes include the apolipoprotein A1 gene, apolipoprotein E4 gene, and glycoprotein IIb/IIIa gene. Familial hypercholesterolemia (FH) is caused by a defective LDL receptor, and this mutation is inherited in an autosomal dominant pattern. In individuals affected by FH, they may have elevated LDL levels, up to double the normal range, which may be seen as early as 2 years of age. Often, signs of CHD can be found by the age of 30 years.

SEX AND LIFE SPAN CONSIDERATIONS

The risk of ischemic heart disease increases with age and when predispositions to atherosclerosis (smoking, hypertension, diabetes mellitus, hyperlipoproteinemia) are present. Nearly 10% of MIs occur in people under age 40 years, however, and 45% occur in people under age 65 years. The incidence of new and recurrent angina increases with age until 85 years, when it declines. Men are at greater risk than women for MI, but the differential progressively declines with advancing age. In people 40 to 74 years old, the age-adjusted prevalence of angina is higher among women than men. In addition, atypical presentations of angina are also more common among women than men. Recent research has been conducted about pain and ischemia in people with no obstructed coronary arteries during angiogram. The findings indicate that this group is predominantly women with vasomotor disorders or coronary microvascular dysfunction. Unique risk factors for women include pregnancy-related disorders, autoimmune dysfunction, chronic inflammation, and psychological risk factors.

HEALTH DISPARITIES AND SEXUAL/GENDER MINORITY HEALTH

The Centers for Disease Control and Prevention reports that 11.5% of White persons, 9.5% of Black persons, 7.4% of Hispanic persons, and 6.0% of Asian persons have heart disease. In people between the ages of 55 and 64 years, new episodes of angina occur in 11.2% of non-Black and 19.3% of Black women and in 11.9% of non-Black and 10.6% of Black men. Prior to age 64 years, the highest prevalence of new angina is in Black women. Significant health disparities exist in the cardiac care of underrepresented groups as compared to White persons. Black, Indigenous, or other people of color are known to receive care less often guided by standard cardiac care guidelines than White persons. Unless patients have health insurance, White patients are more likely to receive coronary angiograms and other coronary interventions than Black and Hispanic patients. Black, Indigenous, or other people of color are also less likely to be referred to cardiologists and cardiac surgeons than White persons (Batchelor et al., 2019).

Transgender is a term used to describe persons whose gender identity is different from their sex assigned at birth. Approximately 1% of the U.S. population identify themselves as transgender. Sexual and gender minority persons have higher odds for multiple chronic conditions, cancer, and poor quality of life, and are more apt to have disabilities than cisgender males and females (cisgender are persons whose gender identity and gender expression are aligned with their assigned sex listed on their birth certificate). Gender-affirming hormone therapy is the use of hormone therapy for gender transition or gender affirmation and can be masculinizing or feminizing. It may also affect cardiovascular health in transgender women. In a large sample, researchers have found that transgender men and women are more likely to be overweight than cisgender women. Compared to cisgender women, transgender women reported higher rates of diabetes, ischemic stroke, angina/coronary disease, and MI. Gender-nonconforming men and women reported higher odds of MI than cisgender women. Transgender women also had higher rates of any cardiovascular disease than cisgender men (Caceres, Jackman, et al., 2020; Connelly et al., 2019). While large-scale studies are not available, these factors may place some sexual and gender minority persons at risk for angina pectoris.

GLOBAL HEALTH CONSIDERATIONS

Heart disease remains the leading cause of death in developed countries but is now also the leading cause of death in low-income countries (India, Pakistan) and middle-income countries (Mexico, Russia). Eastern European countries have among the highest prevalence of heart disease in the world. The reasons for the increase in cardiovascular disease deaths in developing countries are complex but related to improvements in infectious disease management, urbanization with the accompanying lifestyle changes that predispose people to heart disease, and genetic susceptibility of some populations.

ASSESSMENT

HISTORY. Ask the patient to describe past chest discomfort in terms of quality (aching, sharp, tingling, knifelike, choking, squeezing), location and radiation, precipitating factors (activity), duration, alleviating factors (relieved by rest), and associated signs and symptoms during the attack (dyspnea, anxiety, diaphoresis, nausea). Obtain information regarding medications, family history, and modifiable risk factors such as eating habits, lifestyle, and physical activity. If chest discomfort is present at the time of the interview, delay collection of historical data until you implement appropriate interventions for ischemic chest pain and the patient is pain free.

The Canadian Cardiovascular Society grading scale is used to classify the severity of angina: class 0, mild myocardial ischemia with no symptoms; class I, angina only during strenuous or prolonged physical activity (climbing stairs); class II, slight limitation, with angina only when activities are performed rapidly or during vigorous physical activity; class III, symptoms with everyday living activities such as walking one or two blocks; class IV, inability to perform any activity without angina or angina at rest.

PHYSICAL EXAMINATION. During anginal attacks, **chest discomfort** is often described as an ache rather than an actual pain and may be characterized as a **chest heaviness, pressure**, or **tightness**; a squeezing sensation; or indigestion. The discomfort is typically located in the substernal region or across the anterior upper chest. Often, the area of pain is the size of a clenched fist, and the patient may place their fist over the area of discomfort (Levine sign). The sensation may radiate to the neck, jaw, or tongue; to either arm, elbow, wrist, or hand; or to the upper abdomen. Anginal discomfort is typically of short duration, usually 3 to 5 minutes, but can last up to 30 minutes or longer. The discomfort may have been brought on by physical or emotional stress, exposure to extreme temperatures, or eating a heavy meal. Termination of the precipitating factor may bring about alleviation of the discomfort. Frequently, the patient is **anxious, pale, diaphoretic, lightheaded, dyspneic, tachycardic,** and **nauseated**. Upon auscultation, the patient may have atrial or ventricular gallops (S_3, S_4).

PSYCHOSOCIAL. Patients often rationalize that their symptoms are the result of indigestion or overexertion. Denial can interfere with identification of a symptom and be harmful to the patient. Chest pain and all the surrounding implications can be extremely stressful and anxiety producing to the patient and family.

Diagnostic Highlights

Diagnostic data are not collected to diagnose and confirm angina pectoris (a symptom) but rather to diagnose the underlying cause of angina pectoris. Most of the testing is done to determine any damage that may have occurred during an acute anginal episode, such as an MI.

Test	Normal Result	Abnormality With Condition	Explanation
Electrocardiogram (ECG)	Normal PQRST pattern (50% of patients with angina pectoris have normal resting ECGs)	ST segment depression, T-wave inversion; may have transient ST elevation (less frequent)	Assesses the electrical conduction system, which is adversely affected by myocardiac ischemia
Graded Exercise Stress Test	Heart rate reaches 80%–90% of maximal heart rate (target heart, generally 150–200 beats/min for adults or 220 beats/min – age in years) without chest or dysrhythmias other than tachycardia	Pain, hypotension, severe shortness of breath, or cardiac dysrhythmias during exercise	Noninvasive test that assesses cardiac performance related to increased workload
Creatine kinase isoenzyme (MB-CK)	0%–4% to total CK	Elevated in some patients with unstable angina	One-third of patients with unstable angina may have elevations due to tissue damage
Troponin I	< 0.05 ng/mL	Elevated in MI	Differentiates between angina and MI; begins to rise 2–6 hr after MI, peaks 15–24 hr after MI
Troponin T	< 0.1 ng/mL	Elevated in MI	Differentiates between angina and MI; begins to rise 2–6 hr after MI

Other Tests: Chest x-ray is usually normal but may show cardiomegaly or other conditions; stress echocardiography; myocardial perfusion scintigraphy tests (thallium T1 201, technetium-99m sestamibi); cholesterol (total, LDL, high-density lipoprotein); cardiac catheterization (coronary angiography); computed tomography of the chest; blood glucose (see Evidence-Based Practice).

PRIMARY NURSING DIAGNOSIS

DIAGNOSIS. Acute or chronic pain related to narrowing of the coronary artery(ies) and associated with atherosclerosis, spasm, or thrombosis as evidenced by self-reported pain, chest pressure, shortness of breath, and/or tachycardia

OUTCOMES. Cardiac pump effectiveness; Circulation status; Knowledge: Cardiac disease management; Comfort status; Pain control; Pain level; Tissue perfusion: Cardiac; Smoking cessation behavior

INTERVENTIONS. Cardiac care: Acute; Oxygen therapy; Pain management: Acute and chronic; Medication administration; Positioning; Risk identification; Smoking cessation assistance

 PLANNING AND IMPLEMENTATION

Collaborative

For any patient who is experiencing an acute anginal episode, pain management is the priority not only for patient comfort but also to decrease myocardial oxygen consumption. The physician orders selected therapies that either decrease myocardial oxygen demand or increase coronary blood and oxygen supply. These therapies may include medications for pain relief; short-term bedrest; oxygen therapy; cardiac monitoring to prevent potential complications; and small, frequent, easily digested meals. Surgical and other invasive options are discussed under **Coronary Heart Disease**, p. 315.

DIET. A collaborative effort among the patient, dietitian, physician, and nurse plans for a diet low in cholesterol, fat, calories, and sodium. Drinks in the coronary care unit or step-down unit are usually decaffeinated and not too hot or cold.

VITAL SIGNS. During unstable periods, the nurse and physician closely monitor the patient's vital signs and the patient's response to pain-relieving therapies (narcotics, nitrates). Often the patient is placed on a cardiac monitor to determine if life-threatening dysrhythmias occur during an anginal episode, particularly if the angina may be a symptom that the patient is having an MI.

Pharmacologic Highlights

Medication or Drug Class	Dosage	Description	Rationale
Nitroglycerin	0.3–0.6 mg prn SL for stable angina; IV for unstable angina—IV dose varies	Nitrate	Relieves ischemic symptoms by vasodilation of coronary arteries; reduces left ventricular preload and afterload
Antiplatelet agents such as enteric-coated aspirin or clopidogrel	Varies by drug	NSAID and antiplatelet agent	Inhibits platelet aggregation to reduce risk of coronary artery blockage
Ranolazine	500–1,000 mg BID	Antianginal, anti-ischemic agent	Used to treat chronic angina; alters the transcellular late sodium current and indirectly prevents calcium overload
Beta-adrenergic antagonists (atenolol, propranolol, metoprolol, etc.)	Varies by drug	Beta-adrenergic antagonists	Reduce myocardial oxygen demands by decreasing heart rate, blood pressure, and contractility

(highlight box continues on page 102)

Pharmacologic Highlights (continued)

Other Therapies: Goal-directed therapy usually includes beta-adrenergic antagonists, antiplatelet agents, and HMG-CoA reductase inhibitors (statins such as atorvastatin or rosuvastatin). There are numerous drugs to decrease myocardial oxygen consumption: IV NTG by infusion, long-acting nitrates, narcotics for pain control, calcium channel–blocking agents, vasodilators, diuretics, antihypertensive agents, and anticoagulants.

Independent

To decrease oxygen demand, encourage the patient to maintain bedrest until the pain subsides, even though bedrest is usually short term. Encourage rest throughout the entire hospitalization or emergency department visit.

Because anxiety and fear are common among both patients and families, attempt to have them discuss concerns and express their feelings. With the patient and family, discuss the diagnosis, the activity and diet restrictions, and the medical treatment. Refer the patient to a smoking-cessation program or alcohol counseling if appropriate. Numerous lifestyle changes may be needed. Cardiac rehabilitation is helpful in limiting risk factors and providing additional guidance, social support, and encouragement. Adequate education and support are essential if the patient is to adhere to the prescribed therapy and treatment plan.

Evidence-Based Practice and Health Policy

Aggarwal, R., Chiu, N., Pankayatselvan, V., Shen, C., & Yeh, R. (2020). Prevalence of angina and use of medical therapy among U.S. adults: A nationally representative estimate. *American Heart Journal, 228*, 44–46.

* The authors sought to determine the prevalence of angina in the United States and to determine the use of first-line therapy by patients with angina. They used individual patient data from the National Health and Nutrition Examination Survey from 2007 to 2016.
* Of patients with angina, 61.7% were taking beta blockers, 66.8% were on statins, and 54.4% were taking antiplatelet agents. An overall proportion of 32.6% was taking all three first-line medications. The authors encouraged strategies to improve the use of these three medications for patients with angina.

DOCUMENTATION GUIDELINES

* Description of pain: Onset (sudden, gradual), character (aching, sharp, burning, pressure), precipitating factors, associated symptoms (anxiety, dyspnea, diaphoresis, dizziness, nausea, cyanosis, pallor), duration, and alleviating factors of the anginal episode
* Response to prescribed medications
* Reaction to bedrest or limitation in activity

DISCHARGE AND HOME HEALTHCARE GUIDELINES

PREVENTION. Teach the patient factors that may precipitate anginal episodes and the appropriate measures to control episodes. Teach the patient the modifiable cardiovascular risk factors and ways to reduce them. Manage risk factors, including cigarette smoking, alcohol misuse and abuse, hypertension, diabetes mellitus, obesity, and hyperlipidemia.

ACTIVITY. Each person has a different level of activity that will aggravate anginal symptoms. Most patients with stable angina can avoid symptoms during daily activities by reducing the speed of any activity.

MEDICATIONS. Be sure the patient understands all medications, including the dose, route, action, and adverse effects. If the patient's physician prescribes sublingual NTG, instruct the patient to lie in the semi-Fowler position and take up to three tablets 5 minutes apart to relieve chest discomfort. Instruct the patient that if relief is not obtained after ingestion of the three tablets, they should seek medical attention immediately. Remind the patient to check the expiration date on the NTG tablets and to replace the bottle, once it is opened, every 3 to 5 months.

COMPLICATIONS. Teach the patient the importance of not denying or ignoring anginal episodes and of reporting them to the healthcare provider immediately.

Anorectal Abscess and Fistula

DRG Category:	348
Mean LOS:	4.4 days
Description:	SURGICAL: Anal and Stomal Procedures With Complication or Comorbidity
DRG Category:	394
Mean LOS:	3.8 days
Description:	MEDICAL: Other Digestive System Diagnoses With Complication or Comorbidity

An anorectal abscess, sometimes called a *perirectal abscess*, is the formation of pus in the soft tissue that surrounds the anal canal or lower rectum and often arises from the cryptoglandular epithelial lining of the anus. Perianal abscess is the most common form, affecting four out of five patients; ischiorectal (abscess in the ischiorectal fossa in the fatty tissue on either side of the rectum) and submucosal or high intermuscular abscesses account for most of the remaining cases of anorectal abscess. A rare form of anorectal abscess is called pelvirectal abscess, which extends deeply into pelvic regions from the rectum. In approximately half of the cases, fistulas (connection between anal canal and perianal skin) develop without any way to predict them.

Generally, the internal anal sphincter is a protective barrier to infection, preventing bacteria from passing from the gut lumen into the cryptoglandular epithelium that lines the anal canal. When this barrier is interrupted, infection reaches the intersphincteric space, and then moves into the perirectal spaces. Lesions that can lead to anorectal abscesses and fistulas can be caused by infections of the anal fissure; infections through the anal gland; ruptured anal hematoma; prolapsed thrombosed internal hemorrhoids; and septic lesions in the pelvis, such as acute salpingitis, acute appendicitis, and diverticulitis. Anorectal abscesses can lead to anal fistulas, also known as *fistula in ano*. An anal fistula is the development of an abnormal tract or opening between the anal canal and the skin outside the anus. It should not be confused with an anal fissure, which is an elongated ulcer located just inside the anal orifice, caused by the traumatic passage of large, hard stools. Complications include fibrosis, stricture formation, incontinence, sepsis, and septic shock.

CAUSES

Ulcerative colitis and Crohn disease are systemic illnesses that can cause abscesses, and people who are immunosuppressed are more susceptible to abscesses. Patients who are at high risk are people with diabetes, those who engage in receptive anal sex, those who use cathartics habitually, and those with inflammatory bowel disease and immunosuppression.

Other causes include constipation, chronic diarrhea, syphilis, tuberculosis, radiation exposure, and HIV infection.

GENETIC CONSIDERATIONS

No clear genetic contributions to susceptibility have been defined.

SEX AND LIFE SPAN CONSIDERATIONS

The peak incidence occurs in people 20 to 30 years of age, and older adults are also prone to the condition because of their increased incidence of constipation, hemorrhoids, and diabetes mellitus. An anorectal fistula is a rare diagnosis in children, but anorectal abscesses can occur in infants and toddlers, particularly those still in diapers. Anal fistulas are complications of anorectal abscesses, which are more common in men than in women. For anatomical reasons, rectovaginal fistulas are found only in women (see section on Health Disparities and Sexual/Gender Minority Health below).

HEALTH DISPARITIES AND SEXUAL/GENDER MINORITY HEALTH

Transgender is a term used to describe persons whose gender identity is different from their sex assigned at birth. Approximately 1% of the U.S. population identify themselves as transgender. Cisgender is a term used for persons whose gender identity and gender expression are aligned with their assigned sex listed on their birth certificate (Caceres, Jackman, et al., 2020). People who engage in receptive anal sex, both cisgender and transgender individuals, have a higher risk than other groups for anorectal abscesses and fistulas. Transgender men may develop rectovaginal fistulas. Ethnicity and race have no known effect on the risk for anal abscess and fistula.

GLOBAL HEALTH CONSIDERATIONS

No data are available.

ASSESSMENT

HISTORY. Ask the patient to describe the kind of **pain** and the precise location. Determine if the pain is exacerbated by sitting or coughing. Ask if the patient has experienced **rectal itching** or pain with sitting, coughing, or defecating. Elicit a history of signs of infection such as **fever, chills**, nausea, vomiting, malaise, or **myalgia**. Ask the patient if they have experienced constipation, which is a common symptom because of the patient's attempts to avoid pain by preventing defecation.

PHYSICAL EXAMINATION. Inspect the patient's anal region. Note any red or oval swelling close to the anus. Digital examination may reveal a tender induration that bulges into the anal canal in the case of ischiorectal abscess or a smooth swelling of the upper part of the anal canal or lower rectum in the case of submucous or high intermuscular abscess. Digital examination may reveal a tender mass high in the pelvis, even extending into one of the ischiorectal fossae if the patient has a pelvirectal abscess. Examination of a perianal abscess generally reveals no abnormalities. Examination may not be possible without anesthesia. Note any pruritic drainage or perianal irritation, which are signs of a fistula.

On inspection, the external opening of the fistula is usually visible as a red elevation of granulation tissue with purulent or serosanguinous drainage on compression. Palpate the tract, noting whether there is a hardened cordlike structure. Note that superficial perianal abscesses are not uncommon in infants and toddlers who are still in diapers. The abscess appears as a swollen, red, tender mass at the edge of the anus. Infants are often fussy but may have no other symptoms.

PSYCHOSOCIAL. Patients with perirectal abscesses and fistulas may delay seeking treatment because of embarrassment relating to the location, the odor, or the sight of the lesion. Provide privacy and foster dignity when interacting with these patients. Inform the patient of every step of the procedure. Provide comfort during the examination.

Diagnostic Highlights

Test	Normal Result	Abnormality With Condition	Explanation
White blood cell (WBC) count	Adult males and females 4,500–11,100/mL	Elevated	Infection and inflammation may elevate the WBC count; approximately 25% of people with anorectal abscesses and fistulas have normal WBC counts

Other Tests: Endoscopy (sigmoidoscopy or colonoscopy), ultrasound, computed tomography, magnetic resonance imaging, cultures of exudate

PRIMARY NURSING DIAGNOSIS

DIAGNOSIS. Acute pain related to inflammation of the perirectal area as evidenced by self-reported pain, rectal itching, fever, and/or muscle achiness

OUTCOMES. Comfort status; Pain control; Pain level; Tissue integrity: Skin & mucous membranes; Wound healing: Primary intention

INTERVENTIONS. Pain management: Acute; Medication administration; Positioning; Teaching: Prescribed medication

PLANNING AND IMPLEMENTATION

Collaborative

For anal fissures, use the WASH regimen: Warm-water shower or sitz bath after bowel movement, Analgesics, Stool softeners, High-fiber diet. Note that most uncomplicated fissures resolve in 2 to 4 weeks with supportive care, but chronic fissures may require surgical treatment. Some anal fissures are treated with a topical gel that acts as a glue.

SURGICAL. The abscess is incised and drained surgically. For patients with fistulas, fistulotomies are performed to destroy the internal opening (infective source) and establish adequate drainage. The wound is then allowed to heal by secondary intention. Frequently, this procedure requires incision of sphincter fibers. Fistulectomy may be necessary, which involves the excision of the entire fistulous tract. Some surgeons perform a complementary colostomy to manage complex fistulas.

POSTOPERATIVE. Encourage the patient to urinate but avoid catheterization and the use of suppositories. Postoperatively, a bulk laxative or stool softener is often prescribed on the day of the surgery. Intramuscular injections of analgesics are given to control pain. Assess the perirectal area hourly for bleeding for the first 12 to 24 hours postoperatively. When open fistula wounds are left, as in a fistulotomy, the anal canal may be packed lightly with oxidized cellulose.

Encourage the patient to drink clear liquids after any nausea has passed. Once clear liquids have been taken without nausea or vomiting, remove the IV fluids and encourage the patient to begin to drink a full liquid diet the day after surgery. From there, the patient can progress to a regular diet by the third day after surgery. The most common complications are incontinence (if sphincter fibers were incised during surgery) and hemorrhage.

Pharmacologic Highlights

Medication or Drug Class	Dosage	Description	Rationale
Antibiotics	Varies by drug	Antibiotics to cover gastrointestinal infections: ampicillin plus aminoglycosides plus either clindamycin or metronidazole; cefazolin, cefoxitin, or cefotetan alone; aminoglycoside and cefoxitin	Routine use of antibiotics has not been shown to shorten healing time but may be needed in cases of sepsis, cellulitis, diabetes, or immunosuppression. Provide antimicrobials directed against bowel flora, particularly in people who are immunosuppressed.

Independent

POSTOPERATIVE. Immediately following the procedure and before the patient enters the postanesthesia care unit, place a dry, sterile dressing on the surgical site. Provide sitz baths twice a day for comfort and cleanliness, and place a plastic inflatable doughnut on a chair or bed to ease the pain of sitting. As soon as the patient tolerates activity, encourage ambulation to limit postoperative complications.

PATIENT TEACHING. Teach the patient how to keep the perianal area clean; teach the female patient to wipe the perianal area from front to back after a bowel movement in order to prevent genitourinary infection. Teach the patient about the need for a high-fiber diet that helps prevent hard stools and constipation. Explain how constipation can lead to straining that increases pressure at the incision site. Unless the patient is on fluid restriction, encourage them to drink at least 3 L of fluid a day.

Evidence-Based Practice and Health Policy

He, Z., Du, J., Wu, K., Chen, J., Wu, B., Yang, J., Xu, Z., Fu, Z., Pan, L., Wen, K., & Wang, X. (2020). Formation rate of secondary anal fistula after incision and drainage of perianal sepsis and analysis of risk factors. *BMC Surgery, 20*, 1–7.

- The authors observed the formation probability of secondary anal fistula after incision and drainage in patients with perianal sepsis. They also determined factors that contributed to secondary anal fistula formation. They performed a retrospective descriptive analysis of 288 patients with perianal sepsis who were treated with anorectal surgery and followed them for a year after surgery.
- Of the 187 patients who met final inclusion criteria, anal fistula was present in 105 patients, and the rate of formation of secondary anal fistulas was 56%. There was no significant correlation between the location of sepsis and the type of secondary anal fistulas.

DOCUMENTATION GUIDELINES

- Physical findings of perirectal area: Drainage, edema, redness, tenderness
- Response to comfort measures: Sitz baths, inflatable doughnuts, analgesia
- Reaction to ambulation postoperatively
- Presence of surgical complications: Poor wound healing, bleeding, foul wound drainage, fever, unrelieved pain
- Output (stool): Appearance, consistency, odor, amount, color, frequency

DISCHARGE AND HOME HEALTHCARE GUIDELINES

PATIENT TEACHING. Teach female patients to wipe from front to back to avoid the contamination of the vagina or urethra with drainage from the perirectal area. Teach the patient to avoid using bar soap directly on the anus because it can cause irritation to the anal tissue. Teach patients to dilute the soap with water on a washcloth to cleanse the area.

DIET. Explain the need to remain on a diet that will not cause physical trauma or irritation to the perirectal area. A diet high in fiber and fluids will help soften the stools, and bulk laxatives can help prevent straining. Emphasize to the patient the need to avoid spicy foods and hot peppers to decrease irritation to the perirectal area upon defecation.

MEDICATION. Teach the patient the purpose, dosage, schedule, precautions, and potential side effects, interactions, and adverse reactions of all prescribed medications. Encourage the patient to complete the entire prescription of antibiotics that are prescribed.

Anorexia Nervosa

DRG Category:	883
Mean LOS:	8.2 days
Description:	MEDICAL: Disorders of Personality and Impulse Control

Anorexia nervosa (AN) is an eating disorder that is complex and potentially life-threatening. It is an illness of starvation brought on by a severe disturbance of body image and a morbid fear of obesity. The lifetime prevalence for an episode of AN is 2.4% to 4.3%, and tragically, about 5% of those affected die. The mortality rates are significantly higher in the presence of comorbid cluster B personality disorders or substance use disorders. AN has three primary diagnostic criteria: restricted energy intake relative to requirements leading to significantly low body weight (less than minimally expected); intense fear of gaining weight despite weight loss or persistent behavior to prevent weight gain; and a distorted body image or persistent lack of recognition of the seriousness of low body weight.

Weight is accomplished by three different methods: restricting food intake, excessive exercise, or purging either with laxatives or by vomiting. Strategies for weight loss help to define two subtypes of AN. The restricting type is manifested by severe limitation of food. The binge/purging type is manifested by periods of eating followed by self-induced vomiting, laxative or diuretic abuse, and/or excessive exercise. Initially, individuals may receive attention and praise for their extreme self-control over food intake, but as the illness progresses, this attention is replaced by worry and efforts to monitor the patient's food intake. The increased negative attention and attempts to control the patient's food intake often become a source of conflict and a power struggle, typically between parents and their affected child. Adverse consequences of AN include possible atrophy of the cardiac muscle and cardiac dysrhythmias, alteration in thyroid metabolism, and estrogen deficiencies (those with long-standing estrogen deficiencies may develop osteoporosis). Refeeding may lead to slowed peristalsis, constipation, bloating, and fluid retention. Aggressive refeeding increases the risk for electrolyte imbalances including hypophosphatemia, hypocalcemia, hypokalemia, and hypomagnesemia. For many individuals, AN is a chronic or terminal condition. In recent, large follow-up studies, only about 50% of people with AN recovered within 9 years.

CAUSES

The causes of AN are not well understood but are probably a combination of biological, psychological, and social factors. Abnormalities in central neurotransmitter activity are suggested by an alteration in serotonin metabolism. Psychological factors are the most frequently offered explanations. Onset usually occurs during early adolescence, a time when emerging sexuality, individuality, and separation from the family become central issues for the individual. Another theory posits that AN occurs at the time of puberty as a person's way of avoiding adult responsibility and body image. There is insufficient evidence to support the idea that parents of children with eating disorders are over-controlling or rigid and therefore causing pathology in their children. The Academy for Eating Disorders advanced a position statement in 2010 standing firmly against any model suggesting that family influences are the primary cause of eating disorders.

GENETIC CONSIDERATIONS

AN appears to have a complex inheritance pattern, combining mutations in susceptibility genes (several loci have been proposed) and environmental factors. Heritability is estimated between 50% and 70%, while first-degree relatives of individuals with AN have about 12 times the risk of developing AN. Association studies have been performed on over 43 genes, with consistent associations for susceptibility found for agouti-related peptide (*AGRP*), brain-derived neurotropic factor (*BDNF*), catechol-O-methyl transferase (*COMT*), *SK3*, serotonin 5-hydroxytryptamine receptor 2A (*HTR2A*), and opioid receptor delta 1 (*OPRD1*).

SEX AND LIFE SPAN CONSIDERATIONS

AN most often occurs in adolescent females between the ages of 12 and 18 years, usually before the onset of puberty. Onset that occurs prior to age 11 years is associated with a poor prognosis. In the United States, the lifetime prevalence of AN is 1.4% to 1% in females and 0.2% in males. In professions such as ballet and modeling and sports such as running and wrestling, the frequency is much higher for females and males than among the general population. Male athletes with eating disorders may be more difficult to identify and diagnose than females for a variety of reasons associated with differential presentation of symptoms, secretiveness or shame, and sex-related stigma.

HEALTH DISPARITIES AND SEXUAL/GENDER MINORITY HEALTH

AN is most often diagnosed in the White, adolescent population, although it is found in all populations. Experts have found that, when adjusting for income, rates of AN were lower for Black and Hispanic persons as compared to White persons but suggest that it may be underdiagnosed in Black and Hispanic persons because of a low index of suspicion by health providers. Sexual and gender minority persons are disproportionately affected by eating disorders, including AN. Perceived discrimination among sexual and gender minority persons has a significant association with AD. Theories about this association suggest that the occurrence of eating disorders may be associated with being a member of a marginalized and stigmatized group. Experiences with minority stress and stigma may lead to AN as an attempt to regain a sense of control or be related to maladaptive coping as a way to manage emotional distress (Kamody et al., 2019).

GLOBAL HEALTH CONSIDERATIONS

Globally, rates of AN have been on the rise since the 1950s, specifically with increases in developed countries in the West. Estimates are that over 3.3 million healthy life years worldwide are lost due to eating disorders. AN is uncommon in most developing countries.

❊ ASSESSMENT

HISTORY. The patient typically claims to feel well and appears unconcerned about their weight loss. Obtain a diet and weight history. Assess the patient for both gradual and abrupt weight loss, and compare the values with normals for the patient's age and height. Assess the current food intake; develop a diet history; elicit a description of exercise patterns; and assess for the amount and frequency of bingeing, purging, and laxative and diuretic use. Associated symptoms may include reports of cold intolerance, dizziness, chest pain, abdominal bloating, pain, discomfort, constipation, weakness, decreased concentration, and poor memory. Patients with AN should be assessed for infectious diseases since they may have an immune disturbance and a delayed febrile response.

Assess the patient's perception of their body image. Although patients appear emaciated, they view themselves as fat. Hunger is not a complaint. Unlike other starving individuals, people who are anorexic are not fatigued until malnutrition is severe. Most are restless and active, and some exercise excessively. Assess how the patient views food to determine the intensity of the fear of weight gain and the patient's preoccupation with restricting food. Obtain a history of menses in females because usually the patient has a history of amenorrhea or a delayed onset of menses.

PHYSICAL EXAMINATION. On examination, patients appear **extremely thin**—if not emaciated—but animated. Obtain their weight, for which to make a diagnosis should be less than that minimally expected for their age and height. Vital signs often reveal bradycardia, postural hypotension, and hypothermia. The patient's skin may appear dry, pale, and yellow-tinged, and the face and arms may be covered by a fine, downy hair (lanugo). The nails are generally brittle, and there is a loss of or thinning of hair. There is usually delayed sexual maturation. Breasts may be atrophied or poorly developed. Amenorrhea may precede or accompany the weight loss. Bowel sounds may be hypoactive.

PSYCHOSOCIAL. Patients with AN may display traits such as high desire for academic achievement and perfection and lack of age-appropriate sexual behaviors. They may seem developmentally immature and excessively dependent, and they may be socially isolated. Anxiety and depression are common cormorbidities. Some individuals may have symptoms of obsessive-compulsive disorder. Psychosocial assessment should include assessment of self-esteem, peer relationships, changes in school performance, involvement in sports, perception of self as a sexual being, fear of sexual maturity, and perception of body image. Because patients with AN are preoccupied with food, they often isolate themselves from peers and friends. When assessing body image, it is helpful to have the female patient take a female body outline and color in those areas that are pleasing and those that are displeasing.

Assess family communication patterns to determine how decision making and conflict are handled, and how parents view the current problem. Assess recent family crises and recent counseling experiences.

Diagnostic Highlights

General Comments: The diagnosis of AN is made clinically. No laboratory test is able to diagnose AN, but supporting tests are used to follow the response to treatment and the progression of the illness.

Test	Normal Result	Abnormality With Condition	Explanation
Complete blood count and erythrocyte sedimentation rate (ESR) (normals are for adolescent females)	Red blood cells (RBCs) 3.6–5.8 million/mL; white blood cells 4,500–11,100/mL; hemoglobin (Hgb) 11.5–17.3 g/dL; hematocrit (Hct) 36%–52%; reticulocyte count 0.8%–2.5% of total RBCs; platelets 185,000–335,000/mL; ESR 0– 25 mm/hr	Anemia; RBCs < 4.0; hematocrit < 35%; hemoglobin < 12 g/dL; normal ESR	Caused by protracted undernutrition; ESR is checked to identify other conditions that might cause weight loss
Albumin	3.7–5.6 g/dL	May be normal or hypoalbuminemia; albumin < 3.7 g/dL	Caused by protracted undernutrition

(highlight box continues on page 110)

Diagnostic Highlights (continued)

Other Tests: Serum electrolytes may show hypokalemia, hypochloremia, hypomagnesemia, hypocalcemia, or hypoglycemia. Other laboratory tests include cholesterol (elevated), serum amylase (elevated), luteinizing hormone (decreased), testosterone (decreased), thyroxine (mildly decreased), electrocardiogram, and blood urea nitrogen.

PRIMARY NURSING DIAGNOSIS

DIAGNOSIS. Imbalanced nutrition: less than body requirements related to an intense fear of becoming fat, denial of being (too) thin, and/or excessive exercise as evidenced by profound weight loss

OUTCOMES. Nutritional status: Food and fluid intake; Nutritional status: Nutrient intake; Body image; Weight: Body mass; Knowledge: Weight management; Fluid balance; Electrolyte balance

INTERVENTIONS. Eating disorders management; Nutrition management; Nutritional counseling; Nutritional monitoring; Fluid/electrolyte management; Weight management

PLANNING AND IMPLEMENTATION

Collaborative

AN is a complex biological and social-psychological condition that is difficult to treat. Ideally, early diagnosis and treatment in an outpatient setting is the first-line approach for AN. Family-based therapies such as the Maudsley approach are supported in evidence for adolescents with AN. If malnutrition is critical, the patient may need hospitalization. In the early stages of hospitalization, the patient may need tube feedings or total parenteral nutrition when intake is not sufficient to sustain metabolic needs and to prevent malnutrition or death. Usually, the physician prescribes an initial diet of 1,200 to 1,600 kcal/day. A target weight is usually chosen by the treatment team. Calories are increased slowly to ensure a steady weight gain of 2 to 3 pounds per week. IV fluids may be used for severe dehydration to replace vascular volume and total body water. Transfer to an inpatient psychiatric facility may be needed.

The nurse collaborates with the dietitian to determine appropriate weight gain expectations. As refeeding takes place, the patient is involved in group therapy to talk about their feelings, learn new coping behaviors, decrease social isolation, develop a realistic perception of body image, and learn age-appropriate behaviors. Concurrently, both the individual patient and the family are involved in sessions to educate them on the nature and processes of the disease and the prognosis and treatment plan. Family therapy facilitates learning new ways of handling conflict, solving problems, and supporting the patient's move toward independence.

Pharmacologic Highlights

Medication or Drug Class	Dosage	Description	Rationale
Multivitamins	One capsule per day PO	Combination of water and fat-soluble organic substances needed for good nutrition	Provide for growth, reproduction, and health

Other Therapies: Symptoms may be managed with antacids, acetaminophen, bulk laxatives, and stool softeners. Selective serotonin reuptake inhibitor antidepressants have not demonstrated effectiveness in treating AN but may be used to treat comorbid clinical depression; anxiolytic agents may be used to treat comorbid anxiety. Dietary calcium (1,000–1,500 mg/day) and vitamin D (400 IU) may be recommended to reduce bone loss. In acute situations, electrolyte replacement with calcium gluconate, potassium chloride, or potassium phosphate may be necessary along with IV fluid replenishment.

Independent

The primary goal for the nurse is to establish a therapeutic, nonjudgmental, trusting relationship with the patient. The most important nursing intervention is to facilitate refeeding, thus helping patients meet their weight goal and daily nutritional requirements. If tube feedings are needed, use a consistent and matter-of-fact approach. Be alert to possible disconnecting of the tube or signs of suicidal ideation or behavior.

Once tube feedings and total parenteral nutrition are no longer necessary, create a pleasant environment during meals. Smaller meals and supplemental snacks can be an effective strategy. Having a menu available for choice increases a sense of control for the patient. Maintain a regular weighing schedule. To avoid provoking patients' fear of weight gain, weigh patients with their back to the scale. Weigh the patient in a gown rather than in street clothes for consistency. Monitor the exercise program and set limits on physical activities. Work with the patient to develop strategies to stop vomiting and laxative and diuretic abuse as necessary. Usually, strenuous sports activity is limited to reduce energy expenditure, but the disadvantage of curtailing activity is the removal of the patient's coping mechanism, so an activity program needs to be tailored to the individual.

Work with the family individually or in a group to educate about the disease prognosis and treatment process. Parents are educated in ways to encourage their adolescent without limiting their growth and independence. Identify family interaction patterns and educate them about healthy communication patterns. Communicate a message that it is acceptable for family members to be different from each other and that individuation is an important growth step. Assist parents in learning new ways to handle family and marital conflict. Teaching family negotiation skills is important.

Evidence-Based Practice and Health Policy

Solmi, M., Wade, T., Byrne, S., Del Giovane, C., Fairburn, C., Ostinelli, E., De Crescenzo, F., Johnson, C., Schmidt, U., Treasure, J., Favaro, A., Zipfel, S., & Cipriani, A. (2021). Comparative efficacy and acceptability of psychological interventions for the treatment of adult outpatients with anorexia nervosa: A systematic review and network meta-analysis. *The Lancet Psychiatry, 8*, 215–224.

* The authors performed a systematic review of published literature by using electronic databases to determine pharmacologic and nonpharmacologic treatment of adult patients with AN. The primary outcomes were changes in body mass index or global eating disorder psychopathology. Cognitive behavioral therapy (CBT), Maudsley anorexia treatment for adults, family-based treatment, psychodynamic-oriented psychotherapies, a form of CBT targeting compulsive exercise, and cognitive remediation therapy followed by CBT were compared to treatment as usual.
* All psychological therapies demonstrated modest improvements in clinical course and quality of life. No one therapy demonstrated superiority or inferiority over another, although the all-cause dropout rate was lower for CBT than for psychodynamic-oriented treatment approaches. There is an urgent need to fund new research to develop and improve therapies for adults with AN.

DOCUMENTATION GUIDELINES

* Nutrition: Food and fluid intake for each meal; daily weights
* Response to care and teaching: Understanding of the disease process and need for treatment (patient and family); understanding of ways to identify and cope with anxiety and anger; assessment of own body image
* Family meetings: Family interaction patterns
* Verbalizations of increased self-esteem as indicated by positive self-statements concerning appearance, accomplishments, or interactions with peers and family

DISCHARGE AND HOME HEALTHCARE GUIDELINES

Teach the patient how to maintain adequate nutrition and hydration. Explore non-food-related coping mechanisms and ways to have decreased association between food and emotions. Explore ways to recognize maladaptive coping behaviors and stressors that precipitate anxiety. Teach the patient strategies to increase self-esteem and to maintain a realistic perception of body image. Explore ways to maintain increased independence and age-appropriate behaviors.

Aortic Valve Insufficiency

DRG Category:	307
Mean LOS:	3.1 days
Description:	MEDICAL: Cardiac Congenital and Valvular Disorders Without Major Complication or Comorbidity

Aortic insufficiency (AI), also called aortic regurgitation, is the incomplete closure of the aortic valve leaflets, which allows blood to regurgitate backward from the aorta into the left ventricle. The retrograde blood flow occurs during ventricular diastole when ventricular pressure is low and aortic pressure is high. The backflow of blood into the ventricle decreases forward flow in the aorta and increases left ventricular volume and pressure. In compensation, the left ventricle dilates and hypertrophies to accommodate the increased blood volume. Eventually, the increase in left ventricular pressure is reflected backward into the left atrium and pulmonary circulation. Risk of premature death from AI, as well as complications and the chronic need for medication because of congenital heart disease, is approximately 50%.

Most patients with AI experience left ventricular failure. If heart failure is serious, the patient may develop pulmonary edema. If the patient is overtaxed by an infection, fever, or cardiac dysrhythmia, myocardial ischemia may also occur.

CAUSES

AI may result either from an abnormality of the aortic valve or from dilation and distortion of the aortic root. AI can be congenital or acquired. Congenital abnormalities are associated with ventricular septal defect, bicuspid aortic valve (most common), subvalvular aortic stenosis, dysplasia of valve cusps, or the absence of two or three aortic valve leaflets. Acquired AI results from conditions such as infective endocarditis, trauma, systemic diseases such as rheumatic fever or systemic lupus erythematosus, and connective tissue syndromes. Transcatheter aortic valve replacement can also lead to complications including AI.

Dilation or distortion of the aortic root may be due to longstanding systemic hypertension, aortic dissection, syphilis, Marfan syndrome, and ankylosing spondylitis. Rheumatic heart disease and endocarditis cause the valve cusps to become thickened and retracted, whereas an aortic aneurysm causes dilation of the annulus (the valve ring that attaches to the leaflets). Chronic high blood pressure causes an increased pressure on the aortic valve, which may weaken the cusps. All of these conditions inhibit the valve leaflets from closing tightly, thus allowing backflow of blood from the high-pressure aorta.

GENETIC CONSIDERATIONS

AI can occur as a feature of several genetic diseases, including Marfan syndrome (and other connective tissue diseases), Turner syndrome, and velocardiofacial syndrome. Congenital alterations in the aortic valve structure, such as bicuspid aortic valve, have been shown to be heritable. Mutations in the *NOTCH1* gene can lead to aortic valve calcification, among other congenital aortic valve defects, in an autosomal dominant inheritance pattern.

SEX AND LIFE SPAN CONSIDERATIONS

Symptoms do not usually occur until age 40 to 50 years. AI is more common in males. Experts suggest that more males have AI than females because most of the underlying conditions, such as Marfan syndrome, are more common in men. However, when AI is associated with mitral valve disease, it is more common in women. Mild aortic regurgitation is probably quite common in people older than 80 years but is usually overlooked.

HEALTH DISPARITIES AND SEXUAL/GENDER MINORITY HEALTH

Significant health disparities exist in the cardiac care of Black, Indigenous, and other people of color as compared to White persons. The same is true for uninsured persons compared to people with private health insurance. Black, Indigenous, and other people of color are known to receive care less often guided by standard cardiac care guidelines than White persons and are less likely to be referred to cardiologists and cardiac surgeons (Batchelor et al., 2019). Ethnicity, race, and sexual/gender minority status have no known specific effect on the risk for aortic valve insufficiency.

GLOBAL HEALTH CONSIDERATIONS

More than 15 million people worldwide have rheumatic heart disease (RHD). Indigenous peoples such as native Pacific Islanders and Maori have a higher incidence of RHD than do other groups, as do people who live in developing countries, where up to 60% of all admissions for cardiovascular illnesses are related to the condition. Prevalence may be as low as 1 per 100,000 children in Costa Rica to as high as 150 per 100,000 children in China. Areas of particular concern are Southeastern Asia, Central America, North Africa, and the Middle East.

ASSESSMENT

HISTORY. A history of rheumatic fever suggests possible cardiac valvular malfunction; however, many patients who have had rheumatic fever do not remember having the condition. People with AI often have a period of years in which they are asymptomatic, even with exercise. Over time, the most common symptom of AI is **labored breathing on exertion**, which may be present for many years before progressive symptoms develop. **Angina with exertion**, **orthopnea**, and **paroxysmal nocturnal dyspnea** are also principal complaints. Patients with severe AI often complain of an uncomfortable awareness of their heartbeat (palpitations), especially when lying down.

PHYSICAL EXAMINATION. Inspection of the thoracic wall may reveal a thrusting apical pulsation. Palpation of the precordium reveals the apical pulse to be bounding and displaced to the left. Auscultation of heart sounds reveals the classic decrescendo diastolic murmur. The duration of the murmur correlates with the severity of the regurgitation. Auscultation of breath sounds may reveal fine crackles (rales) if pulmonary congestion is present from left-sided heart failure. The pulmonary congestion will vary with the amount of exertion, the degree of recumbency, and the severity of regurgitation. Assessment of vital signs reveals a widened pulse pressure caused by the low diastolic blood pressure (often close to 40 mm Hg). The heart rate may be elevated in the body's attempt to increase the cardiac output and decrease the diastolic period of backflow. A patient with acute AI may have tachycardia, cyanosis, acute pulmonary edema, and peripheral vasoconstriction.

PSYCHOSOCIAL. The symptoms of AI usually develop gradually. Most people have already made adjustments in their lifestyle to adapt, not seeking treatment until the symptoms become debilitating. Assess what the patient has already done to cope with this condition. Heart surgery is a daunting prospect for patients and families, who will require clear explanations and much psychological support.

Diagnostic Highlights

Test	Normal Result	Abnormality With Condition	Explanation
Cardiac catheterization and aortic angiography	Normal aortic valve	Diastolic regurgitant flow from the aorta into the left ventricle; increased left ventricular end-diastolic volume/pressure	Aortic valve is incompetent, and during diastolic phase, blood flows backward into the left ventricle; provides information about severity of AI
Transthoracic echocardiography	Normal aortic valve	Incompetent aortic valve, thickening and flail of valve structures	Aortic valve is incompetent, and during diastolic phase, blood flows backward into the left ventricle; determines optimal time for surgery based on patient condition

Other Tests: Echocardiography to assess aortic valve's structure and mobility electrocardiogram, chest radiography, magnetic resonance imaging, color-flow Doppler, pulse-flow Doppler, continuous-flow Doppler, computed tomography, complete blood count, coagulation profile, blood chemistries, and type and crossmatch for blood before and after surgery.

PRIMARY NURSING DIAGNOSIS

DIAGNOSIS. Decreased activity tolerance related to imbalance between oxygen supply and demand as evidenced by exertional dyspnea and/or exertional chest pain

OUTCOMES. Circulation status; Cardiac pump effectiveness; Respiratory status; Symptom severity; Comfort status: Physical; Self-care status; Ambulation; Rest

INTERVENTIONS. Oxygen therapy; Pain management: Acute and chronic; Medication management; Energy management; Exercise therapy: Ambulation; Self-care assistance

PLANNING AND IMPLEMENTATION

Collaborative

MEDICAL. The treatment of AI depends on the severity of the condition and the severity of the patient's symptoms. If the condition is mild, the patient may be monitored and treated for the underlying cause, such as infective endocarditis or syphilis. Patients are encouraged to limit strenuous physical activity. Fluid restrictions and diuretics may be ordered to reduce pulmonary congestion. Medications may be used to augment cardiac output. Supplemental oxygenation will enhance oxygen levels in the blood to decrease labored breathing and chest pain.

SURGICAL. Many patients can be stabilized with medical treatment, but early elective valve surgery should be considered because the outlook for medically treated symptomatic disease is poor. Recent advances have allowed for percutaneous aortic valve replacement

(PAVR), also known as transcatheter aortic valve implementation. This procedure is a more important therapy for aortic stenosis, but it is also being considered for AI. The approach can be transfemoral, subclavian, aortic (through a minimally invasive incision), and transcaval. Benefits are a reduced short-term risk of death, stroke, renal injury, or bleeding, but an increased risk of heart failure, pacemaker insertion, and the need for reintervention. Five-year survival rates and comparison with surgical replacement of an insufficient aortic valve are not yet known.

Surgical repair or replacement is the most common treatment of AI. The incompetent valve can be repaired (valve-sparing techniques) or replaced with a synthetic or biological valve, such as a pig valve. The choice of valve type is based on the patient's age and potential for clotting problems. The biological valve usually shows structural deterioration after 6 to 10 years and needs to be replaced. The synthetic valve is more durable but also more prone to thrombi formations. Complications include thromboembolism, bleeding, and endocarditis.

Pharmacologic Highlights

Medication or Drug Class	Dosage	Description	Rationale
Digoxin	0.25 mg PO qd	Cardiotonic	Increases force of contraction in people with left ventricular dysfunction
Vasodilators such as nifedipine, diltiazem, hydralazine, prazosin, nitroprusside	Nifedipine, 10–30 mg tid PO or SL	Calcium channel blocker; systemic vasodilators	Decrease afterload (pressure that the left ventricle has to pump against) and decreases regurgitant blood flow
Diuretics	Varies with drug	Thiazides; loop diuretics	Enhance pumping ability of the heart
Angiotensin-converting enzyme (ACE) inhibitors such as captopril, enalapril, lisinopril	Varies with drug	Competitive inhibitors of ACE	Reduces angiotensin II levels and aldosterone secretion to control blood pressure and proteinuria; increases systemic blood flow and reduces potassium loss

Other Medications: Anticoagulation is controversial after surgery unless the patient has comorbidities, but antiplatelet drugs may be prescribed. Patients may be asked to take antibiotics prior to future surgeries and dental procedures. The use of beta blockers is controversial and under investigation. If the patient is critically ill prior to surgery, they may receive a positive inotrope, such as dopamine or dobutamine, and a vasodilator, such as nitroprusside. Angiotensin (losartan, valsartan, azilsartan) receptor blockers may be prescribed.

Independent

Physical and psychological rest decreases cardiac workload, which reduces the metabolic demands on the myocardium. Physical rest is enhanced by providing assistance with activities of daily living and encouraging activity restrictions. Most patients with advanced AI are placed on activity restrictions to decrease cardiac workload. If the patient is on bedrest, advise the patient to use the bedside commode, because research has shown it creates less workload for the heart than using the bedpan. If the patient can tolerate some activities, those that increase isometric work, such as lifting heavy objects, are more detrimental than activities such as walking or swimming.

Encourage the patient to avoid sudden changes in position to minimize increased cardiac demand. If the patient is hospitalized, instruct the patient to sit on the edge of the bed before standing. If pulmonary congestion is present, elevate head of bed slightly to enhance respiration.

Reducing psychological stress is a challenge. Approach the patient and family in a calm, relaxed manner. Decrease the fear of the unknown by providing explanations and current information and encouraging questions. To help the patient maintain or reestablish a sense of control, permit the patient to participate in decisions about aspects of care within the patient's knowledge. If the patient decides to have valve surgery, offer to let them speak with someone who has already had the surgery. Seeing and talking with someone who has undergone surgery and lives with a replacement valve is usually very therapeutic.

Evidence-Based Practice and Health Policy

Sjoding, M., Dickson, R., Iwashyna, T., Gay, S., & Valley, T. (2020). Racial bias in pulse oximetry measurement. *New England Journal of Medicine, 383*, 25–26.

• During medical and surgical treatment for aortic valve insufficiency, pulse oximetry is a useful tool to measure oxygen saturation. The authors studied the accuracy of pulse oximetry measures as compared to the gold standard measure of arterial oxygenation, arterial blood gas (ABG) analysis, in a diverse sample of people. They analyzed 10,789 pairs of measures (pulse oximetry and ABG) in White patients and Black patients. The authors were particularly interested in patients who had a normal to low-normal value of 92% to 96% with oximetry, and yet had occult hypoxemia (<88%) with ABG measurement.

• In patients with a saturation of 92% to 95% with oximetry but lower than 88% with an ABG (the more accurate measure), 11.4% were Black and 4.6% were White. Black patients had nearly three times the frequency of occult hypoxemia that was not detected by pulse oximetry than White patients. These findings indicate that pulse oximetry, a widely used noninvasive measure of oxygenation, is not as accurate in Black patients as in White patients, placing Black patients at risk for undetected low oxygen levels.

DOCUMENTATION GUIDELINES

• Physical findings: Diastolic murmur, bounding apical pulse, rales in the lungs, presence or absence of pain, quality of pulses
• Response to diuretics, cardiotonics, vasodilators, and inotropic agents
• Reaction to activity restrictions, fluid restrictions, and cardiac diagnosis
• Presence of complications: Chest pain, bleeding, fainting, infection, embolic phenomenon

DISCHARGE AND HOME HEALTHCARE GUIDELINES

MEDICATIONS. Be sure the patient understands all medications, including the dose, route, action, adverse effects, and need for routine laboratory monitoring for anticoagulants.

TEACHING. Instruct the patient to report the recurrence or escalation of signs and symptoms of AI, which could indicate that the medical therapy needs readjusting or the replaced valve is malfunctioning. Patients with synthetic valves may hear an audible click like a ticking watch from the valve closure.

PREVENTION OF BACTERIAL ENDOCARDITIS. Patients who have had surgery are susceptible to bacterial endocarditis, which will cause scarring or destruction of the heart valves. Bacterial endocarditis may result from dental work, surgeries, and invasive procedures, so people who have repaired or replaced heart valves should be given antibiotics before and after these treatments.

Aortic Valve Stenosis

DRG Category: 307
Mean LOS: 3.1 days
Description: MEDICAL: Cardiac Congenital and Valvular Disorders Without Major Complication or Comorbidity

Aortic stenosis (AS) is a narrowing of the aortic valve orifice, which obstructs outflow from the left ventricle during systole. The left ventricle must overcome the increased resistance to ejection by generating a higher-than-normal pressure during systole, which is achieved by stretching and generating a more forceful contraction. The blood is propelled through the narrowed aortic valve at an increased velocity. Aortic valve stenosis accounts for approximately 5% of all congenital heart defects. About 4 in 1,000 live births have AS, making this condition a relatively common birth defect. An important contribution of AS is calcification of the aortic valve, which affects up to 3% of the U.S. population over 65 years of age.

As the stenosis in the aortic valve progresses, two sequelae occur. One is that cardiac output becomes fixed, making increases even with exertion impossible. The other is left-sided heart failure. Pressure overload of the heart occurs with concentric hypertrophy of the left ventricle. Left ventricular end-diastolic pressure rises, myocardial oxygen demand increases, and left ventricular mass and wall stress are increased. The increase in left ventricular pressure is reflected backward into the left atrium. Because the left atrium is unable to empty adequately, the pulmonary circulation becomes congested. Eventually, right-sided heart failure can develop as well. If untreated, people who are symptomatic have a 50% mortality rate at 2 years after the onset of symptoms.

CAUSES

The predominant causative factor in AS is congenital malformation of the aortic valve. Congenital causes can lead to unicuspid and bicuspid or malformed valves. When they become calcified, symptoms may occur. Stenosis can also occur with narrowing of the subvalvular outflow tract by fibroelastic membranes or muscle tissue. Acquired valvular stenosis results from rheumatic heart disease and degenerative calcification. Risk factors for degenerative stenosis include advanced age, hypertension, elevated cholesterol, diabetes mellitus, and smoking. The patient's age when the condition manifests itself usually suggests the cause. Congenital stenosis is usually seen in patients younger than 30 years old. In patients between the ages of 30 and 70 years, the cause is equally attributed to congenital malformation and rheumatic heart disease. Atherosclerosis and degenerative calcification of the aortic valve are the predominant causes for stenosis in people older than 70 years.

GENETIC CONSIDERATIONS

Considerable evidence supports a genetic component for congenital AS. A main cause of AS is calcification of a congenital bicuspid, or rarely, a unicuspid aortic valve, which are often caused by genetic mutations in a gene such as *NOTCH1*. Bicuspid aortic valve is often found among relatives of persons affected with other left ventricular outflow tract malformations. AS can occur as a feature of rare genetic diseases such as Williams syndrome, a neurodevelopmental disorder, or Fabry disease, a lysosomal storage disease.

SEX AND LIFE SPAN CONSIDERATIONS

AS can occur at any age, depending on the cause. Among children born with AS, 75% are male, and overall approximately 80% with both congenital and acquired AS are male. Degenerative aortic stenosis is most common in men older than age 75 years. Gender differences occur with treatment. Surgical aortic valve replacement is associated with an elevated risk in the short term for women as compared to men at 30 days after surgery because of an older age and co-occurring conditions. With a newer procedure, transcatheter aortic valve replacement, 30-day outcomes are similar for women and men.

HEALTH DISPARITIES AND SEXUAL/GENDER MINORITY HEALTH

While epidemiology studies are not definitive, experts suggest that Black and Hispanic persons may have a lower prevalence of AS than White persons. There is little debate about the role of health disparities, however. Black and Hispanic patients are less likely to be referred to cardiac surgeons and cardiologists than White patients. Black, Hispanic, and uninsured patients are known to receive care less often guided by standard cardiac care guidelines than White persons. Once selected for surgical procedures, Black and Hispanic patients have similar outcomes to White patients (Batchelor et al., 2019). Sexual and gender minority status has no known specific effect on the risk for aortic valve stenosis.

GLOBAL HEALTH CONSIDERATIONS

Rheumatic heart disease and subsequent valvular disease is a continuing problem in developing countries, where up to 60% of all admissions for cardiovascular illnesses are related to the condition. Prevalence may be as low as 1 per 100,000 children in Costa Rica to as high as 150 per 100,000 children in China. Areas of particular concern are Southeastern Asia, Central America, North Africa, and the Middle East.

ASSESSMENT

HISTORY. A history of rheumatic fever suggests possible cardiac valvular malfunction; however, many patients who have had rheumatic fever do not remember having had the condition. The diagnosis therefore is usually based on symptoms. Some patients describe gradually reducing their activity to avoid symptoms such as angina, syncope, or dyspnea. Given the potential genetic causes, a family history of AS can be significant.

PHYSICAL EXAMINATION. People often have no signs and symptoms for 10 to 20 years. The classic symptoms of aortic stenosis are **chest pain, fainting on exertion (syncope)**, and **labored breathing on exertion** due to heart failure. Patients may be easily fatigued and report difficulty with effort and exercise. Inspection of the thoracic wall may reveal a thrusting apical pulsation. A systolic thrill (vibrations felt from turbulent blood flow) may be palpated over the second intercostal space to the right of the sternum. A lift or heave may be palpated over the apex of the heart.

Auscultation of heart sounds reveals a harsh systolic crescendo-decrescendo murmur. The murmur, referred to as *diamond shaped*, is considered the hallmark of AS and occurs shortly after the first heart sound. Auscultation of breath sounds may reveal fine crackles (rales) if pulmonary congestion is present in left-sided heart failure. The pulmonary congestion will vary with the amount of exertion and severity of stenosis.

PSYCHOSOCIAL. Because the symptoms of AS are usually gradual, most people have already made adjustments in their lifestyle to adapt and do not seek treatment until the symptoms become debilitating. Assess what the patient has already done to cope with this condition. In addition, assess the patient's degree of anxiety about a diagnosed heart condition and potential treatment. Heart surgery is a daunting prospect for patients and families, who will require clear explanations and much psychological support.

Diagnostic Highlights

Test	Normal Result	Abnormality With Condition	Explanation
Cardiac catheterization	Normal aortic valve	Opening in the aortic valve is obstructed and narrowed	Aortic valve is narrowed with the pressure gradient across the valve directly related to the degree of obstruction; indicates severity of stenosis
Two-dimensional and Doppler echocardiography	Normal aortic valve	Stenosed aortic valve	Reveals abnormal blood flow patterns

Other Tests: Echocardiography to assess the aortic valve's structure and mobility, electrocardiogram, chest radiography, radionuclide ventriculography, computed tomography, magnetic resonance imaging, complete blood count, coagulation profile, blood chemistries, and type and crossmatch for blood before and after surgery.

PRIMARY NURSING DIAGNOSIS

DIAGNOSIS. Decreased activity tolerance related to imbalance between oxygen supply and demand as evidenced by chest pain, exertional dyspnea, and/or exertional syncope

OUTCOMES. Circulation status; Cardiac pump effectiveness; Respiratory status; Symptom severity; Comfort status: Physical; Self-care status; Ambulation; Rest

INTERVENTIONS. Oxygen therapy; Pain management: Acute and chronic; Medication management; Energy management; Exercise therapy: Ambulation; Self-care assistance

PLANNING AND IMPLEMENTATION

Collaborative

MEDICAL. Most patients with AS are placed on activity restrictions to decrease cardiac workload. Patients on bedrest should use the bedside commode because research has shown it creates less workload for the heart than using the bedpan. Fluid restrictions and diuretics may be ordered to reduce pulmonary congestion. Supplemental oxygenation will enhance oxygen levels in the blood to decrease labored breathing and chest pain.

SURGICAL. The average survival rate after the appearance of symptoms is less than 5 years for patients with AS who are treated medically. Surgical treatment increases the survival rate dramatically and is the most common treatment of AS. Transcatheter aortic valve replacement (TAVR) has been developed as an alternative to open surgical repair for high-risk and intermediate-risk patients. TAVR is a minimally invasive surgical procedure that repairs the valve without removing the damaged valve by using a catheter that is inserted in the femoral artery (transfemoral) or through a small incision into the chest (transthoracic). The surgeon wedges a bovine replacement valve into the damaged valve's place, pushing the old valve leaflets out of the way and expanding the new valve. Indications for TAVR include symptomatic calcified AS, low-flow stenosis, and the opinion of experts that the patient cannot endure heart surgery because of medical reasons. The procedure is successful in 90% of the cases, and mortality rates are improved over open surgical repair for this high-risk group. Complications include stroke, transient ischemic attack, cardiac dysrhythmias, infection, aortic regurgitation, and renal insufficiency.

The development of symptoms from a stenotic valve is an indiction for replacement, which can be a synthetic valve or a biologic valve, such as a pig valve. The choice of valve type is based on the patient's age and the potential for clotting problems. The biologic valve usually shows structural deterioration after 6 to 10 years and needs to be replaced. The synthetic valve is more durable but also more prone to thrombi formation. Complications include thromboembolism, bleeding, and endocarditis. Surgical mortality is approximately 5%. Five-year survival rate is 80% to 95%. Percutaneous balloon valvuloplasty (valotomy), widening of a stenotic valve using a balloon catheter inside the valve, is an option for patients with a short life expectancy or those who refuse surgery.

Pharmacologic Highlights

Medication or Drug Class	Dosage	Description	Rationale
Digoxin	0.25 mg PO qd	Cardiotonic	May be useful in the presence of heart failure and left ventricular dilation and impaired systolic function; may be used to control the ventricular rate if atrial fibrillation occurs
Beta-adrenergic receptor blockers (esmolol, metoprolol)	Varies with drug	Beta-adrenergic receptor blocker	Used to manage angina or elevated blood pressure in patients who are not candidates for surgery or prior to surgery

Other Therapy: Diuretics, nitrates, and other vasodilators are generally avoided because they reduce filling pressures and may lower systolic blood pressure but may be used for patients with heart failure who are not candidates for surgery. Anticoagulation is controversial after surgery unless the patient has comorbidities, but the patient may be placed on an antiplatelet agent. Patients may be asked to take antibiotics prior to future surgeries and dental procedures.

Independent

Physical and psychological rest decreases cardiac workload, which reduces the metabolic demands of the myocardium. Physical rest is enhanced by providing assistance with activities of daily living and encouraging activity restrictions. Reducing psychological stress can also be difficult. Decrease the fear of the unknown by providing explanations and current information and encouraging questions. To help the patient maintain or reestablish a sense of control, permit the patient to participate in decisions about aspects of care within their knowledge. If the patient decides on surgery, offer to let the patient speak with someone who has already had the surgery.

Discourage sudden changes in position to minimize increased cardiac demand. Instruct the patient to sit on the edge of the bed before standing. Elevate the head of the bed slightly if pulmonary congestion is present, to enhance respiration.

Monitoring physical status is a priority for nursing care. Assess for episodes of dizziness or fainting. The episodes may occur because of decreased cardiac output or cardiac dysrhythmias, so patients should be told to report occurrence of these symptoms promptly. Dizziness and fainting are correlated with sudden death, which, according to recent research, occurs in 10% to 20% of all patients with advanced AS. Maintain a safe physical environment for the patient by removing obstructions in the patient's room.

Evidence-Based Practice and Health Policy

Makkar, R., Thourani, V., Mack, M., Kodali, S., Kapadia, S., Webb, J., Yoon, S., Trento, A., Svensson, L., Herrmann, H., Szeto, W., Miller, D., Satler, L., Cohen, D., Dewey, T., Babaliaros, V.,

Williams, M., Kereiakes, D., Zajarias, A., . . . Leon, M. (2020). Five-year outcomes of transcatheter or surgical aortic-valve replacement. *New England Journal of Medicine, 382,* 799–809.

• The authors studied long-term clinical outcomes and prosthetic valve function in patients (*N* = 2032) with severe aortic stenosis after TAVR as compared to standard surgical valve replacement. They grouped patients according to two surgical routes (transfemoral and transthoracic) and randomly assigned to one of two treatment options: TAVR or surgical replacement. Adverse outcomes included death from any cause or stroke.
• After 5 years, there was no significant difference in death from any cause or disabling stroke between the two groups (47.9% and 43.4%, respectively). Results were similar for the transfemoral-access group, but the incidence of death or disabling stroke was higher after TAVR than after surgery in the transthoracic access group. After 5 years, more patients in the TAVR group had at least mild paravalvular aortic regurgitation, more repeat hospitalizations, and more aortic valve reinterventions.

DOCUMENTATION GUIDELINES

• Physical findings of systolic murmur, systolic thrill, and rales in the lungs
• Response to diuretics, nitrates, and rest
• Reaction to activity restrictions, fluid restrictions, and cardiac diagnosis
• Presence of complications: Chest pain, bleeding tendencies, labored breathing, fainting, infection, embolic phenomenon

DISCHARGE AND HOME HEALTHCARE GUIDELINES

MEDICATIONS. Be sure the patient understands all medications, including the dose, route, action, adverse effects, and need for routine laboratory monitoring for anticoagulants.

TEACHING. Instruct the patient to report the recurrence or escalation of signs and symptoms of AS, which could indicate that the medical therapy needs readjusting or the replaced valve is malfunctioning. Patients with synthetic valves may hear an audible click like a ticking watch from the valve closure.

PREVENTION OF BACTERIAL ENDOCARDITIS. Patients who have had surgery are susceptible to bacterial endocarditis, which will cause scarring or destruction of the heart valves. Because bacterial endocarditis may result from dental work, surgeries, and invasive procedures, people who have repaired or replaced heart valves should be given antibiotics before and after these treatments.

Aplastic Anemia

DRG Category:	812
Mean LOS:	3.4 days
Description:	MEDICAL: Red Blood Cell Disorders Without Complication or Comorbidity

Aplastic, or hypoplastic, anemia is a bone marrow failure characterized by a decrease in all formed elements of peripheral blood and its bone marrow. If all elements are suppressed—resulting in loss of production of healthy erythrocytes, platelets, and granulocytes—the condition is known as *pancytopenia*. Onset is often insidious and may become chronic; however, onset may be rapid and overwhelming when the cause is a myelotoxin (a poison that damages the bone marrow).

With complete bone marrow suppression, leukocytic failure may result in fulminating infections, greatly reducing the chances for complete recovery. Less severe cases may have an acute transient course or a chronic course with ultimate recovery, although the platelet count may remain subnormal, thus requiring a lifetime of precautions against bleeding. Aplastic anemia may produce fatal bleeding or infection, however, especially if it is idiopathic or stems from chloramphenicol or infectious hepatitis. Approximately one-third of patients do not respond to immunotherapy; even the responders risk relapse and late-onset disease, such as leukemia. Depending on the type of treatment, the 10-year survival rate is 68% to 73%. Primary complications are infection and bleeding.

CAUSES

Acquired aplastic anemia develops from an injury or damage to the stem cells, leading to inhibition of red blood cell (RBC) production. Acquired disease occurs in approximately 80% of cases of aplastic anemia. Evidence suggests that it is primarily an autoimmune response. It can also be caused by drugs such as antibiotics and anticonvulsants, toxic agents such as benzene and chloramphenicol, pregnancy, or radiation. The immune mechanism does not explain the bone marrow failure in drug reactions. Drug toxicity seems to occur because of genetically determined differences in metabolic pathways. Other causes include hepatitis, viral illnesses, and preleukemic and neoplastic infiltration of the bone marrow. Approximately 20% of cases of aplastic anemia are congenital (see Genetic Considerations).

GENETIC CONSIDERATIONS

Several inherited conditions can result in aplastic anemia. These include Fanconi anemia (autosomal recessive transmission), dyskeratosis congenita (X-linked recessive is the most common pattern of transmission, but autosomal dominant and autosomal recessive patterns are also seen), Shwachman-Diamond syndrome (autosomal recessive), and reticular dysgenesis (autosomal recessive mutations in the gene *AK2*). Mutations in telomerase reverse transcriptase (*TERT*) or dyskerin (*DKC1*) cause dyskeratosis congenita. Mutations in *TERT* or the telomerase RNA component (*TERC*) can also directly cause aplastic anemia. Polymorphisms in the interferon-gamma gene (*IFNG*), perforin (*PRF1*) gene, nibrin gene (*NBS*), or *SBDS* gene have also been associated with aplastic anemia.

SEX AND LIFE SPAN CONSIDERATIONS

Incidence of the condition is fairly low, without apparent sex or age preference. Congenital hypoplastic anemia occurs in infants in the third month of life, and Fanconi anemia occurs in children under the age of 10 years with a second peak in people who are 20 to 25 years of age.

HEALTH DISPARITIES AND SEXUAL/GENDER MINORITY HEALTH

Ethnicity, race, and sexual/gender minority status have no known effect on the risk for aplastic anemia.

GLOBAL HEALTH CONSIDERATIONS

The annual incidence in both the United States and Europe is 2 to 4 cases per 1 million people. The disease is more common in Asia than in Europe, with rates as high as 14 cases per 1 million people in Japan and 6 cases per million in Thailand. While individuals in Asia are known to have higher rates of aplastic anemia than people in the West, this increase is not found in Asian

Americans and is therefore thought to be related to exposure to environmental factors rather than heredity. In Asia, more males than females are affected.

ASSESSMENT

HISTORY. Although most cases of aplastic anemia are idiopathic, ask the patient for a family and work history (to determine chemical exposure) as well as an environmental history. The patient may report recurrent infections. Determine if the patient has recently been exposed to known risk factors, such as recent treatment with chemotherapeutic drugs or antibiotics known to cause bone marrow suppression, radiation therapy, or accidental exposure to organic solvents. Establish a history of dyspnea, headache, intolerance for activity, progressive fatigue, malaise, chills and possibly fever, easy bruising, or frank bleeding.

PHYSICAL EXAMINATION. Examine the patient's skin for **pallor** or a jaundiced appearance. **Headache, palpitations, shortness of breath,** and **fatigue** are common. Inspect the patient's mucous membranes for bleeding. Inspect the patient's gums and throat for lesions. Palpate the patient's lymph nodes to see if they are enlarged. Palpate the patient's liver and spleen and note any enlargement. Auscultate the patient's chest for tachycardia and adventitious lung sounds. Inherited bone marrow failure may result in a short stature, abnormal skin pigmentation, lack of development of the genitals, and a small head.

PSYCHOSOCIAL. Assess the patient's mental status as an indicator of cerebral perfusion; assess the sensorimotor status to evaluate nervous system oxygenation. Patients may be anxious or fearful because of their low level of energy. Discomfort caused by mouth pain may cause the patient to feel irritable. The parents of an infant with a congenital form of aplastic anemia may be quite agitated over the child's illness.

Diagnostic Highlights

Test	Normal Result	Abnormality With Condition	Explanation
Complete blood count with differential	RBCs 3.6–5.8 million/mcL	Decreased to < 1.0 million/mcL; usually normochromic and normocytic but may be macrocytic (enlarged) and anisocytic (excessive variation in erythrocyte size)	Injury to the stem cells decreases production of blood cells
	White blood cells 4,500–11,100/mcL	Decreased	Injury to the stem cells decreases production of blood cells
	Reticulocyte count 0.8%–2.5% of total RBCs; platelets 150,000–450,000/mcL	Decreased	Injury to the stem cells decreases production of blood cells

Other Tests: Platelets, serum iron, coagulation tests, bone marrow biopsy, hemoglobin electrophoresis, fluorescence-activated cell sorter (FACS) profile of related proteins, transaminase, bilirubin, lactic dehydrogenase, blood urea nitrogen, creatinine, hepatitis testing, peripheral smear. Magnetic resonance imaging of the axial skeleton may be completed.

PRIMARY NURSING DIAGNOSIS

DIAGNOSIS. Risk for infection as evidenced by inadequate secondary defenses and/or immunosuppression

OUTCOMES. Immune status; Knowledge: Infection management; Risk control: Infectious process; Risk detection; Nutritional status; Tissue integrity: Skin and mucous membranes

INTERVENTIONS. Environmental management; Infection control; Infection prevention; Medication management; Nutrition management; Surveillance

☀ PLANNING AND IMPLEMENTATION

Collaborative

MEDICAL. Immunosuppressive therapy using cyclosporine and antithymocyte globulin is considered first-line therapy in patients with severe disease who are older than 50 years and those 35 to 40 years of age with comorbidities. It is also recommended as secondary treatment for younger patients without an appropriate donor. Immunosuppressive therapy has a response rate of approximately 60% to 80% and a 5-year survival rate of 75%. Note that aplastic anemia has a high 10-year mortality rate (> 65%) and should be considered a medical emergency. If anemia is caused by a particular agent or drug, withdrawing it is usually the first step in treatment. Blood component therapy (RBCs, platelets) is initiated based on the patient's clinical status and laboratory values and may be needed until other therapies can be started to manage symptoms (anemia and fatigue) and to prevent bleeding. Clinical research studies have indicated some promising results with colony-stimulating factors (CSFs) such as interleukin-3 to encourage growth of specific blood elements. Oxygen is administered to ensure cellular oxygenation.

SURGICAL. Hematopoietic cell transplantation (HCT) is the treatment of choice for severe aplastic anemia. Protocols may vary slightly but generally indicate that the recipient must have a human leukocyte antigen (HLA) identical to that of the bone marrow donor (such as a sibling or twin) and receive a preparatory regimen of immunosuppression and radiation therapies.

POSTOPERATIVE. Postoperatively, relieve pain with analgesics and ice packs as needed. Monitor the patient for fever or chills, sore throat, or red or draining wounds, and administer prophylactic antibiotics as prescribed. Treat the patient's reactions to postoperative chemotherapy or radiation therapy as prescribed by administering antiemetics to control nausea and vomiting. Postoperative medication management is complex and depends on institutional protocols. Monitor postoperative patients for signs of graft-versus-host reaction, including maculopapular rash, pancytopenia, jaundice, joint pain, and anasarca.

Pharmacologic Highlights

Medication or Drug Class	Dosage	Description	Rationale
Corticosteroids	Varies by drug	Glucocorticoids such as methylprednisolone	Stimulates erythroid production, manages response to anaphylaxis or serum sickness
Antithymocyte globulin	3.5 mg/kg/day for 5 days	Immunoglobulin derived from rabbits	Promotes immunosuppression by depleting T lymphocytes
Cyclosporine	Dosing depends on ideal body weight	Cyclic polypeptide, cyclophilin inhibitor	Suppresses humoral and cell-mediated immunity; used to prepare the body for hematopoietic cell transplantation

Other Therapy: Antibiotics, antifungal agents, and antiviral agents may be given if infection or sepsis is present or to prevent infection. Bone marrow stimulants or growth factors may be prescribed.

Independent

Perform meticulous hand washing before patient contact. If protective isolation is required, use gloves, gown, and mask and make sure that visitors do the same. Report any signs of systemic infection and obtain the prescribed cultures. Provide frequent skin care, oral care, and perianal care to prevent both infection and bleeding. Avoid invasive procedures if possible. When invasive procedures are necessary, maintain strict aseptic techniques and monitor the sites for signs of inflammation or drainage. Teach the patient and significant others symptoms of infection and to report them immediately to healthcare providers. Obtain a nutrition consultation to reduce exposure to bacteria from food such as raw meats, dairy products, fruits, and vegetables that may be colonized with mold, bacteria, or fungi.

To help combat fatigue and conserve patient energy, plan frequent rest periods between activities. Instruct the patient in energy-saving techniques. Encourage the patient to increase activities gradually to the level of maximum tolerance.

Some patients with aplastic anemia undergo bone marrow transplants. Preoperatively, teach the patient about the procedure. Explain that chemotherapy and possible radiation treatments are necessary to remove cells that may cause the body to reject the transplant. Offer support and reassurance.

Evidence-Based Practice and Health Policy

Ahmed, P., Chaudhry, Q., Satti, T., Mahmood, S., Ghafoor, T., Shahbaz, N., Khan, M., Satti, H., Akram, Z., & Iftikhar, R. (2020). Epidemiology of aplastic anemia: A study of 1,324 cases. *Hematology*, *25*, 48–54.

• The authors' purpose was to study the etiology and association of aplastic anemia with various socioeconomic and environmental factors. The study included 1,324 consecutive cases of aplastic anemia at the Armed Forces Bone Marrow Transplant center in Pakistan over 15 years. Patients were interviewed about personal and family medical history, environmental attributes, and other features.

• The patients' average age was 20 years; 997 were male, and 327 were female. The majority of cases were from low- or middle-income families (98.5%). The authors classified the cases as nonsevere (17.4%), severe (45.4%), and very severe (37.4%). Chemical exposure included fertilizers, pesticides, and industrial chemicals. A large number of the cases also identified blood relatives with the condition.

DOCUMENTATION GUIDELINES

• Laboratory findings: Complete blood count, platelet count, coagulation studies
• Physical findings: Degree of fatigue or shortness of breath, signs of infection, skin color, presence of jaundice or ecchymoses, appearance of mouth and throat lesions, vital signs, presence of adventitious breath sounds
• Responses to interventions: Medications, bone marrow transplantation
• Progress toward desired outcomes: Activity tolerance, ability to maintain self-care

DISCHARGE AND HOME HEALTHCARE GUIDELINES

PREVENTION. Teach the patient the importance of avoiding exposure to individuals who are known to have acute infections. Teach the patient to report all episodes of fever. Emphasize the need for preventing trauma, abrasions, and breakdown of the skin. Be sure the patient understands the need to maintain a good nutritional intake to enhance the immune system and resistance to infections. Teach the patient the potential for bleeding and hemorrhage, and offer instruction in measures to prevent bleeding, including the use of a soft toothbrush and an electric razor. Discuss the need for regular dental examinations. Explain the importance of maintaining regular bowel movements to prevent straining and rectal bleeding. Instruct the patient to avoid enemas and rectal thermometers because of the risk of rectal perforation.

MEDICATIONS. Teach the patient the purpose, dosage, schedule, precautions, and potential side effects, interactions, and adverse reactions of all prescribed medications.

POST HCT MANAGEMENT. Provide detailed information about managing discharge after HCT, including housecleaning routines; need for linen changes; air filtration and shower safety; hand-washing procedures; and cooking safety measures. Discuss animal safety measures that help prevent infection. Describe safety measures to limit infection exposure in crowds such as in malls and elevators.

COMPLICATIONS. Teach the patient to recognize the indicators of a systemic infection. Stress that fever and usual wound infection signs may or may not be present because the immune system may be depressed. Instruct the patient about the symptoms that require immediate medical intervention and make sure the patient knows whom to notify. Stress the importance of reporting increased symptoms of anemia, including progressive fatigue, weakness, paresthesia, blurred vision, palpitations, and dizziness.

Appendicitis

DRG Category:	394
Mean LOS:	3.8 days
Description:	MEDICAL: Other Digestive System Diagnoses With Complication or Comorbidity
DRG Category:	338
Mean LOS:	11.4 days
Description:	SURGICAL: Appendectomy With Complicated Principal Diagnosis With Major Complication or Comorbidity
DRG Category:	341
Mean LOS:	7.0 days
Description:	SURGICAL: Appendectomy Without Complicated Principal Diagnosis With Major Complication or Comorbidity

Appendicitis is an acute inflammation of the vermiform appendix—a narrow, blind tube that extends from the inferior part of the cecum. The appendix has no known function but does fill and empty as food moves through the gastrointestinal tract. Appendicitis begins when the inner lining of the appendix becomes inflamed. Irritation and inflammation lead to engorged veins, stasis, and arterial occlusion. Eventually bacteria accumulate, the wall of the appendix becomes ischemic, bacteria invade the organ's wall, and the appendix can develop gangrene. Appendicitis is the most common cause of acute inflammation in the right lower quadrant of the abdominal cavity and is the most common surgical emergency. Patients with appendicitis need urgent referral and rapid treatment.

Experts estimate that appendicitis occurs in approximately 7% of the U.S. population each year and has an overall mortality rate of 0.2% to 0.8%. Mortality is primarily caused by complications of the disease rather than surgical intervention. Complications include ruptured appendix, peritonitis, abscess formation, sepsis, septic shock, and paralytic ileus. At the time of diagnosis, approximately 25% of people will have a perforated appendix.

CAUSES

Appendicitis is generally caused by obstruction. Since the appendix is a small, fingerlike appendage of the cecum, it is prone to obstruction as it regularly fills and empties with intestinal contents. The obstruction may be caused by a fecalith (a hard mass of feces), a foreign body in the lumen of the appendix, fibrous disease of the bowel wall, infestation of parasites, or twisting of the appendix by adhesions. Of all cases, approximately 60% are associated with hyperplasia of the submucosal lymphoid follicles and 35% with fecal stasis or fecalith. It is associated with inflammatory bowel disease, gastrointestinal infection (more common in children and young adults), parasites, foreign bodies, and neoplasms.

GENETIC CONSIDERATIONS

Although exact genetic mechanisms that contribute to susceptibility are unclear, the risk of appendicitis is increased 3- to 10-fold when a first-degree relative is affected, and heritability is estimated at 50%. Familial appendicitis may result from an inherited predisposition to obstructions in the lumen of the appendix.

SEX AND LIFE SPAN CONSIDERATIONS

Appendicitis is rare before the age of 2 years, with the peak incidence of appendicitis occurring between ages 10 and 19 years. In pediatric patients, the mean age for appendicitis ranges between 6 and 10 years. Twice as many young men as young women develop appendicitis; after age 25 years, this ratio gradually diminishes until the gender ratio is even. Appendicitis in the older adult population is being reported with increasing frequency as life expectancy increases. Unfortunately, appendicitis in older adults tends to progress to perforation more rapidly, with fewer symptoms than expected. Older patients usually experience decreased pain sensations, very minor leukocyte elevations, and temperature elevations that are minimal when compared with those in younger patients. Incidence of perforation is higher in patients younger than 18 and older than 50 years. The reasons for this difference in incidence may occur because of delays in diagnosis.

HEALTH DISPARITIES AND SEXUAL/GENDER MINORITY HEALTH

In children with appendicitis, significant health disparities exist in the care of Black and Hispanic children compared to White children. Black and Hispanic children are more likely to have a delayed diagnosis (at least on prior emergency department visit) and less diagnostic imaging (ultrasound, computed tomography) than White children. These disparities may lead to more perforated appendices in Black and Hispanic children as compared to White children (Goyal et al., 2020). Sexual and gender minority status has no known specific effect on the risk for appendicitis.

GLOBAL HEALTH CONSIDERATIONS

Appendicitis is much more common in developed than in developing countries. Experts speculate that the reason for these discrepancies may include a diet low in fiber and high in sugar in developed countries, as well as family history and varying infection exposure depending on geographic region. Dietary habits in Africa and Asia, particularly those with high-fiber diets, are associated with lower rates of appendicitis than occur in Western countries.

☀️ ASSESSMENT

HISTORY. Because of variations in the anatomic position of the appendix as well as age-related differences in clinical presentation, the patient's history may not demonstrate one consistent pattern. Experts note that only 50% of patients have the cardinal symptoms of appendicitis (nausea, right lower quadrant pain, and vomiting). Most patients with appendicitis report a history of **midabdominal pain** that initially comes in waves. In addition, early in the disease process, many patients report a discomfort that creates an **urge to defecate** to obtain relief. As the disease process progresses, patients usually complain of a constant epigastric or periumbilical pain that eventually localizes in the right lower quadrant of the abdomen. Some patients may report a more diffuse lower abdominal pain or referred pain. Should perforation of the appendix occur, pain may subside to generalized abdominal discomfort. In addition to pain, patients often complain of **anorexia, nausea, vomiting**, abdominal distension, and temporary constipation. Temperature elevations may also be reported, usually 100°F to 101°F (37.8°C to 38.3°C). Important differential diagnoses to consider are ectopic pregnancy in females of childbearing age, as well as endometriosis, pelvic inflammatory disease, renal calculi, urinary tract infection, abdominal abscess, cholecystitis, Crohn disease, gastroenteritis, and inflammatory bowel disease.

PHYSICAL EXAMINATION. Rebound tenderness, pain on percussion, and abdominal guarding/rigidity are specific findings in appendicitis. Observe the patient for typical signs of pain, including facial grimacing, clenched fists, diaphoresis, tachycardia, and shallow but rapid respirations. In addition, patients with appendicitis commonly guard the abdominal area by lying still with the right leg flexed at the knee. This posture diminishes tension on the abdominal muscles and increases comfort. Slight abdominal distention may also be observed.

Early palpation of the abdomen reveals slight muscular rigidity and diffuse tenderness around the umbilicus and midepigastrium. Later, as the pain shifts to the right lower quadrant, palpation generally elicits tenderness at the McBurney point (a point midway between the umbilicus and the right anterior iliac crest). Right lower quadrant rebound tenderness (production of pain when palpation pressure is relieved) is typical. Also, a positive Rovsing sign may be elicited by palpating the left lower quadrant, which results in pain in the right lower quadrant.

PSYCHOSOCIAL. The patient with appendicitis faces an unexpected hospitalization and surgical procedure. Assess the patient's coping ability, typical coping mechanisms, stress level, and support system. Also, assess the patient's and family's anxiety level regarding impending surgery and the recovery process.

Diagnostic Highlights

General Comments: Note that the diagnosis of appendicitis is made by clinical evaluation with the diagnostic tests of secondary importance. Prior to radiography, complete a pregnancy test on women of childbearing years.

Test	Normal Result	Abnormality With Condition	Explanation
White blood cell (WBC) count and neutrophil count	WBC count adult males and females: 4,500–11,100/mcL; neutrophil count 40%–75%	Infection and inflammation may elevate the WBC count; 80%–85% of adults have WBC > 10,500/mcL	Leukocytosis may range from 10,500 to 16,000/mcL; neutrophil count is frequently elevated above 75%; in 10% of cases, leukocyte and differential cell counts are normal
Computed tomography of the abdomen with or without contrast	Normal appendix	Enlarged appendix with thickened walls and increased diameter	Inflammation of the appendix leads to enlargement and wall thickening

Diagnostic Highlights (continued)

Test	Normal Result	Abnormality With Condition	Explanation
C-reactive protein	< 1 mg/dL	Elevated within first 12 hr and then returns to normal	Acute-phase reactant synthesized by the liver in response to infection or inflammation

Other Tests: Complete blood cell count; abdominal ultrasonography; flat-plate abdominal x-ray; urinalysis in 25% to 40% of people with appendicitis indicates pyuria, albuminuria, and hematuria; serum electrolytes, blood urea nitrogen, and serum creatinine identify dehydration; barium enema; diagnostic laparoscopy

PRIMARY NURSING DIAGNOSIS

DIAGNOSIS. Acute pain related to inflammation as evidenced by self-report of pain, diaphoresis, tachycardia, and restlessness; Risk for infection as evidenced by fever, wound inflammation, and/or wound swelling

OUTCOMES. Comfort status; Pain control; Pain level; Symptom severity; Immune status; Knowledge: Infection management; Risk control; Risk detection

INTERVENTIONS. Analgesic administration; Anxiety reduction; Environmental management: Comfort; Pain management: Acute and chronic; Medication management; Patient-controlled analgesia assistance; Infection control; Infection protection; Medication prescribing; Surveillance; Wound care; Nutritional management; Fluid/electrolyte management

PLANNING AND IMPLEMENTATION

Collaborative

SURGICAL. Appendicitis is cured only with an appendectomy, but the path to treatment is controversial and may include IV antibiotic therapy followed by an *interval appendectomy*, which would be performed 4 weeks later. IV therapy alone can be used, but approximately 20% to 40% of those patients require an appendectomy within the following year. Both laparoscopic and open appendectomy are options depending on the patient's condition. Appendicitis is a clinical emergency. An appendectomy (surgical removal of the appendix) is the preferred method of management for acute appendicitis if the inflammation is localized. An open appendectomy is completed with a transverse right lower quadrant incision, usually at the McBurney point. A laparoscopic appendectomy may be used in uncomplicated appendicitis, females of childbearing age or who are suspected of being pregnant, those in whom the diagnosis is in question, obese patients, pediatric patients, older adult patients, and patients with perforated appendix. If the appendix has ruptured and there is evidence of peritonitis or an abscess, conservative treatment consisting of antibiotics and IV fluids is given 6 to 8 hours prior to an appendectomy. Generally, an appendectomy is performed within 24 to 48 hours after the onset of symptoms under either general or spinal anesthesia. Preoperative management includes IV hydration; antipyretics; antibiotics; and, after definitive diagnosis, analgesics. Nonsurgical treatment may be required when it is temporarily a high-risk procedure. In this situation, IV antibiotics are administered.

POSTOPERATIVE. Postoperatively, patient recovery from an appendectomy is usually uncomplicated, with hospital discharge in 24 to 48 hours (sometimes sooner depending on the technique). The development of peritonitis complicates recovery, and hospitalization may extend 5 to 7 days. The physician generally orders oral fluids and diet as tolerated within 24 to 48 hours after surgery.

Prescribed pain medications are given by IV or intramuscular route until the patient can take them orally. Antibiotics may continue postoperatively as a prophylactic measure. Ambulation is started the day of surgery or the first postoperative day.

Pharmacologic Highlights

Medication or Drug Class	Dosage	Description	Rationale
Crystalloid IV fluids	100–500 mL/hr IV depending on volume state of the patient	Isotonic solutions such as normal saline solution or lactated Ringer solution	Replace fluids and electrolytes lost through fever and vomiting; replacement continues until urine output is 1 mL/kg of body weight and electrolytes are replaced
Antibiotics (possible choices: metronidazole, gentamicin, cefotetan, cefoxitin, piperacillin, tazobactam sodium, meropenem)	Varies with drug	Broad-spectrum antibiotic coverage	Control local and systemic infection and reduce the incidence of postoperative wound infection

Other Drugs: Analgesics (Several recent research studies have shown that administering opioid analgesics such as morphine sulfate to patients with acute undifferentiated abdominal pain is safe.)

Independent

PREOPERATIVE. Preoperatively, several nursing interventions focus on promoting patient comfort. Avoid applying heat to the abdominal area, which may cause appendiceal rupture. Permit the patient to assume the position of comfort while maintaining bedrest. Reduce the patient's anxiety and fear by carefully explaining each test, what to expect, and the reasons for the tests. Answer the patient's questions concerning the impending surgery, and provide the patient with instructions regarding splinting the incision with pillows during coughing, deep breathing, and moving. Keep the patient NPO until a decision occurs about surgery.

POSTOPERATIVE. Postoperatively, assess the surgical incision for adequate wound healing. Note the color and odor of the drainage, any edema, the approximation of the wound edges, and the color of the incision. Encourage the patient to splint the incision during deep-breathing exercises. Assist the patient to maintain a healthy respiratory status by encouraging deep breathing and coughing 10 times every 1 to 2 hours for 72 hours. Turn the patient every 2 hours, and continue to monitor the breath sounds. Encourage the patient to assume a semi-Fowler position while in bed to promote lung expansion.

Evidence-Based Practice and Health Policy

Patkova, B., Svenningsson, A., Almstrom, M., Eaton, S., Wester, T., & Svensson, J. (2020). Nonoperative treatment versus appendectomy for acute nonperforated appendicitis in children: Five-year follow up of a randomized controlled pilot trial. *Annals of Surgery, 271*, 1030–1035.

- The authors proposed to evaluate the safety and feasibility of nonoperative treatment of acute nonperforated appendicitis in 50 children during 5 years of follow-up. At baseline, the children were randomized to nonoperative treatment with antibiotics or appendectomy. The primary outcome was defined as the need for a secondary intervention under anesthesia that was related to the primary diagnosis of appendicitis.
- In the appendectomy group, there were no children with treatment failure. In the nonoperative treatment group, there were 11 failures, 9 during the first year and 2 that occurred during

years 2 to 5. All patients survived and completed the 5 years of follow-up. The authors concluded that treatment with antibiotics in the intermediate term is safe, but over time, 45% of children treated nonperatively required surgery at a later time.

DOCUMENTATION GUIDELINES

- Location, intensity, frequency, and duration of pain
- Response to pain medication, ice applications, and position changes
- Patient's ability to ambulate and to tolerate food
- Appearance of abdominal incision (color, temperature, intactness, drainage) and any signs of infection

DISCHARGE AND HOME HEALTHCARE GUIDELINES

MEDICATIONS. Be sure the patient understands any pain medication prescribed, including doses, route, action, and side effects. The full course of antibiotic therapy should be completed. Make certain the patient understands that they should avoid operating a motor vehicle or heavy machinery while taking such medication.

INCISION. For open procedures, sutures are generally removed in the physician's office in 5 to 7 days. Explain the need to keep the surgical wound clean and dry. Teach the patient to observe the wound and report to the physician any increased swelling, redness, drainage, odor, or separation of the wound edges. Also instruct the patient to notify the doctor if a fever develops. The patient needs to know these may be symptoms of wound infection. Explain that the patient should avoid heavy lifting and should ask the physician about when lifting can be resumed.

COMPLICATIONS. Instruct the patient that a possible complication of appendicitis is peritonitis. Discuss with the patient symptoms that indicate peritonitis, including sharp abdominal pains, fever, nausea and vomiting, and increased pulse and respiration. The patient must know to seek medical attention immediately should these symptoms occur.

NUTRITION. Instruct the patient that diet can be advanced to their normal food pattern as long as no gastrointestinal distress is experienced.

Arterial Occlusive Disease

DRG Category:	253
Mean LOS:	5.4 days
Description:	SURGICAL: Other Vascular Procedures With Complication or Comorbidity
DRG Category:	299
Mean LOS:	5.1 days
Description:	MEDICAL: Peripheral Vascular Disorders With Major Complication or Comorbidity

Arterial occlusive disease, particularly peripheral arterial occlusive disease (PAOD), is characterized by reduced blood flow through the major blood vessels of the body because of an obstruction or narrowing of the lumen of the aorta and its major branches. More than 10% of the U.S. population older than 65 years have atherosclerosis and an estimated 4% have PAOD. These proportions will only increase as the percentage of the aging population increases. PAOD occurs because of changes in the arterial wall including the accumulation of lipids, calcium, blood components, carbohydrates, and fibrous tissue in the endothelial lining. When a person is at rest, normal blood flow to the muscles of the extremities is 300 to 400 mm/minute, but with exercise, blood flow increases 10 times the normal amount. While patients with PAOD have normal resting blood flow, blood flow to the muscles cannot increase during exercise because of arterial stenoses. Since the metabolic needs of the muscle exceed what the blood flow can deliver, the patient experiences claudication (ischemic muscle pain). Claudication occurs during physical activity such as walking and is relieved by rest. Arterial occlusive disease, which may be chronic or acute, may affect the celiac, mesenteric, innominate, subclavian, carotid, and vertebral arteries. Arterial disorders that may lead to arterial obstruction include arteriosclerosis obliterans, thromboangiitis obliterans, arterial embolism, and an aneurysm of the lower extremity. A sudden occlusion usually causes tissue ischemia and death, whereas a gradual blockage allows for the development of collateral vessels. Usually, arterial occlusive diseases are only part of a complex disease syndrome that affects the entire body. Complications include severe ischemia, skin ulceration, gangrene, leg amputation, and sepsis. In a study over 10 years of people with PAOD, approximately 10% required amputation.

CAUSES

Arteries can become occluded by atherosclerotic plaque, thrombi, or emboli. Single or multiple arterial stenoses produce reduced blood flow to the limbs. Subsequent obstruction and damage to the vessels can follow chemical or mechanical trauma and infections or inflammatory processes. Arteriosclerosis obliterans is marked by plaque formation on the intimal wall of medium-sized arteries, causing partial occlusion. In addition, there is calcification of the media and a loss of elasticity that predisposes the patient to dilation or thrombus formation. Thromboangiitis obliterans (Buerger disease), which is characterized by an inflammatory infiltration of vessel walls, develops in the small arteries and veins (hands and feet) and tends to be episodic. Risk factors include tobacco use (most important risk factor), hyperlipidemia, hypertension, diabetes mellitus, and a sedentary lifestyle.

GENETIC CONSIDERATIONS

Familial forms of arterial occlusive disease have been reported, and genetic risk factors may contribute to the various subtypes of vascular disease. A locus strongly linked to the disease has been identified on chromosome 1. On 15q24, a mutation in the *CHRNA3* gene is associated with arterial occlusive disease, along with a predisposition to nicotine dependence and lung cancer.

SEX AND LIFE SPAN CONSIDERATIONS

Thromboangiitis obliterans (Buerger disease), a causative factor for arterial occlusive disease, typically occurs in male smokers between the ages of 20 and 40 years. Arterial insufficiency usually occurs in individuals over 50 years of age and is more common in men than in women. PAOD affects 4% of people over 65 years of age in the United States.

HEALTH DISPARITIES AND SEXUAL/GENDER MINORITY HEALTH

In a study of more than 1 million patients from 11 countries including the United States, Russia, Germany, and Australia, the authors revealed striking sex differences in treatment for PAOD. Females had fewer interventions such as revascularization as compared to males, and intervention occurred when the disease was at a more advanced stage than in males (Behrendt et al., 2020). This information demonstrates important health disparities for women. In the United States, non-Hispanic Black men are more likely to be affected by PAOD than other groups. Black, Native American, and low-income persons have the highest rates of amputation in patients with PAOD compared to their White counterparts (Barnes et al., 2020). In a series of studies of Veterans Administration patient treatment files, Black and Hispanic veterans with diabetes or PAOD had higher odds of a lower extremity amputation than White patients. Experts suggest that Black and Hispanic persons are less likely to receive a second opinion or having additional diagnostic testing to determine if options other than amputation exist, creating health disparities.

Transgender is a term used to describe persons whose gender identity is different from their sex assigned at birth. Approximately 1% of the U.S. population identify themselves as transgender. Sexual and gender minority persons have higher odds for multiple chronic conditions, cancer, and poor quality of life and are more apt to have disabilities than cisgender males and females (cisgender is a term used for persons whose gender identity and gender expression are aligned with their assigned sex listed on their birth certificate). Gender-affirming hormone therapy is the use of hormone therapy for gender transition or gender affirmation and can be masculinizing or feminizing. It may also affect cardiovascular health in transgender women. In a large sample, researchers have found that transgender men and women are more likely to be overweight than cisgender women and more likely to smoke cigarettes. Compared to cisgender women, transgender women reported higher rates of diabetes, angina/coronary disease, and myocardial infarction. These factors place transgender women at risk for PAOD (Caceres, Jackman, et al., 2020).

GLOBAL HEALTH CONSIDERATIONS

Buerger disease has a high incidence in people from Southeast Asia and Jews of Ashkenazi descent.

ASSESSMENT

HISTORY. Determine the frequency and extent of weekly exercise. Elicit a history of previous illnesses or surgeries that were vascular in nature; ask if the patient has been diagnosed with arterial occlusive disease in the past. Determine if a positive family history exists for hypertension or vascular disorders in first-order relatives. Ask if the patient smokes cigarettes; eats a diet high in fats; leads a sedentary lifestyle; or is subject to emotional stress, anxiety, or ulcers. Determine if the patient has experienced any pain, swelling, redness, or pallor. Establish a history of signs and symptoms that may point to the site of occlusion. Determine if the patient has experienced any transient ischemic attacks (TIAs) because of reduced cerebral circulation. Elicit a history of such signs and symptoms as unilateral sensory or motor dysfunction, difficulty in speaking (aphasia), confusion, difficulty with concentration, or headaches, all of which are signs of possible carotid artery involvement. Ask if the patient has experienced signs of vertebrobasilar artery involvement, such as binocular visual disturbances, vertigo, dysarthria, or episodes of falling down. Determine if the patient has experienced lameness in the right arm (claudication), which is a sign of possible innominate artery involvement.

The specific finding in PAOD is **intermittent claudication**. The **pain** is insidious in onset, **occurring with exercise and relieved by resting for 2 to 5 minutes**; determining how much physical activity is needed before the onset of pain is crucial. The onset of pain is often related to a particular walking distance in terms of street blocks, which helps to quantify patients with some standard measure of walking distance before and after therapy.

Determine if the patient's mesenteric artery is involved by asking if the patient has experienced acute abdominal pain, nausea, vomiting, or diarrhea. Ask the patient if they have experienced numbness, tingling (paresthesia), paralysis, muscle weakness, or sudden pain in both legs, which are all signs of aortic bifurcation occlusion. Determine if the patient has experienced sporadic claudication of the lower back, buttocks, and thighs or impotence in male patients, all of which are indicators of iliac artery occlusion. Elicit a history of sporadic claudication of the patient's calves after exertion; ask if the patient has experienced pain in the feet—these are signs of femoral and popliteal artery involvement.

PHYSICAL EXAMINATION. Observe both legs, noting alterations in color or temperature of the affected limb. Cold, pale legs may suggest aortic bifurcation occlusion. Inspect the patient's legs for signs of cyanosis, ulcers, or gangrene. Limb perfusion may be inadequate, resulting in thickened and opaque nails, shiny and atrophic skin, decreased hair growth, dry or fissured heels, and loss of subcutaneous tissue in the digits. Check the patient's skin on a daily basis.

The most important part of the examination is palpation of the peripheral pulses. Absence of a normally palpable pulse is the most reliable sign of occlusive disease. Comparison of pulses in both extremities is helpful. Ascertain, also, whether the arterial wall is palpable, tortuous, or calcified. Auscultation over the main arteries is useful, as a bruit (sound produced by turbulent flow of blood through an irregular or stenotic lumen) often indicates an atheromatous plaque. A bruit over the right side of the neck is a possible indication of innominate artery involvement.

PSYCHOSOCIAL. Occlusive diseases are chronic or lead to chronic illness. They are usually slow in onset, and much irreversible vascular damage may have occurred before symptoms are severe enough to bring the patient for treatment. Treatment is often long and tedious and brings additional concerns regarding finances, curtailment of usual social outlets, and innumerable other problems. Assess the patient's ability to cope with a chronic illness.

Diagnostic Highlights

Test	Normal Result	Abnormality With Condition	Explanation
Angiography of the peripheral artery system	Normal blood flow to the peripheral arteries of the legs	Stenosis in vascular segments of aorta or lower limb arteries	Identifies location and degree of occlusion in peripheral arteries; usually completed before an endovascular or open surgery is performed
Ultrasound arteriography (Duplex or Doppler ultrasonography)	Negative for presence of aneurysm or atherosclerosis or thrombus; normal blood flow velocity	Narrowed lumen, reduced blood velocity, or both	Reflects the velocity of blood flowing in the underlying vessel, structure, and size
Segmental arterial pressure monitoring	Blood pressure readings in thigh, calf, and ankle are higher than in upper extremities (10 to 20 mm Hg) because of augmentation of the pressure wave as it moves distally from the heart	Blood pressure readings in thigh, calf, and ankle are lower than in upper extremities with the presence of arterial disease	Simultaneous sphygmomanometer readings of systolic pressure placed on the extremities to measure pressure differences between upper and lower and between like extremities
Ankle-brachial index (ABI)	Ratio of the systolic blood pressure at the ankle to the systolic blood pressure in the arm; normal ABI = 0.9–1.1	ABI < 0.9	PAOD reduces arterial blood flow to the extremities

Other Tests: Magnetic resonance angiography, computerized tomographic angiography, plethysmography, ophthalmodynamometry, digital vascular imaging, exercise testing, magnetic resonance imaging

PRIMARY NURSING DIAGNOSIS

DIAGNOSIS. Chronic pain related to narrowing of the peripheral arteries as evidenced by self-reported leg discomfort with physical activity

OUTCOMES. Pain control; Pain: Disruptive effects; Pain level; Knowledge: Peripheral artery disease management; Circulation status; Comfort status; Tissue perfusion: Peripheral; Medication response; Smoking cessation behavior

INTERVENTIONS. Pain management: Chronic; Medication administration; Medication management; Health education; Exercise promotion; Smoking cessation assistance

PLANNING AND IMPLEMENTATION

Collaborative

MEDICAL. Treatment is primarily medical and focuses on slowing the progression of disease and managing the symptoms. Smoking cessation is viewed by experts as the most rapid methods of stopping the progression of PAOD. Generally medications are prescribed to reduce pain and blood clots. Regular exercise is thought to condition muscles and increase collateral vessel formation.

SURGICAL. Surgery is indicated for patients who have advanced arterial disease or for those with severe pain that impairs activities. Surgical procedures include embolectomy, angioplasty, and sympathectomy. Endovascular therapy, with procedures such as stents, balloons, or atherectomy devices, have become more common than open bypass surgeries and amputation for people with PAOD. When lower extremity arterial bypass is performed, the diseased femoropopliteal segment can be bypassed with a synthetic prosthetic material (Teflon or Dacron), or autogenous vein graft, such as with the saphenous vein, can be performed. Care following femoropopliteal bypass is the same as for other arterial surgery.

PERIOPERATIVE CARE. In the preoperative stage, assess the patient's circulatory status by observing skin color and temperature and checking peripheral pulses. Provide analgesia as needed. Use an infusion monitor or pump to administer heparin intravenously. Note any signs of cerebrovascular accident, such as periodic blindness or numbness in a limb.

Pharmacologic Highlights

Medication or Drug Class	Dosage	Description	Rationale
Aspirin	80–325 mg	Antiplatelet	Inhibits prostaglandin synthesis, which prevents formation of platelet-aggregating thromboxane A2
Simvastatin	5–40 mg po QD in evening	Antilipemic agent	Lowers blood cholesterol, thereby reducing risk of vascular events

Other Drugs: Intermittent claudication caused by chronic arterial occlusive disease may be treated with pentoxifylline (Trental), which can improve blood flow through the capillaries by increasing red blood cell flexibility. Antiplatelet agents: dipyridamole, ticlopidine, clopidogrel bisulfate (Plavix), cilostazol (Pletal). Anticoagulant: enoxaparin sodium (Lovenox).

Independent

PREVENTION AND TEACHING. Emphasize to the patient the need to quit smoking or using tobacco and limit caffeine intake. Recommend maintaining a warm environmental temperature of about 70°F (21°C) to prevent chilling. Teach the patient to avoid elevating the legs or using the knee gatch (knee elevation) on the bed to keep legs in a slightly dependent position for periods during the day, to avoid crossing the legs at the knees or ankles, and to wear support stockings. Explain why the patient needs to avoid pressure and vigorous massage on the affected extremity, and recommend the use of padding for ischemic areas.

Stress the importance of regular aerobic exercise to the patient. Explain that activity improves circulation through muscle contraction and relaxation. Exercise also stimulates collateral circulation that increases blood flow to the ischemic area. Recommend 30 to 40 minutes of activity, with warm-up and cool-down activities, on alternate days. Also suggest walking at a slow pace and performing ankle rotations, ankle pumps, and knee extensions daily. Recommend Buerger–Allen exercises if indicated. If intermittent claudication is present, stress to the patient the importance of allowing adequate time for rest between exercise and of monitoring one's tolerance for exercise.

Provide good skin care, and teach the patient to monitor and protect the skin. Recommend the use of moisturizing lotion for dry areas, and demonstrate meticulous foot care. Advise the patient to wear cotton socks and comfortable, protective shoes at all times and to change socks daily. Advise the patient to seek professional advice for thickened or deformed nails, blisters, corns, and calluses. Stress the importance of avoiding the application of direct heat to the skin. The patient also needs to know that arterial disorders are usually chronic. Medical follow-up is necessary at the onset of skin breakdown such as abrasions, lesions, or ulcerations to prevent advanced disease with necrosis.

Evidence-Based Practice and Health Policy

Calanca, L., Lanzi, S., Ney, B., Berchtold, A., & Mazzolai, L. (2020). Multimodal supervised exercise significantly improves walking performances without changing hemodynamic parameters in patients with symptomatic lower extremity peripheral artery disease. *Vascular and Endovascular Surgery, 54*, 605–611.

• The authors evaluated the outcome of supervised exercise training on walking performance and cardiac outcomes in 85 patients with symptomatic peripheral artery disease. The walking program consisted of 36 sessions of 30 to 50 minutes each over a 3-month period under the supervision of an exercise physiologist. The primary method of exercise was using Nordic walking with poles (the study was done in Switzerland).
• Most hemodynamic parameters did not change at the end of the program, nor did body mass index. Walking performance improved in patients with lower extremity peripheral artery disease. Quality of life improved in the areas of physical functioning, social functioning, general mental health, and vitality.

DOCUMENTATION GUIDELINES

• Physical findings: Presence of redness, pallor, skin temperature, peripheral pulses, trophic changes, asymmetrical changes in pulse quality, capillary blanch, condition of skin
• Neurological deficits: Tenderness to touch, lameness, sensory or motor dysfunction
• Response to balanced activity: Lameness, pain, level of activity that produces pain
• Presence of complications: Infection, ulcers, gangrene, loss pulses
• Adherence to the rehabilitation program: Attitude toward exercise, changes in symptoms as response to exercise

DISCHARGE AND HOME HEALTHCARE GUIDELINES

PREVENTION. To prevent arterial occlusive disease from progressing, teach the patient to decrease as many risk factors as possible. Quitting cigarette smoking and tobacco use is of utmost importance and may be the most difficult lifestyle change. Behavior modification techniques and support groups may be of assistance with lifestyle changes.

MEDICATIONS. Be sure the patient understands all medications, including the dosage, route, action, adverse effects, and need for routine laboratory monitoring for anticoagulants.

ADHERENCE TO THE REHABILITATION PROGRAM. Ensure that the patient understands that the condition is chronic and not curable. Stress the importance of adhering to a balanced exercise program, using measures to prevent trauma and reduce stress. Include the patient's family in the plans.

Asthma

DRG Category:	202
Mean LOS:	3.7 days
Description:	MEDICAL: Bronchitis and Asthma With Complication or Comorbidity or Major Complication or Comorbidity

Asthma is classified as an intermittent, reversible, obstructive disease of the lungs. It is a growing health problem in the United States, with approximately 25 million people affected. In the past 20 years, the number of children with asthma has increased markedly, and it is now the leading serious chronic illness in children. Unfortunately, approximately 75% of children with asthma continue to have chronic problems in adulthood. The total deaths annually from asthma have increased by over 100% since 1979 in the United States.

Asthma is a disease of the airways characterized by airway inflammation and hyperreactivity (increased responsiveness to a wide variety of triggers). Hyperreactivity leads to airway obstruction due to acute onset of muscle spasm in the smooth muscle of the tracheobronchial tree, thereby leading to a narrowed lumen. In addition to muscle spasm, there is swelling of the mucosa, which leads to edema. Although asthma can result from infections (especially viral) and inhaled irritants, it often is the result of an allergic response. An allergen (antigen) is introduced to the body, and sensitizing antibodies such as immunoglobulin E (IgE) are formed. IgE antibodies bind to tissue mast cells and basophils in the mucosa of the bronchioles, lung tissue, and nasopharynx. An antigen–antibody reaction releases primary mediator substances such as histamine, slow-reacting substance of anaphylaxis (SRS-A), and others. These mediators cause contraction of the smooth muscle and tissue edema. In addition, goblet cells secrete a thick mucus into the airways that causes obstruction. Intrinsic asthma results from all other causes except allergies, such as infections (especially viral), inhaled irritants, and other causes or etiologies. The parasympathetic nervous system becomes stimulated, which increases bronchomotor tone, resulting in bronchoconstriction.

In asthma, the total lung capacity (TLC), functional residual capacity (FRC), and residual volume (RV) increase, but the hallmark of airway obstruction is a reduction in ratio of the forced expiratory volume in 1 second (FEV1) to the forced vital capacity (FVC). Complications include pneumonia, atelectasis, respiratory failure with hypoxemia, and status asthmaticus (severe and refractory asthma). The classification for asthma is described in Table 1.

• TABLE 1 Classification of Asthma

CLASSIFICATION	DESCRIPTION
Mild intermittent	• Less than twice a week: Cough, wheeze, chest tightness, difficulty breathing • Brief flare-ups with varying intensity; no symptoms between flare-ups • Less than twice a month: Nighttime symptoms • Lung function tests: FEV1 ≥ 80% normal values; peak flow < 20% variability a.m. to a.m. or a.m. to p.m., day to day
Mild persistent	• Three to six times a week: Cough, wheeze, chest tightness, difficulty breathing • Flare-ups may affect activity level • Three to four times a month: Nighttime symptoms • Lung function tests: FEV1 ≥ 80% normal values; peak flow < 20%–30% variability a.m. to a.m. or a.m. to p.m., day to day
Moderate persistent	• Daily: Cough, wheeze, chest tightness, difficulty breathing affecting activity level; symptoms may last for days • Flare-ups may affect activity level • Five or more times a month: Nighttime symptoms • Lung function tests: FEV1 > 60% but < 80% normal values; peak flow > 30% variability a.m. to a.m. or a.m. to p.m., day to day
Severe persistent	• Continual: Cough, wheeze, chest tightness, difficulty breathing that limits activity level • Frequently: Nighttime symptoms • Lung function tests: FEV1 ≤ 60% normal values; peak flow > 30% variability a.m. to a.m. or a.m. to p.m., day to day

CAUSES

The main triggers for asthma are allergies, viral infections, autonomic nervous system imbalances that can cause an increase in parasympathetic stimulation, medications, psychological factors, and exercise. Of asthmatic conditions in patients under 30 years old, 70% are caused by allergies. Three major indoor allergens are dust mites, cockroaches, and cats. In older patients, the cause is almost always nonallergic types of irritants, such as smog. Heredity plays a part in about one-third of the cases.

GENETIC CONSIDERATIONS

The genetic contributions to the development of asthma have been estimated at between 30% and 50% for various asthma phenotypes, and up to 70% for overall IgE levels in plasma. Familial factors thus far appear to be inherited in an autosomal dominant pattern. There are at least 11 candidate genes that contribute to asthma susceptibility. These include *PTGDR*, *GPRA*, *IRAK3*, *CHI3L1*, *HNMT*, *ADRB2*, *IL13*, *SCGB3A2*, *TNF*, *HLA-G*, and *PLA2G7*.

SEX AND LIFE SPAN CONSIDERATIONS

Although the incidence of asthma is estimated at 5% to 10% in the general population, children have a higher incidence of 12%. Children make up one-third of the people with asthma; in the United States, 7 million children are affected, and trends suggest an increasing incidence of asthma in children under the age of 6 years. Asthma is diagnosed more frequently in males under 14 years and over 45 years of age and in females between the ages of 15 and 45 years. Most experts agree that environmental factors play a more important role in asthma etiology than do genetic factors. Approximately 80% to 85% of childhood asthma episodes are associated with a prior exposure to a virus.

HEALTH DISPARITIES AND SEXUAL/GENDER MINORITY HEALTH

The Asthma and Allergy Foundation of America (2020) has written extensively about asthma disparities in the United States. The burden of asthma falls disproportionately on Black, Hispanic, and Native American persons. People from Puerto Rico are two times more likely than White persons to have asthma. Black persons are 1.5 times more likely than White persons to have asthma and are three times more likely to die from asthma than White persons. Black women have the highest death rate from asthma of all groups, and Black children have higher morbidity and mortality rates than White children. Disparities in asthma result from complex factors such as structural determinants (racism, discrimination), social determinants (education, income, neighborhood), biological determinants (ancestry), and behavioral determinants (tobacco use and medication adherence).

Asthma disparities also occur in gender and sexual minority persons. In a study of more than 300,000 youths, scientists found that lesbian, gay, and bisexual youths were more likely to have been diagnosed with asthma compared to heterosexual youth (Curry et al., 2020). Asthma disparities are perpetuated because sexual minority youth receive poor quality of care due to stigma, lack of healthcare providers' awareness, and insensitivity to the unique needs of this community.

GLOBAL HEALTH CONSIDERATIONS

Asthma prevalence varies widely across many countries, with a range from 1% to over 30% in children. Approximately 300 million people globally have asthma, and the prevalence increases by 50% every 10 years. Prevalence is high in developed countries in North America, Europe, and Australia and is increasing in developing countries as they become more industrialized. Examples include increases in South Africa, Eastern Europe, and the Baltic states. The greatest increases are seen in children. The more urbanization and affluence in a country, the higher is the prevalence.

ASSESSMENT

HISTORY. Because patients (especially children) with asthma have a history of allergies, obtain a thorough description of the response to allergens or other irritants. The patient may describe a sudden onset of symptoms after exposure, with a sense of suffocation. Symptoms include dyspnea, wheezing, and a cough (either dry or productive) and also chest tightness, restlessness, anxiety, and a prolonged expiratory phase. Ask if the patient has experienced a recent viral infection. Determine the speed of onset of symptoms, the number of asthma attacks in the past year, and the number of emergency department visits and hospitalizations from asthma in the past year. Children with an impending asthma attack may have been vomiting because of the tendency to swallow coughed up mucus rather than expectorating it.

PHYSICAL EXAMINATION. The most common symptoms are **wheezing, coughing, shortness of breath**, and **chest tightness**. The patient with an acute attack of asthma appears ill, with shortness of breath so severe that they can hardly speak. In acute airway obstruction, patients use their accessory muscles for breathing and are often profoundly diaphoretic. Some patients have an increased anteroposterior thoracic diameter. Children with asthma often prefer standing or sitting leaning forward to ease breathing. As airway obstruction becomes more serious, children may develop sternocleidomastoid contractions that indicate an increased expiratory effort, supraclavicular contractions that indicate an increased expiratory effort, and nasal flaring. If the patient has marked color changes such as pallor or cyanosis or becomes confused, restless, or lethargic, respiratory failure may be on the horizon. Percussion of the lungs usually produces hyperresonance, and palpation may reveal vocal fremitus. Auscultation reveals high-pitched inspiratory and expiratory wheezes, but with a major airway obstruction, breath sounds may be diminished. As the obstruction improves, breath sounds may actually worsen as they can be auscultated throughout the lung fields. During the most severe attacks of asthma, wheezing may be absent because of severe reduction of airflow, or its absence. Usually, the patient also has a prolonged expiratory phase of respiration. A rapid heart rate, mild systolic hypertension, and a paradoxic pulse may also be present.

PSYCHOSOCIAL. The emergency situation and an unfamiliar environment can aggravate the symptoms of the disease, especially if this is the patient's first experience with the condition. If the patient is a child and the parent is anxious, the child's level of anxiety increases and the attack may worsen.

Diagnostic Highlights

Test	Normal Result	Abnormality With Condition	Explanation
FVC: Maximum volume of air that can be forcefully expired after a maximal lung inspiration	4.0 L	Decreased	Airway obstruction decreases flow rates
FEV1: Volume of air expired in 1 second from the beginning of the FVC maneuver	3.0 L	Decreased	Airway obstruction decreases flow rates; hospitalization is recommended if FVC is less than 1 L; FEV1/FVC should be 80% normally, but in asthma, it decreases to as low as 25%
Forced expiratory flow (FEF): Maximal flow rate attained during the middle (25%–75%) of FVC maneuver	Varies by body size	Decreased	Predicts obstruction of smaller airways
RV: Volume of air remaining in lungs at end of a maximal expiration	1.2 L	Increased up to 400% normal	Increased RV indicates obstruction; may remain increased for up to 3 weeks after the attack
FRC: Volume of air remaining in lungs at end of a resting tidal volume	2.3 L	Increased up to 200%	Increased FRC indicates air trapping

Other Tests: Chest x-ray, high-resolution computed tomography (for chronic symptoms), skin testing, pulse oximetry, arterial blood gases, ECG, serum IgE. Peak expiratory flow rates (maximal flow rate attained during the FVC maneuver; decreased from baseline during periods of obstruction) may be used at home daily for patients who require daily medications. When the airways are inflamed, a nitric oxide test may show increased nitric oxide levels. Metacholine challenge is used if the initial lung function test is normal as it is a known asthma trigger and causes airway narrowing.

PRIMARY NURSING DIAGNOSIS

DIAGNOSIS. Ineffective airway clearance related to obstruction from narrowed lumen and thick mucus as evidenced by shortness of breath, wheezing, and/or chest tightness

OUTCOMES. Respiratory status: Airway patency, gas exchange, and ventilation; Symptom severity; Knowledge: Asthma management; Medication response; Comfort status

INTERVENTIONS. Asthma management; Medication administration: Inhalation; Airway management; Anxiety reduction; Oxygen therapy; Airway insertion and stabilization; Cough enhancement; Mechanical ventilation: Invasive and noninvasive; Positioning; Respiratory monitoring

☀ PLANNING AND IMPLEMENTATION

Collaborative

For all but the most seriously ill patients, the primary goal is to prevent symptoms and reduce adverse events when acute episodes occur. Airway obstruction is generally managed with quick relief medications such as short-acting bronchodilators, systemic corticosteroids, and ipratropium (Atrovent). During severe exacerbations, patients may require IV fluid replacement. Unless contraindicated by a cardiac problem, 3,000 to 4,000 mL/day of fluid is usually administered intravenously, which helps loosen secretions and facilitates expectoration of the secretions. Low-flow oxygen therapy based on arterial blood gas results is often administered to treat hypoxemia. For the patient with increasing airway obstruction, endotracheal intubation and perhaps mechanical ventilation may be needed to maintain adequate airway and breathing. Close follow-up is needed when patients are discharged from the hospital because airway hyperactivity usually persists for 4 to 6 weeks after the event. To prevent symptoms, long-term control medications such as inhaled corticosteroids, inhaled cromolyn, long-acting bronchodilators, theophylline, leukotriene modifiers, and anti-IgE antibodies are used.

The National Institutes of Health (NIH, 2020) has developed a stepwise approach for managing asthma for children organized by age with preferred and alternative plans depending on asthma severity, from low to high. For example, the preferred recommendations for children 0 to 4 years of age follows: Step 1 is short-acting beta agonists (SABAs) as needed. Step 2 is low-dose inhaled corticosteroids (ICSs). Step 3 is medium-dose ICSs. Step 4 is medium-dose ICSs and either long-acting beta agonists (LABAs) or montelukast. Step 5 is high dose ICS and either LABA or montelukast. Other directions include to Step Up if needed and reassess in 2 to 6 weeks. Also Step Down if possible (if asthma is well controlled for at least 3 consecutive months). The recommendation is also to consult with an asthma specialist if step 4 or higher is required, and to consider consultation at step 3. Control assessment is a key element of asthma care, involving both impairment and risk. Use of objective measures, self-reported control, and healthcare utilization are complementary and should be employed on an ongoing basis, depending on the individual's clinical situation. NIH also recommends patient education and environmental control at each step.

Pharmacologic Highlights

Medication or Drug Class	Dosage	Description	Rationale
Bronchodilators	Varies by drug	Inhaled beta$_2$-adrenergic agonists by metered-dose inhaler (MDI); albuterol sulfate, pirbuterol acetate, levalbuterol	Reversal of airflow obstruction; relieve reversible bronchospasm by relaxing bronchial smooth muscles; used to treat bronchospasm in acute asthmatic episodes; used to prevent bronchospasm associated with exercise-induced asthma or nocturnal asthma

(highlight box continues on page 142)

Pharmacologic Highlights (continued)

Medication or Drug Class	Dosage	Description	Rationale
Systemic and inhaled corticosteroids	Varies by drug	Methylprednisolone IV; prednisone PO; inhaled corticosteroids (ciclesonide, beclomethasone, fluticasone, budesonide, mometasone)	Decrease inflammatory response; ideal dose is not defined well, but desired outcome is to speed recovery and limit symptoms
Leukotriene antagonists	Varies by drug	Montelukast 10 mg PO daily; zafirlukast 20 mg PO daily	Inhibits leukotrienes, fatty acids that mediate inflammation, from binding to airway smooth muscle cells; prevents rather than reduces symptoms; used for long-term prevention

Other Drugs: Xanthines, such as theophylline, have been used successfully in treating chronic severe steroid-dependent asthmatics. They must be used regularly and not for sudden breathing difficulties to be most effective. Cromolyn sodium decreases bronchospasm, but it is not effective for acute bronchospasms and is used as a preventive measure.

Independent

Maintenance of airway, breathing, and circulation is the primary consideration during an acute attack. Patients should be on bedrest to minimize their oxygen consumption and to decrease the work of breathing. Note that patients usually assume a position to ease breathing; some patients breathe more easily while sitting in an upright position: Do not impose bedrest on a patient who can breathe only in another position. Ask questions that can be answered by nodding or a brief one-word answer so the patient can conserve energy for breathing. If the patient is a child, allow the parents to stay with the child during acute attacks. Have the parents identify a security item that reassures the child, such as a special blanket or toy, and keep the item with the child at all times. Reinforce coping strategies to the parents, and allow them to express any feelings of guilt and helplessness.

For strategies to prevent future attacks, discuss triggers that can induce asthma attacks and ways to avoid them. If the attack is triggered by an allergen, explore with the patient or family the source and discuss possible strategies for eliminating it. Cold air and exercise may increase symptoms. Aspirin and NSAIDs can cause sudden, severe airway obstruction.

Outline the signs and symptoms that require immediate attention. Instruct the patient to notify the physician should they develop a respiratory infection that could trigger an attack. Instruct patients regarding their medications, particularly MDIs, and the indications for use. It is important that the patient uses the bronchodilator MDIs first and then uses the steroid inhalers. Explain to patients on steroid inhalers the need to rinse their mouths out after using them to avoid getting thrush.

Evidence-Based Practice and Health Policy

Wang, L., Timmer, S., & Rosenman, K. (2020). Assessment of a university-based outpatient asthma education program for children. *Journal of Pediatric Health Care, 34,* 128–135.

• The purpose of this randomized intervention/control quality improvement project was to compare outcomes before and after patients and families were offered a home visit to assess environmental asthma triggers. Outcomes number included clinic and/or urgent care visits, emergency department visits, hospitalization, and spirometry results. Of 901 eligible pediatric patients, 458 were randomized to the control and 443 to the intervention groups.

• Of the 443 patients in the control group, 271 received the educational intervention. Only 27 families allowed a home visit, which consisted of education on pathophysiology, self-management techniques, modifications of triggers, and proper use of medications. The results demonstrated a decrease in acute care services after asthma education, but it is important to note only 10% of the intervention group permitted home visitations.

DOCUMENTATION GUIDELINES

• Respiratory status: Patency of airway, auscultation of the lungs, presence or absence of adventitious breath sounds, respiratory rate and depth
• Response to medications, oxygen therapy, hydration, bedrest
• Presence of complications: Respiratory failure, pneumonia

DISCHARGE AND HOME HEALTHCARE GUIDELINES

PATIENT TEACHING. To prevent asthma attacks, teach patients the triggers that can precipitate an attack. In rare instances, asthma can lead to respiratory failure if patients are not treated immediately or are unresponsive to treatment (status asthmaticus). Explain that any dyspnea unrelieved by medications and accompanied by wheezing and accessory muscle use needs prompt attention from a healthcare provider. Encourage patients to identify and avoid things that make their asthma worse and to keep track of their symptoms. The NIH provides excellent information for patient and families about asthma: https://www.nhlbi.nih.gov /health-topics/asthma.

MEDICATIONS. Teach the patient and family the correct use of medications, including the dosage, route, action, and side effects. Provide instructions about the proper use of MDIs. Note that many patients use complementary and alternative medications (CAMs) for asthma or do not use their prescribed dose of medication. Assess the patient's use of CAM therapy and discuss with the patient the long-term consequences.

Atelectasis

DRG Category:	205
Mean LOS:	5.5 days
Description:	MEDICAL: Other Respiratory System Diagnoses With Major Complication or Comorbidity

Atelectasis means "incomplete expansion" (from the Greek words *ateles* and *ektasis*) and is defined as the collapse of lung tissue because of airway obstruction, an abnormal breathing pattern, or compression of the lung tissue. Obstructive atelectasis is the most common type. When the airway becomes completely obstructed, the gas distal to the obstruction becomes absorbed into the pulmonary circulation and the lung collapses. When gas is removed from portions of the lungs, unoxygenated blood passes unchanged through capillaries (a process called *shunting*), and hypoxemia results.

The obstruction, which occurs at the level of the larger or smaller bronchus, can be caused by a foreign body, a tumor, or mucous plugging. When the obstruction is removed, the lungs return to normal unless infection persists.

Nonobstructive atelectasis is caused by loss of contact between the parietal and the visceral pleurae, as well as compression, loss of surfactant, and replacement of parenchymal tissue by scarring or infiltrative disease. Pleural effusions, pneumothorax, blunt trauma, and acute respiratory distress syndrome all are nonobstructive conditions. Abnormal breathing patterns, such as hypoventilation following surgical procedures, can also lead to atelectasis. In such cases, the lung does not fully expand, which causes the lower airways to collapse. Complications of atelectasis include pneumonia and sepsis, bronchiectasis, hypoxemia, pleural effusion, and empyema.

CAUSES

Atelectasis occurs most frequently after surgery and is a major concern for acute care nurses. Patients with abdominal and/or thoracic surgery are the most susceptible, especially in the older age group. The duration of the surgery is also a risk factor. Patients in surgery for more than 4 hours have a 50% incidence of severe atelectasis, compared with a 19% incidence for those in surgery for 2 hours. Other causes of atelectasis are mucous plugs in patients who smoke heavily and inflammation from inflammatory lung disease. Atelectasis also occurs in patients with central nervous system depression following a drug overdose or a critical cerebral event, such as a cerebrovascular accident.

GENETIC CONSIDERATIONS

Atelectasis may be seen as a feature of a number of inherited disorders with pulmonary components, including cystic fibrosis.

SEX AND LIFE SPAN CONSIDERATIONS

Premature infants with idiopathic respiratory distress syndrome develop atelectasis. Atelectasis, however, can occur at any age and equally in men and women. It can occur with a complete obstruction of the lung because of a foreign object, although foreign body aspiration is more common in children under age 4 years than in adults. Generally, however, atelectasis occurs most often in older adults because the aging lung is less compliant.

HEALTH DISPARITIES AND SEXUAL/GENDER MINORITY HEALTH

Ethnicity, race, and sexual/gender minority status have no known effect on the risk for atelectasis.

GLOBAL HEALTH CONSIDERATIONS

While atelectasis occurs around the world, no data are available on incidence.

ASSESSMENT

HISTORY. Assess the patient for such preoperative risk factors as obesity, preexisting respiratory problems, and smoking. Determine if the patient has been febrile since the procedure. Because surgical patients are at risk, be alert for components of the postoperative history that may contribute to atelectasis: a decrease in total lung volume because of pain and splinting, changes in breathing patterns from incisional discomfort or medications, advanced age, and a need for an increased fraction of inspired oxygen (FIO_2). Other factors include use of narcotic analgesics that depress the respiratory drive, immobility, a decrease in consciousness, muscular weakness, hypotension, sepsis, and use of a nasogastric tube.

PHYSICAL EXAMINATION. The patient may appear asymptomatic if small areas of the lung are involved, or they may appear acutely ill with **extreme shortness of breath with pain on the affected side**, fever, clinical signs of oxygen deficit such as **confusion, agitation, rapid heart rate**, and even combative behavior when large areas are affected. Suprasternal, substernal, and intercostal retractions may be present, depending on the severity of atelectasis. Percussion reveals a dullness over the affected lung area. When the patient's breath sounds are auscultated, you may hear decreased breath sounds or even find breath sounds to be absent. In addition, many patients have fine, late inspiratory crackles and coarse crackles or wheezes with airway obstruction.

PSYCHOSOCIAL. The patient with atelectasis may be very anxious if breathing becomes too difficult. If the atelectasis is a result of foreign body aspiration by a child, the parents may be upset and guilty. Determine the patient's and family's ability to cope with the stressful situation.

Diagnostic Highlights

Test	Normal Result	Abnormality With Condition	Explanation
Chest x-ray or computed tomography	Clear lung fields	Areas of increased density at the site of alveolar collapse	Air-filled lungs are radiolucent (x-rays pass through tissue, which appears as a dark area), but collapsed areas appear more dense. Findings may occur on the second day after the occurrence of atelectasis.

Other Tests: Pulmonary function tests (PFTs), arterial blood gases (ABGs), fiberoptic bronchoscopy

PRIMARY NURSING DIAGNOSIS

DIAGNOSIS. Ineffective airway clearance related to obstruction and lung collapse as evidenced by shortness of breath, pain, and/or fever

OUTCOMES. Respiratory status: Gas exchange and ventilation; Symptom control; Infection severity; Comfort status: Physical; Rest

INTERVENTIONS. Airway management; Anxiety reduction; Oxygen therapy; Airway suctioning; Airway insertion and stabilization; Airway management; Cough enhancement; Positioning; Respiratory monitoring

PLANNING AND IMPLEMENTATION

Collaborative

Prevention of postoperative atelectasis is the ultimate goal, which can be met through pain control, early ambulation, adequate fluid intake, coughing and deep-breathing protocols, and the use of incentive spirometry. Patients in pain, especially following abdominal and thoracic surgery, tend to breathe shallowly to decrease their discomfort. Pain medications allow them to breathe more deeply and expand their lungs. Use caution in overmedicating patients, however, because that will reduce respiratory excursion. In the immediate postoperative period, narcotic analgesia is often prescribed because it is readily reversible by naloxone (Narcan).

Incentive spirometry, chest percussion and vibration, and postural drainage may be prescribed by the physician to increase gas exchange and to decrease the risk of atelectasis. Oxygen may be delivered with humidification to improve clearance of mucus. Nebulized bronchodilators and humidity may help liquefy secretions and promote easy removal. If atelectasis lasts more than 24 hours, flexible fiberoptic bronchoscopy will likely be used. If atelectasis persists and hypoxemia becomes life-threatening, noninvasive ventilation or endotracheal intubation and mechanical ventilation with positive-pressure ventilation and positive end-expiratory pressure (PEEP) may be necessary, but these aggressive therapies are usually not needed.

Pharmacologic Highlights

Medication or Drug Class	Dosage	Description	Rationale
Bronchodilators such as albuterol, metaproterenol	Varies with drug	Beta$_2$ agonists	Dilate bronchioles, stimulate cilia, facilitate in removal of secretions

Other: Broad-spectrum antibiotics (cefuroxime, cefaclor) to treat an underlying infection

Independent

Instruct the preoperative patient on coughing and deep-breathing exercises before incisional pain makes learning difficult. Teach the patient breathing exercises, such as pursed-lip breathing and abdominal breathing, to expand the lungs. As soon as the patient is awake and alert after surgery, with a patent airway and adequate breathing, encourage the patient to cough and breathe deeply to help expand the lung. If the patient has abdominal or thoracic incisions, use a pillow to splint the incision to reduce discomfort during breathing exercises. Encourage the patient to use the incentive spirometer at the bedside every 2 hours when the patient is awake. Determine the patient's appropriate level of hydration to ensure liquidation of secretions.

Encourage the patient to ambulate as soon as possible to reduce complications of immobility, which cause retention of secretions and decreased lung volumes. Seating the patient upright allows the patient to breathe more deeply because the lungs can expand better. Turn patients on bedrest at least every 2 hours.

Encourage patients who can expectorate secretions to cough; place a paper bag on the side rails of the bed for sanitary tissue disposal. If the patient is not on fluid restriction, explain that the patient should drink at least 2 to 3 L of fluid a day to liquefy secretions. If the patient is unresponsive, suction the patient endotracheally to remove sputum and to stimulate coughing.

If a child has developed atelectasis because of foreign body obstruction, teach the parents to maintain a safe environment. The most commonly aspirated objects are safety pins and hard foods such as corn, raisins, and peanuts. Parents should not allow children to run or walk while eating because activity predisposes the child to aspiration. Teach the patient and family to evaluate all toys for removable parts; explain that coins are commonly aspirated and should not be given to children. Explain to parents that they should not allow a young child to play with baby powder during diaper changes because if the top is altered and powder spills onto the child's face, the child can inhale it.

Evidence-Based Practice and Health Policy

Sagar, A., Sabath, B., Eapen, G., Song, J., Marcoux, M., Sarkiss, M., Arain, M., Grosu, H., Ost, D., Jimenez, C., & Casal, R. (2020). Incidence and location of atelectasis developed during bronchoscopy under general anesthesia: The I-LOCATE trial. *CHEST, 158,* 2658–2666.

- The authors determined the incidence, anatomic location, and risk factors for developing atelectasis during bronchoscopy under general anesthesia. In 57 patients, they captured images in the right and left bronchi and categorized them as either being aerated lung (snowstorm pattern) or nonaerated (atelectatic pattern). They evaluated eight lung segments.
- Fifty-one patients (89%) had atelectasis in at least one lung segment. Forty-five patients (79%) had atelectasis in at least three segments, 41 patients (72%) had atelectasis in four segments, 33 patients (58%) had atelectasis in five segments, and 18 patients (32%) had atelectasis in at

least six segments. The authors concluded that the incidence of atelectasis during bronchoscopy under general anesthesia in dependent lung zones is high. Risk factors were prolonged time under anesthesia and increased body mass index.

DOCUMENTATION GUIDELINES

• Physiological response: Respiratory status of the patient, vital signs, breath sounds, presence of respiratory distress, arterial blood gases, or pulse oximetry results
• Response to pain medications, respiratory adjuncts, level of hydration
• Ability to cough and breathe deeply, mobilization of secretions

DISCHARGE AND HOME HEALTHCARE GUIDELINES

PREVENTION. To prevent atelectasis, instruct the patient prior to surgery about coughing, deep breathing, and early ambulation. Encourage the patient to request and take pain medications to assist with deep-breathing exercises. Explain that an adequate fluid intake is important to help loosen secretions and aid in their removal.

MEDICATIONS. Instruct patients regarding the use of any medications they are to take at home. Discuss the indications for use and any adverse effects. If patients are placed on antibiotics, instruct them to finish all of the antibiotics even if they feel better before the prescription is completed.

Atrial Dysrhythmias

DRG Category: 309
Mean LOS: 2.9 days
Description: MEDICAL: Cardiac Arrhythmia and Conduction Disorders With Complication or Comorbidity

A cardiac dysrhythmia is any disturbance in the normal rhythm of the electrical excitation of the heart. It can be the result of a primary cardiac disorder, a response to a systemic condition, or the result of an electrolyte imbalance or a drug toxicity. The severity of a dysrhythmia, depending on its hemodynamic effect on the cardiac output, varies on the basis of the cause of the dysrhythmia and the myocardium's ability to adapt. An atrial dysrhythmia arises in the atria of the heart. If the dysrhythmia causes the patient to lose the "atrial kick" (the blood that is ejected into the ventricle during atrial systole), the patient may have more symptoms. The atrial kick provides approximately 35% of the total end-diastolic volume, which is an essential contribution to ventricular filling in individuals with heart disease. Atrial dysrhythmias that cause the loss of the atrial kick include atrial flutter and atrial fibrillation. Figure 1 illustrates types of atrial dysrhythmias in Lead II.

Sinus bradycardia (Figure 2), a heart rate less than 60 beats per minute, has a rhythm that is regular, with the electrical impulse originating in the sinoatrial (SA) node. There is a 1:1 ratio of P waves to QRS complexes, and the P wave and QRS complexes are of normal configuration. Sinus bradycardia is primarily caused by an excessive parasympathetic response. It can be a normal, asymptomatic occurrence in healthy individuals such as athletes or a desired medication effect with drugs such as digoxin and verapamil. Abnormal conditions such as ischemia, hypothermia, pain, anxiety, increased intracranial pressure, or myocardial infarction can also cause sinus bradycardia. Because of its effects on cardiac output, sinus bradycardia can cause symptoms of dizziness, fatigue, palpitations, chest pain, and congestive heart failure. Complications, depending on the type of dysrhythmia, include stroke, thromboembolism, heart failure, hypotension, syncope, and rarely, cardiac arrest.

Sinus tachycardia (Figure 3), a heart rate greater than 100 beats but rarely more than 150 beats per minute, is a regular rhythm whose electrical impulse originates in the SA node. There is a 1:1 ratio of P waves to QRS complexes, and the P wave and QRS complexes are of normal configuration. Sinus tachycardia is generally the result of increased stimulation of the sympathetic nervous system and the resulting release of catecholamines. It can also be a normal response to an increased demand for oxygenation, as in exercise or fever, or in response to a

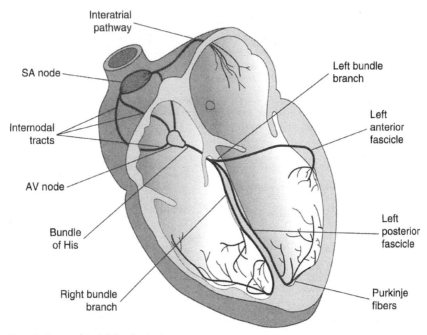

Figure 1 Types of Atrial Dysrhythmias

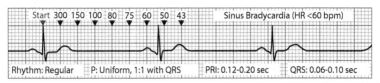

Figure 2 Sinus Bradycardia

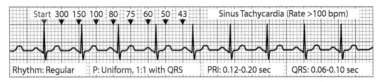

Figure 3 Sinus Tachycardia

decreased cardiac output, as in congestive heart failure or shock syndromes. It can also occur in response to hypoxemia; electrolyte imbalance; acute fluid loss; stress; anxiety; intake of stimulants such as caffeine or nicotine, or anticholinergic medications.

Sinus arrhythmia, defined as a variable rate of impulse discharge from the SA node, occurs when the rhythm is irregular and usually corresponds to the respiratory pattern. The rhythm increases with inspiration and slows with expiration. There is a 1:1 ratio of P waves to QRS complexes, and the P wave and QRS complex are of normal configuration. Sinus arrhythmia can be a normal variation in children. The vagal effect of some medications and of SA nodal disease and conditions that affect vagal tone can be a cause.

Atrial flutter (Figure 4), defined as an abnormally fast, regular atrial rhythm that originates from an ectopic atrial focus, is usually in the range of 250 to 350 beats per minute. It is characterized by regular flutter or sawtooth-appearing waves. The QRS complex appears normal in configuration, and there is not a 1:1 ratio of the P to QRS complex because the ventricle cannot respond to the fast atrial rate. Atrial flutter is seldom seen in a healthy individual. Most frequently, atrial flutter is associated with ischemic myocardial disease, cardiomyopathy, acute myocardial infarction, and rheumatic heart disease. Other associated conditions include mitral valve disease, digitalis toxicity, hyperthyroidism, and chronic obstructive pulmonary disease. The patient is usually asymptomatic because of a controlled ventricular response.

Atrial fibrillation (Figure 5), a rapid and disorganized atrial dysrhythmia, occurs at atrial rates of 300 to 600 beats per minute. There are no clearly discernible P waves, but rather irregular fibrillatory waves. The QRS complex appears normal, but there is a variable, irregular ventricular response because of the atrioventricular (AV) node's ability to respond only partially to this rapid rate. Although atrial fibrillation can occur in healthy individuals, it is generally found in patients with underlying cardiovascular diseases such as ischemic heart disease, mitral valve disease, heart failure, and pericarditis. Other associated conditions include diabetes, hyperthyroidism, hypertension, valvular disease, and obesity.

Premature atrial contractions (PACs), cardiac contractions initiated in the atria, occur earlier than expected. The underlying rhythm is regular, with the early beat producing a slight irregularity. There is usually a 1:1 ratio of P wave to QRS complex unless the P wave is blocked because of the refractory period of the AV node. The P wave of the premature beat may exhibit a slightly different configuration because it does not originate in the SA node but from another area of the atrium. There may be a short "compensatory" pause after the ectopic (electrical stimulation of a cardiac contraction beginning at a point other than the SA node) beat. PACs can be a normal occurrence in all age groups or they can be the result of ischemic heart disease, rheumatic heart disease, stimulant ingestion, or digitalis toxicity.

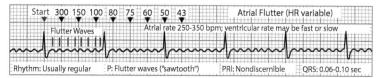
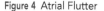

Figure 4 Atrial Flutter

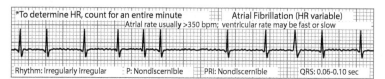

Figure 5 Atrial Fibrillation

Paroxysmal supraventricular tachycardia (PSVT), the sudden onset of a rapid atrial and ventricular rate of 150 to 240 beats per minute, occurs with a regular but aberrant P wave. The P waves are difficult to discern from the preceding T wave, but a P wave precedes each QRS. PSVT occurs when there is an intrinsic abnormality of the AV conduction or in conditions associated with stress, hypoxia, hypokalemia, hypertension, heart disease, or hyperthyroidism. It is also associated with digitalis toxicity, caffeine ingestion, and the use of central nervous system stimulants.

CAUSES

Each type of atrial dysrhythmia has specific causes, as listed previously.

GENETIC CONSIDERATIONS

A number of atrial arrhythmias have been found to run in families. Risk of developing atrial fibrillation (AF) is about 40% higher when there is a history of AF in a first-degree relative. Multiple studies have shown that mutations in ion channel genes such as potassium, sodium, and calcium are linked to AF. Sick sinus syndrome can be caused by a sodium channel mutation (*SCN5A*), via recessive inheritance, or through mutations in the cardiac pacemaker channel gene *HCN4* via dominant inheritance. Wolff-Parkinson-White syndrome can be seen in both autosomal and mitochondrial disease and has been linked to mutations in the *PRKAG2* gene.

SEX AND LIFE SPAN CONSIDERATIONS

The normal aging process is associated with an increase in atrial tachydysrythmias and bradydysrhythmias. They occur in both males and females, but atrial fibrillation and flutter are more common in males, and PSVT is more common in females. Increasing incidence of cardiac diseases, atherosclerosis, and degenerative hypertrophy of the left ventricle that occurs with aging are all contributing factors.

HEALTH DISPARITIES AND SEXUAL/GENDER MINORITY HEALTH

The Centers for Disease Control and Prevention report that 11.5% of White persons, 9.5% of Black persons, 7.4% of Hispanic persons, and 6.0% of Asian persons have heart disease. Black, Indigenous, and other persons of color are known to receive care less often guided by standard cardiac care guidelines than White persons. Unless patients have health insurance, White patients are more likely to receive coronary angiograms and other coronary interventions than Black and Hispanic patients. Black, Indigenous, and other persons of color are also less likely to be referred to cardiologists and cardiac surgeons than White persons (Batchelor et al., 2019).

Transgender is a term used to describe persons whose gender identity is different from their sex assigned at birth. Approximately 1% of the U.S. population identify themselves as transgender. Sexual and gender minority persons have higher odds for multiple chronic conditions, cancer, and poor quality of life and are more apt to have disabilities than cisgender males and females (cisgender is a term used to describe persons whose gender identity and gender expression are aligned with their assigned sex listed on their birth certificate). Gender-affirming hormone therapy is the use of hormone therapy for gender transition or gender affirmation and can be masculinizing or feminizing. It may also affect cardiovascular health in transgender women. In a large sample, researchers have found that transgender men and women are more likely to be overweight than cisgender women. Compared to cisgender women, transgender women reported higher rates of diabetes, angina/coronary disease, and myocardial infarction. Gender nonconforming men and women reported higher odds of myocardial infarction than cisgender women. Transgender women also had higher rates of any cardiovascular disease than cisgender men (Cacerese, Jackman, et al., 2020).

GLOBAL HEALTH CONSIDERATIONS

While atrial dysrhythmias occur around the globe, no data are available on incidence.

ASSESSMENT

HISTORY. Many patients with suspected cardiac dysrhythmias describe a history of symptoms, indicating periods of decreased cardiac output. Although many atrial dysrhythmias are asymptomatic, some patients report a history of **dizziness, fatigue, activity intolerance**, a **"fluttering" in their chest, shortness of breath**, and **chest pain**. They may experience diaphoresis or fainting. In particular, question the patient about the onset, duration, and characteristics of the symptoms and the events that precipitated them. Obtain a complete history of all illnesses, dietary restrictions, and activity restrictions and a current medication history.

PHYSICAL EXAMINATION. Inspect the patient's skin for changes in color or the presence of edema. Auscultate the patient's heart rate and rhythm and note the first and second heart sounds and any adventitious sounds. Auscultate the patient's blood pressure and the strength and regularity of their peripheral pulses. Perform a full respiratory assessment and note any adventitious breath sounds or labored breathing.

PSYCHOSOCIAL. Although not usually life threatening, any change in heart rhythm can provoke a great deal of anxiety and fear. Assess the ability of the patient and significant others to cope with this potential alteration.

Diagnostic Highlights

Test	Normal Result	Abnormality With Condition	Explanation
12-Lead electro-cardiogram (ECG)	Regular sinus rhythm (Fig. 6)	See Figure 1	To detect specific conduction defects and to monitor the patient's cardiac response to electrolyte imbalances, drug effects, and toxicities

Other Tests: Pulse oximetry, echocardiography, continuous ambulatory monitoring to provide a 12- to 24-hour continuous recording of myocardial electrical activity as the patient performs normal daily activities; event recorders for ECG monitoring as long as a month; exercise ECG; electrophysiology study; B-type natriuretic peptide level; cardiac catheterization, thyroid function tests; electrolyte, creatinine kinase, tropinin, and digoxin levels

PRIMARY NURSING DIAGNOSIS

DIAGNOSIS. Risk for decreased cardiac tissue perfusion related to rapid heart rate or the loss of the atrial kick as evidenced by dizziness, fatigue, and/or activity intolerance

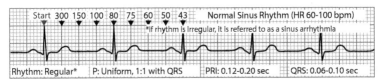

Figure 6 Sinus Rhythm

OUTCOMES. Circulation status; Cardiac pump effectiveness; Knowledge: Cardiac disease management; Tissue perfusion: Cardiopulmonary, Cerebral, Peripheral; Vital signs; Medication response

INTERVENTIONS. Dysrhythmia management; Emergency care; Vital signs monitoring; Cardiac care; Oxygen therapy; Fluid/electrolyte management; Medication administration

☀ PLANNING AND IMPLEMENTATION

Collaborative

The dysrhythmia needs to be identified and appropriate treatment started (Table 1). Trials of various medications or combinations of medications may be used to control the dysrhythmia if the patient is symptomatic. Low-flow oxygen by nasal cannula or mask is often prescribed for patients during tachycardic rhythms. Some patients may require cardioversion, a synchronized countershock for atrial dysrhythmias that are resistant to medical therapy.

• TABLE 1 Treatment of Atrial Dysrhythmias

DYSRHYTHMIA	MANAGEMENT
Sinus tachycardia	• Treat the underlying cause of dysrhythmia
Sinus bradycardia	• Treat only if the patient is symptomatic
	• Determine the underlying cause
	• If appropriate, administer atropine; supplemental oxygen
	• Consider a pacemaker, if appropriate
Atrial flutter	• Convert rhythm to sinus rhythm or controlled ventricular rate to provide adequate cardiac output; supplemental oxygen
	• Rate control: Beta blockers, calcium channel blockers, digitalis; antidysrhythmics such as propafenone, flecainide, amiodarone
	• Anticoagulants to prevent thromboemboli formation
	• Vagal maneuvers, adenosine
	• Other: Cardioversion, atrial-based pacing, atrial defibrillators, catheter ablation, pharmacologic cardioversion: procainamide, dofetilide, ibutilide
Atrial fibrillation	• Convert rhythm to sinus rhythm or controlled ventricular rate to provide adequate cardiac output; supplemental oxygen
	• Use cardioversion (generally successful in acute cases of atrial fibrillation)
	• Rate control: Beta blockers and calcium channel blockers, digitalis if left ventricular function is reduced (used rarely as a single therapy), flecainide, propafenone, sotalol, amiodarone (if unresponsive to other agents)
	• Anticoagulants to prevent thromboemboli formation
	• Other: Atrial-based pacing, atrial defibrillators, catheter ablation
Paroxysmal supraventricular tachycardia	• Attempt noninvasive treatment with stimulation of vagal reflex by Valsalva maneuver or carotid massage (in patients without carotid bruits); supplemental oxygen
	• Treat with IV adenosine or calcium channel blockers; antidysrhythmics such as procainamide, propafenone, flecainide, amiodarone (preferred for patients with heart failure)
	• Synchronized cardioversion
	• Other: Calcium channel blockers such as verapamil or diltiazem or beta blockers such as metoprolol or esmolol, digitalis

Pharmacologic Highlights

Medication or Drug Class	Dosage	Description	Rationale
Calcium channel blockers	Varies by drug	Inhibits influx of calcium through the slow channels into the cells of the myocardial and arterial smooth muscles	Decreases atrioventricular (AV) nodal conduction and prolongs refractory period leading to an antiarrhythmic effect
Beta-adrenergic antagonists	Varies by drug	Blocks beta-adrenergic receptors	May be used to slow the rate in sinus tachycardia if the patient has myocardial ischemia; increases the refractory period of the AV node; may also be used to control a rapid ventricular response in atrial fibrillation
Antidysrhythmics	Varies by drug	Changes the dynamics of automaticity or ions channels related to the myocardial conduction system, which affects the propagation and/or conduction of impulses	Used to restore normal rate and conduction

Independent

Maintain the patient's airway, breathing, and circulation. To maximize oxygen available to the myocardium, encourage the patient to rest in bed until the symptoms are treated and subside. Remain with the patient to ensure rest and to allay anxiety. Discuss any potential precipitating factors with the patient. For some patients, strategies to reduce stress or lifestyle changes help to limit the incidence of dysrhythmias. Teach the patient to reduce the amount of caffeine intake in the diet. If appropriate, encourage the patient to become involved in an exercise program or a smoking-cessation group. Provide emotional support and information about the dysrhythmia, the precipitating factors, and mechanisms to limit the dysrhythmia. If the patient is at risk for electrolyte imbalance, teach the patient any dietary considerations to prevent electrolyte depletion.

Evidence-Based Practice and Health Policy

Choi, Y., Kim, S., Baek, J., Kim, S., Kim, J., Kim, T., Hwang, Y., Kim, J., Jang, S., Lee, M., & Oh, Y. (2021). Acute and long-term outcome of redo catheter ablation for recurrent atrial tachycardia and recurrent atrial fibrillation in patients with prior atrial fibrillation ablation. *Journal of Interventional Cardiac Electrophysiology*, *61*, 227–234.

- The authors analyzed 133 cases of people who underwent previous ablation for atrial fibrillation and returned for a repeat procedure. Atrial tachycardia recurred in 50 patients, and atrial fibrillation recurred in 83 patients.
- The atrial tachycardia group showed a higher success rate (92%) than the atrial fibrillation group (76%) with radiofrequency catheter ablation. The authors concluded that the long-term success rate was superior for the atrial tachycardia group.

DOCUMENTATION GUIDELINES

- Cardiopulmonary assessment: Heart and lung sounds, cardiac rate and rhythm on the cardiac monitor, blood pressure, oxygenation on pulse oximetry; quality of the peripheral pulses, capillary refill, respiratory rate and rhythm

- Activity tolerance, ability to perform self-care, responses to medications
- Complications: Dizziness, syncope, hypotension, electrolyte imbalance, uncorrected cardiac dysrhythmias, ineffective patient or family coping

DISCHARGE AND HOME HEALTHCARE GUIDELINES

PATIENT TEACHING. Explain the importance of taking all medications as prescribed by the physician. If the patient needs periodic laboratory work to monitor the effects of the medications, discuss the frequency of the tests and where to have them drawn. Explain the actions, the route, the side effects, the dosage, and the frequency of the medication. Teach the patient how to take the pulse and recognize an irregular rhythm. Explain that the patient needs to notify the healthcare provider when symptoms such as irregular pulse, chest pain, shortness of breath, or dizziness occur. Emphasize the importance of stress reduction and smoking cessation.

Benign Prostatic Hyperplasia (Hypertrophy)

DRG Category:	713
Mean LOS:	4.0 days
Description:	SURGICAL: Transurethral Prostatectomy With Complication or Comorbidity or Major Complication or Comorbidity
DRG Category:	725
Mean LOS:	5.3 days
Description:	MEDICAL: Benign Prostatic Hypertrophy With Major Complication or Comorbidity

Benign prostatic hyperplasia (BPH; excessive proliferation of normal cells in normal organs) or hypertrophy (an increase in size of an organ) is one of the most common disorders of older men. It is a nonmalignant enlargement of the prostate gland and is the most common cause of obstruction of urine flow in men, resulting in more than 4.5 million visits to healthcare providers annually in the United States. The degree of enlargement determines whether or not bladder outflow obstruction occurs. As the urethra becomes obstructed, the muscle inside the bladder hypertrophies in an attempt to assist the bladder to force out the urine. BPH may also cause the formation of a bladder diverticulum that remains full of urine when the patient empties the bladder. With marked bladder distention, overflow incontinence may occur with any increase in intra-abdominal pressure, such as that which occurs with coughing and sneezing. Complications of BPH include urinary stasis, urinary tract infection, renal calculi, overflow incontinence, hypertrophy of the bladder muscle, acute renal failure, hydronephrosis, and even chronic renal failure.

CAUSES

Because the condition occurs in older men, changes in hormone balances have been associated with the cause. Androgens (testosterone) and estrogen appear to contribute to the hyperplastic changes that occur. Other theories, such as those involving diet, heredity, race, and history of chronic inflammation, have been associated with BPH, but no definitive links have been made with these potential contributing factors. Tobacco and alcohol use have been implicated in some studies.

GENETIC CONSIDERATIONS

When BPH occurs in men under age 60 years and is severe enough to require surgery, chances of a genetic component are high. Autosomal dominant transmission appears likely because a man who has a male relative requiring treatment before age 60 years has a 50% lifetime risk of also requiring treatment. Recently, a variant in the gene *RANBP3L* was found to be associated with BPH risk.

SEX AND LIFE SPAN CONSIDERATIONS

By the age of 60 years, 50% of men have some degree of prostate enlargement, which is considered part of the normal aging process. Many of these men do not manifest any clinical symptoms in the early stages of hypertrophic changes. As men become older, the incidence of symptoms increases to more than 75% for those over age 80 years and 90% by age 85 years. Of those men with symptoms, approximately 50% of men are symptomatic to a moderate degree, and 25% of those have severe symptoms that require surgical interventions.

HEALTH DISPARITIES AND SEXUAL/GENDER MINORITY HEALTH

The prevalence of BPH is similar in White, Hispanic, and Black men, but symptoms of BPH tend to be more severe and progress more quickly in Black men as compared to other populations. One theory is that men with worse symptoms have higher testosterone levels and growth factor activity that lead to an increased rate of prostatic hyperplasia and gland enlargement. Most experts recognize that disparities in patient care for BPH exist for Black and Hispanic men because they receive lower levels of speciality care as compared to White men who are similarly insured.

Transgender is a term used to describe persons whose gender identity is different from their sex assigned at birth. Approximately 1% of the U.S. population identify themselves as transgender. Sexual and gender minority persons have higher odds for multiple chronic conditions, cancer, and poor quality of life and are more apt to have disabilities than cisgender males and females (cisgender is a term used to describe persons whose gender identity and gender expression are aligned with their assigned sex listed on their birth certificate). Gender-affirming hormone therapy is the use of hormone therapy for gender transition or gender affirmation and can be masculinizing or feminizing. Transgender women who take feminizing hormone therapy are not thought to increase the risk of prostate cancer or BPH (Cacerese, Jackman, et al., 2020; Gooren & T'Sjoen, 2018).

GLOBAL HEALTH CONSIDERATIONS

BPH is a significant and widespread international problem that causes symptoms in at least 30 million men globally.

☀ ASSESSMENT

HISTORY. Generally, men with suspected BPH have a history of **frequent urination, urinary urgency, nocturia, straining to urinate, weak stream, hesitancy, dribbling**, and an **incomplete emptying of the bladder**. This group of symptoms is sometimes labeled *LUTS*, or lower urinary tract symptoms. Distinguish between these obstructive symptoms and irritative symptoms such as dysuria, frequency, and urgency, which may indicate an infection or inflammatory process. A "voiding diary" can also be obtained to determine the frequency and nature of the complaints. Elicit a sexual history because LUTS is an independent risk factor for erectile and ejaculatory dysfunctions. Some patients prefer having a male healthcare practitioner take a sexual history. The International Prostate Symptom Score (IPSS) has been adopted worldwide and provides information regarding symptoms and response to treatment (Box 1). Each question allows the patient to choose one of six answers on a scale of 0 to 5 indicating the increasing degree of symptoms; the total score ranges from 0 (mildly symptomatic) to 35 (severely symptomatic). The eighth question, known as the bother score, refers to quality of life.

• BOX 1 The International Prostate Symptom Score (International Prostate Symptom Score. [2021]. Urological Sciences Research Foundation. www.usrf.org/questionnaires/AUA_SymptomScore.html)

1. Incomplete emptying: Over the past month, how often have you had the sensation of not emptying your bladder completely after you have finished urinating? (Not at all = 0, less than one time in five = 1, less than half the time = 2, about half the time = 3, more than half the time = 4, almost always = 5)
2. Frequency: Over the past month, how often have you had to urinate again less than 2 hours after you finished urinating? (Not at all = 0, less than one time in five = 1, less than half the time = 2, about half the time = 3, more than half the time = 4, almost always = 5)
3. Intermittency: Over the past month, how often have you stopped and started again several times when urinating? (Not at all = 0, less than one time in five = 1, less than half the time = 2, about half the time = 3, more than half the time = 4, almost always = 5)
4. Urgency: Over the past month, how often have you found it difficult to postpone urination? (Not at all = 0, less than one time in five = 1, less than half the time = 2, about half the time = 3, more than half the time = 4, almost always = 5)

5. Weak stream: Over the past month, how often have you had a weak urinary stream? (Not at all = 0, less than one time in five = 1, less than half the time = 2, about half the time = 3, more than half the time = 4, almost always = 5)
6. Straining: Over the past month, how often have you had to push or strain to begin urination? (Never = 0, once = 1, twice = 2, three times = 3, four times or more = 4, five times or more = 5)
7. Nocturia: Over the past month, how many times did you most typically get up to urinate from the time you went to bed until the time you got up in the morning? (Not at all = 0, less than one time in five = 1, less than half the time = 2, about half the time = 3, more than half the time = 4, almost always = 5)
8. How would you feel if you were to spend the rest of your life with your urinary condition just the way it is now? (Delighted = 0, pleased = 1, mostly satisfied = 2, mixed = 3, mostly dissatisfied = 4, unhappy = 5, terrible = 6)

PHYSICAL EXAMINATION. Inspect and palpate the bladder for distention. A digital rectal examination (DRE) reveals a rubbery enlargement of the prostate, but the degree of enlargement does not consistently correlate with the degree of urinary obstruction. Some men have enlarged prostates that extend out into soft tissue without compressing the urethra. Determine the amount of pain and discomfort that is associated with the DRE.

PSYCHOSOCIAL. In addition to discomfort, the symptoms are anxiety producing to men. The patient who is experiencing BPH may voice concerns related to sexual functioning after treatment. The patient's degree of anxiety as well as his ability to cope with the potential alterations in sexual function (a possible cessation of intercourse for several weeks, possibility of sterility or retrograde ejaculation) should also be determined to provide appropriate follow-up care.

Diagnostic Highlights

Test	Normal Result	Abnormality With Condition	Explanation
Urinalysis and culture	Minimal numbers of red and white blood cells; no bacteria; clear urine with no occult blood and no protein	Urinary tract infection may occur with the presence of bacteria, blood, leukocytes, protein, or glucose	Urinary retention may lead to infection; voiding may be irritating
Uroflowmetry	Males ages 46–65 years have more than 200 mL of urine at a flow rate of 21 mL/sec	Flow rate is decreased	Prostate inflammation leads to a narrowed urethral channel and obstruction of urine outflow
Prostate-specific antigen (PSA)	Normal: < 4 ng/mL	May be slightly elevated	Screening for prostate cancer remains controversial and should be done if the physician and patient desire. PSA testing may reduce the likelihood of dying from prostate cancer. Patients should be alerted that PSA testing poses the risk of treatment of prostate cancer that would not have caused ill effects if left undetected.

Other Tests: Serum creatinine and blood urea nitrogen, electrolytes, postvoid residual volume, diagnostic ultrasound, cystourethroscopy, abdominal or renal ultrasound, transrenal ultrasound. Note that while BPH does not cause prostate cancer, men at risk for BPH are also at risk for prostate cancer. Screening for prostate cancer remains controversial (see diagnostic highlights above).

PRIMARY NURSING DIAGNOSIS

DIAGNOSIS. Impaired urinary elimination related to urinary retention as evidenced by bladder distention, dribbling of urine, frequent voiding, and/or dysuria

OUTCOMES. Urinary continence; Urinary elimination; Infection severity; Knowledge: Disease process, Medication, Treatment regimen; Symptom control

INTERVENTIONS. Urinary retention care; Bladder irrigation; Fluid management; Fluid monitoring; Medication administration; Infection control; Urinary catheterization; Urinary elimination management; Tube care: Urinary

PLANNING AND IMPLEMENTATION

Collaborative

MEDICAL. Men with mild or moderate symptoms but without complications, and who are not bothered by their symptoms, may be monitored by "watchful waiting." Generally these individuals will have an IPSS score of 8 or less. Most experts suggest that in this situation, the risks of medical treatment may outweigh the benefits, although most experts recommend annual examinations in case their condition changes.

SURGICAL. Those patients with the most severe cases, in which there is total urinary obstruction, chronic urinary retention, and recurrent urinary tract infection, usually require surgery.

Transurethral resection of the prostate (TURP) is the most common surgical intervention. The procedure is performed by inserting a resectoscope through the urethra. Hypertrophic tissue is cut away, thereby relieving pressure on the urethra. Prostatectomy can be performed, in which the portion of the prostate gland causing the obstruction is removed.

The relatively newer surgical procedure called transurethral incision of the prostate (TUIP) involves making an incision in the portion of the prostate attached to the bladder. The procedure is performed with local anesthesia and has a lower complication rate than TURP. The gland is split, reducing pressure on the urethra. TUIP is more helpful in men with smaller prostate glands that cause obstruction and for men who are unlikely to tolerate a TURP. Other minimally invasive treatments for BPH rely on heat to cause destruction of the prostate gland. The heat is delivered in a controlled fashion through a urinary catheter or a transrectal route, has the potential to reduce the complications associated with TURP, and has a lower anesthetic risk for the patient. Minimally invasive procedures include heat from laser energy, microwaves, radiofrequency energy, high-intensity ultrasound waves, and high-voltage electrical energy. Several minimally invasive therapies are continuously being tested and refined to increase efficacy and safety.

POSTSURGICAL. Postsurgical care involves supportive care and maintenance of the indwelling catheter to ensure patency and adequacy of irrigation. Belladonna and opium suppositories may relieve bladder spasms. Stool softeners are used to prevent straining during defecation after surgery. Ongoing monitoring of the drainage from the catheter determines the color, consistency, and amount of urine flow. The urine should be clear yellow or slightly pink in color. If the patient develops frank hematuria or an abrupt change in urinary output, the surgeon should be notified immediately. The most critical complications that can occur are septic or hemorrhagic shock.

NONSURGICAL. In patients who are not candidates for surgery, a permanent indwelling catheter may be inserted. If the catheter cannot be placed in the urethra because of obstruction, the patient may need a suprapubic cystostomy. Conservative therapy also includes prostatic massage, warm sitz baths, and a short-term fluid restriction to prevent bladder distention. Regular ejaculation may help decrease congestion of the prostate gland.

Pharmacologic Highlights

Medication or Drug Class	Dosage	Description	Rationale
Phenoxybenzamine	10 mg PO bid	Alpha-adrenergic blocker	Blocks effects of postganglionic synapses at the smooth muscle and exocrine glands; improvement of urinary flow in 75% of patients
Finasteride	5 mg PO qd	5-alpha reductase inhibitor	Shrinks prostate gland and improves urine flow

Other Drugs: Prazosin, alfuzosin, doxazosin, terazosin, silodosin, tamsulosin, dutasteride

Independent

Patients with severe alterations in urinary elimination may require a catheter to assist with emptying the bladder. Never force a urinary catheter into the urethra. If there is resistance during insertion, stop the catheterization procedure and notify the physician. Monitor the patient for bleeding and discomfort during insertion. In addition, assess the patient for signs of shock from postobstruction diuresis after catheter insertion. Ensure adequate fluid balance. Encourage the patient to drink at least 2 L of fluid per day to prevent stasis and infection from a decreased intake. Encourage the patient to avoid the following medications, which may worsen the symptoms: anticholinergics, decongestants (over-the-counter and prescribed), tranquilizers, alcohol, and antidepressants.

Evaluate the patient's and partner's feelings about the risk for sexual dysfunction. Retrograde ejaculation or sterility may occur after surgery. Explain alternative sexual practices and answer the patient's questions. Some patients would prefer to talk to a person of the same gender/sex when discussing sexual matters. Provide supportive care of the patient and significant others and make referrals for sexual counseling if appropriate.

Evidence-Based Practice and Health Policy

Srinivasan, A., & Wang, R. (2020). An update on minimally invasive surgery for benign prostatic hyperplasia: Techniques, risks, and efficacy. *The World Journal of Men's Health, 38,* 402–411.

* The authors reported on BPH, a common cause of lower urinary tract symptoms in older male adults. While previously BPH was conventionally treated by transurethral resection of the prostate, in recent years minimally invasive therapies (MITs) have become common because of their convenience, safety, and lack of side effects.
* The authors review several novel types of MITs and note their mechanisms of action, contraindications, and advantages. These options personalize the approach to BHP and allow for patient choices depending on the patient's condition. Because there exists a dearth of data testing the long-term effects of these therapies, the authors suggest a series of clinical trials to determine best outcomes.

DOCUMENTATION GUIDELINES

* Presence of urinary discomfort, bleeding, frequency, retention, or difficulty initiating flow
* Presence of bladder distention, discomfort, and incontinence
* Intake and output; color of urine, presence of clots, quality of urine (clear versus cloudy)
* Presence of complications: Urinary retention, bleeding, infection, wound healing
* Reaction to information regarding sexual function

DISCHARGE AND HOME HEALTHCARE GUIDELINES

PATIENT TEACHING. Instruct patients about the need to maintain a high fluid intake (at least 2 L/day) to ensure adequate urine output. Teach the patient to monitor urinary output for 4 to 6 weeks after surgery to ensure adequacy in volume of elimination combined with a decrease in volume of retention. Explain that the patient should not do any heavy lifting or undergo strenuous exercise for several weeks after surgery.

MEDICATIONS. Provide instructions about all medications used to relax the smooth muscles of the bladder or to shrink the prostate gland. Provide instructions on the correct dosage, route, action, side effects, and potential drug interactions and when to provide this information to the physician.

PREVENTION. Instruct the patient to report any difficulties with urination to the physician immediately. Explain that BPH can recur and that he should notify the physician if symptoms of urgency, frequency, difficulty initiating stream, retention, nocturia, or bladder distention recur. A diet low in fat and high in protein and vegetables may reduce the risk of the disorder. Regular alcohol consumption within recommended limits of drinking (no more than two standard drinks per day) is associated with a reduced risk of symptomatic BPH.

POSTOPERATIVE. Encourage the patient to discuss any sexual concerns he or his partner may have after surgery with the appropriate counselors. Reassure the patient that a session can be set up by the nurse or physician whenever one is indicated. Usually, physicians recommend that patients have no sexual intercourse or masturbation for several weeks after invasive procedures.

Bladder Cancer

DRG Category:	656
Mean LOS:	7.5 days
Description:	SURGICAL: Kidney and Ureter Procedures for Neoplasm With Major Complication or Comorbidity
DRG Category:	687
Mean LOS:	4.3 days
Description:	MEDICAL: Kidney and Urinary Tract Neoplasms With Complication or Comorbidity

Cancer of the urinary bladder is the second-most common genitourinary (GU) cancer after prostate cancer. It accounts for approximately 4% of all cancers and 2% of deaths from cancer in the United States. The American Cancer Society estimates that in 2021, there will be approximately 83,000 new cases of bladder cancer, and 17,000 people will die from the disease.

The majority of bladder tumors (> 90%) are urothelial or transitional cell carcinomas (TCC) arising in the epithelial layer of the bladder, although squamous cell carcinomas (SCC) (4%), adenocarcinoma (1% to 2%), and small cell (1%) may occur. Urothelial tumors are classified as invasive or noninvasive and according to their shape (papillary or flat). Noninvasive urothelial cancer affects only the innermost layer of the bladder, whereas invasive urothelial cancer spreads from the urothelium to the deepest layers of the bladder. The deeper the invasion is, the more serious the cancer. Papillary tumors have fingerlike projections that grow into the hollow of the bladder. Flat urothelial tumors involve the layer of cells closest to the inside of the bladder. Metastasis may occur to the sigmoid colon, rectum, and sex organs, and occasionally occurs to the bones, liver, and lungs.

Bladder cancer is staged on the basis of the presence or absence of invasion and is graded (I to IV) on the basis of the degree of differentiation of the cell, with grade I being the best differentiated and slowest growing. Both the stage and the grade of the tumor are considered when planning treatment.

CAUSES

The cause of bladder cancer is not well understood; however, cigarette smoking and occupational exposure to aromatic amines (textile dyes, rubber, hair dyes, and paint pigment) are established risk factors. Given these risks, the following occupations expose people to possible toxic substances: beauticians and barbers, painters, dry cleaners, and people working in the rope and paper industries. Cancer-causing chemicals enter the bloodstream, are filtered through the kidneys, become concentrated in the urine, and then damage the endothelial cells that line the inside of the bladder. Other associated factors include chronic bladder irritation and infection, vesical calculi, and exposure to cyclophosphamide (Cytoxan). Moderate to high amounts of caffeine could also possibly increase risk.

GENETIC CONSIDERATIONS

Although bladder cancer is generally considered to come from somatic (rather than germ line) mutations in bladder cells, mutations in several genes (e.g., *HRAS*, *KRAS*, *RB1*, *OGG1*, *IL31*, and *FGFR3*) have been associated with susceptibility to bladder carcinogenesis.

SEX AND LIFE SPAN CONSIDERATIONS

Bladder cancer occurs most frequently in persons over age 50 years, with more than half of the cases occurring in individuals over age 72 years. It is rare in persons under age 40 years. Bladder cancer is more common in men (1 in 30) than in women (1 in 90). Younger men have reported less impotency following radical cystectomy than have older men.

HEALTH DISPARITIES AND SEXUAL/GENDER MINORITY HEALTH

Incidence is highest among White men, with a rate twice that of Black and Hispanic men and four times that of White women. Women, Black men, and Hispanic men have a lower incidence of bladder cancer but a poorer prognosis than do White men. People with Asian ancestry have the lowest incidence of bladder cancer as compared to other groups. Persons living in urban areas are at higher risk for bladder cancer than persons living in rural areas, possibly from exposure to carcinogens. Sexual and gender minority health is a broad term that includes lesbian, gay, bisexual, trans, intersex, queer, two-spirit, and gender-nonconforming persons. Transgender is a term used to describe persons whose gender identity is different from their sex assigned at birth. Approximately 1% of the U.S. population identify themselves as transgender. Sexual and gender minority persons have higher odds for multiple chronic conditions such as cancer and are more apt to have disabilities than heterosexual persons and cisgender males and females (cisgender is a term used to describe persons whose gender identity and gender expression are aligned with their assigned sex listed on their birth certificate). Compared to cisgender patients, transgender patients are more likely to be diagnosed with advanced stage bladder cancer, and they also have an increased risk of death (Jackson et al., 2021). Sexual and gender minority persons have unique health needs when bladder cancer occurs. Pain during sexual intercourse may occur with receptive sex, and patients may have urinary drainage in place. Cancer-related stress is compounded by the need to adjust to body change that may alter sexual behaviors. Smoking rates are higher in sexual and gender minority persons than other groups, and smoking cessation is an important intervention in bladder cancer. There are limited studies to guide treatment, evaluate the response to bladder cancer, and understand long-term sexual health consequences (Caceres, Jackman, et al., 2020; Vencill et al., 2020).

GLOBAL HEALTH CONSIDERATIONS

The global incidence is 8 per 100,000 males and 2.7 per 100,000 females. Developed countries have an incidence of bladder cancer from 6 to 10 times higher than developing countries and is often related to smoking tobacco. In North and South America, Europe, and Asia, TCC is the most common type of bladder cancer. People in developing countries, particularly in the Middle East and Africa, are more likely to have SCC than TCC because of exposure to *Schistosoma haematobium* infections.

☀ ASSESSMENT

HISTORY. **Gross, painless, intermittent hematuria** is the most frequently reported symptom. Occult blood may be discovered during a routine urinalysis. Ask patients if they are having dysuria and urinary frequency. Burning and pain with urination are present only if there is infection. The patient may not seek medical attention until urinary hesitance, decrease in caliber of the stream, and flank pain occur. Other symptoms may include suprapubic pain after voiding, bladder irritability, dribbling, and nocturia.

PHYSICAL EXAMINATION. The physical examination is usually normal. A bladder tumor becomes palpable only after extensive invasion into surrounding structures.

PSYCHOSOCIAL. After a diagnosis of cancer, treatment with radical cystectomy and creation of a urinary diversion system can threaten the quality of life and sexual functioning of men and women. For women, surgical treatment for bladder cancer can lead to removal of part of the vaginal wall, a shortened vaginal vault, and the potential for pain during vaginal sexual intercourse, reduced desire, pelvic organ prolapse, and fistulas. The procedure can cause impotence in men and a variety of psychological problems for men and women. The psychological impact of a stoma and external urinary drainage system can cause changes in body image and libido.

Diagnostic Highlights

General: Urinalysis generally reveals gross hematuria and occasionally pyuria.

Test	Normal Result	Abnormality With Condition	Explanation
Cystoscopy/ biopsy	Normal view of bladder, free of growths	Suspicious growths are seen; a small piece is removed and biopsied	Biopsy confirms the malignancy
Serum carcinoembryonic antigen (CEA) level	< 2.5 ng/dL in non-smokers; < 5 ng/mL in smokers	Approximately 50% of patients with late-stage bladder cancer have moderately elevated CEA levels	Useful in monitoring response to treatment and extent of disease
Urine cytology	Normal type and amount of squamous and epithelial cells of urinary tract	Abnormal cells are seen under the microscope (tumor and pretumor cells)	Evidence of urinary tract neoplasm

Other Tests: Urine culture, urinalysis with microscopy, IV pyelogram, ultrasonography, pelvic computed tomography scan, magnetic resonance imaging, bone scan, complete blood count, liver and kidney function tests, alkaline phosphatase (bony fraction), urine tumor markers

PRIMARY NURSING DIAGNOSIS

DIAGNOSIS. Risk for impaired urinary elimination as evidenced by dysuria, frequent voiding, and/or hematuria

OUTCOMES. Urinary continence; Urinary elimination; Body image; Knowledge: Disease process and treatment regime; Self-care: Toileting; Self-esteem

INTERVENTIONS. Urinary elimination management; Urinary incontinence care; Body image enhancement; Teaching: Individual; Fluid monitoring; Urinary catheterization; Anxiety reduction; Infection control; Skin surveillance; Tube care: Urinary

PLANNING AND IMPLEMENTATION

Collaborative

Patients with higher stage invasive disease are usually treated with radical curative surgery, whereas patients with lower stage noninvasive disease can be controlled with more conservative measures. Papillary tumors, even when noninvasive, have a high rate of recurrence. Carcinoma in situ (CIS) is usually multifocal and also has a high rate of recurrence.

CONSERVATIVE. Superficial bladder tumors can be treated effectively with conservative measures that consist of surgical removal of the tumor by transurethral resection of the bladder followed by electrical destruction or fulguration, intravesical instillation of chemotherapy or immunotherapy, and frequent follow-up cystoscopic examination. Superficial bladder tumors can also be destroyed with the neodymium:yttrium-aluminum-garnet (Nd:YAG) laser. Patients with multiple superficial bladder tumors receive intravesical instillation of chemotherapy and immunotherapy, such as bacillus Calmette-Guérin (BCG) vaccine. This vaccine is made from a strain of *Mycobacterium bovis* and helps to prevent a relapse.

SURGICAL. Partial or segmental cystectomy may be recommended for patients with diffuse, unresectable tumors or tumors that fail to respond to intravesical therapy. Because tumors are likely to continue to spread and metastasize to distant sites, procedures such as radical cystectomy with creation of a urinary diversion, external radiation therapy, or a combination of preoperative radiation therapy followed by radical cystectomy and urinary diversion are recommended.

The Bricker ileal conduit is the most popular method for creating the urinary diversion. In this procedure, the ureters are implanted into an isolated segment of the terminal ileum. The proximal end of the ileal segment is closed, and a stoma is formed by bringing the distal end out through a hole in the abdominal wall. An external pouch for the collection of urine is worn continuously. Ureteral stents, which are left in place up to 3 weeks after surgery, may be placed during the procedure to promote the flow of urine. An internal continent urinary diversion, commonly known as the *Indiana pouch,* may be created rather than an ileal conduit. The pouch is created from the right colon and terminal ileum. It needs to be emptied by catheterization four to six times a day.

POSTOPERATIVE. Postoperatively, direct nursing care toward providing comfort, preventing complications from major abdominal surgery, and promoting urinary drainage. Monitor the patient's vital signs, dressings, and drains for symptoms of hemorrhage and infection. Monitor the color of the stoma, as well as the amount and color of the urine in the collection pouch, every 4 hours. Urine should drain immediately. Some stomal edema is normal during the early postoperative period, but the flow of urine should not be obstructed.

RADIATION. External beam radiation therapy can be used as both adjuvant and definite treatment for bladder cancer. High-dose, short-course therapy consisting of 16 to 20 Gy can be delivered preoperatively to decrease the size of the tumor(s) and prevent spread during surgery. Radiation therapy with a curative intent may be a treatment option for patients who are opposed to a cystectomy and urinary diversion, but the 5-year survival rate is 20% to 40% as compared to a 90% 5-year survival rate for people with cystectomy. Unfortunately, 30% of patients with invasive bladder cancer eventually relapse.

Pharmacologic Highlights

Medication or Drug Class	Dosage	Description	Rationale
Thiotepa, mitomycin, doxorubicin	Varies with drug	Intravesical chemotherapy	Reduce recurrence in those who had complete transurethral resection
M-VAC (methotrexate, vinblastine, doxorubicin [Adriamycin], cisplatin); GC (gemcitabine, cisplatin)	Varies with drug	Combination systemic antineoplastic chemotherapy	Combination systemic chemotherapy may be effective in prolonging life but is rarely curative

Independent

For patients who require radical cystectomy with urinary diversion, offer support and reinforcement of the information. Ensure that the patient knows what to expect. Involve another family member in the preoperative education. If it is needed, arrange a preoperative visit by someone who has adjusted well to a similar diversion.

If any type of stoma is to be created, arrange for a preoperative visit from the enterostomal therapist. The enterostomal therapist can assist in the selection and marking of the stoma site (although the stoma site is somewhat contingent on the type of urinary diversion to be performed) and can introduce the patient to the external urine collection pouch and related care.

Suggest involvement with community associations such as the United Ostomy Association and the American Cancer Society.

POSTOPERATIVE. Encourage the patient to look at the stoma and take an active part in stoma care as soon as possible. Allow the patient to hold the equipment, observe the amount and characteristics of urine drainage, and empty the urine collection pouch. Implement care to maintain integrity of the skin around the stoma or urinary diversion that has been created. Empty the urinary drainage pouch when it is about one-third full to prevent the weight of the pouch from breaking the skin seal and leaking urine onto the skin. Depending on the type of urinary diversion created, begin teaching stoma care and care of the system 2 to 3 days after surgery.

Be sensitive to the patient's feelings about the potential for altered sexual functioning after radical cystectomy. Listen attentively and answer any questions honestly. Encourage the patient and the patient's partner to explore alternative methods of sexual expression. Consider referral to a sex therapist. If appropriate, suggest that men investigate the possibility of a penile prosthesis with their physician.

Evidence-Based Practice and Health Policy

Vencill, J., Kacel, E., Avulova, S., & Ehlers, S. (2020). Barriers to sexual recovery in women with urologic cancers. *Urologic Oncology.* Advance online publication. https://doi.org/10.1016/j.urolonc.2020.11.011

* Women with urologic cancers undergo treatment that is likely to affect their sexual functioning and well-being. Barriers to sexual recovery include treatment complications such as pain and reduced sexual desire, cancer-related distress, sexual anxiety and avoidance, and relational dynamics.
* The authors suggested that healthcare providers often do not address sexual issues with patients and their partners. Sexual minority women and transgender people have unique sexual needs that remain poorly understood because of the lack of research. In particular, treatments such as pelvic organ-sparing cystectomy need further investigation to determine how they might impact sexual health for sexual minority women and transgender people.

DOCUMENTATION GUIDELINES

* Description of all dressings, wounds, and drainage collection devices
* Physical findings related to the pulmonary assessment, abdominal assessment, presence of edema, condition of extremities, bowel and bladder patterns of voiding
* Response to and side effects experienced related to intravesical instillations of chemotherapy or BCG; systemic chemotherapy
* Teaching performed, the patient's understanding of the content, the patient's ability to perform procedures demonstrated

DISCHARGE AND HOME HEALTHCARE GUIDELINES

PATIENT TEACHING. Following creation of an ileal conduit or continent urinary diversion, teach the patient and significant others how to care for the stoma and/or urinary drainage system. If needed, arrange for follow-up home nursing care or visits with an enterostomal therapist.

Teach the patient the specific procedure to catheterize the continent cutaneous pouch or reservoir. A simple stoma covering made from a feminine hygiene pad can be worn between catheterizations. Stress the need for the patient to wear a medical ID bracelet.

Following orthotopic bladder replacement, teach the patient how to irrigate the Foley catheter. Suggest the use of a leg bag during the day and a Foley drainage bag at night. Once the pouch has healed and the Foley catheter, ureteral stents, and pelvic drain have been removed, teach the patient to "push" or "bear down" with each voiding. Instruct the patient on methods for performing Kegel exercises during and between voidings to minimize incontinence.

Suggest wearing incontinence pads until full control is achieved. Also instruct the patient on self-catheterization techniques in case the patient is unable to void. Instruct patients where to obtain ostomy pouches, catheters, and other supplies. Teach the patient how to clean and store catheters between use following the clean technique.

CARE OF SKIN IN EXTERNAL RADIATION FIELD. Encourage the patient to verbalize concerns about radiation therapy, and reassure the patient that the patient is not "radioactive." Instruct the patient to wash skin gently with mild soap, rinse with warm water, and pat the skin dry each day but not to wash off the ink marking that outlines the radiation field. Encourage the patient to avoid applying any lotions, perfumes, deodorants, or powder to the treatment area. Encourage the patient to wear nonrestrictive soft cotton clothing directly over the treatment area and to protect the skin from sunlight and extreme cold. Stress the need to maintain the schedule for follow-up visits and disease surveillance as recommended by the physician.

Blood Transfusion Reaction

DRG Category:	916
Mean LOS:	2.2 days
Description:	MEDICAL: Allergic Reactions Without Major Complication or Comorbidity

Blood transfusion reactions are adverse responses to the infusion of any blood component, including red cells, white cells, platelets, plasma, cryoprecipitate, or other factors. They may be classified as acute (within 24 hours of administration) or delayed (occurring days, weeks, months, or even years later). They range from mild urticarial reactions that may be treated easily to fatal hemolytic reactions. It is important to note that almost all fatal hemolytic reactions are attributable to human error. Blood transfusion reactions can be mediated by the immune system or by nonimmune factors (Table 1).

• **TABLE 1** Classification of Transfusion Reactions by Type

TYPE AND TIMING	CAUSE	SIGNS AND SYMPTOMS
Allergic; usually occurs within 4 hr	Sensitivity to foreign proteins; immunoglobulin E (IgE)–mediated type 1 hypersensitivity reaction	Mild: Hives, urticaria, fever, flushing, itching
Febrile nonhemolytic transfusion reaction; most common transfusion-related adverse event; occurs within 4 hr of transfusion	Sensitization to donor white blood cell antigens; transfusion of proinflammatory cytokines due to blood component storage	Fever, chills, headache, flushing, muscle aches, respiratory distress, cardiac dysrhythmias
Acute hemolytic transfusion reaction; variable timing	ABO incompatibility reaction to red blood cell antigens; interaction between antigens on donor and/or recipient erythrocytes	Fever, chills, dyspnea, hemoglobinuria, low back pain, flushing, tachycardia, hypotension, vascular collapse, shock, cardiac arrest

(table continues on page 166)

• TABLE 1 Classification of Transfusion Reactions by Type (continued)

TYPE AND TIMING	CAUSE	SIGNS AND SYMPTOMS
Anaphylactic; reactions usually begin within a few seconds or minutes of transfusion	Administration of donor's immunoglobulin A (IgA) proteins to recipient with anti-IgA antibodies; recipient is often IgA deficient	Restlessness, urticaria, wheezing, stridor, angioedema, bronchoconstriction, shock, cardiac arrest
Transfusion-transmitted infections; variable timing	Bacterial or viral infections (West Nile, HIV, cytomegalovirus, viral hepatitis), protozoal infection (malaria), prion disease	Patient develops the symptoms of the disorder; high fever, shock, tachycardia
Transfusion-associated circulatory overload; usually within first 2–6 hr	Infusion of blood at a rapid rate that leads to fluid volume excess and hydrostatic pulmonary edema	Pulmonary congestion, restlessness, cough, shortness of breath, orthopnea, hypoxemia, hypertension, distended neck veins
Transfusion-related lung injury; occurs within 6 hr of transfusion	Antibodies to human leukocytes or neutrophils are present in transfusion components; neutrophils become localized in lung tissue	Hypoxemia, bilateral pulmonary infiltrates, dyspnea, cyanosis, hypotension
Delayed serologic/delayed hemolytic transfusion reactions (DSTR/DHTR); occur 48 hr or more after transfusion	Delayed serologic/hemolytic reactions, post-transfusion purpura, transfusion-related immunomodulation, graft versus host disease	Varies with condition

The immune system recognizes red blood cells, platelets, white blood cells, or immunoglobulins as "non-self" because the donor's blood carries foreign proteins that are incompatible with the recipient's antibodies. Typing, screening, and matching of blood units before administration eliminate most incompatibilities, but all potential incompatibilities cannot be screened out in the matching process. Adverse reactions to transfused blood products in hospital transfusion services are estimated at 282 per 100,000 units transfused. Most deaths are related not to allergic reactions but to circulatory overload or transfusion-related lung injury.

Nonimmune factors are usually related to improper storage. Complications to transfusion reactions include acute bronchospasm, respiratory failure, acute tubular necrosis, and acute renal failure. The most severe reactions can cause anaphylactic shock, vascular collapse, or disseminated intravascular coagulation. Also, current research shows that patients who receive transfusions have an increased risk of infection because the transfusion depresses the immune system for weeks and even months afterward.

CAUSES

The recipient's immune system responds to some transfusions by directing an immune response to the proteins in the donor's blood. Nonimmune factors are involved when the blood or components are handled, stored, or administered improperly. The hemolytic reaction occurs when the donor's blood does not have ABO compatibility with the recipient's blood. Accidental transfusion of red blood cells usually happens either because of misidentification of the patient or blood component or because of confusing two patients with the same or similar names.

Individuals at greatest risk for transfusion reactions are those who receive massive blood transfusions. The transfusions may be administered over a short period of time, such as with trauma victims with severe blood loss or recipients of liver transplants. Individuals who receive a great number of transfusions throughout a more extended period of time, such as people with leukemia or sickle cell disease, are also at greater risk. Over time, they develop more and more protective antibodies after each unit of blood is received. Eventually, they carry so many antibodies in their systems that they react much more readily than a person who is transfusion-naive.

GENETIC CONSIDERATIONS

Blood types are heritable and correspond to antigens present on red blood cells. A person with blood type A must have inherited one or two copies of the A allele. The resulting genotype would be either AA or AO, expressing the A antigen as well as B antibodies. Someone who is blood type B inherited one or two copies of the B allele and could have a genotype of either BB or BO. A person with blood type AB must have both the A and the B alleles, resulting in the AB genotype; the genotype of a person who is type O must be OO. Each parent donates one of their two ABO alleles to each child. The Rh factor allele is inherited independently. An Rh-positive person has one or two Rh-positive alleles with a genotype of Rh+/Rh+ or Rh+/Rh−. An Rh-negative person has a genotype of Rh−/Rh−. A blood transfusion reaction occurs when the transfused blood does not match the person's ABO blood type, and the antibodies they have present react with the antigens on the new blood cells.

SEX AND LIFE SPAN CONSIDERATIONS

Newborns do not form antibodies to ABO blood group antigens during the first 3 months of life. Infants older than 3 to 4 months and older adults are more likely to experience problems of fluid overload with transfusion, and children are more likely to develop transfusion-related HIV infections than are adults. The incidence of transfusion reactions does not appear to be based on gender, although nonhemolytic febrile reactions and extravascular hemolytic reactions are more common in females who have been pregnant.

HEALTH DISPARITIES AND SEXUAL/GENDER MINORITY HEALTH

DHTR occur in patients who have received previous transfusions. They are particularly serious and potentially life threatening for people with sickle cell disease, a blood disorder common in Black people of African origin. They may occur because of differences in red blood cell antigens in White blood donors and Black blood recipients, leading to transfusion reactions and hemolysis. Sexual and gender minority status has no known effect on the risk for transfusion reaction.

GLOBAL HEALTH CONSIDERATIONS

No data are available, but blood transfusion reactions have the potential to occur at any location where blood products are administered.

ASSESSMENT

HISTORY. Individuals who report a history of numerous allergies or previous transfusions should be monitored more carefully because they are at higher risk for transfusion reaction. A history of cardiovascular disease should be noted because those patients need to be monitored more carefully for fluid overload. Note also if a patient has a history of Raynaud syndrome or a cold agglutinin problem because, before being administered and with physician approval, the blood needs to be warmed. Once the transfusion is in process, the patient may report any of the following signs of transfusion reaction: heat or pain at the site of transfusion, **fever, chills, flushing, chest tightness, lower back pain,** abdominal pain, nausea, difficulty breathing, itching, and a feeling of impending doom.

PHYSICAL EXAMINATION. A change in any vital sign can indicate the beginning of a transfusion reaction. Note if the urine becomes cloudy or reddish (hemolysis). Observe any change in skin color or the appearance of hives. Be alert for signs of edema, especially in the oropharynx and face. Auscultate the lungs before beginning the transfusion, and note any baseline adventitious sounds; monitor for crackles or wheezes if the patient shows any signs of fluid overload, and inspect the patient's neck veins for distention.

PSYCHOSOCIAL. Blood bank protocols have lowered the risk of HIV transmission from more than 25,000 cases before 1985. Presently, only 1 in 2 million blood donations might carry HIV and transmit the disease to patients. In spite of the decreased risk, however, many patients worry about contracting HIV when they need blood products. In reality, the risk of hepatitis B and C is much higher; the risk of hepatitis B is 1 per 205,000 donations. If a blood transfusion reaction occurs, the fears and anxieties are compounded and may warrant specific interventions.

Diagnostic Highlights

In the event of a transfusion reaction, immediately stop the transfusion. Send the unit of blood, or empty bag and tubing if the infusion is complete, along with samples of the patient's blood and urine to the laboratory for analysis. Blood type and crossmatching are repeated to determine if mismatched blood was administered.

Test	Normal Result	Abnormality With Condition	Explanation
Free hemoglobin: Urine and plasma	Negative in urine < 3 mg/dL in blood	Free hemoglobin in urine and blood; hemoglobinuria occurs when > 150 mg/dL of free hemoglobin is present in blood	Transfusion reaction leads to escape of hemoglobin from red blood cells during intravascular hemolysis

Other Tests: Blood culture to rule out bacterial infection, urinalysis for presence of protein, serum bilirubin, haptoglobin, complete blood count, prothrombin time, partial thromboplastin time, fibrinogen, calcium, serum electrolytes

PRIMARY NURSING DIAGNOSIS

DIAGNOSIS. Risk for ineffective airway clearance as evidenced by restlessness, wheezing, stridor, dyspnea, and/or angioedema

OUTCOMES. Respiratory status: Airway patency; Respiratory status: Gas exchange; Respiratory status: Ventilation; Comfort status; Infection severity; Knowledge: Treatment regime

INTERVENTIONS. Airway management; Airway insertion and stabilization; Airway suctioning; Anxiety reduction; Oxygen therapy; Respiratory monitoring

PLANNING AND IMPLEMENTATION
Collaborative
PREVENTION. Typing, screening, and matching of blood units before administration eliminate most, but not all, incompatibilities. If a transfusion reaction does occur, stop the transfusion immediately and replace the donor blood with normal saline solution. The severity of the

reaction is usually related to the amount of blood received. Begin an assessment to determine the severity and type of reaction. In minor reactions (urticaria or fever), the transfusion may be restarted after discussion with the physician and after giving the patient an antipyretic, antihistamine, or anti-inflammatory agent. Ongoing monitoring during the rest of the transfusion is essential. If the patient develops anaphylaxis, the patient's airway and breathing are maintained with oxygen supplement, intubation, and mechanical ventilation if needed.

Pharmacologic Highlights

With an acute hemolytic reaction, there are three conditions to consider: renal failure, shock, and disseminated intravascular coagulation (DIC). To counteract shock and minimize renal failure, the physician prescribes aggressive normal saline or colloid IV infusion. Mannitol is often used to promote diuresis. Dopamine may be used if hypotension is a problem. Furosemide (Lasix) may be given to keep urine output at 50 to 100 mL/hr. For pyretic reactions, after the possibility of a hemolytic reaction is ruled out, an antipyretic such as acetaminophen may be given and the transfusion may be restarted with caution. For severe reactions, see the table that follows.

Medication or Drug Class	Dosage	Description	Rationale
Epinephrine	0.1–0.25 mg of 1:10,000 concentration IV over 5–10 min	Sympathomimetic; catecholamine	Given for severe reactions for its pressor effect and bronchodilation
Glucocorticoids	Varies by drug	Corticosteroid	Anti-inflammatory agents that limit laryngeal swelling

Other Drugs: Antihistamines may be given for minor allergic reactions, diuretics may be given to increase renal blood flow in hemolytic transfusion reactions and manage volume overload, and dopamine may be given to maintain cardiac output and renal blood flow.

Independent

Adhere strictly to the policies regarding typing, crossmatching, and administering blood. Check each unit before administration to make sure that it is not outdated, that the unit has been designated for the correct recipient, that the patient's medical records number matches the number on the blood component, and that the blood type is appropriate for the patient. All patients should have their identification band checked by two people before the transfusion is begun. Notify the blood bank and withhold the transfusion for even the smallest discrepancy when checking the blood with the patient identification. If a transfusion reaction occurs, make sure the recipient's blood sample is correctly labeled when it is sent to the laboratory. Maintain universal precautions when handling all blood products to protect yourself and dispose of used containers appropriately in the hazardous waste disposal.

Begin the transfusion at a rate of 75 mL or less per hour. Remain with the patient for the first 15 minutes of the transfusion to monitor for signs of a hemolytic reaction. If the patient develops a reaction, stop the transfusion immediately; evaluate the adequacy of the patient's airway, breathing, and circulation; take the patient's vital signs; notify the physician and blood bank; and return the unused portion of the blood to the blood bank for analysis. If the patient develops chills, monitor the patient's temperature and cover the patient with a blanket unless the temperature is above 102°F (38.9°C). Remain with the patient and explain that a reaction has occurred from the transfusion. If the patient has excessive fears or concerns about the risk of HIV or hepatitis infection, provide specific information to the patient and arrange for a consultation as needed with either a physician or a counselor.

Evidence-Based Practice and Health Policy

Shmookler, A., & Flanagan, M. (2020). Educational case: Febrile nonhemolytic transfusion reaction. *Academic Pathology*. Advance online publication. https://doi.org/10.1177/2374289520934097

- The authors described a case study of a 34-year-old woman who came to the emergency department because of lightheadedness and dizziness. She had a low hemoglobin (6.5 g/dL) and hematocrit (18.5%). Her physician prescribed the transfusion of a unit of red blood cells. Thirty minutes into the transfusion, the patient developed chills and fever.
- The transfusion was stopped immediately. Following a clinical assessment to determine that the patient was stable, the blood bank was alerted to ensure that the appropriate blood product was transfused to the appropriate patient. Following laboratory analysis of the patient's blood and urine, it was determined that she had a febrile nonhemolytic transfusion reaction, which has a risk of 3 per 100 transfusions. Ultimately after further laboratory work, the patient received a different unit of blood without reaction.

DOCUMENTATION GUIDELINES

- Response to transfusion: Description of symptoms; severity of symptoms; adequacy of airway, breathing, and circulation; location and description of any skin changes, vital signs, including temperature; complaints of pain or itching
- Termination of transfusion: Amount infused, amount returned to blood bank, laboratory specimens sent, timing of reaction from start of transfusion

DISCHARGE AND HOME HEALTHCARE GUIDELINES

FOLLOW-UP. Teach the patient to report any signs and symptoms of a delayed reaction, such as fever, jaundice, pallor, or fatigue. Explain that these reactions can occur anytime from 3 days after the transfusion to several months later.

Explain that the patient should notify the primary healthcare provider if they develop any discomfort in the first few months after transfusion. Attributing these signs to specific diseases may make the patient unnecessarily anxious, but the patient should know to notify the healthcare provider for anorexia, malaise, nausea, vomiting, concentrated urine, and jaundice within 4 to 6 weeks after transfusion (hepatitis B); jaundice, lethargy, and irritability with a milder intensity than that of hepatitis B (hepatitis C); or flu-like symptoms (HIV infection).

Bone Cancer

DRG Category:	543
Mean LOS:	4.4 days
Description:	MEDICAL: Pathological Fractures and Musculoskeletal and Connective Tissue Malignancy With Complication or Comorbidity

Bone cancers are sarcomas—that is, cancers of connective tissue. The American Cancer Society estimates that in 2021, about 3,610 new cases of bone cancer will be diagnosed, and 2,060 people will die from the condition. Primary bone cancers are relatively uncommon, constituting less than 0.2% of all cancers. Most (60%–65%) tumors of the bone are secondary, or metastatic, ones from other primary tumors. Cancers originating in the osseous, cartilaginous (chondrogenic), or membrane tissue are classified as bone cancer. Cancers originating from the bone marrow are usually classified as hematological cancers. The most common type of primary bone cancer is osteosarcoma (Table 1). Osteosarcoma and chondrosarcoma are the most common sarcomas of the bone; they comprise 70% of all bone cancers. The remaining 30% of bone cancers are Ewing sarcoma, chordomas, and malignant histiocytoma and fibrosarcomas.

• **TABLE 1** Major Types of Primary Bone Cancer

TYPE AND DESCRIPTION	AGES OF PEAK OCCURRENCE (YEARS)	MAJOR LOCATIONS IN THE BODY	POPULATIONS	COMMENTS
Osteogenic sarcoma or osteosarcoma: Most common malignant bone tumor, arises from bone-forming cells; often a solitary lesion in fast-growing long bones (35% of cases)	10–20; increased incidence during the adolescent growth spurt; a second peak of incidence occurs in adults older than 60	Distal femur, proximal tibia, proximal humerus	Incidence is slightly higher in males as compared to females and slightly higher in Black as compared to White persons	Most common cause of death is pulmonary metastasis; primary treatment is surgical removal of lesion and chemotherapy
Chondrosarcoma: Group of tumors consisting primarily of cartilage (25% of cases)	Peaks at 50–60 but occurs in ages 25–75	Cartilage of pelvis, ribs, ilium, femur, humerus	Incidence is slightly higher in males as compared to females; incidence does not seem to vary among races and ethnicities	Surgery is the primary therapy but chemotherapy or radiotherapy may be used, particularly in palliative care; 5-year survival rate is 50%–60%
Ewing sarcoma: Usually occurs in bone but also arises from soft tissue (16% of cases)	10–20; rare in adults > 30	Long bones of legs and arms; pelvis	Males have a higher incidence than females; incidence is nine times higher in White persons than Black persons	The primary therapy is chemotherapy, but surgery and radiotherapy may be used; overall survival rate is 60%
Fibrosarcoma: Can occur in soft tissue and bone (6% of all cases)	35–55	Bone of leg, arm, jaw	Incidence is slightly higher in males as compared to females; incidence does not seem to vary among races and ethnicities	Primary therapy is surgery, but radiotherapy and chemotherapy may be used; 5-year survival rate is 65%

(table continues on page 172)

• **TABLE 1** Major Types of Primary Bone Cancer (continued)

TYPE AND DESCRIPTION	AGES OF PEAK OCCURRENCE (YEARS)	MAJOR LOCATIONS IN THE BODY	POPULATIONS	COMMENTS
Chordoma: Arises from vertebral column; tumors are slow growing (2%–4% of all cases)	55–65	Sacrum, coccyx, base of skull	Incidence in males is twice that of females; incidence does not seem to vary among races and ethnicities	Primary therapy is surgery, but radiotherapy and chemotherapy are used; 5-year survival rate is 51%

CAUSES

The specific cause of bone cancer is unknown. Evidence links the development of bone cancer with exposure to therapeutic radiation or treatment with some chemotherapeutic agents. A higher incidence has not occurred, however, in populations exposed to other forms of radiation, such as survivors of the atomic bomb. There have been reports of siblings with bone cancer, suggesting genetic influences. Osteogenic sarcoma is most common after puberty, which suggests that hormonal fluctuations and spurts of growth may be involved. Bone cancers tend to be more common in adults who are affected by Paget disease, hyperparathyroidism, and chronic osteomyelitis. The development of bone cancer has also been linked to trauma and sites of old bone infarcts or fractures, multiple exostoses (overgrowth of bone tissue), multiple osteochondromas (benign bone tumor), and bone marrow transplantation.

GENETIC CONSIDERATIONS

Several factors can increase the risk of bone cancer. Families with retinoblastoma (an eye cancer often caused by mutations in *RB1*) have an increased risk for osteosarcoma, as do those with familial cancer syndromes, such as Li-Fraumeni syndrome (from *TP53* and *CHEK2* mutations). The genetic condition of multiple hereditary exostosis (abnormal bone overgrowths) also increases the likelihood of bone cancer, which may be caused by a loss of heterozygosity of a tumor suppressor at 18q21-q22. Rothmund-Thomson syndrome is an autosomal recessive syndrome of congenital bone defects, hair and skin dysplasia, hypogonadism, and cataracts that is also associated with increased risk of osteosarcoma.

SEX AND LIFE SPAN CONSIDERATIONS

Table 1 describes the sex and life span considerations. Children seem particularly susceptible to bone cancer related to exposure to therapeutic radiation or chemotherapeutic agents. Metastatic bone cancer usually appears later in life because it accompanies other cancers, especially lung, breast, prostate, and thyroid cancer.

HEALTH DISPARITIES AND SEXUAL/GENDER MINORITY HEALTH

The National Institutes of Health (https://www.cancer.gov) in the United States provides statistics and information about cancer disparities. Black persons have higher death rates than all other groups for many cancer types. Some forms of cancer have higher rates in Hispanic and Native American persons than White persons. The incidence rates of some types of cancer are much higher in rural Appalachia than urban areas in the same region. Rates of smoking and alcohol use, which increases cancer risk, are higher among sexual and gender minority youths as compared to heterosexual youths. People with low income, low health literacy, long travel distances to cancer screening sites, or who lack health insurance or paid medical leave are less likely to be treated according to cancer care guidelines. People who live in communities that lack clean water and clean air my be exposed to cancer-causing substances. These factors all contribute to inequities in cancer diagnosis, treatment, and outcome. Table 1 describes information on incidence of bone cancer by racial and ethnic groups.

GLOBAL HEALTH CONSIDERATIONS

The overall incidence of bone cancer globally is slightly higher in males than in females and approximately three times higher in developed countries compared with developing countries.

ASSESSMENT

HISTORY. The focus of the assessment should be on gathering data that differentiate bone cancer from arthritic or traumatic pain. The patient usually reports the gradual onset of pain described as a dull or deep ache in the back, pelvis, legs, ribs, and/or arms. The patient often notices a swelling or the inability to move a joint as before. Parents may relate that their child has growing pains or a sprain, which may mimic symptoms of bone cancer. A child may report a history of trauma, which may have links to bone cancer. A distinctive trait of bone cancer pain is its tendency to be worse at night. Generally, it is a localized, aching pain, but it may also be referred from the hip or spine. The sudden onset of pain does not rule out bone cancer, however, because a pathological fracture may be present. If the cancer has spread, the patient may report weight loss and fatigue.

PHYSICAL EXAMINATION. **The most common symptom is pain with activity.** Inspect for any unusual swellings or dilated surface vessels. The patient may walk with a limp or have weakness, or muscle atrophy, of the affected limb. If the tumor has progressed, you may note weight loss or cachexia, fever, and decreased mobility. Perform gentle range-of-motion exercises of all the extremities and document any limitations in joint movement. Note any firm, nontender enlargements in the affected area when it is palpated. Consider, however, that bone tumors are not always visible or palpable. The tumor site may also be tender.

PSYCHOSOCIAL. The impact of a cancer diagnosis is long lasting even after the physical symptoms are treated. Patients have conflicting emotions, including loss, anxiety, fear, despair, hope, and relief. Managing cancer makes transitions necessary. Although some cancers can be cured with treatments that leave no visible signs, primary bone cancer often requires extensive surgical reconstruction or amputation of the affected limb as part of the treatment. Determine the patient's view of their body image and assess whether the impact of the treatment may lead to a body image disturbance.

Diagnostic Highlights

Test	Normal Result	Abnormality With Condition	Explanation
Serum alkaline phosphatase (ALP) and lactic hydrogenase (LDH)	ALP: 25–142 units/L; LDH: 90–203 units/L	Normal to elevated	Elevations occur with formation of new bone by increasing osteoblastic activity; elevated ALP may suggest pulmonary metastases in osteosarcoma; normal LDH may suggest better outcomes

(highlight box continues on page 174)

Diagnostic Highlights (continued)

Test	Normal Result	Abnormality With Condition	Explanation
X-rays and computed tomography (CT); magnetic resonance imaging (MRI); technetium-99 bone scan	No lesions	Visualization of lesions; malignant lesions often have poor margination, irregular new bone growth	Each tumor type has its own characteristic pattern; CT shows extent of soft tissue damage; MRI of primary lesion assesses extent of disease

Other Tests: In Ewing sarcoma and metastatic bone lesions, increases occur in erythrocyte sedimentation rate as well as in leukocytosis and normocytic anemia. Other tests include bone biopsy, serum calcium, complete blood count, liver function tests, serum electrolytes, renal function tests, and urinalysis.

PRIMARY NURSING DIAGNOSIS

DIAGNOSIS. Impaired physical mobility related to activity intolerance and loss of limb as evidenced by self-report of pain with activity, excision of tumors, and/or altered gait

OUTCOMES. Knowledge: Cancer management; Ambulation; Joint movement; Mobility; Self-care: Activities of daily living; Transfer performance; Balance; Muscle rehabilitation participation; Pain level

INTERVENTIONS. Exercise therapy: Ambulation and joint mobility; Positioning; Energy management; Exercise promotion; Self-care assistance; Teaching: Prescribed exercise; Medication management; Pain management: Acute and chronic

PLANNING AND IMPLEMENTATION
Collaborative
MEDICAL. Radiation has variable effectiveness in bone cancer. It is effective with Ewing sarcoma, moderately effective with osteosarcoma, and relatively ineffective in chondrosarcoma. Even when a cure is not possible, radiation is often used to decrease pain and slow the disease process. External beam radiation therapy, where the radiation is delivered from outside of the body, is the type most often used to treat bone cancer. Palliative care becomes important at the end of life.

SURGICAL. Surgery may range from simple curettage (removal of necrotic tissue or tumor with a curet) when primary bone cancer is confined to amputation or extensive resection such as a leg amputation with hemipelvectomy. Ongoing data suggest that for many bone cancers, limb-sparing treatment (surgical removal of only the tumor with chemotherapy and/or radiation) may provide the same cure rate as amputation. Pain is usually managed with narcotic analgesia in the immediate postoperative period. As the patient recovers, prosthetic devices are often fitted after amputations. The patient may have a prosthesis fitted immediately or a more traditional delayed fitting. Usually, a physical therapist works with the patient to help them learn ways to maintain mobility and the appropriate use of appliances and adjuncts.

Pharmacologic Highlights

Medication or Drug Class	Dosage	Description	Rationale
Chemotherapy	Varies by drug	Doxorubicin, vincristine, cyclophosphamide, cisplatin, methotrexate with calcium leucovorin, ifosfamide, etoposide	Chemotherapy is often used preoperatively to reduce the size of the tumor or postoperatively to help eliminate the risk of micrometastasis

Pharmacologic Highlights (continued)

Other Drugs: Immunotherapy, primarily interferon or tumor-specific transfer factor, remains investigational with bone cancer; analgesia. Zoledronic acid is used for the treatment of bone metastases and is superior to the other bisphosphonates in the treatment of pain and skeletal-related events.

Independent

Presurgical preparation is essential. Encourage the patient to eat foods high in protein and vitamins to foster wound healing. Begin teaching the exercises that, after surgery, prevent contractures and strengthen limbs to accept the adjustments in posturing and movement. With extensive resection, the patient is exposed to anesthesia for a longer period of time. Preparation for pulmonary toileting and methods to prevent venous stasis become even more important in those patients. When radiation or chemotherapy is used as well, begin preoperative teaching.

Start exercises within 24 hours after surgery to maintain muscle tone and prevent edema, joint contractures, and muscle atrophy. If a prosthesis is to be fitted after healing, take care to wrap the stump to promote proper shrinking and shaping without compromising the patient's circulation.

Whether the treatment is amputation, resection, chemotherapy, or radiation, the changes in the patient's body create severe emotional stress. Listen to the patient's concerns and support efforts to maintain grooming and hygiene. Provide opportunities for the patient to make treatment decisions and to maintain as much control over their environment as possible. If the patient develops a body image disturbance or ineffective coping, provide referrals for counseling or a support group when required. Acquaint the patient and family with the supports available through the American Cancer Society or hospice.

Evidence-Based Practice and Health Policy

Shinoda, Y., Sawada, R., Yoshikawa, F., Oki, T., Hirai, T., Kobayashi, H., Matsudaira, K., Oka, H., Tanaka, S., Kawano, H., & Haga, N. (2019). Factors related to the quality of life in patients with bone metastases. *Clinical & Experimental Metastasis, 36,* 441–448.

- The authors noted that treatments for bone metastases are focused on preserving patients' quality of life. They studied the clinical factors of quality of life in 174 patients with bone metastasis in different settings and with different treatment statuses. They also collected data on tumor progression, bone metastasis, pain level, and performance status.
- Skeletal-related events (fracture, paralysis, radiation, or surgery), pain, and performance of activities of daily living (ADLs) were related to quality of life, symptoms, and emotional functioning but were not related to prognosis. The authors suggested that the most important focus should not be prognosis but rather level of pain, ability to perform ADLs, and prevention of skeletal-related events to improve quality of life.

DOCUMENTATION GUIDELINES

- Appearance of the surgical incision site: Presence of inflammation, infection, or signs of healing
- Response to chemotherapy or radiation treatments
- Comprehension of treatment plan, including care of surgical site, purpose, and potential side effects of medical treatments
- Reaction to the loss or disfigurement and prognosis
- Readiness to adapt to a prosthetic device and changes in perception of the body
- Presence of complications: Infection, bleeding, poor wound healing, ineffective coping by the patient or significant others

DISCHARGE AND HOME HEALTHCARE GUIDELINES

PREPARATION FOR PROSTHETIC. Teach the patient how to promote healing at the surgical site by keeping the incision clean, dry, and covered. Explain that the stump needs to be wrapped to promote shrinkage and proper shaping for the prosthesis. Teach exercises to maintain strength and range of motion and to prevent contractures. Explain the roles of the interdisciplinary team members in the patient's rehabilitation.

CONTINUING TREATMENT. If the patient receives outpatient chemotherapy or radiation, teach the patient the purpose, duration, and potential complications of those treatments. Refer the patient to hospice or a palliative care specialist if warranted.

Botulism

DRG Category:	868
Mean LOS:	4.6 days
Description:	MEDICAL: Other Infectious and Parasitic Diseases Diagnoses With Complication or Comorbidity

Botulism is a serious neurotoxic disorder caused by the gram-positive, spore-forming bacterium *Clostridium botulinum*, which is found in soil and in the gastrointestinal (GI) tract of birds, fish, and mammals. Although it is usually harmless in the spore state, the organism flourishes in warm anaerobic environments, causing germination with bacterial multiplication and toxin production. Botulism occurs when the bacterium is ingested into the GI tract or enters through an open wound. Once ingested or embedded, the bacterium enters the vascular system. Toxins act at the neuromuscular junction by impairing the release of the neurotransmitter acetylcholine from the presynaptic membrane. Loss of acetylcholine causes paralysis of voluntary and involuntary muscles. Eight distinct toxins are known, including A, B, C alpha, C beta, D, E, F, and G. Each strain of the bacteria produces only a single toxin, and types A, B, E, and rarely F, can affect humans.

Approximately 150 to 200 cases of botulism are reported each year in the United States, of which 25% are food-borne, 72% are infant botulism, and the remainder are from wounds. Botulism has a mortality rate generally reported as 5% to 10%, with death occurring as a result of respiratory failure during the first week. If onset is rapid (< 24 hours) after ingestion of the bacterium, the course of the disease is more severe and potentially fatal. Paralytic ileus is another complication of botulism.

In persons older than 12 months, the spores are unable to germinate in the gut because of the presence of gastric acid. Therefore, the food-borne disease is caused by ingesting a preformed toxin. The spores, however, can germinate in the GI tract of infants younger than 1 year because infants have lower levels of gastric acid, decreased levels of normal flora, and an immature immune system. The GI environment in infants is conducive to toxin production, making infants particularly susceptible to the spores present in unprepared foods.

CAUSES

There are six forms of botulism: food borne, wound borne, infant borne, adult intestinal colonization, infection related, and inhalation. Food-borne botulism occurs when food contaminated with the toxin from the bacteria is ingested. It is caused by the consumption of improperly canned or stored food that is contaminated with spores. Infant botulism occurs when an infant ingests spores in honey or other foods that produce the toxin in the infant's GI tract. Wound botulism occurs from toxin produced in a wound contaminated with *C botulinum*.

GENETIC CONSIDERATIONS

No clear genetic contributions to susceptibility have been defined.

SEX AND LIFE SPAN CONSIDERATIONS

Botulism has been observed in all age groups and equally in both genders; causative factors, however, may differ across the life span. *C botulinum* is usually harmless to adults if ingested while in the spore state, but not so in infants. Botulism occurs most commonly in infants ages 1 week to 11 months; peak susceptibility occurs at 2 to 4 months.

HEALTH DISPARITIES AND SEXUAL/GENDER MINORITY HEALTH

Ethnicity, race, and sexual/gender minority status have no known effect on the risk for botulism.

GLOBAL HEALTH CONSIDERATIONS

Botulism spores from *C botulinum* can be found in the soil throughout the world. In Europe, toxin type B is more common. In Europe, contamination of ham and sausage is the most common mode of transmission. In infants under age 1 year, countries in North America, Western Europe, Japan, China, and Australia have reported the largest number of cases of botulism.

ASSESSMENT

HISTORY. Elicit a history from the patient or parents regarding food consumption for the last 12 to 96 hours. Note that the incubation period ranges between 12 and 36 hours but depends on the amount of toxin the person ingested. Encourage the patient not only to identify the type of food, but also to explain the food preparation, with particular attention to the level of heat to which the food was exposed during preparation. Ask the patient if they have experienced any puncture wounds recently, particularly while gardening or working with soil.

Patients may describe symptoms of botulism within 12 hours of exposure. Initially, patients may describe nausea and vomiting, although often they remain alert and oriented without sensory or neurological deficits. Some patients report diarrhea or constipation, whereas others describe a very dry, sore throat and difficulty swallowing; some may experience GI symptoms prior to neurological symptoms or the symptoms may occur simultaneously. Patients also describe neuromuscular abnormalities. Symptoms usually occur in a descending order from the head to the toes. Ask patients if they have experienced blurred vision, double vision, difficulty swallowing, difficulty speaking, or weakness of the arms and legs.

PHYSICAL EXAMINATION. The most common symptoms in food-borne and wound-borne botulism in adults are **nausea, vomiting**, and **diarrhea**. Cranial nerve involvement occurs early in the disease course and leads to drooping eyelids, double vision, and extraocular muscle paralysis. Most patients lose their gag reflex, and fixed or dilated pupils occur in approximately 50% of patients as the disease progresses. Note if the patient has difficulty speaking. Inspect the symmetry of the facial expression. Evaluate the strength and motion of the extremities because weakness progresses to the neck, arms, thorax, and legs. Ask the patient to shrug the shoulders while you press gently on them to test for strength and symmetry. Check for respiratory depression and apnea. As the disorder progresses, respiratory muscle paralysis occurs from phrenic nerve involvement, and the patient stops breathing.

The most common symptoms of infant botulism are **constipation**, neurological visual deficits (**diplopia, blurred vision**) and **loss of the gag reflex**. Also, infants may have poor feeding, lethargy, ptosis, sluggish pupils, flat facial expression, diminished sucking reflex, and a weak cry. Symptoms may progress to respiratory difficulty and respiratory arrest.

PSYCHOSOCIAL. Because of the potential for lifestyle changes and the lengthy hospitalization, children with botulism are at risk for alterations in growth and development. Assess the growth and development level in all age groups. Parents are understandably worried about the health of their infant or child and need reassurance and possibly counseling.

Diagnostic Highlights

Test	Normal Result	Abnormality With Condition	Explanation
Serum, vomitus or gastric aspiration, suspected food, or stool toxin level	Negative	Positive	C botulinum produces the toxin
Culture and sensitivity from gastric, wound, or stool specimen	Negative	Positive for C botulinum	Bacteria that causes botulism

PRIMARY NURSING DIAGNOSIS

DIAGNOSIS. Ineffective airway clearance related to respiratory muscle paralysis as evidenced by loss of gag reflex

OUTCOMES. Respiratory status: Airway patency, gas exchange, and ventilation; Infection severity; Knowledge: Acute illness management

INTERVENTIONS. Airway insertion and stabilization; Airway management; Airway suctioning; Oral health promotion; Respiratory monitoring; Ventilation assistance

PLANNING AND IMPLEMENTATION

Collaborative

Report cases of botulism toxicity so that others can be protected from the illness; contact the regional Poison Control Center, state health department, or Centers for Disease Control and Prevention Operations Center. Because laboratory results may take time, treatment should be initiated on the basis of symptoms. When botulism poisoning from ingestion is suspected, the patient's stomach is lavaged to remove any unabsorbed toxin; a high colonic enema may also be administered for the same purpose. If impaired swallowing and chewing last longer than 72 hours, enteral feeding via a nasogastric (NG) or nasointestinal tube or total parenteral nutrition is instituted. When infants contract botulism, their course may progress to complete respiratory failure requiring mechanical ventilation.

WOUND CARE. Infected wounds are explored and débrided. Antitoxin can be injected directly into the wound site, and often 3% hydrogen peroxide is applied to produce aerobic conditions. Hyperbaric oxygen therapy may be used. Usually the physician prescribes antibiotics such as penicillin to kill bacteria in the wound. Antibiotic therapy to treat GI infection in infant botulism is contraindicated because the treatment increases toxin release and worsens the condition. Antibiotics may be considered to treat secondary bacterial infections.

SUPPORTIVE CARE. If respiratory paralysis occurs, intubation or tracheotomy and mechanical ventilation are essential to maintain airway and breathing. At least every hour, monitor the patient's breath sounds, placement, and position of the endotracheal tube; the respiratory rate and lung expansion; and the type and characteristics of secretions. A Foley catheter is inserted to monitor urinary output and prevent bladder distention.

Pharmacologic Highlights

Medication or Drug Class	Dosage	Description	Rationale
Trivalent (toxin types A, B, D, E, and F) botulism antitoxin	One vial IM, one vial IV (10,000 IU)	Equine antitoxin	Neutralizes absorbed toxin
Botulism immune globulin IV (human) (Baby-BIG-IV; for infants under the age of 1 year)	50 mg/kg IV as a single dose or a dosage as the package insert recommends	Purified immunoglobulin from adults immunized with botulinum toxoid	Provides antibodies to neutralize circulating toxins

Independent

Other family members who have been exposed to contaminated food should obtain healthcare immediately. Exposed family members should receive an immediate gastric lavage and a high colonic enema to purge their system of the toxin in the bowel if they were exposed.

Patients are not given food, fluids, or medications orally until their swallowing status is normal and they have an active gag reflex. Provide mouth care every 2 hours to improve comfort and to destroy oral flora. Because the patient has difficulty speaking, establish other routes for communication. Explain that the ability to speak returns as the condition resolves.

During periods of impaired mobility, turn patients every 2 hours and monitor their skin for breakdown. Egg crate mattresses or air beds may be useful. At a minimum of every shift, perform active and/or passive range-of-motion exercises for immobile or bedridden patients. Position unconscious patients on their sides to prevent aspiration of stomach contents; tracheal suction and chest physiotherapy may be indicated to maintain pulmonary hygiene.

Offer clarification and support of the information regarding the diagnosis and prognosis to patients and families. Monitor the patient and family to determine if effective coping mechanisms are in place.

Evidence-Based Practice and Health Policy

Panditrao, M., Dabritz, H., Kazerouni, N., Damus, K., Meissinger, J., & Arnon, S. (2020). Descriptive epidemiology of infant botulism in California: The first 40 years. *Journal of Pediatrics, 227*, 247–257.

- The authors proposed to determine the descriptive epidemiology of infant botulism in the first 40 years following initial recognition in 1974 in California counties. They studied cases identified by laboratory identification of botulinum toxin in patients' feces. They located 1,345 cases of infant botulism caused by botulinum toxin types A, B, and F.
- Breastfed infants (83%) were more than twice as old at the onset of disease as formula-fed infants. Approximately 51% were female; 84% were White, 9% were Asian, 3% were Black, and 3% other races. With respect to ethnicity, 30% were Hispanic.

DOCUMENTATION GUIDELINES

- Respiratory assessment: Rate and rhythm, lung expansion, breath sounds, color of skin and mucous membranes, oxygen saturation, patency and placement of artificial airways, response to mechanical ventilation
- Neurological assessment: Level of consciousness, strength and movement, status of cough and gag reflexes, cranial nerve function, ability to swallow
- Cardiovascular assessment: Heart rate and rhythm, blood pressure, peripheral pulses, color of complexion, skin temperature
- Response to medications, intubation, oxygen therapy, mechanical ventilation

- Condition of skin and mucous membranes
- GI assessment: Bowel sounds, presence of abdominal distention, volume and character of NG tube output, stool character, and bowel elimination patterns

DISCHARGE AND HOME HEALTHCARE GUIDELINES

PATIENT AND FAMILY TEACHING. Teach the family that botulism is a preventable disorder. Ensure that any other persons who ate the contaminated food are seen immediately by health providers. Explain that patients should discard any canned food that has a broken seal or an expired date or is swollen. Home-canned foods should be boiled, not warmed, before eating. Boiling for 20 minutes destroys botulism bacteria and spores. Instruct patients living in high altitudes to use a pressure cooker to boil foods adequately. Teach patients to use new cap seals with each canning session if they can at home. Teach the family to recognize the complications of botulism. If the patient survives the poisoning, teach patients and families that residual effects might be present for a year or more. Intensive, multidisciplinary rehabilitation and follow-up may be required to restore full function.

Brain Cancer

DRG Category:	27
Mean LOS:	2.6 days
Description:	SURGICAL: Craniotomy and Endovascular Intracranial Procedures Without Complication or Comorbidity or Major Complication or Comorbidity
DRG Category:	54
Mean LOS:	5.1 days
Description:	MEDICAL: Nervous System Neoplasms With Major Complication or Comorbidity

Adult brain tumors comprise only 2% of cancers in the United States, but brain tumors are the second-most common group of malignancies (after leukemia) that affect children. They account for 2.4% of all cancer deaths. Primary brain tumors develop from various tissue types within the intracranial cavity and are named for the tissue in which they originate (e.g., astrocytomas originate in the astrocytes). Tumors are customarily described as benign or malignant; however, all brain tumors may be considered malignant because without treatment, the patient dies. Even tumors that are well contained may lead to serious consequences because they compress or invade neighboring structures within the enclosed skull. Brain tumors cause their symptoms directly by destroying neurons or indirectly by exerting pressure, displacing brain structures, and increasing intracranial pressure (ICP). Besides primary tumors arising from intracranial tissue, metastatic tumors may also migrate to the area by hematogenous spread. Common sources for brain metastases are the lung, breast, melanoma, and colon. Advances in diagnosis, surgical techniques, and adjunctive therapy have greatly improved the outlook for patients with brain cancer. About 50% are treatable with a hopeful prognosis.

Statistics from the American Cancer Society in 2021 estimated that there would be 24,530 cases of brain and spinal cord tumors diagnosed: 13,840 in men and 10,690 in women. In 2021, approximately 18,600 people will likely die from this disease: 10,500 males and 8,100 females. A person's lifetime risk of developing a brain and spinal cord malignancy is less than 1%.

Because of the difficulty with pathological discrimination and absence of metastasis, the clinical staging method is not used to describe brain cancer. Rather, tumors are classified as low grade or high grade. Although there are a wide variety of histologic types (Table 1), a small number of tumor types account for the most morbidity and mortality. Average survival time for persons with a low-grade astrocytoma is 6 to 8 years; the average survival time for a person with a glioblastoma is 12 months.

• TABLE 1 Primary Intracranial Tumors

TUMOR	PERCENTAGE OF CASES	PEAK INCIDENCE	CLINICAL MANIFESTATIONS	TREATMENT AND PROGNOSIS
Astrocytoma (type of glioma)	30%–35%	30–40 years	Altered mental status; headache, visual disturbances; decreased motor strength and coordination; seizures or altered vital signs	By time of diagnosis, total excision is usually not possible unless there is a cerebellar lesion; variable prognosis; radiotherapy, adjuvant chemotherapy
Glioblastoma multiform (most severe type of astrocytoma; see above)	12%–15% of all intracranial neoplasms; 50%–60% of astrocytic tumors	45–70 years	Twice as common in males; increased ICP with nonspecific mental and behavioral changes at first; later focal signs depending on location	Surgery where possible; poor response to radiation; course is rapidly progressive with poor prognosis
Oligodendroglioma (type of glioma)	5%–19% of all intracranial neoplasms; 25% of gliomas	20–45 years	More common in men; slow growing with gradual development of symptoms; seizures, decreased visual acuity and other visual disturbances	Surgical excision, which is usually successful
Ependymoma (type of glioma)	3%–6%	0–10 years	Similar to oligodendroglioma; increased ICP, hydrocephalus if tumor obstructs cerebrospinal fluid (CSF) pathway, cranial nerve dysfunction, ataxia, papilledema	Surgical excision; usually not radiosensitive

(table continues on page 182)

• TABLE 1 Primary Intracranial Tumors (continued)

TUMOR	PERCENTAGE OF CASES	PEAK INCIDENCE	CLINICAL MANIFESTATIONS	TREATMENT AND PROGNOSIS
Medulloblas-toma	< 5%	0–9 years	Tumor in the cerebellum seen frequently in children; more common in males and White persons than other groups; nonspecific symptoms of increased ICP; local signs vary with location	Surgery combined with radiation and chemotherapy
Meningioma	20%	35–55 years	More common in females and in Black persons; originates from dura or arachnoid; compresses rather than invades structures; headache, vomiting, seizures, mental and behavioral changes	Surgery; may recur if excision is incomplete
Schwannoma (acoustic neuroma, neurilemma)	8%	50–65 years	Higher incidence in women; ipsilateral hearing loss is most common; later may be accompanied by tinnitus, headache	Excision by translabyrinth surgery, craniotomy, or both; usually favorable outcome

CAUSES

Most brain tumors are not associated with any risk factors but rather with individual cell mutations. Evidence suggests that therapeutic radiation for other purposes (e.g., leukemia) may predispose individuals to later development of a brain tumor. Brain tumors are also more common in the immunosuppressed population and patients with HIV infection. Links between cellular telephone use and brain tumors have not been supported scientifically.

GENETIC CONSIDERATIONS

Some rare genetic conditions, including von Hippel-Lindau disease, Turcot syndrome, tuberous sclerosis, Li-Fraumeni, nevoid basal cell carcinoma syndrome, and neurofibromatosis, increase the risk of developing a brain tumor. Abnormalities in over a dozen chromosomal regions have been associated with gliomas, and combinations of both genetic and environmental factors seem to increase susceptibility. Heritability of glioma susceptibility is estimated at 25%. Medulloblastomas are associated with germ line mutations in *SUFU* and *BRCA2* and somatic mutations in *PTCH2*, *CTNNB1*, and *APC*. Neuroblastomas are associated with germ line mutations in *PHOX2B*, *KIF1B*, *ALK*, *NME1*, and *SDHB* genes.

SEX AND LIFE SPAN CONSIDERATIONS

While tumors vary by type, overall tumors are more prevalent in males than females (see Table 1). The greatest difference is in glioblastomas, in which up to 60% are in males. Brain tumors may occur at any age and are fairly common in both children and adults. They are common in children less than age 1 year and then again between ages 2 and 13 years. In children, primary tumors of the brain and spinal column are the second-most common (after leukemias) type of childhood cancer—that is, the most common solid tumor. However, most central nervous system (CNS) tumors occur in patients over age 45 years, with the peak incidence found after age 70 years. More than 50% of these CNS tumors are metastatic rather than primary. The 5-year survival rate decreases with age. For persons ages 15 to 44 years, it is 55%; for those ages 45 to 64 years, it is 16%; and for those over age 65 years, it is 5%.

HEALTH DISPARITIES AND SEXUAL/GENDER MINORITY HEALTH

Gliomas are the most commonly occurring malignant brain tumor in the United States. They occur most often in non-Hispanic White persons, who also have a lower survival rate than other groups. Black women have a slightly higher incidence of meningiomas and pituitary adenomas than do other groups. In children with brain tumors, scientists have determined that, while there do not appear to be disparities at diagnosis, Black and Hispanic children had a greater risk of dying compared with White children. Experts suggest that these differences may depend on implicit bias that made clinicians less willing to take the same risks with children from underrepresented groups, which translated into lack of access to high-quality care for these children (Fineberg et al., 2020). While little is known about health disparities due to brain tumors in sexual and gender minorities, factors such as poverty, stigma, and discrimination affect access to healthcare and may lead to poorer outcomes.

GLOBAL HEALTH CONSIDERATIONS

The global incidence of brain and nervous system cancer is 3.5 per 100,000 males and 2.6 per 100,000 females. Worldwide, the estimates are that each year approximately 250,000 people develop brain and nervous system cancers. Developed countries have rates approximately three times that of developing countries, but those rates may occur because developed countries have more resources for data collection than do developing countries.

ASSESSMENT

HISTORY. Symptoms produced by tumors vary by cell type and location and may cause generalized or focal symptoms. Although clearly every case of headache or dizziness is not a sign of brain tumor, it must always be considered. Determine if any of the following symptoms have occurred: headache, progressive neurological deficit, convulsions (focal or generalized), ataxia, gait disturbance, weakness, increased ICP, and organic mental changes.

The generalized symptoms are usually caused by increased ICP from the tumor, obstruction of the CSF pathways, or cerebral edema. Headache and vomiting are the most common first symptoms of increased ICP. Typically, headache is worse in the morning and may wake the patient from sleep. The patient or significant others may also report personality changes (irritability initially, progressing to apathy and forgetfulness), increased fatigue, decreased endurance, visual disturbances, and a tendency toward social withdrawal. Generalized seizures are the presenting symptoms in 15% of adults and 30% of children.

Focal signs and symptoms result from local pressure or damage to limited parts of the brain and depend on the area of the brain affected. Tumors in the dominant hemisphere produce communication difficulties (aphasia); tumors near an optic tract will produce changes in visual fields. A lesion in the temporal lobe may lead to temporal lobe seizures that are exhibited by unexplained olfactory sensations, visual auras, or psychomotor seizures, all of which may be misdiagnosed as psychological problems or mental illness.

PHYSICAL EXAMINATION. While symptoms vary with brain tumor type or location, common symptoms include **headache**, **visual changes**, **dizziness**, and **seizures**. Inspect the child suspected of a brain tumor before the sutures are closed; there may be head enlargement or bulging of the fontanelles from increased ICP. In rare cases, an adult with meningioma may have skull bulging. The appearance of the optic disk may change; if the tumor compresses the optic nerve, it will remain flat or atrophy. If ICP is increased, papilledema is possible. Perform a thorough neurological examination to identify changes in vision, hearing, sensation, speech, balance, and movement. A tumor may exert local pressure causing apraxia (an inability to use objects), paresthesia (numbness and tingling), paresis (partial or incomplete paralysis), or hyperreflexia.

PSYCHOSOCIAL. Assess for the presence of irritability and personality changes. Changes in a person's mental status and ability to perform various roles are extremely disturbing to patients and significant others. Families and patients often display profound grief, extreme anxiety, and disbelief upon receiving the diagnosis of a brain tumor.

Diagnostic Highlights

Test	Normal Result	Abnormality With Condition	Explanation
Computed tomography and magnetic resonance imaging	No space-occupying lesions	Locates size, location, and extent of tumor	Used for initial evaluation as well as response to treatment
Other Tests: Cerebral angiogram, electroencephalography, lumbar puncture, myelogram, brain scan, positron emission tomography			

PRIMARY NURSING DIAGNOSIS

DIAGNOSIS. Risk for ineffective cerebral tissue perfusion as evidenced by headache, visual changes, dizziness, and/or seizures

OUTCOMES. Neurological status: Consciousness and cranial nerve sensory/motor function; Pain level; Knowledge: Cancer management; Fluid balance

INTERVENTIONS. Cerebral perfusion promotion; Cerebral edema management; Neurological monitoring; Positioning: Neurological; Vital signs monitoring; Medication administration

PLANNING AND IMPLEMENTATION
Collaborative

The type of treatment used for brain cancer depends on the type of tumor (see Table 1). The primary modes of treatment include surgery, radiotherapy, and pharmacologic therapy.

SURGICAL. Surgery remains the primary treatment modality. A craniotomy is done to remove larger tumors. This involves making a surgical opening in the cranium to remove the tumor and inspect various areas of the brain; reconstruction is required. Stereotactic surgery involves insertion of a needle through a small opening in the skull to "suction out" the small tumor. The goals of surgery are (1) total removal of the tumor, (2) subtotal removal to relieve symptoms, or (3) procedures to protect the brain from damage, such as placement of a shunt to relieve hydrocephalus. Other modalities are used in combination. After the surgery, the patient needs careful monitoring for increased ICP. Notify the surgeon if the bone flap becomes elevated, which is a sign of increased ICP. The physician usually manages cerebral swelling and elevated ICP with fluid restriction (usually 1,500 mL or less in 24 hr), steroids, shunt placement, and osmotic diuretics such as mannitol.

RADIATION. For tumors that are not accessible to surgical removal, radiation may be used. Locally contained tumors receive direct-beam radiation focused on the lesion. For multiple lesions, especially metastatic brain lesions, whole-brain radiation therapy (WBRT) is used. Radiation usually is not used in children under age 2 years because of the long-term effects, such as panhypopituitarism, developmental delay, and secondary tumors.

Pharmacologic Highlights

Medication or Drug Class	Dosage	Description	Rationale
Chemotherapy	Varies by drug and tumor type	Some germ cell tumors respond well to a combination of vincristine, bleomycin, methotrexate, and cisplatin	Chemotherapy plays a very minor role in the treatment of brain metastases; the blood-brain barrier prevents delivery to the tumor of the cytotoxic agents in high concentrations
Corticosteroids	Varies by drug	Dexamethasone, prednisone	Used to treat vasogenic cerebral edema to improve endothelial integrity; stabilizes cell membranes; reduces tumor-induced edema; assists with symptom control

Independent

The first priority is to ensure that the airway is patent. Keep equipment to manage the airway (endotracheal tube, laryngoscope, nasal and oral airway) within easy access of the patient. Make sure that working endotracheal suction is at the bedside. Note that an obstructed airway and increased levels of carbon dioxide contribute to increased ICP in patients with a space-occupying lesion. Keep the patient comfortable but not oversedated. If the patient is awake, encourage the patient to avoid the Valsalva maneuver and isometric muscle contractions when moving or sitting up in bed to limit the risk of increased ICP. Perform a serial neurological assessment to watch for sudden changes in mental status. To reduce ICP and optimize lung expansion, place the patient in the semi-Fowler position. Keep the head in good alignment with the body to prevent compression on the veins that allow for venous drainage of the head. Avoid hip flexion. Assist the patient to turn in bed and perform coughing, deep breathing, and leg exercises every 2 hours to prevent skin breakdown as well as pulmonary and vascular stasis. As soon as allowed, help the patient get out of bed and ambulate in hallways three to four times each day. If the patient has sensory or motor deficits, work with the rehabilitation team to encourage activities of daily living and increased independence.

Patients who have been newly diagnosed with brain cancer are often in emotional shock, especially when the disease is diagnosed in the advanced stages or is inoperable. Encourage the patient and family to verbalize their feelings surrounding the diagnosis and impending death.

Assist family members in identifying the extent of home care that is realistically required by the patient. Arrange for visits by a home health agency. Suggest supportive counseling (hospice, grief counselor) and, if necessary, make the initial contact. Local units of the American Cancer

Society offer assistance with home care supplies and support groups for patients and families. Also refer patients to the American Brain Tumor Association and the National Brain Tumor Society. Instruct the patient to use the pain scale effectively and to request pain medication before the pain escalates to an intolerable level. Consider switching as-needed pain medication to an around-the-clock dosing schedule to keep pain under control.

Evidence-Based Practice and Health Policy

Eaton, B., Goldberg, S., Tarbell, N., Lawell, M., Gallotto, S., Weyman, E., Kuhlthau, K., Ebb, D., MacDonald, S., & Yock, T. (2020). Long-term health-related quality of life in pediatric brain tumor survivors receiving proton radiotherapy at < 4 years of age. *Neuro-Oncology, 22,* 1379–1387.

• The authors proposed to determine the long-term quality of life among 59 brain tumor survivors treated with proton therapy under the age of 4 years. The median age was 2.5 years of age at baseline and 9.1 years at follow-up. The two most common diagnoses were ependymoma and medulloblastoma.
• Ninety percent of the children functioned in a regular classroom, 36% required a classroom aid, 23% used an outside tutor, and 46% had an individualized education plan. One-third of the children achieved health-related quality of life levels commensurate with healthy children.

DOCUMENTATION GUIDELINES

• Response to the diagnosis of cancer, the diagnostic tests, and recommended treatment regimen
• Physical responses: Patency of airway, neurological assessments, vital signs, signs of increased ICP or seizure activity, description of all dressings and wounds, appearance of incision
• Response to and tolerance to therapy: Radiotherapy, surgery, chemotherapy
• Presence of complications: Increased ICP, hemorrhage, infection, pulmonary congestion, activity intolerance, unrelieved discomfort
• Activity level, progress in rehabilitation if appropriate, ability to perform independent activities of daily living

DISCHARGE AND HOME HEALTHCARE GUIDELINES

FOLLOW-UP. Consult with occupational and physical therapists to develop an appropriate rehabilitation plan if one is needed. Discuss aids for self-care and mobilization such as wheelchairs, bathroom rails, and speech aids and where and how they can be obtained. Evaluate the home situation before discharge to determine if wheelchair access is available if it is necessary.

Teach the patient and family strategies to avoid exposure to infection. If the patient develops an infection or notes increased bleeding, teach the patient to notify the primary healthcare provider immediately. Teach the patient and significant others the early signs of tumor recurrence so that they can notify the primary healthcare provider if they occur. Instruct the patient on care of the skin in the external radiation field. Arrange for contact with hospice if appropriate. Clarify advance directives and end-of-life care so that these plans are communicated with all family members and the healthcare team.

Stress the need to maintain a schedule for follow-up visits as recommended by the physician.

MEDICATIONS. Explain the purpose, action, dosage, desired effects, and side effects of all medications prescribed by the physician.

Breast Cancer

DRG Category:	582
Mean LOS:	3.5 days
Description:	SURGICAL: Mastectomy for Malignancy With Complication or Comorbidity or Major Complication or Comorbidity
DRG Category:	598
Mean LOS:	4.4 days
Description:	MEDICAL: Malignant Breast Disorders With Complication or Comorbidity

One in eight women in the United States will develop breast cancer in her lifetime. The Centers for Disease Control and Prevention report that breast cancer is the most common cancer among women except for skin cancers and the second leading cause of cancer death after lung cancer for women in the United States. The American Cancer Society (ACS) estimates that there will be 281,550 new cases of invasive breast cancer in women in 2021, 49,290 new cases of ductal carcinoma, and 43,600 deaths from breast cancer. Approximately 2,600 cases of breast cancer are diagnosed in men each year. According to the ACS and the National Institutes of Health, the 5-year survival rate for women with localized (found only in the part of the body where it started) breast cancer is 99%, regional (spread to regional lymph nodes) breast cancer is 86%, and distant (cancer has metastasized) breast cancer is 28%. Carcinoma of the breast stems from the epithelial tissues of the ducts and lobules. Ductal carcinoma is the most common type of breast cancer.

Breast cancer is not one single form of disease but many subtypes of cancer. Subtypes of cancer are classified by the presence or absence of receptors: hormone receptors (HR; both estrogen and progesterone receptors) and human epidermal growth factor receptor 2 tyrosine kinase (HER2). Three of the subtypes include Luminal A subtype (HR+/HER2–), Luminal B subtype (HR+HER+), and HER2-enriched subtype (HR–/HER2+). If none of these receptors is found in women with breast cancer, the patient may have triple negative breast cancer (triple negative because none of the receptors are present, HR–/HER2–), a particularly aggressive disease that comprises 15% to 20% of breast cancers. Inflammatory breast cancer (IBC) is an aggressive form of ductal disease that is often hormone receptor negative. IBC is more commonly diagnosed in young women as compared to other subtypes. The disease progresses rapidly and is often diagnosed late in the disease trajectory.

Breast cancer can also be classified as either noninvasive or invasive. Noninvasive carcinoma refers to cancer in the ducts or lobules and is also called *carcinoma in situ*, or "in its original place" (5% of breast cancers). Invasive carcinoma (also known as *infiltrating carcinoma*) occurs when the cancer cells invade the tissue beyond the ducts or lobules. The rate of cell division of the cancerous growth varies, but it is estimated that the time it takes for a tumor to be palpable ranges from 5 to 9 years. When the cancer cells become invasive, they grow in an irregular or sunburst pattern that is palpated as a poorly defined lump or thickening. As the tumor continues to grow, fibrosis forms around the cancer, causing the Cooper ligaments to shorten, which results in dimpling of the skin. Advanced tumors will interrupt the lymph drainage, resulting in skin edema and an "orange peel" (peau d'orange) appearance. Untreated cancer may erupt on the skin as an ulceration.

CAUSES

The origin of breast cancer is a complex interaction between the biologic and endocrine properties of the person and environmental exposures that may precipitate the mutation of cells to a malignancy. Cancers seem to arise through a series of molecular changes at the level of the cells. These changes result in breast epithelial cells that result in abnormal and uncontrolled growth. The greatest risk by far is family history of breast cancer.

Other risk factors include European ancestry, residence in North America or Europe, an age greater than 40 years, personal history of breast cancer (three- to fourfold increased risk), history of benign breast disease, nulliparity or an age greater than 30 years for first-time pregnancy, menarche before age 12 years, menopause after age 55 years, postmenopausal obesity (especially if the excess fat is in the waist area as opposed to the hips and thighs), and diethylstilbestrol (DES) exposure. Recent studies support an association of breast cancer with moderate alcohol intake, a high-fat diet, smoking and exposure to secondhand smoke, and prolonged hormonal replacement therapy. Other environmental factors include exposure to radiation (during childhood or significant chest radiation) or pesticide residues. Many women with breast cancer have no identifiable risk factors.

GENETIC CONSIDERATIONS

Breast cancer is a feature of several cancer syndromes including Cowden syndrome, Li-Fraumeni syndrome, Peutz-Jeghers syndrome, Bloom syndrome, Werner syndrome, ataxia-telangiectasia, and xeroderma pigmentosum, but these syndromes account for less than 1% of all breast cancers.

More familiar to most people are the nonsyndromic breast cancer susceptibility genes, which account for 5% to 10% of breast cancer cases. The two most widely known genes are *BRCA1* and *BRCA2*, which are both tumor suppressor genes. The lifetime risk of becoming affected by breast cancer for mutation carriers has been estimated to be between 60% and 88%. Breast cancer is considered a complex (multifactorial) disorder caused by both nongenetic and genetic factors. Numerous genes have been shown to contribute to susceptibility. These include the tumor suppressor genes *CHEK2* and *TP53* as well as *BRCA3, BWSCR1A, TP53, BRIP1, RB1CC1, RAD51,* and *BARD1.*

SEX AND LIFE SPAN CONSIDERATIONS

Breast cancer is predominantly a disease of women over the age of 40 years, with incidence rates increasing with age. The mean age of diagnosis for women is 62 years. The probability of being diagnosed with invasive breast cancer is 0.1% at 20 years, 0.5% at 30 years, 1.5% at 40 years, 2.4% at 50 years, 3.5% at 60 years, 4.1% at 70 years, and 3.0% at 80 years (ACS, 2019). Only 1% of breast cancer affects men, and it usually occurs when they are over the age of 60 years. Management of older and younger breast cancer patients is essentially the same.

HEALTH DISPARITIES AND SEXUAL/GENDER MINORITY HEALTH

According to the ACS and the Susan G. Komen Organization (2021), breast cancer rates among women with various races/ethnicities are as follows: non-Hispanic White: 131/100,000; Black: 124/100,000; Asian American/Pacific Islander: 100/100,000; Hispanic: 97/100,000; Native American: 80/100,000. While White women have a higher frequency of breast cancer, Black women are more likely to die from the disease; this difference is attributed to late detection of the cancer and perhaps more aggressive tumors. People with disabilities (such as autism), renal failure, brain injury, ostomy problems, and intellectual disabilities have significantly lower cancer screening participation than those without disabilities, which creates cancer-related disparities.

The National Institutes of Health (https://www.cancer.gov) in the United States provide statistics and information about cancer disparities. People with low income, low health literacy, long travel distances to cancer screening sites, or who lack health insurance or paid medical leave are less likely to be treated according to cancer care guidelines. People who live in communities that lack clean water and clean air may be exposed to cancer-causing substances. These factors all contribute to inequities in breast cancer diagnosis, treatment, and outcome. Cancer disparities are perpetuated because sexual and gender minority people receive poor quality of care due to stigma, lack of healthcare providers' awareness, and insensitivity to the unique needs of this community. Transgender is a term used to describe persons whose gender identity is different from their sex assigned at birth. Approximately 1% of the U.S. population identify themselves as transgender. Sexual and gender minority persons have higher odds for multiple chronic conditions, cancer, and poor quality of life than cisgender males and females (cisgender is a term used to describe persons whose gender identity and gender expression are aligned with their assigned sex listed on their birth certificate.) Female-to-male transgender men who do not have breast surgery may delay or avoid breast cancer screening because of discrimination based on gender identity or the emotional conflict between self-perception and physical anatomy (Gatos, 2018). The current recommendation is that transgender men who have not undergone bilateral mastectomy or who have only undergone breast reduction should follow screening guidelines for cis-female persons. At this time, there is no reliable evidence to guide the screening of transgender men after mastectomy (Sterling & Garcia, 2020). For transgender men who have had breast reduction surgery or mastectomy, little is known about the risk of breast cancer from residual breast tissue.

GLOBAL HEALTH CONSIDERATIONS

Breast cancer (12.3% of all cancers) and lung cancer (12.3% of all cancers) are the most common cancers worldwide (excluding nonmelanoma skin cancer). In developed countries, the incidence of breast cancer is almost three times higher than in developing countries. Rates are higher in developed Western countries likely because of lifestyle factors: dietary patterns, decreased physical activity, high rates of obesity, and the use of exogenous hormones for contraception and menopausal symptoms. In developed countries, screening mammography is used regularly, leading to higher rates of diagnosis and earlier diagnosis. The incidence of breast cancer is increasing in developing countries because of increases in life expectancy, adoption of Western lifestyles, and increased urbanization.

ASSESSMENT

HISTORY. Assess the patient's and family's previous medical history of breast cancer or other cancers. Obtain a detailed history of hormonal and reproductive sequences and medications (specifically hormonal supplements). Assess lifestyle variables such as diet, exercise, alcohol use, smoking, and occupational history. Determine how, when, and by whom the lump was found (breast self-examination [BSE], mammogram, accident) and if any discharge from the breast was noted. Ask how much time elapsed between finding the lump and seeking professional care in order to estimate the length of time the tumor has been present. Proceed with the systemic review with attention to areas where metastasis is common.

PHYSICAL EXAMINATION. Common symptoms include **breast mass, change in breast size or shape, skin dimpling, recent nipple inversion, discharge,** and/or **axillary lumps.** Part of the assessment should occur with the patient upright with arms raised. Inspect the breast skin for signs of advanced disease: the presence of inflammation, dimpling, orange peel effect, distended vessels, and nipple changes or ulceration. Palpate both breasts to evaluate the tissues and identify the mass. Check to see if the breasts are asymmetrical. Examine the axillary and supraclavicular areas for enlarged nodes. You may note the tumor is firm, irregular, and immovable. Assess the patient for pain or tenderness at the tumor site. Signs of metastatic spread include shortness of breath, bone pain, abdominal distention, jaundice, changes in cognition, and headache.

PSYCHOSOCIAL. Patients present a wide range of responses: denial, fighting spirit, hopelessness, stoic acceptance, anxious preoccupation. Elicit a careful and ongoing assessment of the patient's feelings (anger, depression, anxiety, fear) and body image concerns. Identify the patient's perceptions of how breast cancer will affect role relationships, lifestyle, femininity, and sexuality. Be sure to include the partner, significant others, and/or children in the psychological assessment to learn of their emotional needs. While breast cancer is relatively rare in men, the diagnosis is often accompanied by fear, anxiety, and changes in self-concept and body image.

Diagnostic Highlights

General Comments: Because early diagnosis and treatment increase survival, the ACS (November 2020) recommends the following guidelines for early breast cancer detection:

- While recommendations vary, most indicate that women ages 40 to 44 years should have the option for a screening mammogram every 1 year and should continue to do so for as long as they are in good health. At age 55 years and older, they can switch to every 2 years or choose to continue yearly mammograms as long as they are in good health and expect to live another 10 years. The U.S. Preventive Services Task Force (USPSTF) estimates the benefit of mammography to be a 30% reduction in risk of death from breast cancer in women ages 50 to 74 years and a 17% decrease in risk of death for women ages 40 to 49 years.
- Research has not shown a clear benefit for regular breast examinations by either a health professional or by women themselves. The ACS recommends that women be familiar with how their breasts normally look and feel and consult a health provider immediately about any changes.
- Women at high risk for breast cancer should get breast magnetic resonance imaging (MRI) and a mammogram every year, typically starting at age 30 years.

Test	Normal Result	Abnormality With Condition	Explanation
Mammogram	No tumor noted	Radiodense or white mass noted	An x-ray of the breast; can only suggest a diagnosis of cancer
Ultrasound of the breast	No evidence of cyst or tumor	Appearance of a white lesion	Can differentiate between cystic and solid lesions; targets specific area
Biopsy: Fine-needle aspiration, stereotactic core needle, Mammotome, excisional	Benign	Malignant	Confirms the diagnosis

Other Tests: Computed tomography (CT) scan; MRI; estrogen receptor (ER) assay and progesterone receptor (PR) assay; flow cytometry; DNA ploidy; full-field digital mammography (approved by the U.S. Federal Drug Administration but not widely used); computer-aided detection and diagnosis; ductogram

PRIMARY NURSING DIAGNOSIS

DIAGNOSIS. Disturbed body image related to alteration in self-perception as evidenced by partial or complete loss of the breast and/or loss of breast function

OUTCOMES. Body image; Knowledge: Cancer management; Psychosocial adjustment: Life change; Wound healing: Primary intention; Acceptance: Health status

INTERVENTIONS. Body image enhancement; Support group; Support system enhancement; Wound care

▓ PLANNING AND IMPLEMENTATION

Collaborative

Treatment and prognosis for breast cancer are based on the stage of disease at diagnosis according to the TNM classification (T = tumor size and growth into surrounding tissues, N = involvement of regional lymph nodes, M = metastasis to distant sites). Four other aspects of staging include estrogen receptor (ER) status, progesterone receptor (PR) status, HER2 status, and grade (G) of the cancer (how much do the cancer cells look like normal cells?). The ACS Web site explains the categories and subcategories of breast cancer staging (https://www.cancer.org/cancer/breast-cancer/understanding-a-breast-cancer-diagnosis/stages-of-breast-cancer.html). Treatment of breast cancer requires a multimodal approach. Surgery and radiation, either alone or in combination, control cancer in the breast and regional lymph nodes. Chemotherapy and hormonal therapy are intended to provide systemic control. Adjuvant therapy (pharmacologic treatment given to patients with no detectable cancer after surgery) is often recommended because cancer cells can break away from the primary breast tumor and begin to spread through the bloodstream, even in the early stages of disease. These cells cannot be felt or detected on x-ray.

SURGICAL. The goal of surgery is control of cancer in the breast and the axillary nodes. Most women have a choice of surgical procedures, but it depends on the clinical stage, tumor location, contraindications to radiation (pregnancy, collagen disease, prior radiation, multifocal tumors), and the presence of other health problems. Several types of surgical therapy are commonly available, as follows.

MODIFIED RADICAL MASTECTOMY (TOTAL MASTECTOMY). The most common surgical procedure for mastectomy removes the entire breast and some or all of the axillary nodes as well as the lining over the pectoralis major muscle. At times, the pectoralis minor muscle is removed. Contralateral prophylactic mastectomy (Cpm) is being implemented in ductal carcinoma in situ (dcis) to decrease the risk of cancer in the opposite breast. Rates of Cpm have more than doubled in the past 15 years, but Cpm does not improve survival for all patients with breast cancer and should be discussed carefully with an expert physician.

BREAST-CONSERVING SURGERIES. Also called lumpectomy, quadrantectomy, partial mastectomy, or segmental mastectomy, breast-conserving surgery occurs when only the part of the breast with cancer is removed. The goal is to remove the cancer and some surrounding tissue.

In a sentinel lymph node biopsy, a surgeon removes only the lymph nodes under the arm where the cancer would likely spread first. In an axillary lymph node dissection, the surgeon removes many lymph nodes.

COMPLICATIONS OF SURGERY. The complications of breast surgery may be infection, seroma (fluid accumulation at the operative site), hematoma, limited range of motion (ROM), sensory changes, and lymphedema. A seroma is usually prevented with the placement of a gravity drainage device (Hemovac, Jackson-Pratt) in the site for up to 7 days postoperatively. Drains are usually removed when drainage has decreased to about 30 mL per day. ROM exercises for the lower arm are begun within 24 hours postoperation, and full ROM and other shoulder exercises are ordered by the surgeon after the drains are removed. Sensory changes include numbness, weakness, skin sensitivity, itching, heaviness, or phantom sensations that may last a year.

RADIOTHERAPY. Radiotherapy is routinely given 2 to 4 weeks after breast-preserving surgery for early stage breast cancer. Sometimes it is indicated after modified radical surgery if four or more nodes are positive. The incision needs to be healed, and ROM of the shoulder should be restored. Radiotherapy may consist of an external beam to the breast for 4 to 6 weeks, by an experimental method called brachytherapy (interstitial iridium-192 implants) directly to the tumor site, or both. Radiotherapy can be given at the same time as chemotherapy.

CHEMOTHERAPY/HORMONAL THERAPY. Combination chemotherapy is recommended for premenopausal and postmenopausal patients with positive nodes. Hormonal therapy is used to change the levels of hormones that promote cancer growth and increase survival time in women with metastatic breast cancer. Tumors with a positive ER assay (tumors that need estrogen to grow) have a response rate to hormonal therapy of 65% compared with a 10% response rate with a negative ER assay. PR assays that are also positive enhance endocrine therapy response even more. There is a 77% response rate if both ER and PR are positive as compared with a 5% response rate if both are negative. Triple negative breast cancer is managed with cytotoxic chemotherapy (anthracycline, cyclophosphamide, taxane) because hormonal therapy is not effective. Patients with HER2–positive breast cancer, which occurs in 20% of invasive breast cancers, receive chemotherapy directly targeted to HER2 (trastuzumab, neratinib, lapatinib, pertuzumab).

AUTOLOGOUS BONE MARROW TRANSPLANT (ABMT). Certain patients (with chemosensitive tumors) are being treated with high-dose chemotherapy preceded by removal of the patient's bone marrow, which is then restored after chemotherapy.

RECONSTRUCTION. Approximately 30% of women who have mastectomies choose to have breast reconstruction (Table 2).

• TABLE 2 Types of Breast Reconstructive Surgery

TYPE	DESCRIPTION
Saline-filled implants	A tissue expander is placed under the pectoralis muscle and expanded slowly over months with saline injections. The expander is removed and replaced with a permanent saline implant. The expander may be the adjustable type, serving a dual purpose of expanding and permanent implant.
Autologous tissue transfer	Surgical procedure uses the woman's own tissue to form a breast mound. In two procedures (latissimus dorsi flap of the transverse rectus abdominus muscle [TRAM]), the surgeon tunnels a wedge of muscle, fascia, subcutaneous tissue, and skin to the mastectomy site. In free-flap reconstruction (free tissue transfer), the surgeon uses a microvascular technique to transfer a segment of skin and subcutaneous tissue with its vascular pedicle to the chest wall.

Almost all patients who have mastectomies are candidates. It can be immediate (at the time of mastectomy) or delayed for several years.

Postoperatively, use a flowsheet every hour and assess adequate blood supply to the flap and donor site by evaluating the following: color (to verify that it is the same as skin from the donor area [not the opposite breast]), temperature (warm), tissue turgor (to verify that it is not tight or tense), capillary refill (a well-perfused flap will blanch for 1–3 sec), and anterior blood flow using ultrasonic or laser Doppler. Unusual pain or decreased volume of drainage may indicate vascular impairment to the flap. Early detection of impaired circulation can be treated with anticoagulants or antispasmodics and possibly prevent further surgical interventions. Provide emotional support for the patient who is distraught over her appearance to reassure her the breast will look more normal with healing. The nipple and areola can be added 6 to 9 months later.

Pharmacologic Highlights

Medication or Drug Class	Dosage	Description	Rationale
Neoadjuvant (before surgery) and adjuvant (after surgery) chemotherapy often include a combination of two or three of these medications: doxorubicin, epirubicin, paclitaxel, docetaxel, 5-fluorouracil, cyclophosphamide, and/or carboplatin	Depends on drug, stage of cancer, and patient condition	Antineoplastics	Interferes with growth of cancer; often used in combination
Chemotherapy for advanced breast cancer often includes a combination of two or three of these medications: paclitaxel, docetaxel, doxorubicin, epirubicin, cisplatin, carboplatin, vinorelbine, capecitabine, gemcitabine, ixabepilone, eribulin	Depends on drug, stage of cancer, and patient condition	Antineoplastics	Interferes with growth of cancer; often used in combination
Tamoxifen citrate	10–20 mg PO bid or 20 mg PO qd for 5 yr	Antiestrogen	Provides hormonal control of cancer growth; adjuvant treatment after a mastectomy; also used to prevent breast cancer in high-risk women
Trastuzumab (Herceptin)	4 mg/kg loading dose; 2 mg/kg maintenance, IVPB	Recombinant DNA–derived humanized monoclonal antibody	Indicated only for HER2/neu-receptive tumors; decreases breast cancer growth and stimulates immune system to more effectively attack the cancer
Acetaminophen; NSAIDs; opioids; combination of opioid and NSAIDs	Depends on the drug and the patient's condition and tolerance	Analgesics	Choice of drug depends on the severity of the pain

Other Drugs: Methotrexate, raloxifene to reduce breast cancer risk, antiestrogen medications include fulvestrant, letrozole (taken after 5 years of tamoxifen to lower breast cancer reoccurrence)

Independent

The focus of nursing care for a patient with a mastectomy during the 2- to 3-day hospital stay is directed toward early surgical recovery. Teach pain management, mobility, adequate circulation, and self-care activities to prepare the patient for discharge. In the immediate postoperative period, keep the head of the bed elevated 30 degrees, with the affected arm elevated on a pillow to facilitate lymph drainage. Instruct the patient not to turn on the affected side. Place a sign at the head of the bed immediately after surgery with directions for no blood pressures, blood draws, injections, or IV lines on the arm of the operative side; this should help prevent circulatory impairment.

Emphasize the importance of ambulation and using the operative side within 24 hours. Initially, the arm will need to be supported when the patient is out of bed. As ambulation progresses, encourage the patient to hang her arm at her side normally, keeping her shoulders back to avoid the hunchback position and to prevent contractures. Within 24 hours, begin with exercises that do not stress the incision.

Teach the patient how to empty the drainage device (Hemovac or other), measure the drainage accurately, and observe for the color and consistency of the drainage. Create a flowsheet for record-keeping in the hospital, and send it home with the patient to use until the drain is removed. At the dressing change, begin teaching the dressing change procedure and the indications of complications such as infection (purulent drainage, redness, pain), presence of fluid collection, or hematoma formation at the incision. Be sensitive to the patient's reactions upon seeing the incision for the first time with full realization that her breast is gone. Explain that phantom breast sensations and numbness at the operative site along the inner side of the armpit to the elbow are normal for several months because of interruptions of nerve endings.

Women may have feelings of loss not only of their breast but also of lifestyle, social interactions, sexuality, and even life itself. Patients often feel more comfortable expressing their feelings with nurses than with family members or the physician. Effective coping requires expression of feelings. Discuss the services and goals of Reach to Recovery (psychological and physical support from the ACS program that matches volunteers who are breast cancer survivors to patients who desire support). If the patient is willing, arrange for an in-hospital visit or early home visit.

Evidence-Based Practice and Health Policy

Maass, S., Boerman, L., Brandenbarg, D., Verhaak, P., Maduro, J., Bock, G., & Berendsen, A. (2020). Symptoms in long-term breast cancer survivors: A cross-sectional study in primary care. *The Breast, 54,* 133–138.

- The authors proposed to study the symptoms that manifest after breast cancer treatment, and compared them to controls matched by age and primary care physicians. They used a cross-sectional, population-based study with 350 breast cancer survivors and 350 women without cancer. Participants completed a questionnaire and echocardiography.
- Concentration difficulties, forgetfulness, dizziness, and nocturia were more frequent among the breast cancer survivors compared to controls. Differences could not be explained by cardiac dysfunction, cardiovascular diseases, depression, or anxiety. Intermittent claudication and appetite loss were more frequent among breast cancer survivors than controls and associated with cardiac dysfunction, depression, and anxiety.

DOCUMENTATION GUIDELINES

- Response to surgical interventions: Condition of dressing and wound, stability of vital signs, recovery from anesthesia
- Presence of complications: Pain, edema, infection, seroma, limited ROM
- Knowledge of and intent to comply with adjuvant therapies
- Reaction to cancer and body changes
- Knowledge of and intent to comply with incision care, postoperative exercises, arm precautions, follow-up care, and early detection methods for recurrence

DISCHARGE AND HOME HEALTHCARE GUIDELINES

PATIENT TEACHING. The patient can expect to return home with dressings and wound drains. Instruct the patient to do the following: Empty the drainage receptacle twice a day, record the amount on a flowsheet, and take this information along when keeping a doctor's appointment; report symptoms of infection or excess drainage on the dressing or the drainage device; sponge bathe until the sutures and drains are removed; continue with daily lower arm ROM exercises until the surgeon orders more strenuous exercises; avoid caffeinated foods and drinks, nicotine, and secondary smoke for 3 weeks postoperatively. Review pain medication instructions for frequency and precautions.

Teach precautions to prevent lymphedema after node dissection (written directions or a pamphlet from ACS is desirable for lifetime referral):

• Request no blood pressure or blood samples from affected arm.
• Do not carry packages, handbags, or luggage with the affected arm; avoid elastic cuffs.
• Protect the hand and arm from burns, sticks, and cuts by wearing gloves to do gardening and housework, using a thimble to sew, and applying sunscreen and insect repellent when out of doors.
• Report swelling, pain, or heat in the affected arm immediately.
• Put the arm above the head and pump the fist frequently throughout the day.

FOLLOW-UP. Prepare the patient and family for a variety of encounters with healthcare providers (radiologist, oncologist, phlebotomist). Try to provide continuity between the providers (yourself, the clinical nurse specialist, or a nurse consultant system, if available) as a resource for the patient or family to call with questions.

Provide lists and information of local community resources and support groups for emotional support: Reach to Recovery, Y-ME, Wellness Center, Can Surmount, I Can Cope; a list of businesses that specialize in breast prostheses; phone numbers for ACS and the Cancer Information System.

Recurrence is a lifetime threat. Inform the patient that it is necessary to continue monthly BSEs (even on the operative side) and annual mammogram and physician examinations of both the reconstructed and the nonreconstructed breasts. Be certain the patient can demonstrate an accurate BSE.

Bronchiolitis (Respiratory Syncytial Viral Infection)

DRG Category:	202
Mean LOS:	3.7 days
Description:	MEDICAL: Bronchitis and Asthma With Complication or Comorbidity or Major Complication or Comorbidity

Bronchiolitis is a common disease of the lower respiratory tract that is most commonly caused by the respiratory syncytial virus (RSV) and found most often in infants and children 2 to 24 months of age. The infection, which causes inflammation leading to obstruction of the small respiratory airways, can range from a mild infection that lasts only a few days to a serious episode that causes severe respiratory distress. Older children and adults often experience a "mild" upper respiratory infection with RSV because they have larger airways and can tolerate the airway swelling with fewer symptoms than can infants. The virus leads to necrosis of the bronchiolar epithelium, hypersecretion of mucus, and infiltration and edema of the surrounding cells. These changes are further complicated by mucous plugs that obstruct the bronchioles and lead to collapse of the distal lung tissue.

The incubation period is approximately 4 days from the time of exposure to the time of the first manifestation of the illness. Infants shed the virus for up to 12 days, and the spread of infection occurs when large, infected droplets (airborne or through direct contact with secretions) are inoculated in the nose or eyes of a susceptible person. In temperate climates, infants most often contract RSV during the winter months. Mortality of infants with a lower respiratory infection due to RSV is approximately 2%. Young premature infants have a poorer outcome. A significant number of infants who develop bronchiolitis have reactive airway disease later in life. The peak incidence occurs during winter and spring, and bronchiolitis is a major reason for hospital admission for infants less than 12 months of age, particularly children who live in poverty and in urban areas. Bronchiolitis accounts for approximately 4,500 deaths and more than 132,000 hospital admissions each year.

CAUSES

Bronchiolitis has a viral derivation; RSV is responsible for up to 75% of the cases, but other viruses such as the parainfluenza virus (type 3), mycoplasma, human metapneumovirus, or adenoviruses cause the remainder of illnesses. RSV is a medium-sized RNA virus that develops within the infected cell and reproduces by budding from the cell membrane. Generally, the source of the RSV is an older family member with a mild upper respiratory infection. Experts suggest that both intrauterine cigarette smoke exposure and secondhand cigarette smoke exposure may increase the severity of RSV bronchiolitis by reducing the elastic properties of the infant's lung. Children who attend day care and those who are not breastfed also have an increased risk of developing illness.

GENETIC CONSIDERATIONS

An allele of interleukin-8 (*CXCL8*; a neutrophil chemoattractant that causes inflammation) has been associated with determining the severity of RSV infection in children under age 2 years. The walls of airways infected with RSV have high levels of *CXCL8*. Variation in the *CXCL8* promoter region has been associated with increased wheezing in affected children.

SEX AND LIFE SPAN CONSIDERATIONS

Bronchiolitis commonly occurs in the first 2 years of life. Severe infections are rare in children younger than 6 weeks because maternal antibodies have a protective effect during the first weeks of life. Bronchiolitis and pneumonia due to RSV are more common in boys than in girls (ratio 1.5:1).

HEALTH DISPARITIES AND SEXUAL/GENDER MINORITY HEALTH

Hospitalization is more likely to occur in children of families with lower socioeconomic status, and higher rates of hospitalization occur in Native American, Native Alaskan, Black, and Hispanic children (Inagaki et al., 2020). Sexual and gender minority status has no known effect on the risk for bronchiolitis.

GLOBAL HEALTH CONSIDERATIONS

According to the World Health Organization, an estimated 150 million new cases of bronchiolitis occur each year around the world. The global incidence of bronchiolitis in industrialized countries is comparable to the incidence in the United States (11.4% in children younger than

12 months and 6% in children ages 1 to 2 years). RSV peaks in the winter in temperate climates and during the rainy season in tropical climates.

⁂ ASSESSMENT

HISTORY. Ask if any members of the household have had a cold or upper respiratory infection. The infant usually has a history of an upper respiratory infection and runny nose (rhinorrhea) that lasts for several days. Infants may have increasing restlessness or depressed sensorium. Infants often have a moderate fever of approximately 102°F (38.9°C), a decrease in appetite, poor feeding, and gradual development of respiratory distress. A cough usually appears after the first few days of symptoms. Some children wheeze audibly.

PHYSICAL EXAMINATION. The infant or child appears to be in **acute respiratory distress** with a **rapid respiratory rate, air hunger, nasal flaring, tachycardia,** hyperexpansion of the lungs, and even intercostal and subcostal retractions with cyanosis. When you auscultate the infant's chest, you will likely hear diffuse rhonchi, fine crackles, and wheezes. The liver and spleen are easily palpable because they are pushed down by the hyperinflated lungs. Signs of life-threatening respiratory distress include irritability or listlessness, central cyanosis, tachypnea at a respiratory rate of over 70 breaths a minute, and apnea. Usually, the most critically ill infants have greatly hyperexpanded chests that are silent to air movement upon auscultation. Inspect the infant for a rash and conjunctivitis.

PSYCHOSOCIAL. The parents and child will be apprehensive. Assess the parents' ability to cope with the acute or emergency situation and intervene as appropriate. Note that many children are treated at home rather than in the hospital; your teaching plan may need to consider home rather than hospital management.

Diagnostic Highlights

General Comments: Diagnostic testing involves identifying the causative organism, determining oxygenation status, and ruling out masses as a cause of obstruction.

Test	Normal Result	Abnormality With Condition	Explanation
Rapid viral antigen testing for RSV from nasal secretions	Negative	Positive for RSV antigen (available in a few hours)	Detects the antigen of RSV showing the presence of the virus
Pulse oximetry	≥ 95%	< 95%	Low oxygen saturation is present if there is obstruction in the lung passages
Chest x-ray	Normal lung structure	Air trapping or hyperexpansion, peribronchial thickening or interstitial pneumonia, segmental consolidation	Results of inflammation and mucous plugs

Other Tests: Complete blood count, arterial blood gases, differential, C-reactive protein, bacterial cultures, immunofluorescence analysis of nasal washings to detect RSV

PRIMARY NURSING DIAGNOSIS

DIAGNOSIS. Ineffective airway clearance related to bronchial infection and obstruction as evidenced by dyspnea, tachypnea, and/or air hunger

OUTCOMES. Respiratory status: Airway patency; Respiratory status: Gas exchange; Respiratory status: Ventilation; Anxiety level; Fluid balance

INTERVENTIONS. Airway management; Airway suctioning; Respiratory monitoring; Vital signs monitoring; Oxygen therapy; Anxiety reduction; Fluid monitoring

☀ PLANNING AND IMPLEMENTATION

Collaborative

No definitive antiviral treatment is available. The aim of treatment is to maintain a patent airway and provide adequate respiratory exchange. Medical management includes cool, oxygenated mist for severely ill infants who require hospitalization and careful IV hydration. Tube feeding for hydration is preferable to IV therapy if suckling is difficult. Generally, antibiotics are not considered useful and lead to bacterial resistance. Antiviral drugs are used in the most severely ill infants. Frequent suctioning of the nose and mouth will assist in removing thick secretions when the child cannot produce a productive cough independently. Breathing treatments may be ordered for more severe illness.

Measures to ensure prevention are very important. During RSV season, high-risk infants should be separated from those with respiratory symptoms. Careful hand-washing and isolation techniques are important for all healthcare personnel.

Pharmacologic Highlights

Medication or Drug Class	Dosage	Description	Rationale
Albuterol aerosol	Per nebulizer, varies according to size of child	Bronchodilator	Dilates the bronchioles, opening up respiratory passages; used only in those infants with wheezing who seem to benefit from the treatment
Ribavirin	190 mg/L; delivered at a rate of 12.5 L of mist per minute by small particle aerosol for 20 of the 24 hours for 3–5 days	Antiviral	Halts the replication of the RSV by disrupting RNA and DNA synthesis
Palivizumab	15 mg/kg IM q1 month during RSV season	Monoclonal antibodies	Prophylaxis of high-risk infants against RSV infection or for those with chronic lung disease during RSV season
Antipyretics	Varies with drug	Acetaminophen	Reduce fever

Other Drugs: Corticosteroids are used only as a last resort; the use of bronchodilators is controversial.

Independent

Ongoing, continuous observation of the patency of the child's airway is essential to identify impending obstruction. For infants, elevate the crib mattress or place them in an infant seat; older children should have the head of the bed elevated so that they are in Fowler position. Usually, seriously and critically ill infants are hospitalized because their care at home is difficult. Hospitalized infants are usually elevated to a sitting position at 30 to 40 degrees with the neck extended at the same 30- to 40-degree angle.

Children should be allowed to rest as much as possible to conserve their energy; organize your interventions to limit disturbances. Provide age-appropriate activities. Crying increases the child's difficulty breathing and should be limited if possible by comfort measures and the presence of the parents; parents should be allowed to hold and comfort the child as much as possible. If the child is in a cool mist tent, parents may need to be enclosed with the child, or the child may need to be held by the parents with the mist directed toward the child. Children sense anxiety from their parents; if you support the parents in dealing with their anxiety and fear, the children are less fearful. Carefully explaining all procedures and allowing the parents to participate in the care of the child as much as possible help relieve the anxiety of both child and parents.

Provide adequate hydration to liquefy secretions and to replace fluid loss from increased sensible loss (increased respirations and fever). The child might also have a decreased fluid intake during the illness. Apply lubricant or ointment around the child's mouth and lips to decrease the irritation from secretions and mouth breathing.

Evidence-Based Practice and Health Policy

Mansbach, J., Hasegawa, K., Geller, R., Espinola, J., Sullivan, A., Camargo, C., & MARC-35 Investigators. (2020). Bronchiolitis severity is related to recurrent wheezing by age 3 years in a prospective, multicenter cohort. *Pediatric Research, 87*, 428–430.

• The authors enrolled 921 infants hospitalized for bronchiolitis throughout the United States in a prospective cohort study during the 2011 to 2014 winter seasons. The median age of the infants was 3.2 months. They aimed to determine if children with bronchiolitis developed recurrent wheezing by age 3 years and to determine rates of asthma as they grew.
• When the children reached 3 years of age, recurrent wheezing occurred in 32%. Infants who required an intensive care stay had higher rates of wheezing than infants who were not hospitalized in intensive care. They also had higher rates of asthma at age 4 years than infants not hospitalized in intensive care. The authors recommended long-term follow-up for infants hospitalized with bronchiolitis.

DOCUMENTATION GUIDELINES

• Respiratory status: Rate, quality, depth, ease, breath sounds
• Response to treatment: Cool mist oxygen tent, medications, positioning
• Infant's response to illness, feeding, hydration, rest, activity
• Parents' emotional responses and response to teaching

DISCHARGE AND HOME HEALTHCARE GUIDELINES

When the infant is ready for discharge, make sure the caregiver understands any medications that are required at home. Instruct the parents to recognize the signs of increasing respiratory obstruction and advise them when to take the child to an emergency department. Parents should be taught how to safely use the bulb syringe at home. If the child is cared for at home, provide the following home care instructions:

• Prop the infant in a sitting position to ease breathing, not in a flat position.
• Do not use infant aspirin products because of the chance of Reye syndrome.
• Provide a cool mist humidifier. Saline drops may help loosen secretions followed by bulb syringe suction.
• Ensure that parents understand breathing treatments when prescribed for home use.

Bronchitis

DRG Category:	202
Mean LOS:	3.7 days
Description:	MEDICAL: Bronchitis and Asthma With Complication or Comorbidity or Major Complication or Comorbidity

Bronchitis, a form of chronic obstructive pulmonary disease, is an inflammation of the mucous membranes of the bronchi (the air passages that extend from the trachea to the small airways and into the alveoli of the lungs). Each year, over 10 million cases of acute bronchitis occur in the United States. It is a common condition worldwide, and among countries that track health-related data, it is one of the top five reasons for physician visits. Bronchitis is a disease of the larger airways, unlike emphysema, which is a disease of the smaller airways. Inflammation of the airway mucosa leads to edema and the enlargement of the submucosal glands. Damage occurs to cilia and the epithelial cells of the respiratory tract. In addition, leukocytes and lymphocytes infiltrate the walls of the bronchi and lead to inflammation and airway narrowing. Hypersecretion of the submucosal glands leads to obstruction of the airways from excessive mucus. The most prominent symptom is sputum production.

Acute bronchitis has a short, severe course that subsides without long-term effects. People with chronic bronchitis with obstruction generally have a long history of productive cough and late onset of wheezing, and some experts no longer distinguish between chronic bronchitis and asthma. People with chronic mucopurulent bronchitis have persistent or recurrent purulent sputum production in the absence of localized suppurative illness. Chronic bronchitis, which can be reversed after the removal of the irritant, is complicated by respiratory tract infections and can lead to right-sided heart failure, pulmonary hypertension, and acute respiratory failure. Complications include pneumonia, bacterial superinfection, and reactive airway disease such as asthma.

CAUSES

Acute bronchitis is usually caused by respiratory viruses but can also be caused by infections with *Streptococcus pneumoniae* or *Mycoplasma* species. The primary causes of chronic bronchitis are cigarette and marijuana smoking, pipe or cigar smoking, and exposure to some type of respiratory irritant. Established risk factors include a history of smoking, occupational exposures, air pollution, reduced lung function, and heredity. Children of parents who smoke cigarettes are at higher risk for pulmonary infections that may lead to bronchitis. Repeated episodes of gastric reflux can increase a person's risk of developing bronchitis.

GENETIC CONSIDERATIONS

There is recent evidence suggesting that risk for bronchitis is mediated through gene-environment interactions. Polymorphisms in the cytokine gene, *LTA*, and the interleukin genes, *CXCL8* and *IL17A*, have been found to influence susceptibility to bronchitis.

SEX AND LIFE SPAN CONSIDERATIONS

Acute bronchitis can occur at any age, but it is diagnosed most often in children less than age 5 years, and males are diagnosed more often than females. Chronic bronchitis can appear between ages 25 and 50 years, but it is more commonly diagnosed in people older than 50 years. Up to 20% of adult men in the United States have chronic bronchitis.

HEALTH DISPARITIES AND SEXUAL/GENDER MINORITY HEALTH

Some experts reported that Indigenous children and children in low-income families have a higher risk for bronchitis than other children. In adults, the condition occurs more frequently in people with low income and people who live in urban, industrialized areas. Sexual minorities, and lesbian women in particular, reported greater odds of asthma and bronchitis than other groups in national health surveys.

GLOBAL HEALTH CONSIDERATIONS

Bronchitis is one of the top five reasons for seeking healthcare around the world and is most common in underresourced, underdeveloped, and urban parts of the world.

ASSESSMENT

HISTORY. Patients with acute bronchitis usually have a self-limiting upper respiratory infection associated with chills, fever (100°F–102°F [37.7°C–38.9°C]), malaise, substernal tightness and achiness, and cough. The patient describes a painful, dry cough that becomes productive with mucopurulent secretions for several days. The secretions generally clear as the inflammation subsides and the symptoms decrease.

Obtain a smoking and occupational history. Ask about exposures to respiratory irritants or pollutants. Patients generally seek healthcare when they become short of breath, have a cough, or notice increased sputum production. The cough may initially be more common in the winter months and gradually develop into a constant problem regardless of the season. Ask patients if they have experienced fatigue or difficulty with activities of daily living (ADLs) because of shortness of breath. Question their sleep patterns and positions; patients often need to sleep sitting up so that they can breathe better. Request that they explain their eating patterns because often a patient with chronic bronchitis has a poor appetite with difficulty eating because of shortness of breath. A decrease in the patient's weight leads to a decrease in the mass of the diaphragm, which contributes to poor respiratory muscle function.

PHYSICAL EXAMINATION. The most common symptoms are **cough, sputum production**, and **fever**. Patients with acute bronchitis appear acutely ill. Generally, they are febrile and mildly dehydrated, particularly if the bronchitis is associated with influenza or pneumonia. Other symptoms of acute bronchitis include runny nose, headache, sore throat, myalgias, and fatigue. Patients with chronic bronchitis often appear short of breath, a condition that worsens as they speak. To help with breathing, they may use accessory muscles, such as the abdominal muscles, the sternocleidomastoids, and the intercostal muscles. Patients sometimes appear cyanotic. Some with advanced disease have a high $Paco_2$ that leads to disorientation, headaches, and photophobia (eyes are sensitive to light). Expect copious amounts of mucus that is gray, yellow, or white. Chronic bronchitis may lead to signs of right-sided heart failure, such as peripheral edema and neck vein distension. When you auscultate the patient's lungs, you may hear scattered fine or coarse crackles and wheezing, and there may be a prolonged time for expiration.

PSYCHOSOCIAL. The patient with acute bronchitis has a self-limiting disease that lasts approximately 1 to 2 weeks. In contrast, a patient with chronic bronchitis is dealing with a chronic, progressive disease. As the disease progresses, patients become increasingly dependent on others for assistance. They may feel isolated and depressed. Patients are limited in their mobility and are frequently homebound. Others are reluctant to go out if they are dependent on oxygen.

Diagnostic Highlights

Test	Test Results	Abnormality With Condition	Explanation
Sputum culture and sensitivity	Negative	Presence of bacteria or other microorganisms may occur in chronic bronchitis	Common organisms are *S pneumoniae* and *Haemophilus influenzae*

Other Tests: Chest radiography, bronchoscopy, arterial blood gas, complete blood count, procalcitonin levels (to differentiate bacterial from nonbacterial infections), pulmonary function tests. Monitor the patient's PaO$_2$ with a pulse oximeter to determine if the oxygen therapy is maintaining adequate oxygenation.

PRIMARY NURSING DIAGNOSIS

DIAGNOSIS. Impaired gas exchange related to obstructed airways and mucous production as evidenced by cough, shortness of breath, restlessness, and/or fever

OUTCOMES. Respiratory status: Gas exchange; Respiratory status: Ventilation; Fluid balance; Knowledge: Chronic obstructive pulmonary disease; Smoking cessation behavior; Comfort level; Anxiety control

INTERVENTIONS. Airway management; Cough enhancement; Respiratory monitoring; Oxygen therapy; Laboratory data interpretation; Positioning; Smoking-cessation assistance; Ventilation assistance

PLANNING AND IMPLEMENTATION

Collaborative

The focus of treatment is supportive care, managing symptoms, and providing rest. Most hospitalized patients with chronic bronchitis are on low-flow oxygen therapy. If patients retain carbon dioxide, a high level of oxygen shuts off their drive to breathe, and they become apneic. Patients with chronic bronchitis may require chest physiotherapy to help mobilize their secretions. The physician may prescribe postural drainage, chest percussion, and chest vibration to the lobes that are involved several times daily. Schedule the chest physiotherapy sessions so that they occur at least 1 hour before or 2 hours after meals to limit the risk of aspiration.

Pharmacologic Highlights

General Comments: Treatment generally focuses on symptoms such as controlling coughs with preparations such as dextromethorphan and controlling discomfort with analgesics and antipyretics. Routine antimicrobial use is not recommended unless influenza or pertussis is confirmed. Xanthines may also be used to assist with respiratory muscle strength by increasing the contractility of the diaphragm. Steroids are used more often with asthma but may occasionally be used in patients with bronchitis.

Medication or Drug Class	Dosage	Description	Rationale
Antibiotics	Varies with drug	Examples: Amoxicillin and clavulanate; doxycycline, azithromycin, erythromycin	Generally, antibiotics are ineffective unless there is a confirmed pertussis infection or a confirmed bacterial infection. Manage respiratory infections if serious comorbid conditions pose a risk for complications or for older patients.

Pharmacologic Highlights (continued)

Medication or Drug Class	Dosage	Description	Rationale
Bronchodilators	Varies with drug	Ultrasonic or nebulized treatments of medications may be used to open large airways and facilitate clearance of mucus	Relax smooth muscles in the airways and reduce local congestion

Other Drugs: Xanthines such as aminophylline and theophylline are administered to reduce mucosal edema and smooth muscle spasms; cough suppressants; nonsteroidal anti-inflammatory agents to manage symptoms; rimantadine (Flumadine) may be used to inhibit viral replication of influenza A virus subtypes. Other antiviral medications: oseltamivir (Tamiflu), zanamivir (Relenza). Influenza vaccinations may reduce the incidence of acute bacterial bronchitis.

Independent

The patient with bronchitis is often short of breath and fatigued. Space activities to allow frequent rest periods. These patients may be dependent on others for some of their ADLs, especially if they are in the hospital for an exacerbation of their disease. Elevate the head of the bed to allow the patient to assume an easier position for breathing. Patients often assume a tripod position, which is an upright position with arms resting on a table and shoulders hunched forward. Do not impose bedrest on a patient who is short of breath. Patients usually assume the position most advantageous for breathing and, if repositioned, may have worsening gas exchange and even a respiratory arrest. If the patient becomes extremely dyspneic and "air hungry," notify the physician immediately.

If the patient is not on fluid restriction, encourage the patient to drink fluids to replace insensible water losses. Fluid replacement should be based on body weight and the severity of symptoms associated with the illness. A humidifier may help loosen mucus and relieve cough symptoms. Provide frequent mouth care to improve the patient's comfort and to limit the risk of infection. If appropriate, teach a family member or significant other how to perform postural drainage and chest percussion. Encourage the patient to remain recumbent for 10 minutes before the session so that secretions are expectorated more easily after treatment.

Evidence-Based Practice and Health Policy

Balte, P., Chaves, P., Couper, D., Enright, P., Jacobs, D., Kalhan, R., Kronmal, R., Loehr, L., London, S., Newman, A., O'Connor, G., Schwartz, J., Smith, B., Smith, L., White, W., Yende, S., & Oelsner, E. (2020). Association of nonobstructive chronic bronchitis with respiratory health outcomes in adults. *JAMA Internal Medicine, 180*, 676–686.

- The authors aimed to determine whether nonobstructive chronic bronchitis (bronchitis without airflow obstruction or clinical asthma) was associated with adverse respiratory health outcomes in adult smokers and nonsmokers. They enrolled 22,325 adults in a prospective cohort study with bronchitis and without airflow obstruction or clinical asthma at baseline.
- The participants who had nonobstructive chronic bronchitis and were smokers had decreased lung function and increased risk of disease-related hospitalizations and mortality compared to smokers without nonobstructive bronchitis. Similar findings occurred with nonsmokers; nonobstructive bronchitis was associated with poorer long-term outcomes. The authors concluded that nonobstructive bronchitis presents long-term risks to patients not seen in other patients with bronchitis.

DOCUMENTATION GUIDELINES

- Respiratory status of the patient: Respiratory rate, breath sounds, use of oxygen, color of nailbeds and lips; note any respiratory distress
- Response to activity: Degree of shortness of breath with any exertion, degree of fatigue
- Comfort, body temperature
- Response to medications, oxygen, and breathing treatments
- Need for assistance with ADLs
- Response to diet and increased caloric intake, daily weights

DISCHARGE AND HOME HEALTHCARE GUIDELINES

MEDICATIONS. Be sure that the patient understands all medications, including the dosage, route, action, and adverse effects. Patients on aminophylline should have blood levels drawn as ordered by the physician. Before being discharged from the hospital, the patient should demonstrate the proper use of metered-dose inhalers. Recommend that patients receive yearly flu vaccines and all other regular vaccinations unless contraindicated.

COMPLICATIONS. Instruct patients to notify their primary healthcare provider of any change in the color or consistency of their secretions. Green-colored secretions may indicate the presence of a respiratory infection. Recommend that if the patient experiences symptoms that prevent sleep, accompanied by fever or bloody sputum, they should contact their primary care provider. Patients should also report consistent, prolonged periods of dyspnea that are unrelieved by medications.

FOLLOW-UP. Consider that patients with severe disease may need assistance with ADLs after discharge. Note any referrals to social services. Send patients home with a diet, provided by the dietitian and reinforced by the nurse, that provides a high-caloric intake. Encourage the patient to cover the face with a scarf if they go outdoors in the winter. If the patient continues to smoke, provide the name of a smoking-cessation program or a support group. Encourage the patient to avoid irritants in the air.

Bulimia Nervosa

DRG Category:	887
Mean LOS:	4.9 days
Description:	MEDICAL: Other Mental Disorder Diagnoses

Bulimia nervosa (BN) is an eating disorder characterized by repeated episodes of binge eating and recurrent episodes of inappropriate compensatory behaviors to prevent weight gain. During binges, the individual rapidly consumes large amounts of high-caloric food (upward of 2,000–5,000 calories) in a discrete time period, usually in secrecy and accompanied by a sense of loss of control. The binge is followed by self-deprecating thoughts, guilt, and anxiety over fear of weight gain. Compensatory behaviors may include self-induced vomiting, misuse of laxatives, diuretics or other medications, fasting, or excessive exercise. The strict definition used by the *Diagnostic and Statistical Manual of Mental Disorders*, Fifth Edition (*DSM-5*) indicates that a person with BN needs to have at least one binge-eating episode per week for at least 3 months to meet the diagnostic criteria for BN. The individual is caught in a binge-compensation cycle that can recur multiple times each day, several times a week, or at intervals of up to 2 weeks to months. The *DSM-5* further specifies the disorder as *mild, moderate, severe, or extreme* based on the episodes of compensatory behaviors per week. In this classification, individuals with extreme BN have an average of 14 or more episodes of compensatory behaviors per week. Patients with BN experience frequent weight fluctuations of 10 pounds or more, but they are usually able to maintain a near-normal weight.

Individuals with anorexia nervosa (AN) may engage in binge eating and compensatory behaviors similar to those used by individuals with BN. A distinguishing feature, however, is that individuals with BN use compensatory behaviors to stave off weight gain rather than starve themselves, and some individuals with AN will use compensatory behaviors even after consuming small amounts of food. Individuals who have recurrent episodes of binge eating without compensatory behaviors are still identified by the *DSM-5* as having binge eating disorder. In contrast to people with AN, individuals with BN are aware that their behavior is abnormal, but they conceal their illness because of embarrassment. Persons with BN typically have difficulty with direct expression of feelings, are prone to impulsive behavior, and may have problems with alcohol and other substance abuse. Because they can maintain a near-normal weight and, if female, have regular menstrual periods, the problem may go undetected. Bulimic behaviors have been known to persist for decades.

Depending on the severity and duration of the condition, there are significant health consequences. Chronic induced vomiting of stomach contents produces volume depletion and a hypochloremic alkalosis. Dizziness, syncope, thirst, orthostatic changes in vital signs, and dehydration occur with volume depletion. Renal compensation for the metabolic alkalosis and volume depletion leads to further electrolyte imbalances, which may predispose the BN patient to cardiac dysrhythmias, muscle cramps, and weakness. Discoloration of the teeth and dental caries are common because of chronic self-induced vomiting. Laxative abuse is a potentially dangerous form of purging, leading to volume depletion, increased colonic motility, abdominal cramping, and loss of electrolytes in a watery diarrhea. Irritation of intestinal mucosa or hemorrhoids from rapid and frequent stools may cause rectal bleeding. When laxative abuse stops, transient fluid retention, edema, and constipation are common.

CAUSES

The cause of BN is unknown, but it is generally attributed to a combination of psychological, genetic, and physiological influences. Onset occurs in late adolescence or early adulthood when the individual has left or is preparing to leave home. Experts suggest that the stress and depression that accompany this transition lead to bingeing as a way of coping with these changes. Obesity usually precedes the onset of BN, and strict dieting usually triggers the binge–purge cycling. Changes in neurotransmitter metabolism, in particular serotonin, and response to antidepressants suggest a biochemical component to the condition. Cultural pressures toward thinness may also contribute to the onset of BN. BN is more common in people who participate in sports, occupations, or activities in which losing weight rapidly contributes to performance or when slimness and body shape are valued. Sports and activities such as wrestling, bodybuilding, track and field, gymnastics, diving, figure skating, dancing, modeling, and acting are associated with BN.

GENETIC CONSIDERATIONS

There is significant evidence that bulimia runs in families, with a heritability of 55% to 62%. It is most likely that the combined effects of several genes and environment result in the disease. Studies suggest that environmental factors may be less important than the additive effects of genetic mutations. A polymorphism in the *BDNF* gene and an unknown gene on chromosome 10p have been associated with susceptibility to eating disorders in general.

SEX AND LIFE SPAN CONSIDERATIONS

The lifetime prevalence of BN in women is around 2%, and the typical age of onset is adolescence, although it can affect all ages. It is more common in women than men, although men are at risk when they participate in sports or professions with requirements for low body weight or body fat such as wrestling, running, and bodybuilding. Stigma may contribute to underdiagnosis in men.

HEALTH DISPARITIES AND SEXUAL/GENDER MINORITY HEALTH

Experts suggest that people of all races and ethnicities are at risk for BN, although it may be underdiagnosed in Black and Hispanic youth and young adults. Sexual and gender minority persons are disproportionately affected by eating disorders, including BN and AN. Sexual and gender minority youth are at risk for obesity and binge eating disorders compared to their peers. Theories about this association of BN and AN with sexual and gender minority status suggest that the occurrence of eating disorders may be associated with being a member of a marginalized and stigmatized group. Experiences with minority stress, body dissatisfaction, and stigma may lead to BN and AN as an attempt to regain a sense of control or be related to maladaptive coping as a way to manage emotional distress (Kamody et al., 2019).

GLOBAL HEALTH CONSIDERATIONS

In developed countries, eating disorders seem to be more common than in developing countries. Worldwide, the years of living with disability increased by 10% over the last decade for individuals with BN. Mortality risk is estimated at 1.4%.

ASSESSMENT

HISTORY. Patients who are bulimic often report a family history of affective disorders, especially depression. Substance use disorders (particularly stimulants or alcohol misuse) are a common comorbidity as well. The patient may describe patterns of weight fluctuation and frequent dieting, along with a preoccupation with food; this cluster of characteristics may be the first sign of BN. Patients may have dizziness or palpitations due to dehydration. Complaints such as hematemesis, heartburn, constipation, rectal bleeding, and fluid retention may be the initial reasons the patient seeks care from a primary healthcare provider. Patients may also have evidence of esophageal tears or ruptures, such as pain during swallowing and substernal burning. If patients seek treatment for BN, they usually have exhausted a variety of ways to control their bingeing and purging behavior. A detailed history of dieting, laxative and diuretic use, and the frequency and pattern of bingeing and purging episodes is essential. Asking direct questions about bingeing and purging patterns and which foods and situations are most likely to trigger a binge is also essential since patients may not be forthcoming with this information.

The SCOFF screening questionnaire may be helpful during assessment: Do you make yourself SICK because you feel uncomfortably full? Do you worry you have lost CONTROL over how much you eat? Have you recently lost more than ONE stone (14 lb) in a 3-month period? Do you believe yourself to be FAT when others say you are too thin? Would you say that FOOD dominates your life? If these responses are positive, further in-depth assessment is needed.

PHYSICAL EXAMINATION. **Often, no symptoms are noted on the physical examination.** Obtain the patient's weight and compare it with the normal weight range for age and height. In patients with chronic vomiting, you may notice parotid swelling, which gives the patient a characteristic "chipmunk" facial appearance. Assess the patient for signs of dehydration such as poor skin turgor, dry mucous membranes, hair loss, and dry skin. Note dental discoloration and caries from excessive vomiting, scars on the back of the hand from chronic self-induced vomiting, and conjunctival hemorrhages. Poor abdominal muscle tone may be evidence of rapid weight fluctuations. Tearing or fissures of the rectum may be present on rectal examination because of frequent enemas. A neurological assessment is important to rule out possible signs of a brain tumor or seizure disorder. Dehydration may lead to hypotension or tachycardia, and chronic hypokalemia from laxative or diuretic abuse may lead to an irregular pulse or even cardiac arrest and sudden death.

PSYCHOSOCIAL. Assess the patient's current career goals, peer and intimate relationships, psychosexual development, self-esteem, and perception of body image. Pay particular attention to any signs of depression and suicidal ideation and behavior. Assess the patient's ability to express feelings and anger; determine the patient's methods for coping with anxiety as well as the patient's impulse control. Assess the family's communication patterns, especially how the family deals with conflict and solves problems. Assess the degree to which the family supports the patient's growth toward independence and separation.

Diagnostic Highlights

General Comments: The diagnosis of BN is made by clinical assessment. No laboratory test is able to diagnose BN, but supporting tests are used to follow the response to treatment and progression of the illness.

Test	Normal Result	Abnormality With Condition	Explanation
Serum electrolytes and chemistries	Sodium 135–145 mEq/L; potassium 3.5–5.3 mEq/L; chloride 97–107 mEq/L; calcium 8.4–10.2 mEq/L; magnesium 1.6–2.2 mEq/L; glucose 60–100 mg/dL	Hypokalemia, hypochloremia, hypomagnesemia, hypocalcemia, or hypoglycemia	Values reflect loss of electrolytes from vomiting and poor nutrition
Complete blood count	Red blood cells (RBCs) 3.6–5.8 million/mL; white blood cells 4,500–11,100/mL; hemoglobin (Hgb) 11.7–17.3 g/dL; hematocrit (Hct) 36%–52%; reticulocyte count 0.8%–2.5% of total RBCs; platelets 185,000–335,000/mL; ESR 0–25 mm/hr	Anemia; RBCs < 4; Hct < 35%; Hgb < 12 g/dL; bleeding tendencies due to platelets < 150,000/mL	Caused by protracted undernutrition
Amylase	11–300 units/L	Elevated	Elevated levels indicate patient is practicing vomiting behaviors; increases within 2 hr of vomiting and remains elevated for approximately a week
Albumin	3.7–5.1 g/dL	Hypoalbuminemia; albumin < 3.5 g/dL	Caused by protracted undernutrition

Other Tests: Other laboratory tests include arterial blood gases (metabolic alkalosis), blood urea nitrogen (elevated), cholesterol (elevated), luteinizing hormone (decreased), testosterone (decreased), thyroxine (mildly decreased), urinalysis, pregnancy test, electrocardiogram, and chest x-ray.

PRIMARY NURSING DIAGNOSIS

DIAGNOSIS. Imbalanced nutrition: less than body requirements related to recurrent vomiting after eating and/or excessive laxative or diuretic use as evidenced by dental caries, hair loss, and/or weight loss with adequate food intake

OUTCOMES. Nutritional status: Food and fluid intake; Nutritional status: Nutrient intake; Weight: Body mass; Knowledge: Weight management; Fluid balance; Electrolyte balance

INTERVENTIONS. Eating disorders management; Nutrition management; Nutritional counseling; Nutritional monitoring; Fluid/electrolyte management; Weight management

☀ PLANNING AND IMPLEMENTATION

Collaborative

Patients with BN generally do not need hospitalization unless they experience severe electrolyte imbalance, dehydration, or rectal bleeding. BN is usually managed with individual behavioral and group therapy, family education and therapy, medication, and nutritional counseling. Cognitive behavioral therapy (CBT) has been found to be superior to psychoanalytic psychotherapy for improving symptoms. CBT allows the patient to address dysfunctional emotions, maladaptive behaviors, and cognitive processes systematically. It is problem focused (undertaken to address a specific problem, such as purging or bingeing) and action oriented (the therapist tries to help the patient select specific strategies to address bulimia behaviors).

The interdisciplinary team works to coordinate efforts and refer the patient to the physician to evaluate the need for antidepressants and antianxiety medication. The team and patient evaluate the effectiveness of antidepressant or antianxiety medications and explore ways to identify situations that precede depression and anxiety. Collaboration with the dietitian ensures that the patient is educated about appropriate nutrition and dietary intake. Encourage the patient to participate in individual, family, and group sessions to help the patient develop ways to express feelings, handle anger, enhance self-esteem, explore career choices, and develop sexual identity and assertiveness skills.

Pharmacologic Highlights

Medication or Drug Class	Dosage	Description	Rationale
Potassium supplements	20–40 mEq PO	Electrolyte replacement	Replace potassium lost through vomiting

Other Drugs: Drugs that facilitate serotonergic neurotransmission, particularly fluoxetine, may be used. Tricyclic antidepressants (particularly amitriptyline and desipramine), monoamine oxidase inhibitors, and trazodone may also be used. Bupropion is contraindicated related to an increased risk of seizure. Some evidence suggests that topiramate may reduce binge eating episodes.

Independent

Teach the patient to choose correct portion sizes. Encourage the patient to eat slowly and avoid performing other activities, such as reading or watching television, while eating. Most patients are encouraged not to use diet foods or drinks until a stable body weight is established. Encourage the patient to eat a low-sodium diet to prevent fluid retention. Fluid retention is common until the body readjusts its fluid balance; patients may need support if they experience edema of the fingers, ankles, and face. As they begin to eat and drink normally, support patients if they become upset about weight gain and reassure patients that the weight gain and swelling are temporary. Also encourage patients to establish a normal exercise routine but to avoid extremes.

The goals of nursing interventions are to enhance self-esteem, facilitate growth in independence, manage separation from the family, develop sexual identity, and make career choices. Explore ways for the patient to identify and express feelings, manage anger and stress, develop assertive communication skills, and control impulses or delay gratification. Help the patient learn ways other than bingeing and purging to cope with feelings of anxiety and depression. Explore ways to reduce the patient's vomiting, laxative, and diuretic abuse. Some patients respond well to contracting or behavioral management to reduce these behaviors. Educate the family about appropriate nutrition. Explore ways the family can manage conflict and support the patient's move toward independence.

Evidence-Based Practice and Health Policy

Tith, R., Paradis, G., Potter, B., Low, N., Healy-Profitos, J., He, S., & Auger, N. (2020). Association of bulimia nervosa with long-term risk of cardiovascular disease and mortality among women. *JAMA Psychiatry, 77*, 44–51.

• The authors aimed to study the association of BN with long-term cardiovascular disease and mortality in women. The authors followed over 400,000 women hospitalized for BN over 12 years and compared them to women hospitalized for pregnancy-related events. Participants in the BN group needed at least one hospitalization for BN to qualify for the study.
• Patients hospitalized with BN had more than four times the risk for cardiovascular disease and five times the risk for death up to 8 years after the index bulimia-related hospitalization (10.34 per 1,000 person-years) versus those with pregnancy-related events (1.2 per 1,000 person-years). Incidence of future cardiovascular disease was even higher for women with three or more bulimia admissions (25.13 per 1,000 person-years). BN was also associated with almost 22 times the risk for myocardial infarction at 2 years follow-up. Patients with a history of BN should be screened regularly for ischemic cardiovascular disease and may benefit from prevention of and treatment for cardiovascular risk factors.

DOCUMENTATION GUIDELINES

• Nutrition: Diet planning and food intake, frequency and duration of binge–purge episodes
• Volume depletion: Signs of dehydration, pertinent laboratory findings if available
• Response to care and teaching: Understanding of the disease process and the relationship of dehydration and self-induced vomiting, laxative abuse, and diuretic abuse; understanding of ways to identify and cope with anxiety, anger, depression, and own impulses and needs
• Family meeting: Family interactions and support of move toward independence

DISCHARGE AND HOME HEALTHCARE GUIDELINES

Teach the patient ways to avoid binge–purge episodes through a balanced diet. Discuss effective ways of coping with needs and feelings. Explore ways to identify and handle stress and anxiety. Teach the patient strategies to increase self-esteem. Explore ways to maintain increased independence and the patient's own choices.

Burns

DRG Category:	933
Mean LOS:	6.0 days
Description:	MEDICAL: Extensive Burns or Full Thickness Burns With MV > 96 Hours Without Skin Graft
DRG Category:	935
Mean LOS:	5.2 days
Description:	MEDICAL: Non-Extensive Burns

The World Health Organization (WHO, 2022) describes burns as injuries to the skin or other tissues caused by heat, friction, radiation, or chemicals. There are six classifications of burn wounds based on injury mechanism: scalds (by liquids, grease, or steam), contact burns, fire (flash or flame), chemical (caustic acids and bases, chemicals such as bleach, or vesicants such as blistering gases), electrical (high and low voltages, lightning), and radiation (ionizing or ultraviolet). Thermal burns (scalds, contact, fire), which are the most common type, occur because of fires from motor vehicle crashes, accidents in residences, and arson or electrical malfunctions. Burns have a devastating effect on people's quality of life, finances, and relationships as well as create significant suffering and disability. Burns are the third leading cause of accidental death in the United States; approximately 4,000 people die each year from burns. The American Burn Association (ABA) estimates that approximately 500,000 Americans experience burns severe enough to seek medical care each year. Most burn care is delivered in the emergency department, although approximately 40,000 people require hospitalization each year in the United States. The most common place of occurrence for burns is in the home (73%), with less common locations including the workplace (8%), streets or highways (5%), and during recreation or sports (5%). The physiological responses to moderate and major burns are outlined in Table 1. Complications of burns include infection, hypovolemia, hypothermia, respiratory distress and acute respiratory distress syndrome, scarring, and joint contractures. The ABA reports that the survival rate after burns is 96.8%.

• TABLE 1   System Impact of Moderate or Major Burns

SYSTEM	PHYSIOLOGICAL CHANGES
Cardiovascular	Fluid shifts from the vascular to the interstitial space occur because of increased permeability related to the inflammatory response. Hypovolemic shock may result or it may be overcorrected by overzealous fluid replacement, which can lead to hypervolemia. Hypertension occurs in about one-third of all children with burns, possibly caused by stress.
Pulmonary	Pulmonary edema brought about by primary cellular damage or circumferential chest burns limiting chest excursion can occur. Trauma may lead to release of cytokines that damage lung tissue. By-products of combustion may lead to carbon monoxide poisoning. Inhalation of noxious gases (smoke inhalation) may cause primary pulmonary damage or airway edema and upper airway obstructions.

● **TABLE 1** System Impact of Moderate or Major Burns (continued)

SYSTEM	PHYSIOLOGICAL CHANGES
Genitourinary	Potential for renal shutdown brought about by hypovolemia or acute renal failure exists. Massive diuresis from fluid returning to the vascular space marks the end of the emergent phase. Patients may develop hemomyoglobinuria because of massive full-thickness burns or electric injury. These injuries cause the release of muscle protein (myoglobin) and hemoglobin, which can clog the renal tubules and cause acute renal failure.
Gastrointestinal	Paralytic ileus can result from hypovolemia and last 2 or 3 days. Children are particularly susceptible to Curling ulcer, a stress ulcer, because of the overwhelming systemic injury.
Musculoskeletal	Potential exists for the development of compartment syndrome because of edema. Escharatomy (cutting of a thick burn) may be needed to improve circulation. Scarring and contractures are a potential problem if prevention is not started on admission.
Neurological	Personality changes are common throughout recovery because of stress, electrolyte disturbance, hypoxemia, or medications. Children are particularly at risk for postburn seizures during the acute phase.

CAUSES

Most burns result from preventable accidents. Children may be burned when they play with matches or firecrackers or because of a kitchen accident. The percentage of burns caused by abuse is estimated at approximately 10%, but they are some of the most difficult to manage because the causes are complex. Burns occur primarily in the home (73%), followed by occupational burns (8%), burns that occur on the street or highway (7%), and recreational burns (9%). Neglect or inadequate supervision of children is fairly common. Effective prevention and educational efforts such as smoke detectors, flame-retardant clothing, child-resistant cigarette lighters, and the Stop, Drop, and Roll program have decreased the number and severity of injuries.

GENETIC CONSIDERATIONS

No clear genetic contributions to susceptibility have been defined.

SEX AND LIFE SPAN CONSIDERATIONS

Preschool children account for over two-thirds of all burn fatalities. Clinicians use a special chart for children (Lund-Browder chart) that provides a picture and a graph to account for the difference in body surface area by age. Serious burn injuries occur most commonly in males, and, in particular, young adult males ages 20 to 29 years, followed by children under age 9 years. Individuals older than 50 years sustain the fewest number of serious burn injuries. In developed countries, burns occur in males at twice the rate that they occur in females. In developing countries, women have higher rates of burn injury than men, likely because of open fire cooking or unsafe cookstoves.

A young child is the most common victim of burns that have been caused by liquids. Preschoolers, school-aged children, and teenagers are more frequently the victims of flame burns. Young children playing with lighters or matches are at risk, as are teenagers because of carelessness or risk-taking behaviors around fires. Toddlers incur electrical burns from biting electrical cords or putting objects in outlets. Most adults are victims of house fires or work-related accidents that involve chemicals or electricity. Older adults are also prone to scald injuries because their skin tends to be extremely thin and sensitive to heat.

Because of the severe impact of this injury, the very young and the very old are less able to respond to therapy and have a higher incidence of mortality. In addition, when a child experiences a burn, multiple surgeries are required to release contractures that occur as normal growth pulls at the scar tissue of their healed burns. Adolescents are particularly prone to psychological difficulties because of sensitivity regarding body image issues.

HEALTH DISPARITIES AND SEXUAL/GENDER MINORITY HEALTH

The ABA reports that 59% of burns occur in White persons, 20% in Black persons, 14% in Hispanic persons, and 7% in other races and ethnicities. Native American and Black children are more than two and three times more likely than White children to die in a fire. Factors that are associated with increased burn risk include low income and residential overcrowding. Sexual and gender minority status has no known effect on the risk for burns.

GLOBAL HEALTH CONSIDERATIONS

Many developing countries do not track burn rates, but the WHO notes that the majority of burns worldwide occur in low- and middle-income countries in Africa and Southeast Asia. Around the world, an estimated 254,000 deaths occur each year from fires alone. Poverty, overcrowding, lack of water supply, and the lack of a living room in the home are global risks for burn injury. The World Fire Statistics Center reported that the countries with the lowest incidences of fire deaths per 100,000 persons include Singapore, Vietnam, Switzerland, and New Zealand. Those with the highest include Russia, Ukraine, Belarus, and Lithuania. Research in Ireland and Greece suggests that the incidence of burns increases during holidays that feature the use of celebratory fireworks.

ASSESSMENT

HISTORY. The initial triage is done according to ABCDE principles of the primary survey: airway maintenance with stabilization of the cervical spine, breathing and ventilation, circulation with control of hemorrhage, disability assessment and neurological examination, and exposure along with environmental control. The secondary survey is a complete head-to-toe assessment that occurs later as part of the physical assessment. Sometime during the first 48 hours, a tertiary survey is performed to discover any subtle injuries that may have been missed during the initial assessment. Obtain a complete description of the burn injury, including the time, the situation, the burning agent, and the actions of witnesses. The time of injury is extremely important because any delay in treatment may result in a minor or moderate burn becoming a major injury. Elicit specific information about the location of the injury because closed-space injuries are related to smoke inhalation. If abuse is suspected, obtain a more in-depth history from a variety of people who are involved with the child. The injury may be suspect if there is a delay in seeking healthcare, if there are burns that are not consistent with the story, or if there are bruises at different stages of healing. Note whether the description of the injury changes or differs among family or household members.

PHYSICAL EXAMINATION. The most common symptoms are **thermal injury to the skin** and **signs of smoke inhalation (carbonaceous sputum, singed facial or nasal hairs, facial burns, oropharyngeal edema, vocal changes)**. Although the wounds of a serious burn injury may be dramatic, a basic assessment of airway, breathing, and circulation (ABCs) takes first priority. Once the ABCs are stabilized, perform a complete examination of the burn wound to determine the severity of injury. The ABA establishes the severity of injury by calculating the total body surface area (TBSA) of partial- and full-thickness injury along with the age of the patient and other special factors (Table 2).

• TABLE 2 Characteristics of Burns

SUPERFICIAL EPIDERMAL (FIRST DEGREE)	SUPERFICIAL AND DEEP PARTIAL THICKNESS (SECOND DEGREE)	FULL THICKNESS (THIRD AND FOURTH DEGREE)
Erythema, blanching on pressure, mild to moderate pain, no blister (typical of sunburn). Only structure involved is the epidermis.	• Superficial: Papillary dermis is affected with blisters, redness, and severe pain because of exposed nerve endings • Deep: Reticular dermis affected with blisters, pale white or yellow color, absent pain sensation	• Third degree: All levels of the dermis along with subcutaneous fat. Blisters may be absent with leathery, wrinkled skin without capillary refill. Thrombosed blood vessels are visible, insensitive to pain because of nerve destruction. • Fourth degree: Involvement of all levels of dermis as well as fascia, muscle, and bone

The "rule of nines" is a practical technique used to estimate the extent of TBSA involved in a burn. The technique divides the major anatomic areas of the body into percentages: In adults, 9% of the TBSA is the head and neck, 9% is each upper extremity, 18% is each anterior and posterior portion of the trunk, 18% is each lower extremity, and 1% is the perineum and genitalia. Clinicians use the patient's palm area to represent approximately 1% of TBSA. Serial assessments of wound healing determine the patient's response to treatment. Ongoing monitoring throughout the acute and rehabilitative phases is essential for the burn patient. Fluid balance, daily weights, vital signs, and intake and output monitoring are essential to ensure that the patient is responding appropriately to treatment.

PSYCHOSOCIAL. Even small burns temporarily change the appearance of the skin. Major burns will have a permanent effect on the family unit. A complete assessment of the family's psychological health before the injury is essential. Expect preexisting issues to magnify during this crisis, and identify previous ways of coping in order to facilitate dealing with the crisis. Guilt, blame, anxiety, fear, and depression are commonly experienced emotions. Health providers are mandated by state laws to recognize and report suspected abuse. It is important to understand and implement reporting statutes based on the state of residence.

Diagnostic Highlights

Test	Normal Result	Abnormality With Condition	Explanation
Fiberoptic bronchoscopy	Normal larynx, trachea, and bronchi	Thermal injury and edema to oropharynx and glottis	Used to investigate suspected smoke inhalation and damage from noxious gases
Carboxyhemo-globin levels	8%–10% in smokers; < 2% in nonsmokers	10%–20% indicates potential inhalation injury; 20%–30% disturbed judgment, headache, dizziness; 30%–40% dizziness, muscle weakness, visual problems, confusion; 50%–60% loss of consciousness; > 60% death	Carbon monoxide binds to hemoglobin with an affinity 240 times greater than that of oxygen

Other Tests: Because burns are the result of trauma, there are no tests needed to make the diagnosis. Some of the more common tests to monitor the patient's response to injury and treatment are complete blood count, arterial blood gases, serum electrolytes, blood and wound cultures and sensitivities, chest x-rays, urinalysis, and nutritional profiles.

PRIMARY NURSING DIAGNOSIS

DIAGNOSIS. Ineffective airway clearance related to exposure to smoke and airway edema as evidenced by shortness of breath, cough, and/or production of carbonaceous sputum

OUTCOMES. Respiratory status: Airway patency, ventilation, and gas exchange; Symptom control; Mechanical management response; Comfort level: Physical

INTERVENTIONS. Airway insertion and stabilization; Airway management; Oxygen therapy; Anxiety reduction; Airway suctioning; Cough enhancement; Mechanical ventilation management; Positioning; Respiratory monitoring

PLANNING AND IMPLEMENTATION

Collaborative

MINOR BURN CARE. Minor burn wounds are cared for by using the principles of comfort, cleanliness, and infection control. A gentle cleansing of the wound with soap and water two or three times a day, followed with a topical agent such as silver sulfadiazine or mafenide, prevents infection. Minor burns should heal in 7 to 10 days; however, if they take longer than 14 days, excision of the wound and a small graft may be needed. Oral analgesics may be prescribed to manage discomfort, and all burn patients need to receive tetanus toxoid to prevent infection.

MAJOR BURN CARE. For patients with a major injury, effective treatment is provided by a multidisciplinary team with special training in burn care. In addition to the physician and nurse, the team includes specialists in physical and occupational therapy, respiratory therapy, social work, nutrition, psychology, and child life for children. The course of recovery is divided into four phases: emergent-resuscitative, acute-wound coverage, convalescent-rehabilitative, and reorganization-reintegration.

The emergent-resuscitative phase lasts from 48 to 72 hours after injury or until diuresis takes place. If the patient cannot be transported immediately to a hospital, remove charred clothing and immerse the burn wound in cold (not ice) water for 30 minutes. Note that cooling has no therapeutic value if delayed more than 30 minutes after injury. The cold temperature is thought to be related to reduced lactate production, reduced acidosis, and reduced histamine and other mediator release. In addition to ABCs management, the patient receives fluid resuscitation, maintenance of electrolytes, aggressive pain management, and early nutrition. Fluid resuscitation is generally initiated intravenously with lactated Ringer solution based on the Parkland formula (4 mL/kg/% TBSA burned) during the first 24 hours. Patients are monitored carefully for over- and underhydration. Wounds are cleansed with chlorhexidine gluconate, and care consists of silver sulfadiazine or mafenide and surgical management as needed. To prevent infection, continued care includes further débridement by washing the surface of the wounds with mild soap or aseptic solutions. Then the physician débrides devitalized tissue, and often the wound is covered with antibacterial agents such as silver sulfadiazine and occlusive cotton gauze. The nutritional needs of the patient are extensive and complex. Initially metabolic rate is low because of decreased cardiac output, but a severe burn can double the metabolic rate and cause the release of large amounts of amino acids from the muscles. Nutritional assessment and support occur within the first 24 hours after the burn, and feedings are initiated enterally by feeding tube if possible. A nutritional consult is needed to determine exact caloric and nutrient needs.

The acute-wound coverage phase, which varies depending on the extent of injury, lasts until the wounds have been covered through either the normal healing process or grafting. The risk for infection is high during this phase; the physician follows wound and blood cultures and prescribes antibiotics as needed. Wound management includes excision of devitalized tissue, surgical grafting of donor skin, or placement of synthetic membranes. Inpatient rehabilitation takes place during the convalescent-rehabilitative phase. Although principles of rehabilitation are included in the plan of care from the day of admission, during this time, home exercises and wound care are taught. In addition, pressure appliances to reduce scarring, or braces to prevent contractures, are fitted. The reorganization phase is the long period of time that it may take after the injury for physical and emotional healing to take place.

Pharmacologic Highlights

Medication or Drug Class	Dosage	Description	Rationale
Topical antimicrobial agents	Silver sulfadiazine	Cream that lowers bacterial counts, minimizes water evaporation, and decreases heat loss	Antimicrobial agent that is not irritating and has the fewest adverse effects
	Mafenide acetate	Bacterial coverage for gram-negative and anaerobic coverage; deep eschar penetration	Painful but readily absorbed and can lead to metabolic acidosis

Other Drugs: Tetanus prophylaxis, analgesia to manage the severe pain that accompanies thermal injury, other topical applications such as polymyxin B or Acticoat (dressings that release silver ions), H_2 blockers

Independent

The nursing care of the patient with a burn is complex and collaborative, with overlapping interventions among the nurse, the physician, and a variety of therapists. However, independent nursing interventions are also an important focus for the nurse. The highest priority for the burn patient is to maintain the ABCs. The airway can be maintained in some patients by an oral or nasal airway or by the jaw lift–chin thrust maneuver. Patency of the airway is maintained by endotracheal suctioning, the frequency of which is dictated by the character and amount of secretions. If the patient is apneic, maintain breathing with a manual resuscitator bag before intubation and mechanical ventilation.

If the patient is bleeding from burn sites, apply pressure until the bleeding can be controlled surgically. Remove all constricting clothing and jewelry to allow for adequate circulation to the extremities. Implement fluid resuscitation protocols as appropriate to support the patient's circulation. If any clothing is still smoldering and adhering to the patient, soak the area with normal saline solution and remove the material. Wound care includes collaborative management and other strategies. Cover wounds with clean, dry, sterile sheets. Do not cover large burn wounds with saline-soaked dressings, which lower the patient's temperature. If the patient has ineffective thermoregulation, use warming or cooling blankets as needed and control the room temperature to support the patient's optimum temperature. If the patient is hypothermic, limit traffic into the room to decrease drafts and keep the patient covered with sterile sheets. Help the patient manage pain and distress by providing careful explanations and teaching distraction and relaxation techniques.

Depending on the type and extent of injury, dressing changes are generally performed daily; twice-a-day dressing changes may be indicated for infected wounds or those with large amounts of drainage. While dressing protocols vary, one method is to cleanse the wound with sponges saturated with a wound cleanser such as poloxamer 188 to remove the topical antibiotics. Then cover the wound with antibiotic cream. As the wounds heal, use strategies such as tubbing, débridement, and dressing changes to limit infection, promote wound healing, and limit physical impairment. If impaired physical mobility is a risk, place the patient in antideformity positions at all times. Implement active and passive range of motion as needed. Get the patient out of bed on a regular basis to limit physical debilitation and decrease the risk of infection. Implement strategies to limit stress and anxiety.

Evidence-Based Practice and Health Policy

Govender, R., Hornsby, N., Kimemia, D., & Van Niekerk, A. (2020). The role of concomitant alcohol and drug use in increased risk for burn mortality outcomes. *Burns, 46,* 58–64.

- Burn injuries are a major cause of mortality and morbidity in low- and middle-income countries, and the risk may be increased with alcohol and drug use. The authors used a national data set in low- and middle-income countries in Sub-Saharan Africa to explore the risk for burn injuries in adults 18 years and older (*N* = 918).
- Burn victims with full-thickness and partial-thickness burns over more than 30% of TBSA had a risk of mortality 10 times higher when alcohol and drugs were involved as compared to when alcohol and drugs were not involved. The authors concluded that alcohol and drugs may predispose toward more severe burns and a higher risk for sepsis and death.

DOCUMENTATION GUIDELINES

Emergent-resuscitative Phase

- Flow sheet record of the critical physiological aspects of this time period; depending on the patient's condition, documentation times may be established for 15-minute intervals or less for vital signs and fluid balance
- Flow sheet record of information related to the condition of the wound, wound care, and psychosocial issues

Acute-wound Coverage Phase

- The condition of the wound, healing progress, graft condition, signs of infection, scar formation, and antideformity positioning are important documentation parameters
- Psychosocial issues and the family's involvement in care are also important information

Rehabilitative Phase

- Status of healing and the appearance of scars, as well as the patient's functional abilities and their management of body image issues
- Ability of the patient and family to perform the complex care required during the months to come

DISCHARGE AND HOME HEALTHCARE GUIDELINES

Patient teaching is individualized, but for most patients, it includes information about each of the following:

WOUND MANAGEMENT. This includes infection control, basic cleanliness, and wound management.

SCAR MANAGEMENT. Functional abilities, including using pressure garments, exercises, and activities of daily living, must be assessed and taught.

NUTRITION. Nutritional guidelines are provided that maintain continued healing and respond to the metabolic demands that frequently last for some time after initial injury.

FOLLOW-UP. If respiratory involvement exists, include specific teaching related to the amount of damage and ongoing therapy. Teach various techniques for dealing with the reaction of society, classmates, or those in the workplace. Explain where and how to obtain resources (financial and emotional) for assisting the family and patient during the recovery process. Psychological support is essential.

Calculi, Renal

DRG Category:	693
Mean LOS:	5.1 days
Description:	MEDICAL: Urinary Stones With Major Complication or Comorbidity
DRG Category:	694
Mean LOS:	2.7 days
Description:	MEDICAL: Urinary Stones Without Major Complication or Comorbidity

Renal calculi, or nephrolithiases, are stones that form in the kidneys from the crystallization of minerals and other substances that normally dissolve in the urine. Approximately 2 million people seek healthcare for stone disease each year in the United States. Although the reasons are unknown, in the past 30 years, the prevalence of kidney stones has been increasing. The lifetime risk of developing a renal calculi is 8% to 12% in North America and Europe. Renal calculi vary in size, with 90% of them smaller than 5 mm in diameter; some, however, grow large enough to prevent the natural passage of urine through the ureter. Calculi may be solitary or multiple. Approximately 80% of these stones are composed of calcium salts. Other types are the struvite stones (which contain magnesium, ammonium, and phosphate), uric acid stones, and cystine stones. Cystine stones are associated with hereditary renal disease. Having a family member with a history of renal calculi doubles the risk for the condition. Once a person gets more than one stone, others are likely to develop. If the calculi remain in the renal pelvis or enter the ureter, they can damage renal parenchyma (functional tissue). Larger calculi can cause pressure necrosis. In certain locations, calculi cause obstruction, lead to hydronephrosis, and tend to recur. Complications of renal calculi include infection and sepsis, urinary stasis, genitourinary tract injury, and hematuria.

CAUSES

The precise cause of renal calculi is unknown, although they are associated with dehydration, urinary obstruction, calcium levels, and other factors. When high concentrations of stone-forming particles occur in the urine, they form a nidus, or a site for accumulation. Patients who are dehydrated have decreased urine, with heavy concentrations of these calculus-forming substances. Urinary obstruction leads to urinary stasis, a condition that contributes to calculus formation. Any condition that increases serum calcium levels and calcium excretion predisposes people to renal calculi. These conditions include an excessive intake of vitamin D or dietary calcium, hyperparathyroidism, heredity factors, and immobility. Metabolic conditions such as renal tubular acidosis, elevated serum uric acid levels, and urinary tract infections associated with alkaline urine have been linked with calculus formation.

GENETIC CONSIDERATIONS

There are at least 10 different single gene conditions (e.g., primary hyperoxaluria type 1), resulting in familial nephrolithiasis, but these account for less than 2% of persons with renal calculi. Both genetic and environmental factors have been suggested to explain the higher incidence of stone formation in certain geographical areas, including the southeastern United States.

Approximately 50% of individuals who develop calcium stones have hypercalciuria, which often has a familial component. Twin studies estimate a heritability of about 45% for nephrolithiasis, and about 50% for hypercalciuria.

SEX AND LIFE SPAN CONSIDERATIONS

In the United States, approximately 12% of the male population and 7% of the female population develop a stone at some point in their lives. Recent evidence indicates that both incidence and mortality are increasing in women, and experts suggest the narrowing is in part related to increasing rates of obesity in women. Calculi occur more often in men than in women, unless heredity is a factor, and occur most often between ages 30 and 50 years. Individuals living in the South and Southwest in the United States have the highest incidence of stones. When women develop calculi, they are likely to be caused by infection. Children rarely develop calculi.

HEALTH DISPARITIES AND SEXUAL/GENDER MINORITY HEALTH

The prevalence of renal calculi is higher in White and Asian persons than in other populations. Black and Native American persons and those from the Mediterranean region have a lower incidence of stones than other groups. Sex and gender minority status has no known effect on the risk for renal calculi.

GLOBAL HEALTH CONSIDERATIONS

Developed countries have rates of urinary tract stones that are similar to the United States. Although renal calculi occur in all countries, prevalence is lowest in Greenland and parts of Japan. People in Asia have a low lifetime risk as compared to Saudi Arabia and North America. Differences in prevalence are thought to be related to diet.

ASSESSMENT

HISTORY. Symptoms of renal calculi usually appear when a stone dislodges and begins to travel down the urinary tract and enters the ureter. Ask if the patient has a history of renal calculi or urinary tract infection. Establish a history of pain and determine the intensity, duration, and location of the pain. The location of the pain varies according to the position of the stone. The pain usually begins in the flank area but later may radiate into the lower abdomen and the groin. Ask if the pain had a sudden onset. Some stones may cause symptoms of irritation such as urinary frequency and dysuria. Patients may relate a recent history of hematuria, nausea, vomiting, and anorexia. In cases in which a urinary tract infection is also present, the patient may report chills and fever. Determine the patient's history to identify risk factors.

PHYSICAL EXAMINATION. The most typical symptoms of renal calculi are **flank pain radiating to the groin**, **fever**, **hematuria**, **nausea**, and **vomiting**. Inspection reveals a patient in intense pain who is unable to maintain a comfortable position. Assess the patient for bladder distention. Monitor the patient for signs of an infection such as fever, chills, and increased white blood cell counts. Assess the urine for hematuria. Auscultate the patient's abdomen for normal bowel sounds. Palpate the patient's flank area for tenderness. Percussion of the abdominal area is normal, but percussion of the costovertebral angle elicits severe pain.

PSYCHOSOCIAL. Patients with renal calculi may be extremely anxious because of the sudden onset of severe pain of unknown origin. Assess the level of the pain as well as the patient's ability to cope. Because diet and lifestyle may contribute to the formation of calculi, the patient may face lifestyle changes. Assess the patient's ability to handle such changes.

Diagnostic Highlights

General Comments: The physician uses diagnostic tests to eliminate cholecystitis, peptic ulcers, appendicitis, and pancreatitis as the cause of the abdominal pain.

Test	Normal Result	Abnormality With Condition	Explanation
Helical computed tomography scan without contrast	Image of normal abdomen	Calculi present	Visualizes size, shape, relative position of stone; contrast not used; with contrast entire urinary collecting system would appear white, masking the stones
Kidney-ureter-bladder and abdominal x-rays	No renal stones	Presence of renal stones, most of which are radiopaque	Reveals most renal calculi except cystine and uric acid stones
IV pyelography	Normal anatomy of the kidney/collection system	Obstructing stone	Performed when renal colic is severe and obstruction is suspected

Other Tests: Other supporting tests include kidney ultrasonography; urinalysis; complete blood count; serum electrolytes; urine culture and sensitivity; serum calcium and phosphorus levels; 24-hour urine for calcium, oxalate, uric acid, sodium, phosphorus, citrate, magnesium, creatinine, total volume

PRIMARY NURSING DIAGNOSIS

DIAGNOSIS. Impaired urinary elimination related to obstruction of the ureter as evidenced by urinary frequency, dysuria, and/or hematuria

OUTCOMES. Urinary elimination; Knowledge: Medication; Symptom severity; Pain control; Hydration

INTERVENTIONS. Urinary elimination management; Medication prescribing and management; Fluid monitoring; Pain management: Acute; Infection control; Tube care: Urinary

PLANNING AND IMPLEMENTATION

Collaborative

Stones less than 4 mm in diameter will likely pass spontaneously (80% chance), whereas stones larger than 7 to 8 mm in diameter will likely not pass spontaneously (20% chance). In about 80% of cases, renal calculi of 7 to 8 mm or less are treated conservatively with vigorous hydration, which results in the stone passing spontaneously, but supranormal hydration is controversial. Increased fluid intake is ordered orally or IV to flush the stone through the urinary tract. Unless contraindicated, maintain hydration at 200 mL per hour of IV or orally. Strain the patient's urine to detect stones that are passed so they can be analyzed.

Active medical expulsive therapy (MET) reduces the pain of stone passage and the need for surgery for stones 3 to 10 mm in size. Typically, MET includes one to two oral narcotic/acetaminophen tablets every 4 hours and 600 to 800 mg ibuprofen every 8 hours for pain, 30 mg nifedipine extended-release tablet once daily to relax the ureteral smooth muscle, and 0.4 mg tamsulosin once daily or 4 mg of terazosin once daily to relax musculature of the ureter and lower urinary tract. Some protocols include prednisone 20 mg twice a day and the antibiotic trimethoprim/sulfamethoxazole once a day. Generally, MET is limited to a 10- to 14-day course, when most stones will pass.

For calculi larger than 7 to 8 mm or that cannot be passed with conservative treatment, surgical removal is performed. Percutaneous ultrasonic lithotripsy or extracorporeal shock wave lithotripsy (ESWL) uses sound waves to shatter calculi for later removal by suction or natural passage. Calculi in the ureter may be removed with catheters and a cystoscope (ureteroscopy), while a flank or lower abdominal surgical approach may be needed to remove calculi from the kidney calyx or renal pelvis.

Pharmacologic Highlights

General Comments: If nausea and vomiting are present, administer antiemetics as ordered. Diuretics may be ordered to prevent urinary stasis.

Medication or Drug Class	Dosage	Description	Rationale
Analgesia: Primary drugs used are morphine sulfate, butorphanol, and ketorolac (Toradol)	Varies with drug	Narcotics, NSAIDs	To relax the ureter and facilitate passage of stone

Other Drugs: Antibiotics if infection is present (see earlier discussion of MET), antiemetics such as metoclopramide, antidiuretics such as desmopressin

Independent

Initially, the most important nursing interventions concentrate on pain management. Work with the collaborative team to develop an appropriate pain medication regime. Teach relaxation techniques, diversional activities, and position changes. Help promote the passage of renal calculi. Encourage the patient to walk, if possible. Offer the patient fruit juices to help acidify the urine. Make sure the patient understands the urinary straining protocol. Teach the patient the importance of proper diet to help avoid a recurrence of the renal calculi, with particular emphasis on adequate hydration and avoiding excessive salt and protein intake.

To reduce anxiety, give the patient and family all pertinent information concerning the treatment plan and any diagnostic tests. Preoperatively, explain the procedure and what to expect afterward. For patients who are undergoing a flank or abdominal incision, teach deep breathing and coughing exercises. Give postoperative care and monitor for signs of infection or pneumonia. Do not irrigate urinary drainage systems without consulting with the physician.

Evidence-Based Practice and Health Policy

Haas, C., Li, G., Hyams, E., & Shad, O. (2020). Delayed decompression of obstructing stones with urinary tract infection is associated with increased odds of death. *Journal of Urology, 204,* 1256–1262.

- The authors proposed to examine whether a delay in treating obstructive pyelonephritis is an independent predictor of in-hospital mortality and which factors determined delayed versus prompt decompression. The authors identified 300,000 patients from a national sample who were 18 years old or older diagnosed with urinary tract infection and who had either a ureteral stone or kidney stone.
- Although the overall mortality rate in patients with obstructing upper urinary tract is fairly low, the study found that delayed decompression significantly increased the odds of death by 29% and noted a number of factors that led to disparities in the mortality rate. An increased likelihood of delay was associated with weekend admissions, underrepresented minority patients, and patients with low income.

DOCUMENTATION GUIDELINES

• Response to pain relief measures, degree of pain (location, frequency, duration)
• Record of intake and output, daily weights, vital signs
• Presence of complications: Infection, obstruction, hemorrhage, intractable pain
• Observation of color and consistency of urine, presence of stones

DISCHARGE AND HOME HEALTHCARE GUIDELINES

COMFORT MEASURES. Teach the patient to take analgesics as ordered and to use other appropriate comfort measures.

MEDICATION. Be sure the patient understands any medication prescribed, including dosage, route, action, and side effects. If the patient is placed on antibiotics, encourage the patient to complete the entire prescription.

PREVENTION. Instruct the patient to increase fluid intake to enhance the passage of the stone. Instruct the patient to strain all urine and emphasize the importance of returning the stone, if obtained, to the physician for analysis. If the patient has passed the stone and it has been analyzed, teach the necessary dietary changes, fluid intake requirements, and exercise regimen to prevent future stone formation. Patient should drink at least 2.5 L a day of fluid to prevent recurrences unless contraindicated.

COMPLICATIONS. Teach the patient to report any signs of complications, such as fever, chills, or hematuria, as well as any changes in urinary output patterns, to the primary caregiver.

Candidiasis (Moniliasis)

DRG Category:	158	
Mean LOS:	3.5 days	
Description:	MEDICAL: Dental and Oral Diseases With Complication or Comorbidity	
DRG Category:	606	
Mean LOS:	5.9 days	
Description:	MEDICAL: Minor Skin Disorders With Major Complication or Comorbidity	
DRG Category:	868	
Mean LOS:	4.6 days	
Description:	MEDICAL: Other Infectious and Parasitic Diseases Diagnoses With Complication or Comorbidity	

Candidiasis is a yeast infection, an inflammatory reaction caused by *Candida* fungi. Infection occurs when *Candida* fungi penetrate the tissue, colonize, and release toxins that cause an acute inflammatory response. The infection is also termed *moniliasis*, which is a yeast infection of the skin and mucous membranes. Infection is common in the mouth (thrush), esophagus, pulmonary system, vagina (moniliasis), and skin (diaper rash). It is also among the top five causes of nosocomial (hospital-acquired) bloodstream infections in the United States. Most typically, however, *Candida* infections occur in moist areas of the skin such as skin folds, around fingernails, and in mucous membranes, with the most common site being the vulvovaginal area. *Candida* may infect wounds, catheter sites, and IV sites. Infections may take 6 to 8 weeks to resolve. In immunosuppressed patients, candidiasis can become disseminated by entering the bloodstream and causing serious infections in other organs; such infections are difficult to eradicate. *Candida albicans* is a common fungus that causes pathology in patients with HIV, and women with persistent and severe infections should have HIV testing. In recent years, the percentage of non–*Candida albicans* infections has been growing. Most infections do not cause serious consequences or death unless the patient is immunocompromised. In those situations, people with disseminated candidiasis have a 30% to 40% mortality rate. Complications of candidiasis include invasive (disseminated) candidiasis (a systemic infection that can affect the blood, brain, and heart), skin breakdown, gynecological problems, and gastrointestinal (GI) problems.

CAUSES

The *Candida* fungus, which is not pathological under normal conditions, is found normally on the skin and in the GI tract, the mouth, and the vagina. Of the *Candida* species, *C albicans* is common, but other *Candida* species exist, such as *C tropicalis*, *C guilliermondii*, *C krusei*, and *C glabrata*. *C glabrata* and *C krusei* are the leading causes of candidemia (a *Candida* infection of the blood) in patients with malignancy of hematological origin, and *C parapsilosis* is the leading cause of candidemia from medical instrumentation. *Candida* causes infection when a body change permits its sudden proliferation. The most common factor remains the side effects caused by the use of broad-spectrum antibiotics. Changes that contribute to susceptibility to candidiasis include rising glucose levels caused by diabetes mellitus and lowered resistance caused by a disease such as carcinoma, an immunosuppressive drug such as corticosteroids, or radiation therapy. Approximately 14% of patients with immunocompromising illnesses develop systemic candidiasis.

Other associated factors include aging, irritation from dentures, instrumentation (urinary or IV catheters, indwelling foreign bodies), surgery, peritoneal dialysis, and the use of oral contraceptives. Diabetes mellitus is associated with candidemia because of impaired immune responses and the presence of higher glucose levels in the saliva, blood, urine, and feces, which foster colonization with *Candida*.

GENETIC CONSIDERATIONS

Heritable immune responses could be protective or increase susceptibility. Several genes have been linked to an increased susceptibility to fungal infections, including *CARD9*, *STAT1* (causing chronic mucocutaneous candidiasis), and *STAT3* (causing hyper-IgE syndrome).

SEX AND LIFE SPAN CONSIDERATIONS

Candidiasis may occur at any age and under any condition, but it is more common in the genitourinary tract of women than in men. Three-quarters of all women have at least one episode of vulvovaginal candidiasis during their lifetime, and up to 30% have recurrent infections. It commonly occurs during the childbearing years for women when estrogen levels are high, particularly during the use of oral contraceptives and contraceptive devices. The very old and the very young are also likely to have *Candida* infections. In infants, it can cause diaper rash. Older adults and patients with cancer, diabetes mellitus, and HIV infections are most susceptible to infection.

HEALTH DISPARITIES AND SEXUAL/GENDER MINORITY HEALTH

Ethnicity, race, and sexual/gender minority status have no known effect on the risk for candidiasis.

GLOBAL HEALTH CONSIDERATIONS

Candida species is the most common fungus infecting people who are immunocompromised. Women acquire vulvovaginal candidiasis in all parts of the globe. In some cultures, a vaginal infection causes misery, embarrassment, and shame because of stigma.

☀ ASSESSMENT

HISTORY. Question the patient carefully to elicit a history of risk factors or a history of repeated episodes of candidiasis. Factors such as cigarette smoking, tobacco chewing, or pipe smoking are often associated with *Candida* infections. Take a careful medication history and pay particular attention to use of antibiotics, corticosteroids, or other immunosuppressive drugs. A reproductive history, including current pregnancy or oral contraceptive use, is important.

The patient may complain of a burning or painful sensation in the mouth or difficulty in swallowing. The patient also may report regurgitation. Patients with vaginal infections will describe itchiness, irritation, and swelling of the labia. Patients may also describe a white, cheesy vaginal discharge.

PHYSICAL EXAMINATION. Common symptoms include **burning or pain in the mouth or vaginal mucous membranes** and/or **vaginal itchiness and irritation**. Inspect the patient's lips for color, texture, hydration, and lesions. Assess the patient's mouth thoroughly for bleeding, edema, white patches, nodules, or cysts. Inspect the mucosa; the roof and floor of the mouth; the tongue, including under the surface and the lateral borders; the gums; and the throat. Palpate any lesions or nodules. Inspect the patient's nailbeds for swelling, redness, darkening, purulent discharge, or separation from the nails. Inspect the patient's skin for an erythematous, macular rash. Inspect the patient's vagina for vulval rash; erythema; inflammation; cheesy exudate; or lesions of the labia, vaginal walls, or the cervix. Palpate lesions for texture and tenderness.

Systemic infection causes symptoms that can include a high, spiking fever; lowered blood pressure; rashes; and chills. Pulmonary infection may produce a cough. Renal infection may produce painful or cloudy urination and blood or pus in the urine. If the infection occurs in the brain, symptoms can include headache and seizures. Eye infection can cause blurred vision, orbital or periorbital pain, scotoma (blind gap in visual field), and exudate. If the infection occurs in the endocardium, symptoms can include systolic or diastolic murmur or chest pain.

PSYCHOSOCIAL. Because of pain and swelling, severe oral cases may cause the patient to have difficulty eating and drinking, which may contribute to depression. Severe skin and vaginal infections can cause pain, itching, and unsightly lesions that may cause self-consciousness because of a change in body image. Because of painful symptoms, vaginal infection usually affects sexual behavior.

Diagnostic Highlights

Test	Normal Result	Abnormality With Condition	Explanation
T2Candida blood test	Negative	Positive for any of the five species of *Candida* that cause blood infections	Presence of *Candida* in the blood indicates invasive (disseminated) candidiasis
Potassium hydroxide (KOH) cultures of scrapings from skin, vagina, wound or cultures from sputum or blood	Negative	Positive for the organism	Wet mount or scrapings show positive microscopic findings for hyphae (long, branching filamentous structure of a fungus), pseudohyphae, or budding yeast cells).

(highlight box continues on page 224)

Diagnostic Highlights (continued)

Other Tests: Diagnosis relies on signs and symptoms, supported by laboratory cultures. Note that routine laboratory studies are often nonspecific and not very helpful in making the diagnosis.

PRIMARY NURSING DIAGNOSIS

DIAGNOSIS. Impaired oral mucous membrane integrity related to oral swelling and ulcers as evidenced by burning and/or pain

OUTCOMES. Oral health; Tissue integrity: Skin and mucous membranes; Infection severity; Nutritional status; Self-care: Oral hygiene

INTERVENTIONS. Oral health maintenance; Nutrition monitoring; Oral health promotion; Oral health restoration; Pain management: Acute

✳ PLANNING AND IMPLEMENTATION

Collaborative

The first order of treatment, when possible, is to improve any underlying condition that has triggered the onset of candidiasis—for example, discontinuing antibiotic therapy or catheterization or controlling diabetes. The other collaborative interventions are pharmacologic.

Pharmacologic Highlights

Medication or Drug Class	Dosage	Description	Rationale
Antifungal agents: Polyenes	Varies by drug	Topical: Nystatin; IV: amphotericin B	Nystatin is an effective antifungal for superficial candidiasis; prescribed in ointments, creams, powders, oral gels, or oral solutions; increases permeability of fungal cytoplasmic membrane; amphotericin B is given intravenously
Antifungal agents: Echinocandins	Varies by drug	Caspofungin, micafungin, anidulafungin	Inhibit the synthesis of glucan in the cell wall by inhibiting the enzyme 1,3-β glucan synthase
Antifungal agents: Topical azoles, some are troche or lozenge form	Varies by drug	Clotrimazole, butoconazole, miconazole, terconazole, tioconazole	Prescribed for mucous membrane or vaginal infections
Antifungal agents: Oral or IV azoles	Varies by drug	Fluconazole, itraconazole, voriconazole, ketoconazole	Fungistatis activity, slows fungal cell growth
Antifungal agents: Antimetabolites	Varies by drug	Flucytosine	IV therapy may be prescribed for systemic infection

General Comments: Caspofungin is used for invasive candidiasis and is one of a new class of antifungal drugs that are glucan synthesis inhibitors. Premedication with acetaminophen, antihistamines, or antiemetics can help reduce side effects of amphotericin B such as fever, anorexia, nausea, vomiting, or severe chills. IV fluids or total parenteral nutrition therapy may be needed if the patient's fluid and nutritional intake is compromised. A topical anesthetic, such as lidocaine (Xylocaine), may be provided at least 1 hour before meals to alleviate mouth pain.

Independent

The most important nursing intervention for the patient with candidiasis is patient education about the infection and its treatment. Hand hygiene is an effective way to prevent infections. Teach the patient to keep the skin dry and free of irritation and to use a clean towel and washcloth daily. Prescribed creams should be applied to the affected areas until the candidiasis is gone; for those patients with immunosuppression, the creams should be continued for 2 weeks after the symptoms disappear. Encourage the patient to use cold compresses and/or sitz baths to relieve itching. Instruct the patient to wash the hands thoroughly after touching infected areas to prevent the infection from spreading. Recommend nystatin powder or dry padding to obese patients to help avoid irritation in skinfolds. Educate the patient with a vaginal infection to avoid contamination with feces from the GI tract by wiping from front to back after defecation.

If the patient is having difficulty swallowing or chewing that is adversely affecting the patient's nutrition, encourage a soft diet, fluid intake, and small, frequent meals of high-calorie foods. Advise the patient to avoid spicy, hot, or acidic foods that might exacerbate lesions. Explain the need for mouth care before and after meals, recommending the use of a soft gauze pad, rather than a toothbrush, to clean the teeth, gums, and mucous membranes. Advise the patient to avoid mouthwashes with alcohol and to lubricate the lips.

Evidence-Based Practice and Health Policy

Moshfeghy, Z., Tahari, S., Janghorban, R., Najib, F., Mani, A., & Sayadi, M. (2020). Association of sexual function and psychological symptoms including depression, anxiety, and stress in women with recurrent vulvovaginal candidiasis. *Journal of the Turkish German Gynecological Association, 21,* 90–96.

- The authors set out to determine the degree of association of sexual function and psychological factors such as anxiety, stress, and depression in women with recurrent vulvovaginal candidiasis (RVVC). They employed a case-controlled study design that included equal cohorts of women with RVVC and uninfected women, confirmed through microscopic sample analysis, all of whom completed a demographic questionnaire, the Female Sexual Function Index, and Depression Anxiety Stress Scales-21.
- Findings indicated that patients with RVVC experienced less sexual satisfaction and less orgasm and experienced higher levels of depression, anxiety, and stress when compared to healthy individuals. The authors conclude that, given the findings of increased depression, anxiety, and stress concomitant with lowered levels of sexual satisfaction and orgasm, psychological interventions and sexual counseling may be advisable.

DOCUMENTATION GUIDELINES

- Physical findings: Lesions, exudate, rashes, locations of skin irritation or breakdown
- Response to medications: Antifungals, analgesics
- Progressive wound healing
- Presence of complications, spreading, resistance, recurrence

DISCHARGE AND HOME HEALTHCARE GUIDELINES

PREVENTION. Teach the patient to wash hands frequently during the day. Teach the patient to keep the skin clean and dry, especially in skinfolds. Teach the patient to allow the skin to be open to the air, to wear loose-fitting cotton clothing rather than tight-fitting clothing or synthetic fabrics. Teach the patient to maintain good oral care and to correct any ill-fitting dentures that may cause lesions. If the patient is diabetic, provide guidelines on how to maintain good control of blood sugar levels to decrease susceptibility to candidiasis. In recurrent vaginal infections, be sure the patient understands that their sexual partner may need to be treated.

MEDICATIONS. Teach the patient the action, dosage, route, and side effects of all medications.

COMPLICATIONS OF CANDIDIASIS. Patients should understand the symptoms of systemic infection caused by candidiasis, such as a high, spiking fever; chills; cloudy urine or urine with blood or pus; headache or seizures; blurred vision or eye pain. If these symptoms occur, the patient should inform the physician.

Cardiac Contusion (Myocardial Contusion)

DRG Category:	315
Mean LOS:	3.6 days
Description:	MEDICAL: Other Circulatory System Diagnoses With Complication or Comorbidity

Cardiac (myocardial) contusion is a bruise or damage to the heart muscle. Damage to the heart ranges from limited areas of subepicardial petechiae or ecchymoses to full-thickness contusions with fragmentations and necrosis of cardiac muscle fibers. Cellular damage consists of extravasation of red blood cells into and between the myocardial muscle fibers and the selective necrosis of myocardial muscle fibers. Creatine phosphokinase leaks out of the cells into the circulation. Complete healing occurs with little or no scar formation. When myocardial injury is extensive, the pathological changes may resemble those seen in acute myocardial infarction, and the patient may experience some of the same complications associated with it, such as cardiac failure, cardiac dysrhythmias, aneurysm formation, or cardiac rupture. Severe trauma may cause valvular rupture, damage to the coronary arteries, or a fractured sternum.

CAUSES

Cardiac contusion can be caused by any direct traumatic injury to the chest. Most commonly, it is the result of a direct blow to the chest from a steering wheel injury in a motor vehicle crash (MVC), a sports accident, a fall from a high elevation, an assault, or an animal kick. Injury to the myocardium typically occurs as a result of acute compression of the heart between the sternum and the spine. The anterior wall of the right ventricle is most commonly involved because of its location directly behind the sternum.

GENETIC CONSIDERATIONS

No clear genetic contributions to susceptibility have been defined.

SEX AND LIFE SPAN CONSIDERATIONS

Cardiac contusion can occur at any age and in both sexes, although more males than females are involved in traumatic events. Trauma is the leading cause of death between ages 1 and 45 years in the United States and is often preventable. Anyone at high risk for traumatic injuries, such as children and young adults in the first four decades of life, is at high risk for myocardial contusion. Because their bones may be more brittle, older patients also have an increased risk; traumatic injury to the sternum is less tolerated by older as compared to younger patients. Most blunt chest trauma is associated with MVCs, which are two to three times more common in males than in females in the 15- to 24-year-old age group. Men have different patterns of injury than women, and a higher injury severity. Analysis of trauma outcomes indicates that, following traumatic injury, males have higher rates of multiple organ failure, pneumonia, and sepsis than females, creating health disparities for men (Marcolini, 2019). Trauma is the third leading cause of death in people ages 45 to 65 years and the seventh leading cause of death in people older than 65 years.

HEALTH DISPARITIES AND SEXUAL/GENDER MINORITY HEALTH

In recent years, Black persons have been killed in traffic crashes at a rate almost 25% higher than White persons (National Highway Traffic Safety Administration [NHTSA], 2021). Native American persons have the highest rate of MVC injury in the United States, more than twice the rate of Black persons (NHTSA, 2021). Experts have noted that Black and Native American communities tend to be crisscrossed by more dangerous roads than other locations, placing people from those communities at risk for injury. Healthy People 2020 reports that non-Hispanic Black persons have the highest injury death rate in the United States (79.9 injury deaths per 100,000 persons), followed by non-Hispanic White persons (79.2), Native American persons (78.2), Hispanic persons (45.5), and Asian/Pacific Islander persons (25.6). Recent work has shown evidence that rural populations have injury mortality rates that are more than twice as high as urban rates. Many factors contribute to these health disparities, including the risk of traffic injury in narrow rural roads, the lack of graded curves and lighted traffic signals on rural highways, and the distance from major trauma centers. Many of the most dangerous occupations, such as mining and agriculture, are found in rural areas and can result in injury, disability, and death. Sexual and gender minority persons have high risk for dating and interpersonal violence, violence related to bullying, and intentional and unintentional injury (Healthy People 2020).

GLOBAL HEALTH CONSIDERATIONS

While no data are available on the global epidemiology of cardiac contusions, they occur around the world. The World Health Organization (WHO) reports that injuries account for 9% of global mortality, and for the large number of people who survive, there is significant temporary or permanent disability. The WHO estimates that 1.35 million people die each year from MVCs and cost most countries 3% of their gross domestic product. Globally, more than half of all traffic injuries are among vulnerable road users such as pedestrians, cyclists, and motorcyclists. More than 90% of the world's fatalities in traffic injuries occur in low- and middle-income countries. Even in high-income countries, people from lower socioeconomic backgrounds are more likely to be involved in road traffic crashes than other groups.

ASSESSMENT

HISTORY. Elicit a thorough history of the injury event, including the time, place, and description. Discuss any description of the MVC, including the location of the patient in the car and which part of the car was struck, or if the patient was a pedestrian, motorcyclist, or bicyclist. Determine the point of impact and any weapons (baseball bat, brick, fist) used in an assault. Patients usually describe the most common symptom of cardiac contusion—that is, precordial pain resembling that of myocardial infarction. However, coronary vasodilators have little effect in relieving the pain. It is important to note that many patients may be asymptomatic for the first 24 to 48 hours after the chest trauma. In patients with multiple trauma, physical signs may be masked by associated injuries. Note the presence of blunt chest injuries, such as sternal, clavicular, or upper rib fractures; pulmonary contusion; hemothorax; or pneumothorax—all of which raise suspicion for the possibility of a myocardial injury.

PHYSICAL EXAMINATION. Generally, the physical signs of a cardiac contusion are few and nonspecific. Observe the chest wall for the presence of **bruising**, **hematoma**, **swelling**, or the **imprint of a steering wheel** if the patient has been driving a motor vehicle. Note the presence of pain (chest wall or musculoskeletal), dyspnea, tachypnea, tachycardia, and diaphoresis. Be alert for the possibility of cardiac tamponade, active bleeding into the pericardial space that leads to myocardial compression, and cardiogenic shock. Note the presence of hypotension, muffled heart sounds, jugular vein distention, a paradoxic pulse, and shock from potential complications (Table 1).

• **TABLE 1** Complications Associated With Myocardial Contusion

COMPLICATION	SYMPTOMS
Atrial dysrhythmias: Sinus tachycardia, atrial fibrillation, premature atrial contractions	Palpitations, precordial pain, dizziness, faintness, confusion, loss of consciousness
Cardiac tamponade	Hypotension, pulsus paradoxus, muffled heart sounds, pericardial friction rub, anxiety, restlessness, tachypnea, weak to absent pulses, pallor, cyanosis
Heart failure	Orthopnea, tachypnea, crackles, frothy cough, distended neck veins, anxiety, confusion
Pulmonary edema	Pallor, cyanosis, dyspnea
Ventricular aneurysm	Chest pain, dyspnea, orthopnea
Ventricular dysrhythmias: Premature ventricular contractions, ventricular fibrillation	Palpitations, precordial pain, dizziness, faintness, confusion, loss of consciousness

PSYCHOSOCIAL. The patient with a cardiac contusion usually has suffered an unexpected traumatic injury. Because the heart holds many meanings to people (anatomic, romantic, emotional, spiritual), an injured heart may raise significant anxiety. The patient may have numerous other traumatic injuries that accompany the contused heart. Assess the patient's ability to cope with the unexpectedness of the traumatic event. Assess the patient's degree of anxiety regarding the traumatic event, injuries sustained, and the potential implications of the injuries. Note that trauma patients are often teenagers and young adults. During crises, the presence of their parents and peers is essential in their recovery but may challenge the nurse to provide a quiet and stress-free environment for patient recovery. Older patients have more frail bodies than other adults. A traumatic injury is a frightening and painful experience to endure and may lead to anxiety and depression.

Diagnostic Highlights

Test	Normal Result	Abnormality With Condition	Explanation
Transesophageal echocardiogram (TEE)	Normal size, shape, position, thickness, and movement of structures	May identify injury to heart structures, such as echo-free zone anterior to right ventricular wall and posterior wall (cardiac tamponade), wall motion irregularities, aneurysm, or valvular rupture	Probe with an ultrasound transmitter is inserted into the esophagus to record echoes created by deflection of short pulses of ultrasonic beam off cardiac structures. The esophageal approach allows the transducer to rest in close proximity to the heart to capture stronger echocardiogram signals.
Electrocardiogram (ECG)	Normal PQRST pattern	ST segment depression, T-wave inversion; may have transient ST elevation (less frequent); ECG may be normal	Electrical conduction system adversely affected by myocardial ischemia due to injury; 65% of people with myocardial contusion have ECG changes

Diagnostic Highlights (continued)

Test	Normal Result	Abnormality With Condition	Explanation
Creatine kinase isoenzyme (MB-CK)	< 4% of total CK	Elevated in some patients	Some patients with a cardiac contusion have actual tissue damage and therefore would have enzyme elevation
Serum cardiac troponin I	< 0.05 ng/mL	> 0.15 ng/mL	Suggests myocardial damage and necrosis

Other Tests: Supporting tests include aspartate aminotransferase (also known as serum glutamic-oxaloacetic transaminase), lactic dehydrogenase, lactate levels, complete blood count, arterial blood gases, coagulation profile, chest x-ray, computed tomography scans; ultrasonography to evaluate sternal fracture and valvular damage

PRIMARY NURSING DIAGNOSIS

DIAGNOSIS. Acute pain related to chest injury as evidenced by swelling, bruising, and/or hematoma

OUTCOMES. Comfort status; Knowledge: Cardiac disease management; Pain control; Pain level; Symptom severity

INTERVENTIONS. Analgesic administration; Pain management: Acute; Medication management; Cardiac care; Vital signs monitoring

PLANNING AND IMPLEMENTATION

Collaborative

Management of patients with suspected or known cardiac contusion is similar to that of any myocardial ischemic problem. Strategies include oxygen therapy; cardiac and hemodynamic monitoring; analgesics; and, if necessary, antidysrhythmics and inotropic agents. Even in patients without obvious dysrhythmias, maintain IV access for treatment of complications that may be associated with myocardial contusion. Place the patient on continuous cardiac monitoring to assess for dysrhythmias. Perform serial monitoring of vital signs to determine if the patient's heart function is changing. If signs of falling cardiac output occur (confusion or decreased mental status, delayed capillary blanching, cool extremities, weak pulses, pulmonary congestion, increased heart rate, decreased urine output), the physician may insert a pulmonary artery catheter. A pacemaker may be needed for heart block or symptomatic bradycardia. If a blunt pericardial wound occurs, it can be closed by a simple pericardiorrhaphy, be left open, or be repaired with a patch.

One of the more severe complications of myocardial contusion is pericardial tamponade, which can develop more than 1 week after the injury. Immediate surgery is needed for cardiac tamponade. Elective surgery for associated injuries (open reduction of fractures, repair of minor facial fractures) involving general anesthesia may be delayed, if possible, until cardiac function is stable. Delay allows for stabilization and healing of the contusion, which lowers intraoperative and postoperative risk for cardiac complications.

Pharmacologic Highlights

Medication or Drug Class	Dosage	Description	Rationale
Antidysrhythmics	Varies with drug	Amiodarone is the treatment of choice for ventricular tachycardia or fibrillation that persists after defibrillation; others are bretylium, lidocaine, magnesium sulfate, procainamide, atropine, adenosine, esmolol, propagator, acebutolol	Control dysrhythmias; drug depends on type of injury
Inotropic drugs	Varies with drug	Dopamine, dobutamine, amrinone, milrinone	Increase contractility if failure occurs

Other Drugs: IV opiates such as morphine sulfate may be required in the acute phase for comfort and rest; epinephrine depending on advanced cardiac life support guidelines.

Independent

During recovery, nursing interventions focus on conserving the patient's energy. Activity restrictions, including bedrest, may be necessary for a short period of time (usually 48–72 hr) to decrease myocardial oxygen demands and to facilitate healing. Discuss the need for activity restriction with the patient and family.

The young adult trauma patient presents a challenge to the nursing staff. Provide age-appropriate diversionary activities to reduce anxiety. If the patient is a high school student, note that the hospital may be overwhelmed with peers from the local high school who are interested in visiting the patient, particularly if the injury was associated with a school event (prom, football game, party) and if the injury is life threatening. Work with the parents and principal to arrange for a visitation schedule so that both the patient's and the hospital's needs are met.

Evidence-Based Practice and Health Policy

Gao, J., Du, D., Kong, L., Yang, J., Li, H., Wei, G., Li, C., & Liu, C. (2020). Emergency surgery for blunt cardiac injury: Experience in 43 cases. *World Journal of Surgery, 44*, 1666–1672.

- The authors explored the effects of early recognition and expeditious surgical intervention to increase survival in patients experiencing blunt cardiac injury (BCI). They analyzed medical records of 1,903 patients injured over a 15-year period and diagnosed with blunt thoracic trauma. The main cause of injury (48.8%) was traffic accidents, and only 18.3% (348 patients) had BCI.
- Of the 43 patients with BCI who underwent operative treatment, 26 were diagnosed by echocardiography and 17 were diagnosed during surgery. Preoperative pericardiocentesis was not used in anyone. Overall mortality was 32.6%. The authors noted that following blunt chest trauma, a high index of suspicion for BCI is necessary so that early recognition and expeditious thoracotomy can occur. The authors do not recommend preoperative pericardiocentesis.

DOCUMENTATION GUIDELINES

- Detailed observations and assessments of physical findings related to the cardiac system: Heart rate and heart sounds, vital signs, signs of complications (dysrhythmias, chest pain, signs of shock), cardiac rhythm, response to chest pain, response to oxygen therapy
- Detailed assessment findings of respiratory system: Breath sounds, vital signs, signs of complications
- Detailed observations and assessments of physical findings related to traumatic injury: Skin integrity, swelling, fractures, alignment, mental status

DISCHARGE AND HOME HEALTHCARE GUIDELINES

The patient may be sent home on oral analgesics and other medications to manage complications. Be sure the patient understands all medications, including the dosage, route, action, and adverse effects. Educate the patient about the symptoms of potential complications associated with cardiac contusions and instruct the patient to call the physician or go to the emergency department immediately if any of the associated symptoms occur.

Cardiac Tamponade

DRG Category:	315
Mean LOS:	3.6 days
Description:	MEDICAL: Other Circulatory System Diagnoses With Complication or Comorbidity

Approximately 2% of penetrating injuries, such as knife and gunshot wounds, lead to cardiac tamponade. Acute cardiac tamponade is a sudden accumulation of fluid in the pericardial sac leading to an increase in the intrapericardial pressure. It is a medical emergency whose outcome depends on the speed of diagnosis and treatment as well as the underlying cause. The pericardial sac surrounds the heart and normally contains only 10 to 20 mL of serous fluid. The sudden accumulation of more fluid (as little as 200 mL of fluid or blood) compresses the heart and coronary arteries, compromising diastolic filling and systolic emptying and diminishing oxygen supply. The end result is decreased oxygen delivery and poor tissue perfusion to all organs.

The incidence of cardiac tamponade in the United States is approximately two cases per 10,000 individuals. It is a potentially life-threatening condition, needing emergency assessment and immediate interventions. Some patients develop a more slowly accumulating tamponade that collects over weeks and months. If the fibrous pericardium gradually has time to stretch, the pericardial space can accommodate as much as 1 to 2 L of fluid before the patient becomes acutely symptomatic. Three phases of hemodynamic changes occur with acute cardiac tamponade (Table 1). Complications include decreased ventricular filling, decreased cardiac output, cardiogenic shock, and death.

• **TABLE 1** Phases of Cardiac Tamponade

PHASE	DESCRIPTION
Phase 1	As fluid accumulates in the pericardium, it leads to increased ventricular stiffness, which requires a higher filling pressure in both the left and right ventricles
Phase 2	As fluid accumulates further, pericardial pressure increases above the ventricular filling pressure; cardiac output thereby is reduced, leading to phase 3 changes
Phase 3	As the cardiac output decreases, there is equilibration of pericardial and left ventricular filling pressures, and very little blood moves forward into the circulation. Cardiogenic shock may follow.

CAUSES

Cardiac tamponade may have any of a variety of etiologies. Malignant diseases cause more than half of all cases, and renal failure leading to uremic pericarditis is also a leading cause. It can be caused by both blunt and penetrating traumatic injuries and by iatrogenic injuries, such as those associated with removal of epicardial pacing wires and complications after cardiac catheterization and insertion of central venous or pulmonary artery catheters.

Rupture of the ventricle after an acute myocardial infarction or bleeding after cardiac surgery can also lead to tamponade. Other causes include treatment with anticoagulants, viral infections such as HIV, and disorders that cause pericardial irritation such as pericarditis, tuberculosis, or myxedema, as well as collagen diseases such as rheumatoid arthritis or systemic lupus erythematosus.

GENETIC CONSIDERATIONS

Cardiac tamponade is typically not heritable, but it is more common among patients with Marfan syndrome and individuals with heritable connective tissue disorders.

SEX AND LIFE SPAN CONSIDERATIONS

Although a patient of any age can develop a cardiac tamponade, the very young and older adults have fewer reserves available to cope with such a severe condition. Because trauma is the leading cause of death for individuals in the first four decades of life, traumatic tamponade is more common in that age group, whereas the older adult is more likely to have an iatrogenic tamponade. Cardiac tamponade associated with trauma and HIV is more common in young adults, whereas in older adults it occurs more frequently due to malignancy or renal failure.

HEALTH DISPARITIES AND SEXUAL/GENDER MINORITY HEALTH

Males have higher rates of unintentional injury than do females and are more at risk for cardiac tamponade. In children, cardiac tamponade is more common in boys than girls, and more males than females develop pericarditis. Significant health disparities exist in the cardiac care of underrepresented groups as compared to White persons. Non-White persons are known to receive care less often guided by standard cardiac care guidelines than White persons. Unless patients have health insurance, White patients are more likely to receive coronary angiograms and other coronary interventions than Black and Hispanic patients. Non-White persons are also less likely to be referred to cardiologists and cardiac surgeons than White persons (Batchelor et al., 2019). Cisgender men (cisgender are persons whose gender identity and gender expression are aligned with their assigned sex listed on their birth certificate) who have sex with men account for approximately 60% of the persons with HIV in the United States and are at risk for cardiac tamponade if HIV positive. Transgender women have a higher risk for HIV than cisgender women and also are at risk. HIV prevalence in cisgender women who have sex with women is low, but they generally have less access to healthcare than heterosexual women.

GLOBAL HEALTH CONSIDERATIONS

Traumatic injury resulting in pericardial bleeding or tuberculosis resulting in pericardial effusions are the most common causes of cardiac tamponade in developing countries. Pericardial effusions most commonly result from malignancies in developed countries, but motor vehicle crashes and myocardial rupture also contribute to the prevalence.

☀ ASSESSMENT

HISTORY. The patient's history may include metastatic cancer, renal failure, surgery, trauma, cardiac biopsy, viral infection, insertion of a transvenous pacing wire or catheter, or myocardial infarction. Elicit a medication history to determine if the patient is taking anticoagulants or any medication that could cause tamponade as a drug reaction (procainamide, hydralazine, minoxidil, isoniazid, penicillin, methysergide, or daunorubicin). Ask if the patient has renal failure, which can lead to pericarditis and bleeding. Cardiac tamponade may be acute or accumulate over time, as in the case of myxedema, collagen diseases, and neoplasm. The patient may have a history of dyspnea and chest pain that ranges from mild to severe and increases on inspiration. Patients with malignancies or renal failure may have dizziness, weakness, palpitations, weight loss, or fatigue without signs of an acute tamponade. There may be no symptoms at all before severe hemodynamic compromise.

PHYSICAL EXAMINATION. The primary symptoms are related to shock: **dyspnea, tachycardia, tachypnea, pallor,** and **cold extremities**. The patient who has acute, rapid bleeding with cardiac tamponade appears critically ill and in shock. Assess airway, breathing, and circulation (ABCs), and intervene simultaneously. The patient is acutely hypovolemic (because of blood loss into the pericardial sac) and in cardiogenic shock and should be assessed and treated for those conditions as an emergency situation.

If the patient is more stable, when you auscultate the heart, you may hear a pericardial friction rub as a result of the two inflamed layers of the pericardium rubbing against each other. The heart sounds may be muffled because of the accumulation of fluid around the heart. If a central venous or pulmonary artery catheter is present, the mean right atrial pressure (RAP) rises to greater than 12 mm Hg, and the pulmonary capillary wedge pressure equalizes with the RAP. Systolic blood pressure decreases as the pressure on the ventricles reduces diastolic filling and cardiac output. Pulsus paradoxus (> 10 mm Hg fall in systolic blood pressure during inspiration) is an important finding in cardiac tamponade and is probably related to blood pooling in the pulmonary veins during inspiration. Other signs that may be present are related to the decreased cardiac output and poor tissue perfusion. Confusion and agitation, cyanosis, tachycardia, and decreased urine output may all occur as cardiac output is compromised and tissue perfusion becomes impaired.

Assessment of cardiovascular function should be performed hourly; check mental status, skin color, temperature and moisture, capillary refill, heart sounds, heart rate, arterial blood pressure, and jugular venous distention. Maintain the patient on continuous cardiac monitoring, and monitor for ST-wave and T-wave changes.

PSYCHOSOCIAL. Acute cardiac tamponade can be sudden, unexpected, and life threatening, causing the patient to experience fear and anxiety. Assess the patient's degree of fear and anxiety, as well as the patient's ability to cope with a sudden illness and threat to self. The patient's family or significant other(s) should be included in the assessment and plan of care. Half of all patients with traumatic injuries have either alcohol or other drugs present in their systems at the time of injury. Ask about the patient's drinking patterns and any substance use and abuse. Assess the risk for withdrawal from alcohol or other drugs during the hospitalization.

Diagnostic Highlights

Test	Normal Result	Abnormality With Condition	Explanation
Echocardiogram	Normal size, shape, position, thickness, and movement of structures	Echo-free zone anterior to right ventricular wall and posterior to the left ventricular wall; there may also be a decrease in right ventricular chamber size and a right-to-left septal shift during inspiration	Records echoes created by deflection of short pulses of ultrasonic beam off cardiac structures; may also be done as a transesophageal procedure with transmitter inserted into esophagus (transesophageal echocardiogram)

(highlight box continues on page 234)

Diagnostic Highlights (continued)

Other Tests: Prolonged coagulation studies and/or a decreased hemoglobin and hematocrit if the patient has lost sufficient blood into the pericardium; electrocardiogram and chest x-ray; computed tomography; arterial blood gases; creatine kinase and isoenzymes; HIV testing; renal profile; purified protein derivative or blood test for tuberculosis

PRIMARY NURSING DIAGNOSIS

DIAGNOSIS. Decreased cardiac output related to decreased preload and contractility as evidenced by hypotension, dyspnea, tachycardia, tachypnea, and/or pallor

OUTCOMES. Circulation status; Cardiac pump effectiveness; Tissue perfusion: Cardiac, abdominal organs, cerebral, and peripheral; Vital signs status; Fluid balance

INTERVENTIONS. Cardiac care: Acute; Fluid/electrolyte management; Fluid monitoring; Shock management: Volume; Oxygen therapy; Medication administration

☀ PLANNING AND IMPLEMENTATION

Collaborative

The highest priority is to make sure the patient has adequate ABCs. If the patient experiences hypoxia as a result of decreased cardiac output and poor tissue perfusion, oxygen, intubation, and mechanical ventilation may be required. If the symptoms are progressing rapidly, the physician may elect to perform a pericardiocentesis to normalize pericardial pressure, allowing the heart and coronary arteries to fill normally so that cardiac output and tissue perfusion are restored. Assist by elevating the head of the bed to a 60-degree angle to allow gravity to pull the fluid to the apex of the heart if the patient can tolerate it. Leg elevation improved venous return. Emergency equipment should be nearby because ventricular tachycardia, ventricular fibrillation, or laceration of a coronary artery or myocardium can cause shock and death. Pericardiocentesis usually causes a dramatic improvement in hemodynamic status. However, if the patient has had rapid bleeding into the pericardial space, clots may have formed that block the needle aspiration. A false-negative pericardiocentesis is therefore possible and needs to be considered if symptoms continue.

If there is active bleeding into the pericardium, the patient must be taken to surgery after this procedure to explore the pericardium and stop further bleeding. If the patient has developed sudden bradycardia (heart rate < 50 beats per minute), severe hypotension (systolic blood pressure < 70 mm Hg), or asystole, an emergency thoracotomy may be performed at the bedside to evacuate the pericardial sac, control the hemorrhage, and perform internal cardiac massage if needed. The patient may also require fluid resuscitation agents to enhance cardiac output.

Pharmacologic Highlights

Medication or Drug Class	Dosage	Description	Rationale
Sympathomimetics such as dopamine hydrochloride	Varies by drug	Stimulates adrenergic receptors to increase myocardial contractility and peripheral resistance	Supports blood pressure and cardiac output in emergencies until bleeding is brought under control; only used if fluid resuscitation is initiated

Independent

The highest nursing priority is to maintain the patient's ABCs. Emergency equipment should be readily available in case the patient requires intubation and mechanical ventilation. Be prepared to administer fluids, including blood products, colloids or crystalloids, and pressor agents, through a large-bore catheter. Pressure and rapid-volume warmer infusors should be used for patients who require massive fluid resuscitation. A number of nursing strategies increase the rate of fluid replacement. Fluid resuscitation is most efficient through a short, large-bore peripheral IV catheter in a large peripheral vein. The IV should have a short length of tubing from the bag or bottle to the IV site. If pressure is applied to the bag, fluid resuscitation occurs more rapidly.

Emotional support of the patient and family is also a key nursing intervention. If the patient is awake as you implement strategies to manage the ABCs, provide a running explanation of the procedures. If blood component therapy is essential, answer the patient's and family's questions about the risks of hepatitis and transmission of HIV.

Evidence-Based Practice and Health Policy

Dabbagh, M., Aurora, L., D'Souza, P., Weinmann, A., Bhargava, P., & Basir, M. (2020). Cardiac tamponade secondary to COVID-19. *Journal of the American College of Cardiology Case Reports*, *2*, 1326–1330.

• The authors presented a case study of a 67-year-old female to illustrate that coronavirus disease 2019 (COVID-19) can have extrapulmonary consequences that can be identified with physical examination and diagnostic studies. The authors aim to identify COVID-19 as a potential etiology for hemorrhagic pericardial effusion. The authors presented a narrative of the patient's hospitalization including past medical history, differential diagnosis, investigations, management, and follow-up, providing evidence in the form of electrocardiographic videos and readouts.

• The authors reported on a rare presentation of COVID-19 infection complicated by a symptomatic hemorrhagic pericardial effusion and development of cardiac tamponade. The patient's clinical course was complicated by the development of Takotsubo (stress) cardiomyopathy. She was treated with pericardiocentesis, colchicine, corticosteroids, and hydroxychloroquine, with improvement in symptoms, leading to discharge.

DOCUMENTATION GUIDELINES

• Physical findings of cardiovascular and neurological systems
• Adequacy of ABCs, mental status, skin color, vital signs, moisture of mucous membranes, capillary refill, heart sounds, presence of pulsus paradoxus or jugular venous distention, hemodynamic parameters, intake and output
• Response to interventions
• Fluid resuscitation, inotropic agents, pericardiocentesis, surgery
• Presence of complications
• Asystole, ventricular tachycardia, ventricular fibrillation; recurrence of tamponade; infection; ongoing hemorrhage

DISCHARGE AND HOME HEALTHCARE GUIDELINES

MEDICATIONS. Be sure the patient understands all medications, including dosage, route, side effects, and any routine laboratory testing. The patient needs to understand to avoid over-the-counter medications, including aspirin and ibuprofen.

COMPLICATIONS. The patient needs to understand the possibility of recurrence and the symptoms to report to the physician. The patient and significant other(s) also need to understand that symptoms of inadequate tissue perfusion (change in mental status; cool, clammy, cyanotic skin; dyspnea; chest pain) warrant activation of the emergency medical system.

Cardiogenic Shock

DRG Category: 292
Mean LOS: 3.9 days
Description: MEDICAL: Heart Failure and Shock With Complication or Comorbidity

Cardiogenic shock occurs when cardiac output is insufficient to meet the metabolic demands of the body, resulting in inadequate tissue perfusion. It is a medical and nursing emergency. There are four stages of cardiogenic shock: initial, compensatory, progressive, and refractory.

During the initial stage, there is diminished cardiac output without any clinical symptoms. In the compensatory stage, the baroreceptors respond to the decreased cardiac output by stimulating the sympathetic nervous system to release catecholamines to improve myocardial contractility and vasoconstriction, leading to increased venous return and arterial blood pressure. Impaired renal perfusion activates the renin-angiotensin system, whose end product, angiotensin II, causes sodium and water retention as well as vasoconstriction. The progressive stage follows the compensatory stage if there is no intervention or if the intervention fails to reverse the inadequate tissue perfusion. Compensatory mechanisms, aimed at improving cardiac output and tissue perfusion, place an increased demand on an already compromised myocardium. As tissue perfusion remains inadequate, the cells begin anaerobic metabolism, leading to metabolic acidosis and fluid leakage out of the capillaries and into the interstitial spaces. A decrease in circulating volume and an increase in blood viscosity may cause clotting in the capillaries and tissue death.

As the body releases fibrinolytic agents to break down the clots, disseminated intravascular coagulation (DIC) may ensue. Lactic acidosis causes depression of the myocardium and a decrease in the vascular responsiveness to catecholamines, further reducing cardiac output. Blood pools and stagnates in the capillaries, and the continued increase in hydrostatic pressure causes fluid to leak into the interstitium. Severe cerebral ischemia causes depression of the vasomotor center and loss of sympathetic stimulation, resulting in blood pooling in the periphery, a decrease in preload, and further reduction in cardiac output. If there is no effective intervention at this point, the shock will progress to the refractory stage, when the chance of survival is extremely limited. Most experts acknowledge that cardiogenic shock is often unresponsive to treatment and has a mortality rate ranging from 20% to 50% if prompt medical intervention occurs. Complications include cardiopulmonary arrest, dysrhythmias, organ failure, stroke, and death.

CAUSES

The most common cause of cardiogenic shock is acute myocardial infarction (MI) resulting in a loss of more than 40% of the functional myocardium. Cardiogenic shock occurs with 5% to 10% of all hospital admissions for acute MI. Other causes include papillary muscle rupture, left ventricular free wall rupture, acute ventricular septal defect, severe congestive heart failure, end-stage cardiomyopathy, severe valvular dysfunction, acute cardiac tamponade, cardiac contusion, massive pulmonary embolus, or overdose of drugs such as beta blockers or calcium channel blockers.

GENETIC CONSIDERATIONS

While several genetic factors may contribute to susceptibility to cardiogenic shock, no direct genetic link has been documented. Tumor necrosis factor (TNF) alpha (*TNF-alpha*) variants have been associated with severe heart failure. Polymorphisms in several genes may be predictors of survival: *TNF-alpha*, interleukin (IL) 6 (*IL6*), *IL10*, transforming growth factor (TGF) beta (*TGF-beta*), and interferon (IFN)-gamma (*IFNG*) cytokine. Individuals who carry the TNF-2 allele appear to have better outcomes than those with other variants of this gene.

SEX AND LIFE SPAN CONSIDERATIONS

Cardiogenic shock can occur at any age but is more common in middle-aged and older adults. Anyone at risk for coronary artery disease, either male or female, is also at risk for cardiogenic shock as a result of an acute MI. Older adults are at greater risk because of their diminished ability to compensate for an inadequate cardiac output and tissue perfusion; they also have the highest mortality rate (55% for people over 75 years). While the overall incidence of cardiogenic shock is higher in men than in women, the percentage of female patients with MI who develop cardiogenic shock is higher than that of male patients with MI. In cardiogenic shock after MI, women are less likely than men to receive coronary angiography, percutaneous coronary interventions, and mechanical circulatory support despite having higher rates of mortality than men.

HEALTH DISPARITIES AND SEXUAL/GENDER MINORITY HEALTH

The Centers for Disease Control and Prevention report that 11.5% of White persons, 9.5% of Black persons, 7.4% of Hispanic persons, and 6.0% of Asian persons have heart disease. Significant health disparities exist in the cardiac care of underrepresented groups as compared to White persons. Black, Indigenous, and other people of color are known to receive care less often guided by standard cardiac care guidelines than White persons. Unless patients have health insurance, White patients are more likely to receive coronary angiograms and other coronary interventions than Black and Hispanic patients. In cardiogenic shock, temporary mechanical circulatory support such as intra-aortic balloon pump, ventricular assist device, and extracorporeal membranous oxygenation is used more in White patients than in Black patients, and more often in insured patients than in Medicare, Medicaid, or uninsured patients (Thangam et al., 2020). Black, Indigenous, and other people of color are also less likely to be referred to cardiologists and cardiac surgeons than White persons (Batchelor et al., 2019). In cardiogenic shock following MI, hospital-level disparities exist in the management and outcomes. Admissions to urban hospitals have better outcomes and earlier use of technology than admissions to rural hospitals.

Transgender is a term used to describe persons whose gender identity is different from their sex assigned at birth. Approximately 1% of the U.S. population identify themselves as transgender. Sexual and gender minority persons have higher odds for multiple chronic conditions, cancer, and poor quality of life and are more apt to have disabilities than cisgender males and females (cisgender is a term used to describe persons whose gender identity and gender expression are aligned with their assigned sex listed on their birth certificate). Gender-affirming hormone therapy is the use of hormone therapy for gender transition or gender affirmation and can be masculinizing or feminizing. It may also affect cardiovascular health in transgender females. In a large sample, researchers have found that transgender men and women are more likely to be overweight than cisgender women. Compared to cisgender women, transgender women reported higher rates of diabetes, angina/coronary disease, and MI. Gender-nonconforming men and women reported higher odds of MI than cisgender women. Transgender women also had higher rates of any cardiovascular disease than cisgender men (Cacerese, Jackman, et al., 2020).

GLOBAL HEALTH CONSIDERATIONS

European countries have a prevalence of cardiogenic shock similar to that of the United States. For unknown reasons, Asian/Pacific Islanders have a higher incidence of cardiogenic shock than do other groups. No data are available for developing countries.

☼ ASSESSMENT

HISTORY. Cardiogenic shock often occurs after a patient has been admitted to the hospital following an acute MI. The patient is likely to have a history of symptoms of an acute MI, including crushing, viselike chest pain or heaviness that radiates to the arms, neck, or jaw; lasts more than 20 minutes; and is unrelieved by nitroglycerin and rest. Other MI symptoms include shortness of breath, nausea, vomiting, sweating, anxiety, and a sense of impending doom. Determine if the patient has a history of cardiac disease or previous MI, use of cocaine, hypertension, cigarette smoking, or a family history of cardiac disease.

PHYSICAL EXAMINATION. The most common symptoms are **hypotension in the absence of hypovolemia** as well as **oliguria, cyanosis, cool extremities**, and **reduced mental status**. During the initial stage of shock, there are no clinical findings unless the cardiac output can be measured. When the patient has entered the compensatory stage, symptoms may include an altered level of consciousness; sinus tachycardia; the presence of an S_3 or S_4 gallop rhythm; jugular venous distention; hypotension; rapid, deep respirations; pulmonary crackles; venous oxygen saturation (SvO_2) less than 60%; cyanosis; urine output less than 20 mL/hour; decreased urinary sodium; increased urinary osmolarity; peripheral edema; hyperglycemia; hypernatremia; cold, clammy skin; and decreased bowel sounds.

As the patient enters the progressive stage, the symptoms become more pronounced and resistant to treatment. The patient becomes mentally unresponsive; hypotension becomes worse, requiring high doses of positive inotropic agents; metabolic and respiratory acidosis become apparent; oliguria or anuria and anasarca may ensue; and symptoms of DIC may be present. The patient's skin may appear mottled, cyanotic, and ashen with faint peripheral pulses and cold extremities. When the shock reaches the refractory stage, multisystem organ failure is apparent, with the above symptoms unresponsive to treatment.

PSYCHOSOCIAL. The patient in cardiogenic shock is in a life-threatening situation. The chances for survival are reduced, and the patient may experience a sense of impending doom. The impaired tissue perfusion may lead to anxiety and fear. The patient and the patient's family or significant other may be in crisis. Both the patient and the family may be experiencing grief in response to the potential loss of life and need significant emotional support.

Diagnostic Highlights

Test	Normal Result	Abnormality With Condition	Explanation
Hemodynamic monitoring	Right atrial pressure (RAP): 1–8 mm Hg; pulmonary artery occlusion pressure (PAOP): 4–12 mm Hg; cardiac output (CO): 4–7 L/min; cardiac index (CI): 2.5–4 L/min/m²; systemic vascular resistance (SVR): 800–1,200 dynes/sec per cm⁻⁵	RAP: > 6 mm Hg; PAOP: > 18 mm Hg; CO: < 5 L/min; CI: < 2.2 L/min/m²; SVR: >1,200 dynes/sec per cm⁻⁵	Elevated filling pressures in heart and low systolic blood pressure occur in the setting of low cardiac output; arterial constriction occurs as a compensatory mechanism. Hemodynamic monitoring with serial measures of cardiac output is important in the diagnosis of cardiogenic shock.

Other Tests: Compete blood count, serum chemistry tests, electrocardiogram, echocardiogram, transesophageal echocardiography, coronary angiography, cardiac enzymes, lactate levels, troponin T and I levels, arterial blood gases, brain natriuretic peptide, urinalysis, and coagulation studies

PRIMARY NURSING DIAGNOSIS

DIAGNOSIS. Decreased cardiac output related to inadequate cardiac contractility as evidenced by hypotension, oliguria, cyanosis, and/or decreased mental status

OUTCOMES. Circulation status; Cardiac pump effectiveness; Tissue perfusion: Cardiopulmonary, cerebral, abdominal organs, peripheral; Vital signs

INTERVENTIONS. Cardiac care; Emergency care; Vital signs monitoring; Oxygen therapy; Fluid/electrolyte management; Fluid monitoring; Shock management: Volume and cardiac, Medication administration; Resuscitation; Surveillance

☀ PLANNING AND IMPLEMENTATION

Collaborative

Cardiogenic shock is an emergency because of an unstable cardiovascular system that requires immediate intervention to reverse shock before vital organs are damaged. The primary goal in treating cardiogenic shock is to improve tissue perfusion and oxygenation with rapid diagnosis, maintenance of blood pressure and cardiac output with vasoactive medications, and support for airway and breathing. These goals generally are accomplished by coronary reperfusion with medications and percutaneous coronary intervention (coronary angioplasty), or coronary artery bypass surgery within the first 90 minutes after arrival at the hospital. To limit the infarct size and treat the dyspnea, pulmonary congestion, hypoxemia, and acidosis, the physician is likely to prescribe oxygen, intubation, and mechanical ventilation. Further trials are now in progress to determine the role of mechanical circulatory devices such as intra-aortic balloon pulsation, percutaneous mechanical circulatory devices, and extracorporeal membrane oxygenation.

Pharmacologic Highlights

General Comments: Improving cardiac output, which is necessary to improve tissue perfusion, can be accomplished in several ways. If the patient is able to maintain hemodynamic stability, the physician prescribes medications, namely diuretics and nitrates, to reduce preload. Generally, the patient may be too hypotensive to tolerate the vasodilative effects of both diuretics and nitrates. The patient needs improvement in myocardial contractility without adding significant workload on the heart. Dopamine may also be used in an attempt to improve contractility and cardiac output. Other vasoactive drugs, such as milrinone or inamrinone, may also be used to increase contractility. Vasopressors may be used in an attempt to increase the mean arterial blood pressure to a level that provides adequate tissue perfusion (> 70 mm Hg). Several agents that may be administered include dopamine, epinephrine, norepinephrine, and phenylephrine hydrochloride. Antiplatelet agents may also be administered to reduce clotting and opioid analgesics to reduce pain and stress.

Medication or Drug Class	Dosage	Description	Rationale
Dobutamine if the systolic blood pressure is > 80 mm Hg (dopamine is the drug of choice for hypotensive patients)	2–40 mcg/kg/min (but usually in the range of 2–20 mcg/kg/min); milrinone may be added if patients are not responding or are developing tachycardia in response to dobutamine	Sympathomimetic	Dobutamine improves heart contractility without much effect on heart rate; renal function may also improve through increased cardiac output and renal perfusion

(highlight box continues on page 240)

Pharmacologic Highlights (continued)

Medication or Drug Class	Dosage	Description	Rationale
Nitroglycerine	Begin at 5 mcg/min and increase by 5 mcg/min every 3–5 min	Vasodilator	Relax vascular smooth muscle and reduce systemic vascular resistance, thereby increasing cardiac output
Diuretics	Varies by drug	Loop diuretics (preload) diuretics	Reduce venous return

Independent

Patients with cardiogenic shock experience a life-threatening condition that results in multiple complex needs, rapid decision making, and a rapid emergency response. Supporting tissue perfusion and limiting myocardial oxygen consumption are primary concerns. Decreasing oxygen demand may limit ischemia, injury, and infarction. Position the patient to maximize circulation to vital organs. Restrict the patient's activity, and maintain the patient on bedrest. Address the patient's anxiety by explaining all procedures. Permit the family or significant others to remain with the patient as long as their presence does not cause added stress. Maintaining a calm and peaceful environment provides reassurance and reduces anxiety, which in turn reduces myocardial oxygen consumption. Serial vital signs, ongoing surveillance, regular communication with the critical care team, and careful oversight of vasoactive medications are core nursing responsibilities.

Restricted activity could lead to impaired skin integrity, necessitating frequent assessment and care of the skin. Adequate protein and calories are essential for the prevention or healing of impaired skin integrity and should be provided by oral, enteral, or parenteral means.

Evidence-Based Practice and Health Policy

Vallabhajosyula, S., Dunlay, S., Barsness, G., Rihal, C., Holmes, D., & Prasad, A. (2019). Hospital-level disparities in the outcomes of acute myocardial infarction with cardiogenic shock. *American Journal of Cardiology, 124*, 491–498.

- The authors explore whether treatment and outcomes for patients with cardiogenic shock were affected by hospital type (teaching/nonteaching), size (small/large), and location (urban/rural). They examined a large, retrospective cohort of adult admissions from the National Inpatient Sample database during 2000 to 2014 ($N = 362,065$) with a primary diagnosis of acute MI with cardiac tamponade.
- Lower mortality rates were noted among urban nonteaching and urban teaching hospitals as compared with rural hospitals, and lower mortality rates were noted in large hospitals as compared with smaller hospitals. Large and urban hospitals made greater use of early coronary angiography, percutaneous cardiac intervention, and mechanical circulatory support. The authors concluded that the hospital-level disparities in the management and outcomes of acute MI with cardiogenic shock cannot be fully accounted for by differences in patient characteristics, indicating disparities for patients in smaller and rural hospitals.

DOCUMENTATION GUIDELINES

- Physical findings: Cardiopulmonary, renal, neurological, and integumentary systems; skin integrity
- Hemodynamic response to inotropic medications, diuretics, nitrates, mechanical circulatory devices, and oxygen

• Presence of complications: Pulmonary congestion, respiratory distress, unrelieved chest pain, wound infection, thromboses or emboli, and skin breakdown
• Reaction to the crisis and prognosis

DISCHARGE AND HOME HEALTHCARE GUIDELINES

The patient will likely require extensive rehabilitation after a critical illness. Teach the patient how to reduce controllable risk factors for heart disease. Be sure the patient understands the medication prescribed. Discuss smoking cessation programs and support systems.

RECURRENCE OF CHEST PAIN. Teach the patient to call 911 for any chest pain that is not relieved by rest and/or nitroglycerin. Instruct the patient not to ignore the pain or wait to call for assistance.

RECURRENCE OF HEART FAILURE. Teach the patient to restrict fluids to 2 to 2.5 L per day or as prescribed by the physician and to observe sodium restrictions. The patient should report a weight gain of greater than 4 pounds in 2 days to the physician. Finally, teach the patient to monitor for increasing shortness of breath and edema and to report either of those signs or symptoms to the physician. If the patient experiences acute shortness of breath, the patient should call 911 or go to the emergency department immediately.

Cardiomyopathy

DRG Category:	315
Mean LOS:	3.6 days
Description:	MEDICAL: Other Circulatory System Diagnosis With Complication or Comorbidity

Cardiomyopathy is a chronic or subacute disease process that involves the heart muscle and causes systolic dysfunction, diastolic dysfunction, or both; it most commonly involves the endocardium and occasionally the pericardium. Cardiomyopathy is classified as primary when the cause is not known. Secondary cardiomyopathy is a result of some other primary disease process. Three common classifications of cardiomyopathy are dilated, hypertrophic, and restrictive. Dilated cardiomyopathy (DCM) is the most common and is characterized by ventricular dilation, impaired systolic function, atrial enlargement, and stasis of blood in the left ventricle. This form of cardiomyopathy is progressive and leads to intractable heart failure (HF) and death in the majority of patients within 5 years.

Hypertrophic cardiomyopathy (HCM), also known as *hypertrophic obstructive cardiomyopathy* or *idiopathic hypertrophic subaortic stenosis*, consists of ventricular hypertrophy, rapid contraction of the left ventricle, and impaired relaxation. It is commonly the result of hypertension or valvular heart disease. The process may go on for years with no or slowly progressive symptoms, or the first sign of the disease may be sudden cardiac death. Although the patient may live a "normal" life, deterioration usually occurs. The third form of cardiomyopathy, restricted cardiomyopathy, is the least common form. Both ventricles become rigid, which distorts the filling phase of the heart. The contraction phase remains normal. The result is that ventricular walls become fibrotic, cardiac filling diminishes, and cardiac output decreases. Restricted cardiomyopathy has a poor prognosis; many patients die within 1 to 2 years after diagnosis. Complications of cardiomyopathy include heart failure, thromboembolism, valvular regurgitation, cardiac arrest, and sudden death.

CAUSES

The etiology of many cases remains unclear. Cardiomyopathy may occur because of other diseases, such as coronary artery ischemia, hypertension, or valvular disease. Infections such as viruses, bacteria, or fungi may lead to cardiomyopathy, or it may be from a genetic cause. Inflammatory conditions such as rheumatoid arthritis or systemic lupus erythematosus may lead to the condition, or it may result from metabolic and endocrine disorders. Toxins such as alcohol, cocaine, antineoplastic agents, poisons, or anesthesia agents can lead to the condition as well. Cardiomyopathy may also be caused by amyloidosis (restrictive cardiomyopathy), hemochromatosis, metastatic carcinoma affecting the myocardium (restrictive cardiomyopathy), fibrosis secondary to radiation, vitamin deficiencies, or pregnancy.

GENETIC CONSIDERATIONS

There are numerous types of familial cardiomyopathy. Familial DCM is transmitted in an autosomal dominant pattern with age-related penetrance and usually appears in young adulthood. Genetic forms of DCM account for approximately 40% of cases, while many cases are considered idiopathic. Family history accounts for 20% to 25% of cases of idiopathic DCM. Rare cases can result from mutations in the dystrophin gene or in mitochondrial DNA. DCM can be caused by mutations in the lamin A/C (*LMNA*) gene, *PLN* (encodes the protein phospholamban), and the sodium channel gene *SCN5A*. HCM can be inherited in an autosomal dominant fashion with variable penetrance and variable expressivity. About 45% of cases appear to be sporadic. Mutations in genes that code for sarcomeric proteins, including myosin heavy chain, actin, tropomyosin, and titin, have been linked to HCM. Many gene variants have been implicated, some conferring increased risk of severe disease.

SEX AND LIFE SPAN CONSIDERATIONS

Cardiomyopathy may occur at any time from young adulthood to old age. Clinical signs of cardomyopathy appear most often between 20 and 40 years of age. HCM usually occurs in young adults with a family history of the disease. DCM, which is twice as common among men as women, occurs most often in middle age. Women with ischemic cardiomyopathy experience significantly more morbidity and mortality than men because of underlying pathology, delays in both presentation and treatment, and underrepresentation in clinical trials. Women also have higher mortality rates than men while waiting for heart transplants.

HEALTH DISPARITIES AND SEXUAL/GENDER MINORITY HEALTH

Although restrictive cardiomyopathy is not race or ethnicity specific, some of the associated conditions can be seen more frequently in certain races or ethnicities. For example, sarcoidosis is more common in Black females than in other groups. Black, Indigenous, and other children of color hospitalized with cardiomyopathy or myocarditis are more likely to die than their White counterparts, a trend that may be due in part to in-hospital differences in care or response to treatment (Olsen et al., 2021). The Centers for Disease Control and Prevention report that 11.5% of White persons, 9.5% of Black persons, 7.4% of Hispanic persons, and 6.0% of Asian persons have heart disease. Significant health disparities exist in the cardiac care of underrepresented groups as compared to White persons. Black, Indigenous, and other people of color are known to receive care less often guided by standard cardiac care guidelines than White persons. Unless patients have health insurance, White patients are more likely to receive coronary angiograms and other coronary interventions than Black and Hispanic patients. Black, Indigenous, and other people of color are also less likely to be referred to cardiologists and cardiac surgeons compared to White persons (Batchelor et al., 2019).

Transgender is a term used to describe persons whose gender identity is different from their sex assigned at birth. Approximately 1% of the U.S. population identify themselves as transgender. Sexual and gender minority persons have higher odds for multiple chronic conditions,

PRIMARY NURSING DIAGNOSIS

DIAGNOSIS. Decreased cardiac output related to reduced myocardial contractility as evidenced by dyspnea, tachycardia, and/or fatigue

OUTCOMES. Circulation status; Cardiac pump effectiveness; Knowledge: Cardiac disease management; Tissue perfusion: Cardiac, pulmonary, cerebral, abdominal organs, peripheral; Vital signs

INTERVENTIONS. Emergency care; Vital signs monitoring; Cardiac care; Oxygen therapy; Fluid/electrolyte management; Fluid monitoring; Shock management: Volume; Medication administration; Resuscitation; Surveillance

☀ PLANNING AND IMPLEMENTATION

Collaborative

The treatment for cardiomyopathy is usually palliative rather than curative, but more aggressive options exist. Control of the symptoms of HF is the primary goal in treatment. Medical management may vary depending on the type of cardiomyopathy present. Surgical treatment most commonly consists of excision of part of the hypertrophied septum to reduce the outflow obstruction (septal myotomy-myectomy). The patient with restrictive cardiomyopathy usually undergoes surgery to implant a permanent cardiac pacemaker. Technological advances have allowed for treatment options to include left ventricular assist devices as a bridge to transplantation, cardiac resynchronization therapy (biventricular pacing), and automatic implantable cardioverter-defibrillators. Heart transplantation is an option for people with progressive, end-stage heart failure with a poor prognosis.

Pharmacologic Highlights

Medication or Drug Class	Dosage	Description	Rationale
Angiotensin-converting enzyme (ACE) inhibitors and angiotensin II receptor blockers	Varies by drug (enalapril, lisinopril, ramipril, valsartan, losartan)	Inactivates renin-angiotensin system, thereby decreasing vascular resistance and ventricular afterload	ACE inhibitors decrease mortality rates in patients with left ventricular dysfunction; reduce readmissions caused by heart failure
Digoxin	0.25 mg qd	Direct action on cardiac muscle to increase contractility	Idiopathic dilated cardiomyopathy: Improves contractility and slows the renin-angiotensin response
Vasodilators	Varies by drug	Drugs such as nitrates and hydralazine dilate arteries	Reduce both preload and afterload by causing venous and arterial vasodilation

Other Drugs: Beta-adrenergic antagonists (carvedilol, metoprolol) have also been known to be beneficial in the treatment of dilated cardiomyopathy because of the resultant decrease in myocardial oxygen demand, improved ventricular filling, and inhibition of sympathetic vasoconstriction. Medical interventions for HCM are aimed at decreasing the force of ventricular contraction and decreasing the outflow obstruction.

(highlight box continues on page 246)

Pharmacologic Highlights (continued)

Agents commonly used to achieve this goal include beta-adrenergic antagonists or calcium channel blockers. Diuretic treatment is not indicated for HCM because the outflow obstruction requires an adequate preload to maintain sufficient cardiac output. The longer filling time, optimal preload, and decrease in contractility diminish the outflow obstruction by the septum and mitral valve during systole. Calcium channel blockers, most commonly verapamil, are used to promote relaxation of the ventricle, which also results in improved diastolic filling time. Antiarrhythmics are used for patients with supraventricular and nonsustained ventricular tachycardias.

Independent

Elevate the head of the patient's bed 30 to 45 degrees to help alleviate dyspnea. The elevation lowers pressure on the diaphragm, which is caused by the contents of the abdomen, and decreases venous return, thereby decreasing preload. If necessary, assist the patient with the activities of daily living. Although the patient requires frequent rest periods, maintain some level of activity. Prolonged periods of little or no activity can be very difficult to reverse.

Education of the patient and family is most important to prevent exacerbations and frequent hospital visits. HF as a response to cardiomyopathy is managed on an outpatient basis. Teach the patient and family how to prevent exacerbation and worsening of the condition. Explain the disease process clearly, using audiovisual aids whenever possible to help the patient understand the necessity of the prescribed medications, activity restrictions, diet, fluid restrictions, and lifestyle changes. Provide written material for the patient to take home and use as a reference; however, before giving the patient this material, be sure to assess the patient's literacy level.

Teach the patient and family measures to prevent the condition from worsening. Patients and their families may be fearful and anxious, whether this is a new diagnosis or a progression of a chronic condition. The patient and family are required to make many lifestyle changes. Fear, anxiety, and grief can all stimulate the sympathetic nervous system, leading to catecholamine release and additional stress on an already compromised heart. Helping the patient to work through these feelings may improve psychological well-being and cardiac output. Ensure that the patient and family are aware of the growing technological advances that are available to them. If they desire a less aggressive approach, refer them to hospice if that option is appropriate for end-of-life care.

Evidence-Based Practice and Health Policy

Olsen, J., Tjoeng, Y., Friedland-Little, J., & Chan, T. (2021). Racial disparities in hospital mortality among pediatric cardiomyopathy and myocarditis patients. *Pediatric Cardiology, 16*, 59–71.

- Because racially disparate health outcomes exist for a multitude of populations and illnesses, the authors examined the effects of race and ethnicity on mortality for children with cardiomyopathy or myocarditis. The authors conducted a retrospective cross-sectional study using the Kids' Inpatient Database to analyze more than 34,000 hospital admissions for patients 18 years old and younger with cardiomyopathy, myocarditis, or both, and without concomitant congenital heart disease.
- They used multivariate logistic regression models adjusted for age, calendar year, sex, insurance type, diagnostic category, treatment at a pediatric hospital, and noncardiac organ dysfunction and found higher mortality rates for Black and Hispanic children. They concluded that children of racial and ethnic minorities hospitalized with cardiomyopathy or myocarditis were more likely to die than their White counterparts, a trend that may be due in part to in-hospital differences in care or response to treatment.

DOCUMENTATION GUIDELINES

• Physical findings: Vital signs; right atrial pressure, pulmonary artery pressure, pulmonary capillary wedge pressure, cardiac output, systemic vascular resistance, pulmonary vascular resistance; skin temperature, color, dampness; presence or absence of jugular vein distention or hepatojugular reflux, ascites, edema, pulmonary crackles or wheezes, S_3 or S_4, or murmurs; intake and output; daily weight; mental status
• Laboratory results: Electrolyte, complete blood count, and ABG results
• Response to medications such as diuretics, nitrates, inotropes, and oxygen

DISCHARGE AND HOME HEALTHCARE GUIDELINES

PREVENTION. To prevent exacerbations, teach the patient and family to monitor for increased shortness of breath or edema and how to measure fluid intake and output and daily weights. Explain when to notify the physician of changes.

MEDICATIONS. Be sure the patient and family understand all medications, including effects, dosage, route, adverse effects, and the need for routine laboratory monitoring for drugs such as digoxin.

COMPLICATIONS. Instruct the patient to call for emergency assistance for acute shortness of breath or chest discomfort that is not alleviated with rest. Provide hospice information to the patient and family if they require palliative and end-of-life care.

Carpal Tunnel Syndrome

DRG Category:	514
Mean LOS:	2.7 days
Description:	SURGICAL: Hand or Wrist Procedure, Except Major Thumb or Joint Procedures Without Complication or Comorbidity or Major Complication or Comorbidity
DRG Category:	73
Mean LOS:	5.0 days
Description:	MEDICAL: Cranial and Peripheral Nerve Disorders With Major Complication or Comorbidity

Carpal tunnel syndrome (CTS), first described in 1854 as a complication of trauma and again in 1947 as an idiopathic syndrome, is part of a larger group of musculoskeletal alterations called upper extremity repetitive use syndrome, or cumulative trauma disorders. Cumulative trauma disorders involve injury to the tendon, tendon sheath, and related tissues (bones, muscles, and nerves) of the upper extremity. CTS is the most common of the nerve entanglement syndromes; it is a collection of specific symptoms that occur with compression of the median nerve, which carries motor, sensory, and autonomic fibers to the hand within the carpal tunnel. When injured, trauma results in an impairment of sensory and motor function as compression results in slowing of the nerve conduction velocity. CTS has an estimated lifetime risk of 10% in the U.S. population, and the annual incidence is 0.1% among adults. Complications include risks associated with surgery: infection, hemorrhage, and thromboembolic phenomenon.

CAUSES

The cause of CTS is debated, but the most common theory is that patients with CTS have abnormally high carpal tunnel pressures, which cause venous outflow obstruction, edema, and nerve ischemia. Quite a few conditions are associated with the development of CTS. Rheumatoid arthritis, flexor tenosynovitis, severe sprain of the wrist, or dislocation of the wrist are factors that predispose patients to CTS. Other factors include pregnancy, menopause, and hysterectomy. Diabetes mellitus, acromegaly, renal failure, hypothyroidism, tuberculosis, amyloidosis, and myxedema, as well as aging and obesity, are also thought to be contributory factors. CTS is also associated with low aerobic fitness and increased body mass index. Many researchers have reported an occupational link to the performance of certain jobs or ergonomic factors in the workplace. Ultimately, experts suggest that there are complex interactions among genetic, social, vocational, recreational, and demographic characteristics that lead to the syndrome.

GENETIC CONSIDERATIONS

Instances of CTS sometimes cluster in families, but there are also heritable conditions that mimic the symptoms of CTS. These include hereditary neuropathy with liability to pressure palsies, which can be transmitted in an autosomal dominant fashion and often present as peripheral nerve entrapment. A recent genome-wide association study has found 16 susceptibility loci for CTS, as well as a link with short stature. Many of the implicated loci are genes involved in growth and extracellular matrix architecture, which may alter the environment the median nerve transits, contributing to a genetic predisposition.

SEX AND LIFE SPAN CONSIDERATIONS

CTS can occur in both sexes and at any age. However, the highest incidence appears to be in women between the ages of 30 and 49 years. One major study established a mean age for occupational CTS as 37 years, with women being twice as likely as men to develop CTS. The same study found that for nonoccupational CTS, the mean age was 51 years, with women three times as likely as men to develop CTS. Women are more likely than men to have associated muscle atrophy related to CTS.

HEALTH DISPARITIES AND SEXUAL/GENDER MINORITY HEALTH

In the U.S. armed services, White persons have higher rates of CTS than Black persons. Sexual and gender minority status has no known effect on the risk for CTS.

GLOBAL HEALTH CONSIDERATIONS

Developed countries, and specifically North American and European countries, have higher rates of CTS than developing countries, likely because of occupational injury resulting from technical and industrial jobs. Reports of CTS are rare in developing nations.

▓ ASSESSMENT

HISTORY. Elicit a history of hand-related symptoms. Determine the patient's dominant hand and ask if the patient has experienced attacks of painful tingling in the hand(s) at night sufficient to disturb sleep. Ask if the patient has experienced accompanying daytime swelling and numbness of the hands or fingers. Elicit a history of aching, stiffness, and/or burning in the hand(s), fingers, or thumb(s). Ask if the patient has dropped items from the hands without realizing it or has loss of power in the hands. Generally, symptoms are intermittent and associated with activities involving flexion of the hands and wrists (driving, typing on a computer keyboard, playing the piano, knitting, painting, using a walker or wheelchair). Usually, the discomfort is located on the palmar aspect of the thumb and first three fingers and the distal part of the palm.

Establish a history of contributing factors to CTS. Has the patient ever been diagnosed with rheumatoid arthritis, flexor tenosynovitis, diabetes mellitus, hypothyroidism, acromegaly, tuberculosis, amyloidosis, or myxedema? Ask if the patient has sprained or dislocated the wrist. Establish a history of pregnancies, menopause, and/or hysterectomy.

Establish an occupational history. Does the patient's work require use of the hands? Which hand is involved in repetitive movements or the use of tools?

PHYSICAL EXAMINATION. The most common symptoms are **numbness and tingling, pain,** and **hand swelling or tightness.** A two-point discrimination test may be used to locate the areas of sensory loss. Examine the patient's hands and wrists to assess for muscular wasting or weakness. Check the nails for atrophy and ask if the patient can clench the hands into fists. Note the patient's range of motion of the fingers and wrist and the hand strength. Examine the patient for dry, shiny skin.

PSYCHOSOCIAL. Patients with CTS usually have had a progressive, long-term problem that interrupts their activities of daily living and their ability to perform occupational or recreational tasks. Anxiety is a common response. Assess the patient's coping, occupational status, and familial interactions. If an occupational change is necessary, assess the consequences for patient and family.

Diagnostic Highlights

Test	Normal Result	Abnormality With Condition	Explanation
Electromyography (primary diagnostic tool)	Normal conduction	Detects median nerve motor conduction delay of more than 5 msec	The maximum latency difference method, measured by the centrimetric technique ("inching" up the arm), has a high predictive value
Tinel sign (clinical test that is not always predictive)	Negative test	Positive if gentle tapping over the median nerve at the wrist results in pain, tingling, or numbness in the median nerve distribution	Compression of median nerve leads to a positive test result
Finkelstein test (clinical test that is not always predictive)	Negative test	Positive if severe pain at radial styloid (process on distal end of the radium) results from flexing thumb against palm and finger flexed over thumb	Compression of median nerve leads to positive test result
Phalen test (clinical test that is not always predictive)	Negative test	Positive if unforced complete flexion of wrist for 60 sec results in pain, tingling, or numbness over median nerve distribution	Compression of median nerve leads to positive test result

Other Tests: To diagnose CTS, the Occupational Safety and Health Administration requires at least one physical finding (positive Tinel, Finkelstein, or Phalen tests or swelling, redness, deformity, or loss of motion) or at least one subjective complaint (pain, numbness, tingling, aching, stiffness, or burning), resulting in medical treatment, lost work days, or transfer to another job. Nerve conduction studies, however, are considered the best means to determine the presence of CTS. Magnetic resonance imaging is useful preoperatively if a lesion is suspected in the carpal tunnel.

PRIMARY NURSING DIAGNOSIS

DIAGNOSIS. Acute or chronic pain related to nerve compression and injury as evidenced by self-reports of pain, hand and finger numbness, and/or tingling of the hands

OUTCOMES. Comfort status; Pain control; Pain level; Mobility; Musculoskeletal rehabilitation participation

INTERVENTIONS. Pain management: Acute; Analgesic administration; Teaching: Prescribed exercise; Positioning

PLANNING AND IMPLEMENTATION

Collaborative

The most conservative treatment prescribed by physicians is splinting the involved wrist and administering medications. Physical therapy may be prescribed at any point in the treatment process to decrease swelling and promote healing. After 6 weeks of physical therapy, a vocational evaluation is performed to determine the patient's ability to return to their previous job. Vocational retraining may be recommended. If conservative treatment is not successful, the carpal (transverse) ligament is released surgically to relieve compression of the median nerve. The surgeon may also perform neurolysis, a freeing of the nerve fibers, if necessary.

Pharmacologic Highlights

Medication or Drug Class	Dosage	Description	Rationale
NSAIDs	Varies with drug	Includes a number of medications such as naproxen, diclofenac, ibuprofen, indomethacin	Reduce swelling and pain

Other Drugs: Steroid injections are also used to decrease the inflammation of the carpal ligament, celecoxib to reduce inflammation and pain, and hydrochlorothiazide to reduce edema in the carpal tunnel.

Independent

An important focus of nursing interventions is prevention of CTS. Encourage patients to engage in aerobic exercise. Discuss with patients that stationary bike riding and cycling may strain the wrist. When discussing prevention, explain to the patient that people at risk should be rotated into other jobs that do not require similar tasks. Periodic rests should also be taken, accompanied by stretching of the wrist, hand, fingers, and thumbs. If the patient is to wear a splint, teach the proper techniques for applying the splint so that it is not too tight. Teach the patient how to remove the splint in order to exercise and how to perform daily, gentle range-of-motion exercises. If the patient is to wear a sling, instruct the patient to remove it several times daily to perform elbow and shoulder exercises. Advise the patient that occasional exercise in warm water is therapeutic. Encourage the patient to use the hands as much as possible. For patients whose hand use is impaired, assist with bathing and eating tasks. Encourage the patient to verbalize concerns about CTS. Answer questions and arrange for consultations with a licensed physical therapist and a vocational rehabilitation counselor.

Evidence-Based Practice and Health Policy

Fernández-de-las-Peñas, C., Arias-Buría, J., Cleland, J., Pareja, J., Plaza-Manzano, G., & Ortega-Santiago, R. (2020). Manual therapy versus surgery for carpal tunnel syndrome: 4-year follow-up from a randomized controlled trial. *Physical Therapy, 100*, 1987–1996.

- Because previous studies of the effects of manual therapy in CTS were restricted to a period of 1 year or less, the authors compared the effects of manual therapy versus surgery at a 4-year follow-up. They employed a randomized controlled trial design allocating an equal number of women ($N = 120$) to manual therapy (desensitizing maneuvers such as soft tissue mobilization and exercises) or surgery and examined pain intensity, functional status, symptom severity, and self-perceived improvement at baseline, 1 year, and 4 years.
- Between-group changes for all outcomes were not significantly different at 1 year and at 4 years ($N = 87$). No between-group differences (15% physical therapy vs. 13% surgery) in surgery rate were observed during the 4 years. In the long term, manual therapy, including desensitization maneuvers of the central nervous system, resulted in similar outcomes and similar surgery rates compared with surgery in women with CTS.

DOCUMENTATION GUIDELINES

- Physical findings: Hand, wrist, thumb, finger pain; numbness; tingling; burning
- Response to conservative or surgical treatment
- Attendance and response to physical therapy
- Ability to cope with immobility and inability to return to work

DISCHARGE AND HOME HEALTHCARE GUIDELINES

THERAPY. Be sure the patient understands and implements appropriate range-of-motion exercises. Emphasize the need to use the hands as often as possible and the value of warm water exercising.

EQUIPMENT. Teach the patient proper techniques for applying and removing splints and/or slings.

VOCATIONAL COUNSELING. Arrange for the patient to consult with a vocational rehabilitation counselor about returning to work and any modifications that must be made on the job.

Cataract

DRG Category: 117
Mean LOS: 2.7 days
Description: SURGICAL: Intraocular Procedures Without Complication or Comorbidity or Major Complication or Comorbidity

Cataract is the leading cause of preventable blindness among adults in the United States. The incidence of cataract in the United States is 1.2 to 6 cases per 10,000 people. Approximately 3 million people in the United States have cataract surgery each year, and the success rate is 95% reaching 20/20 to 20/40 corrected vision. A cataract is defined as opacity of the normally transparent lens that distorts the image projected on the retina. The lens opacity reduces visual acuity. As the eye ages, the lens loses water and increases in size and density, causing compression of lens fibers. A cataract then forms as oxygen uptake is reduced, water content decreases, calcium content increases, and soluble protein becomes insoluble. Over time, compression of lens fibers causes a painless, progressive loss of transparency that is often bilateral. The rate of cataract formation in each eye is seldom identical. Without surgery, a cataract can lead to blindness.

CAUSES

Cataract has several causes and may be age related, present at birth, or formed as a result of trauma or exposure to a toxic substance. The most common cataract is age related (senile cataract), which is a gradual, progressive visual disorder resulting from genetic, environmental (ultraviolet light exposure), nutritional, and metabolic factors. Traumatic cataract develops after a foreign body injures the lens or a blunt injury of the eye occurs. Work- and sports-related injuries are the most common causes of traumatic cataract. Complicated cataract develops as a secondary effect in patients with metabolic disorders (e.g., diabetes mellitus), radiation damage (x-ray or sunlight), or eye inflammation or disease (e.g., glaucoma, retinitis pigmentosa, detached retina, recurrent uveitis). Toxic cataract results from drug or chemical toxicity. Congenital cataract is caused by maternal infection (e.g., German measles, mumps, hepatitis) during the first trimester of pregnancy.

GENETIC CONSIDERATIONS

Epidemiological studies indicate that cataracts have strong genetic components. Several loci have been identified for an autosomal dominant form of cataracts, including mutations in crystallin genes, a heat-shock transcription factor (*HSF4*), the alpha-8 subunit of the gap junction protein (*GJA8*), and the aquaporin 0 coding *MIP* gene. Mutations in the *NHS* gene cause an X-linked form of congenital cataracts. Congenital cataracts also occur with galactosemia, and these can appear within just a few days of birth. The specific genetic contributions of the more common age-associated cataracts are still unclear.

SEX AND LIFE SPAN CONSIDERATIONS

Age-related (senile) cataract begins to form at age 50 years and is present in 18% of persons ages 65 to 75 years and in 45% to 65% of persons ages 75 to 84 years. Cataracts may be present at birth. Cataract occurs in both men and women, but in the United States, approximately 61% of people with cataract are women. Following cataract surgery, retinal detachment is more common in men than women, a factor that may be due to the longer length of men's eyes.

HEALTH DISPARITIES AND SEXUAL/GENDER MINORITY HEALTH

White persons have a prevalence rate for cataract of 19% as compared to 13% for Black persons and 12% for Hispanic persons. Sexual and gender minority status has no known effect on the risk for cataract.

GLOBAL HEALTH CONSIDERATIONS

Approximately 285 million people have moderate to severe visual impairment and blindness worldwide, and while estimates vary, approximately 50% of the cases can be attributed to cataract. One-third of people with visual impairment have unoperated cataract. It is the world's leading cause of blindness that can be treated. Most people living with visual impairment reside in developing countries, and most impairments can be prevented or cured when technology and medical care are available to them. The highest rate of people living with blindness over 50 years of age is in sub-Saharan Africa.

ASSESSMENT

HISTORY. Changes in vision may go unnoticed for a long time because of the slow progression. Patients frequently complain of problems with reading and night driving. Ask if the patient is color blind, has always worn glasses or contacts, has a history of cataract, or is under the treatment of an eye doctor or optometrist. Generally, patients with cataract report decreasing visual acuity with painless, increasingly blurred vision; visual distortion such as glare, dazzling effects, or dimness; or decrease in color perception and discoloration brought about by changes in lens color to yellow, amber, and finally to brown. Increased glare may occur, particularly with a decrease in contrast sensitivity in brightly lit rooms. Some people report a disabling glare in the dark when driving toward oncoming cars with headlights turned on. The presence of other risk factors, such as trauma, radiation exposure, metabolic disorders, eye infection, and medication history, is important. Ascertain if the patient's mother contracted German measles, mumps, or hepatitis during pregnancy.

PHYSICAL EXAMINATION. Cataract formation causes **decreased visual acuity and blurred vision**, a loss measured by use of the Snellen chart. Cataract is considered relevant to the patient's health and quality of life if visual acuity is altered significantly. Generally, near visual acuity is more affected than distance acuity. Color perception of blue, green, and purple is reported as varying shades of gray. If the cataract is advanced, shining a penlight on the pupil reveals the white area behind the pupil. A dark area in the normally homogeneous red reflex confirms the diagnosis.

PSYCHOSOCIAL. Because the loss of vision is usually gradual, the patient may deny visual dysfunction until it affects the actions of daily life, reading, or driving. Anxiety and fear of losing one's eyesight are common emotional responses. Social isolation may also occur because visual difficulties impede easy movement away from the home, may limit driving, and may cause embarrassment.

Diagnostic Highlights

General Comments: No specific laboratory tests identify cataract. Diagnosis is made by history, visual acuity test, and direct ophthalmoscopic examination.

Test	Normal Result	Abnormality With Condition	Explanation
Ophthalmoscopy or slit-lamp examination	Normal conjunctiva, cornea, crystalline lens, iris, sclera	May reveal a dark area in the red reflex	Microscopic instrument that allows detailed visualization of anterior segment of eye to identify lens opacities and other eye abnormalities

PRIMARY NURSING DIAGNOSIS

DIAGNOSIS. Ineffective protection related to decreased visual acuity as evidenced by blurred vision

OUTCOMES. Vision compensation behavior; Body image; Knowledge: Medication; Personal safety behavior; Anxiety level; Neurological status; Rest

INTERVENTIONS. Communication enhancement: Visual deficit; Medication administration: Eye; Vision screening; Surveillance: Safety

PLANNING AND IMPLEMENTATION
Collaborative
SURGICAL. There is no known medical treatment that cures, prevents, or reduces cataract formation. Surgical removal of the opacified lens is the only cure for cataract. The lens can be removed when the visual deficit is 20/40. If cataract occurs bilaterally, the more advanced

cataract is removed first. Extracapsular cataract extraction, the most common procedure, removes the anterior lens capsule and cortex, leaving the posterior capsule intact. A posterior chamber intraocular lens is implanted where the patient's own lens used to be. Photoemulsification is a type of extracapsular surgery in which the lens is softened with sound waves and then removed through a needle, while the posterior capsule is left intact. Intracapsular cataract extraction removes the entire lens within the intact capsule. An intraocular lens is implanted in either the anterior or the posterior chamber, or the visual deficit is corrected with contact lenses or cataract glasses. A newer surgical method, "small-incision" or "no-stitch" surgery, requires only a very small, 1/8-inch incision. During the procedure, the nucleus is smashed by an ultrasound probe. The benefit of this type of surgery is that healing is faster than with other methods.

COMPLICATIONS. Complications from surgery may include infection, bleeding, retinal disorders, pupillary block, adhesions, acute glaucoma, macular edema, and retinal detachment. Following extracapsular cataract extraction, the posterior capsule may become opacified. This condition, called a *secondary membrane* or *after-cataract*, occurs when subcapsular lens epithelial cells regenerate lens fibers, which obstruct vision. After-cataract is treated by yttrium-aluminum-garnet (YAG) laser treatment to the affected tissue.

Pharmacologic Highlights

Medication or Drug Class	Dosage	Description	Rationale
Acetazolamide	250 mg PO one to four times a day	Carbonic anhydrase inhibitor	Reduces intraocular pressure by inhibiting formation of hydrogen and bicarbonate ions
Phenylephrine	Topical ophthalmic use, 1–2 drops of 0.125% solution every 3–4 hr	Sympathomimetic	Causes abnormal dilation of the pupil, constriction of conjunctival arteries

Other Drugs: Postoperatively, medications in the form of eyedrops are prescribed to reduce infection (gentamicin or neomycin) and to reduce inflammation (dexamethasone). Acetaminophen is prescribed for mild discomfort; tropicamide is prescribed to induce ciliary paralysis.

Independent

If nursing care is provided in the patient's home, structure the environment with conducive lighting for visual safety and to reduce fall hazards. Suggest magnifying glasses and large-print books. Explain that sunglasses and soft lighting can reduce glare. Assist the patient with the activities of daily living as needed to remedy any self-care deficit. Encourage the patient to verbalize or keep a log on their fears and anxiety about visual loss or impending surgery. Help plan events to solve the problems with social isolation.

POSTOPERATIVE HOSPITAL CARE. Postoperative care includes covering the affected eye with an 8- to 24-hour patch and protective shield and positioning the patient supine or on the unoperated side. Apply cool compresses to reduce itching. Monitor and report any drainage, pain, or vital sign alteration. Teach the patient how to administer eyedrops correctly and caution the patient to notify the physician immediately upon experiencing eye pain. During recovery, teach the patient how to adjust home environments and daily activities to promote safety.

Evidence-Based Practice and Health Policy

Qureshi, M., & Steel, D. (2020). Retinal detachment following cataract phacoemulsification—A review of the literature. *Eye, 34,* 616–631.

- The authors wished to learn the incidence of retinal detachment following cataract surgery, whether the risk changes over time postsurgery, and how the risk is modified by intraoperative factors, intrinsic eye-related factors, and patient factors. They also determined how the incidence of retinal detachment postsurgery compares with retinal detachment in the general population. They searched the Medline and Ovid databases for relevant publications from 1990 onward using defined search terms with preplanned inclusion and exclusion criteria.
- The 10-year incidence of retinal detachment postsurgery was identified as being between 0.36% and 2.9%. This decreases over time to 0.1% to 0.2% annually but remains above the general population. The risk is further elevated by (in order of decreasing effect) intraoperative vitreous loss, increasing axial length, younger age, male sex, and trainee operating surgeons. The risk of postsurgical retinal detachment is approximately 10 times the general population's risk. This risk is modified by the interplay of multiple risk factors, of which intraoperative vitreous loss, myopia, age, and sex have the biggest effect.

DOCUMENTATION GUIDELINES

- Presence of complications: Eye discharge, pain, vital sign alterations
- Response to eye medication
- Reaction to supine position

DISCHARGE AND HOME HEALTHCARE GUIDELINES

Be sure the patient understands all medications, including dosage, route, action, adverse effects, and need for postoperative evaluation, usually the next day, by the eye surgeon. Review installation technique of eyedrops into the conjunctival sac. Teach the patient to avoid over-the-counter medications, particularly those with aspirin.

Instruct the patient to report any bleeding, yellow-green drainage, pain, visual losses, nausea, vomiting, tearing, photophobia, or seeing bright flashes of light. Instruct the patient to avoid activities that increase intraocular pressure such as bending at the waist, sleeping on the operative side, straining with bowel movements, rubbing the eyes, lifting more than 15 pounds, sneezing, coughing, or vomiting. The lifting restriction will likely last for a few weeks. Instruct the patient to wear a shield over the operative eye at night to prevent accidental injury to the eye during sleep and to wear glasses during the day to prevent accidental injury to the eye while awake. Notify the patient that swimming or hot tub use for a week should be avoided. Avoid the wind to limit irritants. Recommend that the patient avoid reading for some time after surgery to reduce eye strain and unnecessary movement so that maximal healing occurs.

Advise the patient not to shampoo for several days after surgery. The face should be held away from the shower head with the head tilted back so that water spray and soap avoid contact with the eye.

HOME HEALTH TEACHING. Vacuuming should be avoided because of the forward flexion and rapid, jerky movement required.

Driving, sports, and machine operation can be resumed when permission is granted by the eye surgeon, likely for a few days at least.

Clients fitted with cataract eyeglasses need information about altered spatial perception. The eyeglasses should be first used when the patient is seated, until the patient adjusts to the distortion. Instruct the client to look through the center of the corrective lenses and to turn the head, rather than only the eyes, when looking to the side. Clear vision is possible only through the center of the lens. Hand-eye coordination movements must be practiced with assistance and relearned because of the altered spatial perceptions.

Celiac Disease

DRG Category:	391
Mean LOS:	4.9 days
Description:	MEDICAL: Esophagitis, Gastroenteritis, and Miscellaneous Digestive Disorders With Major Complication or Comorbidity

Celiac disease (CD) is a chronic disease of the gastrointestinal (GI) tract and other body systems resulting from gluten sensitivity that affects approximately 1% of the population of North America. The Celiac Foundation defines gluten as the proteins found in wheat (wheat berries, durum, semolina, spelt, farina, farro), rye, barley, and a combination of wheat and rye called *triticale*. Gluten serves as a glue or structural protein that helps foods maintain their shape and form. CD leads to changes in the GI tract and interferes with the digestion and absorption of macronutrients and micronutrients. When people with CD ingest gluten, an antigen-antibody response leads to damage of the mucosa of their intestines, resulting in poor digestion and malabsorption. Patients with CD generally have increased GI motility and diarrhea, may have weight loss or failure to thrive, or may have only subtle symptoms (atypical CD) or be asymptomatic (silent CD).

Other common complications include anemia, osteopenia, and osteoporosis. Neurological symptoms (weakness and ataxia) and skin disorders may occur. More serious but less common complications include lymphoma and autoimmune diseases, such as type 1 diabetes mellitus and Hashimoto thyroiditis, as well as dermatitis, hormone disorders, and infertility.

CAUSES

CD is an allergic response to a protein found in many grains. Helper T cells mediate the inflammatory response to the antigen. Tissue enzymes transform products of gluten into a negatively charged protein and thereby aggravate cellular allergic reactions. Several changes occur in the intestinal mucosa from the antibody-antigen reaction: destruction of intestinal villi, lengthening of intestinal crypts, and mucosal lesions. As the surface of the intestine is destroyed, maldigestion and malabsorption of the nutrients in food occur. People with type 1 diabetes mellitus, rheumatoid arthritis, Down syndrome, or Turner syndrome have an increased risk of CD, as do children with frequent rotavirus infections.

GENETIC CONSIDERATIONS

CD appears to run in families with a strong hereditary component (heritability estimates range between 57% and 87%). The prevalence of CD in first-degree relatives (parents, offspring, siblings) is approximately 30%. Concordance for the disease in monozygotic twins is about 75%. Approximately 95% of people with CD have the DQ2 or DQ8 isoform of HLA-DQ. However, about 20% to 30% of people with the DQ2 or DQ8 alleles do not develop CD, implicating additional factors in the development of the disease. Numerous other variants (~47) have been shown to influence risk of CD.

SEX AND LIFE SPAN CONSIDERATIONS

Diagnoses are often made during infancy through 40 years of age. Slightly more females than males have CD.

HEALTH DISPARITIES AND SEXUAL/GENDER MINORITY HEALTH

The disorder is more common in White persons, especially with European ancestry, than other groups. Experts suggest that CD is underdiagnosed in Black persons, especially Black persons with diabetes mellitus. Sexual and gender minority status has no known effect on the risk for celiac disease.

GLOBAL HEALTH CONSIDERATIONS

Approximately 6 million people in Europe and the United States have CD, which has its highest prevalence in countries with a mild climate. It is most common in countries with a high proportion of European immigrants, such as Canada, Australia, and the United States. The incidence of CD is increasing in some parts of Africa and Asia.

ASSESSMENT

HISTORY. Patients with CD many have both GI and non-GI symptoms, or they may be asymptomatic. Up to 85% of patients with CD have diarrhea, which may be foul smelling, watery or semiformed, light in color, and/or frothy. Patients may complain of flatulence, abdominal bloating, or stomach growling and grumbling. They also might describe symptoms of malabsorption such as weakness, fatigue, and weight loss. Serious symptoms, which may occur if impaired absorption is longstanding, include severe abdominal pain, increased bleeding tendencies, paresthesia with sensory loss, ataxia, seizures, skin disorders, amenorrhea, and infertility in men and women. Osteoporosis can be severe and is linked to nutritional deficiency and altered calcium transport and binding. Question the patient about a possible lactose intolerance because of its link to CD. Ask the patient if they have a history of unexplained anemia or pathological fractures.

PHYSICAL EXAMINATION. The physical examination may be normal. Common symptoms include **diarrhea, malabsorption of fat, flatulence**, and **weight loss**. Children with frequent diarrhea may have severe dehydration and signs of electrolyte imbalance. Malabsorption of ingested fat (steatorrhea) results in the delivery of excessive dietary fat to the large bowel. This results in the production of hydroxy fatty acids by bacteria, which causes secretion of fluids into the intestine. Tympanic sounds may be heard over loops of filled bowel, and the abdomen may be protuberant due to distention of the intestine with fluids and gas. The patient may appear thin with muscle wasting or loose skinfolds. Other physical signs from malabsorption may include pallor from anemia, skin lesions (dermatitis herpetiformis), orthostatic hypotension, ataxia, peripheral edema, peripheral neuropathy, ecchymoses, and signs of hypocalcemia (Chvostek sign or Trousseau sign).

PSYCHOSOCIAL. Many patients have consulted healthcare providers who fail to take the signs of CD seriously, and patients may receive inappropriate counseling to eat a high-fiber diet, take antidiarrheal agents, and relax. Because the primary management is nutritional, misdiagnosis will prolong the symptoms and may result in anxiety and discouragement with healthcare providers. People with CD often become their own best advocates because of their knowledge of the condition.

Diagnostic Highlights

Test	Normal Result	Abnormality With Condition	Explanation
Antitissue transglutaminase antibody (anti-tTG), IgA by enzyme-linked immunosorbent assay	< 10 units/mL	> 10 units/mL	Most sensitive and specific antibodies to confirm CD; controversial if level correlates with the degree of mucosal damage; IgA level should also be obtained to rule out IgA deficiency
Serum electrolytes, coagulation profile, liver function test, and complete blood count	Normal serum; electrolytes; normal coagulation profile; normal blood count; normal protein and albumin level; alanine aminotransferase/aspartate aminotransferase is commonly elevated	Hypokalemia; hypocalcemia; prothrombin deficiency; anemia; hypoproteinemia and hypoalbuminemia	Impaired absorption of fat; impaired vitamin K, folate, vitamin B_{12}, iron, vitamin D, magnesium, and calcium absorption; rarely, reduced protein absorption
Flexible upper endoscopy with biopsy	Visualization of normal upper GI tract	Biopsy shows atrophied or absent villi of the intestinal tract, decreased villous-to-crypt ratio, and hyperplastic crypts; increased cellularity of the lamina propria with a proliferation of plasma cells and lymphocytes	Damage to intestinal mucosa from immune response
Dual-energy x-ray absorptiometry (DXA)	No bone loss	Bone loss > 3%; T scores are the number of standard deviations (SD) from the mean bone density values in healthy young adults. T score of −1 to −2.5 SD indicates osteopenia; T score of less than −2.5 SD indicates osteoporosis; T score of less than −2.5 SD with fragility fracture(s) indicates severe osteoporosis. Z scores are the number of standard deviations from the normal mean value for age- and sex-matched controls.	Measures bone mineral density (BMD) at several sites; for each SD reduction in BMD, the relative fracture risk increases 1.5–3 times

Note: Some patients may be evaluated with less specific diagnostic tests including antigliadin antibody tests and endomysial antibody tests.

PRIMARY NURSING DIAGNOSIS

DIAGNOSIS. Imbalanced nutrition: less than body requirements related to maldigestion and malabsorption as evidenced by diarrhea, cramping, flatulence, and/or weight loss

OUTCOMES. Knowledge: Celiac disease management; Nutritional status: Food and fluid intake; Nutritional status: Nutrient intake; Nutritional status: Biochemical measures; Energy conservation; Endurance

INTERVENTIONS. Nutrition management; Nutrition therapy; Nutritional counseling and monitoring; Fluid/electrolyte management; Teaching: Prescribed diet

PLANNING AND IMPLEMENTATION

Collaborative

The most important collaborative management strategy is a nutrition consultation. Management involves the complete elimination of gluten-containing grain products (wheat, rye, and barley) as well as oats, which may be contaminated with gluten during factory preparation. After the patient has followed the gluten-free diet for several months, the patient may begin eating oats if they are labeled gluten-free to ensure that factory cross-contamination has not occurred. Avoidance of lactose-containing products (milk, yogurt, cheese, ice cream, cream, salad dressing, mayonnaise) may also improve the symptoms of CD because lactose intolerance often occurs in celiac disease, but dairy products themselves do not cause celiac disease and should be avoided only if they cause symptoms. Healing of the small intestine may take 3 to 6 months once the gluten-free diet is initiated. The gluten-free diet is difficult to maintain because of the presence of flour in many products in the Western diet. Increasing numbers of grocery stores and restaurants, however, are offering gluten-free products.

Dietary changes are a lifetime commitment, and the success of dietary restrictions is monitored by serial anti-tTG levels. Nutritional requirements for restoration of bone health are important and may include dietary sources of calcium and vitamins.

Pharmacologic Highlights

Generally, CD is not treated with medication, but nutritional supplements may be needed to correct malabsorptive deficiencies, such as vitamin D, calcium, and iron. On rare occasions when patients with CD do not respond to a gluten-free diet, corticosteroids may be tried.

Independent

The patient with CD needs encouragement to maintain the gluten-free diet. A gluten-free diet is more expensive than a normal diet and also leads to social challenges for people with CD. Eating out presents multiple difficulties not only because of flour-containing items (which can include common foods and condiments such as sausage, pudding, soy sauce, and salad dressing) but also because of food preparation issues. Avoidance of all gluten-containing grain products takes significant effort, education, and vigilance. Teach patients to use the dishwasher to clean all plates, pans, and utensils that have been exposed to gluten. Several apps, such as AllergyEats Mobile, Dine Gluten Free, and Find Me Gluten Free, are available to guide gluten-free restaurant eating. Many restaurants label gluten-free items on their menu.

During the initial stages of healing, encourage the patient to use safety precautions to reduce the risk of bone fracture if DXA shows decreased bone density. Refer patients to a counselor if anxiety and stress management might help manage the condition. Encourage patients to participate in weight-bearing activities and to maximize health by avoiding alcohol and cigarette smoking.

Evidence-Based Practice and Health Policy

Lojou, M., Sahakian, N., Dutour, A., Vanbiervliet, G., Bege, T., & Gaborit, B. (2020). Celiac disease and obesity: Is bariatric surgery an option? *Obesity Surgery, 30,* 2791–2799.

- In light of the ongoing obesity epidemic, the authors explore the value of bariatric surgery as a treatment for obese patients with celiac disease. The authors undertook a comprehensive review of the literature on celiac disease, its nutritional consequences and complications, the possible impact of bariatric surgery as a treatment, and its effect on the incidence of celiac disease.
- Bariatric surgery is possible and clearly an option in severe obese patients with celiac disease as long as they are compliant with the gluten-free diet and do not have preoperative vitamin deficiencies. However, there are few studies with a long-term follow-up of bariatric operated patients with celiac disease. The authors do not recommend systematic preoperative screening for celiac disease in bariatric patients because it carries a cost, and celiac disease in bariatric surgery is still rare.

DOCUMENTATION GUIDELINES

- Response to nutritional modifications: Ability to maintain gluten restriction, tolerance to food, body weight, appetite, energy level
- Physical response: Hydration, GI assessment, frequency and consistency of bowel movements, skin assessment, level of discomfort
- Emotional response: Level of stress, mood and affect, coping ability

DISCHARGE AND HOME HEALTHCARE GUIDELINES

Explore the patient's dietary patterns and provide a dietary consultation. Provide the patient with a list of support groups and electronic references such as eMedicineHealth (https://www.emedicinehealth.com/celiac_sprue/article_em.htm) and the Celiac Disease Foundation (https://celiac.org). Make sure the patient understands the schedule for repeated blood tests and follow-up appointments.

Cerebral Aneurysm

DRG Category:	27
Mean LOS:	2.6 days
Description:	SURGICAL: Craniotomy and Endovascular Intracranial Procedures Without Complication or Comorbidity or Major Complication or Comorbidity
DRG Category:	70
Mean LOS:	6.2 days
Description:	MEDICAL: Nonspecific Cerebrovascular Disorders With Major Complication or Comorbidity

Cerebral aneurysm is a potentially devastating condition that may lead to life-threatening consequences. Cerebral aneurysm is an outpouching of the wall of a cerebral artery that results from weakening of the wall of the vessel. It is difficult to determine the frequency of cerebral aneurysms because of differences in the definitions of the size of aneurysm and the ways that aneurysms are detected. The prevalence is estimated to range from 5% to 10%; unruptured aneurysms account for approximately 50% of all aneurysms.

Cerebral aneurysms have a variety of sizes, shapes, and causes (Table 1). Most cerebral aneurysms are sacular or berrylike with a stem and a neck. The incidence of cerebral aneurysm has been estimated at 12 cases per 100,000 individuals, with approximately 15% to 25% of patients having multiple aneurysms, often bilaterally in the same location on both sides of the head. Clinical concern arises if an aneurysm ruptures or becomes large enough to exert pressure on surrounding structures. When the vessel wall becomes so thin that it can no longer withstand the surrounding arterial pressure, the cerebral aneurysm ruptures, causing direct hemorrhaging of arterial blood into the subarachnoid space (subarachnoid hemorrhage [SAH]). SAH is a life-threatening situation with a mortality rate of up to 65%.

• TABLE 1 Classification of Cerebral Aneurysms

Size	Small, < 15 mm
	Large, 15–25 mm
	Giant, 25–50 mm
	Supergiant, 50 mm
Shape	Berry: Most common (95%); berry-shaped aneurysm with a neck or stem
	Sacular: Any aneurysm with a sacular outpouching
	Fusiform: Outpouching of an arterial wall but with no stem
Etiology	Traumatic: Aneurysm that results from traumatic (penetrating or closed) head injury
	Charcot-Bouchard: Microscopic aneurysmal formation associated with hypertension; involves the basal ganglia and brainstem
	Dissecting: Related to atherosclerosis, inflammation, or trauma; aneurysm in which the intimal layer is pulled away from the medial layer and blood is forced between the layers

Complications of a ruptured cerebral aneurysm can be fatal if bleeding is excessive. SAH can lead to cerebral vasospasm, cerebral infarction, and death. Rebleeding often occurs in the first 48 hours after the initial bleed but can occur any time within the first 6 months. Other complications include meningeal irritation and hydrocephalus.

CAUSES

Possible causes are congenital structural defects in the inner muscular or elastic layer of the vessel wall; incomplete involution of embryonic vessels; and secondary factors such as arterial hypertension, atherosclerotic changes, hemodynamic disturbances, and polycystic disease. Cerebral aneurysms also may be caused by shearing forces during traumatic head injuries. Associated conditions are arteriovenous malformations, coarctation of the aorta, systemic lupus erythematosus, sickle cell anemia, bacterial endocarditis, and fungal infections. Cigarette smoking and alcohol and drug use and misuse have been linked to cerebral aneurysms.

GENETIC CONSIDERATIONS

Susceptibility to cerebral aneurysm appears to have a genetic component, as individuals with two or more affected family members have a three- to sixfold higher incidence of cerebral aneurysm. Researchers have identified over two dozen variants that may confer susceptibility, but very few specific genes have been identified. The most well replicated is a variant on chromosome 9 near the cyclin-dependent kinase inhibitor genes *CDKN2A* and *CDKN2B*. Other genes that have been associated with aneurysms include perlecan, elastin, collagen I and II, nitric oxide synthase, and endothelin receptor A. There are also rare familial forms of cerebral aneurysm susceptibility, which have unclear patterns of inheritance. In one study of familial inheritance patterns, the autosomal recessive pattern was seen in slightly more than half of the population, and autosomal dominance was seen in just over one-third, with about 5% showing incomplete penetrance. The autosomal dominant disorder polycystic kidney disease has been associated with an increased incidence of intracerebral aneurysm. Other genetic conditions associated with connective tissue disorders have also been associated with increased risk of aneurysms, including neurofibromatosis, Marfan syndrome, multiple endocrine neoplasia, Ehlers-Danlos syndrome, and hereditary hemorrhagic telangiectasia.

SEX AND LIFE SPAN CONSIDERATIONS

The peak incidence of cerebral aneurysm occurs between ages 35 and 60 years. Women in their late 40s through mid-50s are affected slightly more than men. Early age of menopause is associated with the presence of cerebral aneurysm, possibly because of the earlier loss of estrogen. The prognosis of SAH resulting from an aneurysm is worse for women than for men. Cerebral aneurysms rarely occur in children and adolescents, but when they occur, they are often larger than those found in adults; pediatric aneurysms account for approximately 2% of all cerebral aneurysms.

HEALTH DISPARITIES AND SEXUAL/GENDER MINORITY HEALTH

The odds of Black persons having a cerebral aneurysm are approximately twice that of White persons. Black, Hispanic, and uninsured persons are more likely to arrive at the hospital with an aneurysmal subarachnoid hemorrhage (ruptured aneurysm), whereas White persons are more likely to arrive at the hospital with an unruptured aneurysm. Experts suggest that this difference occurs because of reduced access to healthcare by Black, Hispanic, and uninsured persons (Rinaldo et al., 2019).

Transgender is a term used to describe persons whose gender identity is different from their sex assigned at birth. Approximately 1% of the U.S. population identify themselves as transgender. Sexual and gender minority persons have higher odds for multiple chronic conditions, cancer, and poor quality of life and are more apt to have disabilities than cisgender males and females (cisgender is a term used to describe persons whose gender identity and gender expression are aligned with their assigned sex listed on their birth certificate). Gender-affirming hormone therapy is the use of hormone therapy for gender transition or gender affirmation and can be masculinizing or feminizing. It may also affect cardiovascular health in transgender females. In a large sample, researchers have found that transgender men and women are more likely to be overweight than cisgender women. Compared to cisgender women, transgender women reported higher rates of diabetes, ischemic stroke, angina/coronary disease, and myocardial infarction. Gender-nonconforming men and women reported higher odds of myocardial infarction than cisgender women. Transgender women also had higher rates of any cardiovascular disease than cisgender men (Cacerese, Jackman, et al., 2020; Connelly et al., 2019). While large-scale studies are not available, these factors may place some sexual and gender minorities at risk for cerebral aneurysm.

GLOBAL HEALTH CONSIDERATIONS

The estimated frequency of cerebral aneurysm globally is approximately 10 (a range of 4–20) per 100,000 individuals, but it is dependent on location. The highest rates are reported in Japan, China, Sweden, and Finland.

ASSESSMENT

HISTORY. Prior to rupture, cerebral aneurysms are often asymptomatic. The patient is usually seen initially after SAH. Ask about one or more incidences of sudden headache with vomiting in the weeks preceding a major SAH. Other relevant symptoms are a stiff neck, back or leg pain, and photophobia, as well as hearing noises or throbbing (bruits) in the head. "Warning leaks" of the aneurysm, in which small amounts of blood ooze from the aneurysm into the subarachnoid space, can cause such symptoms. These small warning leaks are rarely detected because the condition is not severe enough for the patient to seek medical attention.

Identify risk factors such as familial predisposition, hypertension, cigarette smoking, or use of over-the-counter medications (e.g., nasal sprays or antihistamines) that have vasoconstrictive properties. Ask about the patient's occupation, because if the patient's job involves strenuous activity, there may be a significant delay in going back to work or the need to change occupations entirely.

PHYSICAL EXAMINATION. Common symptoms include **headache, facial pain, visual changes, alterations in consciousness,** and **seizures.** In most patients, the neurological examination does not point to the exact site of the aneurysm, but in many instances, it can provide clues to the localization. Signs and symptoms can be divided into two phases: those presenting before rupture or bleeding and those presenting after rupture or bleeding. In the phase before rupture or bleeding, observe for oculomotor nerve (cranial nerve III) palsy—dilated pupils (loss of light reflex), possible drooping eyelids (ptosis), extraocular movement deficits with possible double vision—as well as pain above and behind the eye, localized headache, or extraocular movement deficits of the trochlear (IV) or abducens (VI) cranial nerves. Small, intermittent, aneurysmal leakage of blood may result in generalized headache, neck pain, upper back pain, nausea, and vomiting. Note if the patient appears confused or drowsy.

PSYCHOSOCIAL. The patient has to cope not only with an unexpected, sudden illness but also with the fear that the aneurysm may rupture at any time. Assess the patient's ability to cope with a sudden illness and the change in roles that a sudden illness demands. In addition, assess the patient's degree of anxiety about the illness and potential complications.

Diagnostic Highlights

Test	Normal Result	Abnormality With Condition	Explanation
Cerebral angiogram	Symmetrical, intact pattern of cerebral vessels	Pooling of contract medium, indicating bleeding or aneurysm	Radiographic views of cerebral circulation show interruptions to circulation or changes in vessel wall appearance
Computed tomography (noncontrast because contrast may obscure SAH)	Intact cerebral anatomy	Identification of size and location of site of hemorrhage	Shows anterior to posterior slices of the brain to highlight abnormalities; identifies SAH in 90%–95% of cases

Other Tests: Noninvasive angiographic methods (computed tomographic angiography and magnetic resonance angiography) allow for detection of aneurysms; lumbar puncture (for patients not at risk for increased intracranial pressure [ICP]), skull x-rays, electroencephalography, transcranial Doppler ultrasonography, single-photon emission computed tomography, positron emission tomography, xenon-CT, cervical spine imaging.

PRIMARY NURSING DIAGNOSIS

DIAGNOSIS. Risk for ineffective cerebral tissue perfusion as evidenced by headache, facial pain, visual changes, and/or alterations in consciousness

OUTCOMES. Circulation status; Cognition; Neurological status; Tissue perfusion: Cerebral; Communication: Expressive, receptive; Vital signs

INTERVENTIONS. Airway management; Cerebral perfusion promotion; Intracranial pressure monitoring; Neurological monitoring; Peripheral sensation management; Vital signs monitoring; Oxygen therapy; Emergency care; Medication management

PLANNING AND IMPLEMENTATION

Collaborative

The first priority is to evaluate and support airway, breathing, and circulation. For patients unable to maintain these functions independently, assist with endotracheal intubation, ventilation, and oxygenation, as prescribed. Monitor neurological status carefully every hour and immediately notify the physician of any changes in the patient's condition.

The management of unruptured cerebral aneurysms is controversial. If there is no history of SAH, aneurysms of less than 10 mm in size have a rupture rate of less than 1% per year. Recent guidelines by expert panels and professional organizations have developed recommendations based on the patient's age, history, and aneurysm size. The choice of surgery versus medical management depends on these parameters as well as on the surgeon's expertise and consideration that mortality rates are 4% and morbidity rates are 16% after surgery. Microsurgery may be used to prevent rupture or rebleeding of the cerebral artery. The decision to operate depends on the clinical status of the patient, including the level of consciousness and severity of neurological dysfunction, the accessibility of the aneurysm to surgical intervention, the skill of the surgeon, and the presence of vasospasm. Surgical procedures used to treat cerebral aneurysms include direct clipping or ligation of the neck of the aneurysm to enable circulation to bypass the pathology. Endovascular coiling of cerebral aneurysms is a minimally invasive technique that may be used in aneurysms with a small neck size (< 4 mm), a luminal diameter < 25 mm, and those that are distinct from the parent vessel. An inoperable cerebral aneurysm may be reinforced by applying acrylic resins or other plastics to the sac. Postoperatively, monitor the patient closely for signs and symptoms of increasing ICP or bleeding, such as headache, unequal pupils or pupil enlargement, onset or worsening of sensory or motor deficits, or speech alterations.

Pharmacologic Highlights

Medication or Drug Class	Dosage	Description	Rationale
Calcium channel blockers	Varies with drugs such as nimodipine, verapamil	Inhibit calcium entry across cell membranes in vascular smooth muscles	Prevent vasospasm and hypertension
Morphine sulfate	5–10 mg IV prn	Opioid analgesic	Drug of choice for pain relief because of reliable effects and ease of reversibility with naloxone

Other Drugs: Antihypertensives such as labetalol may be prescribed for patients with high blood pressure. Antiepileptics such as fosphenytoin are administered for treatment and prevention of seizures. Sedatives may be prescribed to promote rest and relaxation, and aminocaproic acid, a fibrinolytic inhibitor, may be given to minimize the risk of rebleeding by delaying blood clot lysis. The patient may receive colloids such as albumin or plasmanate to decrease blood viscosity and expand the intravascular volume.

Independent

The environment should be as quiet as possible, with minimal physiological and psychological stress. Maintain the patient on bedrest. Limit visitors to immediate family and significant others.

Apply thigh-high elastic stockings and intermittent external compression boots. Discourage and control any measure that initiates Valsalva maneuver, such as coughing, straining at stool, pushing up in bed with the elbows, and turning with the mouth closed. Assist with hygienic care as necessary. If the patient has a facial weakness, assist them during meals.

Preoperatively, provide teaching and emotional support for the patient and family. Position the patient to maintain a patent airway by elevating the head of the bed 30 to 45 degrees to promote pulmonary drainage and limit upper airway obstruction. Suction the patient's mouth and, if needed, the nasopharynx and trachea. Before suctioning, oxygenate the patient well, and to minimize ICP increases, limit suctioning to 20 to 30 seconds at a time. If the patient has facial nerve palsy, apply artificial tears to both eyes. Take appropriate measures to prevent skin breakdown from immobility. Postoperatively, promote venous drainage by elevating the head of the bed 20 to 30 degrees. Emotional support of the patient and family is also important. The patient may be dealing with a neurological deficit, such as paralysis on one side of the body or loss of speech. If the patient cannot speak, establish a simple means of communication such as using a slate to write messages or using cards. Encourage the patient to verbalize fears of dependency and of becoming a burden.

Evidence-Based Practice and Health Policy

Wang, A., Campos, J., Colby, G., Coon, A., & Lin, L. (2020). Cerebral aneurysm treatment trends in National Inpatient Sample 2007–2016: Endovascular therapies favored over surgery. *Journal of NeuroInterventional Surgery, 12*, 957–963.

- The authors studied changes in aneurysm treatment practice patterns in the United States because flow modulation is a new endovascular technique for treatment of cerebral aneurysms as compared to open surgical approaches. Using the National Inpatient Sample Databases (2007–2016), the authors researched patient demographics, hospital characteristics, and clinical outcomes for hospital discharges. They studied patients with unruptured aneurysms (UA), ruptured aneurysms (RA), and/or treatments that included surgical clipping (SC) and/or endovascular treatments (EVT) using the International Classification of Diseases Codes. They also performed 5-year subgroup analyses for treatment differences.
- A total of 39,382 hospital discharges were identified with a significant increase in endovascular techniques over time. Hospitals in the South demonstrated the most significant EVT use. The 5-year subgroup analyses showed that although there was no significant difference in the mean number of cases for the two treatment modalities in the 2007–2011 subgroup, the 2012–2016 subgroup showed that significantly more UA and RA received EVT. The findings illustrated that the standard of care for treatment of cerebral aneurysms is shifting further toward endovascular therapies over open surgical approaches in the United States.

DOCUMENTATION GUIDELINES

- Neurological findings: Level of consciousness; pupillary size, shape, and reaction to light; motor function of extremities; other cranial nerve deficits (blurred vision, extraocular movement deficits, ptosis, facial weakness); aphasia; headache and facial pain; and nuchal rigidity (stiff neck, pain in the neck or back, pain with flexion of the neck, photophobia); deterioration of neurological status
- Response to pain medications and comfort measures

DISCHARGE AND HOME HEALTHCARE GUIDELINES

Prepare the patient and family for the possible need for rehabilitation after the acute care phase of hospitalization. Instruct the patient to report any deterioration in neurological status to the physician. Stress the importance of follow-up visits with the physicians. Be sure the patient understands all medications, including dosage, route, action, and adverse effects, and the need for routine laboratory monitoring if anticonvulsants have been prescribed.

If the patient decides to forgo surgery, the patient and family need to know the warning signs of impending rupture of the aneurysm. The patient and family should discuss quality-of-life issues, including the psychological stresses of living with an unruptured aneurysm. Make sure that the family understands when to schedule follow-up visits and how to support the patient to live a healthy lifestyle.

Cerebral Concussion

DRG Category:	83
Mean LOS:	4.3 days
Description:	MEDICAL: Traumatic Stupor and Coma > 1 Hour With Complication or Comorbidity
DRG Category:	84
Mean LOS:	2.6 days
Description:	MEDICAL: Traumatic Stupor and Coma > 1 Hour Without Complication or Comorbidity or Major Complication or Comorbidity
DRG Category:	955
Mean LOS:	11.0 days
Description:	SURGICAL: Craniotomy for Multiple Significant Trauma

The word *concuss* means "to shake violently." Cerebral concussion is defined as a traumatically induced, transient, temporary, neurogenic disruption caused by mechanical force to the brain. Cerebral concussions, also known as *mild traumatic brain injury* (MTBI), are the most common form of traumatic brain injury (TBI). They account for 15% of all sports-related injuries in high school students. People with concussions may or may not experience loss of consciousness but usually exhibit confusion, delayed responses to questions, a blank facial expression, emotional lability, and headache. Recovery from concussion usually takes minutes to hours. Most concussion patients recover fully within 48 hours, but subtle residual impairment may occur. New research findings indicate that for at least 4 months after an MTBI, the brain continues to display signs of damage even if patients have no symptoms. There is a growing awareness that athletes may not notice mild symptoms or may underreport concussions so that they can continue to play the sport. Repeat concussions are a significant issue for young athletes. Athletes with a history of one or more concussions have a greater risk for being diagnosed with another concussion than those without such a history. The first 10 days after a concussion present the greatest risk for another concussion.

In rare cases, a secondary injury caused by cerebral hypoxia and ischemia can lead to cerebral edema and increased intracranial pressure (ICP). Some patients develop postconcussion syndrome (postinjury sequelae after a mild head injury). Symptoms may be experienced for several weeks and, in unusual circumstances, may last up to 1 year. Chronic traumatic encephalopathy (CTE), a condition in which degenerative changes lead to brain atrophy and protein deposits in the brain, occurs in people with a history of repetitive brain injury. CTE can lead to memory loss, mood disturbances, impaired judgment, and ultimately, dementia. Other complications of cerebral concussion include seizures or persistent vomiting. In rare instances, a concussion may lead to intracranial hemorrhage (subdural, parenchymal, or epidural) or death.

CAUSES

The most widely accepted theory for concussion is that acceleration-deceleration forces cause the injury. Sudden and rapid acceleration of the head from a position of rest makes the head move in several directions. The brain, protected by cerebrospinal fluid (CSF) and cushioned by various brain attachments, moves more slowly than the skull. The lag between skull movement and brain movement causes stretching of veins connecting the subdural space (the space beneath the dura mater of the brain) to the surface of the brain, resulting in minor disruptions of the brain structures. Common causes of concussion are a fall, a motor vehicle crash (MVC), a sports-related injury, and a punch to the head. In high school athletes, the rate of concussions per 1,000 exposures for boys is 0.59 for football, 0.25 for wrestling, and 0.18 for soccer. For girls, the rate of concussions per 1,000 exposures is 0.23 for soccer, 0.09 for field hockey, and 0.16 for basketball. Boxing has the highest rate of head injuries compared to all other sports.

GENETIC CONSIDERATIONS

No clear genetic contributions to susceptibility have been defined.

SEX AND LIFE SPAN CONSIDERATIONS

Cerebral concussions can be experienced by patients of all ages and both sexes, but males are affected at higher rates than females. Recent evidence indicates that females may have a higher rate of sports-related concussions than males, and worse outcomes. Trauma is the leading cause of death between the ages of 1 and 44 years, and falls are the most common cause of TBI, followed by traffic injuries. In children from birth to 4 years of age, assault is the most common cause of concussion. In young adults 15 to 19 years of age, traffic injuries are the leading cause of concussion, followed by sports injuries. Older adults have higher rates of concussion-producing falls than do other age groups.

HEALTH DISPARITIES AND SEXUAL/GENDER MINORITY HEALTH

In recent years, Black persons have been killed in traffic crashes at a rate almost 25% higher than White persons (National Highway Traffic Safety Administration [NHTSA], 2021). Native American persons have the highest rate of MVC injury in the United States, more than twice the rate of Black persons (NHTSA, 2021). Experts have noted that Black and Native American communities tend to be crisscrossed by more dangerous roads than other locations, placing people from those communities at risk for injury. Stark disparities exist with the incidence, management, and rehabilitation of TBI. The Centers for Disease Control and Prevention (CDC) report that Native American children and adults have the highest TBI-related hospitalizations and deaths in the United States. Important health disparities exist in treatment, follow-up, and rehabilitation of TBI. Non-Hispanic Black and Hispanic patients are less likely to receive follow-up care and rehabilitation following TBI and more likely to have poor psychosocial, functional, and employment-related outcomes as compared to non-Hispanic White patients (CDC, 2021).

The CDC report that in the 20 years since the year 2000, more than 400,000 U.S. service members were diagnosed with TBI, including active military service members and Veterans. Approximately 80% of these injuries occurred when the service members were not deployed. These injuries may result in ongoing symptoms, posttraumatic stress disorder, and suicidal thoughts. People in correctional or detention facilities, people who experience homelessness, and survivors of intimate partner violence may have long-term consequences from TBI. People with lower incomes and those without health insurance have less access to TBI care, are less likely to receive surgical procedures and cranial monitoring when indicated, are less likely to receive rehabilitation, and are more likely to die in the hospital. Recent work has shown that rural populations have injury mortality rates that are more than twice as high as urban rates.

Many factors contribute to these health disparities, including the risk of traffic injury on narrow rural roads, the lack of graded curves and lighted traffic signals on rural highways, and the distance from major trauma centers. Many of the most dangerous occupations, such as mining and agriculture, are found in rural areas and can result in injury, disability, and death. People living in rural areas who experience a TBI have more time to travel to get emergency care, less access to high-level trauma care, and more difficulty accessing TBI services. Sexual and gender minority persons have high risk for dating and interpersonal violence, violence related to bullying, and intentional and unintentional injury, and therefore are at risk for TBI (Healthy People 2020).

GLOBAL HEALTH CONSIDERATIONS

TBI contributes to worldwide death and disability more than any traumatic injury. Approximately 69 million individuals sustain a TBI each year. The greatest overall incidence occurs in North America and Europe, in part because they collect higher-quality data, and the least overall incidence occurs in Africa. Southeast Asia and the Western Pacific have the greatest overall burden of disease. The World Health Organization estimates that between 70% and 90% of TBIs are concussions. Falls from heights of less than 5 meters are the leading cause of injury overall, and MVCs are the next most frequent cause. Both have the potential to cause a cerebral concussion.

✳ ASSESSMENT

HISTORY. If the patient cannot report a history, speak to the life squad, a witness, or a significant other to obtain a history. Determine if the patient became unconscious immediately and for how long—a few seconds, minutes, or an hour—at the time of the trauma. Find out if the patient experienced momentary loss of reflexes, arrest of respirations, and possible retrograde or anterograde amnesia. Elicit a history of headache, drowsiness, confusion, dizziness, irritability, giddiness, visual disturbances ("seeing stars"), and gait disturbances.

Other symptoms include memory loss, momentary confusion, residual memory impairment, and retrograde amnesia. The loss of consciousness lasts less than 24 hours if the patient has a concussion (otherwise, the TBI is more serious); the patient usually experiences confusion, disorientation, and amnesia upon regaining consciousness. A postconcussive syndrome that may occur weeks and even months after injury may lead to headache, fatigue, inattention, dizziness, vertigo, ataxia, concentration problems, memory deficits, depression, and anxiety.

PHYSICAL EXAMINATION. The most common symptoms of a concussion include **confusion, emotional lability, pain, dizziness, memory loss**, and **visual disturbances**. First evaluate the patient's airway, breathing, and circulation (ABCs). After stabilizing the patient's ABCs, perform a neurological assessment, paying special attention to early signs of ICP: decreased level of consciousness, decreased strength and motion of extremities, reduced visual acuity, headache, and pupillary changes.

Check carefully for scalp lacerations. Check the patient's nose (rhinorrhea) and ears (otorrhea) for CSF leak, which is a sign of a basilar skull fracture (a linear fracture at the base of the brain). Be sure to evaluate the patient's pupillary light reflexes. An altered reflex may result from increasing cerebral edema, which may indicate a life-threatening increase in ICP. Pupil size is normally 1.5 to 6.0 mm. Several signs to look for include ipsilateral miosis (Horner syndrome), in which one pupil is smaller than the other with a drooping eyelid; bilateral miosis, in which both pupils are pinpoint in size; ipsilateral mydriasis (Hutchinson pupil), in which one of the pupils is much larger than the other and is unreactive to light; bilateral midposition, in which both pupils are 4 to 5 mm and remain dilated and nonreactive to light; and bilateral mydriasis, in which both pupils are larger than 6 mm and are nonreactive to light.

Check the patient's vital signs, level of consciousness, and pupil size every 15 minutes for 4 hours. If the patient's condition worsens, the patient should be admitted for hospitalization. Continue neurological assessment throughout the patient's hospital stay to detect subtle signs of deterioration. Observe the patient to ensure that no other focal lesion, such as a subdural hematoma, has been overlooked.

PSYCHOSOCIAL. The patient with a concussion has an unexpected, sudden illness. Assess the patient's ability to cope with the potential loss of memory and temporary neurological dysfunction. In addition, assess the patient's degree of anxiety about the illness and potential complications. Determine the significant other's response to the injury. Expect parents of children who are injured to be anxious, fearful, and sometimes guilt-ridden. With the growing focus on the long-term consequences of CTE, patients and families will have many questions about the outcomes of the injury. If alcohol or other drugs of abuse were involved at the time of injury, determine if evaluation and follow-up are necessary.

Diagnostic Highlights

Test	Normal Result	Abnormality With Condition	Explanation
Computed tomography	Intact cerebral anatomy	Identification of size and location of site of injury	Shows anterior-to-posterior slices of the brain to highlight abnormalities

Other Tests: Skull x-rays; neuropsychological testing; magnetic resonance imaging; cerebral spine x-rays; and a glucose test, using a reagent strip, of any drainage suspected to be CSF; serum drug and alcohol screens

PRIMARY NURSING DIAGNOSIS

DIAGNOSIS. Risk for acute confusion as evidenced by alterations in cognitive functioning, agitation, alterations in level of consciousness, and/or misperceptions

OUTCOMES. Cognitive orientation; Concentration; Decision making; Information processing; Memory; Neurological status: Consciousness

INTERVENTIONS. Cerebral perfusion promotion; Environmental management; Surveillance; Cerebral edema management; Family support; Medication management

PLANNING AND IMPLEMENTATION

Collaborative

Patients with mild head injuries such as a concussion are often examined in the emergency department and discharged to home, where they usually recover fully in 48 to 72 hours. Most are head-ache free after 4 weeks. The primary foci are cognitive and physical rest during recovery. Generally, a family member is instructed to evaluate the patient routinely and to bring the patient back to the hospital if any further neurological symptoms appear. Parents are often told to wake a child every hour for 24 hours to make sure that the patient does not have worsening neurological signs and symptoms. Treatment generally consists of bedrest with the head of the bed elevated at least 30 degrees if possible, observation, and pain relief. Neurological consultation after 2 to 4 weeks should occur before the athlete resumes a sport, or if there are prolonged symptoms. Patients should be evaluated for a postconcussive syndrome with symptoms such as recurrent headaches, dizziness, memory impairment, ataxia, sensitivity to light and noise, concentration and attention problems, and depression or anxiety.

Pharmacologic Highlights

General Comments: Narcotic analgesics and sedatives are contraindicated because they may mask neurological changes that indicate a worsening condition. There is no indication that medication improves recovery after a concussion.

Medication or Drug Class	Dosage	Description	Rationale
Acetaminophen	325–650 mg PO q 4–6 hr	Nonnarcotic analgesic thought to inhibit prosta-glandin synthesis in the central nervous system	Manages headache

Independent

Generally, patients are not admitted to the hospital for a cerebral concussion. Make sure that before the patient goes home from the emergency department, the significant others are aware of all medications and possible complications that can occur after a minor head injury. Discuss with the patient and family the best ways to maintain cognitive and physical rest. Encourage the patient to avoid activities that require higher-level processes such as reaction time, multitasking, and memory. Patients do not have to remain in bed in a darkened room, but encourage brain rest by having patients stay at home, avoid physical activity, and avoid driving. Children and teenagers should avoid homework until given approval by the healthcare team to resume schoolwork. Most experts recommend avoiding television and electronics such as computers and tablets for several days to rest the brain. Teach the patient and significant others to recognize signs and symptoms of complications, including increased drowsiness, headache, irritability, or visual disturbances that indicate the need for reevaluation at the hospital. Teach the patient that occasional vomiting after sustaining a cerebral concussion is normal. The patient should not go home alone, because ensuing complications are apt to include decreased awareness and confusion.

If the patient is admitted to the hospital, institute seizure precautions if necessary. Ensure that the patient rests by creating a calm, peaceful atmosphere and a quiet environment. Limit visitors to the immediate family or partner and encourage the patient to rest for 24 hours without television or loud music.

Evidence-Based Practice and Health Policy

Hamer, J., Churchill, N., Hutchison, M., Graham, S., & Schweizer, T. (2020). Sex differences in cerebral blood flow associated with a history of concussion. *Journal of Neurotrauma, 37,* 1197–1203.

- The authors evaluated whether cerebral blood flow (CBF) was sex specific by evaluating sex differences in CBF of asymptomatic athletes, with and without a history of concussion (HOC) using arterial spin labeling (ASL). They analyzed 122 athletes: 66 without HOC (33 males/33 females) and 56 with HOC (28 males/28 females).
- Analysis revealed that both females with and without HOC showed no significant differences, although they had significantly higher variability in temporal CBF values in contrast with males with HOC. Males with HOC had lower CBF bilaterally than males without HOC, seen predominantly in the temporal lobes. Additionally, females with multiple concussion had lower CBF posteriorly compared with those with a single concussion, whereas males showed no significant effects. The study demonstrates evidence of sex differences associated with HOC.

DOCUMENTATION GUIDELINES

- Trauma history, description of the event, time elapsed since the event, whether the patient had a loss of consciousness and, if so, for how long
- Adequacy of ABCs; serial vital signs

- Appearance: Bruising or lacerations, drainage from the nose or ears
- Physical findings related to site of head injury: Neurological assessment, presence of accompanying symptoms, presence of complications (decreased level of consciousness, unequal pupils, loss of strength and movement, confusion or agitation, nausea and vomiting)
- Patient's and family's understanding of and interest in patient teaching

DISCHARGE AND HOME HEALTHCARE GUIDELINES

MEDICATIONS. Instruct the patient or caregiver not to administer any analgesics stronger than acetaminophen. Explain that aspirin may increase the risk of bleeding.

COMPLICATIONS. Explain that a responsible caregiver should continue to observe the patient at home for developing complications. Instruct the caregiver to awaken the patient every 1 to 2 hours throughout the night to assess the patient's condition. Explain that the caregiver should check the patient's orientation to place and person by asking "Where are you?" "Who are you?" "Who am I?" Teach the patient and caregiver to return to the hospital if the patient experiences persistent or worsening headache, blurred vision, personality changes, abnormal eye movements, a staggering gait, twitching, or constant vomiting. Teach the patient to recognize the symptoms of postconcussion syndrome, which may last for several weeks and include headache, dizziness, vertigo, anxiety, and fatigue.

PARENT TEACHING. When the patient is a child, teach the parent(s) that it is a common pattern for children to experience lethargy and somnolence a few hours after a concussion, even if they have manifested no ill effects at the time of the trauma. Such responses do not necessarily indicate serious injury. If the symptoms persist or worsen, explain that the parent(s) should notify the healthcare provider immediately.

MANDATORY REPORTING. Healthcare providers are mandatory reporters if they suspect child abuse or neglect. Nurses are responsible to know and follow state laws on mandatory reporting. Generally those laws include reporting suspected abuse to the child protective services office or law enforcement agencies.

Cervical Cancer

DRG Category:	740
Mean LOS:	3.9 days
Description:	SURGICAL: Uterine and Adnexa Procedures for Non-Ovarian and Non-Adnexal Malignancy With Complication or Comorbidity
DRG Category:	755
Mean LOS:	4.1 days
Description:	MEDICAL: Malignancy, Female Reproductive System With Complication or Comorbidity

Cancer of the cervix is one type of primary uterine cancer (the other being uterine-endometrial cancer) and is predominately epidermoid (resembling the cells of the epidermis, or skin). Invasive cervical cancer, that which has spread from the surface of the cervix to tissue deeper in the cervix, is the third-most common female pelvic cancer. The American Cancer Society (ACS) estimates that 14,480 new cases of invasive cervical cancer will be diagnosed in 2021, and

4,290 women are likely to die from the disease. Cervical cancer involves two types of cancer: squamous cell carcinoma (about 85% of cases) and adenocarcinoma (about 10%–15% of cases). Noninvasive cancer is described as carcinoma in situ (CIS), cancer that is only present in the cells where it started, and it is localized or confined at its original place. Generally, noninvasive cervical cancer occurs at four times the rate of invasive cervical cancer. There are descriptors for precancerous types of cervical disease as well. In cervical intraepithelial neoplasia (CIN), the epithelium looks abnormal. In the more serious precancerous condition, low-grade squamous intraepithelial lesion (LSIL), or mild dysplasia, the cells are more abnormal, and the condition may progress to high-grade squamous intraepithelial lesions (HSILs). If untreated, as many as 10 years can elapse between the preinvasive and the invasive stages.

Metastasis occurs through local invasion and by way of the lymphatic ducts. In addition to metastasis (lymph nodes, liver, lung, and bones), other complications include hematuria, constipation, fistulae formation, and obstruction of the urinary system.

CAUSES

Worldwide epidemiological studies suggest that sexually transmitted human papillomaviruses (HPVs) are the primary cause of cervical cancer. HPV viral DNA has been detected in more than 90% of squamous intraepithelial lesions and invasive cervical cancers. HPV infection occurs in a large percentage of sexually active women. Most HPV infections clear spontaneously within months or a year, and only a small proportion progresses to cancer. Other factors influence the progression of LSILs to HSILs, such as the type and duration of viral infection, compromised immunity, multiparity, HIV infection, or poor nutritional status. Risks for cervical cancer include smoking, oral contraceptive use, vitamin deficiencies, age of menarche, age of first intercourse, number and sexual activities of sexual partners, early first pregnancy, postnatal lacerations, grand multiparity, sexual partners with a history of penile or prostatic cancer or those uncircumcised, exposure to diethylstilbestrol (DES) in utero, and a history of cervicitis.

GENETIC CONSIDERATIONS

While most risk factors for cervical cancer are environmental, some studies have found that the daughters and sisters of cervical cancer patients have an increased chance of getting the disease. The increased incidence in families may be due to an inherited vulnerability to HPV infection.

SEX AND LIFE SPAN CONSIDERATIONS

Although cervical cancer can occur from the late teens to old age, it is most often diagnosed in women between the ages of 35 and 44 years, with the average age at diagnosis at 50 years of age. Preinvasive cancer of the cervix is most commonly seen in 25- to 40-year-old women, whereas invasive cancer of the cervix is more common in 40- to 60-year-olds. The ACS notes that 20% of cervical cancer is diagnosed in women over age 65 years, but these cancers are rare when women get regular cancer screening in their earlier years.

HEALTH DISPARITIES AND SEXUAL/GENDER MINORITY HEALTH

Hispanic and Black women are among those with the highest risk for HPV-associated cervical cancer. A likely factor for this health disparity is the decreased access to screening tests and follow-up treatment. In addition, significant disparities exist for sexual minority women, women living in rural areas, women with disabilities, women with obesity, women with low incomes, and women without insurance with respect to cancer screening. Screening is important for all women who have sexual contact with men, and that contact varies by sexual behaviors. Experts report that, because 76% of lesbian adolescent women report male contact, 96% of bisexual adolescent women report male contact, and 98% of heterosexual adolescent women report male contact, adolescents and adult women should be screened for cervical cancer. Transgender is a term used to describe persons whose gender identity is different from their sex assigned at birth. Approximately 1% of the U.S. population identify themselves as transgender. Transgender men need to undergo cervical cancer screening if they have a cervix. For some transgender men, screening is needed even if gender-affirming surgery has occurred. Most female-to-male trans-gender men retain their cervixes but obtain cervical cancer screening less often than cisgender women (cisgender is a term used to describe persons whose gender identity and gender expression are aligned with their assigned sex listed on their birth certificate). Reasons for individuals to delay screening include discrimination based on gender identity and the emotional conflict between self-perception and physical anatomy (Gatos, 2018).

GLOBAL HEALTH CONSIDERATIONS

A significant health disparity exists for women in developed versus developing countries with respect to cervical cancer. It is the third-most common malignancy in women around the world, the second leading cause of cancer-related death for women in developing countries, and the 10th leading cancer-related death for women in developed countries. With routine Papanicolaou (Pap) smears, the incidence of invasive cervical cancer has declined over the past few decades in North America and Western Europe, but rates in Eastern Africa are 10 times the North American rates. Globally, 500,000 new cases are diagnosed each year.

ASSESSMENT

HISTORY. Establish a thorough history with particular attention to the presence of the risk factors and the woman's menstrual history. Determine if and when the patient ever received the HPV vaccine. Establish a history of later symptoms of cervical cancer, including abnormal bleeding or spotting (between periods or after menopause); metrorrhagia (bleeding between normal menstrual periods) or menorrhagia (increased amount and duration of menstrual bleeding); dyspareunia and postcoital bleeding; leukorrhea in increasing amounts and changing over time from watery to dark and foul; and a history of chronic cervical infections. Determine if the patient has experienced weight gain or loss; abdominal or pelvic pain, often unilateral, radiating to the buttocks and legs; or other symptoms associated with neoplasms, such as fatigue.

PHYSICAL EXAMINATION. Early cervical cancer is usually asymptomatic. The first symptom that occurs is usually abnormal vaginal bleeding. Conduct a pelvic examination. Observe the patient's external genitalia for signs of inflammation, bleeding, discharge, or local skin or epithelial changes. Observe the internal genitalia. The normal cervix is pink and non-tender, has no lesions, and has a closed os. Cervical tissue with cervical cancer appears as a large reddish growth or deep ulcerating crater before any symptoms are experienced; lesions are firm and friable. The Pap smear is done before the bimanual examination. Palpate for motion tenderness of the cervix (chandelier sign); a positive chandelier sign (pain on movement) usually indicates an infection. Also examine the size, consistency (hardness may reflect invasion by neoplasm), shape, mobility (cervix should be freely movable), tenderness, and presence of masses of the uterus and adnexa. Conduct a rectal examination; palpate for abnormalities of contour, motility, and the placement of adjacent structures. Nodular thickenings of the uterosacral and cardinal ligaments may be felt.

PSYCHOSOCIAL. Uneasiness, embarrassment about a pelvic examination, or fear of the unknown may be issues for the patient. Determine the patient's level of knowledge about a pelvic examination and what the patient expects. Determine the patient's recommended Pap test screening schedule as well as how the patient obtains the results and their meaning.

If the patient requires follow-up to a positive Pap smear, assess the patient's anxiety and coping mechanisms. Stressors may be fear of the unknown, of sexual dysfunction, of cancer, or of death, or the patient may have self-concept disturbances.

Diagnostic Highlights

Test	Normal Result	Abnormality With Condition	Explanation
Pap smear	No abnormality or atypical cells noted	High-class/high-grade cytological results	Initial screening; indicates a need for further testing
Colposcopy followed by punch biopsy or cone biopsy (via the loop electrosurgical excision procedure [LEEP])	Benign results	Malignant cells	Vaginal vault and cul-de-sac are visualized; malignant diagnosis can be confirmed

Other Tests: Chest x-ray, cystoscopy, proctosigmoidoscopy, IV pyelogram, barium studies of lower bowel, ultrasound, computed tomography, magnetic resonance imaging, and lymphangiography. Visual inspection with acetic acid (vinegar) is being used to identify HPV-positive women in developing countries where a Pap smear is not available.

PRIMARY NURSING DIAGNOSIS

DIAGNOSIS. Acute pain related to postprocedure swelling and nerve damage as evidenced by self-reports of pain, grimacing, protective behavior, and/or diaphoresis

OUTCOMES. Pain level; Pain control; Pain: Disruptive effects; Knowledge: Cancer management; Self-management: Cancer

INTERVENTIONS. Analgesic administration; Pain management: Acute; Transcutaneous electric nerve stimulation (TENS); Heat/cold application

▓ PLANNING AND IMPLEMENTATION

Collaborative

Treatment depends on the stage of the cancer, the woman's age, and concern for future childbearing. Preinvasive lesions (CIS) can be treated by cervical conization, cryosurgery, laser surgery, or simple hysterectomy (if the patient's reproductive capacity is not an issue). All conservative treatments require frequent follow-up by Pap tests and colposcopy because a greater level of risk is always present for the woman who has had CIS. A cone-shaped piece of tissue is removed from the cervix after epithelial involvement is clearly outlined as described with the cone biopsy. The cone includes all the abnormal and some normal tissue. Following this procedure, the woman can still have children. The major complication is postoperative bleeding.

CRYOSURGERY. Cryosurgery is performed 1 week after the patient's last menstrual period (thereby avoiding treatment in early pregnancy). The surgeon uses a probe to freeze abnormal tissue and a small amount of normal tissue.

LASER SURGERY. For laser surgery, a carbon dioxide laser is used. Healing takes place in 3 to 6 weeks, and recurrence rates are lower than with cryosurgery.

HYSTERECTOMY. A hysterectomy, removal of the cervix and uterus, is the definitive therapy for CIS. The risks of general anesthesia and abdominal surgery are present. Major risks are infection and hemorrhage.

INVASIVE CANCER. Invasive cancer (stages I to IV) can be treated with surgery, radiotherapy, or a combination of both (Table 1). Pelvic exenteration can be done for recurrence and/or for advanced stage III or IV. Total exenteration entails the removal of the pelvic viscera, including the bladder, rectosigmoid, and all the reproductive organs. Irradiation of metastatic areas is done to provide local control and decrease symptoms.

• TABLE 1 Treatment Alternatives for Invasive Cervical Cancer

STAGE	TREATMENT ALTERNATIVE
0 (CIS)	May be managed conservatively with cryosurgery, laser ablation, and loop excision followed by lifelong surveillance
I	May be managed conservatively (conization), with simple hysterectomy and close follow-up, or may be treated as stage II; choice of treatment depends on substaging and extent of disease; if the cervix remains in place, patients need lifelong surveillance. Radical vaginal trachelectomy is a fertility-preserving procedure that recently has been used for small invasive cancers.
II	Surgery (total abdominal hysterectomy [TAH] or radical hysterectomy with bilateral pelvic lymphadenopathy) and radiotherapy are treatments of choice; positive pelvic nodes usually receive full pelvic radiation postoperatively.
III	Radiation with chemotherapy (cisplatin)
IV	Radiation alone may be used for palliation or radiation with systemic or regional chemotherapy (paclitaxel and cisplatin, or other agents)

Note that stages have several substages.

RADIATION THERAPY. Radiation therapy may be internal (radium applications to the cervix), external, and interstitial (by the use of cesium). Radiation cystitis, proctitis, and fistula formation (vesicovaginal) are major complications. Radiation sickness (nausea, vomiting, diarrhea, malaise, fever) may be a result of a systemic reaction to the breakdown and reabsorption of cell proteins. Internal radiation results in some cramping because of dilation of the cervix and in a foul-smelling vaginal discharge because of cell destruction. The patient who receives intracavity radiation (brachytherapy) is placed on bedrest and is able only to roll from side to side so as not to dislodge the implant. Vaginal packing, a urinary catheter, and pretreatment enemas plus a low-residue diet are designed to keep healthy tissue from the implant. Smoking increases the side effects from radiation, and patients who smoke are encouraged to stop smoking.

Pharmacologic Highlights

Medication or Drug Class	Dosage	Description	Rationale
Cisplatin, paclitaxel, ifosfamide, topotecan, hydroxyurea, fluorouracil, irinotecan	Depends on the patient's condition, progress of the disease, and if other chemotherapeutic agents are given	Antineoplastic	Used to treat or stabilize the disease; 38% response rate documented; can also be used in combination with other chemotherapeutic agents
Acetaminophen, NSAIDs, opioids, combinations of opioid/NSAIDs	Depends on the drug and the patient's condition and tolerance	Analgesics	Analgesic chosen is determined by the severity of the patient's pain

Independent

Experts note that HPV vaccines prevent HPV infection and are approved for girls and women 9 to 26 years of age and males from 9 to 15 years. Provide information to young women and families when appropriate. Teaching about and providing access to regular Pap screening tests for high-risk and other women are important preventive interventions. The importance of regular Pap smears cannot be overstated because cervical CIS is 100% curable. Embarrassment, modesty, and cultural values may make seeking a gynecological examination more difficult for some women. Provide clear explanations and respect the patient's modesty.

When a patient requires surgery, prepare the patient mentally and physically for the surgery and the postoperative period. Be certain to teach the patient about vaginal discharges that may follow a surgical procedure. Teach the patient that they will probably have to refrain from douching, using tampons, and coitus until healing occurs. Discuss any changes that may affect the patient's sexual function or elimination mechanisms. Explain to the patient that they will feel fatigued and should gradually increase activity but should not do heavy lifting or strenuous or rough activity or sit for long periods. Encourage the patient to explore feelings and concerns about the experience and its implications for the patient's life and lifestyle. Provide the patient who has undergone a hysterectomy with information about what to expect.

If internal radiation (brachytherapy) is the treatment, the primary focus of the nursing interventions is to prepare the patient for the treatment, to promote comfort, and to lessen the sense of isolation during the treatment. Explain to the patient and significant others the reason for the time-restricted visits while the insert is in place. Nursing care is of shorter duration and of essential nature only during this time; therefore, ensure that before the insertion of the implant, the patient has a bath and clean bed linen. Decrease the patient's feelings of isolation by providing diversionary activities and frequent interaction from a safe distance. If the patient has external radiation, teach the patient about how the treatment is given, how the skin is prepared, and how blood tests to monitor white blood cell count are done. Explain that the patient's immunity to common colds and other illnesses is lessened, and teach the proper use of antiemetics and antidiarrheals.

Evidence-Based Practice and Health Policy

Wu, J., Huang, Y., Tergas, A., Melamed, A., Khoury-Collada, F., Hou, J., St. Clair, C., Ananth, C., Hershman, D., & Wright, J. (2020). The effect of guideline-concordant care in mitigating insurance status disparities in cervical cancer. *Gynecologic Oncology, 159*, 309–316.

- The authors evaluated whether the receipt of evidence-based care could mitigate survival disparities among Medicaid recipients and uninsured women with cervical cancer. Using the National Cancer Database to identify women with cervical cancer treated from 2004 to 2016, the authors applied eight quality metrics and examined survival outcomes that were stratified by insurance status and stage. They also compared survival outcomes of the overall cohort to one that was perfectly adherent to all quality metrics. A total of 103,400 patients were identified; 47.0% of patients had private insurance, 21.5% had Medicaid, and 9.2% were uninsured.
- Medicaid and uninsured patients were significantly less likely than privately insured patients to receive timely completion of radiation and timely initiation of treatment, less likely to receive lymph node assessment and primary chemoradiation, and had an increased risk of mortality compared to privately insured patients. Medicaid and uninsured women who received guideline-concordant care were still at an increased risk of death compared to women with private insurance. Additionally, uninsured patients were significantly less likely to receive treatment for locally advanced disease. Medicaid and uninsured patients were less likely to receive evidence-based care and were at increased risk of mortality at all stages compared to privately insured patients. The receipt of quality care does not eliminate insurance status-based disparities among women with cervical cancer.

DOCUMENTATION GUIDELINES

- Physical findings: Pain and discomfort; type, color, and amount of vaginal discharge; appearance of wounds or ulcers; urinary elimination; bowel movement
- Emotional response: Coping, fears, body image, response to examination, strategies to support modesty; partner's response to illness
- Response to treatment: Conization, cryosurgery, laser surgery, hysterectomy; presence of complications

DISCHARGE AND HOME HEALTHCARE GUIDELINES

MEDICATIONS. Be sure the patient and family understand any pain medication prescribed, including dosage, route, action, and side effects.

FOLLOW-UP. Make sure the patient knows all the postprocedure complications. Provide a phone number to call if any complications occur. Ensure that the patient understands the need for ongoing Pap smears if appropriate. Vaginal cytological studies are recommended at 4-month intervals for 2 years, every 6 months for 3 years, and then annually.

Cervical Insufficiency

DRG Category:	833
Mean LOS:	2.6 days
Description:	MEDICAL: Other Antepartum Diagnoses Without Operating Room Procedures Without Complication or Comorbidity or Major Complication or Comorbidity
DRG Category:	819
Mean LOS:	2.3 days
Description:	MEDICAL: Other Antepartum Diagnoses With Operating Room Procedures Without Complication or Comorbidity or Major Complication or Comorbidity

Cervical insufficiency (CI), previously known as cervical incompetence, is a condition in which the cervix spontaneously dilates during the second trimester or early in the third trimester of pregnancy, which results in expulsion of the uterine contents. Because the spontaneous dilation typically occurs in the fourth or fifth month of gestation before the point of fetal viability, the fetus dies unless dilation can be arrested. Incidence of an insufficient cervix has been estimated to be between 0.1% and 2% of all pregnancies. The insufficient cervix has abnormal musculature, with an increased proportion of smooth muscle tissue, which results in a loss of sphincter tone. When the pressure of the expanding uterine contents becomes greater than the ability of the cervical sphincter to remain closed, the cervix suddenly relaxes, allowing effacement and dilation to proceed.

The cervical dilation that occurs with cervical insufficiency is typically rapid, relatively painless, and accompanied by minimal bleeding. These features help distinguish the syndrome clinically from other causes of cervical dilation or bleeding, such as preterm labor, placental abruption, and placenta previa. Complications include premature birth and fetal loss.

CAUSES

Normally in pregnancy, the cervix develops increased tensile strength from fusion and recanalization of a distal duct system by 20 weeks' gestation. Congenital structural defects of the lower genital tract can cause cervical insufficiency depending on the nature of the defect in tensile strength at the cervicoisthmic junction. Such defects were common in women who were exposed to diethylstilbestrol (DES) in utero when their mothers were given the hormone in the 1950s and 1960s to prevent spontaneous abortion. Another important risk for insufficient cervix is previous cervical trauma, such as excessive mechanical dilation during previous obstetric procedures, removal of tissue during previous cervical biopsy, and improperly healed lacerations from previous deliveries. The risk of CI increases with the number of induced abortions. Hormonal factors can also contribute to CI, particularly excessive levels of relaxin, which may cause loss of normal cervical resistance to dilation. Relaxin levels may be higher than usual during some multiple gestations, increasing the risk of CI in these pregnancies.

GENETIC CONSIDERATIONS

Genetic factors may contribute to CI. The HLA-DR genotype has been associated with recurrent late spontaneous abortions and very preterm births related to CI. Recent evidence has shown that single nucleotide polymorphisms in the *IL6* and *MBL2* genes may increase the risk of preterm birth due to cervical insufficiency.

SEX AND LIFE SPAN CONSIDERATIONS

Any woman of childbearing age may experience CI, although older childbearing women may be at greater risk because they are more likely to have experienced previous trauma to the cervix.

HEALTH DISPARITIES AND SEXUAL/GENDER MINORITY HEALTH

In a study of more than 34,000 women in Northern California, the authors found that approximately 1% had CI. Black women had a significantly higher rate of CI (3.2%) as compared to White women (0.9%) as well as higher rates of preterm births. The authors suggested that a higher rate of CI may help explain the higher rates of preterm births among Black women nationally (Tanner et al., 2018). Sexual and gender minority status has no known effect on the risk for cervical insufficiency.

GLOBAL HEALTH CONSIDERATIONS

No data are available.

❖ ASSESSMENT

HISTORY. Obtain a detailed obstetric and medical history. Ask about the date of the last menstrual period to determine the gestational age of the fetus. Inquire about risk factors related to cervical insufficiency. Pregnant people experiencing cervical dilation because of cervical insufficiency may have symptoms that range from feelings of low pelvic pressure or cramping to vaginal bleeding, loss of amniotic fluid, and spontaneous passage of the fetus and placenta. Patients who experience cervical insufficiency frequently report a history of previous second-trimester pregnancy loss, induced abortion, dilation and curettage, cervical biopsy, or prenatal exposure to DES. A history of fertility problems may also be reported.

PHYSICAL EXAMINATION. Many patients are **asymptomatic** until they experience premature rupture of the membranes. Inspect the perineum for bleeding and fluid. Patients may have **pink or dark red spotting, increased vaginal discharge, passage of the mucous plug,** or **leakage of amniotic fluid**. Some report pelvic pressure, cramping, and/or back pain. Cervical insufficiency can be predicted by examining the cervical length with serial transvaginal ultrasound. A cervical length of less than 25 mm between 16 and 24 weeks' gestation indicates potential cervical insufficiency and a risk of preterm birth. A cervical length greater than 35 mm between 18 and 24 weeks' gestation is correlated with preterm birth in 4% of patients. Thus, a shortened cervical length is an excellent predictor of cervical insufficiency and eventual preterm birth, especially in high-risk women. Perform a sterile vaginal examination. The cervix is effaced and dilated, with progression in the absence of painful uterine contractions. A bulging amniotic sac or the fetal presenting part may be palpated through the cervix during the vaginal examination.

PSYCHOSOCIAL. The patient who experiences pregnancy loss because of an insufficient cervix is in a state of psychological crisis. If this is a first episode, the patient is likely to be bewildered because of the rapid progress of dilation and the unexpectedness of the loss. In patients who have experienced infertility or previous fetal loss, psychosocial reactions may be complicated by unresolved feelings or cumulative effects of grief experiences. Anger, fear, numbness, guilt, severe grief, and feelings of loss of control are common in both the pregnant person and significant others.

Diagnostic Highlights

General Comments: Diagnosis is clinically based on a history of habitual second-trimester abortions, painless cervical dilation, and spontaneously ruptured membranes.

Test	Normal Result	Abnormality With Condition	Explanation
Ultrasound (transvaginal)	Long, noneffaced, closed, internal cervical os; cervical length > 35 mm (at 18–24 wk)	Cervix shortening; dilation of the internal os noted; cervical length < 25 mm (at 16–24 wk)	Cervix will usually shorten or efface before dilation; the internal os dilates before the external os; thus, serial imaging can alert one to cervical insufficiency and potential loss

PRIMARY NURSING DIAGNOSIS

DIAGNOSIS. Risk for maladaptive grieving as evidenced by blaming, despair, distress, psychological distress, and/or personal growth

OUTCOMES. Grief resolution; Guilt resolution

INTERVENTIONS. Grief work facilitation: Perinatal death; Guilt work facilitation; Active listening; Presence; Truth telling; Support group

✳ PLANNING AND IMPLEMENTATION

Collaborative

Medical management depends on the degree of cervical dilation that has occurred at the time the patient is examined. In asymptomatic patients with a prior preterm birth, serial transvaginal cervical length screening is performed at 16 weeks' gestation and repeated every 2 weeks until 26 to 28 weeks' gestation. If dilation is progressing rapidly or is complete, preparation is made for delivery of the fetus and placenta. As with any spontaneous abortion, careful evaluation of bleeding is required to detect hemorrhage. Dilation and curettage may be necessary to control bleeding if placental fragments are retained in the uterus.

In less advanced dilation, particularly if the membranes are not ruptured, the patient may be maintained on bedrest in the Trendelenburg position in an attempt to prolong the pregnancy. Usually, if the pregnant person is no more than 23 weeks' gestation, cervical dilation is no greater than 3 cm, the membranes are intact, and bleeding and cramping are not present, a cerclage may be used. In this surgical procedure, a purse-string suture is placed in the cervix at the level of the internal os and tightened to prevent dilation by mechanically closing the os. Either the Shirodkar or the McDonald technique can be used to create the cerclage. Prior to placement of the cerclage, an ultrasound is done to confirm a live fetus and to rule out gross fetal anomalies. In any future pregnancies of women with a history of cervical insufficiency, a cerclage may be placed prophylactically at 14 to 18 weeks' gestation. Prophylactic cerclages have an 85% to 90% success rate of reducing preterm births. For primiparas with risk factors for cervical insufficiency, cervical cerclage may be necessary in only 50% of the cases. All women with risk factors should be assessed with serial transvaginal ultrasound for cervical length. Local anesthesia is usually used during cerclage placement, although regional or light general anesthesia may occasionally be chosen. After a cerclage has been placed, assessment for signs of labor, rupture of membranes, infection in pregnant person, and fetal well-being continues for the remainder of the pregnancy. The cerclage is removed at or near term, with vaginal delivery typically following shortly thereafter. Bleeding, uterine contractions, chorioamnionitis, and ruptured membranes are all contraindications to placement of a cerclage. Transabdominal cerclage is used for patients with extremely short cervixes or those who have had a failed transvaginal cerclage. Robotic-assisted laparoscopic surgery has had some success in preliminary studies.

Recent studies have suggested that intramuscular progesterone supplementation with 17 alpha-hydroxyprogesterone caproate (Makena) may prevent recurrent preterm birth in pregnant people with a history of preterm deliveries. Otherwise, pharmacological management of cervical insufficiency is not indicated until after the loss of the fetus and placenta have occurred.

Pharmacologic Highlights

Medication or Drug Class	Dosage	Description	Rationale
Oxytocin (Pitocin)	10–20 U IV after passage of tissue	Oxytocic	Stimulates uterine contractions to decrease postpartum bleeding
RhD immunoglobulin (RhoGAM)	1,500 IU IV or IM within 72 hr (prepared by blood bank)	Immune serum	Prevents Rh isoimmunizations in future pregnancies; given if pregnant person is Rh-negative and infant is Rh-positive

Independent

Nursing care for patients with cervical insufficiency centers on teaching, psychological support, and prevention of injury to the pregnant person and fetus. If a transvaginal ultrasound is going to be done to measure cervical length, be sure the patient has an empty bladder. Teach the patient about the condition and alert the patient to the potential for injury of the cervix if labor proceeds with a cerclage in place. Symptoms of labor, rupture of the membranes, and infection should be explained to the pregnant person, with emphasis on the need to report such symptoms promptly if they occur. Consider the patient's support systems and coping mechanisms if the pregnancy is continuing. Determine if the patient has the social and financial resources to manage a difficult pregnancy and make appropriate referrals if they are needed.

Evidence-Based Practice and Health Policy

Moore, S., & Cattapan, A. (2020). Women's reproductive health and "failure speak." *Canadian Medical Association Journal, 192*, E325–E326.

- The authors note that patients do not always hear or understand what providers say, and certain words have negative connotations. For pregnant people who have pregnancy challenges, words such as "fertility failure," "failure to progress," and "failure to maintain a pregnancy" can result in confusion, a feeling of being betrayed by one's own body, and disempowerment. The patient may not understand why the patient failed.
- Failure speak can intensify the stigma and alienation for patients having difficulty with becoming pregnant or who have pregnancy complications. Changing medical jargon will take time, but healthcare providers can begin by using alternatives such as the cervix is "weakened," not "incompetent," and the pelvis is "small," not "inadequate." The authors

suggest that such language changes acknowledge patients as authorities and autonomous actors in their experiences of reproductive health.

DOCUMENTATION GUIDELINES

• Continuation of pregnancy: Cervical dilation and effacement; station of fetal presenting part; intactness of membranes; absence of bleeding, contractions, or foul discharge; maternal temperature; fetal heart tones and presence of fetal movement if perceptible
• After spontaneous abortion: Pain; color, odor, and amount of bleeding; firmness and position of fundus; bladder function; vital signs
• Indicators of psychological status: Affect, verbalizations of feelings, grieving behaviors, presence of support people, acceptance of anticipatory guidance and resource materials, effectiveness of coping strategies

DISCHARGE AND HOME HEALTHCARE GUIDELINES

FOLLOWING CERCLAGE PLACEMENT. Be sure the patient understands the importance of immediately reporting any signs of labor or infection. If vaginal rest has been prescribed, teach the patient to avoid vaginal intercourse, orgasm, douching, and tampon use. The patient should also avoid breast stimulation (causes uterine contractions), heavy lifting, and heavy housework. If antibiotics are prescribed, teach the patient to finish the prescription even though the patient feels well. If bedrest has been prescribed, assist the patient and family to develop strategies for maintaining bedrest at home. Ensure that the patient understands and can carry out plans for follow-up surveillance and care. Alert the patient of the signs and symptoms of preterm labor.

FOLLOWING DELIVERY OF VIABLE INFANT. Be sure the patient understands the likelihood of repeated cervical insufficiency and the possibility of prophylactic cerclage placement in future pregnancies.

FOLLOWING PREGNANCY LOSS. Teach the patient to report signs of infection or hemorrhage. Be sure the patient understands the need for pelvic rest until the follow-up gynecological appointment. Provide the patient and family with resources to support grieving, including anticipatory guidance, reading lists or materials, contact information for support groups, and referral to counseling if desired.

Chlamydial Infections

DRG Category:	728
Mean LOS:	3.6 days
Description:	MEDICAL: Inflammation of the Male Reproductive System Without Major Complication or Comorbidity
DRG Category:	758
Mean LOS:	4.4 days
Description:	MEDICAL: Infections, Female Reproductive System With Complication or Comorbidity

Infection with *Chlamydia trachomatis* is the most common sexually transmitted infection (STI) in the United States today, with approximately 4 million cases reported annually (Centers for Disease Control and Prevention [CDC], 2021). While chlamydial infections are reportable in all

50 states, underreporting of this STI is substantial due to the number of individuals who may have the infection and not know it. Because 80% of women and 50% of men with chlamydial infections are asymptomatic, they transmit the disease but are unaware that they harbor the bacteria. Untreated infections in women can result in cervicitis, endometritis, acute salpingitis, bartholinitis, irregular menses, ectopic pregnancy, pelvic inflammatory disease (PID), and infertility. Untreated infections in men can result in nongonococcal urethritis (NGU), epididymitis, or prostatitis. Infections in either gender can result in proctitis; lymphogranuloma venereum (LGV); and, potentially, infertility and sterility.

During pregnancy, *C trachomatis* may be transmitted from pregnant person to fetus, which may cause premature rupture of the membranes, premature labor, and increased fetal morbidity and mortality. Pregnant people who deliver vaginally or by cesarean section can transmit the bacteria to their infants. These newborns can develop otitis media, conjunctivitis, blindness, meningitis, gastroenteritis, respiratory infections, and pneumonia. Because pregnant people are often asymptomatic, medical personnel are unaware that the pregnant person to infant transmission has occurred until infants become very ill.

CAUSES

C trachomatis is an obligate (dependent on the host for energy), gram-negative, intracellular bacterium with several different immunotypes. It is usually spread by sexual activity (oral, anal, or vaginal intercourse) or to the newborn during childbirth. It resembles a virus in that it requires a tissue culture for isolation, but like a bacteria, it has RNA and DNA and is susceptible to antibiotics. The chlamydial infection exists in two forms: The elementary bodies are the infectious particles that enter uninfected cells, and the reticulate bodies are the active forms of the organism that reproduce and form more elementary bodies that are released from the bursting infected cell and can then infect other cells. Replication begins only 12 hours after invasion. The pathogen invades and reproduces inside the cells that line the cervix, endometrium, fallopian tubes, and urethra. Symptoms can occur after a 1- to 3-week incubation period; however, overt symptoms often occur late in the disease.

GENETIC CONSIDERATIONS

Heritable immune responses could be protective or increase susceptibility.

SEX AND LIFE SPAN CONSIDERATIONS

Both men and women are susceptible to chlamydial infection, but their symptoms differ. Although the occurrence of chlamydial infection is related more to sexual practices than to age, many women with chlamydial infection are young, under 25 years of age, and single. With more teens engaging in sexual activity, more male and female adolescents are contracting infections. Depending on the population, 5% to 35% of pregnant people are infected with *C trachomatis*. Hence, the U.S. Preventive Services Task Force recommends that all pregnant people under the age of 25 years be screened for chlamydial infections.

HEALTH DISPARITIES AND SEXUAL/GENDER MINORITY HEALTH

Women living in poverty, who have experienced trauma, or who are homeless with no prenatal care are at high-risk for chlamydial infections. The rate of infection is also highest (17%) in females with a history of gonorrhea or chlamydia in the previous 12 months. Rates are the highest in Black and in Native American/Pacific Islander women, with Black women experiencing a rate six times that of White women (Cha et al., 2019; Lieberman et al., 2020). People involved in sex work, including men who have sex with men, are at high risk for chlamydial infections. The CDC notes that STIs are increasing among gay and bisexual men. The CDC (2021) recommends that gay, bisexual, and other men who have sex with men be tested for rectal chlamydial infection if they have receptive anal sex in the previous year and penal chlamydial infection if they had insertive anal sex or received oral sex in the previous year.

GLOBAL HEALTH CONSIDERATIONS

The World Health Organization (WHO, 2019) reports that more than 1 million STIs are acquired every day, and each year 131 million people are infected with chlamydia. Chlamydia prevalence in women reported by WHO ranges from 7.0% in the region of the Americas (including the United States) to 1.5% in the Southeast Asia region. European prevalence for women is 3.2%.

✖ ASSESSMENT

HISTORY. Although sexual activity is potentially a sensitive topic, it is critical to obtain a detailed sexual and gynecological history. Inquire about the number of partners, use of barrier protection and birth control measures, participation in vaginal, oral, and/or anal intercourse, and previous STIs. Most patients who present with *C trachomatis* have a history of multiple sex partners and engaging in sexual intercourse without the use of barrier protection. Often, patients are simultaneously positive for gonorrhea. Inquire if the patient has any thin or purulent discharge, burning or frequent urination, mucus-covered stools, lower abdominal pain, dyspareunia (painful sexual intercourse), headache, nausea, vomiting, chills, or bleeding after intercourse. Often, patients are asymptomatic, and some may complain only of an increase in vaginal discharge. Male patients may report dysuria, urinary frequency, and pruritus. Ask patients if they are experiencing any diarrhea, tenesmus, or pruritus, any of which indicates that the infection involves the rectum. All pregnant people should be screened for chlamydia.

PHYSICAL EXAMINATION. Patients may be asymptomatic. Common signs are **dysuria, yellow discharge, abnormal vaginal bleeding,** and **pain with sexual intercourse**. For females, inspect the vagina, cervix, and labia and note any mucopurulent discharge. Bartholin glands may be involved. Gently touch the cervix; note any bleeding (friable cervix). Fever usually accompanies PID. Inspect males for purulent discharge at the urinary meatus. Scrotal swelling occurs if the organism has caused epididymitis. Inspect the anus for discharge and excoriation. If LGV is present, ulcerative lesions on the cervix, vagina, labia, anal/rectal area, or penis may occur. Enlarged lymph nodes also can be palpated in the groin. If these nodes rupture, they secrete a thick yellow granular substance.

PSYCHOSOCIAL. Assess the patient's knowledge of STIs and the implications. Assess the patient's ability to cope with having an STI. The diagnosis of an STI can be very upsetting to people who believe they were involved in monogamous or committed relationships. Patients may feel embarrassed and guilty about their condition. Inquire about the patient's ability to obtain condoms. Identify all partners with whom the patient has been sexually active so that they can be examined and treated. Assess the patient's support system; this is especially important if the patient is pregnant. Pregnant people may be concerned about the fetus and need reassurance about the results of treatment.

Diagnostic Highlights

General Comments: The preferred method of testing for chlamydia is the nucleic acid amplification tests (NAATs). These tests have an increased sensitivity and are more comfortable for the patient because the preferred specimen is a first-void urine or vaginal swab. Enzyme-linked immunosorbent assay (ELISA) and antigen detection by direct fluorescent antibody slide staining tissue culture may also be used. The ELISA test has a sensitivity of approximately 85%.

(highlight box continues on page 284)

Diagnostic Highlights (continued)

Test	Normal Result	Abnormality With Condition	Explanation
Cervical tissue culture (females); urethral tissue culture (males)	Negative culture	Positive culture	Growth of the organism confirms the diagnosis
NAATs (urine specimen or vaginal swab)	Negative	Positive signal	Detects chlamydia from DNA/RNA presence

Other Tests: Because symptoms of gonorrhea resemble a chlamydial infection, diagnosis is often made based on a symptomatic patient with a negative gonorrhea culture. HIV testing, Papanicolaou smear, pregnancy test.

PRIMARY NURSING DIAGNOSIS

DIAGNOSIS. Risk for infection as evidenced by dysuria, vaginal discharge, and/or dysparaunia

OUTCOMES. Infection severity; Symptom severity; Immune status; Knowledge: Infection management; Risk control: Sexually transmitted diseases

INTERVENTIONS. Infection control; Infection protection; Teaching: Safe sex; Medication management; Teaching: Prescribed medication; Fertility preservation

PLANNING AND IMPLEMENTATION

Collaborative

Chlamydial infections can easily be cured with oral antibiotics, and patients are rarely hospitalized. Patients need to know to continue to take medication as ordered, even if the symptoms subside. Follow-up with both partners is recommended to ensure that neither partner is still infected. Patients should abstain from sexual intercourse until they are infection free.

Pharmacologic Highlights

Medication or Drug Class	Dosage	Description	Rationale
Doxycycline: Recommended as first-line drug	100 mg PO bid for 7 days	Broad-spectrum antibiotic (tetracycline)	Effective in eliminating C trachomatis
Azithromycin (all patients): Recommended as first-line drug	1 g PO single dose	Antibiotic (macrolide)	As effective as doxycycline
Erythromycin (pregnant people)	400–800 mg PO qid for 7 days	Antibiotic (macrolide)	Safe for pregnant women to take, not as effective as doxycycline in eliminating C trachomatis
Levofloxacin, ofloxacin	Levofloxacin 500 mg PO daily for 7 days; ofloxacin 300 mg PO bid for 7 days	Antibiotic	Treatment of infection
Erythromycin (infants)	Ointment to conjunctiva sac after delivery	Anti-infective	Prophylaxis of neonatal conjunctivitis

Independent

Because patients are often asymptomatic, nurses need to identify those patients at risk for chlamydial infections and recommend screening. Prevention is an important nursing intervention. Explain to patients that monogamous relationships with uninfected partners, use of mechanical barriers, and simultaneously treating the partner to prevent reinfection are ways to prevent transmission of *C trachomatis*. Emphasize that it is possible for them to carry and transmit the bacteria even if they are asymptomatic.

Because a chlamydial infection is easily cured by oral antibiotics, teach the patient about taking the medications properly. Instruct patients to take all medication until the course of treatment is finished even if the symptoms subside. Explain that the patient should abstain from intercourse until all medication is gone to prevent reinfection. For discomfort, teach the patient about warm sitz baths and taking prescribed analgesics as ordered.

Evidence-Based Practice and Health Policy

Dretler, A., Trolard, A., Bergquist, E., Cooper, B., Liang, S., Stoner, B., & Reno, H. (2020). The influence of race and sex on gonorrhea and chlamydia treatment in the emergency department. *American Journal of Emergency Medicine, 38*, 566–570.

- The authors conducted a retrospective chart review and analysis of data from a high-volume emergency department in a Midwestern teaching hospital to determine which patients were undertreated and overtreated. Patients were treated based on symptoms and physical examination and received a gonorrhea/chlamydia nucleic acid amplification test.
- Black patients were more likely to be overtreated as compared to White patients. Females were more likely to be undertreated when positive for infection compared with male patients and less likely to be overtreated when negative for infection. The authors concluded that females with gonorrhea or chlamydia are at a higher risk of not obtaining proper treatment compared to men. The discrepancy may be due to women having more subtle symptoms than men. Consequences of the undertreatment of women can result in pelvic inflammatory disease, chronic pain, and infertility.

DOCUMENTATION GUIDELINES

- Screening done and results if available; note if a female patient is pregnant
- Physical signs and symptoms: Discharge (amount, color, odor, location), pain, bleeding, swelling, dysuria
- Patient's reaction to the diagnosis of an STI
- Patient's understanding of diagnosis, treatment, and prevention

DISCHARGE AND HOME HEALTHCARE GUIDELINES

MEDICATIONS. Be sure the patient understands the correct dosage, route, and time of the medication, as well as the importance of taking all prescribed medication even if the symptoms resolve. Emphasize any dietary restrictions.

PREVENTION. Teach the patient about the importance of barrier contraception, especially latex condoms. Often, patients on oral contraceptives do not realize that although they probably will not get pregnant, they are not protecting themselves from STIs. Educate female patients that contrary to popular belief, douching increases the risk of infection. Emphasize the importance of follow-up visits to ensure that the infection has resolved. Encourage the patient to enforce follow-up of all sexual partners and to refrain from intercourse during antibiotic therapy to prevent reinfection, or for at least 1 week. While experts recommend that all women less than 25 years of age be screened annually for chlamydia, this recommendation for routine screening does not include men. Identification of high-risk groups is important.

There is a direct correlation between gender-based violence and chlamydial infections. Other high-risk groups are teenagers who are incarcerated or detained.

COMPLICATIONS. Teach the patient about potential long-term complications, such as infertility and sterility if reinfection occurs.

Cholecystitis and Cholelithiasis

DRG Category:	412
Mean LOS:	6.4 days
Description:	SURGICAL: Cholecystectomy With Common Duct Exploration With Complication or Comorbidity
DRG Category:	418
Mean LOS:	4.3 days
Description:	SURGICAL: Laparoscopic Cholecystectomy Without Common Duct Exploration With Complication or Comorbidity

Cholecystitis is an inflammation of the gallbladder wall; it may be either acute or chronic. It is almost always associated with cholelithiasis, or gallstones, which most commonly lodge in the cystic duct and cause obstruction. Biliary sludge is a reversible suspension of particles such as crystals and salts that form a thick liquid derived from bile and can lead to cholelithiasis. Silent gallstones may also occur and are so common that most people may have them at some time. Only stones that are symptomatic require treatment. In developed countries, the prevalence is 10% to 20%, and in the United States, approximately 20 million people have gallstones. Cholecystectomy is the most common major surgical procedure performed by general surgeons in the United States.

Gallstones are most commonly made of either cholesterol or bilirubin and calcium. If gallstones obstruct the neck of the gallbladder or the cystic duct, the gallbladder can become infected with bacteria such as *Escherichia coli*. The primary agents, however, are not the bacteria but mediators such as members of the prostaglandin family. The gallbladder becomes enlarged up to two to three times normal size, thus decreasing tissue perfusion. If the gallbladder becomes ischemic as well as infected, necrosis, perforation, pancreatitis, and sepsis can follow.

CAUSES

Cholesterol is the major component of most gallstones in the United States, leading to speculation that a high-fat diet is the explanation for their increased frequency. Supporting theories that point to a high-fat diet note that acute attacks of cholelithiasis may be precipitated by fasting and sudden weight loss. Risk factors include older age, female sex, obesity, weight loss, and pregnancy. Cholecystitis is associated with debilitation, major traumatic stress (injury, sepsis, major surgery), diabetes, sickle cell disease, and HIV infection.

GENETIC CONSIDERATIONS

Cholecystitis and cholelithiasis appear to be caused by the actions of several genes and the environment working together. It is estimated that 50% to 70% of patients with cholecystitis have a positive family history of the disease. Studies suggest that genetic factors account for approximately 30% of susceptibility to gallstone formation. While specific genetic mechanisms have not been elucidated, many candidate genes (e.g., *ABCB4* and *ABCG8*), including those that increase susceptibility to risk factors such as obesity, are under investigation.

SEX AND LIFE SPAN CONSIDERATIONS

The incidence of gallbladder disease increases with age in women and men. Most patients are adult women, often women who have borne several children and gained weight as they grow older. During pregnancy, increased levels of progesterone may lead to biliary stasis and increased rates of gallbladder disease. Because there is a tendency for gallbladder disease to be familial, some young people of both sexes with a familial history as well as young women who have taken oral contraceptives can be affected. Children with sickle cell disease, serious illness, and hemolytic conditions as well as those on total parenteral nutrition are at higher risk for gallbladder disease than other children.

HEALTH DISPARITIES AND SEXUAL/GENDER MINORITY HEALTH

Northern Europeans (Scandinavian) and Hispanic persons have increased prevalence as compared to other groups. Prevalence of gallstones is high in White persons and low in people of Asian and African descent; however, Black individuals with sickle cell disease may have gallstones at a younger age than other groups. Health disparities may exist with respect to the implementation of guidelines for diagnostic testing and standards of care. Female gender, Black race, increased number of morbidities, Medicare payer status, urban-teaching hospital location, and low household income may lead to reduced implementation of standards of care (Chouairi et al., 2021 [see Evidence-Based Practice and Health Policy]). Those factors limit evidence-based care and lead to poorer surgical outcomes. Sexual and gender minority status has no known effect on the risk for cholecystitis and cholelithiasis.

GLOBAL HEALTH CONSIDERATIONS

Several European studies indicate a greater incidence in females and in those older than age 60 years. Cholelithiasis has an increased prevalence among people of Scandinavian, Western European, and Hispanic ancestry and decreased prevalence in people living in Sub-Saharan Africa and Southeast Asia.

✳ ASSESSMENT

HISTORY. Cholecystitis often begins as a mild intolerance to fatty food. The patient experiences discomfort after a meal, sometimes with nausea and vomiting, flatulence, and an elevated temperature. Over a period of several months or even years, symptoms progressively become more severe. Ask the patient about the pattern of attacks; some mistake severe gallbladder attacks for a heart attack until they recall similar, less severe episodes than have preceded it. An acute attack of cholecystitis is often associated with gallstones, or cholelithiasis. The classic symptom is pain in the right upper quadrant that may radiate to the right scapula, called biliary colic. Onset is usually sudden, with the duration from less than 1 to more than 6 hours. If the flow of bile has become obstructed, the patient may pass clay-colored stools and dark urine.

PHYSICAL EXAMINATION. The most common symptom is **upper abdominal pain**. The pain may radiate to the right shoulder or scapula and may be accompanied by **nausea and vomiting**. The patient with an acute gallbladder attack appears acutely ill, is in a great deal of discomfort, and sometimes is jaundiced. A low-grade fever is often present, especially if the disease is chronic and the walls of the gallbladder have become infected. Right upper quadrant pain is intense in acute attacks and requires no physical examination. It is often followed by residual aching or soreness for up to 24 hours. A positive Murphy sign, which is positive palpation of a distended gallbladder during inhalation, may confirm a diagnosis. Older adults may present with vague symptoms such as localized tenderness and without pain and fever. Children may also present without classic findings.

PSYCHOSOCIAL. The patient with an acute attack of cholelithiasis may be in extreme pain and very upset. The experience may be complicated by guilt if the patient has been advised by the physician in the past to cut down on fatty foods and lose weight. The attack may also be very frightening if it is confused with a heart attack.

Diagnostic Highlights

Test	Normal Result	Abnormality With Condition	Explanation
White blood cell (WBC) count	Adult males and females 4,500–11,100/mcL	Infection and inflammation elevate the WBC count	Leukocytosis; WBCs range from 12,000 to 15,000/mcL; if > 20,000, the condition may be associated with gangrene or perforation
Ultrasound scan	Normal gallbladder	Gallbladder wall thickening, peri-cholecystic fluid collections	Sensitive/specific test for cholelithiasis; identifies presence of fluid collection; preferred initial imaging test

Other Tests: Biliary scintigraphy such as hepatobiliary iminodiacetic acid (HIDA) scan can show nonfilling of the gallbladder; biliary scintigraphy and ultrasound are the diagnostic tests most commonly used. HIDA scans have sensitivity of greater than 94% and specificity 65% to 85% for acute cholecystitis. Supporting tests include phosphatase, aspartate amino transferase, lactate dehydrogenase, alkaline phosphatase, serum amylase, and serum bilirubin levels; oral cholecystogram; and computed tomography, with or without contrast. Liver function tests such as alanine aminotransferase (ALT) and aspartate aminotransferase (AST) may be used to assess if hepatitis or common bile duct obstruction are involved. An IV cholangiogram may be used to differentiate cholelithiasis from other causes of extrahepatic obstruction. Additional tests include pregnancy testing and urinalysis.

PRIMARY NURSING DIAGNOSIS

DIAGNOSIS. Acute pain related to obstruction and inflammation as evidenced by self-reports of pain, grimacing, protective behavior, and/or diaphoresis

OUTCOMES. Comfort status; Knowledge: Acute illness management; Pain control; Pain level; Symptom severity; Medication response

INTERVENTIONS. Analgesic administration; Anxiety reduction; Environmental management: Comfort; Pain management: Acute; Medication management; Patient-controlled analgesia assistance

PLANNING AND IMPLEMENTATION

Collaborative

MEDICAL. Antibiotics may be given to manage infection along with bowel rest, IV hydration, correction of electrolyte imbalances, and pain management with follow-up care. Criteria for outpatient treatment include that the patient is afebrile, with no evidence of obstruction on laboratory assessment and sonogram, no underlying medical problems, adequate pain control, and proximity to an acute care facility, if needed, from home. However, given the effectiveness of laparoscopic cholecystectomy, the only patients who will receive medical dissolution are generally those who are nonobese patients with very small cholesterol gallstones and a functioning gallbladder.

SURGICAL. There are several surgical or procedural treatment options. The one seen most commonly today is a laparoscopic cholecystectomy, which is performed early (within 48 hours of acute onset of symptoms) in the course of the disease when there is minimum inflammation at the base of the gallbladder. It is considered the standard of care for the surgical management of cholecystectomy. The procedure is performed with the abdomen distended by an injection of carbon dioxide, which lifts the abdominal wall away from the viscera and prevents injury to the peritoneum and other organs. A laparoscopic cholecystectomy is done either as an outpatient procedure or with less than 24 hours of hospitalization. After the surgery, the patient may complain of pain from the presence of residual carbon dioxide in the abdomen.

The traditional open cholecystectomy is performed on patients with large stones as well as with other abnormalities that need to be explored at the time of surgery. This procedure is particularly appropriate up to 72 hours after onset of acute cholecystitis. Timing of the operation is controversial. Early cholecystectomy has the advantage of resolving the acute condition early in its course.

Pharmacologic Highlights

Medication or Drug Class	Dosage	Description	Rationale
Antibiotics; ciprofloxacin, meropenem, imipenem/cilastatin, ampicillin/sulbactam, piperacillin/tazobactam	Varies with drug	Antibiotic regimen is focused on those appropriate for typical bowel flora (gram-negative rods and anaerobes): third-generation cephalosporin or aminoglycoside with metronidazole	Manage bacteria that are typical bowel flora
Demerol (drug of choice for pain control)	25–100 mg IM, IV	Opiates relieve pain and promote spasms of the biliary duct	Pain is severe; analgesia should be offered only after definitive diagnosis has occurred

Other Drugs: Antiemetics may be administered, particularly promethazine or prochlorperazine. If inflammation of the gallbladder has led to gallstones and obstruction of bile flow, replacement of the fat-soluble vitamins is important to supplement the diet.

Independent

During an acute attack, remain with the patient to provide comfort, to monitor the result of interventions, and to allay anxiety. Explain all procedures in short and simple terms. Provide explanations to the family and significant others.

If the patient requires surgery, the nurse's first priority is the maintenance of airway, breathing, and circulation. Although most patients return from surgery or a procedure breathing on their own, if stridor or airway obstruction occurs, create airway patency with an oral or nasal airway and notify the surgeon immediately. If the patient's breathing is inadequate, maintain breathing with a manual resuscitator bag until the surgeon makes a further evaluation. The incision from a laparoscopic cholecystectomy is small and usually heals without complications. The high incision resulting from an open cholecystectomy may make deep breathing painful, leading to shallow respirations and impaired gas exchange. Splinting the incision while encouraging the patient to cough and breathe deeply helps both pain and gas exchange. Elevate the head of the bed to reduce pressure on the diaphragm and abdomen.

Patients not undergoing surgery or a procedure need clear explanations. Explain the disease process, the possible complications, and all medications. Teach the patient to avoid high-fat foods; dairy products; and, if the patient is bothered by flatulence, gas-forming foods.

Evidence-Based Practice and Health Policy

Chouairi, F., McCarty, T., Hathorn, K., Sharma, P., Aslanian, H., Jamidar, P., Thompson, C., & Muniraj, T. (2022). Evaluation of socioeconomic and healthcare disparities on same admission cholecystectomy after endoscopic retrograde cholangiopancreatography among patients with acute gallstone pancreatitis. *Surgical Endoscopy, 36*, 274–281. https://doi.org/10.1007/s00464-020-08272-2

- Guidelines recommend that patients with acute gallstone pancreatitis receive a cholecystectomy during their initial hospital admission The aim of this study was to investigate the role of clinical and sociodemographic factors in the management of acute gallstone pancreatitis who have same admission cholecystectomy (SAC). Cases from a national database with acute gallstone pancreatitis who underwent endoscopic retrograde cholangiopancreatography (ERCP) during hospitalization between 2008 and 2014 were reviewed and classified by treatment strategy.
- A total of 205,012 cases were analyzed. A majority (53.4%) of cases that did not receive SAC were at urban teaching hospitals. Although length of stay was longer with higher associated costs for patients with SAC, mortality was decreased. Multivariable regression demonstrated female gender, Black race, increased number of morbidities, Medicare payer status, urban teaching hospital location, and household income decreased the odds of undergoing same admission cholecystectomy.

DOCUMENTATION GUIDELINES

- Pain: Location, duration, quality, response to pain medications
- Type and amount of drainage if Penrose drain or T tube is present; vital signs
- Condition of surgical incision and surrounding skin

DISCHARGE AND HOME HEALTHCARE GUIDELINES

PATIENT TEACHING. After a laparoscopic cholecystectomy, provide discharge instructions to a family member or another responsible adult as well as to the patient because the patient goes home within 24 hours after surgery. Explain the possibility of abdominal and shoulder pain caused by the instillation of carbon dioxide so that if the pain occurs, the patient will not experience unnecessary anxiety about a heart attack. Teach the patient to avoid submerging the abdomen in the bathtub for the first 48 hours, to take the prescribed antibiotics to provide further assurance against infection, and to watch the incisions for signs of infection. Following a 3- to 5-day hospital stay for an open cholecystectomy, instruct the patient on the care of the abdomen wound, including changing the dressing and protection of any drains.

POSTOPERATIVE INSTRUCTIONS. Reinforce pain control and deep-breathing exercises until the incision is completely healed. The patient may need instruction on control of elimination after this surgery. The continued use of opiate-type analgesics for 7 to 10 days may necessitate the use of laxatives or suppositories, which are generally prescribed by the physician before discharge. Explain that gradual resumption of both a normal diet and activity aids normal elimination. Instruct the patient to report to the physician if any new symptoms occur, such as the appearance of jaundice accompanied by pain, chills and fever, dark urine, or light-colored stools. Usually, the patient has no complications and is able to resume normal activity within a few weeks.

Chorioamnionitis

DRG Category:	786
Mean LOS:	6.3 days
Description:	SURGICAL: Cesarean Section Without Sterilization With Major Complication or Comorbidity
DRG Category:	787
Mean LOS:	4.0 days
Description:	SURGICAL: Cesarean Section Without Sterilization With Complication or Comorbidity
DRG Category:	807
Mean LOS:	2.2 days
Description:	MEDICAL: Vaginal Delivery Without Sterilization or Dilation & Curettage Without Complication or Comorbidity or Major Complication or Comorbidity

Chorioamnionitis, or intra-amniotic infection (IAI), is an infection of the chorion, amnion, and amniotic fluids that surround the fetus and is characterized by monomorphonuclear and poly-morphonuclear leukocytes invading the membranes. Leukocytes in the membranes originate in the pregnant person; leukocytes in the amniotic fluid (amnionitis) or in the umbilical cord (funisitis) are fetal in origin. Subsequently, the fetus also becomes infected. Chorioamnionitis, which can occur with subtle or acute signs and symptoms, can happen at any time during the prenatal or intrapartum period. It occurs in 0.5% to 10% of all pregnancies and 0.5% to 2% of term pregnancies, most commonly after premature rupture of the membranes. Chorioamnionitis can also cause premature rupture of the membranes and preterm labor. If left untreated, it can lead to sepsis of the pregnant person or fetal demise. In fact, chorioamnionitis is associated with a neonatal mortality rate of 1% to 4% for term infants and up to 10% for preterm infants.

The prognosis for the pregnant person with chorioamnionitis is good. Once the baby is deliv-ered, the source of infection is removed. Rarely does chorioamnionitis lead to septic shock. Occasionally, pelvic inflammatory disease can develop if the infection is not totally resolved. The prognosis for the infant varies depending on the degree of infection that is transmitted to the fetus. Occasionally, no signs of infection develop in the infant, but this is atypical. Another factor involved in the infant's prognosis is prematurity; for the very premature infant, the risk of respiratory distress syndrome may be even greater than the risk of infection. Complications include infection of the pregnant person, infant infection, prematurity, heavy blood loss with labor, thromboembolic events, cesarean delivery, and cerebral palsy.

CAUSES

Chorioamnionitis is usually caused by bacteria that inhabit the genital tract. Less frequently, it can result from pathogens that cross over from the circulation of the pregnant person to the amniotic sac. Rarely, it is caused by the descent of pathogens from the abdominal cavity through the fallopian tubes. Commonly identified pathogens that contribute to chorioamnionitis are *Escherichia coli, Streptococcus faecalis, Neisseria gonorrhea*, group A and B streptococci, *Chlamydia trachomatis*, and *Staphylococcus aureus*.

Risk factors that contribute to chorioamnionitis include poor nutritional status of the pregnant person, young age of the pregnant person, first pregnancy, history of drug abuse, history of multiple sexual partners, premature or prolonged rupture of membranes, prolonged labor, sexually transmitted infections (STIs), the placement of a cerclage (ligature around the cervix to treat cervical incompetence during pregnancy), chorionic villi sampling, intrauterine transfusion, amniocentesis, mechanical cervical ripening for labor induction, and repeated vaginal examinations during labor.

GENETIC CONSIDERATIONS

Although it is not strictly a genetic problem, genetic variants in the cytokine tumor necrosis factor alpha have been associated with an increased risk of chorioamnionitis and fetal morbidity. Additionally, a particular SNP in *IL6* was shown to be associated with decreased expression of placental *IL6*, which may increase susceptibility to microbial infection.

SEX AND LIFE SPAN CONSIDERATIONS

Chorioamnionitis can occur with any pregnancy regardless of the age of the pregnant person. Pregnant teens may be more at risk because they have a high incidence of bacterial vaginosis, urogenital infections, and STIs.

HEALTH DISPARITIES AND SEXUAL/GENDER MINORITY HEALTH

Ethnicity, race, and sexual/gender minority status have no known effect on the risk for chorioamnionitis.

GLOBAL HEALTH CONSIDERATIONS

Countries in North America and Western Europe have relatively similar prevalence. Chorioamnionitis prevalence is high in developing countries with high prevalence of HIV-infected women. In countries such as India and China, the prevalence of group B streptococci infections is lower than in Western countries for unknown reasons.

ASSESSMENT

HISTORY. Ask about the last menstrual period to determine the estimated date of delivery and the gestational age of the fetus. Inquire about any history of vaginal infections or STIs. Question the patient about the presence of any perineal pain, burning, malaise, or chills. Ask if the patient is feeling contractions or has noted any leakage of the amniotic fluid. If the amniotic sac has ruptured, determine the time it occurred, the color of the fluid, and if the patient noted any odor. Also consider any prenatal tests or procedures, such as placement of a cerclage, chorionic villi sampling, intrauterine transfusions, or amniocentesis, which can predispose the patient to developing an intrauterine infection.

PHYSICAL EXAMINATION. Not all patients will have symptoms; however, they may experience signs of infection such as **abdominal tenderness, malaise, fever, tachycardia**, and **foul vaginal discharge**. Early clinical findings in patients with chorioamnionitis may be vague. IAI can be present with no symptoms, and subclinical IAI may be three times more common than IAI with clinical symptoms. Assess the patient's vital signs; patients with chorioamnionitis often display an elevated pulse above 120 beats per minute and temperature above 100.4°F (38°C). Palpate all quadrants of the abdomen for tenderness, noting the response of the pregnant person during examination of each quadrant. Foul odor of the vaginal discharge, color change of amniotic fluid from clear to light yellow to green, and an increase in the purulence of vaginal drainage are all consistent with chorioamnionitis.

Often, preterm labor patients with undiagnosed chorioamnionitis have contractions that do not respond to routine treatments of IV hydration and tocolytic therapy. Evaluate the baseline fetal heart rate. Fetal tachycardia (a heart rate above 160 beats per minute), a decreased fetal heart rate (a heart rate below 110 beats per minute), or decreased variability may be present with chorioamnionitis.

PSYCHOSOCIAL. Increased anxiety is usually present with patients who are experiencing preterm labor, premature rupture of membranes (PROM), or a history of a cerclage placement. Assess the patient's understanding of the situation and encourage the patient to express fears. Also include an assessment of the patient's social support and the response of significant others to the patient's condition.

Diagnostic Highlights

General Comments: Diagnosis may be difficult to establish early on because symptoms are vague. Examination of amniotic fluid is definitive.

Test	Normal Result	Abnormality With Condition	Explanation
Amniocentesis or endocervical culture	No growth	Growth of infecting organism	Culturing the amniotic fluid will reveal the presence of a causative organism, allowing for appropriate choice of antibiotic therapy

Other Tests: Complete blood count with differential, C-reactive protein, group B streptococcal screening, fetal ultrasound, urinalysis, postpartum histological examination of the placenta

PRIMARY NURSING DIAGNOSIS

DIAGNOSIS. Risk for infection as evidenced by abdominal tenderness, malaise, fever, and/or vaginal discharge

OUTCOMES. Infection severity; Immune status; Knowledge: Infection management; Risk control: Infectious process

INTERVENTIONS. Infection control; Infection protection; Medication management; Labor induction; Cesarean birth care

PLANNING AND IMPLEMENTATION
Collaborative

MEDICAL. The medical management of a patient diagnosed with chorioamnionitis is delivery of the infant, regardless of the gestational age. Thus, the current recommendation is to induce labor on all term patients presenting with PROM to decrease the incidence of chorioamnionitis. Delivery benefits the pregnant person by emptying the uterus of all infected material. Once delivered, the infant can then receive the necessary antibiotic therapy and supportive care. Usually, spontaneous labor occurs because of the infection. If an adequate contraction pattern and progressive dilation of the cervix are not noted, contractions can be induced by oxytocin (Pitocin). Broad-spectrum antibiotics administered during labor cross the placenta and achieve peak levels in the fetal circulation within an hour after parenteral administration to the pregnant person. Cesarean section is typically avoided because of the increased risk of spreading the infection; however, if the fetus is showing signs of distress, a cesarean section is performed. If the fetus is preterm, arrange for a neonatologist or pediatrician to speak with the patient before delivery; notification of the nursery is also important. Immediately after delivery, cultures of the placenta and baby are obtained, and the newborn is monitored carefully for signs and symptoms of infection.

Pharmacologic Highlights

Medication or Drug Class	Dosage	Description	Rationale
Ampicillin	1–2 g every 4–6 hr IV	Broad-spectrum penicillin	Broad-spectrum antibiotics are effective against gram-positive, gram-negative, aerobic, and anaerobic organisms; are less toxic; and cross the placenta to help the fetus
Gentamicin	3–5 mg/kg/day IV in divided doses every 8 hr	Extended-spectrum aminoglycoside	Broad-spectrum antibiotics are effective against gram-positive, gram-negative, aerobic, and anaerobic organisms; are less toxic; and cross the placenta to help the fetus

Other Drugs: Other antibiotics such as clindamycin and erythromycin may also be used. Most often combinations of antibiotics are used to treat chorioamnionitis.

Independent

Anticipatory guidance provided by the nurse is beneficial for the patient. Provide information about antibiotic therapy, procedures that occur during labor and delivery, and possible outcomes for the infant. Because the patient's anxiety level is elevated, you may need to repeat information several times. Allow the patient to express fears. Answer the questions of the significant others and take time to listen to their concerns as well.

Monitor the patient for signs of infection after delivery, including the mother's lochia, fundal height, vital signs, and incisional healing. The patient with an intrauterine infection is at a higher risk for a postpartum hemorrhage than are noninfected counterparts. Careful and frequent assessments for vaginal bleeding and firmness of the fundus are critical. If the fundus is "boggy," massage the fundus until firm.

Evidence-Based Practice and Health Policy

Gluck, O., Mizrachi, Y., Herman, H., Bar, J., Kovo, M., & Weiner, E. (2020). The correlation between the number of vaginal examinations during active labor and febrile morbidity, a retrospective cohort study. *BMC Pregnancy and Childbirth, 20*, 246–250.

- The authors noted that the association between the number of vaginal examinations performed during labor and the risk of infection is unclear. They aimed to study this problem in a large cohort ($N = 22,183$) and used a retrospective cohort design. The cohort were grouped according to the number of vaginal examinations performed during labor (up to 4, 5–6, 7–8, and 9 or more). Outcomes included intrapartum febrile morbidity (intrapartum fever and chorioamnionitis), postpartum febrile morbidity (postpartum fever and endometritis), and peripartum febrile morbidity (all of the above).
- The authors concluded that performing five or more vaginal examinations during labor was associated with intrapartum febrile morbidity, postpartum febrile morbidity, and peripartum morbidity. The authors recommended that practitioners carefully consider the benefits and necessity of multiple examinations.

DOCUMENTATION GUIDELINES

• Patient vital signs; fetal heart rate pattern; uterine activity; maternal response to antibiotics; color, odor, and consistency of vaginal discharge

If the Patient Is Delivered
• Patient and infant vital signs; amount and odor of lochia; involution of uterus; assessment of episiotomy or abdominal incision
• Amount of the infant's fluid intake and output, infant's response to antibiotics, daily weight of the baby

DISCHARGE AND HOME HEALTHCARE GUIDELINES

POSTPARTUM COMPLICATIONS IF THE PATIENT IS UNDELIVERED. Instruct the patient to inform the physician if their temperature rises above 100.4°F (38°C). Increased vaginal bleeding, foul odor of the vaginal discharge, increased uterine tenderness, difficulty urinating, the appearance of hardened red areas in the breasts, pain in the calves of the legs, incisional pain, and redness or drainage from the incision are also reasons to notify the physician.

INFANT COMPLICATIONS. Instruct the patient to inform the pediatrician if the baby's rectal temperature is below normal or above 101°F (38.2°C). A decreased interest in feeding, listlessness, increased jaundice, a red or draining umbilical cord or circumcision site, increased irritability, difficulty breathing, lack of a bowel movement in 2 days, and fewer than six wet diapers a day are also reasons to notify the pediatrician.

MEDICATIONS. Instruct the patient to take the entire prescription of antibiotics even if symptoms subside. Encourage the patient to notify the physician if symptoms persist when the prescription has ended.

RESTRICTIONS. Instruct the patient to abstain from sexual intercourse until the 6-week follow-up visit. Teach the patient to resume activity gradually and to limit use of stairs for the first week. Explain that patients should not lift anything heavier than their infant for the first 2 weeks after delivery. Teach vaginally delivered patients to avoid driving for 1 week and cesarean patients to avoid driving until the pain ceases.

Chronic Fatigue Syndrome

DRG Category:	947
Mean LOS:	4.8 days
Description:	MEDICAL: Signs and Symptoms With Major Complication or Comorbidity

Chronic fatigue syndrome (CFS, also known as myalgic encephalomyelitis [ME]) is a unique, controversial, and poorly understood chronic disease that has a sudden onset and lasts for at least 6 months. Some experts recommend that the condition be termed *systemic exertion intolerance disease* (SEID) to reflect the cardinal sign, postexertional malaise. It is a multiple symptom disease that affects the immune and neurological systems and suggests chronic mononucleosis. The pathophysiology of the syndrome is unclear, but the immune system is upregulated, or stimulated, and the levels of antibodies, especially immunoglobulin G, are increased. Experts suggest that an estimated 800,000 to 2.5 million people have CFS in the United States, but most (up to 90%) have not been diagnosed with the condition.

CFS has been mentioned throughout history but only recently has been defined for adults as a distinct disorder. It is characterized by debilitation, chronic fatigue, and a duration of at least 6 months and often much longer; it causes impaired overall physical and mental functioning. The fatigue is not the result of excessive exertion and is not alleviated by rest. People note worsening of symptoms after mental, emotional, or physical exertion. The Centers for Disease Control and Prevention (CDC) criteria have been formulated to standardize diagnosis and include cognitive difficulties, pharyngitis, lymphadenopathy, muscle pain, joint pain, headache, sleep disturbance, poor sleep, and postexercise malaise. Like many chronic illnesses, CFS is often accompanied by depression. People with CFS generally improve over time, although remissions and relapses are common.

CFS is different from but related to fibromyalgia, a condition that generally occurs in young or middle-aged females and is manifested by pain, stiffness, fatigue, disrupted sleep, and problems with cognition. As compared to the development of CFS, fibromyalgia is related to genetic vulnerability and abuse or other traumatic experiences that occur during brain development (childhood) and persistent stress or distress.

CAUSES

The cause of CFS is unknown but is possibly related to an infectious process such as Epstein-Barr viral infection with immune manifestations. Researchers are investigating whether or not the disease is a syndrome triggered by a virus with multiple contributing factors such as age, sex, toxic and environmental exposure, stress, depression, anxiety, and perhaps a precipitating event (recent trauma or surgery).

GENETIC CONSIDERATIONS

CFS appears to have both a genetic and an environmental component, with heritability estimated at 20% to 50%. Several studies have found genetic variants that may influence the development of CFS, but more work is needed to define the pathways that contribute to disease. Several genes have been implicated, including the glutamate receptor ionotropic kinase 2 (*GRIK2*) and neuronal PAS domain protein 2 (*NPAS2*). Additionally, an association has been made with *HLA-C* and *HLA-DQB1* alleles, linking the immune system to CFS pathogenesis.

SEX AND LIFE SPAN CONSIDERATIONS

CFS is more prevalent in females than in males, and it tends to affect persons between the ages of 40 and 60 years. It is more common in adolescents than children. It may be underdiagnosed in children and older adults.

HEALTH DISPARITIES AND SEXUAL/GENDER MINORITY HEALTH

Most people who have been diagnosed with CFS are White persons, but experts suggest that the condition is at least as common among Black and Hispanic persons but is underdiagnosed. While little is known about the numbers of gender and sexual minority persons who have CFS, these individuals are at risk because of issues with healthcare access, the stress of discrimination and violence, and higher odds for depression, multiple chronic conditions, and substance use (Downing & Przedworski, 2018).

GLOBAL HEALTH CONSIDERATIONS

CFS exists worldwide, but the prevalence is uncertain because of the lack of consistent definitions. In the United States, up to 4 million people may have CFS, but more recent statistics indicate that as much as 1% to 2% of the population is affected. Experts believe that this prevalence statistic is likely also applicable to global populations.

ASSESSMENT

HISTORY. Establish a history of the sudden onset of flu-like symptoms accompanied by intense, postexertional fatigue that does not resolve within 6 months. Approximately 25% of patients will acknowledge that they have been bed- or housebound because of symptoms. Ask if the patient has experienced sleep disturbance or fatigue after long periods of rest or sleep. Determine if the patient has experienced any other symptoms of a neurological or psychological nature such as problems with short-term memory or fluency of speech. Ask if the patient has been exposed to a toxin or has recently experienced stress. Determine if the patient's occupation involves interaction with the public leading to viral or environmental exposure. It is important to remember that symptoms can vary widely with CFS.

PHYSICAL EXAMINATION. The most common symptoms include **prolonged fatigue, difficulties with short-term memory**, and **verbal dyslexia** (difficulty speaking accurately and fluently, problems with verbal memory and verbal processing speed). The physical examination may reveal flu-like symptoms such as sore throat, low-grade fever, chills, muscular pain, and swollen, painful lymph nodes. Neurological assessment findings may include sensitivity to light, headache, inability to think clearly or concentrate, short-term memory loss, sleep disorders, equilibrium problems, and depression. Some patients have orthostatic intolerance with symptoms that worsen when they stand upright.

PSYCHOSOCIAL. Patients with CFS are often depressed because of the stress of dealing with a chronic, debilitating illness that affects their total lifestyle and cognition. Anxiety and mood swings are common, and there are increased rates of divorce and suicide among these patients. Assess the effect of the disease on the patient's job and childcare responsibilities.

Diagnostic Highlights

There is no definitive method of diagnosing CFS, but the National Academy of Medicine (formerly the Institute of Medicine) has set forth diagnostic criteria (Box 1). The following diagnostic tests are often drawn: complete blood count, serum electrolytes, liver function tests, thyroid function tests, erythrocyte sedimentation rate, C-reactive protein, creatine kinase, cortisol level, and antinuclear antibody test.

• BOX 1 Criteria for CFS

Diagnosis requires that the patient have the following three symptoms:
1. A substantial reduction or impairment in the ability to engage in preillness levels of occupational, educational, social, or personal activities that persists for more than 6 months and is accompanied by fatigue, which is often profound, is of new or definite onset (not lifelong), is not the result of ongoing excessive exertion, and is not substantially alleviated by rest
2. Postexertional malaise
3. Unrefreshing sleep

At least one of the following two manifestations is also required:
1. Cognitive impairment
2. Orthostatic intolerance

Note that the frequency and severity of symptoms should be assessed. The diagnosis of CFS should be questioned if patients do not have these symptoms at least half of the time with moderate, substantial, or severe intensity.

PRIMARY NURSING DIAGNOSIS

DIAGNOSIS. Activity intolerance related to inflammation as evidenced by muscle and/or joint pain, malaise, and/or fatigue

OUTCOMES. Energy conservation; Coping; Knowledge: Disease process; Mood equilibrium; Symptom severity

INTERVENTIONS. Energy management; Counseling; Exercise promotion; Pain management: Chronic; Activity therapy

PLANNING AND IMPLEMENTATION

Collaborative

Because there is currently no known cure, treatment of CFS focuses on symptom relief. Some patients experience relief of the symptoms by avoiding environmental irritants and certain foods. Exercise therapy has been shown to improve sleep, physical function, and general health as well as to help people feel less fatigued. Current research has not shown that exercise therapy improves pain, quality of life, anxiety, or depression.

Pharmacologic Highlights

Medication or Drug Class	Dosage	Description	Rationale
NSAIDs	Varies by drug	May reduce inflammation, thus reducing symptoms	Efficacy uncertain

Other Medications: Most medications have proved ineffective. Nonsedating antihistamines, antianxiety agents such as alprazolam, and tricyclic antidepressants may be helpful. Experimental treatments include the antiviral acyclovir and selected immunomodulating agents, such as IV gamma globulin, rintatolimod (Ampligen), transfer factor, and others. Doxycycline is used to treat people with elevated immunoglobulin M *C pneumoniae* titers.

Independent

It is important to set realistic goals when planning care with the patient with CFS. Teach patients not to overexert themselves. It is believed that stress can prolong the disease or result in an exacerbation. Relaxation and stress-reducing techniques such as hypnosis, massage, biofeedback, and meditation may be useful if sleep patterns are altered. Explain that although the symptoms tend to wax and wane, they are often debilitating and may last for months or even years. The patient therefore needs to reduce their activities when symptoms are more pronounced but also needs to avoid bedrest, which has no proven therapeutic value for patients with CFS. Encourage a graded exercise program and provide an appropriate referral for continuing exercise. Stress the need to progress slowly with exercise to avoid overfatigue. Referring the patient and family to counseling and support groups may assist in developing appropriate coping skills for dealing with a chronic, debilitating illness.

Evidence-Based Practice and Health Policy

Larun, L., Brurberg, K., Odgaard-Jensen, J., & Price, J. (2019). Exercise therapy for chronic fatigue syndrome. *Cochrane Database of Systematic Reviews.* https://doi.org//10.1002/14651858 .CD003200.pub8

• The authors studied the effects of exercise therapy in adults with CFS. They compared outcomes in three groups: exercise group, any other intervention group, and control group.

Variables were fatigue, adverse outcomes, pain, physical functioning, quality of life, mood disorders, sleep, self-perceived changes in overall health, and health service resources use.

• They located unpublished and ongoing studies through the World Health Organization International Clinical Trials Registry Platform up to May 2014, including randomized controlled trials about adults with a primary diagnosis of CFS. They found that exercise therapy probably has a positive effect on fatigue in adults with CFS compared to other exercises and the control groups. The authors were not able to determine whether exercise therapy reduces depression or the other outcomes.

DOCUMENTATION GUIDELINES

• Physical findings: Activity tolerance, pain, vital signs, range of motion
• Degree of discomfort: Location, frequency, duration, response to analgesia
• Response to medication therapy, rest, and relaxation
• Emotional response: Coping strategies, support from significant others, signs of depression or hopelessness

DISCHARGE AND HOME HEALTHCARE GUIDELINES

Instruct the patient to report any increase in physical symptoms or suicidal thoughts to the primary caregiver. Instruct the patient to obtain assistance as necessary to complete self-care activities and to meet family responsibilities. Teach the patient the proper route, dosage, and side effects to monitor with all medications. Make necessary plans for referrals and follow-up appointments.

Discuss the role of exercise therapy to improve some symptoms.

Cirrhosis

DRG Category:	432
Mean LOS:	6.3 days
Description:	MEDICAL: Cirrhosis and Alcoholic Hepatitis With Major Complication or Comorbidity
DRG Category:	5
Mean LOS:	19.5 days
Description:	SURGICAL: Liver Transplant With Major Complication or Comorbidity or Intestinal Transplant

The Centers for Disease Control and Prevention (CDC) report that 4.5 million people in the United States have liver disease. Cirrhosis along with other chronic liver diseases result in approximately 45,000 deaths annually. In cirrhosis, the damaged liver cells regenerate as fibrotic areas instead of functional cells, causing lymph damage and alterations in liver structure, function, and blood circulation. The major cellular changes include irreversible chronic injury of the functional liver tissue and the formation of regenerative nodules. These changes result in liver cell necrosis, collapse of liver support networks, distortion of the vascular bed, and nodular regeneration of the remaining liver cells.

The classification of cirrhosis is controversial at present. However, most types may be classified by a mixture of causes and cellular changes, defined as follows: alcoholic; cryptogenic and postviral or postnecrotic; biliary; cardiac; metabolic, inherited, and drug related; and miscellaneous. The first three types are the most commonly seen, accounting for 55% to 90% of cases of cirrhosis. Although each of these types has a different etiology, the clinical findings, including portal vein hypertension and eventual liver failure, are much the same. (Box 1 explains the effects of alcohol on the liver.)

• BOX 1 Pathophysiology of Cirrhosis: Progression of Effects

EFFECTS OF OCCASIONAL DRINKING

- Several days after drinking, synthesis of fatty acids and triglycerides increases.
- Fatty acid oxidation decreases.
- Formation and release of lipoproteins decrease.
- Fat appears in the liver.

EFFECTS OF CONTINUAL DRINKING

- Liver cells enlarge because of accumulation of lipids.
- Enlarged liver cells rupture.
- Fatty contents from ruptured liver cells form fatty cysts.
- Cells between adjoining veins in the liver are linked by developing fibrosis.
- Continued scarring and necrosis lead to the liver shrinking.
- Liver function decreases or ceases.
- Obstructed flow of blood leads to increased pressure in the portal vein (portal hypertension).
- Blood backs up in the liver and spleen.
- Veins in the abdomen, rectum, and esophagus dilate.
- The congestion of blood in the liver leads to the leakage of plasma into the peritoneal cavity.
- The liver's production of albumin decreases.
- Decreased serum albumin levels allow more water to move into other body compartments.
- Renin and aldosterone production levels increase, leading to water and sodium retention.
- Ascites, the accumulation of fluid in the peritoneal cavity, results.

CAUSES

Liver cirrhosis is most commonly associated with hepatitis C (26% of cases), alcohol abuse (21%), hepatitis C plus alcohol abuse (15%), cryptogenic causes (etiology not determined; 18%), hepatitis B (15%), and other miscellaneous causes (5%) such as malnutrition, protein deficiency, biliary disease, and chemical toxins. Alcoholic liver disease is also known as Laënnec cirrhosis, portal cirrhosis, nutritional cirrhosis, and fatty cirrhosis. A serious complication is hepatocellular carcinoma. Primary biliary cirrhosis is a chronic and progressive liver disease thought to be of autoimmune derivation. In this condition, a continuous destruction of small and medium bile ducts occurs due to immune effects of complement, a protein that is part of the immune response.

GENETIC CONSIDERATIONS

Cirrhosis is a complex disease including both genetic and environmental factors. The keratin 8 and keratin 18 genes, as well as genes involved in immune signaling, have been implicated in both susceptibility to disease and severity of course. Proinflammatory cytokines have been associated with increased risk of hepatitis and cirrhosis. In addition, several genes have been identified that increase susceptibility to alcoholic liver disease, including higher levels of alcohol dehydrogenase (ADH) and cytochrome P450 2E1 activity, and lower levels of acetaldehyde dehydrogenase (ALDH) activity. Shared environment also contributes to what may at first appear to be genetic transmission.

SEX AND LIFE SPAN CONSIDERATIONS

Cirrhosis is most commonly seen in the middle-aged population; it is the fifth leading cause of death in the population that is 35 to 55 years of age. It is more common in males than in females. Although the cause is obscure, liver disease appears to be more prevalent in preterm infants who have minimum enteral feedings and who were begun on total parenteral nutrition at an early age.

HEALTH DISPARITIES AND SEXUAL/GENDER MINORITY HEALTH

Health disparities exist in the management and outcomes of people treated for cirrhosis. Black persons in the United States have the highest rates of both hospital admission and readmission. Black and Hispanic patients are less likely to receive portosystemic shunts and liver transplantations as compared to White patients (Spiewak et al., 2020). Indigenous peoples, such as Native Americans and Australian Indigenous people, have higher rates of hospital readmissions and poorer survival outcomes after being diagnosed with cirrhosis than other groups. Veterans have higher rates of drinking than their civilian counterparts, likely because of the effect of posttraumatic stress disorder. Not only are there high rates of cirrhosis among Veterans, but also one-third of those diagnosed continue to drink after the diagnosis. Alcohol use disorders, which place people at risk for cirrhosis, are more prevalent in White and Native American persons and younger as compared to older adults. While little is known about the epidemiology of cirrhosis in gender and sexual minority persons, gender and sexual minority youths and young adults have higher rates of alcohol use than their counterparts. Estimates are that 25% of gender and sexual minority adults have moderate alcohol dependency.

GLOBAL HEALTH CONSIDERATIONS

Cirrhosis is among the leading causes of death globally. Half of all cirrhosis-related deaths globally are thought to be related to alcohol consumption. The average global per capita alcohol consumption per year is approximately 6.4 liters The lowest per capita consumption is in the Middle East and Northern Africa, whereas the highest occurs in Russia and Eastern Europe. Primary biliary cirrhosis is more common in Northern Europeans and is less common in people with African ancestry. The World Health Organization reports that the highest death rates occur in Mexico and South America, Central Africa, and Eastern Europe. North American and European countries have lower mortality rates, and rates in Asia vary sharply by country. Hepatocellular carcinoma has the highest prevalence in Asia, South Africa, and some areas of the Middle East. Susceptibility to the disease is believed to be based not on ancestry or nationality but on environmental factors.

ASSESSMENT

HISTORY. Determine if the patient has experienced personality changes such as agitation, forgetfulness, and disorientation. Inquire about fatigue, drowsiness, mild tremors, or flu-like symptoms. Ask about any past or present symptoms that may indicate cirrhosis, such as changes in bowel habits or menstrual irregularities. Elicit a history of easy bruising, nosebleeds, or bleeding gums. Determine the patient's drinking patterns and how long they have existed. Determine if the patient has had early morning nausea and vomiting, anorexia, indigestion, weight loss, weakness, lethargy, epigastric discomfort, or altered bowel habits. Ask about any recent sexual dysfunction.

PHYSICAL EXAMINATION. Common signs and symptoms include **bleeding from esophageal varices, increased bleeding tendencies from coagulopathies, ascites,** and **abdominal pain.** Inspect for signs of muscle atrophy. Note whether the patient's abdomen is protruding. Assess the patient's skin, sclera, and mucous membranes, observing for poor skin turgor, signs of jaundice, bruising, spider angiomas, and palmar erythema (reddened palms). Observe the patient's trunk and note the presence of gynecomastia (enlarged breasts). Observe the abdomen for distention, an everted umbilicus, and caput medusae (a plexus of dilated veins about the umbilicus); measure the abdominal girth.

When assessing the patient's upper extremities, test for asterixis (liver flap or flapping tremor). Have the patient stretch out the arm and hyperextend the wrist with the fingers separated, relaxed, and extended. The patient in stages II (impending) and III (stuporous) of hepatic encephalopathy may have a rapid, irregular flexion and extension (flapping) of the wrist. Note any tenderness or discomfort in the patient's abdomen. Palpate for hepatomegaly by gently rolling the fingers under the right costal margin. The liver is normally soft and usually can be felt under the costal margin. Percuss the patient's abdomen. Note a shifting dullness in the abdomen if ascites is present. Auscultate the abdomen and assess for hypoactive, hyperactive, or normal bowel sounds.

PSYCHOSOCIAL. Cirrhosis is a chronic disease that dictates lifestyle changes for the patient and significant others. Determine the patient's response to the diagnosis and the patient's ability to cope with change. Identify the patient's past ability to cope with stressors and determine if these mechanisms were successful.

Diagnostic Highlights

Test	Normal Result	Abnormality With Condition	Explanation
Percutaneous or laparoscopic liver needle biopsy	Normal hepatocytes	Cellular degeneration	Distinguishes advanced liver disease from cirrhosis; excludes other forms of liver injury such as viral hepatitis
Liver enzymes: Aspartate aminotransferase (AST); alanine aminotransferase (ALT); lactate dehydrogenase (LDH), bilirubin	AST: 10–35 units/L; ALT: 10–40 units/L; LDH: 45–90 units/L; bilirubin < 1.2 mg/dL	Elevated	Liver cellular dysfunction leads to accumulation of enzymes; cirrhosis decreases portal blood flow and hepatic clearance of bilirubin

Other Tests: Ultrasound; computed tomography; magnetic resonance imaging; other supporting tests including antimitochondrial antibodies; serum alkaline phosphate; total serum, serum bilirubin, indirect bilirubin, and urine bilirubin; serum ammonia; and serum albumin, serum total protein, and prothrombin

PRIMARY NURSING DIAGNOSIS

DIAGNOSIS. Excess fluid volume related to retention as evidenced by ascites and/or abdominal pain

OUTCOMES. Fluid balance; Hydration; Nutritional status; Knowledge: Disease process; Knowledge: Treatment regime

INTERVENTIONS. Fluid/electrolyte management; Fluid monitoring; Medication administration; Nutrition management

✖ PLANNING AND IMPLEMENTATION

Collaborative

MEDICAL. Patients will likely undergo a complete nutritional assessment. Protein levels and calorie intake will be determined by the severity of illness, whether or not malnutrition is present, and the patient's level of activity. Frequently, vitamin K injections are ordered to improve blood-clotting factors. If coagulopathies worsen, treatment may require whole-blood or fresh-frozen plasma to maintain the hematocrit and hemoglobin. If alcohol is the primary etiologic factor in liver cirrhosis, strongly encourage the patient to cease drinking. If patients are able to ambulate, they are encouraged to walk as much as possible to prevent muscle wasting.

INTERVENTIONAL RADIOLOGY. A transjugular intrahepatic portosystemic shunt (TIPS) is a bypass used to collect two veins within the liver for patients with portal hypertension and severe ascites. The shunt is placed by an interventional radiologist who uses a guided image to open a pathway to connect the portal vein to the hepatic vein and then threads a stent through the pathway to keep it open. TIPS may reduce internal bleeding in the gastrointestinal (GI) tract and lessen ascites.

SURGICAL. The medical team will consider liver transplantation for patients with decompensated cirrhosis. Candidates for liver transplantation fall into three categories: those with irreversible chronic liver disease, those with malignancies of the liver and biliary tree, and those with fulminant hepatic failure. Approximately 7,000 liver transplants occur each year in the United States. Approximately 15% of patients on the liver transplant waiting list will die while waiting for a transplant because of a shortage of organs. As surgeons have gained more experience with both the surgical procedure and the postoperative management, survival rates have increased. The 1-year survival rate is approximately 90%, and the 5-year survival rate is 70% or more. Patients with alcohol-related liver disease are considered for transplantation after a medical and psychological evaluation that includes the potential for long-term alcohol abstinence. Posttransplantation care is complex and includes careful monitoring for infection, rejection, and hemorrhage as well as assessing the function of the donor liver.

Pharmacologic Highlights

Medication or Drug Class	Dosage	Description	Rationale
Zinc sulfate	220 mg PO BID	Mineral supplement	May improve muscle cramps, stimulate appetite, and improve taste sensitivity

Other Drugs: To remedy itching, an antihistamine can be administered. If a patient has nausea and vomiting, antiemetics may be prescribed. Use caution when administering antiemetics and acetaminophen to patients with liver damage because many medications are cleared through the liver. For primary biliary cirrhosis, the following may be used: ursodeoxycholic acid to slow the progression of the disease; immunosuppressive agents, corticosteroids. For autoimmune hepatitis, prednisone and azathioprine may be used, whereas interferon and other antiviral agents may be used for hepatitis B and C. Patients with chronic liver disease should receive a vaccination to protect against hepatitis A.

Independent

Nursing considerations in the cirrhotic patient are to avoid infection and circulatory problems. Turn the patient and encourage coughing and deep breathing every 2 hours to prevent pneumonia. Because bleeding can occur, monitor the patient closely for signs of hypovolemia. Test any stool and emesis for blood. Follow closely any break in the patient's skin integrity for increased bleeding and apply pressure to injection sites. Warn the patient against straining at stool, blowing the nose, or sneezing too vigorously. Suggest the patient use a soft toothbrush and an electric razor.

Because of fatigue, muscle atrophy, and wasting, the patient needs to rest. Plan activities to include regular rest periods. To prevent breakdown of the skin, place the patient on an eggcrate or air mattress. Avoid using soap to bathe the patient; use moisturizing agents or lubricating lotion and massage areas of the skin that are potential breakdown sites. Use pressure-reducing mattresses or specialty beds to prevent skin breakdown. If patients are strong enough, assist them with ambulation to prevent muscle wasting.

Encourage the patient to verbalize questions, anxieties, and fears. In conversation, note any behavioral or personality changes, including increasing stupor, lethargy, or hallucinations. Arouse the patient periodically to determine the patient's level of consciousness. Emotional and psychological support for the patient and family are important to eliminate anxiety and poor self-esteem. Involve the family members in the patient's care as a means of improving the patient's morale.

Evidence-Based Practice and Health Policy

Bosch, J., Gracia-Sancho, J., & Abraldes, J. (2020). Cirrhosis as new indication for statins. *Gut*, *69*, 953–962.

• The authors noted that in recent years, patients with advanced chronic liver disease have been increasingly treated with statin drugs. With increased use, reports of favorable effects on a range of liver ailments have increased, and the authors aimed to provide an overview of recent developments. The authors reviewed the current knowledge about the applications of statins in chronic liver diseases and described their effects.
• They noted that evidence shows that statins might improve outcomes in cirrhosis, but evidence from randomized trials is limited. Therefore, they note that there is no strong enough evidence for recommending statins for the treatment of cirrhosis.

DOCUMENTATION GUIDELINES

• Physical findings: Bleeding, abdominal enlargement, weight gain or loss, fluid intake and output, easy respirations, breath sounds, heart sounds, level of consciousness, GI status (nausea, vomiting, anorexia, diarrhea), color of skin and sclera
• Laboratory results: White blood cell count, hemoglobin and hematocrit, albumin, serum electrolytes, ALT, AST
• Nutrition: Tolerance of diet, appetite, ability to maintain body weight
• Response to treatment: Medications, surgery, transplantation

DISCHARGE AND HOME HEALTHCARE GUIDELINES

ALCOHOL ABUSE TREATMENT. Emphasize to the patient with alcoholic liver cirrhosis that continued alcohol use exacerbates the disease. Stress that alcoholic liver disease in its early stages is reversible when the patient abstains from alcohol. Encourage family involvement in alcohol abuse treatment. Assist the patient in obtaining counseling or support for their alcoholism.

FOLLOW-UP. Encourage the patient to seek frequent medical follow-up. Visits from a community health nurse to monitor the patient's progress and to help with any questions or problems at home are also helpful. Transplant patients will need lifelong follow-up by a transplant clinic and extensive teaching. When patients are discharged, make sure the patient and family understand all aspects of their medical regime, including medications, nutrition, protection from infection, signs of rejection, activity limits, and schedule of follow-up visits.

SUPPORT GROUPS. Refer the patient to an alcohol support group or liver transplant support group. Refer the patient and family to hospice for palliative care if appropriate in end-stage disease.

Cleft Lip; Cleft Palate

DRG Category:	159
Mean LOS:	2.6 days
Description:	SURGICAL: Dental and Oral Diseases Without Complication or Comorbidity or Major Complication or Comorbidity

Cleft lip (CL) and cleft palate (CP) are facial malformations of the upper lip or palate that are the third most common congenital abnormality in the United States. They may appear separately or, more commonly, together. The malformation is a result of a failure of the maxillary and median nasal processes to fuse during the second month of embryonic development. CL may vary from a small notch to a complete cleft that extends into the base of the nose. When CP occurs alone, it is midline, but when it occurs with CL, it may extend into either side of the soft palate. Combined CL/CP occurs in 50% of cases of this deformity, and isolated CP occurs in 30% of the cases. Related complications of CL/CP include dental malformations, frequent otitis media leading to hearing impairment, speech difficulties, and social isolation due to poor self-image and speech impairments.

CAUSES

A genetic cause for CL/CP is likely; however, environmental exposure to teratogens during critical embryonic development cannot be ruled out. CL with or without CP is etiologically and genetically distinct from isolated CP. Isolated CP has a greater incidence of associated anomalies. CP may also be one of the three signs of Pierre Robin sequence, which also is associated with micrognathia and glossoptosis. There is a twofold increase in the occurrence of clefts with maternal smoking in early pregnancy and a 10-fold increase if the mother has been treated with phenytoin (Dilantin) during pregnancy. Those with prepregnancy diabetes have a higher risk of having a child born with CL/CP than those who do not have diabetes.

GENETIC CONSIDERATIONS

There are more than 400 single-gene, complex disorders or syndromes that include CL and/or CP as features. Overall, CL/CP heritability is estimated at approximately 76%. Approximately 22% of facial clefting can be attributed to single-gene disorders. The gene *IRF6* has been identified as a probable cause in approximately 12% of CLs and may account for familial trends. Familial CP appears to have an autosomal dominant pattern of transmission. Along with the increased risk for CL/CP in some families, those families may have a greater risk genetically for specific types of cancer (e.g., colon) than families who do not have the associated congenital anomalies of CL/CP.

SEX AND LIFE SPAN CONSIDERATIONS

Infant males are more likely to have CL with or without CP, whereas females are more likely to have CP alone.

HEALTH DISPARITIES AND SEXUAL/GENDER MINORITY HEALTH

The incidence of CL with or without CP varies by race, with a higher rate among Japanese and certain groups of Native American persons and a lower rate among Black persons. Sexual and gender minority status has no known effect on the risk for CL/CP.

GLOBAL HEALTH CONSIDERATIONS

A variety of genetic, environmental, and nutritional causes affect global prevalence. People in developing countries with poor nutrition or environmental exposure to toxins may have a higher risk for CL and CP than people in developed countries, as do people with Asian ancestry in Asian countries.

ASSESSMENT

HISTORY. A family history of CL or CP may or may not exist. Identical twins are more likely to share the disorder than are fraternal twins. Inquire about teratogen exposure during the first trimester of pregnancy. If the child has not been followed since birth, question the parents about feeding patterns and any infections that have occurred.

PHYSICAL EXAMINATION. The primary symptoms are **facial malformations of the upper lip or palate.** The CL may vary from a small notch to a widespread open cleft and may be unilateral or bilateral. The CP also varies in the extent of the malformation: It can involve only the uvula; extend into the soft and hard palates; or be unilateral, bilateral, or midline. Assessment for lung aspiration and airway obstruction is critical. Assessment of feeding patterns and infant nutrition is important because of the potential for feeding difficulties. Because otitis media with effusion is common in children with CP, an ear examination by an otolaryngologist is important to evaluate the eustachian tubes for dysfunction.

PSYCHOSOCIAL. Parents' and families' adjustments to an infant with CL or CP may be difficult. The deformity is usually readily observable at birth and often totally unexpected. Support for the family is essential and includes explanations of the surgical procedures and long-term prognosis. The family may find interacting with strangers difficult because of the need to discuss the baby's appearance. Experts suggest that the average lifetime medical cost for one child with CL and CP is $100,000.

Diagnostic Highlights

There are no diagnostic tests for CL or CP. CL is diagnosed by visual inspection. CP is diagnosed by palpating the palate with a gloved finger during the initial newborn assessment at birth. Inspect the palate during crying. It is possible today to diagnose the presence of CL and CP in utero with an ultrasound. Three-dimensional ultrasound can be used to assess fetal faces accurately. Facial x-rays may be used to confirm the extent of bone deformity.

PRIMARY NURSING DIAGNOSIS

DIAGNOSIS. Imbalanced nutrition: less than body requirements related to inadequate intake as evidenced by failure to thrive and/or weight loss

OUTCOMES. Nutritional status; Food and fluid intake; Nutritional status: Nutrient intake; Newborn adaptation; Breastfeeding establishment: Infant; Bottle feeding establishment: Infant

INTERVENTIONS. Nutrition management; Bottle feeding; Infant care; Parent education: Infant

☀ PLANNING AND IMPLEMENTATION

Collaborative

SURGICAL. CL and CP are treated with a combination of surgery, speech therapy, and orthodontic work. Timing for surgery may vary, but a general protocol is used by many medical centers. Surgical repair of a CL is performed 3 months after birth. The repair improves the child's ability to suck. Speech is evaluated at 6 months, speech therapy begins at 9 months, and repair of the CP occurs at 9 to 12 months. Orthodontic treatment begins at 1 year of age and continues through childhood and adolescence as needed. The more extensive the surgery required, the later the surgery may occur. Surgical repair of CL (cheiloplasty) is usually uncomplicated with no long-term intervention other than possible scar revision. Surgical repair of CP (palatoplasty) is more extensive and may require more than one surgery. Anesthesia for repair of CL/CP needs thoughtful consideration due to the proximity of surgery to the airway. If the infant has horseshoe defect, surgery may be impossible. A contoured speech bulb attached to the back of a denture appliance to occlude the nasopharynx may help the child speak.

Pharmacologic Highlights

Medication or Drug Class	Dosage	Rationale
Antibiotics	Depends on the drug and weight of the child	Prevent infection resulting from surgery
Analgesics	Depends on the drug and weight of the child	Relieve surgical pain

Experimental Treatment: Surgical repair of CL in animals in utero demonstrated better healing of the lip than conventional means.

Independent

Because of the long-term, multidisciplinary nature of services needed for the child, assist the parents in accessing appropriate support within the healthcare system. Support the parents before and during the surgical procedure by identifying the positive features of the newborn. Call the infant by name. Current surgical practices provide excellent repairs with minimal scarring. Encourage parents to discuss their feelings about the child's appearance. Sharing pictures of children with successful CL repairs may help the parents cope with their fears and anxieties.

Depending on the severity of the cleft, children with CL/CP may have problems sucking and breastfeeding. Most infants can finish feeding in 30 minutes, but if feeding takes longer than 45 minutes, the infant may become overfatigued. Work with the parents and experiment with devices that will improve nutrition, such as different kinds of nipples. The infant may feed better if the parents use a nipple with a flange that occludes the cleft or a large, soft nipple with large holes. Try holding the infant at different positions during feeding (e.g., at a 60- to 80-degree angle). Breastfeeding can be successfully carried out as long as a seal can be maintained during nursing. In some nursing pairs, the breast tissue may help form the seal. Otherwise, the hand not holding the infant or a molded nipple can be used to form a seal during nursing. Encourage a meeting with a lactation consultant and discharge follow-up to support the breastfeeding parent–baby dyad.

Encourage parents to verbalize fears and anxiety about the deformity. The first time that parents see their baby, they may experience shock, disappointment, or guilt. If you help them see the baby's assets, you encourage bonding and acceptance. Allow ample time for the parents to hold the infant to promote bonding. Explain the surgical procedure and postoperative care to parents.

The postoperative management of an infant with a CL focuses on protection of the operative site. Surgical closure with Dermabond has demonstrated fewer infections and hypertonic scar repair than Steri-Strips. Arm restraints prevent the child from rubbing the site and from self-injury. Hang baby toys within reach of the baby's restrained hands. Many infants are more comfortable in an infant seat rather than lying in a crib. As with all babies, do not place infants on their stomachs for sleep. Pacifiers are contraindicated, and feeding methods should be designed to reduce any tension on the suture line. Use a cotton-tipped applicator and a cleansing solution to clean the suture line. An antibiotic ointment may be prescribed. Pain should be controlled with analgesic medication and nonpharmacologic strategies, such as holding and rocking.

The postoperative management of an infant with a CP centers on prevention of injury and infection to the operative site. Do not place sharp or potentially injurious objects in the child's mouth (spoons, forks, straws, etc.). Feeding may be done from the side, but self-feeding is prohibited. After feeding, make sure to cleanse the child's mouth with water or a cleansing solution.

Evidence-Based Practice and Health Policy

Sparks Lancaster, H., Lien, K., Chow, J., Frey, J., Scherer, N., & Kaiser, A. (2020). Early speech and language development in children with nonsyndromic cleft lip and/or palate: A meta-analysis. *Journal of Speech, Language, and Hearing, 6*, 14–31.

- Authors of this meta-analysis studied early speech and language function in children from birth to 8 years with nonsyndromic CL or CP to their peers without nonsyndromic CL/CP (NSCL/P). Researchers further determined differences in outcomes related to speech articulation (consonant inventory, speech accuracy and speech error type) and expressive and receptive language.
- Findings indicated children with NSCL/P scored significantly lower than their peers in the following measures: consonant inventory, speech accuracy, expressive and receptive language and speech errors. Differences in children with NSCL/P and their peers with typical development narrowed as the children grew up.

DOCUMENTATION GUIDELINES

- Appearance of surgical site: Presence of redness, drainage, swelling; degree of approximation of wound edges
- Response to pain medication and other nonpharmacologic interventions; parents' coping styles
- Ability to feed and maintain weight; parent's and baby's response to feeding

DISCHARGE AND HOME HEALTHCARE GUIDELINES

FEEDING. Teach the parents feeding techniques, how to observe for aspiration, and to bubble the infant frequently. After surgery, teach the parents to avoid putting objects into the infant's mouth.

PREVENTION OF INFECTION. Teach the parents to care for the incision and to assess the incision for infection. Explain the importance of keeping the infant's hands away from the face. Tell the parents that it is important to hold the infant and remove the restraints from time to time.

PAIN CONTROL. Teach the parents the signs of pain in an infant and explore with them nonpharmacologic methods to relieve pain. Review with the parents the analgesic medication dosage, time, and route.

COMPLICATIONS. Instruct parents that the child may have more recurrent middle ear infections than other children. The child may also need orthodontic or speech therapy at some time because of the deformity of the mouth and palate.

Colorectal Cancer

DRG Category:	329
Mean LOS:	13.1 days
Description:	SURGICAL: Major Small and Large Bowel Procedures With Major Complication or Comorbidity
DRG Category:	374
Mean LOS:	7.2 days
Description:	MEDICAL: Digestive Malignancy With Major Complication or Comorbidity

Colorectal cancer is a complex disease that involves genetic, environmental, inflammatory, and nutritional factors. Colorectal cancer is the third most commonly diagnosed cancer for women and men (after lung and breast/prostate cancer). In recent years, both the incidence and the mortality rates have shown a decline, and this is attributed to early identification and improved treatment measures. According to the American Cancer Society (ACS), in 2021, a total of 104,270 new cases of colon cancer and 45,230 new cases of rectal cancer will be diagnosed in the United States. The lifetime risk of colorectal cancer is 4.3% for men and 4.0% for women; the 5-year survival rate is approximately 90% if it is diagnosed at an early stage. The 5-year survival rate drops to 15% if the colorectal cancer spreads to distant organs and lymph nodes.

Of cancers of the colon, 65% occur in the rectum and in the sigmoid and descending colon, 25% occur in the cecum and ascending colon, and 10% occur in the transverse colon. Most colorectal tumors (95%) are adenocarcinomas and develop from an adenomatous polyp. Once malignant transformation within the polyp has occurred, the tumor usually grows into the lumen of the bowel, causing obstruction, and invades the deeper layers of the bowel wall. After penetrating the serosa and the mesenteric fat, the tumor may spread by direct extension to nearby organs and the omentum. Metastatic spread through the lymphatic and circulatory systems occurs most frequently to the liver as well as the lung, bones, and brain.

CAUSES

The cause of colorectal cancer is largely unknown; however, there is much evidence to suggest that incidence increases with age. Risk factors include a family history of colorectal cancer and a personal history of past colorectal cancer, ulcerative colitis, Crohn disease, or adenomatous colon polyps. Persons with familial polyposis coli, an inherited disease characterized by multiple (> 100) adenomatous polyps, possess a risk for colorectal cancer that approaches 100% by age 40 years. Other risk factors include obesity, diabetes mellitus, alcohol usage, cigarette smoking, night-shift work, and physical inactivity.

It has been strongly suggested that diets high in fat and refined carbohydrates play a role in the development of colorectal cancer. High-fat content results in increased amounts of fecal bile acid. It is hypothesized that intestinal bacteria react with the bile salts and facilitate carcinogenic changes. In addition, fat and refined carbohydrates decrease the transit of food through the gastrointestinal (GI) tract and increase the exposure of the GI mucosa to carcinogenic substances that may be present. These physiological changes may also expose people to the risk of colorectal cancer following cholecystectomy. Recent research indicates that aspirin, cytochrome C oxidase (COX)-2 selective NSAIDs, folate, calcium, and estrogen replacement therapy have a potential chemoprotective effect and may prevent colorectal cancer.

GENETIC CONSIDERATIONS

About 75% of colorectal cancers are sporadic; another 25% clearly have genetic contributions. Hereditary nonpolyposis colorectal cancer (HNPCC), or Lynch syndrome, accounts for 5% to 10% of colorectal cancer cases overall. For individuals from families with HNPCC, the lifetime risk of developing colorectal cancer is 70% to 90%, which is several times the risk in the general population. Mutations in several genes, including *MLH1*, *MSH2*, *MSH6*, *EPCAM*, and *PMS2* have been linked to HNPCC, for which genetic testing is available. Colon cancer is also highly penetrant in familial adenomatous polyposis (FAP), which is caused by mutations in the tumor suppressor adenomatous polyposis coli (*APC*). FAP represents about 1% of all colorectal cancer cases. Other genetic risk factors remain unidentified.

SEX AND LIFE SPAN CONSIDERATIONS

Colorectal cancer affects men slightly more than women. The incidence of colorectal cancer is exceeded only by lung cancer in both men and women and by prostate cancer in men and breast cancer in women. There is a slight predominance of colon cancer in women and rectal cancer in men. The incidence increases after age 40 years and begins to decline between ages 65 and 75 years, although 90% of all newly diagnosed cancers are in people older than 50 years. Colorectal cancer can be diagnosed in individuals of any age, but malignancies that occur around age 20 to 30 years are usually difficult to control, diagnosed at a later stage, and signify a poor prognosis.

HEALTH DISPARITIES AND SEXUAL/GENDER MINORITY HEALTH

Black persons have a higher incidence of rectal cancer and higher death rates than non-Hispanic White and Hispanic persons, and are diagnosed at a later (more advanced) stage of the disease. Colorectal cancer is also more common in persons of Alaskan Native background, Jewish people, or people of Eastern European descent than other groups. It is associated with gastric cancer in people with Asian ancestry. Health disparities in colorectal screening exist with people with low income or no insurance. People without insurance are less likely to have colorectal cancer screening. Longer distances between a person's residence and a hospital are also associated with a colorectal cancer diagnosis at a later stage of the disease, raising concern for disparities among rural populations (Schlottmann et al., 2020). While little is known about health disparities due to colorectal cancer in sexual and gender minority persons, factors such as poverty, stigma, and discrimination affect access to healthcare and may lead to poorer outcomes.

GLOBAL HEALTH CONSIDERATIONS

Colorectal cancer is the fourth most common cancer diagnosis around the globe. Approximately one million people die each year from colorectal cancer. Developed countries in North America, Australia, and Western Europe, along with Israel and Japan, have an 8 to 10 times higher incidence of the disease than do developing countries such as China, Algeria, and India. These differences may be associated with cultural differences in diet and patterns of cigarette smoking, alcohol use, and exercise. In developing countries with high levels of poverty, mortality rates for colorectal cancer are higher than in developed countries.

ASSESSMENT

HISTORY. Because of the emphasis on screening, most patients have colorectal cancer detected before they have symptoms. Seek information about the patient's usual dietary intake, family history, and presence of the other major risk factors for colorectal cancer.

In more advanced cases, a change in bowel pattern (diarrhea or constipation), iron deficiency anemia, and the presence of blood in the stool might cause the patient to seek medical attention. Patients may describe fatigue and weight loss. Patients may report that the urge to have a bowel movement does not go away with defecation. Cramping, weakness, and fatigue are also reported. As the tumor progresses, symptoms develop that are related to the location of the tumor within the colon.

When the tumor is in the right colon, the patient may complain of vague cramping or aching abdominal pain and report symptoms of anorexia, nausea, vomiting, weight loss, and tarry-colored stools. A partial or complete bowel obstruction is often the first manifestation of a tumor in the transverse colon. Tumors in the left colon can cause a feeling of fullness or cramping, constipation or altered bowel habits, acute abdominal pain, bowel obstruction, and bright red bloody stools. In addition, rectal tumors can cause stools to be decreased in caliber, or "pencil-like." Depending on the tumor size, rectal fullness and a dull, aching perineal or sacral pain may be reported; however, pain is often a late symptom.

PHYSICAL EXAMINATION. Rectal bleeding, blood in stool, and **changes in bowel habits** are the most common symptoms. Inspect, auscultate, and palpate the abdomen. Note the presence of any distention, ascites, visible masses, or enlarged veins (a late sign due to portal hypertension and metastatic liver involvement). Bowel sounds may be high-pitched, decreased, or absent in the presence of a bowel obstruction. An abdominal mass may be palpated when tumors of the ascending, transverse, and descending colon have become large. Note the size, location, shape, and tenderness related to any identified mass. Percuss the abdomen to determine the presence of liver enlargement and pain. A rectal tumor can be easily palpated as the physician performs a digital rectal examination.

PSYCHOSOCIAL. Individuals who observe healthy lifestyles may feel anger when the diagnosis is made. Treatment for colorectal cancer can result in a colostomy and impotence in men. Many persons have grave concerns about the possibility of these consequences. Assess the patient and significant others' knowledge and feelings related to these issues.

Diagnostic Highlights

General Comments: Pathological results from biopsied tissues provide the definitive diagnosis for cancer.

Test	Normal Result	Abnormality With Condition	Explanation
Hematest (fecal occult blood test)	Negative for blood in stool	Positive guaiac test for occult blood in the stool	An early sign of tumor development is blood in the stool
Endoscopy of the colon	Visualization of normal colon	Visualization of tumor; biopsy	Endoscopy allows for visualization and removal of suspicious polyps or lesions
Serum carcinoembryonic antigen (CEA)	< 2.5 ng/mL (nonsmokers); < 5 ng/dL in smokers	Elevations are associated with tumor recurrence after resection; nonspecific elevations occur with cirrhosis, renal failure, pancreatitis, and ulcerative colitis	Glycoprotein is normally absent in normal adult colonic mucosa

(highlight box continues on page 312)

Diagnostic Highlights (continued)

Other Tests: Complete blood count, barium enema, computed tomography scan, magnetic resonance imaging, and abdominal x-rays to determine abdominal obstruction; fecal immunochemical test (FIT) to identify human hemoglobin to test for occult blood from lower GI lesions; stool DNA test with high sensitivity for cancer

PRIMARY NURSING DIAGNOSIS

DIAGNOSIS. Acute pain related to tissue injury from tumor invasion and the surgical incision as evidenced by self-reports of pain, grimacing, protective behavior, and/or diaphoresis

OUTCOMES. Comfort status; Pain level; Pain control; Pain: Disruptive effects; Knowledge: Medication

INTERVENTIONS. Pain management: Acute; Analgesic administration; Anxiety reduction; Environmental management: Comfort; Patient-controlled analgesia

PLANNING AND IMPLEMENTATION

Collaborative

Although treatment depends on individual patient characteristics, the location of the tumor, and the stage of disease at the time of diagnosis, surgery has been the primary treatment for colorectal cancers. Staging is generally done by the TNM system (T: tumor, N: nodes, M: metastasis) or the modified Duke staging system. Adjuvant chemotherapy and radiation therapy may be used to improve survival or control symptoms. The exact surgical procedure performed depends on the location of the tumor in the colon, the amount of tissue involved, and patient's decisions about preservation of function. When deciding about the nature of surgery, several important considerations exist, including assessment of the likelihood of cure, preservation of anal continence (sphincter-saving procedures are standard of care for patients with colorectal cancer), and preservation of genitourinary functions.

PREOPERATIVE. All patients who are undergoing bowel surgery require careful preoperative care in order to minimize the possibility of infection and promote the adjustment to bodily changes. If nutritional deficits are present, a low-residue diet high in calories, carbohydrates, and protein is given until serum electrolytes and protein levels return to normal. Total parenteral nutrition may be ordered. Twenty-four hours before the scheduled surgery, the physician usually orders a "bowel prep," which consists of a clear liquid diet, a regimen of cathartics and cleansing enema, and oral and IV antibiotics to minimize bacterial contamination during surgery.

POSTOPERATIVE. Postoperatively, direct nursing care toward providing comfort, preventing complications from major abdominal surgery, and promoting the return of bowel function. Monitor vital signs and drainage from wounds and drains for signs of hemorrhage and infection. A nasogastric tube connected to low intermittent or continuous suction is usually present for gastric decompression until bowel sounds return. Note the amount and color of the gastric drainage, as well as the presence of abdominal distention.

Patients who require a colostomy return from surgery with an ostomy pouch system in place as well as a large abdominal dressing. Observe the condition of the stoma every 4 hours. A healthy stoma is beefy red and moist, whereas a dusky appearance could indicate stomal necrosis. A small amount of stomal bleeding is common, but any substantial bleeding should be reported to the surgeon. The colostomy usually begins to function 2 to 4 days after surgery. After surgery, adjuvant radiation therapy to the abdomen or pelvis is used when there is high risk for local recurrence. Adjuvant chemotherapy (5-fluorouracil plus leucovorin) is used when there is high risk or evidence of metastatic disease. Radiation therapy and chemotherapy may be used as palliative measures to reduce pain, bleeding, or bowel obstruction in patients with advanced and metastatic disease.

Pharmacologic Highlights

Medication or Drug Class	Dosage	Description	Rationale
Narcotic analgesic	Varies with drug	Often administered as patient-controlled anesthesia	Manages surgical pain or pain from metastasis
Chemotherapy	Varies with drug	Fluorouracil, vincristine, leucovorin, irinotecan, oxaliplatin, cetuximab, bevacizumab, panitu-mumab, capecitabine, tegafur	Antineoplastic agents to interfere with tumor growth

Independent

Encourage the patient to verbalize fears and clarify the physician's explanation of diagnostic results. Dispel any misconceptions about the need for a permanent colostomy and clarify the purpose of a temporary colostomy if suggested.

If a colostomy is to be performed, encourage the patient and significant other to verbalize concerns about sexual functioning after surgery. Encourage active participation of the patient and family in surgical decisions. Impotence is only a problem after abdominal perineal resection (APR) in men, but the presence of a stoma and a drainage pouch with fecal effluent can affect self-identity and sexual desires in both men and women.

After surgery, discuss methods to decrease the impact of the ostomy during intimate times. After surgery, help the patient avoid complications associated with bowel surgery. Assist the patient to turn in bed and perform coughing, deep breathing, and leg exercises every 2 hours to prevent skin breakdown as well as to avoid pulmonary and vascular stasis. Teach the patient to splint the abdominal incision with a pillow to minimize pain when turning or performing coughing and deep-breathing exercises. The patient who has had an APR may find the side-lying position in bed the most comfortable. Provide a soft or "waffle" pillow (not a rubber doughnut) for use in the sitting position. Change the perineal dressing frequently to prevent irritation to the surrounding skin.

Showing the patient pictures of an actual stoma can help reduce the "shock" of seeing the stoma for the first time. Allow the patient to hold the equipment, observe the amount and characteristics of effluent, and empty the ostomy pouch of contents or gas. When emptying or changing the pouch system, take care to not contaminate the abdominal incision with effluent. Teaching the patient about home care of an ostomy can begin on the second or third postoperative day. Have the patient and a family member demonstrate ostomy care correctly before hospital discharge. Be alert to signs that indicate the need for counseling, and suggest a referral if the patient is not adjusting well.

Evidence-Based Practice and Health Policy

Hofseth, L., Hebert, J., Chanda, A., Chen, H., Love, B., Pena, M., Murphy, E., Sajish, M., Sheth, A., Buckhaults, P., & Berger, F. (2020). Early-onset colorectal cancer: Initial clues and current views. *Nature Reviews of Gastroenterology and Hepatology, 17*, 352–364.

- Because the incidence of early onset colorectal cancer in patients under 50 years of age has increased in recent decades, the authors sought to expand the knowledge of causes and mechanisms of this disease. They then identified inconsistencies in the evidence of the links between behaviors (such as diet and stress) and colorectal cancer that might place nonobese and otherwise healthy people at risk.
- Factors included Westernization of diets (high intake of red and processed meats, high-fructose corn syrup, and unhealthy cooking practices), stress, use of antibiotics and synthetic food dyes, and physical inactivity. The course of the disease and the fact that relevant exposures probably occur in childhood raise important issues for future research.

DOCUMENTATION GUIDELINES

- Response to diagnosis of colorectal cancer, diagnostic tests, and treatment regimen
- Description of all dressings, wounds, and drainage collection devices: Location of drains; color and amount of drainage; appearance of the incision; color of the ostomy stoma; presence, amount, and consistency of ostomy effluent

DISCHARGE AND HOME HEALTHCARE GUIDELINES

PATIENT TEACHING. Teach the patient the care related to the abdominal incision and any perineal wounds. Give instructions about when to notify the physician (if the wound separates or if any redness, bleeding, purulent drainage, unusual odor, or excessive pain is present). Advise the patient not to perform any heavy lifting (> 10 lb), pushing, or pulling for 6 weeks after surgery. If the patient has a perineal incision, instruct the patient not to sit for long periods of time and to use a soft or waffle pillow rather than a rubber ring whenever in the sitting position.

Teach the patient colostomy care and colostomy irrigation.

Give the following instructions for care of skin in the external radiation field: Tell the patient to wash the skin gently with mild soap, rinse with warm water, and pat the skin dry each day; not to wash off the dark ink marking that outlines the radiation field; to avoid applying any lotions, perfumes, deodorants, and powder to the treatment area; to wear nonrestrictive soft cotton clothing directly over the treatment area; and to protect skin from sunlight and extreme cold. Explain the purpose, action, dosage, and side effects of all medications prescribed by the physician.

FOLLOW-UP. Stress the need to maintain a schedule for follow-up visits recommended by the physician. Encourage patients with early stage disease and complete healing of the bowel to eat a diet consisting of a low-fat and high-fiber content with cruciferous vegetables (brussels sprouts, cauliflower, broccoli, cabbage).

Most colorectal tumors grow undetected as symptoms slowly develop. Survival rates are best when the disease is discovered in the early stages and when the patient is asymptomatic. Unfortunately, 50% of patients have positive lymph node involvement at the time of diagnosis. Participation in procedures for the early detection of colorectal cancer needs to be encouraged.

Suggest follow-up involvement with community resources such as the United Ostomy Associations of America and the American Cancer Society.

Coronary Heart Disease (Arteriosclerosis)

DRG Category:	287	
Mean LOS:	3.0 days	
Description:	MEDICAL: Circulatory Disorders Except Acute Myocardial Infarction, With Cardiac Catheterization Without Major Complication or Comorbidity	
DRG Category:	302	
Mean LOS:	3.7 days	
Description:	MEDICAL: Atherosclerosis With Major Complication or Comorbidity	

Coronary heart disease (CHD) is the leading cause of death and illness in Western societies and accounts for approximately one in eight deaths. Someone has a heart attack (myocardial infarction [MI]) every 40 seconds in the United States. According to the American Heart Association (AHA), from 2015 to 2018, almost 130 million people in the United States had some form of heart disease, stroke, and other cardiovascular diseases. A number of conditions result from CHD, including angina, heart failure, MI, and sudden cardiac death. CHD results when decreased blood flow through the coronary arteries causes inadequate delivery of oxygen and nutrients to the myocardium. The lumens of the coronary arteries become narrowed from either fatty fibrous plaques or calcium plaque deposits, thus reducing blood flow to the myocardium, which can lead to chest pain or even MI and sudden cardiac death.

Plaque buildup, known as atheromas, in the coronary arteries is a result of atherosclerosis, defined as thickening of the arterial walls' inner aspect and a loss of elasticity. Lesions resulting from atherosclerosis do not occur randomly but rather are more likely to develop where the arteries branch, which slows blood flow and creates turbulence within the vessel. As the plaque grows in size, inflammation, necrosis, and fibrosis occur, and the arteries may change in form (remodeling). Plaque accumulation reduces the inner arterial lumen and leads to wall thickening, calcification, and reduced blood supply. Complications of CHD include angina, MI, heart failure, stroke, cardiac dysrhythmias, and sudden death.

CAUSES

Atherosclerosis is the most common cause of CHD and is linked to many modifiable risk factors—primarily elevated serum cholesterol levels, elevated blood pressure, cigarette smoking, obesity, lack of physical activity, excessive alcohol use, and mental stress. Blood levels of cholesterol and low-density lipoproteins (LDLs) have been associated with increased risk of CHD. Hypertension places chronic stress on the blood vessels and may initiate plaque deposition. Because smoking increases myocardial oxygen requirements, blood pressure, and heart rate, cigarette smokers are twice as likely to have an MI and four times as likely to have sudden cardiac death. High levels of the following substances are also considered to increase risk for CHD: C-reactive protein; lipoprotein(a); homocysteine; small, dense LDL cholesterol (LDL-C) particles; and fibrinogen. Other risk factors that are not modifiable are older age, family history of heart disease, diabetes mellitus, and race/ethnicity.

GENETIC CONSIDERATIONS

A combination of genetics and environment appears to account for the vast majority of cases of CHD. First-degree relatives of patients with CHD are at higher risk of developing the disease and developing it earlier than the general population. Over 250 different genes have been implicated in the onset of CHD, making it a prime example of the combination of multiple genes and environment seen in complex disease. Defects in genes involved with LDL metabolism, homocysteine metabolism, muscle development, and blood pressure regulation have been associated with CHD. Other genes that have been linked encode the apolipoprotein A1 allele, apolipoprotein E4 allele, and glycoprotein IIb/IIIa. Familial hypercholesterolemia is due to a defective LDL receptor and is inherited in an autosomal dominant pattern. LDL levels elevated to values double that of normal are seen in affected persons as early as 2 years of age, and signs of CHD can be found by the age of 30 years.

SEX AND LIFE SPAN CONSIDERATIONS

According to the AHA, the prevalence of heart disease, coronary artery disease, hypertension, and stroke is higher in males than females. For example, the age-adjusted prevalence of coronary artery disease is 7.2% in males and 4.2% in females. There are differences in clinical presentation, comorbidities, risk factors, and quality of the delivery of care between women and men. Women more frequently than men have atypical chest pain (weakness, breathlessness, malaise). Women have a delay arriving at the emergency department by 1 hour as compared to men, thereby prolonging their time for the start of interventional cardiology. The average age for an MI in men is 65 years; women generally have symptoms 10 years after men and are more apt to have diabetes mellitus and physical frailty than men. Women are more likely than men to have inflammatory diseases such as rheumatoid arthritis or lupus, which double the cardiac risk. Women are also less likely to receive guideline-directed and evidence-based care and percutaneous coronary interventions than men (Mehilli & Presbitero, 2020). In addition, women with symptoms of ischemic heart disease are more likely to have no obstructive coronary disease as compared to men. Approximately 20% of deaths from CHD occur before 65 years of age in men and women.

HEALTH DISPARITIES AND SEXUAL/GENDER MINORITY HEALTH

The Centers for Disease Control and Prevention report that 11.5% of White persons, 9.5% of Black persons, 7.4% of Hispanic persons, and 6.0% of Asian persons have heart disease. Black persons have higher morbidity and mortality rates of CHD, and the burden for Black persons is higher than for White persons because of the prevalence of hypertension, obesity, metabolic syndrome, and decreased physical activity. In people between the ages of 55 and 64 years, new episodes of angina occur in 11.2% of non-Black and 19.3% of Black women and in 11.9% of non-Black and 10.6% of Black men. Prior to age 64 years, the highest prevalence of new angina is in Black women. Significant health disparities exist in the cardiac care of underrepresented groups as compared to White persons. Black, Indigenous, and other people of color are known to receive care less often guided by standard cardiac care guidelines than White persons. Unless patients have health insurance, White patients are more likely to receive coronary angiograms and other coronary interventions than Black and Hispanic patients. Black, Indigenous, and other people of color are also less likely to be referred to cardiologists and cardiac surgeons than White persons (Batchelor et al., 2019). Adults without housing, even when controlling for insurance, are less likely to undergo percutaneous coronary intervention and coronary artery bypass grafting compared with people with a permanent residence. In the United States, Asian Indian persons have a higher prevalence of CHD than White persons.

Transgender is a term used to describe persons whose gender identity is different from their sex assigned at birth. Approximately 1% of the U.S. population identify themselves as transgender. Sexual and gender minority persons have higher odds for multiple chronic conditions, cancer, and poor quality of life and are more apt to have disabilities than cisgender males and females. (Cisgender is a term used to describe persons whose gender identity and gender expression are aligned with their assigned sex listed on their birth certificate.) Gender-affirming hormone therapy is the use of hormone therapy for gender transition or gender affirmation and can be masculinizing or feminizing. It may also affect cardiovascular health in transgender females. In a large sample, researchers have found that transgender men and women are more likely to be overweight than cisgender women. Compared to cisgender women, transgender women reported higher rates of diabetes, ischemic stroke, angina/ coronary disease, and MI. Gender-nonconforming men and women reported higher odds of MI than cisgender women. Transgender women also had higher rates of any cardiovascular disease than cisgender men (Cacerese, Jackman, et al., 2020; Connelly et al., 2019). While large-scale studies are not available, these factors may place some sexual and gender minority persons at risk for CHD.

GLOBAL HEALTH CONSIDERATIONS

Rates of CHD around the developed world are comparable to U.S. rates. Canadian researchers have reported that less than 10% of Canadian adults are in ideal cardiovascular health and that just one in five children has ideal cardiovascular health. England, Scotland, and Finland have similar high rates of CHD. The prevalence of CHD is increasing in the Middle East, India, Russia and other nations from the former Soviet Union, and Central/South America. Some experts suggest that, as Africa becomes more developed and Westernized, the risk of CHD for African people has increased in part because of urbanization. Dietary patterns and alcohol consumption seem to lower rates of CHD in Mediterranean countries, such as France and Greece, and among Alaskan natives.

ASSESSMENT

HISTORY. Discuss with patients any risk factors, paying attention to the quantity and frequency of tobacco and alcohol use as well as family history for cardiac events. Ask about their daily and weekly activity levels. Patients with CHD describe a spectrum of symptoms that varies widely. Some are asymptomatic, and others describe symptoms of myocardial ischemia with stable or unstable angina as the most common symptom. A careful description of the pain, including location, severity, and precipitating factors, is essential. Cardiac pain is usually described as a diffuse aching pain or pressure that is relieved by rest or administration of nitroglycerin. The pain is usually substernal but may radiate to either arm, the neck, or between the shoulder blades. Often, the pain is precipitated by extra physical or emotional demands. Women may describe weakness, breathlessness, and malaise rather than typical chest pain. Atypical pain may originate in the elbow, jaw, or shoulder. The patient may have no pain sensation but may complain of being short of breath or having nausea, vomiting, lightheadedness, or sweating.

Ask patients about symptoms that are more vague than chest pain, such as weakness and fatigue. Patients may report that they are very tired after exercise or activity. They may experience palpitations, leg swelling, or weight gain.

PHYSICAL EXAMINATION. Patients present in a variety of ways, and the physical examination may reveal nothing abnormal. **Chest pain**, **labored breathing**, **pallor**, and **profuse sweating** suggest a possible MI. Other signs of CHD include fatigue, activity intolerance, dizziness, palpitations, swelling of the legs, and weakness. Patients with CHD often have tachycardia, and both hypotension and hypertension may occur. Hypotension in the setting of an acute MI may indicate hemodynamic compromise and more risk. Auscultate the heart sounds carefully to identify accompanying cardiac problems such as valvular dysfunction or heart failure.

There may be evidence of flat or slightly raised yellowish tumors, most frequently found on the upper and lower lids (xanthelasma), or flat, slightly elevated, soft, rounded plaques or nodules, usually on the eyelids (xanthoma). Patients may also have evidence of central obesity (excessive fat around the stomach and abdomen).

PSYCHOSOCIAL. Because the stress in one's life has long been associated with the development of CHD, problem-solving to reduce stress is an important nursing function. Occupational stress or the obligations from multiple roles may vary for female and male patients. Risk of heart disease has many different meanings to people because the heart has many associations, such as courage, strength, romance, and generosity. If parents or siblings have died from heart disease, CHD may also evoke fear or sadness. Individuals whose work involves heavy lifting may require vocational rehabilitation counseling in order to return to work. Continuation of a fulfilling sexual expression requires thoughtful assessment and teaching.

Diagnostic Highlights

Test	Normal Result	Abnormality With Condition	Explanation
Lipid profile	Range varies for age and gender; 140–200 mg/dL; LDL-C: < 100 mg/dL; high-density lipoprotein cholesterol (HDL-C): 40–50 mg/dL (men), 50–60 mg/dL (women); triglyceride 100–150 mg/dL	Total cholesterol level > 200 mg/dL; LDL-C: > 160 mg/dL; HDL-C < 40 mg/dL for men, < 50 mg/dL for women; triglyceride > 200 mg/dL	Elevated levels are associated with CHD
Electrocardiogram (ECG)	Normal ECG with P, Q, R, S, and T waves	Q waves because of a prior MI; resting ST segment depression or elevation; T-wave inversion suggestive of myocardial ischemia	Changes in the electrical activity of the heart are associated with cardiac ischemia, injury, or necrosis

Other Tests: Note that there is no evidence that routine cardiac screening for low-risk adults improves outcomes for patients. Ambulatory electrocardiographic monitoring, exercise echocardiography, stress myocardial perfusion imaging, and cardiac catheterization. Exercise echocardiography is useful in establishing the diagnosis of CHD and allows some determination of risk in patients with angina. Magnetic resonance imaging and computed tomography can depict zones of impaired blood supply and show the coronary anatomy. Electronic beam computed tomography can identify coronary calcification. Complete blood count, blood glucose, hemoglobin A_{1c}, C-reactive protein, troponins, creatine kinase, lactate dehydrogenase, cardiac isoenzymes, B-type natriuretic peptide, homocysteine.

PRIMARY NURSING DIAGNOSIS

DIAGNOSIS. Acute pain related to narrowing of the coronary artery(ies) as evidenced by chest tightness or pressure, shortness of breath, pallor, diaphoresis, and/or palpitations

OUTCOMES. Cardiac pump effectiveness; Circulation status; Comfort status; Pain control; Pain level; Tissue perfusion: Cardiac

INTERVENTIONS. Cardiac care; Oxygen therapy; Pain management: Acute; Medication administration; Anxiety reduction

▓ PLANNING AND IMPLEMENTATION

Collaborative

NONINVASIVE AND INVASIVE PROCEDURES. The primary goal for patients with CHD is to relieve the symptoms and to prevent unstable angina, acute MI, or death from a cardiac event. Many patients with CHD are seen for the first time because of an "index event" such as an acute MI. Some high-risk groups, however, are targeted before such an event occurs, and they will likely be handled with medications (see Pharmacologic Highlights). Drug therapy to lower lipid levels is an important preventative measure. Antiplatelet agents, blood pressure control, control of weight if the patient is overweight or obese, smoking cessation, reduction of alcohol misuse or abuse, and promotion of exercise are important prevention strategies.

Several invasive but nonsurgical procedures can be used to manage CHD. Percutaneous coronary intervention (PCI) includes balloon catheter angioplasty and stenting. A PCI involves an invasive radiographic procedure that is performed under local anesthesia. A balloon-tipped coronary catheter is introduced into a coronary vessel and inflated and deflated in quick succession. The atheroma (fatty lesion) is compressed against the vessel wall, and the stenosis is dilated, which increases coronary blood flow. During the stent procedure, the cardiologist places a small, hollow metal (mesh) tube, or stent, in the artery to keep it open following a balloon angioplasty. Recent research is questioning the use of stents on the basis of long-term outcome data.

CORONARY ARTERY BYPASS GRAFTING (CABG). A patent blood vessel from another part of the body is grafted to the affected coronary artery distal to the lesion. The new vessel bypasses the obstruction. Unfortunately, unless reduction of risks and modification of the lifestyle accompany this procedure, the grafted vessels will also eventually occlude. Vessels commonly used for grafting are the greater or lesser saphenous veins, basilic veins, and right and left internal mammary arteries. Total endoscopic coronary artery bypass surgery is a new procedure used for people who require a single bypass. A surgical robot and computer can be used with the surgeon to perform coronary artery bypass by making small, precise incisions and using three-dimensional views of the arteries. The chest is not opened during the procedure, which allows for a faster recovery, faster resolution of pain, and a shorter hospital stay.

Managing the patient after heart surgery involves complex collaborative strategies among the nurse, surgeon, and respiratory therapist. Usually, a patient leaves the operating room with a systemic arterial and pulmonary artery catheter in place. Fluids and medications are administered according to the patient's hemodynamic response to the surgery. Monitoring for complications is also an essential role. Early complications from heart surgery include hypotension or hypertension (lowered or raised blood pressure), hemorrhage, dysrhythmias, decreased cardiac output, fluid and electrolyte imbalance, pericardial bleeding, fever or hypothermia, poor gas exchange, gastric distention, and changes in level of consciousness.

If the patient has a large amount of drainage from mediastinal tubes, the nurse may initiate autotransfusion. In the immediate postoperative period, patients will need airway management with an endotracheal tube and breathing support with mechanical ventilation. Some patients will also require temporary cardiac pacing through epicardial pacing wires that are inserted during the surgery. Patients will often need fluid therapy with blood, colloids, or crystalloids to replace lost fluids or bleeding.

Pharmacologic Highlights

Medication or Drug Class	Dosage	Description	Rationale
Platelet aggregate inhibitors	Varies by drug	Has an antiplatelet action (aspirin, clopidogrel, abciximab)	Reduces incidence of MI by preventing clots

(highlight box continues on page 320)

Pharmacologic Highlights (continued)

Medication or Drug Class	Dosage	Description	Rationale
Nitrates and other antianginal agents	Varies by drug	Nitrates such as isosorbide and nitroglycerin, beta-adrenergic blockers such as atenolol and propranolol, and calcium channel blockers such as diltiazem, nifedipine, and verapamil	Increase coronary artery blood flow through vasodilation
Antilipemic agents	Varies by drug	Bile-sequestering agents (cholestyramine), folic acid derivatives (gemfibrozil), and cholesterol synthesis inhibitors (lovastatin, rosuvastatin)	Lower excessively high serum lipid levels

Other Drugs: If the patient is having angina, nitrates, beta-blockers, statins, calcium-channel blockers, and ranolazine will be considered. Antihypertensives are also used because hypertension increases stress on damaged blood vessels. A direct vasodilating agent such as hydralazine or sodium nitroprusside may also be used. Angiotensin-converting enzyme inhibitors such as ramipril (altace) and quinapril (accupril) are used to lower blood pressure. Amlodipine (norvasc) relaxes the coronary smooth muscle and produces coronary vasodilation.

Independent

During episodes of chest pain, encourage complete rest and allay the patient's anxiety by remaining close at hand. Monitor the blood pressure and heart rate and initiate collaborative interventions, such as administering nitroglycerin and oxygen. If the pain does not subside, notify the physician. When the episode is over, ask the patient to grade the severity of the pain (1 is low pain and 10 is severe pain), and document it in detail.

Explain strategies to reverse CHD through a program that includes a very low-fat diet, aerobic exercise, and stress-reduction techniques. Information about resumption of sexual activity acceptable for the medical condition is helpful. Patient information literature is abundant and available from cardiac rehabilitation programs as well as from the AHA. Although many patients will be admitted on the day of surgery, preoperative teaching about the intensive care unit environment, the procedure, postoperative coughing and breathing exercises, and postoperative expectations of care is essential. The surgery is a family crisis that may lead to a long recovery, patient dysfunction, and even death. The family needs emotional support and constant information about the patient's progress.

Evidence-Based Practice and Health Policy

Hamad, R., Penko, J., Kazi, D., Coxson, P., Guzman, D., Wei, P., Mason, A., Wang, E., Goldman, L., Fiscella, K., & Bibbins-Domingo, R. (2020). Association of low socioeconomic status with premature coronary heart disease in U.S. adults. *JAMA Cardiology, 5,* 899–908.

• The authors estimated the excess CHD burden among individuals in the United States with low socioeconomic status (SES) and the proportions attributable to traditional risk factors added to other factors associated with low SES. They created a computer simulation study, using the Cardiovascular Disease Policy Model, a model of CHD and stroke incidence, prevalence, and mortality among adults in the United States, to project the excess burden of early CHD.

• Compared with individuals with higher SES, the group with lower SES had double the rate of MIs, 40% of which were explained by a higher burden of traditional SES risk factors, and 60% of which were attributable to other factors associated with low SES. The authors concluded that for approximately one-quarter of U.S. adults aged 35 to 64 years, low SES was substantially associated with early CHD burden. Disease burden disparities by SES may remain without addressing SES itself.

DOCUMENTATION GUIDELINES

• Episodes of angina describing character, location, and severity of pain; precipitating or mitigating factors; interventions; and evaluation
• Patient teaching about disease process and planned treatments, including medication regimen, healthy lifestyles, smoking cessation, drinking alcohol within recommended limits, exercise planning
• Perioperative hemodynamic response: Pulmonary and systemic arterial pressures, presence of pulses, capillary refill, urine output
• Pulmonary assessment: Breath sounds, ventilator settings, response to mechanical ventilation, secretions
• Complications: Bleeding, blood gas alterations, fluid volume deficit, hypotension, dysrhythmias, hypothermia
• Coping: Patient and family
• Mediastinal drainage and autotransfusion

DISCHARGE AND HOME HEALTHCARE GUIDELINES

PREVENTION. Review the risk factor and lifestyle modifications that are acceptable to the patient and the patient's family members.

MEDICATIONS. Be certain that the patient and appropriate family members understand all medications, including the correct dosage, route, action, and adverse effects.

PERIOPERATIVE
Care of Incision. Often the incision heals with no home healthcare, but the patient needs to know the signs of infection.

Activity Restrictions. The activity recommendations will depend on the type and extent of the patient's underlying condition. Instruct patients on when they can resume exercise and the intensity of the exercise.

Cor Pulmonale

DRG Category: 315
Mean LOS: 3.6 days
Description: MEDICAL: Other Circulatory System Diagnoses With Complication or Comorbidity

Cor pulmonale is a disorder of the structure and function of the right side of the heart caused by a disease of the respiratory system, primarily pulmonary hypertension. Cor pulmonale is estimated to cause approximately 5% to 7% of all types of heart disease in adults, and chronic obstructive pulmonary disease (COPD) due to chronic bronchitis or emphysema is the causative factor in more than 50% of people with cor pulmonale. While it is difficult to know how many people in the United States have cor pulmonale, experts estimate that 15 million people have the condition. The right ventricle is a thin-walled chamber as compared to the left ventricle and is more responsive to volume changes. With increased resistance in the pulmonary system, the right side of the heart works harder, the systolic pressure rises, the right ventricle dilates, and ultimately, right-sided heart failure occurs.

A number of physiological changes lead to poor gas exchange. Alveolar wall damage results in anatomic reduction of the pulmonary vascular bed as the number of pulmonary capillaries are reduced and the vasculature stiffens from pulmonary fibrosis. Constriction of the pulmonary vessels and hypertrophy of vessel tissue are caused by alveolar hypoxia and hypercapnia. Abnormalities of the ventilatory mechanics bring about compression of pulmonary capillaries. Cor pulmonale accounts for approximately 25% of all types of heart failure. Complications of cor pulmonale include biventricular heart failure, hepatomegaly, pleural effusion, and thromboembolism related to polycythemia.

CAUSES

In addition to COPD, acute cor pulmonale is produced by a number of other pulmonary and pulmonary vascular disorders but primarily by acute respiratory distress syndrome (ARDS) and pulmonary embolism. Two factors in ARDS lead to right ventricular overload: the disease itself and the high transpulmonary pressures that are needed to treat ARDS with mechanical ventilation. In the United States, approximately 25,000 sudden deaths occur per year from heart failure associated with pulmonary emboli. Other conditions can also lead to cor pulmonale. Respiratory insufficiency—such as chest wall disorders, upper airway obstruction, obesity hypoventilation syndrome, and chronic mountain sickness caused by living at high altitudes—can also lead to the chronic forms of the disease. It can also develop from lung tissue loss after extensive lung surgery. A contributing factor is chronic hypoxia, which stimulates erythropoiesis, thus increasing blood viscosity. Cigarette smoking is also a risk factor.

GENETIC CONSIDERATIONS

No clear genetic contributions to susceptibility have been defined.

SEX AND LIFE SPAN CONSIDERATIONS

Middle-aged and older men are more likely to experience cor pulmonale, but incidence in women is increasing. In children, cor pulmonale is likely to be a complication of cystic fibrosis, hemosiderosis, upper airway obstruction, scleroderma, extensive bronchiectasis, neurological diseases that affect the respiratory muscles, or abnormalities of the respiratory control center.

HEALTH DISPARITIES AND SEXUAL/GENDER MINORITY HEALTH

The Centers for Disease Control and Prevention report that 11.5% of White persons, 9.5% of Black persons, 7.4% of Hispanic persons, and 6.0% of Asian persons have heart disease. Significant health disparities exist in the cardiac care of underrepresented groups as compared to White persons. Black, Indigenous, and other people of color are known to receive care less often guided by standard cardiac care guidelines than White persons. Unless patients have health insurance, White patients are more likely to receive coronary angiograms and other coronary interventions than Black and Hispanic patients. Black, Indigenous, and other people of color are also less likely to be referred to cardiologists and cardiac surgeons than White persons (Batchelor et al., 2019). COPD is a leading cause of hospitalization for Veterans. During military deployment, soldiers are often exposed to dust, chemicals, smoke, and fumes for long periods of time. Cigarette smoking rates are high among active and retired military.

Transgender is a term used to describe persons whose gender identity is different from their sex assigned at birth. Approximately 1% of the U.S. population identify themselves as transgender. Sexual and gender minority persons have higher odds for multiple chronic conditions, cancer, and poor quality of life, and are more apt to have disabilities than cisgender males and females (cisgender is a term used to describe persons whose gender identity and gender expression are aligned with their assigned sex listed on their birth certificate). Gender-affirming hormone therapy is the use of hormone therapy for gender transition or gender affirmation and can be masculinizing or feminizing. It may also affect cardiovascular health in transgender females. In a large sample, researchers have found that transgender men and women are more likely to be overweight than cisgender women. Compared to cisgender women, transgender women reported higher rates of diabetes, ischemic stroke, angina/coronary disease, and myocardial infarction. Gender-nonconforming men and women reported higher odds of myocardial infarction than cisgender women. Transgender women also had higher rates of any cardiovascular disease than cisgender men (Cacerese, Jackman, et al., 2020; Connelly et al., 2019). While large-scale studies are not available, these factors may place some sexual and gender minority persons at risk for cor pulmonale.

GLOBAL HEALTH CONSIDERATIONS

The prevalence of cor pulmonale around the world depends on the prevalence of cigarette smoking and other tobacco use, air pollution, toxic exposure, and other risk factors for lung diseases. Global data are not available from developing countries.

ASSESSMENT

HISTORY. Ask the patient to describe any history or cardiopulmonary disease. Determine if the patient has experienced orthopnea, cough, fatigue, epigastric distress, anorexia, or weight gain or has a history of previously diagnosed lung disorders. Discuss the patient's occupational and military service history to determine if they experienced environmental or toxic exposure. Ask if the patient smokes cigarettes, noting the daily consumption and duration. Ask about the color and quantity of the mucus the patient expectorates. Determine the amount and type of dyspnea and if it is related only to exertion or is continuous.

PHYSICAL EXAMINATION. The patient may appear acutely ill with **severe dyspnea at rest** and visible **peripheral edema**. Observe if the patient has difficulty in maintaining breath while the history is taken. Evaluate the rate, type, and quality of respirations. Examine the underside of the patient's tongue, buccal mucosa, and conjunctiva for signs of central cyanosis, a finding in congestive heart failure. Oral mucous membranes in dark-skinned individuals are ashen when the patient is cyanotic. Observe the patient for dependent edema from the abdomen (ascites) and buttocks and down both legs.

Inspect the patient's chest and thorax for the general appearance and anteroposterior diameter. Look for the use of accessory muscles in breathing. If the patient can be supine, check for evidence of normal jugular vein protrusion. Place the patient in a semi-Fowler position with the head turned away from you. Use a light from the side, which casts shadows along the neck, and look for jugular vein distention and pulsation. Continue looking at the jugular veins and determine the highest level of pulsation using your fingers to measure the number of finger-breadths above the angle of Louis.

While the patient is in semi-Fowler position with the side lighting still in place, look for chest wall movement, visible pulsations, and exaggerated lifts and heaves in all areas of the precordium. Locate the point of maximum impulse (at the fifth intercostal space, just medial of the midclavicular line) and take the apical pulse for a full minute. Listen for abnormal heart sounds. Hypertrophy of the right side of the heart causes a delayed conduction time and deviation of the heart from its axis, which can result in dysrhythmias. With the diaphragm of the stethoscope, auscultate heart sounds in the aortic, pulmonic, tricuspid, and mitral areas. In cor pulmonale, there is an accentuation of the pulmonic component of the second heart sound. The S_3 and S_4 sounds resemble a horse gallop. The presence of the fourth heart sound is found in cor pulmonale. Auscultate the patient's lungs, listening for normal and abnormal breath sounds. Listen for bibasilar rales and other adventitious sounds throughout the lung fields.

PSYCHOSOCIAL. The patient has had to live with the anxiety of shortness of breath for a long time. Chronic hypoxia can lead to restlessness and confusion, and the patient may seem irritated or angry during the physical examination.

Diagnostic Highlights

Test	Normal Result	Abnormality With Condition	Explanation
Chest x-rays	Normal heart size and clear lungs	Enlarged right ventricle and pulmonary artery; may show pneumonia	Demonstrate right-sided hypertrophy of heart and possibly pulmonary infection with other underlying pulmonary abnormalities
Electrocardio-gram (ECG)	Normal electro-cardiographic wave form with P, Q, R, S, T waves	To reveal increased P-wave amplitude (P-pulmonale) in leads II, III, and a ventricular failure seen in right-axis devi-ation and incomplete right bundle branch block	Changes in cardiac conduction due to right-sided hypertrophy
Echocardiography (two dimensional and Doppler)	Normal heart size	To show ventricular hypertro-phy, decreased contractility, and valvular disorders in both right and left ventricular failure	Demonstrates heart hypertrophy and tricus-pid valve malfunction if present

Other Tests: Magnetic resonance imaging; ultrafast, ECG-gated computed tomogra-phy scanning; ventilation/perfusion (V/Q) lung scanning; complete blood count, coag-ulation profile, arterial blood gases; brain natriuretic peptide (may be elevated due to elevated pulmonary hypertension and right-sided heart failure or in decompensated left ventricular heart failure)

PRIMARY NURSING DIAGNOSIS

DIAGNOSIS. Decreased cardiac output related to an ineffective ventricular pump as evidenced by dyspnea at rest and/or peripheral edema

OUTCOMES. Cardiac pump effectiveness; Circulation status; Tissue perfusion; Fatigue level; Knowledge: Chronic disease management; Vital signs; Electrolyte and acid-base balance; Endurance; Energy conservation; Fluid balance

INTERVENTIONS. Cardiac care; Fluid/electrolyte management; Medication administration; Medication management; Oxygen therapy; Vital signs monitoring

PLANNING AND IMPLEMENTATION
Collaborative

The primary goals of treatment for cor pulmonale are to manage the underlying lung disease, improve oxygenation, and increase right ventricular contractility. The patient with an acute exacerbation of cor pulmonale requires mechanical ventilation and is usually admitted to an intensive care unit. Patients admitted with heart failure related to ARDS or pulmonary embolism who require specialized treatment, such as hemodynamic monitoring, may also be admitted to a special care unit.

Specific medical treatment for cor pulmonale consists of reversing hypoxia with low-flow oxygen and improving right ventricular function, depending on the underlying cause. In the case of acute cor pulmonale associated with pulmonary emboli, higher concentrations of oxygen may be used. The physician seeks to correct fluid, electrolyte, and acid-base disturbances and may prescribe fluid and sodium restrictions to reduce plasma volume and the work of the heart. In the setting of right ventricular failure, therapies may include vasopressor medications and fluid loading to maintain blood pressure. Single-lung or double-lung transplantation may be considered for people with terminal disease.

SUPPORTIVE CARE. Respiratory therapists provide bronchodilator therapy and may need to teach or reinforce the patient's use of breathing strategies. Therapists may also teach energy conservation. A dietitian confers with the patient and family about the need for low-sodium foods and small, nutritious servings. Specific nutritional deficiencies may need to be corrected as well. Depending on the derivation of cor pulmonale, fluids need to be limited to 1,000 to 1,500 mL per day to prevent fluid retention. Social service agencies will probably be needed for a consultation as well because cor pulmonale creates long-term disability with the likelihood that the patient has not been employed for some time. Unless the patient is old enough to receive Medicare, hospitalization costs are a serious concern.

Pharmacologic Highlights

Medication or Drug Class	Dosage	Description	Rationale
Calcium channel blockers	Varies with drug	Nifedipine, diltiazem	Lower pulmonary pressures
Bronchodilators	Varies with drug	Beta$_2$-adrenergic agonists, anticholinergics	Relieve bronchospasm

Other Drugs: Diuretics are used when right ventricular pressures are elevated, but they are used cautiously so that cardiac output does not decrease. Massive pulmonary embolism may require thrombolytic agents. Oxygen therapy, vasodilators, low-dose digitalis, theophylline, antidysrhythmic agents, prostacyclin analogues and receptor agonists, endothelin receptor antagonists, and anticoagulation therapy may be used in long-term management.

Independent

The patient requires bedrest and assistance with the activities of daily living if hypoxemia and hypercapnia are severe. Provide meticulous skin care. Reposition the bedridden patient frequently to prevent atelectasis. Reinforce proper breathing strategies for the patient: breathe in through the nose and out slowly through pursed lips, using abdominal muscles to squeeze out the air; inhale before beginning an activity and then exhale while doing the activity, such as walking or eating.

Nurses can teach patients to control their anxiety, which affects their breathlessness and fear. Teach the patient the use of relaxation techniques. Because patients are continually breathless, they become anxious if they feel rushed; focus on providing a calm approach. Help reduce the patient's fear of exertional dyspnea by providing thoughtful care that builds trust. Encourage the patient to progress in small increments.

Because of the exertion that talking requires, many patients with cor pulmonale may not be able to respond adequately in conversation. Try to understand the patient's reluctance to "tire out" and become familiar with reflective techniques that allow a patient to respond briefly. Integrate your teaching into the care to avoid the need to give the patient too much information to assimilate at the time of discharge.

Evidence-Based Practice and Health Policy

Mandoli, G., Sciaccaluga, C., Bandera, F., Cameli, P., Esposito, R., D'Andrea, A., Evola, V., Sorrentino, R., Malagoli, A., Sisti, N., Nistor, D., Santoro, C., Bargagli, E., Mondillo, S., Galderisi, M., & Cameli, M. (2021). Cor pulmonale: The role of traditional and advanced echocardiography in the acute and chronic settings. *Heart Failure Reviews, 26,* 263–275.

- The authors explained the value of echocardiography in diagnosing cor pulmonale and creating a therapeutic plan. They provided an overview of the current standards of an echocardiographic evaluation in both acute and chronic cor pulmonale, focusing also on the findings in the most common pathologies causing this condition.
- Although the distinction between acute and chronic cor pulmonale is primarily based on taking the patient's history and performing a clinical examination, echocardiography can provide additional information about right ventricular morphology and function. In the context of both acute and chronic cor pulmonale, echocardiography also can provide information to help in determining particular treatments as well as evaluating their success.

DOCUMENTATION GUIDELINES

- Physical findings: Vein distention, presence of peripheral edema, cardiopulmonary assessment
- Responses to activity, treatments, and medications
- Understanding of and willingness to carry out prescribed therapy

DISCHARGE AND HOME HEALTHCARE GUIDELINES

COMPLICATIONS. Teach the patient and family the signs and symptoms of infection, such as increased sputum production, change in sputum color, increased coughing or wheezing, chest pain, fever, and tightness in the chest. Teach the patient how to recognize signs of edema. Make sure the patient knows to call the physician upon recognizing these signs.

MEDICATIONS. Be sure the patient understands any pain medication prescribed, including dosage, route, action, and side effects.

NUTRITION. Explain the importance of maintaining a low-sodium diet. Review nutrition counseling and the prescribed fluid intake.

ONGOING OXYGEN THERAPY. If the patient is going home with low-flow oxygen, ensure that an appropriate vendor is contacted. Determine whether a home care agency needs to evaluate the home for safety equipment and pollution factors.

Crohn Disease

DRG Category:	329
Mean LOS:	13.1 days
Description:	SURGICAL: Major Small and Large Bowel Procedures With Major Complication or Comorbidity
DRG Category:	386
Mean LOS:	4.3 days
Description:	MEDICAL: Inflammatory Bowel Disease With Complication or Comorbidity

Crohn disease (CD), also known as *granulomatous colitis* or *regional enteritis*, is a chronic, nonspecific inflammatory disease of the bowel that occurs most commonly in the terminal ileum, jejunum, and colon, although it may affect any part of the gastrointestinal (GI) system from the mouth to the anus. In the United States, approximately 800,000 people have CD; the annual incidence of CD is estimated between 1 and 10 cases per 100,000 people. Like ulcerative colitis, CD is marked by remissions and exacerbations, but, unlike ulcerative colitis, it can affect any portion of the tubular GI tract.

Because of chronic inflammation of T cells, tissues in the GI tract are injured because of cytokines such as interleukin-12 and tumor necrosis factor alpha that are released during the inflammatory response. The cytokines recruit inflammatory cells that release substances that directly injure the intestine. The disease creates deep, longitudinal mucosal ulcerations and thickening of the mucosa called *granulomas*, which give the intestinal wall a cobblestone appearance and may alter its absorptive abilities. The inflamed and ulcerated areas occur only in segments of the bowel, and normal bowel tissue segments occur between the diseased segments. Eventually, thickening of the bowel wall, narrowing of the bowel lumen, and strictures of the bowel are common. Also, fistulae that connect to other tissue—such as the skin, bladder, rectum, and vagina—often occur. Other complications include GI obstruction, colon cancer, and perforated abdomen. Some patients develop musculoskeletal diseases such as arthritis and fibromyalgia and dermatologic conditions.

CAUSES

Research has not established a specific cause for CD, but experts suggest that it may be an imbalance between proinflammatory and anti-inflammatory mediators. Some experts suggest that patients have an inherited susceptibility for an abnormal immunological response to one or more of these factors: infectious agents such as a virus or bacterium, an autoimmune reaction, environmental factors such as geographic location, individual factors such as smoking and dietary exposure, and genetic factors. Researchers now believe that emotional stress and psychological changes are results of the chronic and severe symptoms of CD rather than causes of the disease.

GENETIC CONSIDERATIONS

There is no clear agreement on how genetic and environmental factors lead to the tissue damage in inflammatory bowel disease. A sibling of an affected person has a 30% higher risk of developing the disease than someone from the general population. Mutations in the gene encoding NOD2 (nucleotide-binding oligomerization domain protein 2) may result in CD by altering intestinal production of antimicrobial proteins. Recent evidence indicates that the *GLI1* gene appears to be important for an appropriate inflammatory response, and the *CCDC88B* gene is necessary for colitis to occur. Variants in these genes have been linked to CD.

SEX AND LIFE SPAN CONSIDERATIONS

CD may occur at any age in both men and women, with rates slightly higher in males; it is generally first diagnosed between the ages of 15 and 30 years, although CD is increasingly being diagnosed in children. Reports indicate that the number being diagnosed at age 55 years and older is growing; thus, the age distribution is bimodal (15–30 and 55–70). Two factors that may predispose older adults to CD are an increased vulnerability to infection and a susceptibility to inadequate blood supply to the bowel because of the aging process.

HEALTH DISPARITIES AND SEXUAL/GENDER MINORITY HEALTH

CD is more common in White than Black or Asian persons in the United States, and there is a two- to fourfold increase of the prevalence of CD in Jewish persons in the United States and Europe as compared with other groups. Children from low-income families or who are Black or Hispanic are less likely to undergo major operative procedures to manage CD as compared to higher-income or White children (McLoughlin et al., 2020). Black children also have more active disease than White children and therefore carry a heavier disease burden. While sexual and gender minority persons have no known specific risk for CD, they are at risk for multiple chronic conditions, difficulty accessing high-quality healthcare, and mental health risks due to stress, bullying, discrimination, and stigma, all which may be related to risk.

GLOBAL HEALTH CONSIDERATIONS

Western developed countries seem to have a similar prevalence of CD. In Western Europe and North America, the more temperate the climate and the more urban the environment, the higher are the rates of CD. Urban areas with high social deprivation and low incomes are associated with higher levels of CD. Rates are lower in Asia and the Middle East as compared to North America and Western Europe, and people from South America and Africa have the lowest rates.

ASSESSMENT

HISTORY. Obtain a complete family, medical, and surgical history. With children, obtain a nutritional and growth history from the parents. Patients initially report insidious symptoms such as nonbloody diarrhea (three to five semisoft stools per day), fatigue, anorexia, weight loss, and vague, intermittent abdominal pain. Some patients may have nausea and vomiting. As the disease progresses, they complain of more severe, constant abdominal pain that typically localizes in the right lower quadrant, more severe fatigue, and moderate fever. Some patients may also report mucus and/or pus in the stool as well as skin breakdown in the perineal and rectal areas.

PHYSICAL EXAMINATION. Most common symptoms include **low-grade fever**, **diarrhea with abdominal pain**, **weight loss**, and **fatigue**. Because CD is a chronic disease that affects the GI system and causes anorexia and multiple episodes of diarrhea, common problems are malnutrition and dehydration. Inspect for hair loss, dry skin, dry and sticky mucous membranes, poor skin turgor, muscle weakness, and lethargy. The patient may have oral ulcers. Also, inspect the patient's perianal area for signs of fistula formation.

Palpate the patient's abdomen for pain, tenderness, or distention. Generally, pain localizes in the right lower quadrant, but note the location, intensity, type, and duration of discomfort. Auscultate the patient's abdomen for bowel sounds. Often, hyperactive sounds will be noted during an acute inflammatory episode.

PSYCHOSOCIAL. The effects of chronic illness and debilitating symptoms, along with frequent hospitalizations, often result in psychological problems and social isolation. In the past, experts suggested that emotional stress and psychological changes caused CD, but current thinking is that mental distress is the result of trying to cope with chronic and severe symptoms. Assess the coping mechanisms as well as the patient's support system.

Diagnostic Highlights

Test	Normal Result	Abnormality With Condition	Explanation
Sigmoidoscopy or colonoscopy	Normal GI tract on direct visualization	To detect location of illness as well as early mucosal changes, inflammation, strictures, and fistulae	May help differentiate CD from ulcerative colitis and allows for biopsy
Imaging studies (plain radiography, computed tomography, computed enterography, magnetic resonance imaging)	Normal GI tract without bowel obstruction, inflammation, fibrosis, fistulae, abscesses	To determine the location and extent of rectal involvement, including inflammation strictures, perianal disease, and fistulae	To differentiate among pathologies and extent of disease

Diagnostic Highlights (continued)

Other Tests: Low-radiation protocols are used by many centers to reduce radiation exposure to younger patients and children. Complete blood count, serum albumin, cholesterol, electrolytes (particularly calcium and magnesium), C-reactive protein, orosomucoid (a globulin in blood plasma), sedimentation rate; culture of stool specimens for routine pathogens, ova, parasites, *Clostridium difficile* toxin; perinuclear antineutrophil cytoplasmic antibody (a myeloperoxidase antigen more commonly found in ulcerative colitis) and antibodies to the yeast *Saccharomyces cerevisiae* (anti–*S cerevisiae* antibodies), which are more commonly found in CD; ultrasound.

PRIMARY NURSING DIAGNOSIS

DIAGNOSIS. Imbalanced nutrition: less than body requirements related to anorexia, abdominal pain, and/or diarrhea as evidenced by weight loss

OUTCOMES. Nutritional status: Food and fluid intake; Nutritional status: Nutrient intake; Energy conservation; Bowel elimination; Endurance

INTERVENTIONS. Nutrition management; Nutrition therapy; Nutritional counseling and monitoring; Fluid/electrolyte management; Medication management; Enteral tube feeding; IV therapy; Total parenteral nutrition administration

PLANNING AND IMPLEMENTATION

Collaborative

MEDICAL. Much of the medical management centers on medications. New therapies, including biological anti–tumor necrosis factor (anti-TNF) agents, have improved medical management. During acute exacerbations, bowel rest is important to promote healing; bowel rest can be achieved by placing the patient NPO with the administration of total parenteral nutrition to supply the required fluids, nutrients, and electrolytes. Once the acute episode has subsided and symptoms are relieved, a diet high in protein, vitamins, and calories is prescribed. The patient's diet should be balanced, and supplements of fiber may be beneficial for colonic disease; a low-roughage diet is usually indicated for patients with obstructive symptoms. In addition, a low-residue, milk-free diet is generally well tolerated.

SURGICAL. Surgery, although not a primary intervention, may be necessary for patients who develop complications such as bowel perforation, abscess, intestinal obstruction, fistulae, or hemorrhage and for those who do not respond to conservative management such as nutritional and drug therapy. Unfortunately, there is a 60% recurrence of the disease process after surgical intervention. Multiple resections also may lead to short-bowel syndrome, defined as malabsorption of fluids, electrolytes, and nutrients, which leads to nutritional deficiencies. The syndrome occurs when less than 150 cm of functional small bowel remains.

Pharmacologic Highlights

Medication or Drug Class	Dosage	Description	Rationale
Mesalamine (5-ASA; see description) (Asacol, Pentasa)	800–1,600 mg PO tid	Anti-inflammatory agent, 5-ASA	5-ASA preparations such as mesalamine have become treatment of choice; can be used in people who cannot tolerate sulfasalazine

(highlight box continues on page 330)

Pharmacologic Highlights (continued)

Medication or Drug Class	Dosage	Description	Rationale
Biological anti–TNF agents (infliximab, adalimumab, certolizumab pegol, natalizumab)	Varies with drug	Monoclonal antibodies	Improves likelihood of induction and maintenance of remission; used in severe disease unresponsive to other therapies
Other anti-inflammatories	Varies with drug; sulfasalazine: 0.5–1 g PO qid; prednisone: 10–40 mg PO tid; methylprednisolone: 20–40 mg IV q 12 hr; hydrocortisone: 100 mg IV q 6 hr	Sulfasalazine (Azulfidine) and corticosteroids	Slow the inflammatory process; sulfasalazine is not used in treatment of disease confined to small intestine; glucocorticoids such as prednisone are used in acute exacerbations. Agents are administered until clinical symptoms subside, at which time steroidal agents are tapered off
Antidiarrheal agents	Varies with drug	Example: loperamide (Imodium)	Alleviate symptoms of abdominal cramping and diarrhea in patients with mild symptoms or postresection diarrhea
Metronidazole (Flagyl)	250 mg PO tid	Antibacterial agent	Effective in colon disease; treats infections with fistulae and perianal skin breakdown; beneficial in patients who have not responded to other agents
Immunosuppressive agents	Varies with drug	Azathioprine (Imuran) 6-mercaptopurine, methotrexate	Decrease inflammation and symptoms if steroids fail or decrease steroid requirements

Other Drugs: Abdominal cramps may be treated with propantheline, dicyclomine, or hyoscyamine, but these drugs should not be used if a bowel obstruction is possible. Some patients who are suffering with severe abdominal pain may require narcotic analgesics such as meperidine (Demerol). Also, patients who develop deficiencies because of problems of malabsorption may require vitamin B_{12} injections monthly or iron replacement therapy. Other nutritional supplements include calcium, magnesium, folate, and other micronutrients.

Independent

Nursing care focuses on supporting the patient through acute episodes of inflammation and teaching measures to prevent future inflammatory attacks. Maintaining patient fluid and electrolyte balance is particularly important. Encourage the patient to drink 3,000 mL of fluid per day, unless it is contraindicated. Implement measures to prevent skin breakdown in the perianal area.

Provide frequent rest periods. Maintain adequate nutritional status using calorie counts. Other measures include assisting the patient with frequent oral hygiene; providing small, frequent meals with rest periods interspersed throughout the day; monitoring IV fluids and total parenteral nutrition as prescribed; and noting the patient's serum albumin levels.

Encourage patients to express their feelings and refer them for more extensive counseling as needed. Also, discuss measures to diminish stressful life situations with the patient and family.

Evidence-Based Practice and Health Policy

Sandall, A., Wall, C., & Lomer, M. (2020). Nutrition assessment in Crohn's disease using anthropometric, biochemical, and dietary indexes: A narrative review. *Journal of the Academy of Nutrition and Dietetics, 120*(4), 624–640.

• The authors evaluated existing evidence for nutrition assessment of patients with CD compared with healthy controls with the goal of providing a comprehensive guide with relevant measures for clinical practice. The authors conducted a literature search using Medline, Embase, and Scopus from inception to October 1, 2018. They focused on 41 articles that assessed body composition, muscle strength, micronutrient status, and/or dietary intake in adults with CD compared with age- and sex-matched healthy individuals.

• While only a single article reported a clinically significant difference for body mass index, significant deficits in fat mass, fat-free mass, and muscle strength were observed in patients with CD compared with healthy controls. The studies also reported significantly lower serum micronutrients, lower intake of micronutrients, and lower fruit and vegetable intake in patients with CD.

DOCUMENTATION GUIDELINES

• Evidence of stability of vital signs, hydration status, bowel sounds, and electrolytes
• Response to medications; tolerance of foods; ability to eat and select a well-balanced diet and weight gains or losses
• Location, intensity, and frequency of pain; factors that relieve pain
• Number of diarrheal episodes and stool characteristics
• Presence of complications: Fistulae, skin breakdown, abscess formation, infection

DISCHARGE AND HOME HEALTHCARE GUIDELINES

Emphasize measures that will help prevent future inflammatory episodes, such as getting plenty of rest and relaxation, reducing stress, and maintaining proper diet (high protein, low residue). Teach the patient to recognize the signs of incipient inflammatory attacks. Explain all the prescribed medications, including the actions, side effects, dosages, and routes. Be certain the patient understands signs of possible complications, such as an abscess, fistula, hemorrhage, or infection, and the need to seek medical attention if any of them occurs. Caution the patient to be vigilant with skin care, especially in the perianal area. Instruct the patient to assess frequently for breakdown in this area and seek medical attention if it should occur.

Cushing Syndrome

DRG Category:	644
Mean LOS:	4.3 days
Description:	MEDICAL: Endocrine Disorders With Complication or Comorbidity

Cushing syndrome (CS) is defined as the clinical effects of increased glucocorticoid hormone. It can be characterized by an excess production of glucocorticoids (primarily cortisol) by the cortex of the adrenal gland, but it is most commonly due to therapy with glucocorticoid drugs. Cortisol is an essential hormone for many body functions, including maintaining normal electrical excitation of the heart, blood glucose level, nerve cell conduction, and adequate circulatory volume, and for metabolizing proteins, fats, and carbohydrates.

Overproduction of glucocorticoids leads to a host of multisystem disorders in metabolism, water balance, wound healing, and response to infection. Complications affect almost every system of the body. Increased calcium resorption from bones may lead to osteoporosis and bone fractures. A blunted immune response causes a high risk for infection as well as poor wound healing. CS may also mask life-threatening infections. Gastrointestinal (GI) irritation may lead to peptic ulcers, and both insulin resistance and glucose intolerance can cause hyperglycemia.

CAUSES

The causes are divided into three categories: iatrogenic, primary, and secondary. More than 99% of CS is due to iatrogenic causes (disorder caused by medical treatment), the result of excessive cortisol levels from chronic therapy with glucocorticoids. This type of CS is also called *exogenous (external) CS*. Primary and secondary CS are from endogenous (internal) causes. When cortisol-producing tumors occur in adrenal glands, they cause primary CS. These tumors have a high risk of malignancy, particularly in children. Most secondary CS in adults is caused by excessive adrenocorticotropic hormone (ACTH) production from pituitary adenomas. Overproduction of ACTH leads to overproduction of cortisol from the adrenal glands. Other tumors can also produce ACTH, particularly in the lung, with the same resulting overproduction of cortisol by the adrenal glands.

GENETIC CONSIDERATIONS

Most cases of Cushing syndrome (CS) are sporadic and therefore not inherited. However, CS can occur in other inherited conditions that affect endocrine function. These include multiple endocrine neoplasia type I (MEN I), McCune-Albright syndrome, Li-Fraumeni syndrome, Beckwith-Wiedeman syndrome, and Carney complex.

SEX AND LIFE SPAN CONSIDERATIONS

While 90% of cases of CS occur in adults, in infants it usually results from adrenal carcinoma. Primary disease is often linked to a familial autoimmune disorder and is seen in children and young adults of both sexes. Secondary disease is more common than primary disease in children older than 6 or 7 years and, as in adults, is usually the result of overproduction of ACTH. In adults, secondary CS that results from pituitary disease is most common in females aged 30 to 50 years. Secondary CS that results from ACTH-secreting tumors outside of the pituitary is more common in males, possibly because of the higher incidence of bronchogenic carcinomas caused by smoking.

HEALTH DISPARITIES AND SEXUAL/GENDER MINORITY HEALTH

Ethnicity, race, and sexual/gender minority status have no known effect on the risk for CS.

GLOBAL HEALTH CONSIDERATIONS

Incidence of adrenal tumors is greater in some regions of the world, such as South America and Japan, but it is unclear whether these differences are caused by environmental or genetic factors.

ASSESSMENT

HISTORY. Question whether the patient is taking corticosteroid medications, and if so, for how long. Generally, the symptoms of CS do not occur until the individual has taken the medications for at least a month. Ask if the patient has had recent changes in memory, attention span, or behavior. Discuss the patient's sleep-wake pattern, and evaluate the patient for sleep disturbances. Family members may comment on the patient's changed affect, short-term memory, emotional instability, and ability to concentrate.

Some patients describe gastric pain or irritation of ulcers. Other signs include weakness, fatigue, back pain, general discomfort, difficulty completing activities of daily living, and changes in urinary output. Be sure to question the patient about weight gain and changes in body proportions between the shoulders. Patients may report that their face is more rounded ("moon face"). Patients may also notice changes in their appetite and thirst. Other changes in appearance include hirsutism, oily skin, acne, purple striae, and poor wound healing. Women may have noted changes in menstruation, and both men and women may note changes in libido and in their feelings about themselves.

PHYSICAL EXAMINATION. Most common symptoms include **muscle weaknesses, visual disturbances**, and **truncal weight gain**. Changes in fat metabolism lead to generalized obesity, a round ("moon") face, a hump in the interscapular area, and truncal obesity. Hyperpigmentation of skin and mucous membranes may be present as a result of increases in ACTH. Because of alterations in protein metabolism, loss of collagen support in the skin leaves the skin more fragile and easily bruised. Both males and females experience changes in secondary sexual characteristics and body hair distribution, along with an increase in acne. Some patients have peripheral edema from water and sodium retention. Muscle wasting, especially in extremities, leads to difficulty in getting up and down from a sitting position, difficulty in climbing stairs, or generalized weakness and fatigue. Note if the extremities are thin with atrophied muscles.

Auscultate the patient's blood pressure; most patients are hypertensive because of increased circulating volume or increased sensitivity of the arterioles to circulating catecholamines. Neck vein distention may be present.

PSYCHOSOCIAL. A diagnosis of CS can be devastating depending on the underlying cause. Determine the patient's response to the disease and the effect the disease has had on the patient's sexuality, body image, and relationships with others.

Diagnostic Highlights

Abnormal blood chemistries are common, including hypokalemia, hypochloremia, and metabolic alkalosis because of increased excretion of potassium and chloride. Random cortical tests are not useful for diagnosis because of the wide range of normal values.

Test	Normal Result	Abnormality With Condition	Explanation
24-hr urine testing for urinary free cortisol	Urinary free cortisol: > 70 mg/ 1.73 m²/24 hr	Elevated	Increased production or ingestion of glucocorticoids
Overnight dexamethasone suppression test: 1 mg given PO at 11 p.m.; plasma cortisol levels are measured at 8 a.m. the next morning	Plasma cortisol level: 5 mcg/dL	Elevated above 5 mcg/dL	Failure to suppress normal cortisol response is diagnostic of CS; abnormal results indicate need for low-dose dexamethasone suppression test
Low-dose dexamethasone suppression test; 0.5 mg dexamethasone given PO q 6 hr for 48 hr	Urine cortisol: 20 mcg/dL for 24 hr	Elevated above 20 mcg/dL for 24 hr	Failure to suppress normal cortisol response is diagnostic of CS; testing should not be done during severe illness or depression, which may lead to false-positive results; phenytoid therapy alters dexamethasone metabolism and may lead to false results

(highlight box continues on page 334)

Diagnostic Highlights (continued)

Test	Normal Result	Abnormality With Condition	Explanation
Adrenocorticotropic hormone level	< 80 pg/mL in a.m.; < 50 pg/mL in p.m.	Results vary; see explanation	Elevated with high cortisol levels if ACTH-producing tumor; decreased with high cortisol levels if adrenal adenoma or carcinoma is present

Other Tests: Complete blood count, computed tomography scan, bone age, bone mineral density, pituitary magnetic resonance imaging, ultrasound, and angiogram

PRIMARY NURSING DIAGNOSIS

DIAGNOSIS. Excess fluid volume related to abnormal retention of sodium and water as evidenced by weight gain

OUTCOMES. Fluid balance; Hydration; Electrolyte balance; Nutritional status; Knowledge: Treatment regime

INTERVENTIONS. Fluid/electrolyte management; Fluid monitoring; Medication administration; Weight management

PLANNING AND IMPLEMENTATION

Collaborative

The main focus is to find the primary cause of the cortisol excess and remove it if possible. In the case of iatrogenic CS, care is focused on alleviating as many of the signs and symptoms as possible when the therapy cannot be discontinued. If the patient has primary CS from an adrenal tumor, the tumor is removed surgically. Even if the tumor is unilateral, the patient is treated for adrenal insufficiency after the surgery because the high levels of cortisol from the tumor may have caused the unaffected adrenal gland to atrophy. Patients with adrenal carcinoma are treated postoperatively with mitotane to treat metastases. Throughout the patient's recovery, fluid, electrolyte, and nutritional assessment and balance are essential.

For secondary CS from a pituitary tumor, the preferred option is a transsphenoidal adenectomy, a procedure that explores the pituitary gland to find microadenomas. It is successful in 20% to 70% of patients. A second option is the transsphenoidal hypophysectomy, a procedure that removes the entire pituitary gland and leads to a cure in 100% of patients. It is usually used for more invasive tumors and requires lifelong hormone replacement (glucocorticoids, thyroid hormone, gonadal steroids, and antidiuretic hormone). In a newer procedure, surgeons use endoscopic surgery, operating through a fiberoptic device that has been inserted through an incision in the lining of the nose. This procedure takes less time and causes fewer complications than transsphenoidal hypophysectomy. A third alternative is bilateral total adrenalectomy, which cures the signs and symptoms of excess cortisol but does not decrease ACTH secretion. The patient requires lifelong replacement therapy with glucocorticoids and mineralocorticoids. If the patient has secondary CS because of ectopic production of ACTH from a nonendocrine tumor, the first concern is to remove the source of the ectopic secretion of ACTH. If this is not possible, mitotane (see Pharmacologic Highlights) decreases cortisol production in the adrenal gland but may cause damage to the gland and is used with caution. Radiation therapy is used when the patient either has no defined tumor or needs an adjunct to tumor removal.

POSTOPERATIVE. Patients with pituitary surgery need careful management of airway, breathing, and circulation. In the first postoperative hours, serial neurological examinations are important to identify the risk for increased intracranial pressure from edema. The incision is generally performed through the upper gum line; ask the surgeon about the procedure for oral hygiene. Nasal packing is removed after 2 days in most patients. At that time, observe for rhinorrhea, and ask the patient to report a "runny" nose. Teach the patient to avoid coughing, sneezing, or blowing the nose immediately after surgery.

Pharmacologic Highlights

Medication or Drug Class	Dosage	Description	Rationale
Mitotane	2–16 g per day in divided doses PO	Antineoplastic	Inhibits activity of adrenal cortex; used to treat inoperable adrenocortical carcinomas and CS

Other Drugs: Etomidate is an ultra short-acting nonbarbiturate hypnotic that blocks steroid production. Ketoconazole is an antifungal agent that also blocks steroid production. Aminoglutethimide inhibits cholesterol synthesis, and metyrapone partially inhibits adrenal cortex steroid synthesis. These drugs may be used in conjunction with surgery or radiation if the tumor is not completely resectable or if complete remission is not expected.

Independent

An important goal is to limit the risk of infection for the patient. Note, document, and report any signs of skin or pulmonary infection. Restrict visitors with upper respiratory infections. Unless contraindicated after surgery, encourage the patient to cough and deep breathe, turn in bed at least every 2 hours, and use good oral hygiene. Focus on helping the patient deal with changes in body image, sexuality, and self-esteem. Let the patient know that many of the body changes are reversible with treatment; this information allows the patient to focus on setting goals. Include the patient's partner in all education. Patient and family teaching occurs throughout the patient's hospitalization and after discharge. Provide information about patient care and activity restrictions. Explanations of all diagnostic tests and their findings, as well as the treatment plan, are important. The patient and family often require time to consider treatment options. As time progresses, the patient and family need information about the disease process and lifelong management with medication and diet changes.

Evidence-Based Practice and Health Policy

Palen-Tytko, J., Przybylik-Mazurek, E., Rzepka, E., Pach, D., Sowa-Staszczak, A., Gillis-Januszewska, A., & Hubalewska-Dydejczyk, A. (2020). Ectopic ACTH syndrome of different origin: Diagnostic approach and clinical outcome: Experience of one clinical centre. *PLOS ONE, 15*(11), e0242679. https://doi.org/10.1371/journal.pone.0242679

- The authors aimed to present a 20-year experience with 24 patients with ectopic Cushing syndrome (EAS) in a single clinical center. The diagnosis of EAS was based on the clinical presentation, imaging, and diagnostic tests to find the source.
- Half of the patients were diagnosed with neuroendocrine tumors, and in these patients muscle weakness was the leading symptom. Typical cushingoid appearance was seen in only a few patients, and more patients had weight loss than weight gain. Patients with neuroendocrine tumors had significantly higher midnight cortisol levels, and patients with infections had higher cortisol levels as well.

DOCUMENTATION GUIDELINES

- Physical response: Vital signs, neurological assessment, cardiopulmonary assessment, wound healing, signs of infection (fever, wound drainage, productive cough), important laboratory deviations (serious electrolyte imbalances, alterations in glucose levels)
- Nutrition: Daily weights, appetite, food tolerance, food preference, response to diet teaching, calorie count if indicated
- Emotional response: Concerns over body image, self-concept, mood, affect

DISCHARGE AND HOME HEALTHCARE GUIDELINES

Describe the pathophysiology of the disease. Identify factors that aggravate the disease (stress, changes in diet, injury) as well as the signs and symptoms. Explore complications of the disease and ask whom to notify if they occur. Describe the treatment plan and expected effects as well as possible complications. Describe all medications, including the name, dosage, action, side effects, route, and importance of lifelong dosing if indicated.

Cystic Fibrosis

DRG Category:	640
Mean LOS:	4.5 days
Description:	MEDICAL: Miscellaneous Disorders of Nutrition, Metabolism, Fluids, and Electrolytes With Major Complication or Comorbidity

Cystic fibrosis (CF) is a multisystem genetic disease of the exocrine glands—those glands with ducts such as the mucous, salivary, and sweat-producing glands. CF, originally called CF of the pancreas, is also associated with the glands of the respiratory system and the skin, and it has the potential for multiple organ involvement. More than 30,000 people in the United States have CF, and 1,000 new cases are diagnosed annually. In the 1950s, babies had a short life expectancy of approximately 5 years. Because of scientific advancements, recent studies report an average survival age of 56 years for males and 49 years for females. The lungs are most frequently affected, but the gastrointestinal (GI) tract (including the small intestine and pancreatic and bile ducts) and eventually the reproductive organs are affected as well.

CF leads to an increase in viscosity of bronchial and pancreatic secretions, which obstruct the glandular ducts. Secretions have less chloride and increased reabsorption of sodium and water. These changes decrease hydration of mucus, create mucus that clings to bacteria, and promote infection and inflammation. As thick secretions block the bronchioles and alveoli, the patient develops severe atelectasis (lung collapse) and emphysema. The GI effects of the disease lead to deficiency in the enzymes trypsin, amylase, and lipase. With enzyme deficiency, the conversion and absorption of fats and proteins are altered, and vitamins A, D, E, and K are not properly absorbed. Pancreatic changes include fibrosis, cyst formation, and the development of fatty deposits that lead to pancreatic insufficiency and decreased insulin production. Intelligence and cognitive function are typically not affected.

Complications of CF can be life threatening. Respiratory complications include lung collapse, pneumothorax, airway collapse, and pneumonia. GI complications include dehydration, malnutrition, gastroesophageal reflux, and rectal prolapse.

CAUSES

The responsible gene, the CF transmembrane conductance regulator (*CFTR*), is mapped to chromosome 7 (see Genetic Considerations). The underlying defect of this autosomal recessive condition involves a defective protein that interferes with chloride transport, which in turn makes the body's secretions very thick and tenacious. The ducts of the exocrine glands subsequently become obstructed.

GENETIC CONSIDERATIONS

CF is caused by mutations in the *CFTR* gene, which are inherited in an autosomal recessive pattern. Over 1,000 different mutations have been reported. Unaffected parents of an affected child are obligate carriers (heterozygotes). Disease carriers are asymptomatic, but rarely, a parent may be found to have a mild case after the diagnosis of the child is made. With two carrier parents, each sibling of the proband has a 25% chance of being affected. A symptomatic sibling has a two-thirds chance of being a carrier.

SEX AND LIFE SPAN CONSIDERATIONS

Females have persistent disadvantages as compared to men with respect to clinical outcomes and life expectancy. Experts suggest this difference may be related to female sex hormones, which may reduce mucus clearance in the airways, reduce immunity, and increase airway infection. Female airways are also more narrow than airways in males. Pulmonary function declines are steeper in females than males, adherence to therapy is lower in females than males, and females report a poorer quality of life and a stronger emotional impact on their lives than males. Adolescence tends to exacerbate symptoms, and it is often during this period that the number of hospitalizations to treat a pneumonia or "clean out" the lungs increases significantly. During adolescence, the progression of the disease is manifested in delayed menses, delayed development of secondary sex characteristics, and decreased fertility as a result of the thickened cervical mucus in females. In the event the female patient does conceive, the pregnancy is more difficult to maintain as a result of the stress on the already taxed respiratory and cardiac systems of the CF patient. Sterility is also likely in 99% of males, as the vas deferens is obstructed, preventing sperm from entering the semen. Males may produce offspring with reproductive technologies; the decision to reproduce generally occurs with the assistance of genetic counseling. In about 3% of the cases, diabetes mellitus occurs, and these children or young adults are insulin dependent. There is no cure for CF.

HEALTH DISPARITIES AND SEXUAL/GENDER MINORITY HEALTH

CF is the most common fatal genetic disease of White children with European ancestry in the United States (1 case per 3,200). Hispanic (1 case per 9,200), Black (1 case per 15,000), and Asian (1 case per 31,000) children have lower prevalence rates. A number of disparities exist with Hispanic and Black children because of complex social and environmental factors that influence health. Hispanic persons have higher rates of mortality than non-Hispanic persons. Black persons have more severe respiratory symptoms at diagnosis than non-Black persons. Hispanic and Black persons with CF have worse pulmonary function than White persons with CF. These differences may be related to unconscious bias or discrimination in healthcare, lack of access to specialty care, or other unknown factors. Sexual and gender minority status has no known effect on the risk for CF.

GLOBAL HEALTH CONSIDERATIONS

Northwestern European countries have a greater prevalence of CF than Southeastern countries such as India. In the United States, Asian American and Black people have higher rates of CF than people born in Asia and Africa, probably reflecting the influence of multiracial parentage.

While little is known about the incidence in developing countries, in European populations, the overall rate is approximately 1 case per 2,000 to 4,000 individuals, with England and Scotland reporting the highest rates.

☀ ASSESSMENT

HISTORY. CF has a highly variable presentation and course, ranging from mild to severe. The average age of diagnosis is 6 to 8 months of age. Parents often report that the child's skin has a characteristic taste of salt when they kiss the child. Hence, this classic early symptom is referred to as the "kiss of salt." In addition, during the first year or two of life, the child may experience repeated upper respiratory infections such as nasopharyngitis, croup, bronchiolitis, and pneumonia. Although the child has a voracious appetite, the child does not gain weight and has steatorrhea (frequent foul-smelling, fatty stools). Moreover, the child may not achieve developmental milestones, particularly in the area of gross motor skills.

PHYSICAL EXAMINATION. Primary symptoms depend on the age of the child. The newborn may have a **meconium ileus**; this finding occurs in about 10% to 15% of the newly diagnosed cases. The infant or child may be classified as exhibiting organic **failure to thrive** and may fall below the 10th percentile. Early in the disease, the lungs have many adventitious breath sounds, such as **coughing, rales, rhonchi**, and **wheezes**. The anterior-posterior to lateral diameter begins to increase as the disease progresses so that the child appears barrel chested. Older children may present with **chronic cough** and **sputum production**. The patient may be in acute respiratory distress with retractions or cyanosis. Clubbing of the nails is indicative of advanced progression of the disease and may be noted in a toddler or a preschooler who has a severe form of the disease. GI findings may include abdominal distension, vitamin deficiencies, or rectal prolapse.

PSYCHOSOCIAL. Children or adolescents with CF deal with a chronic illness that makes them unique from their peers. They need to feel as if they have a degree of control in their lives; this need may be manifested in refusing to take their enzymes with their meals or their insulin if they become diabetic. Body image is especially critical because of their short stature and small body structure. Many adolescents are embarrassed and try to cover up a protuberant abdomen with baggy clothing and large shirts or to disguise the clubbing of their nails with dark nail polish. In addition, the patients often learn early to achieve a sense of competency by performing well in their academics or becoming computer "wizards" because they are unable to compete in sports. Developmental tasks for children, adolescents, and young adults who have a shortened life take on a different framework from that of children who have an average life expectancy. Patients and families who receive treatment at specialized CF centers have an opportunity to receive psychological support from a team of specialists who understand the children's unique challenges across their life span. End-of-life planning and palliative care are important.

Diagnostic Highlights

General Comments: Prenatal and genetic tests are performed to identify fetal disease and carrier status. Failure to thrive and frequent upper respiratory infections often lead to diagnostic testing to confirm the CF diagnosis.

Test	Normal Result	Abnormality With Condition	Explanation
Quantitative sweat electrolyte test (pilocarpine iontophoresis)	Cl: < 40 mEq/L; Na: < 70 mEq/L	Cl > 60 mEq/L (40–60 mEq/L is highly suggestive); > 90 mEq/L (70–90 mEq/L is highly suggestive)	Almost all patients with CF have increased chloride and sodium in their sweat

Diagnostic Highlights (continued)

Test	Normal Result	Abnormality With Condition	Explanation
Genotyping	No mutations	Probes identify the most common 87 of the 900 known mutations; finding of two *CFTR* mutations along with clinical symptoms is diagnostic for the condition; negative results on genotype analysis do not exclude the diagnosis of CF	Genotyping identifies genetic alterations

Other Tests: Serum electrolytes, chest x-ray, arterial blood gases, pulmonary function tests, semen analysis, nasal potential difference measurement of the nasal mucosa, bronchoalveolar lavage, sputum microbiology

PRIMARY NURSING DIAGNOSIS

DIAGNOSIS. Ineffective airway clearance related to excess tenacious mucus as evidenced by coughing, rales, rhonchi, and/or wheezing

OUTCOMES. Respiratory status: Airway patency; Respiratory status: Gas exchange; Respiratory status: Ventilation; Infection severity; Fluid balance

INTERVENTIONS. Chest physiotherapy; Positioning; Airway management; Surveillance; Fluid management

PLANNING AND IMPLEMENTATION

Collaborative

The major goals of treatment are to improve pulmonary, GI, and pancreatic function; support nutrition; and manage complications. These goals are achieved through a combination of medications, nutrition, and exercise regimens. If antibiotics are given to prevent and treat pneumonia, the physician and pharmacist monitor therapeutic blood levels of the antibiotics to determine the peak and trough levels. To help prevent the recurrence of pneumonia, chest physiotherapy (CPT) is performed in the home or hospital four times a day before meals to avoid emesis or after an aerosol treatment. A ThAIRapy vest, a device that provides high-frequency chest wall oscillations to loosen secretions, may also be used.

Maintain calorie counts on daily meal plans; supplement nutritional needs with high-calorie feedings. A patient may also have nasogastric feedings to which pancreatic enzymes are added to ensure the digestion and absorption of fats, protein, and carbohydrates. The physician may also prescribe total parenteral nutrition and fat-soluble vitamins (A, D, E, and K).

Exercise, including mobility and muscle-strengthening exercises, should be encouraged on a regular basis. Exercise helps maintain physical wellness and supplements the patient's airway clearance strategies by helping to loosen pulmonary secretions.

Some patients develop right-sided heart failure, and if this occurs, most of them die within a year. They may require the use of home portable oxygen therapy and receive digoxin and/or diuretics. As the disease progresses toward the terminal phase, hemoptysis is present, and cyanosis is markedly apparent.

Pharmacologic Highlights

Medication or Drug Class	Dosage	Description	Rationale
Ibuprofen	High doses	NSAID	Reduces inflammation that causes damage to lung tissue; slows lung deterioration
Ivacaftor; lumacaftor; tezacaftor; elexacaftor	Varies by drug	CFTR	Potentiates CFTR protein, a chloride channel present at the surface of epithelial cells, and thereby facilitates increased chloride transport
Trimethoprim sulfame-thoxazole (Bactrim DS); gentamicin; ciprofloxacin; aztreonam; tobramycin; chloramphenicol; clinda-mycin; piperacillin; ceph-alexin; ceftazidime; other aerosol antibiotics	Depends on drug and patient	Antibiotic	Prevent and treat lung infections
Dornase alfa recombinant	2.5 mg inhaled once daily using a recommended nebulizer	Enzyme, mucolytic	Breaks down the DNA from neutrophils, loosening secretions
Pancrelipase	Enteric-coated pancreatic enzyme microspheres	Digestant	Aids in digestion of fats and proteins

Other Drugs: Supplement of fat-soluble vitamins (A, D, E, K) is necessary for biological pathways. Bronchodilators such as albuterol help open airways. Experimental Therapies: New peptide antibiotics (PA-1420, IB-357, IB-367, and SMAP-29) are being investigated as treatment for resistant bacteria. Gene and lung transplants are also being studied, and families should be informed of these options.

Independent

Educate to reinforce the importance of regular CPT and expectoration of the mucus. Encourage increased fluid intake to loosen the secretions and provide frequent mouth care before meals. Teach the parents not to offer cough suppressants, which can lead to obstruction, lung collapse, and infection.

Support the child's or adolescent's body image concerns; compliment the patient on their strengths. Encourage the child to develop in as many areas as possible. Very often, other CF patients become a significant support group as the child matures. The child is always dramatically affected when another peer with CF dies. Plan group discussions with the patients, and have a psychiatric nurse clinical specialist serve as facilitator of this grief work for both patients and staff. In addition, siblings often worry that they may contract the disease or they may exhibit feelings of jealousy of the attention given to the sibling with CF. A referral to a social worker or the Cystic Fibrosis Foundation may be needed.

Counsel couples on the risk that subsequent pregnancies may result in a child with CF, since there is a one in four chance with any pregnancy that a child could have CF if both parents are carriers. Discuss the role of amniocentesis and the difficult issues surrounding terminating a pregnancy if CF is confirmed prenatally.

Evidence-Based Practice and Health Policy

Hewer, S., Smyth, A., Brown, M., Jones, A., Hickey, H., Kenna, D., Ashby, D., Thompson, A., & Williamson, P. (2020). Intravenous versus oral antibiotics for eradication of *Pseudomonas aeruginosa* in cystic fibrosis (TORPEDO-CF): A randomised controlled trial. *The Lancet Respiratory Medicine, 8,* 975–986.

- Chronic pulmonary infection with *Pseudomonas aeruginosa* is an important cause of mortality and morbidity in people with CF. Antibiotics need to be started early in the course of illness. The authors aimed to compare the effectiveness and safety of IV ceftazidime and tobramycin versus oral ciprofloxacin to eliminate an infection with *P aeruginosa*. The authors conducted a multicenter, parallel group, open-label, randomized controlled trial in 72 CF centers in the United Kingdom and Italy.
- While a higher percentage of participants receiving antibiotics orally achieved the primary outcome, the differences were not statistically significant, and the same percentage of participants in both groups experienced serious adverse events. These results do not support the use of IV antibiotics to manage this condition.

DOCUMENTATION GUIDELINES

- Physical response: Pulmonary assessment; color, odor, character of mucus; cardiac and GI assessment; pulse oximetry
- Nutritional data: Weight, use of enzymes, adherence to supplemental feedings
- Emotional response: Patient's feelings about dealing with a chronic illness, patient's body image, parents' coping ability, siblings' response

DISCHARGE AND HOME HEALTHCARE GUIDELINES

Teach the patient and family how to prevent future episodes of pneumonia through CPT, expectoration of sputum, and avoidance of peers with common colds and nasopharyngitis. Explain that medications need to be taken at the time of each meal, especially pancreatic enzymes and supplemental vitamins. Teach the parents protocols for home IV care, as needed. Teach parents when to contact the physician when temperature is elevated over 100.5°F (38.1°C), sputum has color to it, or the child complains of increased lung congestion or abdominal pain. Also educate parents on the need to keep routine follow-up appointments for medication, laboratory, and general checkups. Teach the patient or parents proper insulin administration and the appropriate signs and symptoms of high and low glucose levels.

Cystitis

DRG Category:	689
Mean LOS:	4.8 days
Description:	MEDICAL: Kidney and Urinary Tract Infections With Major Complication or Comorbidity

Cystitis is an inflammation of the bladder wall, which may be acute or chronic. It is generally accepted to be an ascending infection, with entry of the pathogen via the urethral opening. Noninfectious cystitis is referred to as interstitial cystitis (IC), but this is a poorly understood disorder with an uncertain cause. In this condition, in spite of symptoms of cystitis, the urine is sterile. The person develops a decreased bladder capacity, possibly because of the healing of bladder ulcers (called *Hunner ulcer*) that leave behind scar tissue. If IC is associated with chemical agents that lead to bleeding, it is termed *hemorrhagic cystitis*; otherwise, IC may also be termed *painful bladder disease* (PBD).

Although cystitis occurs in both men and women, the incidence in women is significantly higher. Sexually active women have 50 times more cystitis than men in general. In the United States, approximately 20% to 40% of young adult women have had cystitis at some point in their lives. Females are more susceptible to cystitis because of their short urethra, which is 1 to 2 inches long, as contrasted with the male urethra, which is 7 to 8 inches in length. The placement of the female urethra, which is closer to the anus than the male urethra, increases the risk of infection from bacteria in the stool. Complications of cystitis include pyelonephritis, urinary sepsis, and septic shock.

CAUSES

The most common pathogen that leads to bladder infection is *Escherichia coli*, which accounts for about 80% of cases of cystitis. Other common pathogens include *Proteus*, *Klebsiella*, and *Enterobacter*. Three main mechanisms lead to bladder infections: colonization of the lower urinary tract that ascends to the bladder, spread of infection from the bloodstream, and spread of infection from the peri-urogenital area. Predisposing factors are urethral damage from childbirth, catheterization, or surgery; decreased frequency of urination; other medical conditions such as diabetes mellitus; and, in women, frequent sexual activity and some forms of contraceptives (poorly fitting diaphragms, use of spermicides). No one is certain about the frequency of viral and herpetic cystitis because culture results are sometimes negative even when the patient has the condition. A large number of people probably have asymptomatic infections initially with herpes simplex viruses, so the incidence of herpetic cystitis may be higher than culture-positive results indicate. Hemorrhagic cystitis may also occur owing to adenoviral infections, particularly in people who are immunocompromised, such as patients with bone marrow transplantation or AIDS.

The cause of IC is unknown but has been linked to chemical agents such as some medications (cyclophosphamide) and radiation therapy. Some experts suggest that IC is an autoimmune response, a result of pelvic floor dysfunction, neural hypersensitivity, and/or disruptions of the layers of the bladder. The incidence of IC is higher in women with systemic lupus erythematosus than other women, showing the possible association of IC and autoimmune responses.

GENETIC CONSIDERATIONS

Heritable immune responses could be protective or increase susceptibility.

SEX AND LIFE SPAN CONSIDERATIONS

Cystitis is uncommon in young children and teenagers. Pregnancy increases the risk of infection because of hormonal changes in women and because the enlarging uterus restricts the flow of urine and creates urinary stasis and bacteria proliferation. Although at one time IC was considered a disease of menopause, experts note that it is most common in middle-aged rather than older women. As women age, vaginal flora and lubrication change; decreased lubrication increases the risk of urethral irritation in women during intercourse. Men, on the other hand, secrete prostatic fluid that serves as an antibacterial defense. As men age past 50 years, however, the prostate gland enlarges, which increases the risk for urinary retention and infection. By age 70 years, prevalence is similar for men and women, but prior to that, cystitis is three times as common in women than men.

HEALTH DISPARITIES AND SEXUAL/GENDER MINORITY HEALTH

Cystitis and urinary tract infections (UTIs) occur across all population groups. IC occurs primarily in women and is more common in Jewish women, and prevalence is higher among

U.S. women than among women in Europe and Japan. Sexual and gender minority status has no known effect on the risk for cystitis.

GLOBAL HEALTH CONSIDERATIONS

Some European countries have rates of cystitis higher than the U.S. rates. In most developed countries, 20% to 40% of women have cystitis at some point in their lives. Schistosomiasis and tuberculosis resulting in cystitis are more common in developing countries and countries with warm climates than in developed countries with temperate climates.

ASSESSMENT

HISTORY. Question the patient with cystitis about the presence of urinary symptoms, including frequency, urgency, pain, a sensation of incomplete emptying of the bladder, and blood or pus in the urine. The patient may have a low-grade fever but generally does not have other systemic symptoms. Consider the patient's previous history of urinary infections, vaginal discharge, and chronic conditions such as diabetes mellitus, pregnancy, or neurological problems. Ask about recent sexual activity and previous sexually transmitted infections. Ask if the patient has experienced severe lower abdominal or pelvic pain, nocturia, urinary urgency, and excessive (up to 60 times a day) urinary frequency. Some women describe dyspareunia (painful sexual intercourse).

PHYSICAL EXAMINATION. Common symptoms are **urinary frequency**, **urgency**, and **pain** with **blood or pus in the urine**. Many people have suprapubic tenderness. Generally, the physical examination is unremarkable. Examine the patient to determine the presence of abdominal pain or costovertebral angle tenderness, which may indicate pyelonephritis. The examination should include surveillance for sexually transmitted infections (STIs).

PSYCHOSOCIAL. Cystitis is typically an acute illness with rapid response to prescribed therapy. The patient usually does not experience a disruption of normal activity. Women with IC, however, must learn to manage not only a chronic disease but also one that physicians may have either ignored, labeled as "psychosomatic," or related to hormonal changes that occur during menopause.

Diagnostic Highlights

Test	Normal Result	Abnormality With Condition	Explanation
Urine dip	Negative	Positive (purple shade)	Presence of leukocyte esterase indicates UTI; 90% accurate in detecting white blood cells (WBCs) in the urine
Urine culture and sensitivity	< 1,000 colony-forming units (CFU)/mL	> 1,000 CFU/mL	Identifies causative organism; determines appropriate antibiotic; pyelonephritis is diagnosed if the result is > 10,000 CF/mL
Urinalysis	WBCs 0–4/mL; red blood cells (RBCs) ≤ 2 mL; nitrites—none; pH 4.6–8; crystals—none; clear, aromatic	WBCs > 10/mL	Increased WBCs in urine reflect the response to infection

Other Tests: In severe or recurrent cases of cystitis, an IV pyelogram, voiding cystourethrogram, retrograde pyelogram, or cystoscopy could be done to discover factors contributing to cystitis. Urodynamic evaluation, cystoscopy, and a bladder biopsy may be performed to diagnose IC.

PRIMARY NURSING DIAGNOSIS

DIAGNOSIS. Impaired urinary elimination related to irritation of bladder mucosa as evidenced by urgency, pain, pyuria, and/or hematuria

OUTCOMES. Urinary elimination; Knowledge: Medication; Knowledge: Symptom control; Medication response; Infection severity

INTERVENTIONS. Medication prescribing; Medication administration; Urinary elimination management; Infection control

✴ PLANNING AND IMPLEMENTATION

Collaborative

Bacterial cystitis is usually treated with a brief course of antibiotics, generally including nitrofurantoin monohydrate/macrocrystals (5- to 7-day course), trimethoprim-sulfmethoxazole (3-day course), or fosfomycin (single dose). Generally patients are treated as outpatients. Hospital admission may occur if structural abnormalities such as obstruction or calculi are involved, if the patient is immunocompromised, or if the patient has a disease such as diabetes mellitus or renal insufficiency.

A variety of treatments have been used for IC, including dietary and fluid management, time and stress management, and behavioral modification. Foods that may aggravate symptoms of IC include coffee, alcoholic beverages, tomatoes, vinegar, carbonated beverages, spicy food, and chocolate. Other interventions that have been used with varying success are biofeedback and pelvic floor rehabilitation, such as Kegel exercises, and bladder training programs. Generally, treatments are initiated in a progressively more invasive fashion until symptomatic relief is obtained.

Pharmacologic Highlights

General Comments for IC: Antibiotics worsen the symptoms of patients with IC by irritating the bladder. The treatment of IC is controversial, and no single treatment is accepted as best. Commonly used medications include anti-inflammatories, antispasmodics, tricyclic antidepressants, and antihistamines, which are used with varying success. Other treatments include instillations of preparations such as sodium oxychlorosene (Clorpactin), silver nitrate, and dimethylsulfoxide (DMSO) directly in the bladder to promote healing and relief of pain. Sodium pentosan polysulfate (Elmiron) is used orally to create a protective mucin layer in the bladder.

Medication or Drug Class	Dosage	Description	Rationale
Cotrimoxazole; trimethoprim and sulfamethoxazole (Bactrim, Septra)	800 mg sulfamethoxazole and 160 mg trimethoprim q 12 hr for 3 days	Anti-infective, sulfonamide	Bacteriocidal
Nitrofurantoin (Macrodantin)	100 mg PO bid for 5–7 days	Urinary antiseptic	Bacteriocidal; concentrates in the urine and kidneys to kill bacteria
Fosfomycin	3 gm PO one dose	Antibacterial	Bacteriocidal
Cefaclor	500 mg tid PO for 7 days	Second-generation cephalosporin	Bacteriocidal; used if other recommended agents cannot be used
Ciprofloxacin	250 mg bid PO for 3 days	Fluoroquinolone	Bacteriocidal; usually used for complicated cystitis
Phenazopyridine (Pyridium)	100–200 mg PO tid until pain subsides	Urinary analgesic	Relieves pain

Independent

Reinforce the need for patients to complete the medication therapy. Inform women that they may develop a vaginal yeast infection during therapy, and review preventive measures. Encourage patients with infections to increase fluid intake to promote frequent urination. Recommend strategies to limit infection recurrence, such as wiping from front to back after a bowel movement (women), avoiding tub and bubble baths, wearing cotton underwear, and avoiding tight clothing such as jeans. Assess patients' voiding patterns and encourage them to empty their bladder frequently, both during the acute phase of the infection and also when uninfected. There is some support for reducing the risk of recurrent UTI in older hospitalized patients by drinking 10 to 16 ounces of cranberry juice daily.

Encourage patients with IC to eat a healthy diet. Certain foods such as coffee, caffeinated tea, carbonated beverages (including colas and noncolas, diet, and decaffeinated), alcohol, tomatoes, fruits and fruit juices (grapefruit, cranberry, lemon, orange, pineapple), vinegar, chocolate, artificial sugars, and highly spiced foods may aggravate symptoms of IC. Patients with IC present a challenge to the nurse because no clear treatment exists for the condition. Provide information about the condition and validate that the symptoms are indeed shared by many other patients. Listen to the patient's feelings and provide the patient with a list of national and local resources that can provide further support. The IC network provides helpful information on their Web site: https://www.ic-network.com/interstitial-cystitis.

Evidence-Based Practice and Health Policy

Nace, D., Hanlon, J., Crnich, C., Drinka, P., Schweon, S., Anderson, G., & Perera, S. (2020). A multifaceted antimicrobial stewardship program for the treatment of uncomplicated cystitis in nursing home residents. *JAMA Internal Medicine*, *180*, 944–951.

- The authors studied the effect of a quality improvement intervention to reduce unnecessary antimicrobial use for unlikely cystitis in noncatheterized nursing home residents. Unlikely cystitis was defined as nonspecific symptoms and positive culture results with asymptomatic bacteriuria or a urine sample improperly collected for culture. Using published guidelines, the authors initiated a multifaceted intervention to encourage application of standards of care on antibiotic use for cystitis. The incidence of antibiotic treatment for unlikely cystitis was the primary outcome. Secondary outcomes included overall antibiotic use as well as all-cause hospitalizations and death. They used cases of cystitis in 12 intervention and 13 control nursing homes.
- Fewer unlikely cystitis cases were treated with antibiotics in intervention facilities compared with control facilities. Overall antibiotic use for any type of UTI was 17% lower in the intervention facilities as compared to the control facilities. There was no increase in all-cause hospitalizations or deaths due to the intervention in either group. A low-intensity intervention was associated with improved antibiotic prescribing for uncomplicated cystitis.

DOCUMENTATION GUIDELINES

- Physical response: Pain, burning on urination, urinary frequency; vital signs; nocturia; color and odor of urine; patient history that may place the patient at risk
- Location, duration, frequency, and severity of pain; response to medications
- Absence of complications such as pyelonephritis

DISCHARGE AND HOME HEALTHCARE GUIDELINES

Explain the proposed therapy, including the medication name, dosage, route, and side effects. Explain the signs and symptoms of complications such as pyelonephritis and the need for follow-up before the patient leaves the setting. Explain the importance of completing the entire course of antibiotics, even if symptoms decrease or disappear. Encourage the patient with GI discomfort to continue taking the medications with a meal or milk unless contraindicated. Warn the patient that drugs with phenazopyridine turn the urine orange.

Encourage the patient to drink adequate fluids every day and empty the bladder at least every 4 hours and after sexual intercourse. Recommend that they wipe their genitourinary area from front to back. Encourage the patient to avoid irritating feminine products. Note that some experts recommend that people consume a cranberry supplement or drink cranberry juice daily.

Cytomegalovirus Infection

DRG Category:	866
Mean LOS:	3.4 days
Description:	MEDICAL: Viral Illness Without Major Complication or Comorbidity

Cytomegalovirus (CMV) is a member of the human herpesvirus group. The virus, transmitted by human contact, results in an infection so mild that it is usually overlooked because no symptoms are present. Approximately 80% of the general population experience a CMV infection by the time they reach middle age. Immunosuppressed patients, however, and particularly patients who have received transplanted organs, are highly susceptible to CMV, with estimates as high as 90% of such patients contracting a CMV infection. Generally, the CMV infection occurs 4 to 6 weeks after the implementation of increased doses of immunosuppressive drugs to treat rejection. CMV infection is also present in at least 80% of patients with AIDS, causing serious problems such as encephalitis, retinitis, pneumonia, and esophagitis in 30% of them.

The virus generally inhabits the salivary glands in a latent infection that is reactivated by pregnancy, blood transfusions, or immunosuppressive medications. While it is benign in people with normal immune systems, the virus can be devastating to an unborn fetus (leading to developmental defects and sensory loss) or a person with immunosuppression. The virus is spread throughout the body by the white blood cells (lymphocytes and mononuclear cells) to organs such as the liver, lungs, gastrointestinal (GI) tract, and central nervous system (CNS), leading to cellular inflammation and possibly organ dysfunction. Complications include pneumonia, hepatitis, encephalitis, neuropathy, myelitis, and uveitis (infection of the middle layer of tissue in the eye wall), and in immunocompromised people, mononucleosis syndrome, Guillain-Barré syndrome, pericarditis, thrombocytopenia, and anemia. CMV retinitis is a serious complication that occurs in immunocompromised people and may lead to visual loss and blinding. In both solid organ and bone marrow transplants, CMV causes serious illness, and if interstitial pneumonia occurs, mortality can be as high as 70% in some recipients.

CAUSES

CMV is transmitted by contact with the fluids that contain the virus, such as saliva, urine, breast milk, cervical mucus, and semen. It can be transmitted during sexual intercourse or pregnancy from a primary or reactivated CMV infection. It can be transmitted during delivery from contact with cervical secretions or after delivery in the breast milk. The virus may be present for years after the primary infection.

GENETIC CONSIDERATIONS

Heritable immune responses could be protective or increase susceptibility.

SEX AND LIFE SPAN CONSIDERATIONS

Seropositivity is the presence of antibodies or other immune markers in serum that indicate exposure to an organism or antigen. In the United States, half of young adults are CMV seronegative (no presence of CMV antibodies), and the incidence increases with age. Across the life span, fetuses and infants are at particular risk because intrauterine CMV infection is the most common congenital infection; it occurs in 0.5% to 3% of all live births, or approximately 8,000 newborns each year in the United States. Infection of the fetus by CMV may not be recognized until birth or several years after birth because pregnant women with CMV infections may not have clinical symptoms. Infants who have been infected with CMV during gestation may have intrauterine growth retardation, microcephaly (small head size), or hydrocephaly (increased cerebrospinal fluid in the brain).

In adults, CMV may be serious and can cause blindness or a mononucleosis-type infection. CMV mononucleosis is the most common form of CMV infection, and it occurs at about 25 to 30 years of age. Adults over the age of 80 years have a seropositivity rate of over 90%.

HEALTH DISPARITIES AND SEXUAL/GENDER MINORITY HEALTH

While all people are susceptible to CMV infection, people who have immigrated from developing countries have a higher CMV seropositivity rate than people born in the United States. Hispanic and Black persons have a higher rate of CMV seropositivity than other groups, possibly because of the effects of immigration among their groups. Men who have sex with men are considered a high-risk group and have a CMV seropositivity rate of at least 90%. Other high-risk groups are people who spend time at day-care centers, have sex with multiple sex partners, and receive blood transfusions.

GLOBAL HEALTH CONSIDERATIONS

The global prevalence of CMV varies widely. Infants and children in developing countries tend to acquire CMV early in their lives because few women in those countries are seronegative. In comparison, in developed countries, half of young adults are seronegative. In countries with low resources, permanent hearing loss from congenital CMV infections is a particular problem.

ASSESSMENT

HISTORY. Ask about immunosuppressive conditions such as recent traumatic injury that may have required multiple blood transfusions, organ transplantation, or HIV infection. Note that many people are infected with CMV with no symptoms or with mild flu symptoms. The episode may be labeled a "fever of unknown origin." The patient may describe a recent viral infection with symptoms such as sore throat, tiredness, joint and muscle aches, and headache. Some patients will remember an episode that lasted approximately 3 weeks with high fevers as the only symptom. In an immunosuppressed patient, there may be specific organ involvement, such as the lungs (dry cough, difficulty breathing), the GI tract (watery diarrhea, bloody diarrhea, nausea, vomiting, and cramping), and the CNS (blurred vision, headache, neck rigidity, tremors, lethargy, and even seizures and coma).

PHYSICAL EXAMINATION. Common signs and symptoms include **fever**, **sore throat**, **tiredness and fatigue**, and **headache**. Infants may show signs of delayed development and may show signs of jaundice, petechial rash, respiratory distress, and permanent hearing loss.

With adults, assess all body systems, but the most severe signs and symptoms occur with lung, CNS, or liver involvement. Evaluate patients for signs of fever, pallor, changes in the lymph node tissue, and pharyngitis. Auscultate the patient's lungs to assess for crackles. Note decreased breath sounds, cough, shortness of breath, and symptoms of pneumonia.

Patients may also have mental status changes such as irritability, lethargy, and even seizures and coma. Patients may evidence hyperactive bowel sounds, tenderness to palpation of the stomach, and possible distention. Assess for neck rigidity, pupil changes, motor weakness, positive Babinski reflex, and tremors. Perform an eye examination to identify changes in the eye grounds, initially with small, white, cotton-wool spots with irregular borders on the retina that enlarge to fluffy white exudates and visible hemorrhages, causing vision loss progressing to blindness.

PSYCHOSOCIAL. Assess the patient's or the patient's parents' ability to cope. The unborn child's parents will need counseling and support to deal with the possible effects of CMV on their unborn infant. Families of infants with CMV infection will need emotional support. Answer questions about CMV infection, symptoms, complications, and treatment. People who are immunocompromised may have higher levels of anxiety about a CMV infection because of the complications that may occur.

Diagnostic Highlights

General Comments: A viral culture is the most sensitive diagnostic laboratory procedure. Cultures, however, take 3 to 7 days and cannot differentiate acute from chronic infection.

Test	Normal Result	Abnormality With Condition	Explanation
Antigen testing and polymerase chain reaction	Negative for CMV antigens or CMV genetic material in leukocytes	Positive	Detects the presence of antigens against the virus or genetic material from the virus
Culture of the urine, sputum, or mouth swab	Virus not isolated	Virus isolated	Presence of virus confirms the diagnosis
IgM antibodies	Antibodies not present	CMV antibodies present	Indicates a recent infection

Other Tests: Virus isolation of samples from cervix, semen, breast milk, white blood cells, and biopsy specimens; shell vial assay; because cultures of CMV may grow slowly and require up to 6 weeks of incubation, this assay is an adaptation of tissue culture technique that provides results more rapidly. It is described as the centrifugation enhancement monoclonal-antibody culture technique, or the shell-vial assay. Complement-fixation tests, indirect immunofluorescent antibody (IFA) tests.

PRIMARY NURSING DIAGNOSIS

DIAGNOSIS. Risk for infection as evidenced by fatigue, fever, sore throat, tiredness, and/or headache

OUTCOMES. Infection severity; Rest; Fatigue level; Thermoregulation; Knowledge: Infection management; Knowledge: Medication; Risk control: Infectious process; Risk detection

INTERVENTIONS. Infection protection; Risk identification; Surveillance; Teaching: Individual; Temperature regulation

PLANNING AND IMPLEMENTATION
Collaborative

INFANTS. Infants with congenital abnormalities require careful monitoring of growth and developmental patterns throughout infancy. Parents may need referrals for information on special education, physical therapy, audiology services, and social services.

ADULTS. Treatment focuses on preventing complications and relieving symptoms; treatment varies depending on the type and degree of infection. Patients with a generalized infection receive antipyretics for fever and analgesics for aching and sore throat. Such patients need rest, good nutrition, and adequate fluid intake for chronic fatigue. Other, more severe infections are usually treated with antiviral medications. The amount and duration of medication depend on the severity of the infection. Organ system complications are managed based on the symptoms.

Pharmacologic Highlights

Medication or Drug Class	Dosage	Description	Rationale
Ganciclovir; valganciclovir for solid organ transplantation; letermovir; acyclovir	Varies by drug	Antiviral	Inhibits DNA production in CMV
Foscarnet	60 mg/kg q 8 hr or 90 mg/kg q 12 hr for 2–3 wk, then 90–120 mg/kg per day of IV	Antiviral	Inhibits replication of virus

Other Drugs: Immunoglobulins may also be used as passive immunization for the prevention of CMV disease. Valganciclovir is used for the prevention of CMV infection in transplant patients.

Independent

Important priorities are to maintain an adequate level of functioning, prevent complications, support the recuperative process, and provide information about the disease process, prognosis, and treatment. Patients, and caregivers in the case of infants, need to be educated about decreasing the risk of spreading CMV infection. Secretions, particularly in infants, are apt to contain the virus.

Patients and caregivers need to wash their hands with soap and water for at least 30 seconds after each contact. CMV can also survive on plastic and latex; explain that these surfaces should be cleaned with a mild disinfectant or alcohol-based sanitizer when in contact with secretions or saliva. Teach adult patients about the CMV infection, the need for adequate rest, exercise, good nutrition, and fluid intake.

Evidence-Based Practice and Health Policy

Chatzakis, C., Ville, Y., Makrydimas, G., Dinas, K., Zavlanos, A., & Sotiriadis, A. (2020). Timing of primary maternal cytomegalovirus infection and rates of vertical transmission and fetal consequences. *American Journal of Obstetrics & Gynecology, 223,* 870–883.

- The aim of this meta-analysis was to explore fetal and maternal rates of cytomegalovirus (CMV) infection in order to calculate rates of transmission and fetal impairments depending on the timing of primary maternal infection. The authors identified 17 studies by consulting multiple library sources and calculated pooled rates of primary maternal infection at the preconception period, periconception period, first trimester, second trimester, and third trimester. They also studied fetal infection and impairment.
- The pooled rates of transmission were 5.5% at the preconception period, 21% at the periconception period, 37% at first trimester, 40% at second trimester, and 66% at third trimester. Transmission of CMV infection from mother to baby increased with advancing pregnancy, starting from the preconception period. The most severe fetal impairments are rare unless the mother is infected during the first trimester of pregnancy.

DOCUMENTATION GUIDELINES

- Physical changes, such as enlarged lymph nodes, GI symptoms, pulmonary symptoms, funduscopic abnormalities
- Response to medications and treatments
- Complications, resistance, recurrence of symptoms

DISCHARGE AND HOME HEALTHCARE GUIDELINES

PREVENTION. Teach the patient's caregiver to handle diapers carefully, washing hands for 30 seconds to prevent the spread of CMV. In the hospital, universal precautions are needed for women of childbearing potential. Frequent funduscopic examinations are imperative in HIV-positive and AIDS patients to assess for CMV retinitis. Female healthcare workers who are attempting pregnancy may wish to have CMV titers drawn to identify their risk for the disease. Pregnant people working in day-care centers or hospital nurseries need to avoid caring for infected infants and to use universal precautions.

MEDICATIONS. Teach the patient information about the prescribed dosage, route, action, and follow-up laboratory work needed for all medications. Teach the patient the appropriate use of antipyretics for fever and analgesics for pain and discomfort.

COMPLICATIONS. Inform the patient that signs of a relapse or complications may occur after an initial improvement. The patient should be instructed to report visual changes; changes in GI function, such as weight loss, nausea, vomiting, and anorexia; continued fever; and pulmonary symptoms (cough, shortness of breath, chest tightness). If these complications occur, teach the patient to seek medical attention.

Diabetes Insipidus

DRG Category: 644
Mean LOS: 4.3 days
Description: MEDICAL: Endocrine Disorders With Complication or Comorbidity

The disorder diabetes insipidus (DI) is characterized by the excretion of large amounts of dilute urine (> 3 L/24 hr). DI can be of central (neurogenic) or renal (nephrogenic) origin. In central DI, excess urine is caused by insufficient amounts of antidiuretic hormone (ADH, also known as *plasma vasopressin* or arginine vasopressin [AVP]). Renal DI occurs when the kidney has a decreased responsiveness to ADH. DI can also occur during pregnancy as gestational DI because of a deficiency in ADH, but the deficiency is not because of a neurogenic or nephrogenic defect. The overall incidence of DI in the general population is approximately three cases per 100,000 individuals.

Normally, body water balance is partially regulated by ADH, which is produced in the hypothalamus and is released from the posterior pituitary gland when body fluids become more concentrated than usual (serum osmolarity > 283 mOsm/L). ADH causes water reabsorption in the distal portions of the nephron of the kidney by increasing the number of pores in the distal tubular system to allow for water reabsorption. ADH deficiency leads to little or no reabsorption; as a consequence, dilute urine formed in more proximal parts of the nephron is excreted essentially unchanged. The loss of solute-free water causes mild dehydration, a rise in plasma osmolality, and the stimulation of thirst.

Complications are most likely in patients with decreased mental alertness because their impairment makes it less likely they will drink in response to their stimulated thirst. The most serious complication of untreated DI is hypovolemia, which may lead to hyperosmolarity, loss of consciousness, circulatory collapse, shock, and central nervous system (CNS) damage.

CAUSES

The cause of approximately 30% to 50% of central DI is familial or idiopathic (from unknown causes). Trauma because of brain surgery and head injury accounts for approximately 35% of central DI, and neoplasms of the brain or pituitary cause approximately 25% of the cases. The brain swelling that accompanies anoxic brain death may also lead to central DI. Other causes of central DI include trauma to the pituitary gland, infection/inflammation, lung cancer, anorexia nervosa, and vascular changes such as stroke and aneurysm. Renal DI is caused by drugs (lithium, demeclocycline, methoxyflurane, or amphotericin), hyperglycemia, hypokalemia, hypercalcemia, and other metabolic and disease conditions such as sickle cell disease and amyloidosis. In addition, congenital DI in neonates occurs as a result of malformation of the CNS. Depending on the underlying illness, most patients recover from DI. Some have permanent DI requiring chronic treatment.

GENETIC CONSIDERATIONS

Nephrogenic DI can be transmitted in either an X-linked recessive (via mutations in the vasopressin V2 receptor) or autosomal dominant pattern (via mutations in the aquaporin-2 water channel). A large number of variants in the *AVP* gene have been associated with both the autosomal dominant and the autosomal recessive patterns of transmission for familial neurohypophyseal DI.

SEX AND LIFE SPAN CONSIDERATIONS

DI may occur at any age and in both sexes, depending on the underlying cause. Females and males have approximately the same susceptibility. Infants and older adults exhibit more symptoms because they are less able to adjust to changes in fluid status. A temporary form of DI can occur during the fifth or sixth month of pregnancy but usually disappears spontaneously after delivery.

Primary neonatal DI occurs as a result of a congenital defect in newborns and can be central or renal in origin. In children, DI is most frequently caused by tumors of the hypothalamus (craniopharyngiomas in particular). In children, a history of ocular abnormalities or growth failure can suggest a midbrain tumor that leads to DI. Enuresis (involuntary discharge of urine after a child is toilet trained), irritability, excessive thirst, and a preference for ice water in children are all signs of DI.

HEALTH DISPARITIES AND SEXUAL/GENDER MINORITY HEALTH

Ethnicity, race, and sexual/gender minority status have no known effect on the risk for DI.

GLOBAL HEALTH CONSIDERATIONS

DI is relatively uncommon around the globe. No prevalence data are available.

☀ ASSESSMENT

HISTORY. Generally, patients with suspected DI complain of excessive urination (polyuria), excessive thirst (polydipsia), and nocturia (excessive urination at night). The onset is often abrupt. Urinary output is usually in the range of 4 to 15 L per day but can be as high as 30 L per day. Assess the patient for a history of known causative factors: recent surgery, head trauma, or medication use. The patient may also report a history of weight loss, lightheadedness, weakness, intolerance to activity, and constipation. Parents may notice that children are more irritable than usual and may have sleep disturbances and anorexia.

PHYSICAL EXAMINATION. The most common symptoms are **polyuria**, **polydipsia**, and **nocturia**. DI is associated with few physical signs. If the patient has not urinated recently, the bladder may be enlarged. Except in unusual cases, dehydration is not sufficient to be evident on the physical examination. Unless water is restricted or the patient is not alert enough to respond to thirst, patients maintain their fluid balance by drinking. In patients who are not mentally alert, look for signs and symptoms of dehydration: decreased tear formation, dry lips and mouth, complaints of excessive thirst, skin tenting, and dizziness. In spite of signs of dehydration, urine is clear or pale yellow and in copious amounts. You may note tachycardia, orthostatic changes in blood pressure, and decreased muscle strength.

PSYCHOSOCIAL. Assess the patient's ability to cope with a chronic illness and the financial resources to manage a chronic illness.

Diagnostic Highlights

Test	Normal Result	Abnormality With Condition	Explanation
Urine osmolality (osmolality refers to a solution's concentration of solute particles per kilogram of solvent)	200–1,200 mOsm/L	< 250 mOsm/L	Excretion of dilute urine in spite of dehydration and hypernatremia due to underproduction of ADH
Blood osmolality	275–295 mOsm/L	> 300 mOsm/L	Water loss in the urine and hemoconcentration; levels > 320 mOsm/L are considered "panic levels" and require immediate intervention
Serum sodium, serum glucose	Sodium: 135–145 mEq/L; fasting glucose: 70–100 mg/dL	Sodium: > 145 mEq/L; fasting glucose > 126 mg/dL	Water loss in the urine leads to hemoconcentration; elevated glucose level may indicate other conditions

Other Tests: Serum electrolytes; urine specific gravity and urine electrolytes; urine specific gravity of the first morning urine determines the kidney's ability to concentrate urine; dilute urine with a high serum sodium and serum osmolarity effectively establishes the diagnosis; brain or pituitary magnetic resonance imaging; circulating pituitary hormone levels, plasma antidiuretic hormone level

PRIMARY NURSING DIAGNOSIS

DIAGNOSIS. Impaired urinary elimination related to hormonal imbalances as evidenced by polyuria, polydipsia, and/or nocturia

OUTCOMES. Urinary elimination; Urinary continence; Fluid balance; Electrolyte balance; Knowledge: Disease process; Medication response; Neurological status; Symptom control; Symptom severity

INTERVENTIONS. Fluid management; Fluid monitoring; Electrolyte management; Urinary elimination management; Medication prescribing

PLANNING AND IMPLEMENTATION

Collaborative

The most important aspect of DI treatment is to treat the underlying cause. The treatment of DI is primarily pharmacologic. In addition to medication, fluid replacement to maintain vascular volume is essential. Rapid correction of hypernatremia is potentially dangerous because of the possibility of a rapid shift of water into brain cells, which increases the risk of seizures or cerebral edema. The water deficit is corrected gradually over 2 to 3 days with water by mouth, gastric feeding tube, or intravenously with dextrose in water or half- or quarter-isotonic saline. If IV fluids are needed, usually they are administered at rates of 500 to 750 mL/hour, with the rate guided by the serum sodium.

Pharmacologic Highlights

Medication or Drug Class	Dosage	Description	Rationale
Desmopressin (aqueous vaso-pressin* may be used)	1–2 mcg IV bid (vasopressin dose: 5–10 units IV or SC two to three times a day); may also be given nasally; an oral preparation is also available in tablet form (starting dose 50 mcg)	Synthetic antidiuretic hormone (vasopressin is a vasopressor and antidiuretic)	Supplement to pro-vide hormone in ADH deficiency; given for central DI
Chlorpropamide (Diabinese)	250–500 mg daily	Sulfonylurea	Reduces urine output by 30%–70%
Thiazide diuretics	Varies by drug	Decreases polyuria	Effective when the kidney does not respond to vasopressin-like sub-stances; given for renal DI

*Note: Vasopressin tannate (suspended in oil) is an intramuscular preparation that is given as a one- to five-unit injection. The oil-based preparation may have a duration of action as long as 96 hours, whereas the aqueous form lasts from 3 to 6 hours. Desmo-pressin acetate (DDAVP), a synthetic analog of vasopressin, can also be given intrana-sally in a dosage of 10 to 25 units twice a day.

Independent

The most important nursing interventions focus on maintaining an adequate balance of fluid intake and output. Discuss dietary restriction of salt with the patient and family. The patient should also avoid coffee, tea, or other caffeinated substances because caffeine has exaggerated diuretic effects. The patient needs easy access to the bathroom, bedpan, or urinal. If the patient has muscle weakness or impaired mobility, make sure the pathway for ambulation to the bath-room is free from all obstructions to limit the risk of patient falls.

Monitor the response to all medications and treatments by daily measuring the urine specific gravity as part of assessment data. Normal specific gravity is greater than 1.010. To identify the intake and output balance, monitor and carefully record the oral fluid intake and urine volume over a 24-hour period.

Encourage the patient to wear a medical identification bracelet and to carry any medications at all times. Note that some medications needed for a chronic disease, such as desmopressin, are quite expensive. If the family does not have insurance coverage that includes medications, explore methods to obtain the needed medications. Refer the family to social service if neces-sary. Urge the patient and family to express their feelings about the patient's condition; if they are having difficulty in coping, arrange for a counseling session.

Evidence-Based Practice and Health Policy

Refardt, J., Winzeler, B., & Christ-Crain, M. (2020). Diabetes insipidus: An update. *Endocrinol-ogy & Metabolism Clinics of North America*, *49*, 517–531.

- The authors provide a scientific review of DI. They describe the different types and etiolo-gies of DI and then focus on new procedures in the differential diagnosis. They identify three types of polyuria polydipsia syndrome: central DI, nephrogenic DI, and primary polydipsia. In addition, they note that gestational DI can occur during pregnancy due to increased AVP metabolism.

• Copeptin, which is part of the arginine molecule, can be measured with osmotic or nonosmotic stimulation and can thereby improve the diagnosis of DI. The treatment of choice for central DI remains desmopressin, either by the oral or nasal route of administration.

DOCUMENTATION GUIDELINES

• Physical response to treatment: Skin turgor, urinary output, color of urine
• Fluid balance: 24-hour intake and output, maintenance of body weight
• Urinary response to prescribed medications: Specific gravity
• Understanding of and interest in patient teaching
• Response (of patient and family) to chronic illness, if appropriate

DISCHARGE AND HOME HEALTHCARE GUIDELINES

PREVENTION. To prevent dehydration, teach the patient to use the thirst mechanism as a stimulus to drink oral fluids. To prevent polyuria, teach the patient to restrict salt and to avoid caffeine-containing products.

MEDICATIONS. Be sure the patient understands all medications, including the dosage, route, action, adverse effects, and the need for routine laboratory monitoring for DDAVP (plasma osmolarity). Ensure that the patient has access to the appropriate medications.

Diabetes Mellitus

DRG Category:	637
Mean LOS:	5.0 days
Description:	MEDICAL: Diabetes With Major Complication or Comorbidity

Diabetes mellitus (DM) is a chronic disorder of carbohydrate, protein, and fat metabolism in which there is a discrepancy between the amount of insulin required by the body and the amount of insulin available. The Centers for Disease Control and Prevention (CDC) state that more than 120 million people in the United States are living with DM or prediabetes. Almost 10% of the U.S. population has DM. The 88 million people who have prediabetes will likely have DM within 5 years if they are not treated, and more than half of the people with that condition are unaware that they are prediabetic. The health-related problems of DM are extensive in lives lost and money spent. It is the seventh leading cause of death in the United States. DM is classified into several categories (Table 1).

• TABLE 1 Types of Diabetes Mellitus

TYPE	DESCRIPTION
1	Patients are dependent on insulin for prevention of hyperglycemia or ketosis Formerly referred to as *insulin-dependent DM* Estimates are that 1.6 million people in the United States have type 1 DM The most serious life-threatening problem is diabetic ketoacidosis Time of onset is usually under age 20 years but may occur in adults 30–40 years Beta cells of pancreas have insulitis (pancreatic inflammatory response) with beta cell destruction

• TABLE 1 Types of Diabetes Mellitus (continued)

TYPE	DESCRIPTION
2	Patients are not dependent on insulin but ultimately may require insulin therapy to manage blood glucose control
	Patients have insulin resistance, impaired insulin secretion, and/or inappropriate glucagon secretion
	Formerly referred to as non-insulin-dependent DM
	Most common type of DM: Approximately 80%–90% of patients with DM have this type
	Most serious problem is the development of hyperosmolar hyperglycemic nonketotic syndrome
	Time of onset is usually over age 40 years
	Beta cells have no insulitis; resistance to insulin occurs at the target cell receptor
Gestational DM (GDM)	Patients develop glucose intolerance during pregnancy
Other types of diabetes	Diabetes develops secondary to other conditions, including pancreatic, hormonal, or endocrine disease and insulin resistance, or it is drug induced
Malnutrition-related DM	Occurs in underdeveloped countries to individuals with a history of malnutrition

The beta cells of the pancreas produce insulin and a protein called C-peptide, which are stored in the secretory granules of the beta cells and are released into the bloodstream as blood glucose levels increase. Insulin transports glucose and amino acids across the membranes of many body cells, particularly muscle and fat cells. It also increases the liver storage of glycogen, the chief carbohydrate storage material, and aids in the metabolism of triglycerides, nucleic acids, and proteins. In type 1 DM, beta cells of the pancreas have been infiltrated by lymphocytes and destroyed by autoimmune processes, whereas in type 2 DM, relative insulin deficiency occurs accompanied by resistance to the actions of insulin in muscle, fat, and liver cells. Insulin resistance is associated with increased levels of free fatty acids in the blood, reduced glucose transport in muscle cells, elevated hepatic glucose production, and increased breakdown of fat. For type 2 DM to occur, both insulin resistance and inadequate insulin secretion must occur.

Long-term complications, such as disease of the large and small blood vessels, lead to cardiovascular disease (coronary artery disease, peripheral vascular disease, hypertension), retinopathy, renal failure, and premature death. Diabetic patients also have nerve damage (neuropathy) that can affect vision and the peripheral nerves, resulting in numbness and pain of the hands or feet. The novel coronavirus 2019 disease (COVID-19) was linked to poorer outcomes for diabetic patients than for other patients. Experts suggest that the reasons for a worse prognosis is related to comorbidities such as hypertension and cardiovascular disease, obesity, and a proinflammatory state.

Because diabetic patients are hyperglycemic, they are at higher risk for infection because an elevated glucose encourages bacterial growth. The combination of peripheral neuropathies with numbness of the extremities, peripheral vascular disease leading to poor tissue perfusion, and the risk for infection makes the diabetic patient prone to feet and leg ulcers.

CAUSES

The cause of DM is not known, but genetic, autoimmune, viral, environmental, and socioeconomic factors have all been implicated in the development of the disease. Type 1 DM is most likely an autoimmune response in patients with genetic susceptibility. Following an environmental stimulus, such as a virus or bacteria, antibodies attack the beta cells of the pancreas and cause insulitis—inflammation and destruction of the beta cells. When 80% to 90% of the beta cells are destroyed, the patient develops hyperglycemia. It is thought that type 2 DM is caused by hereditary insulin resistance or abnormal insulin production. It is generally considered to involve complex interactions between heredity and environmental factors. If insulin resistance is acquired rather than inherited, it is usually the result of obesity. Experts note that approximately 90% of individuals with type 2 DM are overweight or have obesity. Other factors related to the development of type 2 DM include age older than 45 years, weight greater than 120% of desirable body weight, family history of type 2 diabetes, environmental pollutants, low birth weight, and an energy-dense diet.

GENETIC CONSIDERATIONS

DM is a complex disorder, with several genes and the environment working together. Type 1 DM is an autoimmune disease with approximately 30% to 50% twin concordance rate in monozygotic twins. Variants in the HLA allele (DR3, DR4) account for more than 50% of cases, but recent studies have found over 40 chromosomal regions that confer risk for type 1 diabetes. Type 2 DM is a heterogeneous disease with both a genetic and an environmental component (heritability estimates vary from 20% to 80%). Individuals with one affected parent have a 40% chance of developing type 2 DM, while those with two affected parents have a 70% chance. There is also varied genetic linkage in different populations (e.g., loci on chromosomes 2 and 11 are linked in Mexican Americans, whereas different loci on chromosomes 12 and 7 are implicated in Finns and Pima Indians, respectively). There are now over 100 loci associated with type 2 DM risk. The strongest and most consistent risk gene is *TCF7L2*, which encodes a signaling protein active in beta cells. Single-gene disorders of the beta cell can also cause familial DM. Maturity-onset diabetes of the young (MODY) is associated with autosomal dominant inheritance. MODY has the following characteristics: onset in at least one family member younger than 25 years old, the absence of autoantibodies and ketosis, and correction of fasting hyperglycemia without insulin for at least 2 years.

SEX AND LIFE SPAN CONSIDERATIONS

Approximately 1.6 million people have type 1 DM in the United States, where it is more common in males than females. Type 1 most commonly develops in childhood or before age 20 years but can occur at any age. Onset is often very abrupt. Because of the early age of onset, teenagers often deal with the long-term complications of the disease.

Type 2 DM usually occurs after age 40 years, particularly in individuals who are overweight or have hereditary factors, and occurs in males and females approximately equally. Type 2 DM is becoming increasingly common in all groups because DM prevalence increases with age and people are living longer than in past centuries. In addition, it is more frequent in younger people in accordance with the rising prevalence of childhood obesity. GDM, which is present during pregnancy, occurs in 3% to 10% of pregnant women, usually in those older than age 30 years.

HEALTH DISPARITIES AND SEXUAL/GENDER MINORITY HEALTH

The prevalence of type 2 DM in the United States varies by race and ethnicity. The American Diabetes Association reports the prevalence is 14.8% in Native American persons, 12.5% in Hispanic persons, 11.7% in Black persons, 7.4 in White persons, and 5.6% to 12.6% (depending on ancestry) in Asian persons. Asian persons are at risk for type 2 DM at lower weights than other persons. Non-Hispanic Black and Hispanic persons bear a disproportionate burden of type 2 DM when compared to non-Hispanic White persons. They also have higher rates of retinopathy, end-stage renal disease, and limb amputation than White persons. Experts suggest that these disparities occur for biological (genetic predisposition and fat distribution) as well as social factors such as income, language and literacy barriers, and limited access to and discrimination during healthcare. Several other factors lead to health disparities in persons with diabetes. Those with private insurance have been found to have better control of conditions such as blood pressure and visual disturbances related to DM as compared to persons who are uninsured, possibly because of improved diabetes management. Persons living in rural America have a higher prevalence of obesity and type 2 diabetes than urban populations and less access to behavioral programs to manage risks. Disparities in developing GDM also exist for foreign-born pregnant people. The relative risk for foreign-born versus U.S.-born pregnant people is higher across most ethnic groups.

Transgender is a term used to describe persons whose gender identity is different from their sex assigned at birth. Approximately 1% of the U.S. population identify themselves as transgender. Sexual and gender minority persons have higher odds for multiple chronic conditions, cancer, and poor quality of life, and are more apt to have disabilities than cisgender males and females (cisgender is a term used to describe persons whose gender identity and gender expression are aligned with their assigned sex listed on their birth certificate). Gender-affirming hormone therapy is the use of hormone therapy for gender transition or gender affirmation and can be masculinizing or feminizing. It may also affect cardiovascular health in transgender females. In a large sample, researchers have found that transgender men and women are more likely to be overweight than cisgender women. Compared to cisgender women, transgender women reported higher rates of diabetes, ischemic stroke, angina/coronary disease, and myocardial infarction. Gender-nonconforming persons reported higher odds of myocardial infarction than cisgender women. Transgender women also had higher rates of any cardiovascular disease than cisgender men (Cacerese, Jackman, et al., 2020; Connelly et al., 2019). Transgender persons are more prone to DM as they age than other groups (Gooren & T'Sjoen, 2018).

GLOBAL HEALTH CONSIDERATIONS

DM is a global epidemic, with the number of people with DM exceeding 422 million. The International Diabetes Federation states that by 2045, the number will exceed 700 million, and the countries with the most cases include the most populous countries of the world as well as Western Europe. Some experts note that type 1 DM is increasing by up to 5% each year in the Middle East, Western Europe, and Australia. Scandinavian countries have the highest prevalence rates for type 1 DM, while China and Japan have the lowest prevalence.

Type 2 DM is more common in developed countries than in developing countries. Experts suggest that in developing countries, and particularly in Africa, people ingest fewer calories and have higher levels of activity (less sedentary) than in North America and Western Europe. As countries become more developed, however, the prevalence of weight gain and type 2 DM increases dramatically. Africa will likely be the location for the largest increase in people with type 2 DM in the next decade. Screening for GDM occurs less often in developing countries than developed countries, decreasing the opportunity for early management.

ASSESSMENT

HISTORY. The timing of symptom appearance is important in DM. Type 1 DM often occurs suddenly, and patients may report symptoms of only days in duration. Establish a history of the patient's usual weight gains and losses; weight loss is common in type 1 DM. Determine if the patient has been under stress, had an infection, feels fatigued, had muscle cramping, or had nausea or blurred vision. Ask if the patient has experienced excessive thirst (polydipsia), excessive urination (polyuria), or excessive hunger (polyphagia). The most common symptom of DM is fatigue; determine if the patient has experienced fatigue out of the ordinary. Ask females of childbearing age if they are pregnant. Establish a history of using medications that antagonize the effects of insulin.

Patients with type 2 DM may not report these symptoms. However, ask whether the patient has experienced any recent itching or blurred vision or frequent infections, which are common complaints with type 2 DM. Question if the patient has experienced any visual difficulties, kidney problems, or changes in circulation and sensation to the extremities, such as numbness or tingling (paresthesia) or pruritus.

PHYSICAL EXAMINATION. The most common symptoms are **polydipsia**, **polyuria**, and **polyphagia**. Appearance may be entirely normal, or the patient with type 1 DM may have weight loss, muscle wasting, muscle cramping, and loss of subcutaneous fat. They may experience nausea, abdominal pain, and changes in bowel patterns. The patient with type 2 DM, by contrast, may have thin limbs with fatty deposits around the face, neck, and abdomen. Observe the color of the skin and note any changes in sensation of temperature, touch, and pain. Examine both feet closely, including the spaces between the toes, for signs of skin ulcers or infection. Assess the legs and feet to identify any unhealed wounds or ulcers. Check the temperature of the skin, which often feels cool, and the skin turgor, which is often poor.

When assessing vital signs, you may note hypertension, a common complication in diabetic patients. Palpate the peripheral pulses to determine their strength, regularity, and symmetry. During the neurological examination, use an ophthalmoscope to evaluate the patient for retinopathy or cataracts. Assess the patient for any signs and symptoms of hypoglycemia or hyperglycemia (Table 2).

• TABLE 2 Signs, Symptoms, and Treatment of Hypoglycemia and Hyperglycemia

HYPOGLYCEMIA

Cause: Usually secondary to excess insulin, exercise, or not enough food

Signs and Symptoms

Nervousness	Irritability
Diaphoresis (heavy sweating)	Hunger
Weakness	Tachycardia
Fatigue	Hypotension
Palpitations	Tachypnea
Tremors or shaking	Pallor
Blurred or double vision	Incoherent speech
Headache	Numbness of tongue and lips
Confusion	Coma

Treatment

Provide rapidly absorbed source of glucose:
• Fruit juice
• Graham crackers
• Sugar cubes, sugar packets
• Hard candy

As symptoms improve:
• Provide a meal or source of complex protein or carbohydrates
• Provide emotional support

HYPERGLYCEMIA

Cause: Usually secondary to insufficient insulin, illness, or excess food

Signs and Symptoms

Nausea	Confusion
Vomiting	Irritability
Anorexia	Fatigue
Abdominal cramping	Weakness
Thirst	Numbness
Lethargy	Tachycardia
Kussmaul breathing	Hypotension
Increased temperature	Decreased level of consciousness
Flushed or dry skin	Coma
Poor skin turgor	Fruity breath
Dry mucous membranes	

● **TABLE 2** Signs, Symptoms, and Treatment of Hypoglycemia and Hyperglycemia (continued)

HYPOGLYCEMIA

Treatment (requires hospitalization)
- Restore fluid balance
- Replace electrolytes
- Lower blood glucose with regular insulin
- Monitor level of consciousness, vital signs, intake and output, and electrolytes
- Provide emotional support

PSYCHOSOCIAL. Management of DM is a lifelong endeavor with multiple consequences related to mental and physical health. The need for daily management with medications, diet, and exercise repeatedly reminds the individual of the illness. In addition, the reality of a long-term illness may affect individuals' view of themselves, resulting in lower self-esteem. Young people with type 1 DM may have trouble managing developmental tasks and a chronic disease simultaneously. Parents may become overprotective, and children may have delayed emotional maturation.

Diagnostic Highlights

Test	Normal Result	Abnormality With Condition	Explanation
Fasting (no food for at least 8 hr before measurement) plasma glucose (FPG)	70–100 mg/dL	> 126 mg/dL	Insufficient insulin is available to transport insulin into body cells
Glucose tolerance test (2 hr after oral ingestion of 75 g of glucose; glucose is given after an overnight fast)	< 140 mg/dL	> 200 mg/dL; levels from 140 to 200 mg/dL indicate impaired glucose tolerance	Insufficient insulin is available to transport insulin into body cells
Hemoglobin A$_{1c}$	4%–6%	> 8% poorly controlled diabetics; < 7% well-controlled diabetics; initial diagnosis is made when level reaches 6.5%	Integrated measure of blood glucose profile over the preceding 2–3 mo; A$_{1c}$ is formed when glucose in the blood binds irreversibly to hemoglobin; since normal life span of red blood cells is 90–120 days, A$_{1c}$ is eliminated only when the red cells are replaced

Other Tests: Urinalysis (glycosuria). Note: The diagnosis of DM is made when FPG is greater than or equal to 126 mg/dL on two occasions or random glucose is greater than or equal to 200 mg/dL along with the classic symptoms of DM (polyuria, polydipsia, polyphagia, weight loss). The goal of treatment is to lower and maintain blood glucose levels into the following range: preprandial blood glucose levels of 90 to 130 mg/dL and HbA$_{1c}$ levels of less than 7%.

PRIMARY NURSING DIAGNOSIS

DIAGNOSIS. Imbalanced nutrition: less than body requirements related to decreased oral intake, nausea, vomiting, and/or insulin deficiency as evidenced by weight loss

OUTCOMES. Nutritional status: Food and fluid intake; Nutritional status; Biochemical measures; Fluid balance; Knowledge: Diabetes management; Medication response

INTERVENTIONS. Nutrition management; Nutrition therapy; Nutritional counseling and monitoring; Fluid/electrolyte management; Medication management

⚛ PLANNING AND IMPLEMENTATION

Collaborative

There is no known cure for DM, although pancreatic transplantation is available in some medical centers and is usually accomplished when patients also require a kidney transplant for end-stage renal disease. Continuous glucose monitoring (CGM) checks glucose levels regularly, and standard blood glucose meters use a drop of blood to check glucose levels. Management of the disease focuses on lifelong control of the serum glucose level to prevent or delay the development of complications. Individuals with type 1 DM require subcutaneous insulin administration. Insulin may be rapid, intermediate, or slow acting and may be delivered by multiple daily injections, or continuous subcutaneous insulin infusion with a battery pump. Technology is rapidly changing to better serve patients' needs for glucose monitoring and insulin pumps. The diabetes team assists patients to select the best systems for themselves. Ideally, blood glucose should be maintained at near normal levels and hemoglobin A_{1c} at levels under 7%. Patients learn to self-monitor to adjust their insulin dose as indicated. They also need to test for urine ketones when they have high or fluctuating levels of blood glucose or develop symptoms of a cold or other illnesses.

Patients with mild DM and those with type 2 DM or GDM may be able to control the disease by diet management alone. A diabetic diet attempts to distribute nutrition and calories throughout the 24-hour period. Daily calories consist of approximately 50% carbohydrates and 30% fat, with the remaining calories consisting of protein. The total calories allowed for an individual within the 24-hour period are based on age, weight, activity level, and medications.

In addition to strict dietary adherence to control blood glucose, obese patients with type 2 DM also need weight reduction. The dietitian selects an appropriate calorie allotment depending on the patient's age, body size, and activity level. A useful adjunct to the management of DM is exercise. Physical activity increases the cellular sensitivity to insulin, improves tolerance to glucose, and encourages weight loss. Exercise also increases patients' sense of well-being concerning their health.

Pharmacologic Highlights

Medication or Drug Class	Dosage	Description	Rationale
Insulin	Varies with severity to maintain pre-meal blood glucose of 80–130 mg/dL and HbA$_{1c}$ < 7%	Hormone; hypoglycemic	Hormonal supplement to replace deficient or absent levels of insulin; can be rapid acting (genetically engineered preparations: lispro, glulisine, and aspart), short acting (regular insulin: zinc insulin crystals in solution), intermediate acting (NPH [neutral protamine Hagedorn]: crystalline suspension of human insulin with protamine and zinc), long acting (glargine, insulin detemir)

Pharmacologic Highlights (continued)

Medication or Drug Class	Dosage	Description	Rationale
Antidiabetics	Varies with drug	Several groups of medications besides insulin are available in the treatment of DM: sulfonylureas, alpha-glucosidase inhibitors, biguanides, meglitinide derivatives, thiazolidinediones	Varies by drug; sulfonylureas stimulate release of insulin from beta cells of pancreas; alpha-glucosidase inhibitors slow carbohydrate breakdown in small intestine; biguanides decrease hepatic glucose output, enhance peripheral glucose uptake; meglitinide derivatives are short-acting insulin secretagogues; thiazolidinediones are insulin sensitizers
Exenatide (Byetta)	5 mcg SC bid within 1 hr before meals in the morning and evening	Incretin mimetic agent	Mimics glucose-dependent insulin secretion, suppresses elevated glucagon secretion, delays gastric emptying; used to improve glycemic control for type 2 diabetics

Other Drugs: Insulin pumps for type 1 DM: Continuous subcutaneous insulin infusion by battery-operated pump allows for a continuous subcutaneous infusion of rapid-acting insulin. The pump provides a programmed dose of insulin that also can be administered as a bolus dose before a meal. The patient self-monitors glucose levels and adjusts the bolus dose. The pump method provides better glucose control than multiple injections. Other therapies for type 2 DM: dipeptidyl peptidase IV inhibitors, glucagonlike peptide. Rapid-acting insulin aspart (Fiasp) is a human insulin analog formulated with niacin to speed absorption and can be used to treat adults.

Independent

If the patient has recently been diagnosed with DM, explain the disease process, the goals of management, and strategies to limit complications. Use simple explanations for clarity, answer questions, and provide written information for the patient to refer to between teaching sessions. In addition to general information on the disease process and reinforcement of collaborative teaching about medications and nutrition, the patient needs specific information about foot and vision care.

Explain that all cuts and blisters need to be cleaned and treated with an antiseptic preparation. If a cut or blister begins to appear infected (warmth, pain, swelling) or has drainage, encourage the patient to notify the primary healthcare provider immediately. Teach the patient to avoid constricting clothing such as constricting stockings, garters, girdles, or elastic slippers. If the patient needs to be on bedrest, encourage the patient to keep bed linens loose over the feet and legs. Instruct the patient to avoid very hot baths if peripheral neuropathy causes decreased temperature sensation.

If the patient is a child or teenager, recognize that a diagnosis of DM changes a family permanently. Parents usually expect their child to be healthy and often react with shock and disbelief. The impact on the child depends on the child's age. School-age children may be impressed with the new "condition" and may be challenged by the new skills it involves. Adolescents, in comparison, may feel unfairly victimized and respond by becoming depressed, resistant, uncooperative, or insecure. Work with the entire family to support their adaptation to the illness. Introduce the family to other families with the same problem. If the problems are abnormal, make a referral to a counselor.

Evidence-Based Practice and Health Policy

Rosenstock, J., Bajaj, H., Janež, A., Silver, R., Begtrup, K., Hansen, M., Jia, T., & Goldenberg, R. (2020). Once-weekly insulin for type 2 diabetes without previous insulin treatment. *New England Journal of Medicine, 383*, 2107–2116.

- The authors explored whether reducing the frequency of basal insulin injections by using insulin icodec (a basal insulin analogue designed for once-weekly administration) would encourage treatment acceptance and adherence among patients with type 2 diabetes. The authors conducted a 26-week, randomized trial to investigate the efficacy and safety of once-weekly insulin icodec as compared with once-daily insulin glargine U100 in patients who had not previously received long-term insulin treatment. Patients whose type 2 diabetes was inadequately controlled (glycated hemoglobin level, 7.0%–9.5%) were selected. The primary endpoint was the change in glycated hemoglobin level from baseline to 26 weeks. The authors enrolled 247 patients.
- A total of 247 participants were randomly assigned to two groups with similar characteristics, one of which received icodec and the other received glargine insulin. There were no differences in the groups in the change from baseline in glycated hemoglobin level and at 26 weeks. There were no differences in adverse events between the groups. The authors concluded that once-weekly treatment with insulin icodec had glucose-lowering efficacy and a safety profile similar to once-a-day glargine insulin.

DOCUMENTATION GUIDELINES

- Results of urine and blood tests for glucose
- Physical findings: Visual problems, skin problems or lesions, changes in sensation or circulation to the extremities
- Patient teaching, return demonstrations, patient's understanding of teaching
- Response to insulin

DISCHARGE AND HOME HEALTHCARE GUIDELINES

MEDICATIONS. Patients need to understand the purpose, dosage, route, and possible side effects of all prescribed medications. If the patient is to self-administer insulin, have the patient demonstrate the appropriate preparation and administration techniques.

PREVENTION. The patient and family require instruction in the following areas to minimize or prevent complications of DM.

Diet. Explain how to calculate the American Diabetic Association exchange list to develop a satisfactory diet within the prescribed calories. Emphasize the importance of adjusting diet during illness, growth periods, stress, and pregnancy. Encourage patients to avoid alcohol and refined sugars and to distribute nutrients to maintain a balanced blood sugar throughout the 24-hour period.

Insulin. Patients need to understand the type of insulin prescribed. Instructions should include onset, peak, and duration of action. Stress proper timing of meals and planning snacks for the time when insulin is at its peak and recommend an evening snack for those on long-acting insulins. Reinforce that patients cannot miss a dosage, and there may be a need for increasing dosages during times of stress or illness. Teaching regarding the proper preparation of insulin, how to administer, and the importance of rotating sites is necessary.

Urine and Blood Testing. Teach patients the appropriate technique for testing blood and urine and how to interpret the results. Patients need to know when to notify the physician and increase testing during times of illness.

Skin Care. Stress the importance of close attention to even minor skin injuries. Emphasize foot care, including the importance of properly fitting shoes with clean, nonconstricting socks; daily washing and thorough drying of the feet; and inspection of the toes, with special attention paid to the areas between the toes. Encourage the patient to contact a podiatrist as needed. Because of sensory loss in the lower extremities, teach the patient to test the bath water to prevent skin trauma from water that is too hot and to avoid using heating pads.

Circulation. Because of the atherosclerotic changes that occur with DM, encourage patients to stop smoking. In addition, teach patients to avoid crossing their legs when sitting and to begin a regular exercise program.

Diffuse Axonal Injury

DRG Category:	84
Mean LOS:	2.6 days
Description:	MEDICAL: Traumatic Stupor and Coma > 1 Hour Without Complication or Comorbidity or Major Complication or Comorbidity
DRG Category:	86
Mean LOS:	4.0 days
Description:	MEDICAL: Traumatic Stupor and Coma < 1 Hour With Complication or Comorbidity
DRG Category:	955
Mean LOS:	11.0 days
Description:	SURGICAL: Craniotomy for Multiple Significant Trauma

A diffuse axonal injury (DAI), the most severe of all traumatic brain injuries (TBIs), occurs when nerve axons are stretched, sheared, or even torn apart during trauma. A DIA generally consists of tears in the white matter of the brain that measure 1 to 15 mm in size. The severity and outcome of a DAI depend on the extent and degree of damage to brain structures and can be classified as mild, moderate, or severe DAI. All types of DAI are associated with an immediate and prolonged (> 6 hr) coma. Mild DAI is associated with a coma that lasts from 6 to 24 hours and has a 15% mortality rate; 80% of patients experience a good recovery. Moderate DAI, the most common form, is associated with a coma that lasts 24 hours or more, decerebration (extension posturing), and decortication (flexion posturing). Approximately 25% of patients with moderate DAI die. Severe DAI, which has a mortality rate of 50%, occurs when there is an extensive disruption of axons in the white matter of the central nervous system. People who emerge from coma usually do so in the first 3 months after injury, but many of those who live remain in a persistent vegetative state. DAI is more likely to cause morbidity than other types of TBI.

The pathophysiology of DAI is based on a model of shear injury; the TBI occurs because of sudden acceleration-deceleration impact, which can produce rotational forces that affect the brain. The injury to tissue is greatest in areas where the density difference in the brain is greatest, so most DAI lesions occur at the junction of gray and white matter. Injury results in edema and axonal tearing, and the severity of injury depends on the distance from the center of rotation, the arc of rotation, and the duration and intensity of the force. Complications include posttraumatic coma, disability, persistent neurovegetative state, and death.

CAUSES

The predominant causes of injuries that lead to DAI are high-speed motor vehicle crashes (MVCs), motorcycle crashes, and automobile-pedestrian crashes. The severity of the MVC is correlated with the severity of DAI. While there is some uncertainty, experts suggest that DAIs can result from explosion injuries and incendiary weapons.

GENETIC CONSIDERATIONS

No clear genetic contributions to susceptibility have been defined.

SEX AND LIFE SPAN CONSIDERATIONS

DAIs can be experienced by patients of all ages and both sexes, but males are affected at higher rates than females. Trauma is the leading cause of death between the ages of 1 and 44 years, and high-speed MVCs are the most common cause of DAI followed by sports injuries. In children from birth to 4 years of age, assault is the most common cause of TBI. In people recovering from DAIs, younger age is associated with a more favorable recovery.

HEALTH DISPARITIES AND SEXUAL/GENDER MINORITY HEALTH

In recent years, Black persons have been killed in traffic crashes at a rate almost 25% higher than White persons (National Highway Traffic Safety Administration [NHTSA], 2021). However, Native American persons have the highest rate of MVC injury in the United States, more than twice the rate of Black persons (NHTSA, 2021). Experts have noted that Black and Native American communities tend to be crisscrossed by more dangerous roads than other locations, placing people from those communities at risk for injury. Healthy People 2020 reports that non-Hispanic Black persons have the highest overall injury death rate in the United States (79.9 injury deaths per 100,000 people), followed by non-Hispanic White persons (79.2), Native American persons (78.2), Hispanic persons (45.5), and Asian/Pacific Islander persons (25.6). Stark disparities exist with the incidence, management, and rehabilitation of TBI and DAI. The Centers for Disease Control and Prevention (CDC) report that Native American children and adults have the highest TBI-related hospitalizations and deaths in the United States. Important health disparities exist in treatment, follow-up, and rehabilitation of TBI. Non-Hispanic Black and Hispanic patients are less likely to receive follow-up care and rehabilitation following TBI and more likely to have poor psychosocial, functional, and employment-related outcomes as compared to non-Hispanic White patients (CDC, 2021).

The CDC reports that in the 20 years since the year 2000, more than 400,000 U.S. service members were diagnosed with TBI, including active military service members and Veterans. Approximately 80% of these injuries occurred when the service members were not deployed. These injuries may result in ongoing symptoms, posttraumatic distress syndrome, and suicidal thoughts. People in correctional or detention facilities, people who experience homelessness, and survivors of intimate partner violence may have long-term consequences from TBI. People with lower incomes and those without health insurance have less access to TBI care, are less likely to receive surgical procedures and cranial monitoring when indicated, are less likely to receive rehabilitation, and are more likely to die in the hospital. Recent work has shown that rural populations have injury mortality rates that are more than twice as high as urban rates. Many factors contribute to these health disparities, including the risk of traffic injury in narrow rural roads, the lack of graded curves and lighted traffic signals on rural highways, and the distance from major trauma centers. Many of the most dangerous occupations, such as mining and agriculture, are found in rural areas and can result in injury, disability, and death. People living in rural areas who experience a TBI have more time to travel to get emergency care, less access to high-level trauma care, and more difficulty accessing TBI services. Sexual and gender minority persons have high risk for dating and interpersonal violence, violence related to bullying, and intentional and unintentional injury and therefore are at risk for TBI (Healthy People 2020).

GLOBAL HEALTH CONSIDERATIONS

DAI is a diagnosis made primarily in Western countries by radiography. Few epidemiological data are available internationally or in developing countries. However, developing countries have a growing health crisis as MVCs increase, and violence/war is an ongoing, serious issue in many parts of the developing and developed world.

ASSESSMENT

HISTORY. If the patient has been in an MVC, determine the speed and type of the vehicle, the patient's position in the vehicle, whether the patient was restrained, and whether the patient was thrown from the vehicle on impact. If the patient was injured in a motorcycle crash, determine if the patient was wearing a helmet. Determine if the patient experienced momentary loss of reflexes, momentary arrest of respiration, loss of consciousness, and the length of time the patient was unconscious. Determine if the patient has been experiencing excessive sweating (hyperhidrosis) or hypertension since the injury.

PHYSICAL EXAMINATION. The primary symptom of DAI is **decreased neurological status with loss of consciousness**. The initial evaluation is focused on assessing the airway, breathing, circulation, and disability (neurological status). Exposure (undressing the patient completely) is incorporated as part of the primary survey. The secondary survey, a head-to-toe assessment, including vital signs, is then completed. Note a very high fever, hyperhidrosis, or hypertension. Observe posturing for flexion or extension.

The initial and ongoing neurological assessment includes monitoring of the vital signs, assessment of the level of consciousness, examination of pupil size and level of reactivity, and assessment of the Glasgow Coma Scale (GCS), which evaluates eye opening, best verbal response, and best motor response. Clinical findings may include a rapidly changing level of consciousness from confusion to coma, ipsilateral pupil dilation, hemiparesis, and abnormal posturing that includes flexion and extension. A neurological assessment is repeated at least hourly during the first 24 hours after the injury.

Examine the patient for signs of a basilar skull fracture: periorbital ecchymosis (raccoon's eyes), subscleral hemorrhage, retroauricular ecchymosis (Battle sign), hemotympanum (blood behind the eardrum), and leakage of cerebrospinal fluid from ears (otorrhea) or nose (rhinorrhea). Gently palpate the entire scalp and facial bones, including the mandible and maxilla, for bony deformities or step-offs. Examine the oral pharynx for lacerations, and check for any loose or fractured teeth.

PSYCHOSOCIAL. A DAI will likely alter an individual's ability to cope effectively and may be a life-changing injury. It may lead to significant cognitive and behavioral disabilities. Although it is not possible to assess the comatose patient's coping strategies, it is important to assist the family or significant others.

Diagnostic Highlights

Test	Normal Result	Abnormality With Condition	Explanation
Magnetic resonance imaging	Normal brain and spinal cord	Cerebral edema, damage to brain structures	More valuable than CT scanning in diagnosing DAI; preferred method of diagnosis over other procedures, especially with gradient-echo sequences
Computed tomography (CT) scan	Normal brain and spinal cord	Cerebral edema, damage to brain structures	Identifies structural lesions in patients with head injuries

Other Tests: Skull and cervical spine x-rays, arterial blood gases, complete blood count

PRIMARY NURSING DIAGNOSIS

DIAGNOSIS. Ineffective airway clearance related to hypoventilation, accumulation of secretions, loss of gag reflex, and/or airway obstruction as evidenced by alterations in respiratory effort, dyspnea, lack of chest/diaphragmatic excursion, and/or apnea

OUTCOMES. Respiratory status: Airway patency; Respiratory status: Gas exchanges; Respiratory status: Ventilation; Comfort level

INTERVENTIONS. Airway management; Oxygen therapy; Airway suctioning; Airway insertion and stabilization; Anxiety reduction; Cough enhancement; Mechanical ventilation management: Invasive; Positioning; Respiratory monitoring

PLANNING AND IMPLEMENTATION

Collaborative

Most patients with severe injury will require endotracheal intubation and mechanical ventilation to ensure oxygenation and ventilation and to decrease the risk of pulmonary aspiration. A Pao_2 greater than 100 mm Hg and a $Paco_2$ between 28 and 33 mm Hg may be maintained to decrease cerebral blood flow and intracranial swelling. Fluid administration guided by intracranial pressure (ICP), cerebral perfusion pressure (CPP; calculated number CPP = MAP − ICP; MAP is mean arterial pressure), arterial blood pressure, and saturation of mixed venous blood (SvO_2) is critical.

ICP monitoring may be used in patients with severe head injuries who have a high probability of developing intracranial hypertension. Some physicians use a GCS score of less than 7 as an indicator for monitoring ICP. The goal of this monitoring is to maintain the ICP at less than 10 mm Hg and the CPP at greater than 80 mm Hg. Management of intracranial hypertension can also be done by draining cerebrospinal fluid through a ventriculostomy.

Some patients may have episodes of agitation and pain, which can increase ICP. Sedatives and analgesics can be administered to control intermittent increases in ICP, with a resulting decrease in CPP. Additionally, some patients with severe head injuries may require chemical paralysis to improve oxygenation and ventilation. Other complications are also managed pharmacologically, such as seizures (by anticonvulsants), increased ICP (by barbiturate coma), infection (by antibiotics), and intracranial hypertension (by diuretics). While corticosteroids have been used to reduce swelling and improve outcomes after DAI, several randomized controlled trials have shown that they are not beneficial in DAI.

Pharmacologic Highlights

Medication or Drug Class	Dosage	Description	Rationale
Sedatives and chemical paralytics	Varies by drug	Short-acting: Midazolam (Versed); propofol (Diprivan)	Control intermittent increases in ICP with a resultant decrease in CPP; improve oxygenation and ventilation
Analgesics	Varies by drug	Fentanyl (Sublimaze)	Control intermittent increases in ICP with a resultant decrease in CPP

Independent

The highest priority is to maintain a patent airway, appropriate ventilation and oxygenation, and adequate circulation. Make sure the patient's endotracheal tube is anchored well. If the patient is at risk for self-extubation, maintain the patient in soft restraints. Note the lip level of the endotracheal tube to determine if tube movement occurs. Notify the physician if the patient's Pao_2 drops below 80 mm Hg, if $Paco_2$ exceeds 40 mm Hg, or if severe hypocapnia ($Paco_2$ < 25 mm Hg) occurs.

Serial assessments of the patient's neurological responses are of the highest importance. When a patient's assessment changes, timely notification to the trauma surgeon or neurosurgeon can save a patient's life. The patient with DAI is dependent on nurses and therapists for maintaining muscle tone, joint function, bowel and bladder function, and skin integrity. Consult the rehabilitation department early in the hospitalization for evaluation and treatment. Frequent turning, positioning, and use of a pressure-release mattress help prevent alterations in skin integrity. Keep skin pressure points clean and dry.

Provide the family with educational tools about head injuries. Referrals to clinical nurse specialists, pastoral care staff, and social workers are helpful in developing strategies to increase education and support. Establish a visiting schedule that meets the needs of the patient and family while providing adequate time for patient care and rest. The mortality of patients with diffuse axonal injury ranges from 15% to 51%, with a wide variation in the level of cognitive functioning that the patient can reach through intensive rehabilitation. Education and support for the family are critical in assisting them in coping with the severity of this injury.

Evidence-Based Practice and Health Policy

Lohani, S., Bhandari, S., Ranabhat, K., & Agrawal, P. (2020). Does diffuse axonal injury MRI grade really correlate with functional outcome? *World Neurosurgery, 135,* e424–e426.

• The authors examined the association of DAI grades with the extended Glasgow Outcome Scale (GOSE). The authors performed a medical record review of a cohort of patients discharged with the diagnosis of DAI with a focus on GCS, DAI grade, length of hospital stay, and occurrence of posttraumatic seizures. They contacted patients 6 months after treatment to assess their GOSE.
• Nine patients (23%) had posttraumatic seizures. Mean GCS at admission was 9.67; mean length of hospital stay was 24.12 days. Mean GOSE after 6 months was 6.10. Mortality rate was 12.5%. Patients with low mean GCS had significant unfavorable outcomes, but higher DAI grades were not associated with unfavorable outcomes. The authors concluded that mean GCS at presentation is a better predictor of outcome after DAI than its grade.

DOCUMENTATION GUIDELINES

• Trauma history, description of the event, time elapsed since the event, whether or not the patient had a loss of consciousness, and if so, for how long
• Physical findings related to the site of head injury: Neurological assessment, presence of accompanying symptoms, presence of complications (decreased level of consciousness, unequal pupils, loss of strength and movement, confusion or agitation, nausea and vomiting), CPP, ICP, appearance, bruising or lacerations, drainage from the nose or ears
• Signs of complications: Seizure activity, infection (fever, purulent discharge from any wounds), aspiration pneumonia (shortness of breath, pulmonary congestion, fever, productive cough), increased ICP
• Response to medications used to control pain and increase ICP

DISCHARGE AND HOME HEALTHCARE GUIDELINES

Many patients require extensive rehabilitation and may be discharged there. If the patient is going home, families may have a significant caregiving burden. Teach the patient and significant others the purpose, dosage, schedule, precautions, and potential side effects, interactions, and adverse reactions of all prescribed medications. Teach the patient and family the strategies required to prevent complications of immobility. Encourage participation in physical, occupational, and speech therapy. Verify that the patient and family have demonstrated safety in performing the activities of daily living.

Review with the patient and family all follow-up appointments that are necessary. If outpatient or home therapies are needed, review the arrangements. If appropriate, assist the patient and family in locating ongoing psychosocial support to cope with this injury.

Dislocation; Subluxation

DRG Category:	480	
Mean LOS:	7.3 days	
Description:	SURGICAL: Hip and Femur Procedures Except Major Joint With Major Complication or Comorbidity	
DRG Category:	538	
Mean LOS:	2.9 days	
Description:	MEDICAL: Sprains, Strains, and Dislocations of Hip, Pelvis, and Thigh Without Complication or Comorbidity or Major Complication or Comorbidity	
DRG Category:	566	
Mean LOS:	3.0 days	
Description:	MEDICAL: Other Musculoskeletal System and Connective Tissue Diagnoses Without Complication or Comorbidity or Major Complication or Comorbidity	

Dislocation and subluxation describe the anatomic displacement of a bone from its normal position in the joint. Dislocation is the complete separation of the bone from the articular surfaces of the joint, whereas subluxation is only a partial displacement in the joint. Both dislocations and subluxations refer to the position of the distal bone in relation to its proximal articulation. Although dislocation or subluxation can affect any joint, the most frequently occurring sites are the finger, thumb, wrist, elbow, shoulder, knee, and hip. The shoulder is the most commonly dislocated joint in the body.

When dislocation or subluxation is a result of trauma, there are generally associated injuries to the blood vessels, nerves, ligaments, and soft tissues that surround the joint. In addition to the actual damage at the joint, tissue death from circulatory compromise to the distal extremity or permanent nerve damage from edema can occur. Other complications include arthritis in the affected joint, avascular necrosis (death of bone cells because of inadequate blood supply), and repeated injury from recurrent instability.

CAUSES

Sports-related injuries, occupational injuries, and motor vehicle crashes are common causes of dislocations to the thumb or finger, wrist, elbow, shoulder, knee, hip, or other joints. Dislocations and subluxations can occur as a result of injury or developmental dysplasia of the hip (DDH), previously referred to as *congenital hip dysplasia*. DDH can also lead to dislocations and subluxations, and there tends to be an increase in occurrence of DDH within families that have had other children with the condition. In addition, dislocations and subluxations may be acquired as a result of chronic conditions such as rheumatoid arthritis.

GENETIC CONSIDERATIONS

A genetic predisposition to dislocation is seen in connective tissue disorders, such as Marfan syndrome and Ehlers-Danlos syndrome. Both can produce joint laxity. It is likely that genetic factors contribute to the occurrence of nonsyndromic dislocations as well. Congenital dysplasia of the hip (associated with the hormone relaxin) has a high incidence of hip dislocation.

SEX AND LIFE SPAN CONSIDERATIONS

Trauma is the leading cause of death during the first four decades of life. In general, more men than women are injured in violent events. Traumatic dislocations occur most frequently in persons under age 20 years as a result of their involvement in sports or risk-taking activities. The recurrence of a dislocation is very high in people who experience the first injury when they are under the age of 20 years, and males have higher rates of recurrence than females. If the first injury occurs when the person is aged 30 to 40 years, the potential for a repeat dislocation decreases. Displacements as a result of chronic conditions are more prevalent with people of advanced age. DDH, as compared with unintentional injuries, is usually diagnosed in the newborn period or early childhood years.

HEALTH DISPARITIES AND SEXUAL/GENDER MINORITY HEALTH

Ethnicity, race, and sexual/gender minority status have no known effect on the risk for dislocations and subluxation.

GLOBAL HEALTH CONSIDERATIONS

While no data are available about global prevalence, injury is a concern that occurs in all parts of the world, particularly during the first four decades of life.

ASSESSMENT

HISTORY. When the condition is a result of injury, elicit complete details of the injury from the patient, significant others, or life squad. Note the time of injury as well as the description, angle of force, and patient's immediate sensations. Always ask if the patient felt any numbness immediately after the injury. In an acquired dislocation or subluxation, note a complete history of recent alterations in mobility, pain, or any other changes. For traumatic or acquired displacements, it is important to obtain information about any previous dislocations of this joint or any other joint.

DDH can range from a minor instability to total dislocation. In moderate to severe DDH, diagnosis can be made at birth during the physical examination. However, for less severe conditions, symptoms may not occur until the child starts to crawl or walk. Elicit a developmental history from the parents covering the child's mobility.

PHYSICAL EXAMINATION. The most common symptoms are **pain and inability to move or use the involved extremity**. With traumatic or acquired dislocation, the immediate clinical manifestations may include severe pain, inability to move the extremity, change in the length of the extremities, abnormal contour of the joint, and ecchymosis (bruising). The symptoms of subluxation are the same but usually less severe. Make sure to remove all of the patient's clothing to observe skin surfaces. Assess joint range of motion unless there is suspected cervical spine injury. In that situation, defer motion until radiographs are completed. Palpate all extremities and note pain, crepitus, instability, and deformity.

Monitor the neurovascular status of the patient with a dislocation before and after reduction or other interventions. Impairment in circulation or neurological deficits may occur during injury, before the reduction because of pressure from bleeding or edema, and after the reduction or as a result of interventions. The impairment may occur at the joint, but it may also occur distal to the injury. Serial neurovascular assessment includes critical data related to the five Ps: pain, pallor, paralysis, paresthesia, and pulselessness. Normal pulses do not rule out compartment syndrome.

Signs of DDH include asymmetry of gluteal and thigh folds, limited hip abduction, and apparent shortening of the femur with knees in flexion. If the child is beginning to walk, gait abnormalities occur. In the infant, a positive Ortolani-Barlow maneuver is an indication of dislocation. This maneuver involves placing the hands on the knees of the baby with fingers on the upper portion of the femur and abducting the hips while the infant lies on its back. Resistance to abduction, or the presence of a click as the femur slips out of the acetabulum, is considered a positive response.

PSYCHOSOCIAL. If the dislocation resulted from an injury, the sudden impact may have disrupted the individual's routines and created certain losses. If dislocation or subluxation is a result of a chronic disease process, the deficit may be a reminder of the deterioration of the body; depression may follow as a result of the decreased mobility or role change. With any congenital or developmental problem, parents may experience anxiety, guilt, or depression.

Diagnostic Highlights

Test	Normal Result	Abnormality With Condition	Explanation
Radiological examination: chest, pelvis, lateral cervical (all cervical vertebrae including C7–T1 junction) spine x-rays	Normal bone, joint, and soft tissue structure	Dislocations and subluxations; assessment of fractures or dislocations should include two views (90 degrees to each other, and of affected area with joints above and below)	If the patient is unconscious, spinal and pelvic injuries need to be ruled out

Other Tests: Supporting tests include computed tomography scan, magnetic resonance imaging, and ultrasound.

PRIMARY NURSING DIAGNOSIS

DIAGNOSIS. Acute pain related to lack of the continuity of the bone to joint, edema, and/or muscle spasms as evidenced by self-reports of pain and/or inability to move the involved extremity

OUTCOMES. Comfort status; Pain control; Pain level; Symptom severity; Body mechanics performance

INTERVENTIONS. Analgesic administration; Anxiety reduction; Environmental management: Comfort; Pain management: Acute; Medication management

PLANNING AND IMPLEMENTATION
Collaborative

If the joint remains unreduced (to reduce is to restore the components of the joint to their usual relationships), the patient is at greater risk for avascular necrosis. The primary goal for therapeutic management is to realign the bones of the joint to their normal anatomic position. With injuries or chronic conditions, the physician will generally use a closed reduction (manually placing the bone into the joint) after giving the patient a sedative or a local or general anesthetic. The decision for a closed reduction depends on the person's age, condition, and severity of the injury. If the same joint has repeatedly become dislocated or if the condition is severe, an open reduction or arthroscopy may be required. Open reduction requires general anesthesia or an anesthetic block and involves surgical intervention for repositioning the bones and repairing ligaments. Once the proper position has been achieved, the physician may use pins or screws to maintain alignment.

After the open or closed reduction is accomplished, the physician immobilizes the joint to allow for healing through slings, taping, splints, casts, or traction devices. Treatment of subluxation is similar to that of a dislocation, but subluxation generally requires less healing time. Patients require a carefully regulated exercise program to restore the joint to its original range of motion without causing another dislocation.

The goal for treating DDH is the same as for other dislocations or subluxations. However, the age of the child and the developmental nature of the condition alter the intervention. Treatment approaches vary according to the child's age. Infants under 3 months of age may simply require a triple diapering technique. This procedure abducts (by use of the thick diapers) the baby's legs, positioning the femoral head into the acetabulum as the baby grows. Skin traction such as Bryant or split Russell may be used for the baby over 3 months of age. These procedures relocate the femur to the acetabulum while gently stretching the ligaments and muscles around the joint. For 3- to 6-year-old patients, serial casting (the placement of several casts over time as the child grows or as realignment is required) or open reduction with casting may be needed.

Pharmacologic Highlights

Medication or Drug Class	Dosage	Description	Rationale
NSAIDs	Naproxen, 500 mg PO followed by 250 mg q 6–8 hr; also may use ibuprofen, ketoprofen	Analgesic, anti-inflammatory and anti-pyretic activities	Uncertain mechanism of action; may inhibit cyclo-oxygenase activity and prostaglandin synthesis
Analgesics and sedatives	Varies with drug	Analgesia: Narcotics such as morphine, hydroco-done, codeine, or fentanyl (Sublimaze); sedation: midazolam (Versed)	To achieve easily arous-able analgesia and sedation so that ongoing assessments can occur

Independent

Before reduction of the joint, direct nursing care to relieve pain and protect the joint and extremity from further injury. Maintain proper positioning and alignment to limit further injury. Accompanying soft tissue injuries are treated by rest, ice, compression bandage, and elevation (RICE) therapy with or without immobilization.

The patient and family need support to cope with a sudden injury. Allow time each day to listen to concerns, discuss the patient's progress, and explain upcoming procedures. They may be concerned about recurrent injuries and how they might affect the use of the joint. Older patients may experience depression and loss if the injury has long-term implications on self-care. Use social workers and advanced-practice nurses for consultation if the patient's anxiety or fear is abnormal. Immobilization involving the whole person rather than one extremity requires aggressive prevention of the hazards of immobility. Motivate and educate patients to help them prevent complications. Encourage a balanced diet that contains foods that promote healing, such as those that have protein and vitamin C. Stimulation of the affected area by isometric and isotonic exercises also helps promote healing.

Evidence-Based Practice and Health Policy

Erickson, B., Chalmers, P., Dernard, P., Lederman, E., Horneff, G., Werner, B., Provencher, M., & Romeo, A. (2021). Does commercially available shoulder arthroplasty preoperative planning software agree with surgeon measurements of version, inclination, and subluxation? *Journal of Shoulder and Elbow Surgery, 30,* 413–420.

- The authors noted that preoperative planning with imaging software can improve decision making during shoulder arthroplasty. Four software programs were used to measure shoulder inclination, version, and subluxation of the humerus. Those measurements were compared with the measurements made by five surgeons with special training.
- The authors found significant differences between the software measurements and the surgeon measurements; therefore, the software should be used cautiously. The surgeons' measurements had high interrater reliability. The authors suggested that reoperative planning software for shoulder arthroplasty has limited agreement, whereas surgeons' measurements had high reliability.

DOCUMENTATION GUIDELINES

- Restrictions of movement before and after reduction, level of discomfort, pain relief, neurovascular assessment (pain, pallor, paresthesia, paralysis, pulselessness)
- Response to treatment (open or closed procedure), understanding of aftercare guidelines

DISCHARGE AND HOME HEALTHCARE GUIDELINES

Be certain the patient and/or family understands the importance of the prescribed rehabilitation. For children, outline the appropriate activities to maintain growth and development. Demonstrate the adaptations required for patients with casts. Discuss the need to report any changes in pain, numbness, or other signs of neurovascular compromise. Make certain the patient or parents and family understand the signs and symptoms of suture line infections if open reduction has been accomplished and that odors or drainage from a cast should have immediate attention. If antibiotics have been ordered, stress the importance of completing the course as prescribed. Discuss the potential for repeat dislocations and the need for protection during sports or other activities.

Disseminated Intravascular Coagulation

DRG Category:	813
Mean LOS:	4.9 days
Description:	MEDICAL: Coagulation Disorders

Disseminated intravascular coagulation (DIC) is a life-threatening hemostatic disarray in which bleeding and clotting occur simultaneously. The International Society on Thrombosis and Haemostasis defines DIC as the following: "DIC is an acquired syndrome characterized by the intravascular activation of coagulation with loss of localization arising from different causes. It can originate from and cause damage to the microvasculature, which, if severe, can produce organ dysfunction." DIC is also called *consumptive coagulopathy* and *defibrination syndrome*. Some experts estimate that DIC occurs in up to 1% of hospitalized patients. The pathophysiology involves an overactivation of the clotting mechanisms with both enhanced fibrin production leading to small clots and fibrinolysis leading to enhanced bleeding. As its name implies, tiny clots accumulate in the microcirculation (capillaries) throughout the body, depleting the blood supply of its clotting factors. These microemboli interfere with blood flow and lead to ischemia and organ damage. As the clots begin to lyse, fibrin degradation products (FDPs), which have an anticoagulant property of their own, are released. The FDPs, along with decreased levels of clotting factors in the bloodstream, lead to massive bleeding internally from the brain, kidneys, adrenals, heart, and other organs or from any wounds and old puncture sites. Because DIC is somewhat difficult to diagnose, the following definition may be helpful in understanding the disorder: It is a systemic thrombohemorrhagic coagulation disorder associated with well-defined clinical situations (see Causes) and laboratory evidence of coagulant activation, fibrinolytic activation, inhibitor consumption, and biochemical evidence of end-organ damage. Morbidity and mortality depend on the underlying disease that initiates DIC and the severity of coagulopathy. In people who are severely injured, the presence of DIC generally doubles the mortality rate. Complications include hemorrhage, impaired peripheral circulation leading to gangrene and loss of fingers or toes, acute kidney injury, acute liver injury, cardiac tamponade, hemothorax, intracerebral hematoma, shock, and death.

CAUSES

DIC always occurs in response to another type of disease or trauma. DIC is usually an acute syndrome, although it may be chronic in patients with cancer or more longstanding conditions. Sepsis is the most common cause of DIC, with a prevalence of 7% to 50%.

Conditions that may precede its development are cardiac and peripheral vascular disorders, transfusion reactions, sepsis, septic shock, and severe infection, viremias, organ destruction such as liver and pancreatic disease, transplant rejection, leukemia, metastatic cancer, burn injuries, and obstetric complications (abruptio placentae, pregnancy-induced hypertension, saline abortion, amniotic fluid embolism, or a retained dead fetus). It is not known how these disorders trigger the onset of DIC, but they activate the intrinsic or extrinsic pathway of the coagulation cascade. Some experts suggest that these disorders cause a foreign protein to be released into the circulation and that the vascular endothelium is injured. Others note that one of the following clinical situations needs to be present in order for DIC to occur: arterial hypotension, hypoxemia, acidemia, and stasis of capillary blood flow.

GENETIC CONSIDERATIONS

Alterations in production of components of clotting and thrombolysis (e.g., factor V deficiency, protein C deficiencies) are heritable and can contribute to DIC. Protein C deficiency has been linked to over 160 mutations and is usually inherited as an autosomal dominant trait and is associated with an increased risk of venous thrombosis.

SEX AND LIFE SPAN CONSIDERATIONS

DIC can occur any time during the life span. Women of childbearing age who develop pregnancy-induced hypertension and the HELLP syndrome (hemolysis, elevated liver, low platelet) are potential candidates to develop DIC. Other high-risk patients are those with neoplasms (often older adults), sepsis, or traumatic injuries (often young adult males) such as burns and crush injuries.

HEALTH DISPARITIES AND SEXUAL/GENDER MINORITY HEALTH

Postpartum complications sometimes result in DIC. Experts note that Black women have the highest risk of complications from postpartum hemorrhage and the occurrence of DIC, are more likely to undergo hysterectomy as a postpartum outcome, and have a higher risk of death than other groups of women (Gyamfi-Bannerman et al., 2018). Sexual and gender minority status has no known effect on the risk for DIC.

GLOBAL HEALTH CONSIDERATIONS

DIC is recognized globally, but no data on prevalence are available.

☀ ASSESSMENT

HISTORY. Obtain a history specific to the precipitating disorder. If the patient is alert, ask if the patient has any chest, joint, back, or muscle pain, which is often severe in DIC. Recognize that the patient may be confused and disoriented as a result of blood loss or the underlying condition, so that historic information may not be accurate and may need to come from others.

PHYSICAL EXAMINATION. The most common symptoms are **blood loss from wounds, gums, and gastrointestinal tract**, **bleeding into the skin**, **hematuria**, and/or **epistaxis**. Some experts note that bleeding from at least three unrelated body sites increases the suspicion for DIC. Assess the patient's skin for any petechiae, ecchymoses, hematoma formation, epistaxis, bleeding from wounds, vaginal bleeding in the labor or postpartum patient, hematuria, conjunctival hemorrhage, and hemoptysis. Bruising can occur anywhere in the body. In addition, assess the patient's skin for bleeding or oozing at any IV, intramuscular, or epidural sites. The patient may have signs of diffuse or localized thrombosis with decreased tissue perfusion. Assess the patient's vital signs. If the patient is hypovolemic, expect to find a decreased blood pressure, rapid thready pulse, increased respiratory rate, and respiratory distress. The patient may be restless, agitated, confused, or even unconscious. Measure the abdominal girth to obtain a baseline for further assessments. Note the presence of oliguria and compare current urine output with previous readings.

PSYCHOSOCIAL. Patients may feel a sense of "impending doom," and the family is probably fearful of losing a loved one. This situation is intensified if the patient is a young pregnant or newly delivered parent. Note that increased blood or bleeding is associated with death and dying for many people; the visible presence of multiple bleeding or oozing sites and the need for multiple transfusions will likely also be a source of anxiety.

Diagnostic Highlights

Test	Normal Result	Abnormality With Condition	Explanation
Antithrombin III	Child: 82%–139% of normal; Adult: 80%–120% of normal	Decreased	Irreversible complexing of thrombin and circulating coagulation factors with antithrombin lower this level
D-dimer	0–0.5 mcg/mL fibrinogen equivalent units (FEU)	Elevated > 500 mcg/mL FEU indicates DIC	Fibrin degradation fragment; measured amount of clot breakdown products specific for cross-linked fragments derived from fibrin; in DIC, extensive fibrinolysis occurs
FDPs	< 5 mcg/mL	Elevated > 40 mcg/mL indicates DIC	Seven split products are formed from splitting fibrin as a result of plasmin during dissolution of fibrin clots; FDP quantifies amount of split products present in blood; in DIC, extensive breakdown of clots occurs
Fibrinogen	200–400 mg/dL	Decreased < 50 mg/dL	Decreased levels of fibrinogen (factor I) occur due to depletion of clotting factors; low fibrinogen not seen in all cases of DIC

Diagnostic Highlights (continued)

Test	Normal Result	Abnormality With Condition	Explanation
Partial thromboplastin time (activated; APTT)	Varies by laboratory; generally 25–35 sec	Prolonged; may be prolonged > 80 sec	Indicates how long it takes for recalcified, citrated plasma to clot after partial thromboplastin is added; screens for deficiencies in all factors except VII and XIII; factors are depleted, causing prolonged APTT
Platelet count	150,000–450,000/ mm^3	> 100,000/mm^3	Platelets are consumed during clot formation
Prothrombin time (PT)	Varies by laboratory; generally 10–13 sec	Prolonged > 15 sec	Prothrombin is a vitamin K–dependent glycoprotein necessary for firm clot formation; converts to thrombin in clotting cascade; in DIC, clotting factors are depleted and PT is prolonged

Other Tests: INR (international normalized ratio; more appropriate to evaluate anticoagulation medication); factors: Decrease in factors II, V, and VIII; prothrombin fragments 1 and 2 and fibrinopeptide A (through enzyme-linked immunosorbent assay). A DIC risk assessment has been developed by the International Society on Thrombosis and Haemostasis. The scale involves calculating a score based on the laboratory coagulation tests: platelet count, D-dimer, FDP, fibrinogen, PT, and APTT. The scoring is as follows: platelet count: > 100 = 0 points, < 100 = 1 point, < 50 = 2 points; elevated fibrin marker: no elevation = 0 points, moderate increase = 2 points, strong increase = 3 points; prolonged PT: < 3 seconds = 0 points, > 3 to < 6 =1 point, > 6 = 2 points; fibrinogen level: > 1 g/L = 0 points, < 1 = 1 point. A score greater than or equal to 5 is compatible with overt DIC, and a score less than 5 suggests nonovert DIC. The patient should also be assessed to determine if an underlying disorder such as trauma or sepsis exists.

PRIMARY NURSING DIAGNOSIS

DIAGNOSIS. Deficient fluid volume related to coagulation dysfunction as evidenced by abnormal blood loss in the urine or stool, bleeding from the gums and/or nose, and/or bruising

OUTCOMES. Fluid balance; Blood loss severity; Circulation status; Cardiac pump effectiveness; Hydration; Knowledge: Disease process

INTERVENTIONS. Bleeding reduction; Fluid resuscitation; Blood product administration; IV therapy; Shock management: Volume

PLANNING AND IMPLEMENTATION

Collaborative

Because DIC always occurs in association with another condition, medical treatment focuses on correcting the underlying disorder. In addition, the physician seeks to return the patient to normal hemostasis. Active bleeding is managed by blood component therapy. To ascertain the success of cell and factor replacement, constant surveillance of laboratory values is critical to determine which blood components should be administered. In general, packed red blood cells are used to improve oxygen delivery by increasing the hemoglobin content of the blood. Fresh-frozen plasma replaces many of the clotting factors, whereas cryoprecipitate is the best source of fibrinogen and factors VIII and XIII. Platelet transfusion is used when the platelet count falls below 100,000/mm³.

If the patient is critically ill, the physician may place a pulmonary artery catheter (PAC) to monitor the patient's hemodynamic status. Note that increased bleeding tendencies make the insertion time of central access devices important; central catheters such as a PAC should be placed when the coagulation profile has been corrected with blood component therapy to prevent dangerous bleeding into the cardiopulmonary system.

If the patient is pregnant, fetal monitoring is continuous; notify the physician of late decelerations, decreased variability, or bradycardia. Keep the patient on the left side and administer oxygen by mask at a rate of 10 L per minute. Turn and reposition the patient frequently and gently to avoid further bleeding. The goal is to keep the fetus oxygenated while stabilizing the patient so that a cesarean section can be done.

Pharmacologic Highlights

Medication or Drug Class	Dosage	Description	Rationale
Heparin	Varies with patient; patient-based dosing is common, with a starting bolus of 80 units/kg and an infusion of 18 units/kg per hr. Then dosage is calculated based on APTT results.	Anticoagulant	Inactivates thrombin and factors IX and X by antithrombin III; note that use is controversial but experts generally agree it is indicated for obvious thromboembolic events or with fibrin deposition
Antithrombin III	Total doses equals: (desired level – initial level) × (0.6 × total body weight kg) IV q 8 hr with a desired level > 125% loading dose of 100 units/kg IV over 3 hr followed by continuous infusion of 100 units/kg per day	Anticoagulant	Replacement; used for moderately severe to severe DIC; increases effects of heparin
Drotrecogin alfa activated (Xigris); activated protein C (APC)	24 mcg/kg per hr IV by continuous infusion over 96 hr	Recombinant form of human APC	Antithrombotic effect; inhibits factors Va and VIIIa with indirect profibrinolytic activity
Analgesics	Varies with drug	Narcotics such as morphine and fentanyl	Relieve pain of hemarthrosis

Other Drugs: Tissue factor pathway inhibitor

Independent

When a bleeding disorder occurs in addition to another condition, the patient's and significant others' coping skills and resiliency may be at a low point. During this time, the patient and significant others need accurate information, honest reports about the patient's condition and prognosis, and an attentive nurse to listen to their concerns. Provide emotional support and educate them as to the interventions and expected outcomes. Help them understand the severity of the condition and the treatments and present realistic and factual information. Offer to call a chaplain or religious counselor if needed. The patient is usually maintained on complete bedrest. Pad the side rails to help prevent injury. Reposition the patient every 2 hours and provide skin care. Gently touch the skin when repositioning and bathing; vigorous rubbing could dislodge a clot and initiate fresh bleeding. Crusted blood can be gently cleaned with a mixture of hydrogen peroxide and water and cotton. If the patient has experienced hemarthrosis (bleeding into the joints), the condition is very painful. Manipulate any joint gently and with great care to minimize discomfort and to limit further bleeding.

Inform all healthcare personnel coming in contact with the patient about the patient's bleeding tendency. Place notations on the chart cover and at the head of the bed to alert caregivers to the patient's bleeding condition. Keep all venipunctures to a minimum and hold pressure to any puncture site for at least 10 minutes.

Evidence-Based Practice and Health Policy

Ikezoe, T. (2021). Advances in the diagnosis and treatment of disseminated intravascular coagulation in haematological malignancies. *International Journal of Hematology, 113*, 34–44.

- Hematological malignancies such as acute leukemia and non-Hodgkin lymphoma frequently cause DIC. DIC is an acquired thrombotic disorder that reflects the severity of the underlying disease and is associated with a poor prognosis. In Japan, recombinant human soluble thrombomodulin is most frequently used to treat DIC caused by hematological malignancies. DIC improvement parallels the improvement of the underlying hematological diseases, and some question if the treatment of DIC would improve the long-term prognosis of patients.
- Innovative therapies also include stem cell transplantation as well as the recently introduced chimeric antigen receptor (CAR)-T-cell therapy, which are innovative therapies to produce a cure in a subset of patients with malignancies. These treatments need to be studied more completely to understand outcomes and complications.

DOCUMENTATION GUIDELINES

- Physical responses: Amount of blood loss, location of bleeding; fluid intake and output; condition of skin (oozing of puncture sites, bruising, petechiae); vital signs, including hemodynamic monitoring results if appropriate; patency of airway and adequacy of gas exchange
- Response to therapy: Fluid replacement, blood component therapy, heparin
- Laboratory findings: Coagulation profile
- Signs and symptoms of systems complications: Hemorrhage, hypovolemic shock, transfusion reaction
- Condition of newborn if recently delivered

DISCHARGE AND HOME HEALTHCARE GUIDELINES

Teach the patient and significant others about the disorder and that it is unlikely that it will recur in the future. If the patient required blood component therapy, provide information about the risk of hepatitis or HIV transmission. Check with the patient's obstetrician to determine if the patient can nurse the infant and resume unprotected sexual relations. Provide discharge instructions related to the patient's primary diagnosis. Teach the patient to notify the physician of any uncontrollable bleeding or syncope.

Diverticular Disease

DRG Category:	329
Mean LOS:	13.1 days
Description:	SURGICAL: Major Small and Large Bowel Procedures With Major Complication or Comorbidity
DRG Category:	391
Mean LOS:	4.9 days
Description:	MEDICAL: Esophagitis, Gastroenteritis, and Miscellaneous Digestive Disorders With Major Complication or Comorbidity

Diverticular disease has two clinical forms, diverticulosis and diverticulitis. People with diverticulosis have multiple, noninflamed diverticula (outpouches of the intestinal mucosa through the circular smooth muscle of the bowel wall). Usually, diverticulosis is asymptomatic and does not require treatment. Diverticulitis, in contrast, occurs when the diverticula become inflamed or microperforated. Diverticular disease usually occurs in the descending and sigmoid colon and is accompanied by signs of inflammation.

Mortality and morbidity are related to complications of diverticulosis such as diverticulitis and lower gastrointestinal (GI) bleeding, which occur in 10% to 20% of patients with diverticulosis during their lifetime. The lifetime recurrence is 20% to 30% after the first episode of diverticulitis and 35% to 50% after a second episode. Complications include fistula or abscess formation, scar tissue formation, intestinal obstruction, intestinal perforation, and peritonitis. Complications may be more severe in people who are immunocompromised, such as people with HIV, those following organ transplantation, or people taking long-term corticosteroid treatment.

CAUSES

Patients with diverticular disease generally have increased muscular contractions in the sigmoid colon that produce muscular thickness and increased intraluminal pressure. This increased pressure, accompanied by a weakness in the colon wall, causes diverticular formations. There is a significant risk of diverticular disease in people who are obese, and diet may be a contributing factor. A diet with insufficient fiber reduces fecal residue, narrows the bowel lumen, and leads to higher intra-abdominal pressure during defecation. Diverticulitis is caused when stool and bacteria are retained in the diverticular outpouches, leading to the formation of a hardened mass called a fecalith. The fecalith obstructs blood supply to the diverticular area, leading to inflammation, edema of tissues, and possible bowel perforation and peritonitis.

GENETIC CONSIDERATIONS

The heritability of diverticulosis is estimated to be about 40%. Diverticula can also occur as a feature of other genetic disorders, including type IV Ehlers-Danlos syndrome and autosomal dominant polycystic kidney disease. Genetic contributions to isolated diverticula are suggested by the ethnic distribution.

SEX AND LIFE SPAN CONSIDERATIONS

Only 20% of those with diverticular disease are under 40 years of age. When the disorder does occur before age 40 years, it can usually be attributed to a congenital predisposition. From 30%

to 60% of people with diverticular disease are between ages 60 and 80 years. As people age, structural changes in both genders occur in the muscular layers of the colon, which places older adults at risk for the disease. By the age of 85 years, two-thirds of the population has the condition. The male-to-female ratio is approximately equal, although women have poorer surgical outcomes and a higher mortality rate than men.

HEALTH DISPARITIES AND SEXUAL/GENDER MINORITY HEALTH

Health disparities related to diverticular disease exist with several aspects of the disease. Better surgical outcomes occur with planned, elective surgery than emergency surgery, which has higher rates of complications than elective surgery. Older adults, people with more severe disease, people living in rural areas, and uninsured people have decreased odds of having elective surgical procedures such as minimally invasive procedures to manage the disease (Lemini et al., 2019). Emergency rather than elective surgical care was most likely to occur in uninsured persons, Black persons, obese persons, and persons with multiple comorbidities, increasing their risk for complications. White persons have higher rates of diverticular disease than other groups. Sexual and gender minority status has no known effect on the risk for diverticular disease.

GLOBAL HEALTH CONSIDERATIONS

Diverticular disease is a disease of industrialized Western countries, probably because diet influences the prevalence, and data are not always recorded in developing countries. For unknown reasons, Asian populations have a tendency toward right-sided diverticula as compared to other groups, who have more left-sided disease. Globally, most experts suggest that the international incidence likely parallels that in the United States, which is 6% to 22% of the population. In recent years, the prevalence has increased in Japan, possibly because of changes in diet and lifestyle.

ASSESSMENT

HISTORY. Patients with diverticulosis are generally asymptomatic but may report cramping abdominal pain in the left lower quadrant of the abdomen that may radiate to the back and may be relieved with episodes of flatulence and a bowel movement. Occasional rectal bleeding may also be noted. Patients frequently describe episodes of constipation and diarrhea, low-grade fever, chills, weakness, fatigue, nausea, vomiting, abdominal distention, flatulence, and anorexia. Patients may report that symptoms often follow and are accentuated by the ingestion of foods such as popcorn, celery, fresh vegetables, whole grains, and nuts. Symptoms are also aggravated during stressful times.

PHYSICAL EXAMINATION. The most common symptoms are **left lower quadrant pain**, **cramping**, and **change in bowel habits**. Abdominal distention, a tender mass if an abscess has formed, and hyperactive or hypoactive bowel sounds may be present. Because diverticular disease is a chronic disorder that generally alters a patient's nutritional intake, inspect for malnutrition symptoms such as weight loss, lethargy, brittle nails, and hair loss. Assess vital signs because temperature and pulse elevations are common. Palpate the patient's abdominal area for pain or tenderness over the left lower quadrant. Palpate for a mass in this area, which may indicate diverticular inflammation.

PSYCHOSOCIAL. The discomfort of diverticular disease is a stressful situation, and stress can lead to further inflammation. Stress reduction strategies such as meditation or yoga may help to reduce stress. Managing a chronic disease can be difficult; determine the patient's coping mechanisms and what type of support system is available.

Diagnostic Highlights

Test	Normal Result	Abnormality With Condition	Explanation
Computed tomography (test of choice) and magnetic resonance imaging	No abnormalities	Diverticula, localized colonic wall thickening (> 5 mm)	Abnormalities such as diverticula, abscesses, fistulas, and pericolic fat inflammation can be located; excludes other pathologies
Technetium-99m sodium pertechnetate (gastric or Meckel) scan	Normal gastric mucosa	May demonstrate diverticula	Highlights the presence of mucosal abnormalities
Abdominal x-rays: Acute abdominal series with flat and upright abdominal imaging	Normal abdomen	Identifies perforation in lower quadrant mass	May show signs of free air if the GI tract has perforated; identifies signs of intestinal irritation (ileus), volvulus, bowel obstruction

Other Tests: Stool specimen, angiography if bleeding is occurring, and complete blood count. Barium enema usually fails to identify diverticulum. Lipase/amylase and liver function tests, ultrasound, sigmoidoscopy, and double-contrast enema.

PRIMARY NURSING DIAGNOSIS

DIAGNOSIS. Acute pain related to inflammation and swelling as evidenced by self-reports of pain or cramping, facial grimacing, and/or protective behavior

OUTCOMES. Comfort status; Pain control; Pain level; Symptom severity; Symptom control

INTERVENTIONS. Analgesic administration; Anxiety reduction; Pain management: Acute; Medication management

☀ PLANNING AND IMPLEMENTATION

Collaborative

MEDICAL. For uncomplicated diverticulosis, a diet high in vegetable fiber is recommended. If constipation is a problem, bulk-forming laxatives and stool softeners are often prescribed to decrease stool transit time and minimize intraluminal pressure. For diverticulitis, care centers on resting the bowel until the inflammatory process subsides. Bedrest is recommended to decrease intestinal motility, and oral intake is restricted, with supplemental IV fluid administration followed by a liquid diet and, eventually, a bland, low-residue diet. After the inflammatory episode resolves, the patient is advanced to a high-fiber diet to prevent future acute inflammatory attacks.

SURGICAL. Surgical intervention may be required if the diverticular disease becomes symptomatic and is not relieved with conservative treatment. Elective minimally invasive surgery has lower rates of complications and for that reason is preferred over emergent surgery, which is mandatory if complications develop, such as hemorrhage, bowel obstruction, abscess, or bowel perforation. A colon resection with temporary colostomy placement may be necessary until the bowel heals. Elective resection of the bowel is recommended after three episodes of diverticulitis to prevent further exacerbations and serious complications.

Pharmacologic Highlights

Medication or Drug Class	Dosage	Description	Rationale
Anticholinergic drugs	Varies with drug	Diminishes colon spasms	Control pain by decreasing spasms
Oral antibiotics (metronidazole, ciprofloxacin, amoxicillin/clavulanate, sulfamethoxazole and trimethoprim, ceftriaxone, cefotaxime, moxifloxacin)	Varies with drug	Kills invading bacteria	Control the spread of infection when a fever is present

Other Drugs: Analgesics may also be ordered. Generally, meperidine (Demerol) is preferred, because morphine increases intracolonic pressure, thus creating more discomfort and possibly intestinal perforation.

Independent

For uncomplicated diverticulosis, nursing interventions focus on teaching measures to prevent acute inflammatory episodes. Explain the disease process and the strong connection between dietary intake and diverticular disease. Instruct the patient that a diet high in fiber—such as whole grains and cereals, fresh fruits, fresh vegetables, and potatoes—should be followed. Caution the patient to avoid foods with seeds or nuts, which may lodge in the diverticula and cause inflammation.

Teach the patient about prescribed medications. In addition, discuss measures to prevent constipation. Instruct the patient to avoid activities that increase intra-abdominal pressure, such as lifting, bending, coughing, and straining with bowel movements. Instruct the patient about relaxation techniques. Discuss symptoms that indicate an acute inflammation, which would require prompt medical attention.

For patients with diverticulitis, provide supportive care to promote bowel recovery and provide comfort. As the inflammation subsides, teach the patient measures to prevent inflammatory recurrences. Instruct the patient about the purpose of any diagnostic procedures ordered. Should surgery be required, instruct the patient preoperatively about the procedure and postoperative care, leg exercises, deep-breathing exercises, and ostomy care when appropriate. Postoperatively, meticulous wound care must be provided to prevent infection.

Evidence-Based Practice and Health Policy

Patel, S., Hendren, S., Zaborowski, A., & Winter, D. (2020). Evidence-based reviews in surgery: Long-term outcome of surgery versus conservative management for recurrent and ongoing complaints after an episode of diverticulitis: Five-year follow-up results of a multicenter randomized controlled trial (DIRECT-Trial). *Annals of Surgery, 272*, 284–287.

- The authors aimed to determine whether surgery or conservative management of recurring diverticulitis results in a higher quality of life (QoL) at 5-year follow-up. They conducted a randomized controlled trial at multiple locations of patients (18–75 years of age) with ongoing abdominal complaints and/or more than two episodes of left-sided diverticulitis.
- They compared those who received elective sigmoid resection within 6 weeks with those who received conservative management as measured by the Gastrointestinal Quality of Life Index at the 5-year level. The surgical group had a higher QoL score than the conservative group, but the findings did not reach statistical significance. The study results demonstrate that health-related quality of life at 5-year follow-up may be improved in patients undergoing surgical resection.

DOCUMENTATION GUIDELINES

• Presence of abdominal pain, nausea and vomiting, and diarrhea or constipation
• Patient's ability to cope with the stoma
• Appearance of abdominal wound and stoma
• Ability to manage a colostomy, if appropriate

DISCHARGE AND HOME HEALTHCARE GUIDELINES

Be sure the patient understands any prescribed medications, including purpose, dosage, route, and side effects. Explain the need to keep the wound clean and dry. Teach the patient any special care needed for the wound. Review stoma care with the patient. Teach the patient to observe the wound and report any increased swelling, redness, drainage, odor, separation of the wound edges, or duskiness of the stoma. Review with the patient measures for preventing inflammatory recurrences. Discuss the signs of diverticular inflammation, such as fever, acute abdominal pain, a change in bowel pattern, and rectal bleeding. Explain that such symptoms require prompt medical attention.

Ectopic Pregnancy

DRG Category:	817
Mean LOS:	6.4 days
Description:	MEDICAL: Other Antepartum Diagnoses With Operating Room Procedures With Major Complication and Comorbidity
DRG Category:	818
Mean LOS:	4.0 days
Description:	MEDICAL: Other Antepartum Diagnoses With Operating Room Procedures With Complication and Comorbidity
DRG Category:	819
Mean LOS:	2.3 days
Description:	MEDICAL: Other Antepartum Diagnoses With Operating Room Procedures Without Major Complication and Comorbidity

An ectopic pregnancy is an implantation of the blastocyst (a solid mass of cells formed by rapid mitotic division of the zygote that eventually form the embryo) in a site other than the endometrial lining of the uterus. It is the leading cause of pregnancy-related death in the first trimester of pregnancy. In more than 95% of ectopic pregnancies, this implantation occurs somewhere in the fallopian tubes, hence the term "tubal pregnancy." The fallopian tube lacks a submucosal layer, which allows the ovum to burrow through the epithelium. Fertilization occurs, and the zygote lies within the muscular wall of the tube, drawing its blood supply from parental vessels. The ampullary portion of the tube is the most common site (80%), followed by the isthmic portion (12%) and the fimbria (5%). The cornual and interstitial regions of the tube have lower (2%) prevalence but a higher risk of mortality. Nontubal sites are rarer and include abdominal, ovarian, and cervical locations.

After the blastocyst implants in the tube, it begins to grow and can cause bleeding into the abdominal cavity. Eventually, the ovum becomes too large, and the tube can rupture, causing further bleeding that can lead to shock and death. Heterotopic pregnancies, in which there is an ectopic and a uterine pregnancy at the same time, occur at a rate of 1:10,000. The frequency of ectopic pregnancy has increased fourfold since 1970, owing to the increase in sexually transmitted infections (STIs), better diagnostic techniques, increased use of artificial reproductive technology, and increased use of tubal surgeries to treat infertility. Ectopic pregnancy accounts for 3% to 4% of all pregnancy-related deaths and reduces the chance of future pregnancy because of tubal damage; approximately one-third of those who experience an ectopic pregnancy subsequently give birth to a live infant. Hemorrhage, peritonitis, and infertility are the main complications.

CAUSES

The major cause of ectopic pregnancy is previous tubal damage, which can result from pelvic inflammatory disease, previous pelvic or tubal surgery, or endometriosis. Other causes may be hormonal factors that impede ovum transport and mechanically stop the forward movement of the egg in the tube, congenital anomalies of the tube, and a blighted ovum. Pelvic infections and STIs, specifically chlamydia and gonorrhea, are often involved. Other risk factors include advanced age of the pregnant person, smoking, diethylbestrol exposure, T-shaped uterus, certain intrauterine devices (IUDs), and a ruptured appendix. Approximately 90% of ectopic pregnancies occur in women who are multigravidas.

GENETIC CONSIDERATIONS

No clear genetic contributions to susceptibility have been defined.

SEX AND LIFE SPAN CONSIDERATIONS

Women over age 40 years have three times the likelihood of ectopic pregnancy as compared to their younger counterparts. Aging may result in progressive loss of myoelectrical activity responsible for moving the egg through the fallopian tube. Also, ectopic pregnancy often occurs in teens who have engaged in high-risk sexual practices that have resulted in frequent pelvic infections. Men have a role in ectopic pregnancies. In a large study of approximately 1 million pregnancies, less healthy men had a higher risk of siring a pregnancy ending with ectopic pregnancy than healthy men (Kasman et al., 2020).

HEALTH DISPARITIES AND SEXUAL/GENDER MINORITY HEALTH

In the United States, ectopic pregnancy is most often seen in Black women, Indigenous women, and women of color over age 35 years. Black and Hispanic females have a mortality rate from ectopic pregnancy almost seven times higher than that of White females. Health disparities exist in the management of ectopic pregnancy. In a large study, Black and Hispanic patients were less likely to have tubal conserving surgery, and uninsured patients were less likely to have conservative management. Both of these disparities may affect the risk for complications as well as future childbearing potential (Hsu et al., 2017). These findings were replicated in studies of the U.S. military, where Black women are less likely than White women to receive laparoscopy as compared to more invasive surgeries. Sexual and gender minority status has no known effect on the risk for ectopic pregnancy.

GLOBAL HEALTH CONSIDERATIONS

In developing countries, deaths from ectopic pregnancy are 10 times higher than those reported in developed countries. Several reasons may contribute to this disparity, including increased prevalence due to untreated STIs and lack of prompt identification and intervention when an ectopic pregnancy occurs.

ASSESSMENT

HISTORY. Women in their childbearing years, including teens, should be evaluated for an ectopic pregnancy any time they are evaluated for abdominal pain, cramping, or vaginal bleeding. Elicit a history about the onset of menses, gynecological disorders, pattern of sexual practices and birth control, and past pregnancies. Patients with an ectopic pregnancy often have some history of tubular damage because of infections or endometriosis. They may also have had tubal surgeries. Often, patients describe a history of using an IUD, and some may report a history of infertility. Question the patient about their last menstrual period to determine the onset, duration, amount of bleeding, and whether it was a "normal" period for the patient. This description is important because although amenorrhea may be present in many cases of ectopic pregnancy, uterine bleeding that occurs with ectopic pregnancy may be mistaken for a menstrual period. In addition to amenorrhea, the patient may exhibit other signs of pregnancy, such as breast tenderness, nausea, and fatigue.

PHYSICAL EXAMINATION. The most common symptoms include **abdominal pain, amenorrhea**, and **vaginal bleeding**. An undocumented ectopic pregnancy is a life-threatening emergency. Assess vaginal bleeding for the amount, color, and odor; if none is noted, bleeding may be concealed. Bleeding can occur as vaginal spotting, as a "slow leak," or as a massive hemorrhage depending on the gestational age and whether the tube has ruptured. Usually, the bleeding is slow, and the abdomen can become rigid and tender. Sometimes, vaginal bleeding is present with the death of the embryo. If internal hemorrhage is profuse, the patient experiences signs and symptoms of hypovolemic shock (restlessness, agitation, confusion, cold and clammy skin, increased respirations and heart rate, delayed capillary blanching, hypotension).

Evaluate the patient's pain; it can range from a feeling of fullness in the rectal area and abdominal cramping to excruciating pain. Often, the pain is one-sided and increases when the cervix is moved during a vaginal examination. Some women do not feel any pain until the tube is about to rupture, usually at the third month of gestation. If the tube ruptures, the woman experiences sharp, one-sided, lower abdominal pain and syncope. The pain may radiate to the shoulders and neck and is aggravated by situations that cause increased abdominal pressure, such as lifting or having a bowel movement.

PSYCHOSOCIAL. Often, the patient experiences anger, grief, guilt, and self-blame over the loss of the fetus. The patient may also be anxious about their ability to conceive in the future. Because much anxiety may stem from lack of information about the condition, assess the patient's learning needs. Determine the ability of the other parent and family members to cope and support the patient.

Diagnostic Highlights

General Comments: Diagnosis is based on a positive pregnancy and inability to visualize the embryo in the uterus. Have a high index of suspicion for any female patient in her reproductive years who reports abdominal pain, cramping, or vaginal bleeding. All these females should be screened for ectopic pregnancy.

Test	Normal Result	Abnormality With Condition	Explanation
Transvaginal ultrasonography	Intrauterine gestational sac is visualized	Unable to visualize intrauterine sac	This result, combined with a positive pregnancy test (elevated hCG), confirms the diagnosis
Human chorionic gonadotropin (hCG)	Normally is not present in nonpregnant women	The level is above the discriminatory zone of 1,500 m International Units	hCG doubles every 2 days during the first 40 days of pregnancy; failure to do so is evidence of abnormality

Diagnostic Highlights (continued)

Test	Normal Result	Abnormality With Condition	Explanation
Progesterone level (not accurate if fertility drugs were used)	> 25 ng/L	< 5 ng/L (values between 5 and 25 are inconclusive)	Progesterone increases with normal pregnancy

Other Tests: Laparoscopic examination of the abdominal cavity (used only in confusing cases), color flow Doppler ultrasound (used in cases when the gestational sac is questionably empty), Rh antibody screen and blood type, complete blood count and coagulation studies, culdocentesis

PRIMARY NURSING DIAGNOSIS

DIAGNOSIS. Risk for bleeding as evidenced by active or occult hemorrhage, tachycardia, hypotension, and/or pallor

OUTCOMES. Blood loss severity; Fluid balance; Hydration; Circulation status

INTERVENTIONS. Bleeding reduction; Blood product administration; Fluid monitoring; IV therapy; Shock prevention; Shock management: Volume

PLANNING AND IMPLEMENTATION

Collaborative

MEDICAL. Medical management of a tubal pregnancy depends on the patient's condition, fetus's gestational age and size, and whether the fallopian tube has ruptured. If the tube is intact, the gestation is less than 6 weeks, the fertilized mass is less than 3.5 cm in diameter, and the patient is hemodynamically stable with normal liver and renal function; methotrexate, a chemotherapeutic agent that inhibits cell division, may be ordered. The patient must also be committed to coming in for follow-up appointments, which are critical to the patient's well-being and to assessing the effectiveness of treatment. The hCG levels and fetal cardiac activity are monitored with methotrexate therapy; success of treatment is based on these two assessments (hCG should decrease 15% by day 4, and fetal cardiac activity should cease by day 7). If the tube is damaged or ruptured, surgical management is indicated immediately.

SURGICAL. Laparoscopic laser surgery is usually performed, but if the tube has already ruptured, a laparotomy may be indicated. A salpingectomy (removal of the tube), salpingostomy (incision and evacuation of tubal contents), salpingotomy (incision and closure of the tube), or segmental resection and anastomosis can be performed. The goal is to salvage the tube, especially in women who desire future pregnancy.

Postoperative care includes monitoring vital signs and observing for other signs of shock. Monitor the fluid intake and output as well and note the color and amount of vaginal bleeding. Observe the incision for any signs and symptoms of infection. Administer analgesics and assess the patient's level of pain relief from the medication.

Pharmacologic Highlights

Medication or Drug Class	Dosage	Description	Rationale
Methotrexate sodium (Folex)	50 mg/m² IM	Antineoplastic, acts as a folic acid antagonist	Inhibits the growth of the pregnancy by interfering with DNA, RNA, and protein synthesis

(highlight box continues on page 386)

Pharmacologic Highlights (continued)

Medication or Drug Class	Dosage	Description	Rationale
Analgesics	Varies by drug	Narcotics, NSAIDs; drug used depends on the level of pain	Relieve pain
RhoD immunoglobulin (RhoGAM)	1,500 International Units IM within 72 hr	Immune serum	Given only if pregnant person is Rh-negative and other parent is Rh-positive; prevents the antigen-antibody response leading to Rh iso-immunization in future pregnancies

Independent

Provide emotional support, using therapeutic communication techniques to relieve the patient's anxiety. Emotional support of this patient is important because the termination of any pregnancy causes a host of psychological and physiological changes. Inform the patient of perinatal grief support groups.

The patient may be concerned about infertility. Provide information and clarify the physician's explanations if needed. If necessary, provide a referral for a clinical nurse specialist or counselor.

Evidence-Based Practice and Health Policy

Wall-Wieler, E., Robakis, T., Lyell, D., Masarwa, R., Platt, R., & Carmichael, S. (2020). Benzodiazepine use before conception and risk of ectopic pregnancy. *Human Reproduction*, *37*, 1685–1692.

- The purpose of the study was to determine if women who fill a benzodiazepine prescription for anxiety or insomnia before conception are at increased risk of ectopic pregnancy. The researchers relied on outpatient prescription data and insurance medical claim codes for data on approximately 1.7 million pregnancies.
- The authors found that 1.1% of the sample filled at least two benzodiazepine prescriptions for a 10-day supply in the 90 days before conception. Women with a benzodiazepine prescription before conception had an increased risk of ectopic pregnancy compared with women who did not have a benzodiazepine prescription.

DOCUMENTATION GUIDELINES

- Physical responses: Amount and character of blood loss, vital signs, abdominal assessment (presence and description of pain, response to analgesics)
- Serial laboratory values: Hemoglobin and hematocrit, coagulation profile, white blood cell count; results of Rh test
- Response to treatments: Surgery, laparoscopy, fluid or blood replacement, medications
- Emotional status and coping abilities, partner's response
- Presence of complications: Hemorrhage, hypovolemic shock, infection

DISCHARGE AND HOME HEALTHCARE GUIDELINES

PATIENT TEACHING. If the patient is receiving methotrexate on an outpatient basis, teach the patient that more severe pain may indicate treatment failure and that the patient needs to notify the physician. The patient should not drink alcohol or take vitamins containing folic acid if methotrexate is prescribed. The patient may experience anorexia, nausea and vomiting, mouth ulcers, and sensitivity to sunlight as side effects of methotrexate. The patient also needs to follow up with scheduled hCG testing.

If a salpingectomy was done, explain to the patient that becoming pregnant again may be difficult. Fertilization takes place only on the side of the remaining tube after ovulation of the ovary on the same side. If a tubal repair was done, the patient is at a higher risk for a subsequent ectopic pregnancy as well as infertility. Educate the patient to recognize the signs and symptoms of ectopic pregnancy and to notify the doctor immediately if these should occur.

To prevent recurrence, advise the patient to engage in safe sexual practices. Teach the patient strategies to avoid STIs and pelvic infections that could cause further damage to the fallopian tubes.

POSTOPERATIVE INSTRUCTIONS. Give the patient the following instructions: Limit activity and get plenty of rest. Increase fluid intake. Keep the incision clean. Refrain from sexual intercourse for 2 weeks until the follow-up appointment with the physician occurs. Delay pregnancy for at least 3 months to allow for tubal healing. Determine that the patient has a method of birth control prior to leaving the hospital.

REFERRAL. If the patient is having difficulty dealing with the perinatal loss, referring the patient to a support group is appropriate. Often, follow-up by the hospital perinatal grief counselor is done. Referral to a fertility specialist is indicated if the patient is having difficulty conceiving for 6 months after tubal surgery.

Eczema

DRG Category:	606
Mean LOS:	5.9 days
Description:	MEDICAL: Minor Skin Disorders With Major Complication or Comorbidity

Eczema, or atopic dermatitis, is used to describe a group of chronic conditions associated with skin inflammation or irritation. The term *atopic* is used because the disease is often inherited, and people with eczema often develop other allergic conditions, such as asthma and hay fever. The prevalence of some form of eczema is approximately 10% of the U.S. population. The National Eczema Association identifies eight types of eczema: atopic dermatitis, contact dermatitis (result of skin touching an allergen), dyshidrotic eczema (occurs on feet and hands with blisters), hand eczema (combination of genetic and irritant causes), lichen simplex chronicus (thick, scaly patches), nummular eczema (round lesions caused by allergens), superrich dermatitis (white, greasy patches near oil-producing glands), and stasis dermatitis (poor circulation to the legs). For the diagnosis to be made, the skin condition must have the following characteristics: pruritus; xerosis (dry skin); flexural lichenification (thick, leathery skin along the skin folds, such as at the groin or under the breasts in women); and lichenification on the hands, nipples, or eyelids. Complications include sleep problems because of itching, bacterial skin infections, viral and fungal infections, and atopic dermatitis flares; 50% of children with severe atopic dermatitis develop asthma, and 75% develop allergic rhinitis.

CAUSES

Atopic dermatitis is immunologically mediated. A large proportion of people with eczema have elevated concentrations of serum immunoglobulin E (IgE). Two causes seem possible. First, an immune dysfunction resulting in IgE sensitization may lead to a problem with the skin's function as an epithelial barrier. Second, there may be a genetic defect in epithelial cells leading to a defective barrier problem, entry of antigens, and production of inflammatory cytokines. Risk factors are extremes of climate (very hot or very cold), co-occurrence of food allergies or asthma, and frequent skin infections. Triggers are thought to include frequent bathing, swimming, and hand washing; contact with soaps, detergents, deodorants, and cosmetics; and contact with secondhand cigarette smoke. Dust mites are a possible trigger.

GENETIC CONSIDERATIONS

A strong familial inheritance pattern exists, with a heritability of approximately 75%. Several genes have been linked to atopic eczema, with the strongest association in the gene encoding filaggrin (*FLG*), which is mutated in 20% to 30% of people with eczema. Filaggrin is a protein in the epidermal granular layer that functions in skin development and maintenance. Eczema has also been associated with mutations in the *CARD11* gene, which is inherited in an autosomal dominant pattern. Associations have also been found in several interleukin genes (*IL4*, IL4 receptor, *IL13*).

SEX AND LIFE SPAN CONSIDERATIONS

Eczema is more common in young children and infants than in other age groups. About 60% of all people with the condition have their first outbreak by age 1 year and 90% by age 5 years. While many infants who develop the condition outgrow it by their second birthday, some people continue to experience symptoms in adulthood. Females seem to have more severe symptoms than males.

HEALTH DISPARITIES AND SEXUAL/GENDER MINORITY HEALTH

Black, Native American, and Asian/Pacific Islander children have the highest eczema prevalence. The severity of the disease and the length of the outbreak tend to be greater in Black and Hispanic children as compared to White children. In adults, people who are multiracial have the highest eczema prevalence. Sexual and gender minority status has no known effect on the risk for eczema.

GLOBAL HEALTH CONSIDERATIONS

Developed countries, particularly those in the West, have an increasing prevalence of atopic dermatitis and other atopic diseases, such as asthma. People who live in Asia have much lower disease prevalence, but when they migrate to areas of higher prevalence, they are more likely to develop dermatitis than if they had not migrated. This change supports the theory that there are important environmental factors related to atopic dermatitis.

ASSESSMENT

HISTORY. Assess the patient for a personal or family history of dermatitis, itchy skin lesions, dry skin, lichenification of the hands and feet, asthma, or hay fever. Find out how often flares occur and the location of flares. Question the patient to determine if the skin is raw, sensitive, swollen, or seeping. Ask the patient if they have nipple eczema, susceptibility to skin infections with *Staphylococcus aureus* or herpes simplex virus, erythroderma (inflammatory redness of the skin), recurrent conjunctivitis, orbital darkening, or food intolerance.

PHYSICAL EXAMINATION. The most common symptoms are **itchy skin lesions** and **skin thickening**. Inspect the patient for rough, red plaques on the face (cheeks, forehead, scalp), neck, and upper trunk. Acute lesions appear as erosions with seeping of serous fluid or intensely itchy papules and vesicles on a reddened base. Less acute lesions are scaly, with excoriated papules or plaques with a reddened base. Check the skinfolds under the arms and breasts and the inner surfaces of the elbows and knees. In patients with dark skin, the lichenified areas may have lighter pigmentation. During an acute episode of atopic dermatitis, the patient may have redness over 90% of the body with weeping wounds or in discrete plaques.

PSYCHOSOCIAL. Assess the person's ability to deal with a skin condition that is visible on the face. The lesions may cause embarrassment or anxiety. Determine the patient's willingness to follow primary prevention strategies and to institute changes that decrease the risk of skin breakouts. Children with eczema have higher rates of depression, anxiety, and conduct disorder than other children and may have trouble coping with body image issues. There is an association between eczema and autism spectrum disorder and between eczema and attention deficit-hyperactivity disorder.

Diagnostic Highlights

General Comments: Generally, no laboratory testing is necessary. A swab of infected skin may help with the isolation of specific bacteria if infection is suspected. Allergy testing is of little value. Tests to determine if eosinophilia and increased IgE levels are present are usually not completed. A skin biopsy may be performed to complete histological studies.

PRIMARY NURSING DIAGNOSIS

DIAGNOSIS. Impaired skin integrity related to inflammation and irritation as evidenced by self-reports of itching and/or skin thickening

OUTCOMES. Tissue integrity: Skin and mucous membranes; Wound healing: Primary intention; Medication response; Knowledge: Treatment regimen and treatment behavior

INTERVENTIONS. Wound care; Skin surveillance; Medication administration: Skin; Infection control; Allergy management

PLANNING AND IMPLEMENTATION

Collaborative

Moisturization and topical steroids are the most typical treatments. People with the condition often benefit from lukewarm baths, adding apple cider vinegar or emulsifying oils to bathwater. The body should be left wet after bathing and the bath followed by the application of a moisturizer, such as white petrolatum, to seal in moisture and allow water to be absorbed through the stratum corneum. Note that these patients have hyperirritable skin. Anything that dries or irritates their skin, such as low humidity, seasonal changes, and very hot and cold temperatures, may trigger an episode of atopic dermatitis. The American Academy of Dermatology recommends using a diluted bleach bath with warm water to prevent flares by decreasing skin bacteria twice a week.

Phototherapy with ultraviolet light therapy is successful in some people with eczema, but it has several drawbacks. It is an expensive treatment and increases the risk for melanoma and nonmelanoma skin cancer.

Pharmacologic Highlights

Medication or Drug Class	Dosage	Description	Rationale
Topical steroids	Topical application; varies by drug; dose should be tapered when lesions clear to prevent side effects of corticosteroids	Hydrocortisone 1%; triamcinolone; betamethasone valerate	Reduces inflammation of the skin
Prednisone	20 mg PO for 7 days	Systemic corticosteroid	Controversial because it only temporarily reduces inflammatory response; generally, symptoms return once the course is completed

Independent

Nursing care focuses on prevention strategies, skin hydration, and nutritional considerations. Recommend taking short baths and showers with gentle soaps rather than deodorant soaps and antibacterial soaps (see Collaborative section for recommendations on bleach bathing). If bathing is done daily, teach the patient to use emulsifying oils and to pat the skin dry and then immediately apply emollients such as Aquaphor, Eucerin, Cetaphil, or Vaseline. Creams are preferred because they have lower water content and will remain longer on the skin. Teach the patient to avoid situations in which clothing is irritating or leads to sweating, which can worsen the skin reaction. The clothing that touches the skin should be soft and light, such as natural cotton fabrics. Cool temperatures will reduce sweating and itching. Cool mist prevents excess drying of the skin and is helpful to hydrate the skin year round. Teach the patient to wash clothes in a mild detergent without bleach or fabric softener. Encourage the patient to avoid outdoor activities that cause excessive sweating.

Foods can trigger allergic reactions and atopic dermatitis. Common foods to avoid include peanuts and peanut butter, eggs, seafood, milk, chocolate, wheat products, and soy products. If some foods are irritating, advise patients to apply a barrier of petroleum jelly around the mouth before eating irritating foods, such as tomatoes and oranges. Animal dander, dust, and pollen can also trigger a reaction.

Nighttime itching can be problematic for children. Recommendations include cutting nails short or placing gloves over the child's hands to prevent nighttime scratching. Antihistamines may be recommended for those patients who are unable to sleep due to aggravated symptoms of itching. However, there are no data to support that the medications actually stop the itching.

Evidence-Based Practice and Health Policy
Nakamichi, M., & Madi, D. (2020). Intestinal microbiota and child health: A review of the literature. *Pediatric Nursing, 46*, 125–137.

• Twenty-five articles were included in this systematic literature review to determine if intestinal microbiota in children with specific chronic health conditions effects illness. Supplementation with probiotics and prebiotics was also explored to determine any protective effects on various illnesses, including eczema, when given to mothers during pregnancy, while breastfeeding, or directly to the mother during breastfeeding. Additional supplementation was explored during the use of antibiotic administration.
• The review indicates that mothers should be encouraged to breastfeed, increase intake of dietary fiber and yogurt/kefir foods, and increase probiotic use prenatally, postnatally, and in childhood as adjunctives to current prevention strategies. These actions may help reduce and prevent chronic health conditions, such as eczema, in children.

DOCUMENTATION GUIDELINES

• Physical findings related to eczema: Location and description of lesions, degree of healing, level of discomfort from itching
• Patient's history related to eczema and associated risk factors
• Psychological response: Psychosocial state related to diagnosis; self-esteem, body image, level of anxiety, coping ability
• Response to diagnostic and treatment interventions: Ability to manage self-care

DISCHARGE AND HOME HEALTHCARE GUIDELINES

MEDICATIONS. Be sure the patient understands all topical medications, including the dose, route, action, adverse effects, and the need to taper them as the skin improves.

PREVENTION. Teach the patient primary prevention strategies:
• Perform self-skin assessments
• Manage skin hydration procedures: Bathing, application of moisturizers, use of cool mist

- Manage environmental temperature and humidity, provide clothing and activity recommendations
- Manage physical activity
- Avoid allergy triggers: Food (peanuts, eggs, seafood, milk, soy, and chocolate), detergents, cigarette smoke, animal dander, dust mites

---

Emerging Infectious Diseases (COVID-19)

DRG Category:	177
Mean LOS:	6.9 days
Description:	MEDICAL: Respiratory Infections and Inflammations With Major Complication or Comorbidity (DRGs are assigned for COVID-19. If the patient develops another infectious disease, the disease type will determine the DRG assigned.)
DRG Category:	178
Mean LOS:	5.1 days
Description:	MEDICAL: Respiratory Infections and Inflammations With Complication or Comorbidity
DRG Category:	179
Mean LOS:	3.8 days
Description:	MEDICAL: Respiratory Infections and Inflammations Without Complication or Comorbidity or Major Complication or Comorbidity
DRG Category:	207
Mean LOS:	13.9 days
Description:	MEDICAL: Respiratory System Diagnosis With Ventilator Support > 96 Hours
DRG Category:	208
Mean LOS:	6.7 days
Description:	MEDICAL: Respiratory System Diagnosis With Ventilator Support ≤ 96 Hours

Emerging infectious diseases are defined by the Centers for Disease Control and Prevention (CDC, 2018) as those infectious diseases whose incidence in humans has increased in the past two decades or threatens to increase in the near future. They are outbreaks of previously unknown diseases that have newly appeared or have existed but are rapidly increasing in incidence or geographic scope (National Institutes of Health [NIH], 2018). They persist in an uncontrolled manner and respect no national boundaries. They threaten the health and safety of all people because prevention and control recommendations may not be immediately available when the disease appears (CDC, 2018). Recent outbreaks of emerging infectious diseases include H1N1 influenza virus (swine flu, 2009), avian influenza (2013), chikungunya virus (2013), Ebola virus (2013), Zika virus (2015), and the novel coronavirus disease 2019 (COVID-19), the primary focus of this entry.

An outbreak of novel coronavirus infections was first reported to the World Health Organization (WHO) on December 31, 2019. The virus was termed "severe acute respiratory syndrome coronavirus-2" (SARS-CoV-2), more commonly known as COVID-19, and WHO declared a global pandemic on March 11, 2020 (Majumder & Minko, 2021). By early February 2020, a vaccine candidate had been designed and manufactured, and by March 2020, the first clinical trials were beginning. Authorization for emergency use was granted by the U.S. Food and Drug Administration in December 2020 for vaccines (NIH, 2021). As of March 2, 2022, the WHO reported 437,333,859 confirmed cases of COVID-19; 5,960,972 deaths; and 10,585,766,316 vaccine doses administered (https://covid19.who.int).

COVID-19 is a respiratory disease spread through droplets produced when an infected person coughs, sneezes, or talks. Symptoms appear 2 to 14 days after exposure. Complicating the risk for transmission, approximately 10% to 30% of people with COVID-19 remain asymptomatic (Marian, 2021). Although most patients have mild or moderate disease, up to 10% have severe and even life-threatening symptoms, and mortality is approximately 1% to 2%. Lung changes in people with serious disease include formation of hyaline membranes (fibrous layers that settle in the alveoli and prevent oxygen absorption), interstitial and alveolar edema, hemorrhage, microthrombi, and inflammatory activation.

Because COVID-19 is a novel coronavirus, humans had no prior exposure and no prior immune response, making the world's entire population susceptible until either a vaccine was developed or herd immunity was achieved. Complications include acute respiratory distress syndrome, cardiac arrhythmias, acute cardiac injury, heart failure, stroke, Guillain-Barré syndrome, and acute kidney injury. Long-term complications, sometimes called long COVID, occur when health issues continue for more than 4 weeks after diagnosis. Symptoms of long COVID include fatigue, rapid heart rate, chest pain, fever, shortness of breath, oxygen dependence, cough, joint pain, muscle pain, memory or concentration problems, anxiety, depression, headache, sleep difficulty, loss of smell and taste, and dizziness (Desai et al., 2022).

CAUSES

Infection with SARS-CoV-2 causes COVID-19. The reproduction number, or R, is defined as the average number of people whom someone with the virus will infect. The R value for the seasonal flu is approximately 1.3, and the R value for COVID-19 has been estimated at 3. Transmission also likely depends on the viral load, or the quantity of the virus in a given volume of fluid or droplets, after an infected person coughs or sneezes, or even exhales. The virus enters the uninfected person through the mouth or nose and latches onto the ACE2 (angiotensin-converting enzyme) receptor, which is a protein that breaks down angiotensin. It then merges with the cell membrane and releases its genetic material into the healthy cell of the respiratory tract in the uninfected person, who thereby becomes infected.

Variants of a virus occur as viruses mutate, and different variants emerge over time. A variant of concern is generally considered to be more infectious, more likely to cause reinfections, and more likely to lead to breakthrough infections in people who are vaccinated. With the emergence of alpha and beta variants, new waves of infections occurred around the world in 2020 (Karim & Karim, 2022). In 2021 the delta variant rapidly became dominant and appeared to be more transmissible than other variants (CDC, 2021). On November 25, 2021, omicron was reported as a new variant of concern when vaccine immunity from COVID-19 was more common around the world (Karim & Karim, 2022). Making COVID-19 disease even more complicated, variants such as omicron may have subvariants (BA.1 virus, BA.2 virus) that may have different transmission rates, degrees of severity rates, or responses to treatment (Chen & Wei, 2022). While scientists continue to investigate the omicron variant, experts suggest that not only may it be even more transmissible than previous variants, but also other variants are likely to emerge in the next months and years. The CDC lists the following characteristics and medical conditions that place people at risk for severe illness from COVID-19: older age; smoking; having cancer, diabetes mellitus, chronic liver disease, HIV disease, chronic heart disease, chronic lung disease, chronic kidney disease, dementia, Down syndrome, or tuberculosis; being overweight or obese, immunocompromised, or pregnant; and having a history of organ transplant, stroke, or substance use disorder. Being uninsured or underinsured is also a risk factor for COVID-19.

GENETIC CONSIDERATIONS

The clinical manifestations of the disease caused by the SARS-CoV-2 virus can vary widely in severity; some patients have no or mild symptoms, while others develop rapid respiratory failure. Studies have identified two genomic regions that are associated with the development of more severe disease progression. These include a six gene region on chromosome 3. Five of the six genes (*LZTFL1, CCR9, CXCR6, XCR1*, and *FYCO1*) are involved in T-cell and dendritic-cell function, while the sixth gene (*SLC6A20*) is regulated by ACE2 (the SARS-CoV-2 receptor). Another study demonstrated an association with the ABO blood group locus on chromosome 9. Patients with blood group A had an increased risk of severe COVID-19, and those with blood group O had a decreased risk. However, future studies will need to be conducted to further elucidate the mechanism of this genetic risk.

SEX AND LIFE SPAN CONSIDERATIONS

The severity and mortality of COVID-19 are higher in males than females, possibly because viral clearance is slower in males, and females have a stronger response to pathogens (Pradhan & Olsson, 2020). In a study of 16 countries with a total population of 2.4 billion, mortality rates were 77% higher in men than women. In addition, mortality was eight times higher in people 55 to 64 years old as compared to those 54 years old and younger. People 65 years old and older had mortality rates 62 times higher than those 54 years old and younger (Yanez et al., 2020). Thus, being male and being 65 years old or older are risk factors for severe illness and death from COVID-19. There is some evidence suggesting that pregnant women with COVID-19 are more likely to deliver before week 37 of gestation and more at risk for pregnancy loss. Pregnant or postpartum individuals with COVID-19 also have a higher risk of mortality or serious morbidity from obstetric complications as compared to individuals without the infection (Metz et al., 2022). Although COVID-19–associated hospitalizations and deaths occur more frequently in adults than children, who usually experience milder illness than adults, it can cause severe illness in children and adolescents. The highly transmissible delta variant caused increased COVID-19 hospitalizations for children across the United States during 2021 (CDC, 2021).

HEALTH DISPARITIES AND SEXUAL/GENDER MINORITY HEALTH

The role of race and ethnicity with respect to hospitalization and mortality rates is complicated. The U.S. Commission on Civil Rights (2021) reported that COVID-19 has had a disproportionate toll on Native American communities. They note that the Navajo Nation experiences one of the highest infection rates in the United States. With respect to other groups, in a study of 7,868 patients age 18 years and older with COVID-19 across 88 hospitals in the United States, the authors found a disproportionate number of the patients were Hispanic and Black (33% Hispanic, 26% Black, 6% Asian, and 35% White). More than half of the deaths occurred in Hispanic and Black patients. When considering the racial/ethnic breakdown of the U.S. population in 2020 (White 58%, Hispanic 19%, Black 12%), Hispanic and Black patients bore a disproportionate representation with respect to mortality and morbidity from COVID-19 (Rodriguez et al., 2021). The reasons for this discrepancy may include inequities in COVID-19 testing and the fact that Hispanic and Black persons are overrepresented in the essential workforce leading to higher risk for exposure. Additionally, discrimination in healthcare and living in urban areas may increase risk for exposure. There is some evidence that Hispanic and Black pregnant women may be at higher risk for severe disease than White pregnant women. Because sexual and gender minority persons have been historically affected disproportionately by lack of health insurance, poverty, discrimination, mental health disorders, and substance use disorders as compared to nongender and sexual minorities, COVID-19 presents additional burdens for them.

GLOBAL HEALTH CONSIDERATIONS

COVID-19 is a worldwide epidemic. As of March 2, 2022, the WHO reports approximately 450,000,000 confirmed cases of COVID-19 and approximately 6 million deaths. The United States has the highest number of confirmed cases, followed in order by India, Brazil, France, the United Kingdom, the Russian Federation, and Germany.

ASSESSMENT

HISTORY. Determine if the patient has a history of travel to areas of high contagion and has been in close contact (within 6 feet) of a known COVID-19–positive person or someone who has been exposed to the illness. Determine the length of time since the exposure. Ask about the nature of the patient's employment, with particular attention to high-risk positions such as healthcare workers or workers in emergency or essential services such as transportation, food service, or sales. Solicit a history of the patient's symptoms, with particular attention to a history of fever, fatigue, and nonproductive cough. The patient may also report body aches, shortness of breath, and diarrhea. If the patient is stable enough to take a history, determine any comorbid conditions, such as diabetes mellitus and obesity, and whether the patient has taken preventive measures such as masking and social distancing. Ask if the patient has received a vaccine against COVID-19, the type of vaccine, the date received, and any booster doses. Ask if the patient has self-medicated to manage the symptoms of COVID-19 or to try to prevent the infection.

PHYSICAL EXAMINATION. Examination should occur with staff wearing personal protective equipment (PPE) and, if possible, in a private room with negative pressure to prevent viral transmission. **Fever** is the most common symptom of COVID-19, followed by **cough, dyspnea, fatigue,** and **diarrhea.** New onset of **dysgusia** (loss of taste) and **anosmia** (loss of smell) may occur. The patient may have tachycardia and tachypnea, and early assessment with pulse oximetry is important to identify hypoxemia, a sign of pending respiratory failure. Further respiratory symptoms include increased work of breathing, use of accessory muscles to breathe, and mild expiratory wheezes. Patients also may have circumoral cyanosis and confusion as their oxygen levels decrease. Repeat examinations are necessary as the disease progresses to a more serious or critical stage. Consider a COVID-19 diagnosis for people presenting with conditions such as septic shock, acute kidney injury, diabetic ketoacidosis, or acute cardiac disease.

PSYCHOSOCIAL. COVID-19 is a life-threatening illness whose prevention and treatment have been surrounded by healthcare-related and social controversies. The family's response depends on their view of the disease and treatment and may range from extreme anxiety to concern to guilt to a more confrontational approach. The potential for other family members to contract the disease makes interactions more complex. Ultimately, the family may be faced with the death of a loved one and personal COVID-19 diagnosis. Continuously assess the coping mechanisms and anxiety levels in both patients and families.

Diagnostic Highlights

Test	Normal Result	Abnormality With Condition	Explanation
SARS-CoV-2 reverse-transcription polymerase chain reaction assay	Negative	Positive for SARS-CoV-2 genetic material (RNA)	Test of secretions from a nasal swab can identify small amounts of viral RNA

Diagnostic Highlights (continued)

Test	Normal Result	Abnormality With Condition	Explanation
Chest x-ray, computed tomography of chest	Clear lung fields	Ground glass opacity (hazy opacification) due to air displacement by fluid; bilateral infiltrates without cardiomegaly or pulmonary vascular redistribution; peribronchial thickening	Findings reflect noncardiogenic pulmonary edema, viral infection, and inflammation
Arterial blood gases (ABGs)	Pao_2 80–95 mm Hg; $Paco_2$ 35–45 mm Hg; SaO_2 > 95%	Pao_2 < 80 mm Hg; $Paco_2$ varies; SaO_2 < 95%	Poor gas exchange leads to hypoxemia and, as respiratory failure progresses, to hypercapnea. When the $Paco_2$ is divided by the Fio_2, the result is 200 or less. Patients with COVID-19 may have "silent hypoxemia," low levels of oxygenation without difficulty breathing (Tobin et al., 2020).

PRIMARY NURSING DIAGNOSIS

DIAGNOSIS. Impaired gas exchange related to increased alveolar-capillary permeability, interstitial edema, and decreased lung compliance as evidenced by abnormal ABGs, dyspnea, abnormal breathing pattern, confusion, hypoxemia, and/or irritability

OUTCOMES. Respiratory status: Gas exchange; Respiratory status: Ventilation; Respiratory status: Airway patency; Mechanical ventilation response: Adult; Fluid balance; Comfort status: Physical; Vital signs; Anxiety level

INTERVENTIONS. Airway insertion and stabilization; Airway management; Respiratory monitoring; Oxygen therapy; Mechanical ventilation management; Vital signs monitoring; Anxiety reduction; Fluid management

PLANNING AND IMPLEMENTATION

Collaborative

Key management principles include early diagnosis, immediate patient isolation, and supportive care with fluids, nutrition, respiratory support, and oxygenation (Majumder & Minko, 2021). To date, there is no effective treatment for COVID-19 although multiple drugs are currently undergoing randomized controlled trials. A series of antiviral therapies have been developed and tested. The corticosteroid dexamethasone has become a mainstay of treatment by reducing deaths by one-third in patients with COVID-19 on mechanical ventilation (https://www.recoverytrial.net). Baricitinib and tocilizumab, drugs used to manage inflammation due to rheumatoid arthritis, may help control the exaggerated inflammatory response resulting from COVID-19. Recent findings indicate that they may reduce deaths of hospitalized patients (https://www.recoverytrial.net). A monoclonal antibody combination has been found to reduce deaths for patients who are hospitalized with COVID-19 who have not mounted an immune response (https://www.recoverytrial.net).

Critically ill patients may develop cardiopulmonary failure, which is treated with oxygen therapy and noninvasive or invasive mechanical ventilation, vasoactive medications, and if needed, extracorporeal membrane oxygenation. Other modalities of mechanical cardiopulmonary support such as left ventricular assist device may be warranted. Prone positioning is considered standard of care for patients with both acute respiratory distress syndrome (ARDS) and severe hypoxemic respiratory failure with COVID-19 (Rajagopal et al., 2020). Just as in ARDS, severity of respiratory failure due to COVID-19 is determined by the ratio of Pao_2 to inspired oxygen concentration (Fio_2) when the patient is on at least 5 cm H_2O of positive end-expiratory pressure (PEEP) or continuous positive airway pressure (CPAP). Three categories of ARDS severity are mild (ratio = 200–300), moderate (ratio = 100–200), and severe (ratio of ≥100). As of early 2022, the care of people with severe COVID-19 remains challenging and an area of intensive investigation to determine an effective treatment.

Rehabilitation after an acute infection with COVID-19 focuses on patients who have experienced physical, mental, and cognitive impairments that threaten the return to their previous circumstances. Plans for rehabilitation need to occur early in the recovery phase with consultation from a multidisciplinary team collaborating with the acute care team. Occupational and physical therapy for positioning and splinting followed by passive range of motion and using communication devices can occur early in the disease course when the patient is no longer unstable. When the patient's sedation level allows for it, active range of motion, bed mobility, sitting on the edge of the bed, and cognitive stimulation continue rehabilitation care until the patient is transferred to a less-intensive care environment.

Pharmacologic Highlights

Medication or Drug Class	Dosage	Description	Rationale
Antivirals (remdesivir, ritonavir-boosted nirmatrelvir, sotrovimab, molnupiravir)	Varies by drug	Anti-SARS-CoV-2 therapies	Inhibit viral replication (Singh & de Wit, 2020)
Dexamethasone	6 mg daily PO or IV	Synthetic corticosteroid	Anti-inflammatory that reduces mortality in mechanically ventilated patients and those requiring oxygen (Marian, 2021)
COVID-19 mRNA vaccine	Varies by drug	mRNA vaccine	Induces cells to make a protein that then stimulates the immune system to develop antibodies to COVID-19; only effective prophylactically; not administered during an acute viral infection
Anti-SARS-CoV-2 monoclonal antibodies (combination of casirivimab and imdevimab)	Varies by drug	Monoclonal antibodies are proteins genetically engineered from a single clone and consisting of identical antibody molecules; used for patients with mild to moderate infection hospitalized for a reason other than COVID-19	Should be started as soon as patient has positive SARS-CoV-2 reverse-transcription polymerase chain reaction assay and within 10 days of symptom onset (https://www.recoverytrial.net)
Immunomodulators (baricitinib, tocilizumab)	Varies by drug	May control the inflammatory response to COVID-19	Reduces deaths in patients hospitalized with COVID-19 (https://www.recoverytrial.net)

Other Drugs: Anticoagulation, inhaled pulmonary vasodilators, neuromuscular blocking agents. Research continues to determine the role of antiviral medications, convalescent plasma, immunotherapy (Majumder & Minko, 2021).

Independent

Providing acute and critical care to patients with COVID-19 is challenging because it involves the maintenance of airway, breathing, and circulation simultaneously with protecting caregivers with PPE. Patients may develop rapidly developing respiratory failure, septic shock, metabolic acidosis, coagulation disorders, and multiple organ failure (Yuan et al., 2020), and the protocol for donning and removing several levels of protective equipment is a time-consuming and necessary addition to acute and critical care management. In addition to oxygen therapy and either noninvasive ventilation (CPAP or bilevel positive airway pressure [BiPAP]) or invasive mechanical ventilation, current expert opinion is to place the patient in the prone position for up to 16 of 24 hours with repositioning every 2 hours (Makic, 2020; Rajagopal et al., 2020). Patients have better outcomes if prone position is used in the initial hours of severe hypoxia. However, prone position presents challenges such as inadvertent dislodgement of IV lines and endotracheal tubes, concerns about aggravating hemodynamic instability, skin injury, gastroesophageal reflux, and the physical difficulties of rotating patients (three to five persons are needed). Prior to proning, protective dressings of the feet, knees, hips, shoulders, and face should be placed along with eye lubrication and taping to protect the corneas. Correct patient selection for prone position and timely initiation when warranted are important. Contraindications include extreme obesity, pregnancy, unstable spine, seizures, elevated intracranial pressure, facial surgery, and hemodynamic instability (Makic, 2020).

To augment gas exchange, the patient needs periodical endotracheal suctioning. Prior to suctioning, hyperventilate and hyperoxygenate the patient to prevent the ill effects of suctioning, such as cardiac dysrhythmias or hypotension. As the patient improves, get them out of bed for brief periods, even if they are intubated and on a ventilator. Provide passive range-of-motion exercises every 8 hours to prevent contractures. Communication with family is challenging because of infection control protocols. Arrange communication mechanisms that protect patients, families, and staff from COVID-19 exposure. Explain the critical care environment and technology, but emphasize the importance of the patient's humanness over and above the technology. Maintain open communication among all involved. Answer all questions, and provide methods for patients and families to communicate. Patients and families are likely to be fearful and anxious. Families are well-aware that with a COVID-19 diagnosis, intubation indicates a worsening condition and may indicate that the patient has a terminal illness. Acknowledge their fear without providing false reassurance.

Evidence-Based Practice and Health Policy

Coppo, A., Bellani, G., Winterton, D., Di Pierro, M., Soria, A., Faverio, P., Cairo, M., Mori, S., Messinesi, G., Contro, E., Bonfanti, P., Benini, A., Valsecchi, M., Antolini, L., & Foti, G. (2020). Feasibility and physiological effects of prone positioning in non-intubated patients with acute respiratory failure due to COVID-19 (PRON-COVID): A prospective cohort study. *Lancet Respiratory Medicine*, 8(8), 765–774.

- The authors initiated a study of patients 18 to 75 years of age (*N* = 56) hospitalized with a confirmed diagnosis of COVID-19–related pneumonia receiving supplemental oxygen or noninvasive CPAP. Patients were helped into the prone position, which was maintained for a minimum of 3 hours. Clinical data were collected at baseline, after 10 minutes of prone positioning, and 1 hour after returning to supine position.
- Oxygenation substantially improved from supine to prone position. After resuming the supine position, improved oxygenation occurred in 50% of the patients. Patients with improved oxygenation had shorter time between admission and prone positioning. The authors encouraged further investigation of the prone position in COVID-19 patients.

DOCUMENTATION GUIDELINES

- Respiratory status of the patient: Respiratory rate, breath sounds, and the use of accessory muscles; vital signs; ABG levels; pulse oximeter and chest x-ray results

- Responses to treatment, mechanical ventilation, immobility, prone position, and bedrest
- Response to medications, level of pain, level of consciousness, level of anxiety; presence of any complications or long COVID
- Family response, family understanding of patient's condition and infection control measures

DISCHARGE AND HOME HEALTHCARE GUIDELINES

PREVENTION. Rationale and timing for COVID-19 vaccinations, prompt attention for any infections

COMPLICATIONS. If the patient survives COVID-19, physical, mental, and cognitive residual effects often occur, as can long COVID. If the patient has experienced a critical illness, arrangement for extensive rehabilitation is likely, and planning needs to occur with the entire healthcare team and family together.

Emphysema

DRG Category:	190
Mean LOS:	4.5 days
Description:	MEDICAL: Chronic Obstructive Pulmonary Disease With Major Complication or Comorbidity

Emphysema is a chronic obstructive pulmonary disease (COPD) characterized by permanent enlargement of the air spaces beyond the terminal bronchioles. In addition to this abnormality, destruction of respiratory walls occurs. The syndrome includes both chronic bronchitis and emphysema, both of which are airflow-limited states; some experts do not distinguish between the two conditions. COPD affects more than 15 million people and is the fourth leading cause of death overall in the United States. Approximately 5% to 6% of male adults and 1% to 3% of female adults in the United States have emphysema.

In emphysema, the affected terminal bronchioles contain mucous plugs that, when enlarged, eventually result in the loss of elasticity of the lung parenchyma, causing difficulty in the expiratory phase of respiration. The alveolar walls are destroyed by abnormal levels of enzymes (proteinases) that break down respiratory walls. Gas exchange is impaired by the reduced surface area that results from the destruction of alveolar walls.

Four types of emphysema have been identified: paraseptal emphysema, which affects the periphery of the lobule; panacinar or panlobular emphysema, which affects the lower anterior segments or the entire lungs; centriacinar or centrilobular emphysema, the most common form, which destroys respiratory bronchioles and is associated with chronic bronchitis and cigarette smoking; and bronchiectasis or chronic necrotizing infection that leads to abnormal and permanent bronchial dilation, which occurs rarely. Complications from emphysema include cor pulmonale, respiratory failure, pneumothorax, and recurrent respiratory tract infections. Emphysema is the most common cause of death from respiratory disease in the United States.

CAUSES

Cigarette smoking strongly contributes to emphysema and leads to neutrophil activation and retention in the lung functional tissue. Up to 80% of people with emphysema have a history of smoking. Approximately 20% of people with emphysema have chronic occupational exposure to inhaled mineral fumes or dusts, organic dusts from wood or grains, or fumes from exhausts or chemical vapors. Enzymes, primarily proteinases and elastases, destroy the extracellular matrix of the lung and cause emphysema. Normally, plasma proteinase inhibitors in lung tissue prevent proteolytic enzymes from digesting structural proteins of the lungs, but if an excess of proteinase occurs, the defenses cannot manage the enzymes, and destruction occurs. Emphysema is the result of an imbalance between the proteinases and antiproteinases, with an excess of proteinases.

Risk factors for the development of emphysema include cigarette smoking, living or working in a highly polluted area, a family history of pulmonary disease, and substance use (cocaine, IV drug use with methadone and methylphenidate). HIV infection is also an independent risk factor for emphysema.

GENETIC CONSIDERATIONS

Emphysema has both genetic and environmental components. Emphysema is most often caused by smoking, but susceptibility may be influenced by genetics. Heritability is estimated at 30% to 50%. There is also a rare form of familial emphysema caused by mutations in the *SERPINA1* gene, leading to alpha-1 antitrypsin (AAT) deficiency. These mutations are inherited in an autosomal codominant pattern, meaning that two different gene alleles are expressed, and both contribute to the development of the trait. The M allele is most common and results in production of normal levels of AAT. People who are homozygous normal have copies of the M allele from both parents. The two variants (S and Z) cause production of low or moderately low amounts of AAT. Persons with the ZZ or SZ genotype are most likely to develop AAT deficiency. Persons with an MS or SS genotype usually produce enough AAT to protect the lungs. There is an increased risk of emphysema for those who carry the MZ alleles, particularly if they are smokers. Familial factors predisposing to emphysema in the absence of AAT deficiency are also likely.

SEX AND LIFE SPAN CONSIDERATIONS

Symptoms of emphysema may begin in the third or fourth decade of life but usually become severe during the fifth decade or later, which is when they are most likely to come to the attention of a healthcare provider. Previously, experts noted that emphysema occurs more often in males than in females, but as smoking rates have increased in women, the rates have equalized. Currently, women are dying from COPD more frequently than men and developing severe COPD earlier than men.

HEALTH DISPARITIES AND SEXUAL/GENDER MINORITY HEALTH

Black persons bear a significant burden of lung disease. Black patients with emphysema have worse symptoms, poorer quality of life, and increased complications as compared to White patients. Additionally, when neighborhood-level factors (neighborhood walkability, access to healthcare, socioeconomic level) were considered, Black patients continued to have increased risk of exacerbation and worse outcomes (Ejike et al., 2020). Multiple studies have indicated that education and income have a protective effect on lung health, but White persons have an even stronger protective effect from those factors than Black and Hispanic persons, creating additional disparities. Sexual and gender minority persons have higher odds for multiple chronic conditions, cancer, and poor quality of life and are more apt to have disabilities than cisgender males and females (cisgender is a term used to describe persons whose gender identity and gender expression are aligned with their assigned sex listed on their birth certificate) (Cacerese, Jackman, et al., 2020; Connelly et al., 2019). Gender and sexual minority persons also smoke more than their heterosexual and cisgender counterparts. While large-scale studies are not available, these factors place sexual and gender minority persons at risk for emphysema.

GLOBAL HEALTH CONSIDERATIONS

Research from Latin America, specifically, and likely around the globe, has shown higher prevalence of emphysema than the United States. Because more than 1.2 billion humans smoke cigarettes, prevalence is climbing. Results from pooled data suggest that the global prevalence of COPD is approximately 10% in adults over age 40 years; chronic bronchitis prevalence alone is 6%, and emphysema alone is 2% in adults.

☀ ASSESSMENT

HISTORY. Establish a history of dyspnea, determining if it has increased over time. Ask if the dyspnea is extreme during exertion and present even during rest. Ask if wheezing occurs during exertion. Determine if the patient has experienced anorexia, weight loss, and weakness. Ask if the patient has had a cough (often described as a "smoker's cough") and, if so, for how long. Determine if there are signs of oxygen deficiency; ask significant others if the patient has been restless or confused or has experienced changes in mental status. Ask if the patient lives or works in a highly polluted area. Establish cigarette smoking habits, including how long, how many, and whether they are unfiltered. Elicit a history of family pulmonary disease or frequent childhood pulmonary infections.

PHYSICAL EXAMINATION. The chief symptom is **dyspnea with exertion and rest**. Patients experience a limitation of expiratory air flow, meaning that it takes patients longer to exhale than inhale. Inspect the patient for a decreased muscle mass and increased anteroposterior diameter (also known as barrel chest). Observe respirations for the use of accessory muscles, such as the sternocleidomastoid and pectoral muscles, as well as pursed-lip breathing during expiration. Assess the patient's respirations for rate, rhythm, and quality. Inspect the patient for neck vein distention or liver congestion. Note signs of oxygen deficiency, such as restlessness, changes in mental status, confusion, and tachycardia.

A cough may be present during the later stages of the disease; the small amount of sputum it produces is usually mucoid. Upon palpation, note decreased tactile fremitus. Percussion may elicit a diffusely hyperresonant sound. Auscultate for decreased or absent breath sounds, distant heart sounds, wheezes, and possibly crackles. Examine the patient for peripheral cyanosis or clubbing of the fingers.

PSYCHOSOCIAL. Patients with emphysema may be anxious or restless depending on the degree of dyspnea and hypoxemia they are experiencing. Emphysema may necessitate role or occupational changes, or even retirement, and that could lead to multiple stresses and even depression. Emphysema is a risk factor for suicide, and statements about suicide should be taken seriously. Assess the patient's and family's emotional, financial, and social concerns to help support the best strategies to manage a chronic disease.

Diagnostic Highlights

Test	Normal Result	Abnormality With Condition	Explanation
AAT (alpha-1–antitrypsin) level	> 11 mmol/L	< 11 mmol/L	Genetic variants of AAT-level deficiency are associated with serum levels below the protective threshold of 11 mmol/L; the diagnosis of severe AAT deficiency is confirmed when the serum level falls below the protective threshold value of 3–7 mmol/L

Diagnostic Highlights (continued)

Test	Normal Result	Abnormality With Condition	Explanation
Forced vital capacity (FVC): Maximum volume of air that can be forcefully expired after a maximal lung inspiration	4.0 L	50% of the predicted value	Air trapping and obstruction with plugs decrease flow rates
Forced expiratory volume in 1 sec (FEV1): Volume of air expired in 1 sec from the beginning of the FVC maneuver	3.0 L or 84% of FVC1	25%–35% of the predicted value	Air trapping and airway obstruction with plugs decrease flow rates
Forced expiratory flow (FEF): Maximal flow rate attained during middle (25%–75%) of FVC maneuver	Varies by body size	25% of the predicted value	Predicts airway trapping and obstruction of smaller airways
Residual volume (RV): Volume of air remaining in lungs at end of a maximal expiration	1.2 L	Increased up to 400% of normal	Increased RV indicates air trapping and obstruction
Functional residual capacity (FRC): Volume of air remaining in lungs at end of a resting tidal volume	2.3 L	Increased up to 200% of normal	Increased FRC indicates air trapping

Other Tests: Chest x-ray, chest computed tomography, pulse oximetry, arterial blood gases, complete blood count, and electrocardiogram. Peak expiratory flow rates (PEFRs; maximal flow rate attained during the FVC maneuver; decreased from baseline during periods of obstruction) may be used at home daily for patients who require daily medications.

PRIMARY NURSING DIAGNOSIS

DIAGNOSIS. Impaired gas exchange related to destruction of alveolar walls as evidenced by dyspnea and/or wheezing

OUTCOMES. Respiratory status: Gas exchange; Respiratory status: Ventilation; Comfort status; Anxiety level

INTERVENTIONS. Airway management; Cough enhancement; Respiratory monitoring; Oxygen therapy; Laboratory data interpretation; Positioning; Smoking cessation assistance; Ventilation assistance

PLANNING AND IMPLEMENTATION

Collaborative

Viral or bacterial infections may lead to bronchospasm or increased mucous secretions. Acute exacerbations are accompanied by dyspnea, fatigue, and even respiratory failure. Low-flow oxygen therapy based on arterial blood gas results is often administered to treat hypoxemia. For the patient with increasing airway obstruction and plugging, noninvasive or invasive mechanical ventilation may be needed to maintain adequate airway and breathing, followed by pulmonary rehabilitation. Adequate hydration is also necessary to help liquefy secretions. A smoking cessation program is the most important collaborative intervention that is needed for long-term health and the most effective intervention for most patients. Refer the patient to a smoking cessation counselor.

Surgical options exist for patients with emphysema with the goal of restoring function and improving symptoms. Surgery is discussed carefully because it is linked with significant morbidity, and patients are chosen who will receive the greatest benefit. Types of procedures that are considered include bullectomy (removal of giant bullae), lung volume reduction surgery (resection of the most diseased portions of the lungs), and lung transplantation, which improves quality of life but does not prolong it.

Pharmacologic Highlights

Medication or Drug Class	Dosage	Description	Rationale
Bronchodilators: Anticholinergic agents	Varies by drug	Atropine sulfate, ipratropium bromide	Reversal of bronchoconstriction
Bronchodilators: Beta$_2$-adrenergic agents	Varies by drug	Inhaled beta$_2$-adrenergic agonists by metered-dose inhaler (MDI) such as albuterol, metaproterenol, or terbutaline	Reversal of bronchoconstriction
Tiotropium	Two oral inhalations of an 18-mcg capsule daily with inhaler	Quaternary ammonium compound; long-acting muscarinic agent with anticholinergic and antimuscarinic effects; has an inhibitory effect on M$_3$ receptors in airway smooth muscle	Long-lasting bronchodilation (24 hr)
Systemic corticosteroids (oral and inhaled)	Varies by drug	Methylprednisolone IV; prednisone PO; may also add inhaled fluticasone, inhaled budesonide	Decrease inflammatory response and improve airflow in some patients for a few days during acute exacerbations; should only be added if patient is also on a long-acting bronchodilator

Other Drugs: Bronchodilators, which are used for prevention and maintenance therapy, can be administered as aerosols or oral medications. Generally, inhaled anticholinergic agents are the first-line therapy for emphysema, with the addition of beta-adrenergic agonists added in a stepwise fashion. Antibiotics are ordered if a secondary infection develops. As a preventive measure, influenza and pneumonia vaccines are administered.

Independent

Smoking cessation is the most effective therapy for patients. The healthcare team needs to coordinate the approach to smoking cessation, often introduced by the physician but implemented by the nurse, who may develop the smoking cessation plan. Experts suggest multiple interventions and multiple settings such as group programs and one-to-one counseling and teaching sessions. When the patient is acutely ill, maintaining a patent airway is a priority. Use a humidifier at night to help the patient mobilize secretions in the morning. Encourage the patient to use controlled coughing to clear secretions that might have collected in the lungs during sleep. Instruct the patient to sit at the bedside or in a comfortable chair, hug a pillow, bend the head downward a little, take several deep breaths, and cough strongly.

Place patients who are experiencing dyspnea in a high Fowler position to improve lung expansion. Placing pillows on the overhead table and having the patient lean over in the orthopneic position may also be helpful. Teach the patient pursed-lip and diaphragmatic breathing. To avoid infection, screen visitors for contagious diseases and instruct the patient to avoid crowds. Conserve the patient's energy in every possible way. Plan activities to allow for rest periods, eliminating nonessential procedures until the patient is stronger. It may be necessary to assist with the activities of daily living and to anticipate the patient's needs by having supplies within easy reach. Refer the patient to a pulmonary rehabilitation program if one is available in the community. Patient education is vital to long-term management. Teach the patient about the disease and its implications for lifestyle changes, such as avoidance of cigarette smoke and other irritants, activity alterations, and any necessary occupational changes. Provide information to the patient and family about medications and equipment.

Evidence-Based Practice and Health Policy

Lim, E., Sousa, I., Shah, P., Diggle, P., & Goldstraw, P. (2020). Lung volume reduction surgery: Reinterpreted with longitudinal data analyses methodology. *Annals of Thoracic Surgery, 109*, 1496–1502.

- The authors reevaluated the National Emphysema Treatment Trial (NETT) in order to report longer-term outcomes of lung volume reduction surgery (LVRS). The authors analyzed trial data released by the U.S. National Heart, Lung, and Blood Institute to ascertain the difference in lung function variables between patients receiving LVRS and patients receiving medical care out to 5 years.
- For the outcome of forced expiratory volume in 1 second in patients randomized to LVRS, there was an immediate improvement compared with medical therapy, with an estimated decline to baseline approximately 5 years after randomization. Five years after surgery, physiological function improved in the areas of shortness of breath, well-being, and exercise performance in the surgical group. LVRS improved lung function and exercise workload that returned to baseline within a 5-year period. Although LVRS may not improve survival, the procedure improved dyspnea as far out as 5 years after surgery.

DOCUMENTATION GUIDELINES

- Rate, quality, and depth of respirations; vital signs
- Physical findings: Dyspnea, cyanosis, decreased muscle mass, cough, increased anteroposterior chest diameter, and use of accessory muscles during respiration; characteristics of sputum
- Activity tolerance, ability to perform self-care
- Signs and symptoms of infection; response to pharmacologic therapy, response to oxygen therapy

DISCHARGE AND HOME HEALTHCARE GUIDELINES

MEDICATION AND OXYGEN. Be sure the patient and family understand any medication prescribed, including dosage, route, action, and side effects. Arrange for return demonstrations of equipment used by the patient and family. If the patient requires home oxygen therapy, refer the patient to the appropriate rental service and explain the hazards of combustion and increasing the flow rate without consultation from the primary healthcare provider.

PREVENTION. Instruct the patient to report any signs and symptoms of infection to the primary healthcare provider. Explain necessary dietary adjustments to the patient and family. Recommend eating small, frequent meals, including high-protein, high-density foods. Recommend smoking cessation programs and provide materials to make follow-up easy.

REST AND NUTRITION. Encourage the patient to plan rest periods around their activities, conserving as much energy as possible.

Encephalitis

DRG Category: 98
Mean LOS: 7.1 days
Description: MEDICAL: Non-Bacterial Infections of Nervous System Except Viral Meningitis With Complication or Comorbidity

Encephalitis, or inflammation of the brain, usually occurs when the cerebral hemispheres, brainstem, or cerebellum is infected by a microorganism. Approximately 2,000 cases of encephalitis are reported each year in the United States, but this is probably only a fraction of the cases. Most forms have mortality rates of less than 10%, with the exception of eastern equine encephalitis (EEE), for which mortality is as high as 50%. Determining the true incidence is impossible because reporting policies are neither standardized nor rigorously enforced.

When the virus invades the brain, it enters neural cells, which leads to interrupted function of the cells, congestion, hemorrhage, and an inflammatory response. When the brain becomes inflamed, lymphocytes infiltrate brain tissue and the meninges of the brain. Cerebral edema results, and ultimately, brain cells can degenerate, leading to widespread nerve cell destruction.

Encephalitis has two forms: primary and postinfectious (or para-infectious). The primary form of the disease occurs when a virus invades and replicates within the brain. Postinfectious encephalitis describes brain inflammation that develops in combination with other viral illnesses or following the administration of vaccines such as measles, mumps, and rubella. In that case, encephalitis occurs because of a hypersensitivity reaction that leads to demyelination of nerves. Complications from encephalitis can be short term or lifelong. Bronchial pneumonia and respiratory tract infections may complicate the course of encephalitis. Patients may go into a coma and experience all the complications of immobility, such as contractures and pressure ulcers. Other complications include epilepsy, parkinsonism, behavioral and personality changes, syndrome of inappropriate antidiuretic hormone secretion, and mental retardation. A comatose state may last for days, weeks, or months after the acute infectious state.

CAUSES

Most cases of encephalitis are related to viruses, and the most common cause is herpes simplex virus-1 (HSV-1) in adults. HSV-2 is more common in neonates and may be transmitted from a mother infected with genital herpes during childbirth. Herpes encephalitis has a range of clinical presentations and can be transmitted during birth, through the blood, or by neuronal transmission. Neuronal transmission often occurs from the peripheral neuron in retrograde fashion to the brain. Arboviruses are also common causes of encephalitis; although most people bitten by arbovirus-infected insects do not develop the disease, approximately 10% have overt symptoms. Transmission of arboviruses requires an insect vector and usually occurs in the Northern Hemisphere between June and October. The two most common arboviruses cause La Crosse encephalitis and St. Louis encephalitis. In the United States, most cases of nonepidemic encephalitis are caused by the La Crosse virus, are most common in rural areas of the Midwest, and affect children. Epidemics of both St. Louis encephalitis (found mostly in the East and Midwest) and western equine encephalitis (WEE; found across North America) have contributed a large number of the total cases since 1955. Many sources cite the St. Louis encephalitis virus as the most common form in this country, although many forms of the disease exist.

Although relatively uncommon, the deadliest arbovirus is EEE, which is mostly encountered in the New England region. Other viruses include WEE (most common in rural communities west of the Mississippi River), Powassan (POW) virus, the only arbovirus known to be transmitted by ticks, Epstein-Barr virus, and cytomegalovirus. Encephalitis has also been associated with many other diseases, including Creutzfeldt-Jakob disease, HSV (specifically HSV-1), kuru, malaria, mononucleosis, rabies, trichinosis, and typhus.

GENETIC CONSIDERATIONS

Heritable immune responses could be protective or increase susceptibility. Susceptibility to herpes simplex encephalitis is linked to mutations in *TLR3* and *UNC93B1*.

SEX AND LIFE SPAN CONSIDERATIONS

Encephalitis may occur at any age. However, people at the extremes of age (the very old and the very young) are most at risk as are people with weak immune systems. Encephalitis caused by HSV-1 is most common in children and young adults. La Crosse encephalitis is most common in children from age 5 to 10 years. EEE commonly occurs in children younger than age 10 years and in older adults, whereas WEE occurs in infants under a year old and in older adults. St. Louis encephalitis is seen most often in adults older than age 35 years.

HEALTH DISPARITIES AND SEXUAL/GENDER MINORITY HEALTH

Ethnicity and race have no known effect on the risk for encephalitis. People who have infections with HIV are immunosuppressed and are more at risk for encephalitis than people with normal immune systems.

GLOBAL HEALTH CONSIDERATIONS

The Japanese virus encephalitis is the most common cause of encephalitis worldwide outside the United States. It is a common infection in Japan, China, Southeast Asia, and India.

ASSESSMENT

HISTORY. Obtain a history of recent illnesses, which may include an upper respiratory infection or a minor systemic illness that caused headache, muscle ache, malaise, sore throat, and runny nose. Note if the patient has other sites of infection, such as a recent skull fracture or head injury, middle ear infection, or sinus infection. Ask if the patient has had a recent immunization, exposure to mumps or HSV, animal bites, recent travel, or exposure to epidemic outbreaks or mononucleosis. Ask if a child has been playing in a rural area where exposure to ticks or mosquitoes was possible.

Encephalitis typically has an abrupt onset. The patient, parents, or family may describe altered respiratory patterns, fever, headache, nuchal (neck) rigidity, and vomiting. Neurological symptoms generally follow 24 to 48 hours after the initial onset; often, a seizure is the initial presenting symptom. The family may describe personality changes and sensitivity to light. The patient and family may describe other symptoms such as facial palsies, difficulty speaking, and decreased movement and sensation of the extremities.

PHYSICAL EXAMINATION. The most common symptoms are **decreased level of consciousness, personality changes, seizure activity, neck stiffness**, and **photophobia**. The patient appears acutely ill with an altered mental status that may range from mild confusion to delirium and coma, or they may have generalized or focal seizures. The patient may have tremors, cranial nerve palsies, and absent superficial or exaggerated deep tendon reflexes. There may be a decrease in sensation, along with weakness and lethargy or even flaccid paralysis of the extremities. The patient may have no sense of taste or smell and may have difficulty speaking and swallowing. Heart and respiratory rates may be rapid. The patient's skin is often warm because of fever. Some patients have headache and others backache.

PSYCHOSOCIAL. Encephalitis can be life threatening and lead to permanent disability; therefore, determine the patient's and family's ability to cope with sudden illness, anxiety, and stress as well as disability. If the patient is a child, the parents may be excessively anxious. Analyze the family structure, the number of children, the financial resources, and the role of parental support systems to determine the extent of the problem.

Diagnostic Highlights

Test	Normal Result	Abnormality With Condition	Explanation
Lumbar puncture and cerebrospinal fluid (CSF) analysis	Pressure: 70–180 mm H$_2$O Glucose: 45–80 mg/dL Protein: 15–45 mg/mL	Slight to moderate increase in proteins and white blood cells in the CSF; normal glucose level; CSF pressure is often normal or slightly increased; if the patient has HSV, the CSF may contain red blood cells	Encephalitis is usually caused by viral rather than bacterial infections, hence the normal CSF glucose
Polymerase chain reaction (PCR)	Negative for HSV	Positive for HSV	Produces relatively large numbers of copies of DNA from a source to determine if HSV is present in the sample; negative PCR does not completely rule out HSV encephalitis

Other Tests: Electroencephalogram, computed tomography scan, magnetic resonance imaging, CSF cultures, and radionuclide scans; complete blood count, platelet count, blood urea nitrogen and creatinine, liver function tests

PRIMARY NURSING DIAGNOSIS

DIAGNOSIS. Risk for infection as evidenced by decreased consciousness, neck stiffness, and/or photophobia

OUTCOMES. Risk control: Infectious process; Infection severity; Risk detection; Cognition

INTERVENTIONS. Infection protection; Medication administration; Temperature regulation; Teaching: Disease process

PLANNING AND IMPLEMENTATION

Collaborative

To maintain a patent airway, many patients require endotracheal intubation, oxygen therapy, and mechanical ventilation if gas exchange is impaired. One of the most important roles of the nurse and physician is ongoing neurological assessment. Using serial assessments, the healthcare team documents changes in the patient's condition and initiates proper care immediately. Pupil size and reaction, level of consciousness, strength and motion of the extremities, and the patient's response to noxious stimuli are all essential for patient assessment and management. Intracranial pressure monitoring may be necessary to manage severe encephalitis. Collect all laboratory samples prior to the start of antiviral agents. Management of fever, pain, and complications such as hypotension, shock, hypoxemia, and seizures is important for recovery.

Pharmacologic Highlights

Medication or Drug Class	Dosage	Description	Rationale
Antiviral agents	Adults: Acyclovir 10 mg/kg q 8 hr; infuse IV over at least 1 hr for 7–10 days; children: 250 mg/m² q 8 hr; infuse IV over at least 1 hr for 7–10 days; vidarabine (ARA-A) 15 mg/kg per day infused IV over 12 hr	Interferes with DNA synthesis and viral	Combat herpes simplex encephalitis

Other Drugs: Foscarnet, an antiviral, may be considered for HIV-positive patients. Patients may receive corticosteroids such as dexamethasone or diuretics such as furosemide to manage brain inflammation, but little data support their use in this situation.

Independent

The maintenance of airway, breathing, and circulation is the foremost concern for the patient with encephalitis. If the patient is unable to clear secretions or maintain a patent airway as the disease progresses, notify the physician immediately and prepare for endotracheal intubation. The family is likely to be anxious and need a great deal of support should intubation and mechanical ventilation be necessary. Once the airway is in place, maintaining an open airway with suctioning as needed is a primary nursing responsibility.

Always take into account patient safety and weigh it against the possibility of the patient's further increase in intracranial pressure. Manage fever and pain to reduce the effects of increased intracranial pressure. Alterations can occur in thought processes when intracranial pressure begins to increase and the level of consciousness begins to decrease. Elevate the head of the bed, keep the neck in appropriate alignment, and perform serial neurological assessments, including pupillary responses. Reorient the patient to time, place, and person as needed. Keep familiar objects or pictures around the patient. Implement measures to limit the effects of immobility, such as skin care, range-of-motion exercises, and a turning and positioning schedule. Note the effect of position changes on intracranial pressure and space activities as necessary.

The patient and significant others need assistance in learning about the disease process and treatments. The patient's behavioral and communication changes are often the most difficult to face and understand. Allow visitation of significant others. Establish alternative means of communication if the patient is unable to maintain verbal contact (e.g., the patient who needs intubation).

Evidence-Based Practice and Health Policy

McKnight, C., Kelly, A., Petrou, M., Nidecker, A., Lorincz, M., Altaee, D., Gebarski, S., & Foerster, B. (2017). A simplified approach to encephalitis and its mimics: Key clinical decision points in the setting of specific imaging abnormalities. *Academic Radiology*, *24*, 667–676.

• The authors aimed to develop a systematic approach that considers both the clinical manifestations and the imaging findings of infectious encephalitis and the diseases it resembles. They sought to determine if the approach can contribute to more accurate and timely diagnosis. They examined their hospital imaging database to generate a list of adult and pediatric patients who had imaging to evaluate possible cases of encephalitis. They combined clinical and imaging findings to generate useful flowcharts, and key imaging features were placed in the context of the flowcharts.

• Four flowcharts based on the primary anatomic site of imaging were created and used to demonstrate similarities and key differences. The authors proposed that the flowcharts could enable clinicians and radiologists to differentiate encephalitis from diseases that mimic the disease, thereby improving patient care.

DOCUMENTATION GUIDELINES

• Physical responses: Adequacy of airway, breathing, circulation; serial neurological assessments; signs of increased pressure; vital signs; seizures
• Ability to respond to environment, need for restraints, level of orientation, response to family

DISCHARGE AND HOME HEALTHCARE GUIDELINES

Although most patients recover fully before being discharged from the hospital, some have lifelong deficits following encephalitis. If the patient needs supportive care, teach the family, significant others, and caregivers how to plan and administer hygiene, nutrition, and medications. If arrangements need to be made for a nursing home or long-term facility, work with the family and social service to arrange for a careful transition.

Teach the patient and family about the disease process and signs of recurrence. Make sure the patient and family know when the follow-up visit with the healthcare provider is scheduled. Teach the patient and family about the route, dosage, mechanism of action, and side effects of all medications. Provide written information so the patient and family have a permanent record of the communication.

Endometriosis

DRG Category:	742
Mean LOS:	3.8 days
Description:	SURGICAL: Uterine and Adnexa Procedures for Non-Malignancy With Complication or Comorbidity or Major Complication or Comorbidity
DRG Category:	761
Mean LOS:	2.2 days
Description:	MEDICAL: Menstrual and Other Female Reproductive System Disorders Without Complication or Comorbidity or Major Complication or Comorbidity

Endometriosis is a hormonal and immune system disease characterized by a benign growth of endometrial tissue that occurs atypically outside of the uterine cavity. Although endometriosis can grow anywhere in the body, it is typically found in the ovaries, fallopian tubes, uterosacral ligaments, retrovaginal septum, sigmoid colon, round ligaments, and pelvic peritoneum. During the reproductive years, the atypical endometrial tissue responds the same to hormonal stimulation as does the tissue within the uterus. Thus, the tissue grows during the proliferative and secretory phase of the woman's menstrual cycle and bleeds during or immediately after it. This bleeding drains into the peritoneal cavity and causes an inflammatory process with subsequent fibrosis and adhesions. Such scarring may lead to blockage or distortion of any of the surrounding organs.

The primary complication of endometriosis is infertility, which results from adhesions and scarring that are caused by bleeding from the atypical endometrial tissue. These adhesions may occur around the uterus and fix it into a retroverted position. They may also block the fallopian tubes or the fimbriated ends, preventing the ovum from being carried into the uterus. Endometriosis can also lead to spontaneous abortion and anemia.

CAUSES

The cause of endometriosis is not known. The most predominant theory is the retrograde menstruation theory, which suggests that endometriosis results from a backflow of endometrial tissue from the uterus into the pelvic cavity during menstruation. This flow starts through the fallopian tubes and passes into the peritoneal cavity, where it implants to form atypical (ectopic) sites of endometrial tissue. Other theories of endometrial etiology posit that cells lining the peritoneum undergo metaplastic transformation and give rise to the endometrial lesions; tissue spreads via the vascular and lymphatic systems; and also, that dormant, immature cells spread during the embryonic period and that metaplasia then occurs in adulthood. Endometriosis may also have an autoimmune and genetic component. Studies have found immunoglobulins in the peritoneal fluid of infertile patients with endometriosis, and an altered immune response to the displaced endometrial tissue may occur. Risk factors include family history, early age of menarche, short menstrual cycles less than 27 days, long duration of menstrual flow of greater than 7 days, heavy bleeding during menses, delayed childbearing, uterine or fallopian tube defects, and hypoxemia and/or anemia.

GENETIC CONSIDERATIONS

Endometriosis has both genetic and environmental components, with an estimated heritability of 50%. Several genes have been implicated to confer risk, with the most robust being *WNT4* (Wnt family member 4) and *VEZT* (vezatin, adherens junctions transmembrane protein).

SEX AND LIFE SPAN CONSIDERATIONS

Endometriosis is estimated to occur in 7% to 10% of women of reproductive age in the United States. It can occur at any age after puberty, although it is most commonly found in women ages 30 to 40 years. For patients operated on for the first time for endometriosis, age at menarche is not associated with the disease phenotype. There is a higher incidence of endometriosis in persons who bear children later in their lives. The course of the disease is individual and may worsen with each repeated cycle, or patients may remain asymptomatic throughout the reproductive years. Endometriosis is an estrogen-based disease; therefore, the symptoms and progression of the disease stop after menopause.

HEALTH DISPARITIES AND SEXUAL/GENDER MINORITY HEALTH

Most of the research on endometriosis has been focused on White women, but experts suggest that all women are likely at similar risk for endometriosis (Bougie et al., 2019). Evidence exists that women without private insurance and Black, Hispanic, and Native American women are less likely to receive laparoscopy and more likely to be treated in the emergency department rather than by obstetricians and gynecologists. These issues lead to health disparities and inequities of care. Transgender is a term used to describe persons whose gender identity is different from their sex assigned at birth. Approximately 1% of the U.S. population identify themselves as transgender. Gender-affirming hormone therapy is the use of hormone therapy for gender transition or gender affirmation and can be masculinizing or feminizing. Evaluation for endometriosis is underutilized by transgender transmasculine persons. Testosterone treatment can resolve symptoms, but additional treatment for endometriosis may be needed for transmasculine persons (Shim et al., 2020).

GLOBAL HEALTH CONSIDERATIONS

Prevalence statistics in the United States reflect those in other developed countries. No data are available for most developing countries.

ASSESSMENT

HISTORY. Elicit a complete history of the patient's menstrual, obstetric, sexual, and contraceptive practices. Endometriosis is difficult to diagnose because some of its symptoms are also manifestations of other pelvic conditions, such as pelvic inflammation, ovarian cysts, and ovarian cancers. A thorough description of the patient's symptoms becomes important, therefore, in the early diagnosis of the condition. Symptoms of endometriosis vary with the location of the ectopic tissue. Some patients may even be asymptomatic during the entire course of the disease. The classic triad of symptoms of endometriosis are dysmenorrhea, dyspareunia (painful sexual intercourse), and infertility.

The symptoms may also change over time. The major symptom is dysmenorrhea (pain associated with menses) that is different from the normal uterine cramping during the patient's menstrual cycle. This cramping has been referred to as a deep-seated aching, pressing, or grinding in the lower abdomen, vagina, posterior pelvis, and/or back. It usually occurs 1 to 2 days before the onset of the menstrual cycle and lasts 2 to 3 days. Other possible symptoms are pain during a bowel movement around the time of menstruation, a heaviness noted in the pelvic region, menorrhagia, nausea, diarrhea, and pain during sexual intercourse (dyspareunia) or exercise. Some patients may have no symptoms at all, and endometriosis is diagnosed during infertility testing.

PHYSICAL EXAMINATION. Common symptoms include **pain with menstruation**, **abdominal/pelvic tenderness and aching**, and **dyspareunia**. During a pelvic examination, the cervix may be laterally displaced to the left or right of the midline. Palpation of the abdomen may uncover nodules in the uterosacral ligament, with tenderness in the posterior fornix and restricted movement of the uterus. Palpation may also identify ovarian enlargement that was caused by the presence of ovarian cysts. Speculum examination may reveal bluish nodules on the cervix or posterior wall of the vagina.

During acute flare-ups of the disease, an internal pelvic examination may cause the patient excruciating suprapubic and abdominal pain. The acute disease may be difficult to distinguish from appendicitis or other conditions that lead to an "acute abdomen." The patient may have a rigid abdomen, abdominal guarding, and a low-grade fever.

PSYCHOSOCIAL. Endometriosis is a chronic, long-term condition, with symptoms that occur every month for 2 to 3 days until menopause. Severe discomfort, interferences with activities of daily living or leisure activities, impaired sexual function, and the disappointments of infertility can contribute to depression in patients with this chronic disease. Inquire about the level of partner support.

Diagnostic Highlights

General Comments: Endometriosis is often first diagnosed when the person seeks help for infertility.

Test	Normal Result	Abnormality With Condition	Explanation
Laparoscopy	No ectopic tissue is visualized	Ectopic tissue is visualized	Presence of ectopic tissue confirms the diagnosis; laparoscopy is the gold standard for diagnosis or endometriosis
Transvaginal ultrasound (or abdominal pelvic ultrasound if the patient is a teenager or not sexually active)	No ectopic tissue is visualized	Ovarian or rectal endometrioma	Can diagnose or exclude ovarian or rectal endometriomas
Biopsy	N/A	Identifies the tissue as benign endometrial tissue	Rules out malignancy, confirming the diagnosis

PRIMARY NURSING DIAGNOSIS

DIAGNOSIS. Chronic pain related to internal bleeding, swelling, and inflammation during the menstrual cycle as evidenced by self-reports of pain, self-reports of abdominal cramping, and/or protective behavior

OUTCOMES. Comfort status; Pain control; Pain level; Symptom severity; Symptom control; Knowledge: Pain management; Knowledge: Medication; Knowledge: Disease process

INTERVENTIONS. Pain management: Chronic; Analgesic administration; Teaching: Prescribed medication; Teaching: Disease process

PLANNING AND IMPLEMENTATION

Collaborative

MEDICAL. Patients are prescribed birth control or gonadotropin-releasing hormone antagonists because suppressing ovulation may decrease the pain. Patients who are nearing menopause are usually treated prophylactically until they enter menopause. If the patient is in no distress and is approaching menopause, no treatment will be necessary except observing the progression of the disease. By contrast, a younger patient who wishes to become pregnant may be treated more aggressively.

Some patients may be instructed to get pregnant as quickly as possible if they wish to have children. Pregnancy and lactation suppress menstruation and result in shrinkage of the endometrial tissue implants. Relief from symptoms has been noted to persist years after the pregnancy.

SURGICAL. Surgery is performed conservatively by laparoscopy or laparotomy using laser via the laparoscope. The goal is to remove as much of the ectopic endometrial tissue as possible and retain the patient's reproductive ability. In older patients with severe symptoms who have completed childbearing, or as a last resort in childbearing-aged patients, a hysterectomy may be the surgery of choice with or without a bilateral salpingo-oophorectomy. The decision whether to have medical treatment or surgery depends on symptoms, medical history, and the patient's desire to preserve reproductive potential. Patients who opt for medical treatment have a higher rate of recurrent pain (53%) than patients who opt for surgery (44%).

Pharmacologic Highlights

Medication or Drug Class	Dosage	Description	Rationale
Oral contraceptives with low-dose estrogens, progestins (medroxyprogesterone acetate)	1 tab per day or 400 mg IM per month (maintenance)	Hormonal therapy	Halts the spread and shrinks the endometrial implant, suppresses ovulation, prevents dysmenorrhea
Danazol (Danocrine)	200–800 mg per day in two divided doses for 3–9 mo	Gonadotropin inhibitor; synthetic androgenic steroid similar to testosterone	Suppresses follicle-stimulating hormone (FSH) and luteinizing hormone (LH), suppressing ovulation, resulting in atrophy of the endometrial tissue
Nafarelin (Synarel) Leuprolide (Lupron) Goserelin (Zoladex)	Metered nasal spray bid 3.75 mg IM daily/ monthly (or 11.25 mg q 3 mo) Subcutaneous implant	Gonadotropin (Gn)–releasing hormone agonist	Restricts the secretion of Gn hormones and the production of FSH, LH, and estrogen; produces a "pseudomenopause"

(highlight box continues on page 412)

Pharmacologic Highlights (continued)

Medication or Drug Class	Dosage	Description	Rationale
LNG-IUS (Mirena intrauterine device [IUD])	IUD inserted for 6 mo	Releases levonorgestrel	Reduces pain, suppresses ovulation, shrinks endometrial implant
Acetaminophen, various narcotics	Varies by drug	Over-the-counter and prescription pain-relieving drugs	Relieve discomfort but do not affect the progress of the disease; NSAIDs are not contraindicated but they may increase bleeding

Independent

Unless a total hysterectomy is done, the patient needs to understand that all other treatments offer relief and not cure. Careful discussions about the patient's desire to preserve or not to preserve their reproductive potential are important with respect to treatment decisions. The nurse needs excellent communication skills to teach, inform, and support the patient. Care focuses on strategies to relieve pain and discomfort, to support the patient during a stressful time, and to provide patient education. The pain of endometriosis can be mild or severe. Unless the patient has other underlying diseases, the patient will generally be managed on an outpatient basis until surgical intervention is needed. To relieve pain, instruct the patient that over-the-counter analgesics such as acetaminophen are preferable to NSAIDs and aspirin because of the latter's tendency to increase bleeding. Some patients obtain relief from cramping by lying on the side with the legs bent, taking warm baths, or using a heating device on the lower abdomen. Make sure the patient uses heating devices on a low setting to prevent burns. Caution the patient with acute abdominal pain from unknown causes not to use a heating pad because of the risk of a perforated appendix, ectopic pregnancy, and hemorrhagic ovarian cysts.

Assess the patient's cultural and ethnic influences, which will play a part in the patient's understanding and subsequent coping with endometriosis. Be emotionally supportive. Provide interested couples with information on the Endometriosis Association, Resolve (a support, education, and research group for infertile couples), and newer techniques for infertility management. Encourage the couple to talk openly about the disease and its effects on their sexual compatibility and urge the patient to tell their partner about any discomfort during sexual intercourse to minimize misunderstandings. Encourage the couple to try different positions during sexual intercourse to find those most comfortable for the patient.

Evidence-Based Practice and Health Policy

Rea, T., Giampaolino, P., Simeone, S., Pucciarelli, G., Alvaro, R., & Guillari, A. (2020). Living with endometriosis: A phenomenological study. *International Journal of Qualitative Studies on Health and Well-being, 15.* https://doi.org/10.1080/17482631.2020.1822621

• The purpose of this study was to understand the lived experiences of women with endometriosis. The investigators enrolled 25 women after they indicated their interest in participation to their healthcare providers. The investigators adopted Cohen's phenomenology as the method for the study. Participants were interviewed in their homes and were asked one question: Could you kindly describe your experience living with endometriosis?
• The data analysis identified four main themes: delay in diagnosis, worsening of one's life, disastrous intimate life with one's partner, uncertainty about being able to have one's own children. Delay of diagnosis and treatment of endometriosis has physical and psychosocial consequences regarding women's quality of life. Understanding how it affects women can lead to targeted intervention programs.

DOCUMENTATION GUIDELINES

- Physical symptoms: Pain, cramping, abdominal guarding, degree of menstrual flow
- Response to interventions for relief of pain and treatment modalities
- Response of the partner to the disease process, possible changes in sexual practices, possibility of infertility
- Ability to carry out activities of daily living and other desired activities

DISCHARGE AND HOME HEALTHCARE GUIDELINES

MEDICATIONS. Ensure that the patient understands the dosage, route, action, and side effects before going home.

FOLLOW-UP. Encourage the patient to be alert to their emotions, behavior, physical symptoms, diet, rest, and exercise. Encourage the patient to maintain open communication with their significant other and family to discuss concerns the patient may have about the disease process.

Epididymitis

DRG Category:	728
Mean LOS:	3.6 days
Description:	MEDICAL: Inflammation of the Male Reproductive System Without Major Complication or Comorbidity

Epididymitis is an infection or inflammation of the epididymis—a coiled duct that is responsible for nutrition and maturation of the sperm. The epididymis carries sperm from the testicle to the urethra. Epididymitis, the most common intrascrotal infection, is usually unilateral. Epididymitis needs to be differentiated from testicular torsion (when the spermatic cord twists and cuts off blood supply to the testicle), tumor, and trauma. If it is left untreated, epididymitis may lead to orchitis, an infection of the testicles, which may lead to sterility. The incidence of epididymitis is less than 1 in 1,000 males each year. Complications include infertility, duct obstruction, erectile dysfunction, and sepsis.

CAUSES

Infection that results in epididymitis is usually caused by prostate obstruction, a sexually transmitted infection (STI), or another form of infection. STIs leading to epididymitis include infection by *Neisseria gonorrheae, Chlamydia trachomatis,* and syphilis. STIs lead to an ascending infection, are the most common cause of epididymitis, and can lead to both an acute reduction in sperm and a chronic reduction leading to infertility. Epididymitis may be a complication of prostatitis or urethritis, or it may be associated with chronic urinary infection caused by *Escherichia coli,* pseudomonas, or coliform pathogens. Strain or pressure during voiding may force urine that is harboring pathogens from the urethra or prostate through the vas deferens to the epididymis, leading to inflammation and infection.

Urological abnormalities due to structural alterations are common in children, who may have an ectopic ureter, ectopic vas deferens, prostatic utricle, urethral duplication, posterior urethral valves, urethrorectal fistula, detrusor sphincter dyssynergia, or vesicoureteral reflux. Common structural abnormalities in men older than age 40 years include bladder outlet obstruction or urethral stricture.

GENETIC CONSIDERATIONS

Heritable immune responses could be protective or increase susceptibility.

SEX AND LIFE SPAN CONSIDERATIONS

Epididymitis commonly occurs in men ages 18 to 50 years and is the fifth most common urological diagnosis in that age group. It rarely occurs in those who have not reached puberty. The average age of people diagnosed with chronic epididymitis is 49 years. In men under age 35 years, the most common cause is an STI. Generally, epididymitis in men over age 35 years is from other bacterial causes or from obstruction.

HEALTH DISPARITIES AND SEXUAL/GENDER MINORITY HEALTH

While ethnicity and race have no known effect on the risk for epididymitis, several factors are important for sexual and gender minority health. Transgender is a term used to describe persons whose gender identity is different from their sex assigned at birth. Approximately 1% of the U.S. population identify themselves as transgender. Sexual and gender minority persons have higher odds for multiple chronic conditions than cisgender males and females (cisgender is a term used to describe persons whose gender identity and gender expression are aligned with their assigned sex listed on their birth certificate). Transgender women may engage in "tucking," a practice that involves displacing the testes upward and positioning and affixing the penis and scrotal sac between the legs and rearward. For many, this practice is gender-affirming but may result in traumatic or mechanical injury and may lead to epididymitis and other infections. The Centers for Disease Control and Prevention report that sexually active gay, bisexual, and other men who have sex with men are at greater risk for STIs than other men, and thereby also have a higher risk for epididymitis than other men.

GLOBAL HEALTH CONSIDERATIONS

While no data are available, epididymitis occurs in men around the world.

ASSESSMENT

HISTORY. Establish a history of sudden scrotal pain, redness, swelling, and extreme scrotal and groin tenderness. In 90% of the cases, the symptoms are unilateral. Determine if the patient has experienced fever, chills, or malaise. Ask if the patient has experienced nausea and vomiting. Elicit a history of prostatitis, urethritis, or chronic urinary infections. Determine if the patient has experienced urethral discharge prior to the onset of symptoms. Ask if the patient has been diagnosed with tuberculosis. Determine if the patient has undergone a prostatectomy or has had a traumatic injury to the genitalia. Take a sexual history to determine if the patient has had unprotected sex with a partner who may have had an STI.

PHYSICAL EXAMINATION. The most common symptom is **scrotal pain**. Inspect the patient's scrotum, noting any marked induration, edema, or redness. Evaluate if the patient has scrotal cellulitis. Gently palpate the scrotum for tenderness or pain. Observe any urethral discharge. Observe the patient's gait; patients with epididymitis often assume a characteristic waddle to protect the groin and scrotum.

PSYCHOSOCIAL. Patients may be concerned about their sexuality. They may be fearful of becoming sterile or impotent and anxious about whether they can continue to have sexual relationships. If the patient is transgender, making a decision about changing practices that help them affirm their gender is likely to be distressing. The patient may express anger or feelings of victimization if the condition was caused by an STI. Be familiar with your local and state requirements on reporting of STIs to the department of health, and alert the patient of your responsibilities.

Diagnostic Highlights

General Comments: Diagnosis is made based on visual symptoms and isolation of infective organisms.

Test	Normal Result	Abnormality With Condition	Explanation
Urinalysis	Clear, no pus	Pyuria; white blood cell count > 10,000 mm³	A urinary tract infection can contribute to epididymitis
Urine culture and sensitivity tests	< 10,000 bacteria/mL	> 10,000 bacteria/mL; pathogen is identified	A urinary tract infection can contribute to epididymitis
Cultures for STIs	Negative culture	Positive for STI	An STI can lead to epididymitis
Prehn sign	N/A	Pain is relieved when the scrotum is lifted onto the symphysis	Testicular torsion may be present if pain is not relieved when the scrotum is lifted onto the symphysis

Other Tests: An ultrasound to rule out testicular torsion, which presents with similar symptoms and is a medical emergency; white blood count; gram stain of urethral discharge; testing for HIV and syphilis

PRIMARY NURSING DIAGNOSIS

DIAGNOSIS. Acute pain related to swelling and inflammation of the scrotum as evidenced by self-reports of pain, facial grimacing, and/or protective behavior

OUTCOMES. Pain level; Pain control; Pain: Disruptive effects; Rest; Knowledge: Disease process

INTERVENTIONS. Analgesic administration; Medication administration; Heat/cold application; Positioning; Teaching: Individual; Teaching: Sexuality

PLANNING AND IMPLEMENTATION

Collaborative

The goal of treatment is to combat infection and reduce pain and swelling. This is usually accomplished through the use of pharmacologic agents. Sexual activity is not recommended during the treatment process, and all sexual partners need to be treated. If epididymitis is recurrent, an epididymectomy under local anesthesia or a vasectomy may be indicated, and this will result in sterility.

Pharmacologic Highlights

Medication or Drug Class	Dosage	Description	Rationale
Antibiotics	Depends on drug	Antibiotic used is determined by its ability to eliminate the pathogen	Appropriate antibiotic is needed to eliminate infective organism
Antipyretics	Depends on drug	Preparation to reduce fever	Fever often is present with epididymitis
Analgesics and anti-inflammatories	Depends on drug	Analgesic used depends on the severity of the pain	Decreases pain, discomfort, and inflammation

Independent

The most important interventions are pain control and emotional support. Lifting of the scrotum often relieves the pain in epididymitis; elevating the testicles on a towel eases tension on the spermatic cord and reduces pain. Ice packs to the scrotum also relieve pain, but a barrier between the scrotum and the ice pack is necessary to prevent frostbite or the ascension of the testes into the abdominal cavity. Encourage oral fluids of up to 2 to 3 L per day. As patients heal, they can resume walking but should wear an athletic supporter or other support.

Encourage patients to verbalize their fears and concerns. Answer questions nonjudgmentally. Point out that the patient's sexual partners are at risk if the condition was caused by an STI; urge the patient to notify all partners of the condition and follow the regulations of the state department of health with respect to reporting STIs. The underlying STI can be transmitted to female sexual partners. For patients who face the possibility of sterility, suggest professional counseling.

Evidence-Based Practice and Health Policy

Wenzel, M., Deuker, M., Welte, M., Hoeh, B., Preisser, F., Homrich, T., Kempf, V., Hogardt, M., Mandel, P., Karakiewicz, P., Chun, F., & Kluth, L. (2020). Catheter management and risk stratification of patients with inpatient treatment due to acute epididymitis. *Frontiers in Surgery*. Advance online publication. https://doi.org/10.3389/fsurg.2020.609661

- The authors evaluated catheter management in patients with acute epididymitis ($N = 334$) requiring inpatient treatment and developed risk factor classification predicting severity of the disease, including residual urine, fever, C-reactive protein (CRP), and white blood cell count. One hundred and seven patients (32%) of the total received either a transurethral or suprapubic catheter.
- Median length of stay was longer in the catheter group (7 versus 6 days), while the need for surgery for abscesses or recurrent epididymitis did not differ. According to risk scores, 44% of patients had low risk factors, and 56% had high risk factors. In the high-risk group, patients received a catheter significantly more often than the low-risk group. Catheter patients were older, had more comorbidities, and had higher CRP and white blood cell levels. The authors concluded that patients who received a catheter upon admission were older, had more morbidities, and have more severe symptoms.

DOCUMENTATION GUIDELINES

- Physical findings: Swelling, redness, and tenderness of the scrotum; urethral discharge
- Color, odor, and consistency of urine
- Activity tolerance during ambulation
- Response to antibiotic therapy, analgesics, and other treatments; acceptance of need to notify sexual partners according to state law
- Acceptance and understanding of sterility as a result of infection or epididymectomy

DISCHARGE AND HOME HEALTHCARE GUIDELINES

PREVENTION. Teach the patient to use a condom and spermicide for sexual encounters to prevent STIs. Encourage the patient to continue to increase fluid intake and to empty the bladder frequently.

POSTOPERATIVE TEACHING. If the patient had an epididymectomy, teach the patient to report incisional bleeding, unusual difficulty in starting the urine stream, blood in the urine, or increasing pain and swelling. Remind the patient of the postoperative appointment and that sexual activity is discouraged until after the postoperative checkup. Suggest the patient use an ice pack and athletic supporter to relieve minor discomfort from the surgery. Tepid sitz baths may also help relieve pain. Remind patients to avoid strenuous activity and heavy lifting until they are seen by the physician for a postoperative evaluation.

COMPLICATIONS. Teach the patient to report problems of impotence to the physician immediately.

MEDICATIONS. Be sure the patient understands any medication prescribed, including dosage, route, action, and side effects. Emphasize the need to complete the course of antibiotic medications even if symptoms have diminished.

Epidural Hematoma

DRG Category:	70
Mean LOS:	6.2 days
Description:	MEDICAL: Nonspecific Cerebrovascular Disorders With Major Complication or Comorbidity
DRG Category:	955
Mean LOS:	11.0 days
Description:	SURGICAL: Craniotomy for Multiple Significant Trauma

An intracranial epidural hematoma is a rapidly accumulating mass of blood, usually clotted, or a swelling confined to the space between the skull and the dura mater. It is usually found in the temporoparietal region where a skull fracture will cross the path of the middle meningeal artery or the dural branches. It occurs in approximately 2% of people with traumatic brain injuries (TBIs) and 5% to 15% of people with fatal brain injuries; estimates are that up to 20% to 50% of people die after an epidural hematoma. If an epidural hematoma expands rapidly, such as when the bleeding is arterial in origin, the injury is potentially fatal. The accumulation of blood rapidly displaces brain tissue and can result in cerebral herniation downward into the posterior fossa or toward the midline into the tentorial notch. Skull fractures occur in approximately 90% of adults with an epidural hematoma. If the hematoma is evacuated and bleeding is controlled promptly, the patient's prognosis is good. An epidural hematoma may also occur along the spine.

Generally, TBI involves both a primary injury and a secondary injury. The primary injury results from the initial impact, which causes immediate neurological damage and dysfunction. The secondary injury follows the initial trauma and probably stems from cerebral hypoxia and ischemia, which lead to cerebral edema, increased intracranial pressure (ICP), and brain herniation.

CAUSES

The injuries that cause the condition are a strong direct force to the head or an acceleration-deceleration force, which can occur in motor vehicle crashes (MVCs), automobile-pedestrian crashes, falls, and assaults. TBI causes a linear fracture of the temporal lobe in many patients. The bone fracture lacerates the middle meningeal artery or veins. Bleeding from these vessels leads to the accumulation of the hematoma within the extradural portion of the skull.

GENETIC CONSIDERATIONS

Although many vascular problems are related to trauma, vascular malformations and coagulopathies can be familial and can potentially lead to spontaneous epidural hematomas.

SEX AND LIFE SPAN CONSIDERATIONS

TBI is the leading cause of all trauma-related deaths. Most are associated with MVCs, which in the 15- to 24-year-old age group are three times more common in males than in females. The age group younger than 20 years accounts for 60% of epidural hematoma occurrence. Some experts suggest that the pediatric population may have improved neurological outcomes after head injuries compared to adults. Epidural hematoma is relatively uncommon in older adults because, as people age, the dura is strongly adhered to the skull.

HEALTH DISPARITIES AND SEXUAL/GENDER MINORITY HEALTH

In recent years, Black persons have been killed in traffic crashes at a rate almost 25% higher than White persons (National Highway Traffic Safety Administration [NHTSA], 2021). Native American persons have the highest rate of MVC injury in the United States, more than twice the rate of Black persons (NHTSA, 2021). Experts have noted that Black and Native American communities tend to be crisscrossed by more dangerous roads than other locations, placing people from those communities at risk for injury. Stark disparities exist with the incidence, management, and rehabilitation of TBI. The Centers for Disease Control and Prevention (CDC) report that Native American children and adults have the highest TBI-related hospitalizations and deaths in the United States. Important health disparities exist in treatment, follow-up, and rehabilitation of TBI. Non-Hispanic Black and Hispanic patients are less likely to receive follow-up care and rehabilitation following TBI and more likely to have poor psychosocial, functional, and employment-related outcomes as compared to non-Hispanic White patients (CDC, 2021).

The CDC reports that in the 20 years since the year 2000, more than 400,000 U.S. service members were diagnosed with TBI, including active military service members and Veterans. Approximately 80% of these injuries occurred when the service members were not deployed. These injuries may result in ongoing symptoms, posttraumatic distress syndrome, and suicidal thoughts. People in correctional or detention facilities, people who experience homelessness, and survivors of intimate partner violence may have long-term consequences from TBI. People with lower incomes and those without health insurance have less access to TBI care, are less likely to receive surgical procedures and cranial monitoring when indicated, are less likely to receive rehabilitation, and are more likely to die in the hospital. Recent work has shown that rural populations have injury mortality rates that are more than twice as high as urban rates. Many factors contribute to these health disparities, including the risk of traffic injury in narrow rural roads, the lack of graded curves and lighted traffic signals on rural highways, and the distance from major trauma centers. Many of the most dangerous occupations, such as mining and agriculture, are found in rural areas and can result in injury, disability, and death. People living in rural areas who experience a TBI have more time to travel to get emergency care, less access to high-level trauma care, and more difficulty accessing TBI services. Sexual and gender minority persons have high risk for dating and interpersonal violence, violence related to bullying, and intentional and unintentional injury; therefore, they are at risk for TBI (Healthy People 2020).

GLOBAL HEALTH CONSIDERATIONS

Internationally, falls from heights of less than 5 meters are the leading cause of injury overall, and automobile crashes are the next most frequent cause. Both have the potential to cause an epidural hematoma.

🔲 ASSESSMENT

HISTORY. Obtain a detailed description of the initial injury. Determine if the patient experienced momentary loss of reflexes or momentary arrest of respiration. Be sure to determine if the patient was unconscious at any time and, if so, for how long. Determine if the patient experienced nuchal rigidity, a seizure, photophobia, nausea, vomiting, dizziness, convulsions, decreased respirations, or progressive insensitivity to pain (obtundity). Ask if the individual had urinary or fecal incontinence. Note that approximately one-third of patients with an epidural hematoma have initial unconsciousness followed by a period of lucidity and then subsequent unconsciousness. Some experienced clinicians suggest the initial period of unconsciousness is brought about by a concussion. The patient awakens, only to become unconscious again because of epidural bleeding. Children may be difficult to diagnose; in addition to neck sensitivity, parents may describe irritability or other unspecific symptoms.

PHYSICAL EXAMINATION. The most common symptoms are **headache, nausea and vomiting, seizures**, and **changes in mental status**. The initial evaluation is centered on assessing the airway, breathing, circulation, and disability (neurological status). Exposure (undressing the patient completely) is incorporated as part of the primary survey. The secondary survey, a head-to-toe assessment including vital signs, is then completed.

The initial neurological assessment of the patient includes monitoring vital signs, assessing the level of consciousness, examining pupil size and level of reactivity, and assessment using the Glasgow Coma Scale (GCS), which evaluates eye opening, best verbal response, and best motor response. The neurological signs and symptoms depend on the location, rapidity, and source of bleeding. More than half of patients develop symptoms within the first 6 hours. Common symptoms include pupil dilation, hemiparesis, seizures, and decerebrate posturing (extension). A neurological assessment is repeated at least hourly during the first 24 hours after the injury.

Examine the entire scalp and head for lacerations, abrasions, contusions, or bony abnormalities. Take care to maintain cervical spine immobilization during the examination. Patients may have associated cervical spine injuries or thoracic, abdominal, or extremity trauma. Examine the patient for signs of basilar skull fractures, such as periorbital ecchymosis (raccoon eyes), subscleral hemorrhage, retroauricular ecchymosis (Battle sign), hemotympanum (blood behind the eardrum), and leakage of cerebrospinal fluid from the ears (otorrhea) or nose (rhinorrhea). Gently palpate the facial bones, including the mandible and maxilla, for bony deformities or step-offs. Examine the oral pharynx for lacerations, and check for any loose or fractured teeth.

Ongoing assessments are important throughout the trauma resuscitation and during recovery. Assess the patient's fluid volume status, including hemodynamic, urinary, and central nervous system (CNS) parameters, on an hourly basis until the patient is stabilized. Cardiovascular changes may include bradycardia or hypertension if ICP is elevated. Notify the physician of any early indications that volume status is inadequate, such as delayed capillary refill, tachycardia, or a urinary output less than 0.5 mL/kg per hour. Monitoring urinary specific gravity, serum sodium, potassium, chloride, and osmolarity is helpful in assessing volume status. Infection surveillance is accomplished by assessing temperature curves, white blood cell counts, and the entrance sites of monitoring devices.

PSYCHOSOCIAL. Epidural hematoma is the result of a sudden, unexpected traumatic injury and may alter an individual's ability to cope effectively. The patient may be anxious during intervals of lucidity. Expect parents of children who are injured to feel anxious, fearful, and sometimes guilty. Note if the injury was related to alcohol consumption (approximately 40% to 60% of head injuries occur when the patient has been drinking), and elicit a drinking history from the patient or significant others. Assess the patient for signs of alcohol withdrawal 2 to 14 days after admission.

Diagnostic Highlights

Test	Normal Result	Abnormality With Condition	Explanation
Computed tomography scan	Normal brain structures	Structural abnormalities, including skull fractures, soft tissue abnormalities, hemorrhage, cerebral edema, and shifting brain structures	Provides rapid, accurate diagnostic evaluation of a suspected epidural hematoma
Radiological examination: Skull, chest, and cervical (all cervical vertebrae including C7-T1 junction) spine x-rays with anteroposterior, lateral, and open-mouth view	Normal bone, joint, and soft tissue structure	Accompanying structural abnormalities	If the patient is unconscious, skull, chest, and spinal injuries need to be ruled out

Other Tests: Transcranial Doppler ultrasound and arterial blood gases, complete blood count, coagulation studies, serum drug and alcohol screens, magnetic resonance imaging

PRIMARY NURSING DIAGNOSIS

DIAGNOSIS. Ineffective airway clearance related to hypoventilation or airway obstruction as evidenced by reduced chest excursion and/or apnea

OUTCOMES. Respiratory status: Airway patency; Respiratory status: Gas exchange; Respiratory status: Ventilation; Comfort level

INTERVENTIONS. Airway management; Oxygen therapy; Airway suctioning; Airway insertion and stabilization; Anxiety reduction; Cough enhancement; Mechanical ventilation; Positioning; Respiratory monitoring

PLANNING AND IMPLEMENTATION

Collaborative

Endotracheal intubation and mechanical ventilation may be necessary to ensure oxygenation and ventilation and to decrease the risk of pulmonary aspiration. A Pao_2 greater than 100 mm Hg and $Paco_2$ between 28 and 33 mm Hg can decrease cerebral blood flow and intracranial swelling. If the patient is treated medically, serial neurological assessments are essential so that if neurological deterioration occurs, treatment can be initiated immediately.

The decision to treat surgically as compared to conservative medical treatment generally depends on the size of the hematoma and the severity of symptoms. Surgical evaluation of the clot, control of the hemorrhage, and resection of nonviable brain tissue may be warranted as soon as possible. A Jackson-Pratt drain may be used for 24 to 48 hours to drain the site. Complications include intracranial hypertension, re-accumulation of the clot, intracerebral hemorrhage, and the development of seizures. If surgical evacuation is not possible and the patient has a rapidly deteriorating status, the surgeon may place a burr hole on the same side as a dilated pupil or on the opposite side of motor deficits and the hematoma.

ICP monitoring may be used in patients who have a high probability of developing intracranial hypertension along with osmotic diuretics, hyperventilation, and elevation of the head of the bed. The goal of monitoring is to maintain the ICP at less than 10 mm Hg and the cerebral perfusion pressure (CPP) at greater than 80 mm Hg. Intermittent or continuous draining of cerebrospinal fluid through a ventriculostomy can be used to reduce ICP.

Pharmacologic Highlights

Medication or Drug Class	Dosage	Description	Rationale
Sedatives, analgesics, anesthetics	Varies with drug	Midazolam (Versed); propofol (Diprivan); fentanyl (Sublimaze)	Control intermittent increases in ICP with a resultant decrease in CPP; the drugs are short acting so that they can be temporarily stopped for intermittent neurological assessment
Chemical paralytic agents	Varies with drug	Mivacurium (Mivacron); atracurium (Tracrium); vecuronium (Norcuron)	Neuromuscular blocking agent to provide muscle relaxation is needed to improve oxygenation and ventilation; sedation must accompany paralysis

Other Drugs: Seizure activity can elevate ICP and increase oxygen demand. Phenytoin (Dilantin) or fosphenytoin may be used prophylactically, but the overall effectiveness has yet to be determined. Persistently elevated ICP, despite routine therapeutic interventions, may be managed by inducing a barbiturate coma to reduce the metabolic rate of brain tissue. Pentobarbital is commonly used. Before beginning this therapy, it is critical to determine adequate volume status to prevent hypotension and to ensure adequate tissue perfusion caused by the drug's depressant effect on myocardial contractility. Broad-spectrum antibiotic therapy is used to treat meningitis until culture and sensitivity results are available. Commonly prescribed diuretics (furosemide and mannitol) may be used to assist in managing intracranial hypertension, although their use remains controversial. Fever needs to be treated promptly with acetaminophen. Methylprednisolone may be administered to decrease inflammation, particularly if the spinal cord is involved.

Independent

The highest management priority is maintaining a patent airway, appropriate ventilation and oxygenation, and adequate circulation. Make sure the patient's endotracheal tube is anchored well. If the patient is at risk for self-extubation, use soft restraints. Note the lip level of the endotracheal tube to determine if tube movement occurs. Notify the physician if the patient's Pao_2 drops below 80 mm Hg, $Paco_2$ exceeds 40 mm Hg, or severe hypocapnia ($Paco_2$ < 25 mm Hg) occurs.

Avoid body temperature elevations and flexing, extending, or rotating the patient's neck to prevent a sudden increase in ICP. Maintain the patient in a normal body alignment to prevent obstruction of venous drainage. Generally, the head of the bed is elevated to reduce ICP. Maintain a quiet, restful environment with minimal stimulation. Time nursing care activities carefully to limit prolonged ICP elevations. When suctioning, hyperventilate the patient beforehand and suction only as long as necessary. When turning the patient, prevent Valsalva maneuver by using a draw sheet to pull the patient up in bed. Instruct the patient not to hold on to the side rails.

Provide support and encouragement to the patient and family. Provide educational tools and teach the patient and family appropriate rehabilitative exercises. Provide diversionary activities appropriate to the patient's mental and physical abilities. Head injury support groups may be helpful. Referrals to clinical nurse specialists, pastoral care staff, and social workers are helpful in developing strategies for support and education.

Evidence-Based Practice and Health Policy

McClung, C., Anshus, J., Anshus, A., & Baker, S. (2020). Bedside craniostomy and serial aspiration with an intraosseous drill/needle to temporize an acute epidural hemorrhage with mass effect. *World Neurosurgery, 142,* 218–221.

- The authors report on a technique for an immediate mechanical intervention using a familiar tool for emergency physicians and trauma surgeons to manage acute epidural bleeding with mass effect. They describe a case study of a 38-year-old male with active extradural hemorrhage and expanding hematoma who was treated at the bedside with an intraosseous drill to perform a craniostomy.
- This procedure allowed for serial aspirations of continued bleeding and immediate management of a large epidural hemorrhage. The technique can be applied by emergency physicians or trauma specialists when neurosurgical consultation is delayed.

DOCUMENTATION GUIDELINES

- Trauma history, description of the event, time elapsed since the event, whether or not the patient had a loss of consciousness and, if so, for how long
- Adequacy of airway, breathing, circulation; serial vital signs
- Appearance, bruising or lacerations, drainage from the nose or ears
- Physical findings related to the site of head injury: Neurological assessment, presence of accompanying symptoms, presence of complications (decreased level of consciousness, unequal pupils, loss of strength and movement, confusion or agitation, nausea and vomiting), CPP, ICP
- Signs of complications: Seizure activity, infection (fever, purulent discharge from any wounds), aspiration pneumonia (shortness of breath, pulmonary congestion, fever, productive cough), increased ICP
- Response to surgery: Stabilization of vital signs, changes in neurological status
- Response to medications used to control pain and increase ICP

DISCHARGE AND HOME HEALTHCARE GUIDELINES

Review with the patient and family proper care techniques for wounds and lacerations. Discuss the recommended activity level, and explain rehabilitative exercises. Teach the patient and family to recognize symptoms of infection or a deteriorating level of consciousness, and stress the need to contact the physician if such signs or symptoms appear. Teach the patient the purpose; dosage; schedule; precautions; and potential side effects, interactions, and adverse reactions of all prescribed medications. Review with the patient and family all follow-up appointments that have been arranged. Review with the patient and family information regarding the use of safety restraints. If the injury was related to alcohol or other drugs of abuse, make appropriate referrals for follow-up.

Epilepsy

DRG Category:	100
Mean LOS:	5.9 days
Description:	MEDICAL: Seizures With Major Complication or Comorbidity

Epilepsy is a paroxysmal neurological disorder characterized by a predisposition to generate recurrent episodes of convulsive movements or other motor activity, loss of consciousness, sensory disturbances, and other behavioral abnormalities. It has not only neurological consequences but cognitive, psychological, and social consequences as well. Because epilepsy occurs in more than 50 diseases, it is considered a syndrome rather than a disease. It is the fourth most common neurological problem (after migraine, stroke, and Alzheimer disease) in the United States.

Approximately 1% of the U.S. population (2 to 3 million people) has been diagnosed with epilepsy. Each year, approximately 150,000 new cases of epilepsy occur.

Convulsive seizures are the most common forms of attacks of epilepsy. Seizures occur with abnormal electrical discharges from brain cells, and these discharges are caused by the movement of ions across the cell membrane. Although seizures are the dominant manifestation of epilepsy, patients can have a seizure and not have epilepsy. For over 35 years, a classification system was used to characterize seizures on the basis of whether the person was conscious during the seizure and whether one or two sides of the body were involved. A new classification system was announced in 2017 by the International League Against Epilepsy. The new system is based on the location in the brain where the seizure begins, the level of awareness during a seizure, and other features of the seizure. The Epilepsy Foundation provides an explanation of the new classification at https://epilepsy.com, which is incorporated in Table 1.

• TABLE 1 Classification of Seizure Types, 2017

FEATURES	DESCRIPTION
Where they begin	Focal seizures: Seizure involves one side of the brain at onset • Generalized seizure: Seizure involves both sides of the brain at onset • Unknown onset • Focal to bilateral seizure: Seizure starts on one side and spreads to both sides
Level of awareness	Focal aware: Awareness remains intact • Focal impaired awareness: Awareness is impaired • Awareness unknown • Generalized seizure: Presumed to affect awareness or consciousness
Other features	Describing motor and other symptoms in focal seizures • Focal motor seizure: Some form of movement occurs during the seizure • Focal nonmotor seizure: Other symptoms occur before movement • Auras: Symptoms the person may feel at the beginning of the seizure; are not in the above descriptions Describing generalized onset seizures • Generalized motor seizure: Generalized tonic-clonic seizure • Generalized nonmotor seizure: Absence seizures with brief change of awareness, staring, and possibly automated movements

Status epilepticus is defined as more than 30 minutes of unconsciousness with continuous or intermittent convulsive seizure activity. Usually, status epilepticus results when more than six seizures occur in 24 hours or when the patient progresses from one seizure to the next without resolution of the postictal period. Pseudoseizures are the physical appearance of seizure activity without the cerebral electrical activity. Complications include pulmonary aspiration; airway occlusion; injury to the head, extremities, or tongue; memory loss or personality changes after seizures; cardiac changes (blood pressure instability, cardiac dysrhythmias, cardiac arrest); and status epilepticus.

CAUSES

The cause of epilepsy is often unknown, but there are also many genetic disorders that lead to seizure activity (see Genetic Considerations). Seizures may be caused by primary central nervous system (CNS) disorders, metabolic or systemic disorders, or idiopathic origins. Primary CNS disorders include any potential mass effect (tumor, abscess, atrioventricular malformation [AVM], aneurysm, or hematoma) and all types of strokes, especially those that are embolic. Metabolic and systemic causes include acute overdose, acute drug withdrawal (especially CNS depressants, alcohol, benzodiazepines, and barbiturates), febrile states, hypoxia, hyperosmolarity, hypertensive encephalopathy, hyperthermia, and a multitude of electrolyte disturbances. A seizure occurs when there is a sudden imbalance of the electrical properties of the cerebral cortex, leading to neural excitation and decreased inhibition.

GENETIC CONSIDERATIONS

Epilepsy is a broad condition that includes several disorders that have different etiologies. Overall, epilepsy has a significant genetic component, with heritability estimated at 77% to 85%. The most significant genetic association with epilepsy is the gene *SCN1A*, which encodes for a sodium channel protein. Mutations in *SCN1A* are usually inherited in an autosomal dominant pattern and can cause several different epileptic disorders. There are also many diseases and disorders that include propensity for seizures as a feature. Some examples include tuberous sclerosis and fragile X syndrome.

SEX AND LIFE SPAN CONSIDERATIONS

Epilepsy affects males and females equally. The incidence is approximately 1 in every 100 to 300 persons. Although epilepsy can occur in any age group, usually the onset is before age 20. Different age groups have distinct associated causes. In newborns up until 6 months of age, seizures are generally caused by birth trauma or metabolic disturbances, such as hypoxemia, hypoglycemia, and hypocalcemia. In children from 6 months to 5 years of age, etiology is related to febrile episodes or metabolic disturbances such as hyponatremia or hypernatremia, hypoglycemia, or hypocalcemia. In the 5- to 20-year-old age group, seizures are primarily idiopathic (50%). In adults from 20 to 50 years of age, a new onset of seizures is almost exclusively caused by trauma or tumors. In older adults, seizures are generally caused by vascular disease and cardiac dysrhythmias.

HEALTH DISPARITIES AND SEXUAL/GENDER MINORITY HEALTH

Native American and Alaskan Native persons have the longest time lapse between a seizure and the diagnosis of epilepsy, which leads to important disparities in health outcomes. People with epilepsy who have low incomes have also been found to have more frequent visits to emergency departments for the management of seizures, more adverse effects from medications, higher levels of depression and anxiety, worse quality of life, and are less likely to be seen by an epilepsy provider than those with high incomes.

Transgender is a term used to describe persons whose gender identity is different from their sex assigned at birth. Approximately 1% of the U.S. population identify themselves as transgender. Sexual and gender minority persons have higher odds for multiple chronic conditions, cancer, and poor quality of life and are more apt to have disabilities than cisgender males and females. (Cisgender is a term used to describe persons whose gender identity and gender expression are aligned with their assigned sex listed on their birth certificate.) Gender-affirming hormone therapy is the use of hormone therapy for gender transition or gender affirmation and can be masculinizing or feminizing. Antiepileptic drugs (AEDs) may interact with the hormones that are used for gender-affirming therapy for both transwomen (male-to-female transgender persons) and transmen (female-to-male transgender persons) and may thereby change the effective dose of both the AEDs and hormones (Johnson & Kaplan, 2017).

GLOBAL HEALTH CONSIDERATIONS

In many parts of the world, having epilepsy leads to stigmatization, presents barriers to marriage, and may limit employment or education. Based on the principles of social justice, the World Health Organization is attempting to remedy the stigma associated with the condition. Epilepsy affects people of all global regions, whether they are high- or low-resourced countries. Of the 50 million people affected with epilepsy, almost 90% live in developing countries, and of those people, 75% have not received the treatment they require to manage the disorder.

ASSESSMENT

HISTORY. To obtain a history, it is helpful to interview both the individual who experienced the seizure and also people who observed the person during the seizure. Obtain a thorough patient and family history of past illnesses and surgeries. Lifestyle changes, medications or vaccinations, and history of past head injury may be significant. Obtain data about the age of onset and the frequency, duration, and severity of the seizures. Ask patients if they experienced any type of aura or prodromal symptoms before the seizure or if there are any precipitating factors such as dizziness, palpitations, flashing lights, or fatigue. Discuss with patients if they had any recollection of the seizure or had any sensation during the seizure. A history of seizure activity is crucial from persons who have witnessed the activity. Elicit information about eye movements, body movements, level of consciousness, and presence of urinary or fecal incontinence. Ask observers to describe the patient's postictal state.

PHYSICAL EXAMINATION. The most common symptom of untreated epilepsy is **seizure activity**, which has varying characteristics depending on the type of seizure (see Table 1). A thorough neurological examination includes assessing changes in mental status, cranial nerve function, muscular tone and strength, sensations, reflexes, and gait. Describe in detail any seizure activity that may occur during the physical examination. Assess the initial manifestations, motor activity, pupil size, gaze, incontinence, and duration of the seizure. Assess what the patient is like in the postictal state. Because the patient may bite the tongue during the seizure, assess the patient for mouth and tongue injury.

PSYCHOSOCIAL. A diagnosis of epilepsy is life changing and can have significant psychological impact. Depression is the most frequent comorbidity in people with epilepsy and occurs in up to 35% of people with the disorder. When it is poorly controlled, epilepsy may be seriously debilitating and can challenge plans for schooling and career. Attending school or going to work may be a serious trial for the person with poorly controlled epilepsy. Vocational rehabilitation may support patients having to make career changes. Mobility is frequently disturbed because of the inability to drive. Lifestyle precautions also include caution when ascending heights, working with fire or cooking, using power tools, bathing, and swimming. Seizure activity in public is embarrassing, poorly understood by the public, and upsetting to patients.

Diagnostic Highlights

Test	Normal Result	Abnormality With Condition	Explanation
Magnetic resonance imaging	Normal brain structures	Structural brain changes such as sclerosis, tumors, infarcts, or atrophy can lead to seizures	Assesses the CNS for changes in brain structure, such as atrophy of certain areas or brain tumors
Electroencephalogram	Normal patterns of electrical activity	Abnormal patterns of electrical activity, reflecting seizure activity	Recording of electrical potentials based on distribution of waveforms generated by cerebral cortex of brain; waveforms demonstrate abnormal patterns during seizures; they are not useful in the acute management of status epilepticus

Other Tests: Computed tomography scans (often done upon emergency admission), positron emission tomography, and skull x-rays; serum laboratory data to explore possible causes include glucose, calcium, blood urea nitrogen, and electrolyte, toxic, and metabolic screens

PRIMARY NURSING DIAGNOSIS

DIAGNOSIS. Ineffective airway clearance related to clonic-tonic motor activity and tongue obstruction as evidenced by reduced chest excursion and/or apena

OUTCOMES. Respiratory status: Airway patency; Respiratory status: Gas exchange; Respiratory status: Ventilation; Neurological status: Risk control; Knowledge: Epilepsy management

INTERVENTIONS. Airway insertion; Airway management; Airway suctioning; Oxygen therapy; Respiratory monitoring; Ventilation assistance

☀ PLANNING AND IMPLEMENTATION

Collaborative

MEDICAL. In general, the management of seizures is done pharmacologically. The patient with status epilepticus is considered a medical emergency. Airway management is critical, often endotracheal intubation is needed, and IV medications are administered. If there is a delay in treatment or if the patient is unresponsive to treatment, irreversible brain damage, coma, or death can occur.

SURGICAL. Over 200,000 people in the United States have intractable epilepsy, and at least 50% of these people are potential surgical candidates. Left untreated, they are at risk for sudden death and personal injury and are less likely to be employed as compared to people with controlled seizures. Surgical management results in an excellent prognosis for seizure control and has low surgical morbidity, improved quality of life, and improved occupational outcomes. In some cases, the epileptogenic zone is mapped using video-EEG monitoring or intracranial electrodes. Examples of common surgical techniques include anteromedial temporal resection (AMTR; most common surgery for medial temporal lobe epilepsy): corpus callosotomy (surgery for generalized epilepsy syndromes); modified hemispherotomy; and multiple subpial transection (MST; newer type of epilepsy surgery with limited applications). Vagal nerve stimulation is a palliative strategy that involves implanting a stimulating device to treat refractory focal-onset epilepsy.

Pharmacologic Highlights

Medication or Drug Class	Dosage	Description	Rationale
Anticonvulsants	Varies with drug	Multiple drug therapies are available: Phenytoin sodium (Dilantin), carbamazepine, lacosamide, felbamate, perampanel, valproate, lamotrigine, gabapentin; phenobarbital, lorazepam (Ativan), diazepam (Valium)	Lorazepam (Ativan) or diazepam (Valium) may be used to stop seizures quickly; phenytoin (Dilantin) is the preferred maintenance anticonvulsant for status epilepticus; a newer drug, fosphenytoin (Cerebyx), has been developed that is safer for parenteral administration; phenobarbital may be given if seizures occur after phenytoin loading

Other Drugs: Thiamine 100 mg and 50 mL of 50% dextrose in water may be administered in an emergency to rule out seizures because of thiamine deficiency or hypoglycemia.

Other Information About Anticonvulsants: The primary treatment for epilepsy is one or more of the multitude of AEDs or anticonvulsants. The choice of AED or combination of AEDs depends on seizure type, patient tolerance, and cost. Carbamazepine (Tegretol) is a widely used and cost-effective anticonvulsant. Valproic acid, primidone

(Mysoline), clonazepam, and ethosuximide are prescribed depending on the seizure type. Lamotrigine (Lamictal), levetiracetam, and gabapentin are among the AEDs approved for partial seizures.

Independent

The most important nursing interventions are to maintain adequate airway, breathing, and circulation during the seizure and to prevent injury. Have an oral airway and suction apparatus at the bedside at all times. A patient who begins a seizure should not be left alone. If in the hospital setting, use the call light to obtain assistance, and if the patient is upright, gently ease the patient to the floor. Position the patient to maintain the airway, but do not force anything into the patient's mouth if the teeth are clenched. If the patient's mouth is open, protect the patient's tongue by placing a soft cloth or a well-padded tongue blade between the teeth. Help the patient to a lying position, remove constricting clothing, and place a pillow or sheet under the patient's head to cushion the patient from injury. Clear the area of objects that are hard or sharp. Do not restrain the patient's movement during the seizure. Assist the patient with hygiene and linen changes should incontinence occur during the seizure.

To lower the risk of injury, provide a safe environment at all times. Pad and raise the side rails, but do not use pillows for padding because of the possibility of suffocation. The extent of seizure precautions should be consistent with the type of seizures. Good oral hygiene is important. Also observe for signs of infection if there is any damage to the tongue and oral mucosa.

Educate the patient and family about providing care during a seizure, the medication schedule and side effects, and the importance of regular follow-up. Involve the family as much as possible in patient care. Use patient and family teaching to dispel any myths and misconceptions about epilepsy. Assure the family that most patients can control the syndrome if they follow the prescribed routine. Because epilepsy can be a debilitating, restrictive disease, provide support and encouragement. Refer patients to national organizations (Epilepsy Foundation of America) and local support groups.

Evidence-Based Practice and Health Policy

Jothi, A., Ramamoorthy, L., & Nair, P. (2020). The effect of comprehensive video assisted epilepsy education on drug adherence and self-care in people with epilepsy. *Journal of Neurosciences in Rural Practice, 11*, 538–544.

- The authors set out to determine the effectiveness of video-assisted epilepsy education on drug adherence and self-care in patients with epilepsy. They used a single group, experimental design (pretest-posttest) to evaluate the effect of a video-assisted teaching program on self-care efficacy and level of knowledge of patients with epilepsy.
- At 3 months, the levels of drug adherence, self-care, and knowledge were assessed. Following video-assisted teaching, the proportion of participants with adequate knowledge increased, the percentage of participants who had good drug adherence increased, and the percentage of participants who had a high level of self-care increased. The authors recommended that people with epilepsy should be personally educated to increase their knowledge of drug adherence and self-care.

DOCUMENTATION GUIDELINES

- Seizure activity: Events preceding and following seizure, type, length, progression, airway maintenance, ability to follow commands, ability to respond verbally, and memory of events
- Complications: Airway compromise, extremity injury, tongue laceration, lowered self-esteem
- Institution of safety precautions
- Response to AEDs: Drug levels and side effects, response to treatment
- Understanding of and interest in patient teaching

DISCHARGE AND HOME HEALTHCARE GUIDELINES

Be sure that the patient understands all medications, including the dosage, route, action, adverse effects, and need for routine laboratory monitoring of AEDs. Stress the need for taking medications as prescribed even if seizure activity is under control. Ensure that the patient has basic epilepsy safety information, such as no tub baths, no swimming, and no driving without seizure control for at least 1 year. Family members should be able to verbalize what to do during a seizure. Patients should wear jewelry identifying them as having epilepsy. Make sure patients and family understand what laboratory tests are needed depending on their medications.

HOME CARE. Emphasize the following management strategies:
• Maintain adequate rest and nutrition; check with a physician before dieting
• Limit alcohol intake
• Report infections promptly
• Avoid trigger factors (flashing lights, hyperventilation, loud noises, video games, television)
• Brush the teeth regularly with a soft toothbrush
• Avoid activities that precipitate seizure activity
• Keep follow-up appointments
• Lead as normal a life as possible

Esophageal Cancer

DRG Category:	326
Mean LOS:	13.2 days
Description:	SURGICAL: Stomach, Esophageal, and Duodenal Procedures With Major Complication or Comorbidity
DRG Category:	375
Mean LOS:	4.7 days
Description:	MEDICAL: Digestive Malignancy With Complication or Comorbidity

Carcinoma is the most common cause of obstruction of the esophagus. Approximately half of all esophageal cancers are squamous cell carcinomas, which usually occur in the middle and lower two-thirds of the esophagus and are often associated with alcohol and tobacco use. The remaining 50% are adenocarcinomas, which generally begin in glandular tissue of the esophagus. Adenocarcinomas are associated with Barrett esophagus, a condition that occurs because of continued reflux of fluid from the stomach into the lower esophagus. Over time, reflux changes the cells at the end of the esophagus. Adenocarcinomas may invade the upper portion of the stomach.

Esophageal tumors begin as benign growths and grow rapidly because there is no serosal layer to inhibit growth. Because of the vast lymphatic network of the esophagus, esophageal cancers spread rapidly, both locally to regional lymph nodes and distantly to the lungs and liver. Complications include pulmonary problems that result from fistulae and aspiration; invasion of the tumor into major vessels, causing a massive hemorrhage; and obstruction and compression of the other structures in the head and neck. Although survival rates are improving, esophageal cancer is usually diagnosed at a late stage, and most patients die within 6 months of diagnosis. The American Cancer Society (ACS) estimates that 19,260 new cases of esophageal cancer will be diagnosed in 2021, and approximately 15,530 people will die from the disease. The 5-year survival rate for localized disease is 41%, and it is 18% for people with all stages of the disease.

CAUSES

Although its etiology is unknown, experts believe that the exposure of the esophageal mucosa to toxins results in cellular changes that lead to cancer. For many years in the United States, the primary risk factors were alcohol and tobacco use. Alcohol and tobacco together seem to have a synergistic effect on esophageal cancer development; because alcohol is a solvent of fat-soluble compounds, it seems to allow carcinogens associated with tobacco to penetrate esophageal tissues more easily. Squamous cell carcinoma is the cancer type associated with smoking, alcohol use, poor nutrition, exposure to toxins, and infection. Recently, oral exposure of the human papillomavirus (HPV) infection has also been identified as a risk factor. In parts of the world where it is most common (Southeast Asia, the Middle East, and South Africa), the disease has been linked to nitrosamines and other contaminants in the soil. It has also been found to have a higher incidence in individuals whose diets are chronically deficient in fresh fruits, vegetables, vitamins, and proteins. Other risk factors include caustic injuries from lye ingestion and occupational exposure to perchloroethylene, which is used in the automotive and dry cleaning industries. Squamous cell carcinoma is also associated with drinking scalding beverages. Other types of esophageal cancer occur as well. In recent decades, there has been a progressive increase in adenocarcinoma of the esophagus related to gastroesophageal reflux disease (GERD) because of irritation from reflux of acid and bile. Obesity also is associated with adenocarcinoma, likely because of release of inflammatory mediators and the potential for metabolic syndrome.

GENETIC CONSIDERATIONS

Although the exact cause of esophageal cancer is not clear, environmental risk factors (such as smoking and alcohol consumption) appear to be predominant. Epidemiological studies in Chinese populations have found that variants in the low-molecular-weight polypeptide (LMP) genes, which function in immunological surveillance, increase risk for esophageal squamous cell carcinoma. These variants are likely inherited in autosomal recessive patterns, although the combination of genes and environmental factors is the most likely etiology of esophageal cancer.

SEX AND LIFE SPAN CONSIDERATIONS

Cancer of the esophagus usually occurs in men between the ages of 50 and 70 years. The disorder affects men in a 3:1 ratio to women.

HEALTH DISPARITIES AND SEXUAL/GENDER MINORITY HEALTH

The ACS notes that adenocarcinoma is more common in White persons, and squamous cell carcinoma is more common in Black persons. Although treatment guidelines indicate that management of esophageal cancer should include surgery, Black persons are less likely than White persons to undergo surgery. Persons with low income and patients with no private insurance also have lower rates of surgery than other groups. Importantly, patients who do not receive surgery when indicated have higher mortality rates (Savitch et al., 2021), leading to health disparities for Black, low income, and uninsured patients. Gender and sexual minorities have several risk factors for esophageal cancer. They smoke more than their heterosexual and cisgender counterparts, increasing the risk for esophageal cancer. In addition, HPV is present in approximately 65% of gay men overall and 95% of gay men with HIV, also increasing risk. While little is known about health disparities due to esophageal cancer in sexual and gender minorities, factors such as poverty, stigma, and discrimination affect access to cancer screening and healthcare, which may lead to poorer outcomes.

GLOBAL HEALTH CONSIDERATIONS

The global incidence of esophageal cancer is 10 per 100,000 males and 5 per 100,000 females, but in some countries with high soil contamination, rates are as high as 800 per 100,000 individuals. In developing countries, females have a higher incidence of the condition than in developed countries, whereas the male incidence of esophageal cancer is approximately the same across countries. Esophageal cancer is more common in Iran, India, China, Southern Russia, and southern and eastern Africa than in the United States. Incidence is low in central Africa and South/Central America.

ASSESSMENT

HISTORY. Obtain an accurate history of risk factors, including race, cultural background, use of cigarettes and alcohol, pneumonia or HPV infections, and any esophageal problems. Dysphagia is usually experienced when at least 60% of the esophagus is occluded. Initially, it is mild and intermittent, and it occurs only with solid foods. Patients may report a sensation that "food is sticking in their throat." Patients may describe hoarseness and a persistent cough. If the disease is untreated, symptoms soon progress to the inability to swallow semisoft or liquid food, and the patient experiences a severe weight loss, as much as 40 to 50 pounds over 2 to 3 months. Eventually, the patient is unable to swallow saliva. Also inquire about regurgitation, vomiting, chronic hiccups, odynophagia (painful swallowing), and dietary patterns. Patients may report pain radiating to the neck, jaw, ears, and shoulders.

PHYSICAL EXAMINATION. Dysphagia is the most common symptom and **weight loss** is the second most important symptom. Observe the patient's ability to swallow food. Note any chronic coughing and increased oral secretions. Listen to the patient's voice: Tumors in the upper esophagus can involve the larynx and cause hoarseness. Place the patient in the recumbent position; pain, hoarseness, coughing, and potential aspiration often occur in this position. Weigh the patient and determine the patient's strength and motion of the extremities. Severe weight loss and weakness are common symptoms. Except for weight loss, the physical examination may be normal.

PSYCHOSOCIAL. The patient needs to make a psychological adjustment to the diagnosis of a chronic illness that is often terminal, particularly if it is diagnosed at an advanced stage. Evaluate the patient for evidence of altered mood (e.g., depression or anxiety), and assess the coping mechanisms and support systems.

Diagnostic Highlights

Test	Normal Result	Abnormality With Condition	Explanation
Esophagogastro-duodenoscopy	Visualization of a normal esophagus and stomach	Direct visualization of tumor or fistula	Locates the tumor for a biopsy

Other Tests: Computed tomography scan, endoscopic ultrasound, thoracoscopy, laparoscopy, liver scan, bronchoscopy, magnetic resonance imaging, positive emission tomography

PRIMARY NURSING DIAGNOSIS

DIAGNOSIS. Imbalanced nutrition: less than body requirements related to dysphagia as evidenced by weight loss

OUTCOMES. Nutritional status: Food and fluid intake; Nutrient status: Biochemical measures; Self management: Cancer; Knowledge: Cancer management

INTERVENTIONS. Nutrition management; Nutrition therapy; Nutritional monitoring; Nutritional counseling; Fluid/electrolyte management; Medication management

PLANNING AND IMPLEMENTATION

Collaborative

Surgery, radiotherapy, chemotherapy, laser therapy, and endoscopic therapy are all options for treating cancer of the esophagus, and they may be used alone or in combination. Early stage patients may be treated with endoscopic therapies, such as endoscopic mucosal resection or endoscopic submucosal dissection. Trimodal therapy, which includes chemotherapy and radiotherapy (chemoradiation), followed by surgery is recommended for those who can tolerate this rigorous treatment regime. Preoperative chemotherapy followed by surgery has poorer patient outcomes than trimodal therapy. Two surgical procedures are commonly performed: esophagectomy (removal of all or part of the esophagus with a Dacron graft replacing the part that was removed) and esophagogastrectomy (resection of the lower part of the esophagus together with a proximal portion of the stomach, followed by anastomosis of the remaining portion of the esophagus and stomach). Postoperatively, monitor the nasogastric (NG) tube for patency. Expect some bloody drainage initially; within 24 to 48 hours, the drainage should change to a yellowish-green. Do not irrigate or reposition the NG tube without a physician's order. Fluid and electrolyte balance as well as intake and output should be monitored carefully. Monitor the patient who has had an anastomosis for signs and symptoms of leakage, which is most likely to occur 5 to 7 days postoperatively. These include low-grade fever, inflammation, accumulation of fluid, and early symptoms of shock (tachycardia, tachypnea).

For patients who are not candidates for surgery but rather for palliation, chemotherapy, radiotherapy, and laser therapy, reduce the size of the tumor and provide some relief to the patient. Usually, external beam radiation therapy is used. Normal esophageal tissue is also affected by the radiation, which is given over a 6- to 8-week period to minimize the side effects. Side effects include edema, epithelial desquamation, esophagitis, odynophagia, anorexia, nausea, and vomiting. Although radiation by itself does not cure esophageal cancer, it eases symptoms such as pain, bleeding, and dysphagia.

Pharmacologic Highlights

Medication or Drug Class	Dosage	Description	Rationale
Chemotherapy	Varies by drug	Combinations: Paclitaxel and carboplatin; fluorouracil and cisplatin; fluorouracil and oxaliplatin; irinotecan and cisplatin; paclitaxel and fluoropyrimidine. Other types of chemotherapy: 5-fluorouracil, capecitabine, docetaxel, bleomycin, mitomycin, doxorubicin, methotrexate, vinorelbine, topotecan, mitoguazone, epirubicin, porfimer	Kills cancer cells; primary chemotherapy will not cure esophageal cancer unless surgery and/or radiation is also used; preoperatively, chemotherapy may be given to reduce tumor size; approximately 10%–40% of patients will have a significant shrinking of the tumor from these drugs

Independent

Carefully monitor the patient's nutritional intake and involve the patient in planning their diet. Maintain a daily record of caloric intake and weight. Monitor the skin turgor and mucous membranes to detect dehydration. Keep the head of the bed elevated at least 30 degrees to prevent reflux and pulmonary aspiration. If the patient is having problems swallowing saliva, keep a suction catheter with an oral suction at the bedside at all times. Teach the patient how to clear the mouth with the oral suction.

When appropriate, discuss expected preoperative and postoperative procedures, including information about x-rays, IV hydration, wound drains, NG tube and suctioning, and chest tubes. Immediately after surgery, implement strategies to prevent respiratory complications.

Provide emotional support. Focus on the patient's quality of life and discuss realistic planning and end-of-life care with the family. Involve the patient as much as possible in decisions concerning care. If the patient is terminally ill, encourage the significant others to involve the patient in discussions about funeral arrangements and terminal care, such as hospice care. Provide a referral to the patient to the American Cancer Society, support groups, and hospice care as appropriate.

Evidence-Based Practice and Health Policy

Findlay, M., Purvis, M., Venman, R., Luong, R., & Carey, S. (2020). Nutritional management of patients with oesophageal cancer throughout the treatment: Benchmarking against best practice. *Supportive Care in Cancer, 28,* 5963–5971.

• The study benchmarks current nutrition management of patients with esophageal cancer against best practice recommendations. The authors identified critical points in the treatment trajectory where nutritional status is compromised and service gaps occur. The authors collected demographic, medical, and nutritional data from medical records of 37 patients who received curative treatment for esophageal cancer at a tertiary referral hospital.

• The authors found that nutritional care was inconsistent across different treatment stages, weight declined over the course of treatment, and malnutrition led to unplanned readmission. While best practice recommendations were met for aspects of the immediate postoperative period, the authors identified service gaps that remained during preoperative and postdischarge care.

DOCUMENTATION GUIDELINES

• Physical assessment data: Ability to eat and swallow, patency of airway, regularity of breathing, temperature, daily weights, breath sounds, intake and output, calorie counts
• Chronological record of symptoms and response to interventions
• The nature, location, duration, and intensity of pain; response to pain medication or other interventions
• Patient's emotional response to a poor prognosis and treatment modalities

DISCHARGE AND HOME HEALTHCARE GUIDELINES

MEDICATIONS. The patient should be able to state the name, purpose, dosage, schedule, common side effects, and importance of taking their medications.

COMPLICATIONS. Teach the patient to report any dysphagia or odynophagia, which may indicate a regrowth of the tumor. Teach the patient to inspect the wound daily for redness, swelling, discharge, or odor, which indicates the presence of infection.

HOME CARE. Teach family members to assist the patient with ambulation, splinting the incision, and chest physiotherapy. Educate caregivers on nutritional guidelines, food preparation, tube feedings, and parenteral nutrition, as appropriate. Inform the patient and family about the availability of high-caloric, high-protein, liquid supplements to maintain the patient's weight.

RESOURCES. Provide patients with a list of resources for support after discharge: Visiting nurses, American Cancer Society, hospice, support groups.

Esophageal Diverticula

DRG Category:	394
Mean LOS:	3.8 days
Description:	MEDICAL: Other Digestive System Diagnoses With Complication or Comorbidity
DRG Category:	326
Mean LOS:	13.2 days
Description:	SURGICAL: Stomach, Esophageal, and Duodenal Procedures With Major Complication or Comorbidity

Esophageal diverticula, or herniations of the esophageal mucosa, are hollow outpouchings of the esophageal wall that occur in three main areas of the esophagus: proximally near the anatomic hypopharyngeal sphincter (Zenker diverticulum, the most common location), near the midpoint of the esophagus (a midesophageal or midthoracic diverticulum), and just above the lower esophageal sphincter (an epiphrenic diverticulum, the least common location). A single diverticulum ranges from 1 to 4 inches in diameter. Food, fluids, and secretions accumulate in these dilated outpouchings, creating discomfort and dysphagia (difficulty swallowing). Over time, esophageal diverticula enlarge, gradually producing more symptoms. Regurgitation often occurs at night when an individual is lying down, and patients may have difficulty with a choking sensation that interrupts sleep. Complications include aspiration pneumonia, bronchitis, bronchiectasis, and lung abscess, which may be the result of regurgitating contents of the esophageal diverticula. Esophageal diverticula may also lead to esophageal perforation and, rarely, esophageal cancer.

CAUSES

Esophageal diverticula develop from weakened esophageal musculature (congenital and acquired), traumatic injury, and scar tissue associated with chronic inflammation. Developmental muscle weakness of the posterior pharynx above the border of the cricopharyngeal muscle leads to Zenker diverticulum. Pressure caused by swallowing and contraction of the pharynx before the sphincter relaxes aggravates the muscle weakness and results in the development of diverticula. A response to scarring and pulling on esophageal walls by an external inflammatory process, such as tuberculosis, or by traction from old adhesions may lead to midesophageal diverticula. Other causes of esophageal diverticula include motor disturbances, such as achalasia (absence of normal peristalsis in esophageal smooth muscle and elevated pressure at the physiological cardiac sphincter), diffuse esophageal spasms, and reflux esophagitis.

GENETIC CONSIDERATIONS

Esophageal diverticula appear to run in families. They are also a feature of autosomal dominantly inherited polycystic kidney disease.

SEX AND LIFE SPAN CONSIDERATIONS

Infants and children have been known to have esophageal diverticula, although the disorder predominantly occurs in adults beyond midlife after they reach age 50 years. It affects men three times as often as women. Epiphrenic diverticula usually occur in middle-aged men. Zenker diverticulum occurs most often in men over age 60 years.

HEALTH DISPARITIES AND SEXUAL/GENDER MINORITY HEALTH

While there do not seem to be racial or ethnic differences in the prevalence of esophageal diverticuli, Black and Hispanic patients have higher rates of postoperative complications than White patients. Sexual and gender minority status has no known effect on the risk for esophageal diverticula.

GLOBAL HEALTH CONSIDERATIONS

While esophageal diverticula likely occur around the world, no epidemiological data are available to describe prevalence.

ASSESSMENT

HISTORY. Establish a recent history of weight loss, which is generally attributed to difficulty in eating. Determine if the patient has experienced subtle, gradually progressive esophageal dysphagia that primarily affected the swallowing of solid foods. Patients may describe chest pain. Achalasia ("failure to relax"; refers to inability of the lower esophageal sphincter to open so that food may pass into the stomach) can lead to dysphagia. Ask if the patient has experienced gagging, gurgling, or a sense of fullness in the throat as if something were "stuck." Inquire whether the patient has regurgitated food particles and saliva soon after eating. Determine if the patient has experienced an unpleasant taste and nocturnal coughing with regurgitation of retained secretions and undigested foods. Establish a history of heartburn following ingestion of coffee, alcohol, chocolate, citrus juices, or fatty foods, particularly when the patient was bending over or lying down within 2 hours of intake. These indicators suggest that the esophageal diverticula are secondary to achalasia.

PHYSICAL EXAMINATION. The most common symptoms are **dysphagia**, **achalasia**, **weight loss**, and **regurgitation**. Assess the patient's appearance, noting apparent weight loss or the malnourished look that is associated with anorexia. Note halitosis, a common sign of esophageal diverticula. Inspect the patient's neck for visible signs of esophageal distention that has been caused by food trapped in the diverticula.

PSYCHOSOCIAL. The patient may experience self-imposed social isolation because of feelings of embarrassment that are caused by noisy swallowing, unusual facial expressions during eating, or halitosis. The patient may become depressed because of the loss of pleasure and socialization connected with eating, along with grieving over the loss of dietary preferences. The patient's family may be anxious about the social effects of the patient's disease as well.

Diagnostic Highlights

Test	Normal Result	Abnormality With Condition	Explanation
Esophageal manometry	Multilumen esophageal catheter is introduced through the mouth, and pressures along the esophagus are measured during swallowing: normal contractions, swallowing, peristalsis	Abnormal contractions, swallowing, and peristalsis	Assesses and diagnoses dysphagia, esophageal reflux, spasm, motility abnormalities, hiatal hernia
Barium swallow with computed tomography scanning	Normal esophagus	Identifies irregular or abnormal areas of the esophagus	Locates and describes irregularities in the esophageal wall
Esophagoscopy	Visualization of a normal esophagus	Direct visualization of diverticula	Locates esophageal diverticula

PRIMARY NURSING DIAGNOSIS

DIAGNOSIS. Risk for aspiration as evidenced by choking, gagging, dysphagia, and/or regurgitation

OUTCOMES. Knowledge: Disease process; Respiratory status: Ventilation; Nutritional status: Food and fluid intake; Oral health; Self-care: Eating

INTERVENTIONS. Airway suctioning; Surveillance; Respiratory monitoring; Feeding; Positioning

PLANNING AND IMPLEMENTATION

Collaborative

MEDICAL. When diverticula are symptomatic, they do not require treatment. When achalasia is implicated, pharmacologic therapy may be chosen as the first option. It can also be treated with pneumatic dilation or botulinum toxin injection (onabotulinumtoxinA, or Botox) into the lower esophageal sphincter during endoscopy. Assess the effects of treatments because the drugs may worsen the diverticula by relaxing an already weakened esophageal musculature.

SURGICAL. Surgical techniques are rapidly changing as minimally invasive endoscopic treatments and laparoscopic approaches become more common. Endoscopic treatment is typically completed for relief of symptoms. Laparoscopy to repair diverticula has the lowest complication rates when performed by an experienced surgeon and lower morbidity because of no thoracotomy incisions, but complications have been reported in as many as 20% of the cases. The choice of surgical option (less or more invasive) is controversial. More invasive procedures such as an esophagomyotomy (incision into the esophageal musculature) and diverticulectomy (surgical removal of the diverticulum) may be warranted, particularly for patients with Zenker diverticulum. A cricopharyngeal myotomy, a procedure in which the surgeon divides the cricopharyngeal muscle, involves cutting the muscle to make it incompetent so that when the individual swallows, the muscle relaxes and allows food to pass through. Postoperative care is determined by the incisional approach. With a cervical approach, a drain is commonly inserted in the neck to diminish edema at the incisional site. A chest incision (thoracic approach) requires care associated with a thoracotomy. Postoperative care is directed at monitoring the patency of the airway, maintaining pulmonary ventilation by chest drainage with chest tubes, monitoring neck drainage with either gravity drainage or low suction, and preventing aspiration.

Pharmacologic Highlights

Medication or Drug Class	Dosage	Description	Rationale
Onabotulinum-toxinA (Botox)	80–100 units, 20–25 units in each of four quadrants	Neuromuscular blocking agent	Inhibits acetylcholine, relaxes smooth muscles, and reduces lower esophageal sphincter resting pressure
Antacids	Varies with drug	Amphojel, AlternaGEL, Gelusil, Maalox, Mylanta	Neutralize gastric acid and reduce symptoms, especially with midesophageal or epiphrenic diverticula, because they usually do not produce complications

Independent

Care focuses on maintaining a patent airway, preventing aspiration of regurgitated food and mucus, providing emotional support, and providing adequate nutrition. Implement interventions to maintain airway patency if there is any suspicion it is at risk. Use the jaw thrust or chin lift or insert an oral or nasal airway. Prevent aspiration of regurgitated food and mucus by positioning the patient carefully, with the patient's head elevated or turned to one side. Recommend that the patient sleep with the head elevated (using pillows or bed blocks) to reduce esophageal reflux and nocturnal choking. Show the patient how to use massage to empty any visible outpouching to the neck to prevent aspiration during sleep.

Education, rather than medical or surgical intervention, may become the treatment of choice. Provide the patient with information on lifestyle changes to reduce symptoms. Teach appropriate nutrition. Advise the patient to explore textures and quantities of foods to determine which cause the least discomfort. Recommend that the patient consider bland, semisoft and soft foods, and advise adding fiber to the diet to stimulate peristalsis of the gastrointestinal (GI) system, reducing lower GI tract pressure on the esophagus. Recommend food supplements between meals to prevent weight loss and malnourishment, and advise the patient to drink fluids intermittently with meals to aid in propulsion of the food bolus through the esophagus. Teach the patient to concentrate on the act of eating to maximize each phase of the process of ingesting food and fluids, moistening the mouth before eating to facilitate chewing and swallowing. Explain how to use Valsalva maneuver to increase esophageal pressure, thus facilitating food bolus movement beyond the hypopharyngeal sphincter. Recommend that the patient sit upright when eating or drinking to facilitate gravitational flow through the esophagus, and advise remaining upright for at least 2 hours after eating.

Advise taking adequate fluids (> 15 mL) with medications to prevent chemical esophageal irritation. Recommend eliminating oral drugs immediately before bedtime to decrease the risk of deposits in diverticula that can create ulceration. Advise the patient to avoid food and fluids within 3 to 4 hours of bedtime to reduce nocturnal symptoms.

Evidence-Based Practice and Health Policy

Crawley, B., Dehom, S., Tamares, S., Marghalani, A., Ongkasuwan, J., Reder, L., Ivey, C., Amin, M., Fritz, M., Pitman, M., Tulunay-Ugur, O., & Weissbrod, P. (2019). Adverse events after rigid and flexible endoscopic repair of Zenker's diverticula: A systematic review and meta-analysis. *Otolaryngology–Head and Neck Surgery, 161,* 388–400.

- The authors aimed to determine adverse events after endoscopic flexible versus endoscopic rigid cricopharyngeal myotomy for treatment of Zenker diverticulum. They completed a structured literature search, seeking only studies that provided data for a minimum of 10 adults patients who had undergone treatment. Additional studies were identified from review citations and a by-hand search of manuscripts referencing Zenker diverticulum. They applied Methodological Index for Non-randomized Studies (MINORS) criteria to assess study quality, including all reported adverse events, recurrences, follow-up, and operative times.
- In total, 115 studies were included, divided into three different forms of repair (rigid endoscopic stapler repair, rigid laser repair, and repair with other rigid endoscopic instruments). Mortality, infection, and perforation were not significantly more likely in either the rigid or the flexible group, but bleeding and recurrence were more likely after flexible endoscopic techniques. Dental injury and vocal fold palsy were reported rarely in the rigid endoscopic groups. The authors concluded that adverse events are rare, and the flexible approach minimized exposure limitations.

DOCUMENTATION GUIDELINES

- Physical findings: Rate and depth of respirations; breath sounds; presence of dysphagia, choking, or regurgitation
- Changes (improvement or lack of improvement) of symptoms
- Halitosis, dysphagia, regurgitation, gurgling with swallowing, coughing, persistence of a bad taste in the mouth
- Complications: Airway swelling, fever, productive cough, respiratory distress, weight loss, poor wound healing, wound infection

DISCHARGE AND HOME HEALTHCARE GUIDELINES

PATIENT TEACHING. Teach the patient methods to reduce symptoms, prevent malnutrition and weight loss, and improve sleep and rest. Make sure the patient understands the dosage, route, action and purpose, side effects, and contraindications of the prescribed medications. Explain the potential for aspiration, respiratory impairment, weight loss or malnourishment, and sleep deprivation. Remind the patient to see the physician if symptoms of esophageal diverticula return or worsen.

Fat Embolism

DRG Category:	175
Mean LOS:	5.1 days
Description:	MEDICAL: Pulmonary Embolism With Major Complication or Comorbidity or Acute Cor Pulmonale

An embolism is any undissolved mass that travels in the circulation and occludes a blood vessel. A fat embolism, which is an unusual complication from a traumatic injury, occurs when fat droplets enter the circulation and lodge in small vessels and capillaries, particularly in the lung and brain. Two theories exist that explain the pathophysiology of fat emboli: the mechanical theory and the biochemical theory. The mechanical theory states that trauma disrupts fat cells and tears veins in the bone marrow at the site of a fracture. Fat droplets enter the circulation because of increased pressure of the interstitium at the area of injury. The biochemical theory states that a stress-related release of catecholamines after trauma mobilizes fat molecules from a tissue. These molecules group into fat droplets and eventually obstruct the circulation through an inflammatory response and the release of local toxic mediators. In addition, free fatty acids destroy pulmonary endothelium, increase capillary permeability in the lungs, and lead to pulmonary edema.

The result of either theory is the accumulation of fat droplets that are too large to pass easily through small capillaries, where they lodge and break apart into fatty acids, which are toxic to lung tissues, the capillary endothelium, and surfactant. Pulmonary hypertension, alveolar collapse, and even noncardiac pulmonary edema follow. If the patient has a patent foramen ovale (an opening in the wall between the right and left atria), the embolus may pass into the systemic circulation and affect the brain or kidneys. Mortality rates are approximately 10% to 20%. Patients with increased age, underlying medical conditions, and poor physiological reserves have poorer health outcomes than other patients.

CAUSES

Fat embolism is associated with severe traumatic injury with accompanying long-bone (tibial or femoral) or pelvic fractures and generally occurs within 3 days of the fracture. It has also been reported in patients with severe burns, head injury, or severely compromised circulation. Nontraumatic disease states that have occasionally been associated with fat embolism include acute pancreatitis, alcoholism, diabetes mellitus, sickle cell disease, and osteomyelitis. Procedures such as liposuction, orthopedic surgery, joint replacement, abdominal surgery, and cardiac massage (closed chest) are also associated with fat embolism. It is also associated with parenteral lipid infusion and corticoid administration. Fat embolisms are the most common nonthrombotic cause of pulmonary emboli.

GENETIC CONSIDERATIONS

No clear genetic contributions to susceptibility have been defined.

SEX AND LIFE SPAN CONSIDERATIONS

Many patients who develop the disorder are under age 30 years and have severe associated traumatic injuries. Males are more likely than females to have a significant traumatic injury. Older adults have a poorer outcome than their younger counterparts.

HEALTH DISPARITIES AND SEXUAL/GENDER MINORITY HEALTH

Ethnicity, race, and sexual/gender minority status have no known effect on the risk for fat embolism.

GLOBAL HEALTH CONSIDERATIONS

While no global data are available, developed countries have a continuing problem with motor vehicle crashes leading to significant traumatic injuries. The surgeries that present risks for fat emboli are more common in developed countries than in developing countries. Traffic crashes are a growing problem in developing countries as more vehicles crowd roads that are not always well constructed. Around the world, fat emboli are common occurrences following trauma.

◼ ASSESSMENT

HISTORY. Elicit a history of recent traumatic injury, particularly blunt trauma leading to long-bone or pelvic fractures. In most patients, the injury is obvious because of the presence of wounds, fractures, casts, or traction devices. Some patients exhibit changes in mental status such as restlessness, delirium, or drowsiness progressing to coma and even seizures. Others complain of fever, anxiety, unexplained discomfort, or respiratory distress (shortness of breath, cough).

Fat embolization may be classified into three distinct forms based on the patient's progression of symptoms: subclinical, classic, and fulminant. Approximately half of patients with uncomplicated fractures have subclinical fat emboli, which resolve spontaneously within a few days. Patients with the classic form generally have a latent period of 1 to 2 days, followed by the development of symptoms that include mental status changes, shortness of breath, fever, tachycardia, and petechiae. The fulminant form is characterized by an early onset of neurological and respiratory deterioration as well as the onset of signs of right ventricular failure (distended neck veins, liver congestion, peripheral edema). A rapid onset of neurological deterioration in patients who sustained severe injuries and multiple fractures but who were initially conscious suggests a fat embolism.

PHYSICAL EXAMINATION. The most common symptoms are related to cardiopulmonary function and include **tachycardia, dyspnea, fever**, and **signs of hypoxemia**, including restlessness, agitation, confusion, or even stupor. Some patients may have a seizure. Note that neurological changes usually occur 6 to 12 hours before respiratory system changes and rarely without impending respiratory involvement.

Inspect the patient's skin for petechiae, a classic sign that appears 1 to 2 days after injury in more than half of patients with fat embolism. Petechiae are of short duration, last only 4 to 6 hours, and appear most commonly on the neck, upper trunk, conjunctivae, or retina. An ophthalmic examination may reveal fat globules in the retinal vessels. Approximately half of the patients who display neurological symptoms also develop microinfarcts of the retina. When auscultating the patient's heart and lungs, a rapid heart rate and respiratory rate with rales, rhonchi, and possibly a pleural friction rub are usually heard.

PSYCHOSOCIAL. Because fat embolism is a complication of other disease processes or traumatic injuries, the addition of another life-threatening complication could be the final breaking point for the family or significant others involved. Evaluate the patient's social network to determine what support is available during the acute illness.

Diagnostic Highlights

Test	Normal Result	Abnormality With Condition	Explanation
Platelet count	150,000–450,000/mm³	Decreased < 15,000 mm³	Platelets are used up in the clotting process
Pao₂	80–95 mm Hg	< 60 mm Hg	Hypoxemia occurs because of problems with ventilation and perfusion due to obstruction of pulmonary circulation
Electrocardiogram	Normal rate; rhythm; and P, Q, R, S, and T waves	Tachycardia, right bundle branch block, depressed ST segments	Obstruction of the pulmonary circulation leads to right heart strain

Other Tests: Increased serum lipase, fat in the urine, fibrinogen, complete blood count, patchy infiltrates on chest x-ray, ventilation perfusion scans, computed tomography and magnetic resonance imaging, pulse oximetry to detect arterial oxygen saturation, transesophageal echocardiography, calcium levels, arterial blood gas analysis

PRIMARY NURSING DIAGNOSIS

DIAGNOSIS. Impaired gas exchange related to pulmonary capillary inflammation and arteriovenous shunting as evidenced by dyspnea, restlessness, and/or agitation

OUTCOMES. Respiratory status: Gas exchange; Respiratory status: Ventilation; Symptom control; Symptom severity; Comfort level

INTERVENTIONS. Airway management; Anxiety reduction; Oxygen therapy; Airway suctioning; Airway insertion and stabilization; Cough enhancement; Mechanical ventilation: Invasive and noninvasive; Positioning; Respiratory monitoring

PLANNING AND IMPLEMENTATION

Collaborative

SUPPORT FOR AIRWAY, BREATHING, AND CIRCULATION. Management of the patient with severe symptoms of fat emboli almost always requires support of the patient's airway and breathing with supplemental oxygen, airway pressure release ventilation, and possibly endotracheal intubation and mechanical ventilation. Patients with a deteriorating mental status, dropping arterial oxygen saturations, and decreasing levels of Pao₂ (less than 50 mm Hg) may need positive pressure ventilation with positive end-expiratory pressure and possibly pressure control ventilation. Serial monitoring with pulse oximetry is important. Tachycardia may resolve with treatment of hypoxemia, but if hypotension and circulatory depression occur, fluid resuscitation, blood transfusion, and vasoactive medications may be required. However, volume overload may worsen hypoxemia, so volume is administered judiciously, and pulmonary artery catheterization may be necessary.

The nurse and trauma surgeon or orthopedist work together to prevent fat emboli whenever possible by encouraging adequate gas exchange; this entails clearing secretions and promoting good ventilation. Discuss the patient's activity restrictions with the physician. To limit the effects of immobilization, turn the patient frequently and, when the patient is ready, get the patient out of bed. If the injuries allow, encourage dangling or ambulation. Maintain the patient's hydration by IV or enteral fluids, as prescribed, and provide prophylaxis for deep venous thrombosis and stress-related gastrointestinal bleeding. Hematological laboratory measures are followed carefully to determine the need for blood component therapy.

PHARMACOLOGIC. Diuretics may be needed if pulmonary edema develops. Many experts recommend prophylactic use of corticosteroids, particularly methylprednisolone, for patients at high risk for fat emboli, but they seem less effective after fat emboli develop. Some experts suggest that the introduction of steroids may help treat pulmonary manifestations by decreasing the inflammatory response of the pulmonary capillaries as well as by stabilizing lysosomal and capillary membranes; corticosteroid use is not supported by randomized controlled trials. Analgesics are also necessary to manage the pain of the traumatic injury.

The best treatment of fat emboli is preventing their occurrence. Surgical stabilization of extremity fractures to reduce bone movement probably minimizes the release of fatty products from the bone marrow. The location of the fracture determines whether the surgeon uses internal or external fixation techniques.

Pharmacologic Highlights

General Comments: Medications provide supportive management rather than curative measures.

Medication or Drug Class	Dosage	Description	Rationale
Corticosteroids, often methylprednisolone	Varies with drug	Anti-inflammatories	Decrease inflammatory response of pulmonary capillaries; stabilize lysosomal and capillary membranes; use is controversial

Other Drugs: Analgesics are also necessary to manage the pain of the traumatic injury.

Independent

The highest priority is maintaining the airway and breathing to reduce the effects of hypoxemia. Ongoing monitoring of the pulmonary system is essential, coupled with interventions such as suctioning and placement of an oral airway. Serial assessments of the heart rate and blood pressure are important to ongoing assessment of the circulatory system. If the cardiopulmonary system becomes compromised (ongoing hypoxemia, unresolved tachycardia, persistent hypotension), further consultation with the trauma service is essential.

Patients need to be active participants in their care. Before they undergo activity or coughing and deep-breathing exercises, make sure that the patient's pain is controlled. In addition to administering prescribed medications, explore nonpharmacologic alternatives to pain management, such as diversionary activities and guided imagery.

The patient's and family's level of anxiety is apt to be exacerbated by the critical care environment. Explain all the equipment and answer questions honestly and thoroughly. If the patient has to undergo endotracheal intubation, provide a method for communication, such as a magic slate or point board. Work with the family to allow as much visitation as the patient's condition allows. Remember that although young people in their late teens often appear to be adults, they often regress during a serious illness and need a great deal of support from their parents and significant others.

Evidence-Based Practice and Health Policy

Tsitsikas, D., Bristowe, J., & Abukar, J. (2020). Fat embolism syndrome in sickle cell disease. *Journal of Clinical Medicine, 9,* 3601–3616.

• Fat embolism syndrome is a severe complication of sickle cell disease that results from bone marrow necrosis. It is associated with high mortality rates, and survivors often have severe neurological consequences. Red blood cell exchanges and transfusions improve mortality. The authors reviewed the cases of eight patients and also discussed the current literature on the subject.

• All eight patients developed respiratory failure and neurological involvement, and there was a 100-fold increase of the serum ferritin from baseline. All received either red cell exchange transfusion, simple blood transfusion, or therapeutic plasma exchange. Two patients died, two patients suffered severe neurological impairment, and one had mild neurological impairment on discharge. One-third of the patients made a complete recovery. Immediate red cell exchange transfusion can be life-saving and should be instituted as soon as fat embolism syndrome is suspected.

DOCUMENTATION GUIDELINES

• Physical responses: Vital signs, cardiopulmonary assessment, neurological assessment, mental status, presence or absence of petechiae
• Emotional response: Coping strategies, mood, affect, flexibility, cooperation
• Presence of complications: Fever, infection, skin breakdown, loss of consciousness
• Ongoing monitoring: Pulse oximetry or arterial blood gases results that are abnormal, abnormal laboratory findings
• Response to treatment: Mechanical ventilation, response to fluid replacement and medications, response to supplemental oxygen

DISCHARGE AND HOME HEALTHCARE GUIDELINES

A patient who has recovered from the underlying disease process or injury is no longer at risk for developing fat embolism and can be discharged. Teach the patient about any medications and treatments needed before the patient leaves the hospital. Explain the disease process and how it occurred, and note that recurrence is doubtful unless the patient experiences another traumatic injury. Arrange for any follow-up care with the primary healthcare provider.

Fetopelvic Disproportion

DRG Category:	806
Mean LOS:	2.7 days
Description:	MEDICAL: Vaginal Delivery Without Sterilization or Dilation & Curettage With Complication or Comorbidity

Fetopelvic disproportion (FPD), also known as *cephalopelvic disproportion* (CPD), refers to the inability of the fetal head to pass through the parental pelvis; it occurs in 1% to 3% of all primigravidas. The size differential can be related to pelvic capacity or fetal factors. In absolute FPD, the fetal head is too large for the parental pelvis so that vaginal birth cannot be safely achieved, and cesarean delivery is required. Normally, the fetus delivers in the occiput-anterior position, assuming a flexed attitude, and with a suboccipitobregmatic diameter of 9.5 cm. If the fetal head takes other positions (occiput-posterior, brow), the delivering diameter of the head is larger, with a size of 11.5 cm and 13.5 cm, respectively. Most fetuses presenting with this larger diameter will not fit through the parental pelvis.

Any contraction of the pelvis will impede the passage of the fetus through the birth canal. The parental pelvis can be contracted at the inlet (defined as a diagonal conjugate of < 11.5 cm), at mid-pelvis (defined as < 15.5 cm; the sum of the interischial spinous and posterior sagittal diameters of the midpelvis), or at the pelvic outlet (defined as an interischial tuberous diameter of 8 cm or less). In relative FPD, the fetus may be delivered vaginally if a favorable combination of other factors can be achieved, including efficient uterine contractions; favorable fetal attitude, presentation, and position; maximization of parental pelvic diameters; adequate molding of the fetal head; adequate expulsive efforts by the patient; and adequate stretching of parental soft tissues.

FPD can lead to prolonged labor, with delayed engagement of the fetal head in the pelvis and increased risk of umbilical cord prolapse. Prolonged labor can place the patient at risk for complications such as dysfunctional uterine contractions, fluid and electrolyte imbalance, exhaustion, hypoglycemia, uterine rupture, need for operative delivery, and postpartum hemorrhage. Risks to the fetus include hypoxia, hypoglycemia, acidemia, and infection. Vaginal delivery may be difficult in these patients, with increased risk of parental vaginal, cervical, and perineal lacerations; fractured sacrum or coccyx; fetal birth asphyxia; shoulder dystocia (difficult delivery because of fetal shoulder position); and traumatic birth injuries, especially cervical spine, nerve, clavicle, and cranial injuries. Some patients who experience FPD that resulted in a cesarean delivery with one infant can deliver a subsequent infant vaginally.

CAUSES

The cause of FPD can be attributed to both parental and fetal factors. Parental factors include inability of the pelvic soft tissues to stretch adequately and inadequate diameters of the parental bony pelvis. Contractures of the parental pelvis may occur in one or more diameters of the pelvic inlet, midpelvis, or pelvic outlet. Fetal macrosomia (fetal weight > 4,000 g), incomplete flexion of the fetal head onto the chest, occiput-posterior or transverse fetal position, and inability of the fetal head to mold to the parental pelvis all contribute to the syndrome. Studies show that pregnant persons with body mass indices in the obese range are more predisposed to cesarean deliveries related to dystocia, large for gestational age (LGA) fetuses, and fetal macrosomia, which is consistent with FPD.

GENETIC CONSIDERATIONS

Dystocia is considered a complex disorder with both genetic and environmental components. Heritability for dystocia has been estimated at 28%, and six loci have been implicated for increased risk, but more research is needed to confirm these findings. Predictors for FPD, such as maternal height and shoe size, are quantitative genetic traits that are influenced by many genes. Other risk factors with genetic contributions include paternal height and large head-to-height ratios in both parents.

SEX AND LIFE SPAN CONSIDERATIONS

Any woman of childbearing age may experience FPD, although women who have already delivered one or more infants vaginally have less risk of FPD than those having their first vaginal delivery. Teenagers under the age of 18 years have an increased risk of FPD because their pelvic growth may not be fully completed.

HEALTH DISPARITIES AND SEXUAL/GENDER MINORITY HEALTH

Ethnicity, race, and sexual/gender minority status have no known effect on the risk for FPD.

GLOBAL HEALTH CONSIDERATIONS

The World Health Organization (WHO) recommends that the optimal cesarean section rate is 15% of deliveries. Those countries with cesarean rates under 10% are underusing the technique. The U.S. national cesarean section rate is over 30%, which is considered by the WHO as overuse of the technique. There has been a striking increase in cesarean sections in medium- and high-income countries around the world, which most experts agree increases complications for both mothers and babies. Parental and perinatal deaths following caesarean sections are disproportionately high in low- and middle-income countries.

☀ ASSESSMENT

HISTORY. Patients may have a family history of fetal macrosomia or pelvic contractures. Any personal history of rickets, scoliosis, pelvic fracture, or excessive weight gain during pregnancy should also be noted. Gestational diabetes, which may contribute to fetal macrosomia, may be present. Ask the patient about prior deliveries to ascertain whether the patient has delivered an infant vaginally before.

PHYSICAL EXAMINATION. Determine the pelvic type of the patient. Android and platypelloid pelvic classifications are not favorable for a vaginal birth; the gynecoid and anthropoid pelvis classifications are present in 75% of all women and are favorable for a vaginal birth. Perform an internal examination; the following findings indicate a contracted pelvis and a potential for FPD to occur if the patient becomes pregnant: ability to touch the sacral promontory with the index finger; significant convergence of the side walls; forward inclination of a straight sacrum; sharp ischial spines with a narrow interspinous diameter; and a narrow suprapubic arch.

Common assessment findings with FPD during labor include **delayed engagement of the fetal head, lack of progress in cervical effacement,** and **dilation in the presence of adequate uterine contractions.** If FPD is suspected during labor, physical assessment should include pelvic size and shape; fetal presentation, position, attitude, and presence of molding or caput succedaneum of the fetal head (swelling on the presenting part of the fetal head during labor); fetal activity level; maternal bladder distention and presence of stool in rectum; duration, frequency, and strength of contractions; effacement and dilation of the cervix; and descent of the fetal head in relation to the patient's ischial spines. If fetal hypoxia or hypoglycemia occurs, loss of fetal heart rate variability, late decelerations, or fetal bradycardia may be seen on the electronic fetal monitor. Fetal scalp stimulation may fail to elicit heart rate acceleration, and fetal capillary blood pH obtained by scalp sampling may indicate acidosis.

PSYCHOSOCIAL. Assess the patient and partner (or other labor support people present) for the ability to cope with the difficult labor and ability to maintain a positive self-concept and role performance. Assess the presence of anxiety or fear related to the patient's or baby's well-being or to medical interventions, such as forceps or vacuum extractor use or cesarean delivery. Answer all questions honestly and explain all procedures to the patient and support persons. Feelings of exhaustion, disappointment, or failure are common during a difficult labor and birth.

Diagnostic Highlights

General Comments: FPD cannot be diagnosed except in rare cases without allowing labor to proceed for several hours. In labor, the pubic symphysis and other pelvic joints gain mobility under the influence of high levels of relaxin and other hormones. Therefore, evidence of lack of progressive dilation and fetal descent in labor is usually considered more important than pelvic measurement in diagnosing FPD. During the second stage of labor, if there is progress in fetal descent, cesarean sections can be delayed up to 4 hours if there are no other fetal or parental implications.

Test	Normal Result	Abnormality With Condition	Explanation
Clinical pelvimetry	Diagonal conjugate >11.5 cm; outlet > 8 cm	Diagonal conjugate < 11.5 cm; outlet < 8 cm	An adequate pelvic inlet and outlet are needed for a vaginal delivery

PRIMARY NURSING DIAGNOSIS

DIAGNOSIS. Risk for injury of mother or fetus as evidenced by maternal bleeding, fetal hypoxemia, and/or fetal demise

OUTCOMES. Risk control; Risk detection; Fetal status: Intrapartum; Maternal status: Intrapartum; Maternal status: Postpartum

INTERVENTIONS. Intrapartal care: High-risk delivery; Electronic fetal monitoring: Intrapartum

PLANNING AND IMPLEMENTATION
Collaborative
MEDICAL. Medical management of FPD can include the use of Pitocin to induce or augment labor contractions. Assisting the patient into a squatting position during pushing helps to enlarge the pelvis to allow passage of the head. Manual or forceps rotation of the fetus into an occiput-anterior position, and vaginal delivery assisted by outlet forceps or vacuum extractor may be required. The cutting of a midline or mediolateral episiotomy is often necessary. If shoulder dystocia occurs, the McRoberts maneuver (extreme flexion of the mother's legs at the hips) and firm suprapubic pressure may accomplish delivery. In some cases, intentional fracture of the infant's clavicle is used to accomplish delivery in the presence of severe shoulder dystocia. When vaginal delivery appears to be impossible or likely to be very traumatic, cesarean delivery is indicated.

Labor patients using analgesia or anesthesia require careful monitoring. The healthcare provider may allow the epidural to wear off to allow the patient to push. For patients using narcotic analgesics, monitor pulse, blood pressure, and respirations. Watch for signs of respiratory depression. Because IV narcotics readily cross the placenta, observe the fetal heart rate; often, a temporary loss of variability is seen. For patients using regional anesthesia, monitor pulse, blood pressure, and respirations. Check the patient's blood pressure every 1 to 5 minutes for 15 minutes after the epidural or spinal bolus dosage and then every 30 minutes. Watch for lowered blood pressure.

Pharmacologic Highlights

Medication or Drug Class	Dosage	Description	Rationale
Opioid analgesics; anesthetics	Varies with drug, usually given IV push or via epidural	Pain relievers	Labor is difficult and prolonged; often, back pain is increased owing to the position of the fetus; episiotomy repair and forceps or vacuum extraction require anesthesia
Oxytocin (Pitocin)	Mix 10 units in 500 mL of IV solution, begin infusion at 1 mU/min; increase 1–2 mU/min q 15–30 min until adequate labor is established	Oxytocic	Appropriate to induce labor or to give the patient a trial labor; should be discontinued upon a definitive diagnosis of FPD, requiring a cesarean section

Independent
Have the laboring patient change positions frequently (approximately every half hour) to encourage movement of the fetal head into a favorable position for delivery. Sitting, squatting, positioning on hands and knees, or side lying (alternating sides) may be used. Avoid supine positioning. To encourage rotation of a fetus from a posterior position, suggest lying on the same side as the fetal limbs or position the patient on hands and knees. Pelvic rocking exercises may be helpful. Encourage periods of ambulation as long as the membranes are not ruptured or the fetal head is well applied to the cervix.

Keeping the bladder and rectum empty allows maximum pelvic space for the descent of the fetal head. Fluid and caloric intake should be attended to during labor. In some delivery settings, however, patients may receive IV solutions for electrolyte, fluid, and/or glucose intake. In other settings, ice chips, clear liquids, or a light diet may be encouraged.

In the second stage of labor, instruct the laboring patient to use the diaphragm and abdominal muscles to bear down during contractions. Help the patient find a comfortable and effective position for pushing, such as supported squatting, semi-sitting, side lying, or sitting upright in bed or on a chair, birthing stool, or commode. Perineal massage during pushing will help decrease the likelihood of an episiotomy or decrease the degree of episiotomy needed.

Provide encouragement of the patient's coping strategies and assistance with pain management. Nonpharmacologic aids that can be offered include breathing techniques, massage, sacral counterpressure, rocking chair, application of heat or cold, visualization or relaxation techniques, therapeutic touch, music, showering or bathing, companionship, and encouragement. Provide emotional support; families are often unprepared to deal with an unplanned, unwanted cesarean birth.

Evidence-Based Practice and Health Policy

Mendez-Dominguez, N., Vazquez-Vasquez, G., Lavida-Molina, H., Inurreta-Diaz, M., Fajardo-Ruiz, L., & Azcorra, H. (2020). Cephalopelvic disproportion as primary diagnosis for cesarean section: Role of neonatal birthweight in relation to maternal height at a hospital in Merida, Mexico. *American Journal of Human Biology, 33,* e1–e7.

- The authors aimed to analyze the association between newborn and maternal characteristics and the risk for cesarean section due to CPD and non-CPD causes. They analyzed a sample of 3,453 single term infants and their mothers. Variables included mode of delivery, maternal height and weight, number of previous vaginal deliveries, and newborn data.
- Mothers who had cesarean section due to CPD weighed more at the end of their pregnancy and were shorter. Maternal age and weight increased the risk for having cesarean section, and the number of previous vaginal deliveries reduced the risk for experiencing cesarean due to CPD. The relative risk was higher when considering both neonatal birth weight and maternal height index. Cephalopelvic disproportion is the result of the interrelation of the variables of maternal height, weight, and fetal size, not just fetal size. Patients should be advised to maintain healthy weight gain in pregnancy and avoid gaining too much weight, which could increase the risk of CPD in childbirth.

DOCUMENTATION GUIDELINES

- Progress in labor: Cervical effacement and dilation, station of fetal head, presence of molding or caput, contraction pattern
- Factors contributing to FPD: Pelvic size and shape; fetal presentation, position, and attitude; maternal position; bladder and bowel fullness; duration, frequency, and strength of contractions
- Indicators of fetal well-being: Fetal baseline heart rate, variability, presence of accelerations and decelerations; fetal activity level; response to scalp stimulation
- Indicators of maternal well-being: Tolerability of labor pain, effectiveness of coping strategies, presence of support people, indicators of psychological status, vital signs

DISCHARGE AND HOME HEALTHCARE GUIDELINES

BIRTH INJURIES. Be sure the patient understands the nature of and care of any birth injuries sustained by the infant. Ensure that plans for follow-up care can be carried out by the family.

POSTPARTUM SELF-CARE. Review use of any pain medication prescribed as well as nonpharmacologic comfort measures for episiotomy, lacerations, and hemorrhoid care. Instruct the patient to report any increase in perineal or uterine pain, foul odor, fever or flu-like symptoms, or vaginal bleeding that is heavier than a menstrual period. Patients with longer labors have an increased risk for postpartum infection. Sadness or mood swings that persist beyond 4 weeks should be reported to the physician.

Fibrocystic Breast Condition

DRG Category: 601
Mean LOS: 3.0 days
Description: MEDICAL: Non-Malignant Breast Disorders Without Complication or Comorbidity or Major Complication or Comorbidity

Fibrocystic breast condition (sometimes called fibrocystic complex) is the most common type of benign breast disorder. It was previously referred to as fibrocystic breast disease. Fibrocystic breast condition is a catchall diagnosis used to describe the presence of multiple, often painful, benign breast nodules. These breast nodules vary in size and blend into surrounding breast tissue. However, the histological changes responsible for the breast nodules could belong to one of several different categories.

The College of American Pathologists has categorized the types of fibrocystic breast condition according to the associated increased risk for subsequent invasive breast cancer and the particular histological (microscopic) change that is present: no increased risk (nonproliferative changes, including microcysts, adenosis, mild hyperplasia, fibroadenoma, fibrosis, duct, apocrine metaplasia, and gross cysts); slightly increased risk (relative risk, 1.5 to 2; proliferative changes without atypia, including moderate hyperplasia and papilloma); moderately increased risk (relative risk, 4 to 5; proliferative changes with atypia or atypical hyperplasia); and significantly increased risk (relative risk, 8 to 10; ductal and lobular carcinoma in situ). A complication of fibrocystic breast condition is atypical hyperplasia, but fibrocystic breast disease is usually not associated with breast cancer.

CAUSES

The monthly variations in the circulating levels of estrogen and progesterone are thought to account for most fibrocystic breast changes. Although the exact contribution of each hormone is not well understood, it is believed that an excess amount of estrogen over progesterone results in edema of the breast tissue. At the onset of menses, hormone levels decrease, and the fluid responsible for the breast edema is removed by the lymphatic system. All the fluid in the breast may not be removed; eventually, the fluid accumulates in the small glands and ducts of the breast, allowing cyst formation.

GENETIC CONSIDERATIONS

Having a family history of cyst formation is common among women with fibrocystic breast disease. It is thought that changes in estrogen levels, which could be influenced by genetics, may play a role in cyst formation.

SEX AND LIFE SPAN CONSIDERATIONS

Fibrocystic changes that cause premenstrual pain, tenderness, and increased tissue density usually begin when a woman reaches her mid-20s to early 30s. Cysts occur most frequently in women in their 30s, 40s, and early 50s. Advanced stages can occur during the mid- to late 40s. Symptoms should resolve and cysts should disappear once menopause is complete. However, symptoms may persist in women who are taking hormone replacement therapy for menopausal discomfort. Breast cysts are uncommon in women who are 5 years postmenopause and are not undergoing hormone replacement therapy. Therefore, the possibility of a more serious breast problem in any woman who is more than 5 years postmenopause and who presents with a breast mass should be carefully investigated.

HEALTH DISPARITIES AND SEXUAL/GENDER MINORITY HEALTH

Ethnicity, race, and sexual/gender minority status have no known effect on the risk for fibrocystic breast condition.

GLOBAL HEALTH CONSIDERATIONS

Limited data are available internationally. Some evidence exists that rates among Japanese women are lower than other groups of women because they consume a diet high in iodine from seafood intake.

ASSESSMENT

HISTORY. Elicit a reproductive history. Patients with a fibrocystic breast condition may have a history of spontaneous abortion, shortened menstrual cycles, early menarche, and late menopause. Patients are frequently nulliparous and have not taken oral contraceptives. Cyclic, premenstrual breast pain and tenderness that last about a week are the most common symptoms. With time, the severity of the breast pain increases, and onset occurs 2 to 3 weeks before menstruation. In advanced cases, the breast pain can be constant rather than cyclic.

Fibrocystic breast changes usually occur bilaterally and in the upper outer quadrant of the breast. A patient may appear with gross nodularity or with one or more defined lumps in the breast. The abnormality may be described as a hardness or a thickening in the breast. The areas are usually tender and change in size relative to the menstrual cycle (becoming more pronounced before menstruation and decreasing or disappearing by day 4 or 5 of the cycle). Approximately 50% of patients have repeated episodes of breast cysts.

PHYSICAL EXAMINATION. The most common symptoms include **premenstrual breast pain and tenderness**. The breasts should be inspected in three positions: with the patient's arms at the side, raised over the head, and on the hips. Instruct the patient to "press in" with the hands on the hips to contract the chest muscles. Compare the breasts for symmetry of color, shape, size, surface characteristics, and direction of nipple. Patients with deep or superficial cysts or masses may have some distention of breast tissue in the affected area, but often, no changes are noted on examination. Dimpling, retraction, scaling, and erosion of breast tissue indicate more serious breast conditions, and none of these disfigurations are usually found in fibrocystic breast condition.

Palpate the breasts in both the sitting and the supine positions. Use the pads of the three middle fingers to palpate all breast tissue, including the tail of Spence, in a systematic fashion. Breast cysts are filled with fluid and feel smooth, mobile, firm, and regular in shape. Superficial cysts are often resilient, whereas deep cysts often feel like a hard lump. Cystic lesions vary from 1 to 4 cm in size, can appear quickly, are often bilateral, and occur in mirror-image locations.

To conclude palpation of the breasts, gently squeeze the nipple. About one-third of patients with advanced fibrocystic change experience nipple discharge. Nipple discharge in benign conditions is characteristically straw-yellowish, greenish, or bluish in color. A bloody nipple discharge often signals the presence of ductal ectasia or intraductal papillomatosis and should be further evaluated.

PSYCHOSOCIAL. Finding a lump or irregularity in the breast is distressing. The almost "overnight" appearance of cysts can make a patient doubt the validity of a recent negative physical examination or mammogram. In addition, the pain associated with advanced fibrocystic changes can be debilitating. Assess the patient's prior experience with breast problems and the patient's use of coping strategies.

Diagnostic Highlights

General Comments: Diagnostic testing is needed to rule out malignancy as well as to confirm the diagnosis. Some 80% of breast lumps are found to be benign.

Test	Normal Result	Abnormality With Condition	Explanation
Fine-needle aspiration (FNA)	Not applicable	Green, brown, or yellow fluid obtained	Confirms diagnosis; bloody fluid is suspicious and should be sent to pathology
Mammogram	No tumor noted	Well-rounded mass with a discrete border noted (cyst); vague, asymmetrical radiodensity (white)	Confirms diagnosis
Ultrasound or magnetic resonance imaging	No abnormalities seen	Will show a fluid-filled mass, which is consistent with a cyst (not a solid mass, which is consistent with a malignant lump)	Confirms diagnosis
Biopsy	Benign	Benign	Performed to diagnose cancer if a lump remains after an FNA

PRIMARY NURSING DIAGNOSIS

DIAGNOSIS. Acute and chronic pain related to edema and nerve irritation as evidenced by self-reports of pain and/or reports of a pinching sensation in the breast

OUTCOMES. Comfort status; Pain control; Pain: Disruptive effects; Knowledge: Acute illness management; Anxiety level

INTERVENTIONS. Analgesic administration; Pain management: Acute and chronic; Medication administration

PLANNING AND IMPLEMENTATION

Collaborative

The physician will attempt an FNA of a breast mass that appears to be cystic. Once the fluid is removed, the cyst collapses and the pain is relieved. Medical therapies may be used in an effort to decrease breast nodularity and relieve breast pain and tenderness.

Pharmacologic Highlights

Medication or Drug Class	Dosage	Description	Rationale
Low-estrogen, high-progesterone oral contraceptives	Estrogen and progesterone dosages vary; 1 tab daily	Estrogen-progesterone combination	Successful in 60%–70% of young women; relieves pain during the first cycle and improves the condition in 6 mo
Danazol (Danocrine)	50–200 mg PO bid or tid, until desired response, then wean	Synthetic androgen (gonadotropin inhibitor)	Effective with 70%–90% of women with repeat episodes
Tamoxifen (Nolvadex)	10 mg PO daily	Antiestrogen	Prescribed for perimenopausal women

Pharmacologic Highlights (continued)

Controversial Therapy: The efficacy of vitamins E and A in reducing the symptoms of fibrocystic changes has been reported with conflicting results. Likewise, the benefit achieved by decreasing or eliminating the intake of methylxanthine (caffeine) has met with controversy. Injection of omega-3 fatty acids is now being investigated as an anti-inflammatory and antiproliferative compound to reduce nonproliferative breast disease. Iodine intake has also been implicated as a protective mechanism to promote breast health. Ibuprofen and acetaminophen usually relieve pain and tenderness.

Independent

Patients who are undergoing evaluation for a breast lump need support and understanding, especially if it is the patient's first experience with the condition. Encourage patients to express their feelings. Explain the purpose and procedure of diagnostic studies and surgical techniques (FNA, excisional biopsy). Encourage patients to request information as to the exact nature of a benign breast lump (such as whether it was nonproliferative or proliferative), and explain the actual risk for malignant breast disease that is associated with the various histological changes.

Advise the patient to wear a brassiere that offers good support. Assess the amount of caffeine and salt present in the diet. Help the patient identify foods that are high in these substances and adopt measures to reduce their dietary intake. Other suggested dietary patterns that may decrease fibrocystic breast are supplementing diet with vitamin B_6 and evening primrose oil, eating organic foods, and avoiding unnecessary chemicals, although clinical trials do not support these recommendations. Some organic topical substances such as soothing oils and poultices may provide pain relief.

Evidence-Based Practice and Health Policy

Balci, F., Uras, C., & Feldman, S. (2020). Clinical factors affecting the therapeutic efficacy of evening primrose oil on mastalgia. *Annals of Surgical Oncology, 27,* 4844–4852.

- Mastalgia (breast tension, discomfort, and pain) is often mild, but up to 10% of women who experience it have severe pain. The authors enrolled 1,015 women and randomized them into one group treated with acetaminophen and one group treated with evening primrose oil, which is thought to restore the fatty acid balance and decrease sensitivity to steroidal hormones or prolactin. They measured the response to treatment through a visual analog scale at baseline, 2 weeks, and 6 weeks.
- Patients who received the evening primrose oil reported higher therapeutic effect than those on acetaminophen. Patients rarely reported side effects such as allergy, anxiety, blurred vision, constipation, and nausea. Hormone replacement therapy, iron deficiency, hypothyroidism, and thyroiditis affected the efficacy of evening primrose oil.

DOCUMENTATION GUIDELINES

- Description of breast lump or any breast abnormality: Location, size, texture; color and amount of any nipple discharge
- Characteristics, location, intensity, duration of breast pain, and whether pain relief is achieved

DISCHARGE AND HOME HEALTHCARE GUIDELINES

CARE OF THE PUNCTURE SITE. Leave the bandage in place for 24 hours; report any pain, warmth, severe ecchymosis, or drainage. Emphasize to the patient that it is not uncommon for more cysts to form.

CARE OF INCISION. Leave the dressing in place until the sutures are removed; clean the site gently with soap and water once sutures are removed; teach the patient how to empty the drains if any are present.

MEDICATIONS. Explain the purpose, action, dosage, desired effects, and side effects of all medications that have been prescribed by the physician.

FOLLOW-UP VISITS. Patients with gross cysts or solid masses in the breast are often seen every 6 months for repeat physical examinations.

EARLY DETECTION PROCEDURES. Assess the patient's knowledge and performance of breast self-examination (BSE); reinforce and teach the BSE technique as indicated. Explain the importance of adhering to the follow-up visit schedule as recommended by the physician and to the American Cancer Society's recommendations for screening mammography: first screening by age 40 years, mammography repeated every 1 to 2 years from ages 40 to 49 years, and mammography repeated every year over age 50 years. The following should be reported to the physician if they occur: new or unusual lumps, redness or puckering of the breast skin, new discharge from the nipples (clear or bloody), indentation or flattening of the nipple.

Gallbladder and Biliary Duct (Biliary System) Cancer

DRG Category:	412
Mean LOS:	6.4 days
Description:	SURGICAL: Cholecystectomy With Common Duct Exploration With Complication or Comorbidity
DRG Category:	415
Mean LOS:	5.9 days
Description:	SURGICAL: Cholecystectomy Except by Laparoscope Without Common Duct Exploration With Complication or Comorbidity
DRG Category:	436
Mean LOS:	4.5 days
Description:	MEDICAL: Malignancy of Hepatobiliary System or Pancreas With Complication or Comorbidity

Gallbladder cancer and biliary duct cancer are relatively rare and account for fewer than 1% of all cancers. The American Cancer Society estimated that in 2021, there will be 11,980 new cases of gallbladder and ductal cancer diagnosed. Of those diagnosed, 4,310 people will die from the disease. The average age of diagnosis is 73 years. Most cancers of the gallbladder and biliary tract are inoperable at the time of diagnosis because of their late diagnosis, and the disease progresses rapidly. At early stages, the 5-year survival rate is 50% to 80%, whereas at stage 4, the 5-year survival rate ranges from 2% to 4%. If the cancer has been found incidentally at the time of a cholecystectomy, longer survival may be possible. More than 75% of gallbladder cancers are nonpapillary adenocarcinomas, and approximately 6% are papillary adenocarcinomas; a small number are squamous cell, adenosquamous cell, mucinous, or small cell carcinomas. Papillary cancers have a better prognosis and grow along the connective tissue and blood vessels; they are not as likely to metastasize to the liver and lymph nodes. Adenocarcinomas occur most frequently at the bifurcation in the common bile duct.

Biliary system cancer is insidious and metastasizes via the lymphatic and blood systems and by direct extension to the liver, pancreas, stomach, and duodenum. Invasion of the gastrointestinal (GI) tract can cause complete obstruction of the extrahepatic bile ducts with intrahepatic biliary dilation and enlargement of the liver. If the tumor is restricted to one hepatic duct, biliary obstruction is incomplete, and jaundice may not be present. Inflammatory disorders such as cholangitis (bile duct inflammation) and peritonitis often obscure an underlying malignancy. Complications include infection, which also often accompanies cancer of the gallbladder, and ulcerative colitis, which may accompany bile duct cancers.

CAUSES

The cause of biliary system cancer is unknown, although a possibility is that gallstones and chronic inflammation cause bile to be released slowly. If the bile contains carcinogens, the gallbladder tissue is exposed to these carcinogens for a longer period of time. Approximately 1% of all cholecystectomy specimens are found to be cancerous. Because of the risk of cancer, even for asymptomatic cholelithiasis, a cholecystectomy is recommended. Primary carcinoma of the gallbladder is rare and is usually associated with cholecystitis. Most biliary cancer is from metastasis, commonly from the head of the pancreas. Risk factors for biliary system cancer include gallstones, porcelain gallbladder (calcification of the gallbladder wall), obesity, aging, choledochal cysts, bile duct abnormality, gallbladder polyps, and exposure to industrial and environmental chemicals. Approximately a third of gallbladder cancers are attributed to obesity.

GENETIC CONSIDERATIONS

Familial clustering is apparent in both of these cancers. A recent study found polymorphisms in the ATP binding cassette subfamily B genes, *ABCB1* and *ABCB4*, increase risk for gallbladder cancer. It is likely that environmental factors also influence the risk for these cancers. Recent genome-wide association study has demonstrated that different risk alleles may stratify by population or ethnic group.

SEX AND LIFE SPAN CONSIDERATIONS

Biliary system cancer occurs most commonly in individuals older than 64 years of age. It occurs two times more frequently in women than in men and is rare prior to age 40 years.

HEALTH DISPARITIES AND SEXUAL/GENDER MINORITY HEALTH

Gallbladder cancer is more prevalent in Native American and Hispanic persons and less so in Black persons; the disease occurs in Native American persons four times more often than in White persons. Barriers to screening in Native American persons are thought to contribute to high rates of gallbladder cancer. Factors include language issues, expense of screening, distance to screening sites, lack of information, and skepticism related to Western medicine (Bea et al., 2020). People with disabilities, such as autism, renal failure, brain injury, ostomy problems, and intellectual disabilities, have significantly lower cancer screening participation than those without disabilities. While little is known about health disparities due to gallbladder and biliary duct cancer in sexual and gender minorities, factors such as poverty, stigma, and discrimination affect access to healthcare and may lead to poorer outcomes. Sexual minority women have higher rates of obesity than heterosexual women (Caceres, Ancheta, et al., 2020), which may contribute to gallbladder and biliary duct cancer risk.

GLOBAL HEALTH CONSIDERATIONS

In those regions where people with mixed ancestries of Indigenous and Spanish heritage live (Colombia, Ecuador, Peru, Bolivia, and Chile), prevalence is higher than in most other regions.

It is also more common in India, Pakistan, and Central Europe than in Western Europe and Scandinavia, which have some of the lowest prevalence rates globally.

ASSESSMENT

HISTORY. Most patients do not have symptoms until late in the disease. Patients may describe symptoms similar to those of cholelithiasis or cholecystitis, because they are similar to symptoms resulting from obstruction and inflammation of the biliary tree. The most common symptom is intermittent to steady pain in the upper right abdomen. Mild pain in the epigastric area may also be reported. GI symptoms are related to the blockage of bile. Patients may complain of anorexia, nausea, vomiting, belching, diarrhea, and weight loss. Diarrhea may be related to steatorrhea, and weight loss can be as much as 14 to 28 pounds. Because of frequent metastasis to the liver and pancreas, patients may describe clinical manifestations of cancer in those organs such as itchy skin, jaundice, and dark urine.

PHYSICAL EXAMINATION. The most common symptom is **right-sided abdominal pain**. Patients with extensive disease may appear thin and malnourished because of anorexia, nausea, or vomiting. Determine if the patient is jaundiced from an enlarging tumor that is pressing on the extrahepatic ducts, but note that jaundice may be delayed if only one main duct is involved. Inspect for skin irritation and skin trauma because of pruritus. If the tumor is of sufficient size, an abdominal mass may be palpated; this mass in the gallbladder area feels hard and is sometimes tender. Intrahepatic metastases are not usually palpable. If the abdomen is distended, individual organs may be difficult to palpate. The liver may be very large and smooth, 5 to 12 cm below the costal margin.

PSYCHOSOCIAL. Because the prognosis of biliary cancer is poor, determine how much the patient understands. Determine the patient's and family's desire for end-of-life care, and support discussions about funeral arrangements, pain management, do-not-resuscitate orders, and hospice care.

Diagnostic Highlights

Test	Normal Result	Abnormality With Condition	Explanation
Computed tomography scan	Normal gallbladder and duct system	Presence of tumor(s)	Detects site and size of tumor(s)
Ultrasonography	Normal gallbladder and duct system	Presence of tumor(s), thick gallbladder wall	Detects site and size of tumor(s)

Other Tests: Tests include serum bilirubin level, urinalysis, serum alkaline phosphatase and aspartate aminotransferase levels, carcinoembryonic antigen and cancer antigen 19-9 (tumor markers), serum mitochondrial antibody test, renal function tests, complete blood count, and liver biopsy. Radiological studies include upper GI barium studies, endoscopic retrograde cholangiopancreatography, cholangiography, magnetic resonance imaging, angiography, cholecystogram, and laparoscopy.

PRIMARY NURSING DIAGNOSIS

DIAGNOSIS. Acute pain related to obstruction of the biliary tree as evidenced by self-reports of pain, facial grimacing, and/or protective behavior

OUTCOMES. Comfort status; Pain control; Pain level; Symptom severity; Knowledge: Disease process

INTERVENTIONS. Analgesic administration; Anxiety reduction; Pain management: Acute; Medication management; Patient-controlled analgesia assistance

☀ PLANNING AND IMPLEMENTATION

Collaborative

MEDICAL. Most medical treatment is aimed at supportive care, such as managing pain and controlling the GI symptoms and the discomforts of jaundice.

SURGICAL. A cholecystectomy is done as soon as possible after the cancer is detected, although the cancer may have been found by doing the surgery for cholecystitis. Surgery may include removal of a section of the liver. Internal radiotherapy, using iridium-129 wire or radium needles, may be combined with biliary drainage. Some surgeons recommend chemotherapy and radiation after surgery. Chemotherapy has not been shown to be particularly effective against this cancer, although the following drugs may be administered: gemcitabine, cisplatin, 5-fluorouracil, capecitabine, and oxaliplatin. External radiation and chemotherapy may be used palliatively for cancer of the bile duct but are not effective against gallbladder cancer. If the tumor is inoperable or increases in size after surgery and is occluding any of the bile ducts, palliative measures may be taken to allow the bile to flow into the duodenum. Drainage of the bile can be accomplished by an external system, similar to that of a T-tube, or an internal stent that drains directly into the duodenum. As an alternative to surgery, a stent made of specialized plastic or steel is placed either by endoscopy or percutaneously through the tumor to allow drainage of the trapped bile. Complications include cholangitis and obstruction and dislocation of the stent.

DIETARY. Dietary changes are similar to those needed by patients with cholelithiasis, except the emphasis is on gaining weight rather than on weight reduction. A diet balanced with high calories and protein and low fat helps control the GI symptoms. Each individual needs to determine what foods are best tolerated. Medications to control nausea may be needed before meals, and the patient usually needs a pain-control regimen.

Pharmacologic Highlights

Medication or Drug Class	Dosage	Description	Rationale
Narcotic analgesia	Varies with drug	Drugs such as morphine sulfate, Demerol, or oxycodone may be used to control pain after surgery and during end-of-life care	Controls pain

Independent

The nurse has an important role in maximizing the patient's comfort. To augment the pain control obtained from analgesia, initiate nonpharmacologic strategies. Allow the patient to participate in the activities of daily living as much as possible. Assist with personal hygiene as much as needed and include significant others in learning the process. The itching associated with pruritus can be controlled by maintaining skin integrity; using soft, dry linens and cloths; and using warm water for bathing. Keep the area around all surgical incisions and drainage devices clean and dry. A large number of support groups exist to help patients and families manage cancer. Listen to the patient's concerns. Give the patient and family the number for the American Cancer Society and hospice care if appropriate.

Evidence-Based Practice and Health Policy

Nara, S., Esaki, M., Ban, D., Takamoto, T., Shimada, K., Ioka, T., Okusaka, T., Ishii, H., & Furuse, J. (2020). Adjuvant and neoadjuvant therapy for biliary tract cancer: A review of clinical trials. *Japanese Journal of Clinical Oncology, 50*, 1353–1363.

- The authors reviewed the evidence available from clinical trials of adjuvant and neoadjuvant therapy for biliary tract cancer and described ongoing clinical trials. A literature search was performed using the National Library of Medicine's PubMed database for studies published since January 1, 2000. The search identified five phase I, eleven phase II, and nine phase III clinical trials of adjuvant therapy, as well as two phase I, four phase II, and one phase III clinical trials of neoadjuvant therapy, and these studies were included in the analysis in the review.
- Recent clinical studies have demonstrated the promising efficacy of adjuvant or neoadjuvant therapy for biliary tract cancer. Considering the low completion rate of adjuvant chemotherapy, neoadjuvant therapy may be a promising option. However, the accumulated evidence is scarce, and further clinical studies are necessary to establish a standard adjuvant or neoadjuvant therapy regimen for biliary tract cancer.

DOCUMENTATION GUIDELINES

- Physical findings: Signs of blocked bile ducts (pain, nausea and vomiting, jaundice, brown urine, and gray or white stools), skin color and integrity, vital signs, signs of infection (fever, abdominal guarding, increasing white blood cell count)
- Pain control: Response to analgesics, response to nonpharmacologic strategies, location of pain, duration of pain, precipitating factors
- Postoperative assessment of incision, GI functioning, drainage devices (amount and color of drainage)
- Nutrition: Daily weights, appetite, food intake, tolerance to food, presence of nausea and vomiting
- Psychosocial: Response to poor prognosis, support systems

DISCHARGE AND HOME HEALTHCARE GUIDELINES

DRAINAGE SYSTEM. Whether the tube is internal or external, teach the patient the signs and symptoms of a blocked tube. If the drainage system is external, teach the patient how to care for the tube, including emptying the bag, irrigating the tube, periodic clamping of the tube, and managing skin care around the tube.

COMPLICATIONS. Teach the patient to report signs of infection, excessive drainage, leakage, and obstruction to the physician. Provide the patient with a contact phone number.

PRURITUS. Teach the patient methods to control itching.

MEDICATIONS AND DIET. Teach the patient about each medication, including the purpose and correct dosages, along with any potential side effects. Explain the requirements for a low-fat, high-calorie, and high-protein diet.

END-OF-LIFE. Explain ways that the patient can be kept as comfortable as possible and can participate in their own care. Make sure that the family understands all the support systems available through the American Cancer Society, hospice, religious groups, and social services.

Gastric Cancer

DRG Category:	326
Mean LOS:	13.2 days
Description:	SURGICAL: Stomach, Esophageal, and Duodenal Procedures With Major Complication or Comorbidity
DRG Category:	375
Mean LOS:	4.7 days
Description:	MEDICAL: Digestive Malignancy With Complication or Comorbidity

Gastric cancer is a relatively uncommon malignancy, accounting for approximately 2% of all cancers in the United States. While reports vary, the World Health Organization states that it is the fourth-most common cancer worldwide with approximately 754,000 deaths a year. The American Cancer Society (ACS) estimates that in the United States, 26,560 cases of gastric cancer will be diagnosed in 2021, and 11,180 people will die. This type of cancer, like lung cancer, is primarily found in the seventh decade of life. Because it is often found in advanced stages, in both developed and developing regions of the world, it is difficult to cure. Depending on the stage of cancer at the time of diagnosis, the 5-year survival rate ranges from 70% for localized disease to 6% in distant disease.

Nearly 95% of gastric neoplasms are classified as adenocarcinomas; these tumors develop from the epithelial cells that form the innermost lining of the stomach's mucosa. The most common sites for cancer in the stomach include the antrum, the pylorus, and along the area of lesser curvature. According to the Lauren classification, gastric adenocarcinomas are divided into two main histological types: diffuse and intestinal. The diffuse type is ill defined, infiltrates the gastric wall, and lacks a distinctive mass. The intestinal type, by contrast, is composed of neoplastic cells that cluster together, resembling glands; it is associated with a better prognosis, as are tumors along the area of lesser curvature. A poor prognosis is associated with tumors of the cardia or the fundus.

Metastasis occurs via the lymphatics and the blood vessels by seeding of peritoneal surfaces or by direct extension of the tumor. Sites of metastasis are the liver, lungs, bone, adrenals, brain, ovaries, colon, and pancreas. Intestinal tumors are more likely to spread to the liver, whereas diffuse-type tumors are more likely to spread along peritoneal surfaces. Other complications include malnutrition, gastrointestinal (GI) obstruction, iron deficiency anemia, pleural and peritoneal effusions, jaundice from hepatomegaly, and cachexia.

CAUSES

A probable factor in developing gastric cancer is a *Helicobacter pylori* infection leading to atrophic gastritis (inflammation and damage to the inner layer of the stomach). Dietary factors linked to gastric cancer are associated with either gastric irritation or exposure to mutagenic or carcinogenic compounds. They include a high intake of smoked foods, salted fish and meat, nitrite-preserved foods, starch, and fat, along with a low intake of fruits, vegetables, and animal proteins. Associated environmental factors include exposure to ionizing radiation and being employed in metal products or chemical industries. Physiological factors are related to a rise in gastric pH or the formation of mutagenic or carcinogenic compounds. Obesity is also a risk factor for gastric cancer. Other associated conditions include gastric ulcers, gastric polyps, pernicious anemia, intestinal metaplasia, achlorhydria, hypochlorhydria, gastric atrophy, and chronic peptic ulcers. Similarly, patients who have undergone a partial gastrectomy for benign gastric disease are predisposed to developing gastric cancer.

GENETIC CONSIDERATIONS

Most gastric cancer is not hereditary, with only 1% to 3% of gastric cancers resulting from hereditary syndromes. One such syndrome, called hereditary diffuse gastric cancer, is caused by mutations in the *CDH1* gene, which encodes for the protein E-cadherin. Mutations in *CDH1* are transmitted in an autosomal dominant pattern, and carriers have a 56% to 70% chance of developing gastric cancer during their lifetime. Other genetic factors that are linked to an increased incidence of gastric cancer include a family history of stomach cancer and type A blood. Recently, *PALB2* (partner and localizer of *BRCA2*) has been implicated as a new familial gastric cancer gene.

SEX AND LIFE SPAN CONSIDERATIONS

The average age at diagnosis is 68 years, and only 2% of cases occur in people under 35 years. Two-thirds of the patients with gastric cancer are older than 65 years. More men than women die of gastric cancer.

HEALTH DISPARITIES AND SEXUAL/GENDER MINORITY HEALTH

Black, Asian, and Hispanic persons as well as Hawaiian/Pacific Islander persons have approximately twice the rate of gastric cancer diagnosis and death as compared to White persons. Studies in California show that Asian American persons with Korean or Japanese ancestry have a particularly high risk for gastric cancer. The ACS notes that GI cancer deaths for Black men and women are up to 20% higher than for White men and women. Experts note that Black patients do not receive surgery as often as White patients for GI cancer, and the receipt of surgery is the strongest predictor for survival. Therefore, if Black patients do not receive surgery, they are undertreated for GI cancer, have lower survival rates than White patients, and have a significant health disparity (Bliton et al., 2021 [see Evidence-Based Practice and Health Policy]). People with disabilities, such as autism, renal failure, brain injury, ostomy problems, and intellectual disabilities, have significantly lower cancer screening participation than those without disabilities and are at risk for gastric cancer. While little is known about health disparities due to gastric cancer in sexual and gender minority persons, factors such as poverty, stigma, and discrimination affect access to healthcare and may lead to poorer outcomes. Sexual minority women have higher rates of obesity than heterosexual women (Caceres, Ancheta, et al., 2020), which may contribute to gastric cancer risk. Gender and sexual minority persons are a vulnerable group because people with low income, long travel distances to cancer screening sites, or who lack health insurance or paid medical leave are less likely to be treated according to cancer care guidelines (National Institutes of Health, 2021).

GLOBAL HEALTH CONSIDERATIONS

Gastric cancer is the sixth-most common cancer worldwide (after lung, breast, prostate, skin, colon, and rectal cancer). It has relatively low rates in Northern Europe and North America and rates as high as 80 per 100,000 individuals per year in Southeast Asia, South America, and some Eastern European countries, particularly Russia. The highest rates are in Iran, Turkmenistan, and Kyrgyzstan. Developing countries have higher rates of gastric cancer than do developed countries.

ASSESSMENT

HISTORY. Gastric cancer may not produce symptoms until the disease is very advanced. About one-third of the patients report a long history of dyspepsia (painful digestion) and sense of fullness after eating. Patients may describe difficulty swallowing, loss of appetite, and gas pains. Patients may also report experiencing unusual tiredness, constipation, weight loss, and a bad taste in the mouth. Massive GI bleeding is unusual, although chronic bleeding may occur, which results in a positive occult blood test. Patients with advanced gastric cancer report the classic symptoms of anemia, such as fatigue and activity intolerance, as well as vomiting (coffee ground or sometimes containing frank blood), anorexia, abdominal pain, and dyspepsia.

PHYSICAL EXAMINATION. In the early stages of gastric cancer, the patient usually appears healthy. The most common initial symptoms are **mild epigastric discomfort, dysphagia** (difficulty swallowing), **loss of appetite, nausea,** and a **sense of fullness or gas pains.** In later stages, patients may appear weak, pale, dyspneic, and fatigued from anemia; they are thin and seem to be malnourished. Only 37% of patients have a palpable abdominal mass. Observe for abdominal swelling and ascites (poor prognostic sign) and palpate for hepatomegaly secondary to liver or peritoneal metastases. Some patients may have palpable lymph nodes, especially the supraclavicular and axillary nodes. Gastric cancer is frequently staged using the TNM classification system (T: primary tumor, N: lymph node, M: distant metastasis).

PSYCHOSOCIAL. Survival rates after treatment for gastric cancer remain discouraging (the 5-year survival rate is 32% for all gastric cancers), and patients with gastric cancer have special psychosocial concerns. Assess their support systems and their ability to cope with major lifestyle changes. As appropriate, assess the patient's and family's transition through the end of life and the availability of hospice care if needed.

Diagnostic Highlights

General Comments: The presence of lactic acid and a high lactate dehydrogenase level in the gastric juice are suggestive of cancer. Often, in patients with gastric cancer, plasma tumor markers (carcinoembryonic antigen [CEA], cancer antigen [CA] 19-9) are elevated. Positive fecal occult blood tests are associated with the chronic bleeding that is related to gastric cancer.

Test	Normal Result	Abnormality With Condition	Explanation
Esophagogastro-duodenoscopy	Normal stomach	Visualization of cancer in the stomach	Visualizes tumor for biopsy; has a diagnostic accuracy of 95%

Other Tests: Cytology studies of the specimens obtained; computed tomography scan (chest, abdomen, pelvic); positron emission tomography, abdominal ultrasonography, and laparoscopy; complete blood count, blood chemistries, CEA, cancer antigen 19-9 (CA19-9)

PRIMARY NURSING DIAGNOSIS

DIAGNOSIS. Acute pain related to gastric erosion as evidenced by self-reports of pain, facial grimacing, and/or protective behavior

OUTCOMES. Comfort status; Pain level; Pain control; Knowledge: Cancer management; Medication response

INTERVENTIONS. Analgesic administration; Anxiety reduction; Pain management: Acute; Medication management; Patient-controlled analgesia assistance

PLANNING AND IMPLEMENTATION

Collaborative

Treatment includes surgery, chemotherapy, and radiation. If the cancer is resected before it has invaded the stomach wall, the 5-year survival rate is about 90%. The deeper the cancer invades the stomach wall, the poorer is the prognosis. Endoscopic mucosal resection or surgery with a complete en bloc resection of an early, localized tumor is the only cure. Most patients undergo a subtotal gastrectomy, after which GI continuity can be restored by either a Billroth I (gastroduodenostomy) or a Billroth II (gastrojejunostomy) procedure. Intraoperative radiotherapy with a high dose to avoid unaffected body structures is showing promising long-term outcome results. After such gastric surgery, patients are prone to vitamin B_{12} deficiency and megaloblastic anemia from lack of intrinsic factor; monthly vitamin B_{12} replacement is therefore necessary. For patients who undergo a Billroth I procedure, postprandial dumping syndrome is a problem. For patients who undergo a Billroth II procedure, postoperative intestinal obstruction is a concern. In addition, transfusions of packed red blood cells are given to patients to correct anemia.

For patients with advanced disease, palliative subtotal or total gastrectomies may be performed to alleviate gastric symptoms, such as bleeding or obstruction. After surgery, chemotherapy or radiation, or both, may be provided.

Pharmacologic Highlights

Medication or Drug Class	Dosage	Description	Rationale
Chemotherapeutic agents	Varies with drug	Used as adjuvant (in addition to) or neoadjuvant (before surgery) often in combination: fluorouracil, leucovorin, doxorubicin, methyl-1-(2-chloroethyl)-3-cyclohexyl-1-nitrosourea (CCNU), cisplatin, epirubicin, docetaxel, methotrexate, etoposide; trastuzumab combined with cisplatin and capecitabine or 5-FU (for people who have not had previous chemotherapy)	Treat cancer that has metastasized to organs beyond stomach; shrink tumors before surgery
Vitamins	Tablets come in various sizes	Vitamin B complex	Combat vitamin B_{12} deficiency and megaloblastic anemia from lack of intrinsic factor
Narcotic analgesics	Varies with drug	Manage pain, side effects of treatment drugs such as morphine, meperidine	Increase patient comfort during end-stage disease

Other Drugs: Antiemetics may be used to control nausea, which increases as the tumor enlarges. In the advanced stages, the physician may prescribe sedatives, narcotics, and tranquilizers to increase the patient's comfort. Antispasmodics and antacids may also help relieve GI discomfort.

Independent

PREOPERATIVE. Explain all preoperative and postoperative procedures. Preoperative needs include nutritional adequacy, IV fluids, and prophylactic bowel preparation. Inform the patient about the need for GI decompression via a tube for 1 to 3 weeks postoperatively. Explain the amount of pain that should be anticipated, and reassure the patient that analgesia provides relief. Teach coughing and deep-breathing exercises and have the patient practice them.

POSTOPERATIVE. Maintain wound care, provide adequate fluid and nutrition, manage pain, and control symptoms. Monitor the patient for complications such as hemorrhage, intestinal obstruction, and infection. Teach wound care and the signs and symptoms of infection. Teach nonpharmacologic pain management techniques. As indicated, teach the signs and symptoms of "dumping syndrome": epigastric fullness, nausea, vomiting, abdominal cramping, and diarrhea that occur within 30 minutes of eating. Teach patients that they may also experience sweating, dizziness, pallor, and palpitations related to the dumping syndrome. To relieve the symptoms, teach patients to avoid drinking fluids within a half hour of meals and to eat small meals that are low carbohydrate, high fat, and high protein.

Evidence-Based Practice and Health Policy
Bliton, J., Parides, M., Muscarella, P., Papalezova, K., & In, H. (2021). Understanding racial disparities in gastrointestinal cancer outcomes: Lack of surgery contributes to lower survival in African American patients. *Cancer, Epidemiology, Biomarkers & Prevention, 30*, 529–538.

- The authors point out that there are race/ethnicity differences in rates of cancer surgery and cancer mortality for people with GI cancers. They used the National Cancer Database to estimate the extent to which differences in surgical rates explain disparities in cancer survival in more than 600,000 patients, 12% of which had esophageal or gastric cancer. The authors used mediation analysis to identify variables influencing the relationship between race/ethnicity and mortality.
- The operative rates for Black as compared to White patients were low, and two factors that were related to survival were the receipt of surgery and socioeconomic factors. The authors concluded that Black patients are undertreated as compared to White patients, and the low operative rates contribute to low survival rates for Black as compared to White patients.

DOCUMENTATION GUIDELINES

- Physical findings related to gastric cancer: Epigastric discomfort, dyspepsia, anorexia, nausea, sense of fullness, gas pains, unusual tiredness, abdominal pains, constipation, weight loss, vomiting, hematemesis, blood in the stool, dysphagia, jaundice, ascites, bone pain
- GI decompression data: Irrigation and patency of tube, assessment of bowel sounds and passage of gas, complaints of nausea, amount and description of gastric fluid output
- Presence of postoperative complications: Hemorrhage, obstruction, anastomotic leaks, infection, peritonitis
- Presence of postoperative dumping syndrome and associated patient symptoms

DISCHARGE AND HOME HEALTHCARE GUIDELINES

Teach the patient the importance of compliance with palliative and follow-up care. Be sure the patient understands all medications, including the dosage, route, action, and adverse effects. Teach the patient the signs and symptoms of infection and how to care for the incision. Instruct the patient to notify the physician if signs of infection occur. Encourage the patient to seek psychosocial support through local support groups (e.g., I Can Cope), clergy, or counseling services. If appropriate, suggest hospice services. Teach the patient methods to enhance nutritional intake to maintain ideal body weight. Several small meals a day may be tolerated better than three meals a day. Take liquid supplements and vitamins as prescribed. Refer the patient to the dietitian for a consultation. Teach family members and friends prevention strategies. Strategies include increasing the intake of fresh fruits and vegetables that are high in vitamin C; maintaining adequate protein intake; and decreasing intake of salty, starchy, smoked, and nitrite-preserved foods.

Gastritis

DRG Category: 391
Mean LOS: 4.9 days
Description: MEDICAL: Esophagitis, Gastroenteritis, and Miscellaneous Digestive Disorders With Major Complication or Comorbidity

Gastritis is any inflammatory process of the mucosal lining of the stomach. The inflammation may be contained within one region or be patchy in many areas. Gastric structure and function are altered in either the epithelial or the glandular components of the gastric mucosa. The inflammation is usually limited to the mucosa, but some forms involve the deeper layers of the gastric wall. Gastritis is classified into acute and chronic forms.

ACUTE. Two categories of acute gastritis occur. In acute erosive gastritis, or acute hemorrhagic gastritis, the erosions are limited to the mucosa, which has edema and sites of bleeding. Erosions can be diffuse throughout the stomach or localized to the antrum. Erosion occurs because of gravity, because irritating substances lie on the greater curvature of the stomach. Substances such as certain medications, alcohol, cocaine, and bile reflux irritate the mucosa. Acute nonerosive gastritis is usually caused by *Helicobacter pylori*, which can also lead to chronic gastritis.

CHRONIC. The type of chronic gastritis associated with *H pylori* develops in two patterns. Antral predominant gastritis is characterized by inflammation primarily located in the antrum of the stomach. People with this pattern may develop peptic ulcers. Multifocal atrophic gastritis involves the corpus and gastric antrum and ultimately leads to gastric atrophy, the loss of gastric glands, and replacement of the glands by epithelium. Individuals who develop gastric carcinoma and gastric ulcers have this pattern. Chronic gastritis can also occur from bile reflux, NSAIDs, infectious agents, radiation, autoimmunity, or an allergic response. Complications of gastritis include bleeding, anemia, ulcers, and cancerous and noncancerous growths.

CAUSES

ACUTE GASTRITIS. Alcohol abuse and ingestion of aspirin or other NSAIDs are the most common causes. Other causes are steroid or digitalis medications; ingestion of corrosive agents such as lye or drain cleaners; ingestion of excessive amounts of tea, coffee, mustard, cloves, paprika, or pepper; chemotherapy or radiation to the upper abdomen; severe stress related to critical illness; staphylococcal food poisoning; and infections (candida, cytomegalovirus, herpesvirus) in immunosuppressed patients. These conditions and substances disrupt the gastric mucosal barrier and make it vulnerable to normal gastric secretions.

CHRONIC GASTRITIS. The primary cause of chronic gastritis is *H pylori*, which colonizes the deep layers of the mucosa and the protective gel that coats the gastric mucosa. This disruption damages the mucosal protective properties. Experts suggest that cigarette smoking may have a synergistic effect along with *H pylori* to worsen symptoms or may contribute to the persistence of the infection.

GENETIC CONSIDERATIONS

The autoimmune form of gastritis has a strong genetic predisposition. Gastritis is associated with polymorphisms in genes involved in inflammatory responses (ILB, TLR), and detoxification enzymes (CYP450). Genetic variations in immune factors leading to an increased susceptibility to infection with *H pylori* will also increase risk.

SEX AND LIFE SPAN CONSIDERATIONS

Acute gastritis occurs in men more than in women, whereas chronic gastritis occurs more frequently in women than in men. The incidence is highest between the ages of 50 and 70 years. The incidence increases with age from 10% to 20% in persons in their 30s to over 45% in persons over age 70 years.

HEALTH DISPARITIES AND SEXUAL/GENDER MINORITY HEALTH

Autoimmune gastritis occurs more often in persons who are White, particularly of northern European descent, and Black persons. Approximately 35% of adults in the United States are infected with *H pylori*, but the prevalence of infection in minority groups and people who come to the United States from developing countries is much higher than other groups. Children in developing countries are much more likely than children in developed countries to acquire the infection. Age is the most important factor relating to the prevalence of *H pylori* infection. People born before 1950 have a significantly higher rate of infection than people born thereafter and are therefore at risk for gastritis. Sexual and gender minority status has no known effect on the risk for gastritis, although some subgroups have higher rates of cigarette use and alcohol consumption as compared to their heterosexual or cisgender counterparts, which may place them at risk for or worsen the symptoms of gastritis.

GLOBAL HEALTH CONSIDERATIONS

The prevalence of gastritis is increasing in developing countries and decreasing in developed countries.

ASSESSMENT

HISTORY. Obtain a detailed history of past illnesses as well as the onset, duration, and aggravating and relieving factors of any symptoms. Common symptoms include epigastric pain, changes in stool color, nausea and vomiting (emesis may be bright red, coffee ground, or bile colored), and appetite and weight changes. Assess the patient's usual daily diet, including fish, alcohol, tea, and coffee ingestion. Obtain a complete medication profile that includes both prescribed and over-the-counter (OTC) drugs, particularly NSAIDs and corticosteroids. Patients with gastritis may have only mild epigastric discomfort or intolerance for spicy or fatty foods. Patients with atrophic gastritis may be asymptomatic.

PHYSICAL EXAMINATION. The most common symptom is **burning epigastric pain**. The patient may appear normal or may seem to be in discomfort, with facial grimaces and restlessness. Inspect for signs of dehydration or upper GI bleeding, which may be the only sign of acute gastritis. Bleeding can range from a sudden hemorrhage to an insidious blood loss that can be detected only by stool guaiac testing for occult blood or an unexplained anemia. Pallor, tachycardia, and hypotension occur with dramatic GI bleeding accompanied by hematemesis and melena.

Auscultate for decreased bowel sounds, which may or may not accompany gastritis. Palpate the abdomen to evaluate the patient for distention, tenderness, and guarding. Epigastric pain and abdominal tenderness are usually absent with patients who have GI bleeding. Gastritis caused by food poisoning and corrosive agents (ingestion of strong acids) results in epigastric pain, nausea, and vomiting.

PSYCHOSOCIAL. Assess the patient's and family's anxiety and ability to cope with the fears that are associated with hemorrhage if that has occurred. Assess the patient's understanding of disease management and coping abilities to participate in lifestyle modifications. Because stress is an important risk for gastritis, consider the patient's level of stress, how the medical condition might contribute to stress, and how the patient and family respond to stress. Assess whether the patient is willing to consider smoking cessation and, if the patient is misusing alcohol, to decrease drinking.

Diagnostic Highlights

Test	Normal Result	Abnormality With Condition	Explanation
Esophagogastro-duodenoscopy with biopsy	Visualization of normal stomach; biopsy results show normal cells	Visualization of inflamed gastric mucosa; biopsy results show the specific type of gastritis	Demonstrates location and depth of inflammation of stomach lining and rules out gastric cancer

Other Tests: Supporting tests include upper GI x-rays, serum tests, biopsy to determine histological evidence of *H pylori*, and enzyme-linked immunosorbent assay for *H pylori* immunoglobulins.

PRIMARY NURSING DIAGNOSIS

DIAGNOSIS. Acute pain related to gastric erosion or inflammation as evidenced by self-reports of pain, facial grimacing, and/or protective behavior

OUTCOMES. Comfort status; Pain level; Pain control; Knowledge: Disease process; Symptom severity; Medication response

INTERVENTIONS. Analgesia administration; Medication management; Anxiety reduction; Pain management: Acute

▓ PLANNING AND IMPLEMENTATION

Collaborative

The immediate treatment for acute gastritis is directed toward alleviating the symptoms and withdrawing the causative agents. The physician usually prescribes an H_2 antagonist. The medical goal is to maintain the pH of gastric contents above 4. Acute hemorrhagic gastritis may disappear within 48 hours because of rapid cell proliferation and restoration of gastric mucosa. If the bleeding is profuse and persistent, blood replacement is necessary. An infusion of vasopressin (Pitressin) or embolization of the left gastric artery is used to halt hemorrhage. Surgical intervention is not performed unless hemorrhage is uncontrollable. In this rare situation, vagotomy with pyloroplasty is usually performed.

There is no known treatment that will reverse the pathogenesis of chronic gastritis. Eradication of *H pylori* bacteria halts active gastritis in approximately 92% of the cases unless there is permanent damage to the gastric epithelium. The medical regimen for eradicating *H pylori* is a combination of bismuth salts and two antibiotics over a 10-day to 2-week period. Omeprazole may be added in addition to these three medications. An important part of management of patients with chronic gastritis is long-term follow-up for early detection of gastric cancer. Patients who have chronic gastritis may develop pernicious anemia; destruction of parietal cells in the fundus and body of the stomach leads to inadequate vitamin B_{12} absorption.

Pharmacologic Highlights

Medication or Drug Class	Dosage	Description	Rationale
Omeprazole	20–40 mg PO daily	Proton pump inhibitor	Inhibits the protein pump that produces acid in the stomach; used with antibiotics to treat *H pylori*
Vasopressin (Pitressin)	0.2–0.4 units/min with progressive increases to 0.9 units/min IV	Vasopressor, antidiuretic	Halts acute hemorrhage from gastritis

Pharmacologic Highlights (continued)

Medication or Drug Class	Dosage	Description	Rationale
Antibiotics to treat H pylori	Varies with drug	Clarithromycin, amoxicillin, metronidazole, tetracycline, and furazolidone	Cure rates from a single antibiotic are low; regimens vary but may include bismuth, metronidazole, tetracycline; or clarithromycin plus omeprazole

Other Drugs: Bismuth subsalicylate (Kaopectate); antacids used as buffering agents to neutralize gastric acid and maintain gastric pH above 4 include aluminum hydroxide with magnesium hydroxide (Maalox, Mylanta) or aluminum hydroxide (Amphojel); vitamin B_{12} prevents pernicious anemia; H_2 antagonist, cimetidine

Independent

Encourage the patient to avoid aspirin and NSAIDs (indomethacin and ibuprofen) unless they have been prescribed. Reinforce the need to take these medications with food or to take enteric-coated aspirin. Other drugs that may contribute to gastric irritation include chemotherapeutic agents, corticosteroids, and erythromycin. Explain the importance of reading the labels of OTC drugs to identify those that contain aspirin. Instruct the patient about the action, dosage, and frequency of the medications (antacids, H_2 antagonists, antibiotic regimen) that are administered while the patient is in the hospital. Discuss the possible complications that can develop with acute or chronic gastritis (hemorrhage, pernicious anemia, iron deficiency anemia, or gastric cancer). Explain the pathophysiology and treatment of each possible complication. Discuss how ingestion of caffeine and spicy foods results in irritation and inflammation of the mucosa of the stomach.

Be sure the patient understands how smoking and alcohol aggravate gastritis and that abstaining from both will facilitate healing and reduce recurrence. Provide information about various smoking cessation and alcohol rehabilitation programs available in the community. Explain the rationale for the need for support during this very difficult lifestyle change for permanent abstinence.

Assist the patient in identifying the patient's personal physical and emotional stressors. Review coping skills that the patient has used previously to change behaviors. Talk about how to adapt the environment to which the patient must return in order to meet the needs of lifestyle changes. Involve the family in assisting with the patient's needed changes. Assess the family's response and ability to cope.

Evidence-Based Practice and Health Policy

Lahner, E., Conti, L., Annibale, B., & Corleto, V. (2020). Current perspectives in atrophic gastritis. *Current Gastroenterology Reports, 22,* 1–8.

- The authors aimed to provide a review that would update current knowledge and progress on atrophic gastritis. They note that atrophic gastritis affects mostly adults with persistent dyspepsia, deficient anemia, autoimmune disease, long-term proton pump inhibitor use, and a family history of gastric cancer. Gastric biopsies represent the gold standard for diagnosis and cancer risk stage.
- Electronic chromoendoscopy has allowed targeted biopsies of intestinal tissue to determine the bacteria that may lead to gastric cancer. They conclude that there is a multifaceted clinical presentation of atrophic gastritis, and it should be monitored by endoscopy and gastric biopsies. Autoimmune and *H pylori*–induced atrophic gastritis have different gastric microbial profiles that play different roles in the origin of gastric tumors that need to be recognized.

DOCUMENTATION GUIDELINES

- Assessment findings: Epigastric discomfort, nausea, vomiting, hematemesis, melena, anemia, dehydration
- Response to medications: Antacids, H_2 antagonists, antibiotics
- Reaction to emotional and physical rest
- Presence of complications: Anemia, hemorrhage, pernicious anemia

DISCHARGE AND HOME HEALTHCARE GUIDELINES

Instruct the patient to avoid caffeinated drinks, hot and spicy foods, identified aggravating foods, alcohol, smoking, and aspirin and other OTC NSAIDs. Provide a written list of symptoms of GI bleeding and pernicious anemia (weakness, sore tongue, numbness and tingling in the extremities, anorexia, weight loss, angina, shortness of breath, palpitations). Inform the patient of the need for lifetime vitamin B_{12} intramuscular injections if pernicious anemia develops. Reinforce the need for follow-up for early detection testing for gastric cancer. Review medication action, dosage, frequency, and side effects. Make referrals to smoking and alcohol cessation programs of the patient's choice. Reinforce relaxation exercises and stress management techniques.

Gastroenteritis

DRG Category:	391
Mean LOS:	4.9 days
Description:	MEDICAL: Esophagitis, Gastroenteritis, and Miscellaneous Digestive Disorders With Major Complication or Comorbidity

Gastroenteritis is an inflammation of the stomach and the small bowel. It can occur because of bacterial and viral infections and is a very common problem in both primary and emergency care. Estimates are that bacterial gastroenteritis causes 5% of pediatric office visits and 10% of hospitalizations of children annually in the United States. In adults, it accounts for 8 million doctor visits and 250,000 hospitalizations each year. A number of viruses cause gastroenteritis, resulting in millions of cases and thousands of hospitalizations in children and adults each year in the United States. Norovirus alone causes 19 to 20 million cases a year in the United States, mainly in young children, and causes 500 to 1,000 deaths in primarily children and older adults. It is more common in autumn and winter than in the warmer seasons.

Gastroenteritis is a self-limiting disease that is also called *intestinal flu, traveler's diarrhea, viral enteritis,* or *food poisoning*. The viral or bacterial organisms enter the intestinal tract and cause inflammation to the intestinal lining and diarrhea by one of the following means: (1) Enterotoxins are released from the organism and stimulate the intestinal mucosa to secrete increased amounts of water and electrolytes into the intestinal lumen. (2) The organisms either infiltrate the intestinal wall, causing cell destruction of the lining, or attach themselves to the epithelium, causing cell destruction of the intestinal villae. The stomach and small bowel react to any of the causative agents with inflammation and increased gastrointestinal (GI) motility, leading to severe diarrhea. Gastroenteritis ranks second to the common cold as a cause of sick days among U.S. workers. Complications include dehydration, hypotension, electrolyte imbalances, sepsis, inflammatory responses (particularly joints and skin), renal failure, and irritable bowel syndrome.

CAUSES

The majority of organisms, such as *Salmonella*, that cause intestinal infections are acquired through contaminated food and water. The major risk factor for gastroenteritis caused by food poisoning is improper handling and storage of food. Bacterial or viral food poisoning usually occurs within 16 hours after eating contaminated food. Some infections are transmitted by person-to-person contact. Fecal-oral transmission is a result of poor hygiene.

The viral forms are rotavirus gastroenteritis and outbreaks of epidemic viral gastroenteritis. Rotavirus is responsible for about 50% of all cases of acute gastroenteritis in developed countries and 5% to 20% of cases of diarrhea in developing countries. Rotaviruses are transmitted via the fecal-oral or possibly fecal-respiratory route; the incubation period is 24 to 72 hours. Noroviruses cause 80% of all outbreaks of food-borne gastroenteritis in developed countries. It is a common cause in settings such as nursing homes, other healthcare settings, and cruise ships.

There are several forms of bacterial gastroenteritis: *Campylobacter* enteritis (traveler's diarrhea), *Escherichia coli* diarrhea (also known as traveler's diarrhea), and shigellosis (bacillary dysentery). Since 2000, the number of cases of *Clostridium difficile* infection (CDI) has increased greatly, occurring primarily in hospitalized patients or patients recently discharged. Factors that contribute to the host's susceptibility to the agent are an elevated pH with the use of antacids; decreased production of gastric acid; or excessive intake of high-fat foods, which protect the microbe from gastric acid. Also, slow small-bowel motility increases the time the pathogen is in contact with the lumen of the bowel, which aids in the development and duration of symptoms. Normal intestinal flora protect a person from pathogenic organisms.

GENETIC CONSIDERATIONS

Heritable immune responses could be protective or increase susceptibility.

SEX AND LIFE SPAN CONSIDERATIONS

Children under age 2 years are more susceptible than older children to infectious gastroenteritis because their immune system is not yet fully developed. Rotavirus gastroenteritis is usually confined to infants and children under 3 years of age. By age 3 years, most children develop antibodies against the rotaviruses. People with low levels of antibody can be infected, particularly family members of affected infants. Severe, prolonged diarrhea may be fatal in older persons and infants when severe fluid and electrolyte imbalance occurs. Infants become dehydrated very rapidly.

HEALTH DISPARITIES AND SEXUAL/GENDER MINORITY HEALTH

Ethnicity and race have no known effect on the risk for gastroenteritis. Men who have sex with men are at risk for sexual transmission of organisms that lead to gastroenteritis. They may also experience multiresistant strains of organisms, which makes the illness more difficult to treat (Newman et al., 2020). A focus on prevention and condom use is important for this group of persons.

GLOBAL HEALTH CONSIDERATIONS

Gastroenteritis is a common disease throughout the world, and outbreaks often occur in epidemics, especially among people who are living in crowded conditions. It is a major cause of mortality and morbidity in developing countries, and up to 5 billion cases of acute diarrhea occur in the world each year. The World Health Organization estimates that more than 500,000 children under 5 years of age die from diarrheal diseases each year. Acute diarrhea is also a leading cause of malnutrition in children. Experts suggest that as many as 50% of visitors to developing countries experience diarrhea. During November to April, outbreaks of virally induced gastroenteritis tend to occur in locations with cooler climates such as Northern Europe; the American

Northeast; St. Petersburg, Russia; and Canada. In recent years, outbreaks of norovirus infection on cruise ships have had significant human and economic costs.

ASSESSMENT

HISTORY. Determine the frequency, color, consistency, and amount of bowel movements. The epidemic viral diarrhea lasts only 24 to 48 hours, whereas rotaviral infection may last up to 7 days. Nausea and vomiting are usually confined to the first 48 hours of illness. Ask if cramping, pain, nausea, or vomiting has accompanied the diarrhea.

Fever often occurs with bacterial intestinal infections. Flu symptoms (malaise, headache, myalgia [muscle achiness]) are associated with the epidemic viral gastroenteritis. Determine if other family members or coworkers have the same symptoms. It is important to determine if the gastroenteritis is communicable from contaminated food or water so that the community health department can be notified. Inquire about recent travel and food intake. Investigate what and where the patient has eaten in the last 2 days. Note if the patient has recently been discharged from the hospital.

PHYSICAL EXAMINATION. Diarrhea is the cardinal symptom of gastroenteritis, but the severity varies with the causative organism. **Dehydration** is the primary cause of complications from the diarrhea. Viral infections are accompanied by mild fever; vomiting; and watery, nonbloody diarrhea. *Campylobacter* enteritis results in 20 to 30 foul-smelling stools per day for as long as a week. *E coli* may cause blood and mucus in the stool, with a duration of 7 to 10 days. Diarrhea from shigellosis is greenish in color, may last from 2 to 20 days, and also contains blood and mucus. The patient generally appears acutely ill, with dry skin and poor skin turgor. Inspect the mouth and note that the mucous membranes are usually dry, the tongue is furrowed, and salivation is decreased. Other signs include flattened neck veins, redness of the perianal area, decreased urine volume (< 20 mL/hr or 480 mL in 24 hr), and increased urine concentration (a dark, concentrated color). When performing auscultation, check for hyperactive bowel sounds. The patient may have abdominal distention with diarrheal stools that are liquid, green, foul-smelling, and bloody or mucus filled.

PSYCHOSOCIAL. Identify the patient's perception of the threat of the symptoms. The discomfort from repetitive diarrhea will likely make the patient upset, anxious, and irritable. The patient has likely had problems sleeping. Identify coping skills the patient is using, such as problem-solving, anger, and daydreaming.

Diagnostic Highlights

Test	Normal Result	Abnormality With Condition	Explanation
Stool culture and Gram stain	Negative for pathogens; normal stool flora	Presence of enteric pathogens; enterotoxigenic *E coli*; pus cells, white blood cells and shigella; white blood cells, red blood cells, and *Campylobacter*	Demonstrate presence of pathogens or the effect of pathogens

Other Tests: Laboratory testing may not be necessary because the clinical presentation of viral gastroenteritis is generally definitive. Blood chemistries to identify dehydration, complete blood count, stool pH, electron microscopy and immunoassay for epidemic viral or rotavirus gastroenteritis.

PRIMARY NURSING DIAGNOSIS

DIAGNOSIS. Diarrhea related to increased intestinal motility as evidenced by bowel urgency, loose/liquid stools, and/or cramping

OUTCOMES. Bowel elimination; Electrolyte and acid/base balance; Fluid balance; Hydration; Infection severity; Nutritional status: Food and fluid intake

INTERVENTIONS. Diarrhea management; Fluid/electrolyte management; Fluid monitoring; Perineal care; Skin surveillance; Medication management

PLANNING AND IMPLEMENTATION

Collaborative

Many intestinal infections are short lived (24–48 hr) and are adequately treated by resting the colon and with rehydration and electrolyte supplementation, particularly potassium. The patient is instructed to take nothing by mouth until vomiting stops. Early fluid and electrolyte replacement is critical for debilitated, aged, and very young patients. Clear liquids are started slowly until tolerance is evaluated. Gatorade or other drinks with electrolytes are preferred to water. Oral rehydration therapy with products such as Resol may be used for older patients. The patient may advance to bland solids within 24 hours. Some experts recommend the BRAT diet (bananas, rice, applesauce, toast) during early recovery, but when tolerated the patient should progress to lean meats and clear fluids when possible. When rapid dehydration occurs, the patient is admitted to the hospital for IV fluid replacement with solutions such as half-strength normal saline solution to prevent serious complications or possible death. Electrolytes such as potassium may be added to IV solutions depending on the patient's blood chemistry results.

It is mandatory to notify the local health department of cases of shigellosis and, in some areas, of *Campylobacter* enteritis. Check with the local and state health department guidelines for reporting gastroenteritis.

Antiemetics and anticholinergics are contraindicated because they slow the motility of the bowel, which interferes with evacuating the causative organism. The longer the infectious agent is in contact with the intestinal wall, the more severe the infection.

Pharmacologic Highlights

Medication or Drug Class	Dosage	Description	Rationale
Anti-infectives	Varies with drug	Trimethoprim-sulfamethoxazole (Bactrim, Septra)	Combat shigellosis enteritis
Antibiotics	Varies with drug	Ampicillin, tetracycline, cefixime, ceftriaxone, cefotaxime, erythromycin, vancomycin, rifaximin	Combat infection if leukocytes are present in stools

Depending on the type of organism, antidiarrheal agents may be used in adults but not in children. Probiotics are live but nonpathogenic microorganisms that may provide beneficial effects to decrease the severity of infectious gastroenteritis. They improve the balance of the intestinal flora, possibly by suppressing the growth of bacteria and improving intestinal barrier function. These preparations have entered mainstream healthcare and are thought to affect immune function by alleviating inflammation. Preparations include *Lactobacillus casei* strain GG and *Saccharomyces boulardii*.

Independent

Provide for periods of uninterrupted rest, which often helps decrease the patient's symptoms. The patient with gastroenteritis is anxious and weak from vomiting and diarrhea. Explain the rationale for the treatment regimen of having no oral intake, maintaining bedrest, and administering IV fluids. Measure all urine, emesis, and loose stools. Tell the patient to call for assistance to use the bathroom and explain the use of the commode "hat" for the purpose of measuring output. Try to place the patient in a private room to decrease embarrassment about the frequent, foul-smelling stools and to limit cross-contamination. Encourage the patient to wash hands carefully after each stool and after performing perianal care; make sure all staff use good hand-washing techniques and universal precautions when dealing with stool and vomitus to prevent disease transmission. Follow infection control procedures based on the type and nature of the invading organism.

To prevent excoriation, provide skin protective agents and creams (petroleum jelly, zinc oxide) to apply around the anal region. Teach the patient to cleanse with water or barrier cleanser spray, wipe with cotton pads, and apply the cream after each bowel movement. Inspect the perineal area daily for further breakdown. Sitz baths for 10 minutes two to three times per day are helpful for perianal discomfort.

Evidence-Based Practice and Health Policy

Sandelius, S., & Wahlberg, A. (2020). Telenurses' experiences of monitoring calls to parents of children with gastroenteritis. *Scandinavian Journal of Caring Sciences, 34*, 658–665.

• The authors aimed to describe telenurses' experiences with telephone advice to parents of children with gastroenteritis. Nineteen telenurses from two healthcare call centers in Sweden were interviewed. Data were analyzed using inductive qualitative content analysis.
• The telenurses focused on increasing parent's feeling of security and on the child's safety. Monitoring calls also provided a learning opportunity for parents and telenurses, and the possibility of relieving pressure on in-person healthcare services. The authors concluded that the use of monitoring calls might be an effective strategy in helping insecure parents care for their child with gastroenteritis.

DOCUMENTATION GUIDELINES

• Frequency and characteristics of bowel movements: Number, presence of blood and mucus, color, consistency (formed, watery), response to antibiotic therapy
• Comfort: Presence of abdominal colicky pain, cramping
• Nutrition and fluid balance: Response to fluid and electrolyte replacement, intake and output, signs of dehydration, tolerance of fluids and food
• Complications: Increased abdominal discomfort or bleeding, uncorrected dehydration, skin breakdown
• Prevention: Understanding of measures to prevent transmission of infections

DISCHARGE AND HOME HEALTHCARE GUIDELINES

The primary goal of discharge teaching is to educate the patient and family about reducing the risk of transmitting the organisms that cause gastroenteritis. Demonstrate hand-washing techniques. Instruct the patient and family to use an antibacterial soap, such as liquid Dial, for hand washing after toileting. Stress the importance of daily bathing and meticulous personal hygiene with a focus on perianal cleansing. Frequent cleansing of the commode with an antibacterial cleanser is necessary to avoid exposure of stools to others. The patient should not handle food that will be eaten by others. Discuss the need for the patient to have their own toothpaste, towel, and washcloth and not to share dishes, utensils, or drinking glasses. Provide these instructions in written form; explain that they are to be carried out for at least 7 weeks or, in the case of shigellosis, for several months.

The patient may be discharged with a prescription for antibiotics or anti-infective agents. Teach the patient to continue the medications for the full length of therapy. Tell the patient to space the medication evenly around the clock; take with a full glass of water; and report symptoms of rash, fever, bleeding, bruising, or other new symptoms. Instruct the patient to report recurring symptoms of diarrhea, fever, vomiting, or any change in frequency and appearance of stool.

Gastroesophageal Reflux Disease

DRG Category: 328
Mean LOS: 2.9 days
Description: SURGICAL: Stomach, Esophageal and Duodenal Procedures Without Complication or Comorbidity or Major Complication or Comorbidity

DRG Category: 391
Mean LOS: 4.9 days
Description: MEDICAL: Esophagitis, Gastroenteritis, and Miscellaneous Digestive Disorders With Major Complication or Comorbidity

Gastroesophageal reflux disease (GERD) is a syndrome caused by esophageal reflux, or the backward flow of gastroesophageal contents into the esophagus, causing troubling symptoms and other complications. It is a common syndrome that is experienced by up to 40% of people at some point in their lives, and approximately 10% experience it daily. GERD occurs because of inappropriate relaxation of the lower esophageal sphincter (LES) in response to an unknown stimulus. Reflux occurs in most adults, but if it occurs regularly, the esophagus cannot resist the irritating effects of gastric acid and pepsin because the mucosal barrier of the esophagus breaks down. Without this protection, tissue injury, inflammation, hyperemia, and even erosion occur.

As healing occurs, the cells that replace the normal squamous cell epithelium may be more resistant to reflux but may also be a premalignant tissue that can lead to adenocarcinoma. Repeated exposure may also lead to fibrosis and scarring, which can cause esophageal stricture to occur. Stricture leads to difficulty in swallowing. Chronic reflux is often associated with hiatus hernia.

Barrett esophagus is a condition thought to be caused by the chronic reflux of gastric acid into the esophagus. It occurs when squamous epithelium of the esophagus is replaced by intestinal columnar epithelium, a situation that may lead to adenocarcinoma. Barrett esophagus is present in approximately 10% to 15% of patients with GERD. Other complications include esophagitis, esophageal bleeding, esophageal ulcer, esophageal stricture, scarring, tooth decay, sleep apnea, and respiratory difficulty (cough, hoarseness, wheezing, asthma, bronchitis, laryngitis, and pneumonia).

CAUSES

The causes of GERD are not well understood. Many patients with GERD have normal resting LES pressure and produce normal amounts of gastric acid. Possible explanations for GERD include delays in gastric emptying, changes in LES control with aging, and obesity. Environmental and physical factors that lower tone and contractility of the LES include diet and drugs (see Assessment section for listing).

GENETIC CONSIDERATIONS

Family history appears to be a significant risk factor for GERD, as heritability is estimated at 43%. Recent studies have identified more than 30 loci that associate with GERD, but more research is needed to identify the causal genes. Barrett esophagus most likely has a genetic component as well because its incidence associated with GERD is highly variable.

SEX AND LIFE SPAN CONSIDERATIONS

GERD occurs at any age but is most common in people over age 40 years. It occurs in both men and women, and it is a common disorder that affects as much as 40% of the total population.

HEALTH DISPARITIES AND SEXUAL/GENDER MINORITY HEALTH

Although White males are more at risk than other populations for Barrett esophagus and adenocarcinoma, no sex or racial and ethnic considerations are reported for other types of GERD. White persons and persons with private insurance are more likely to receive surgical repair for GERD than persons of other groups, creating disparities in the availability of healthcare services. Sexual and gender minority status has no known effect on the risk for GERD.

GLOBAL HEALTH CONSIDERATIONS

While the global prevalence of GERD is unknown, heartburn is a common problem in North America and Western Europe, with approximately 10% of the population reporting daily symptoms.

☀ ASSESSMENT

HISTORY. Elicit a history of contributing factors, including the regular consumption of fatty foods, caffeinated beverages, chocolate, nicotine, alcohol, or peppermint. Take a drug history to determine if the patient has been taking drugs that may contribute to GERD: beta-adrenergic blockers, calcium channel blockers, nitrates, theophylline, diazepam, anticholinergic drugs, estrogen, and progesterone. Inquire about smoking habits, which may contribute to the disease.

Little relationship appears to occur between the severity of symptoms and the degree of esophagitis. Some patients have minimal evidence of esophagitis, whereas others with severe, chronic inflammation may have no symptoms until stricture occurs. Patients may describe the characteristic symptom of heartburn (also known as *pyrosis* or *dyspepsia*). The discomfort is often a substernal or retrosternal pain that radiates upward to the neck, jaw, or back. They may have a sensation that food is stuck in the retrosternal area. Patients describe a worsening pain when they bend over, strain, or lie flat. With severe inflammation, discomfort occurs after each meal and lasts for up to 2 hours. Patients may describe coughing, hoarseness, or wheezing at night.

Patients may also report regurgitation, with a sensation of warm fluid traveling upward to the throat and leaving a bitter, sour taste in the mouth. Other symptoms may include difficulty swallowing (dysphagia) and painful swallowing (odynophagia) during eating, as well as eructation, flatulence, or bloating after eating. Atypical symptoms include ear pain from otitis media and tooth decay from regurgitation.

PHYSICAL EXAMINATION. The most common symptoms are **heartburn**, **regurgitation**, and **dysphagia**. Generally, the patient's physical appearance is unchanged by GERD. On rare occasions, some patients may experience unexplained weight loss. Their voice may be hoarse from irritated vocal cords due to gastric reflux, and they may have a repetitive dry cough or experience wheezing.

PSYCHOSOCIAL. Psychosocial assessment should include assessment of the degree of stress the person experiences and the strategies the person uses to cope with stress. Severe GERD is painful and interferes with quality of life if untreated. The patient may find ongoing symptoms and the inability to eat favorite foods discouraging.

Diagnostic Highlights

Test	Normal Result	Abnormality With Condition	Explanation
Esophagogastro-duodenoscopy	Normal squamous epithelial lining of the esophagus	People with GERD may have a normal endos-copy result; changes may be classified according to metaplasia, ulceration, stricturing, and erosions (MUSE)	Metaplasia is abnormal changes with replacement of normal stratified squamous epithelial lining of the esoph-agus with goblet cells due to chronic exposure to acid from reflux
Esophageal pH monitoring	> 5	< 5	Presence of gastric contents in the esophagus decreases pH
Esophageal manometry	Congruent esophageal pres-sures bilaterally; competent LES	Abnormal contractions and peristalsis; incom-petent LES; low resting pressure of LES	Multilumen esophageal cathe-ter introduced through mouth; used to measure esophageal pressures during a variety of swallowing maneuvers

Other Tests: Barium esophagogram, scintigraphy, gastroesophageal reflux scintigra-phy, Bernstein test (acidic solution infused into stomach causing heartburn in patients with GERD)

PRIMARY NURSING DIAGNOSIS

DIAGNOSIS. Acute pain related to esophageal reflux and esophageal inflammation as evi-denced by self-reports of pain, facial grimacing, and/or protective behavior

OUTCOMES. Comfort status; Pain control; Pain level; Knowledge: Disease process; Symptom severity; Medication response

INTERVENTIONS. Medication administration; Medication management; Pain management; Positioning; Nutritional monitoring; Weight management

PLANNING AND IMPLEMENTATION

Collaborative

Although diet therapy alone can manage symptoms in some patients, most patients can have their GERD managed pharmacologically. Dietary modifications that may decrease symptoms include reducing intake of fatty foods, caffeinated beverages, chocolate, nicotine, alcohol, and peppermint. Reducing the intake of spicy and acidic foods (citrus foods and juices, chocolate, onions, tomato-based products) lets esophageal healing occur during times of acute inflamma-tion. Encourage the patient to eat five to six small meals during the day rather than large meals. Ingestion of large amounts of food increases gastric pressure and thereby increases esopha-geal reflux. Limiting alcohol use is an important lifestyle modification. Both weight loss and smoking-cessation programs are also important for any patients who have problems with obesity and tobacco use.

Surgical procedures to relieve reflux are generally reserved for those otherwise healthy patients who have not responded to medications because they may develop complications such as strictures or Barrett esophagus. The most common surgical repair is the Nissen fundoplication, in which the surgeon wraps fundus of the stomach around esophagus to anchor the LES area below the diaphragm. More than half of fundoplication surgeries in the United States are now done by laparoscopic techniques. Long-term evaluation of patients who have had this surgery indicates that 90% of patients no longer have to take antireflux medications at 10 years after surgery.

Pharmacologic Highlights

Medication or Drug Class	Dosage	Description	Rationale
Antacids	Usually 30 mL between meals and as needed PO	Aluminum or magnesium salts	Neutralize gastric acid and relieve heartburn
Proton pump inhibitors (thought to be more effective) or H$_2$ receptor antagonists	Varies with drug; routes vary	Decrease gastric acid production; omeprazole, lansoprazole, cimetidine, famotidine, nizatidine	Proton pump inhibitors are the most powerful medications available; used when GERD is well documented; proton pump inhibitors block final step in the H$^+$ ion secretion by the parietal cell, have few adverse effects, and are well tolerated
Metoclopramide	10 mg PO tid before meals	GI stimulant	Improves gastric emptying and increases LES pressure

Independent

Many patients experience nighttime reflux because of the recumbent position and infrequent swallowing. Changing the patient's position by elevating the head of the bed during sleep may mitigate symptoms. Place 6-inch blocks under the head of the bed or place a wedge under the mattress to enhance nocturnal acid clearance. Encourage the patient to avoid food for 3 hours before going to sleep and advise the patient to eat slowly and chew food thoroughly. Encourage patients to avoid large meals.

Lifestyle modifications are important in the management of GERD. Lifestyle changes to reduce intra-abdominal pressure may be helpful to relieve symptoms. Encourage the patient to avoid the following: restrictive clothing, lifting heavy objects, straining, working in a bent-over position, and stooping. Support the patient's efforts to stop smoking, lose weight, reduce stress, and follow dietary guidelines. Make appropriate referrals to the dietitian to provide the knowledge essential for weight control and dietary management.

Evidence-Based Practice and Health Policy

Yadlapati, R., & Pandolfino, J. (2020). Personalized approach in the work-up and management of gastroesophageal reflux disease. *Gastrointestinal Endoscopy Clinics of North America, 30,* 227–238.

- GERD is associated with reduced quality of life and increased healthcare expenditure. The authors present a stepwise framework to phenotype GERD to manage care and minimize risk and cost. They characterized the symptom profile and the patient's response to proton pump inhibitor therapy. When the patient's symptom response is inadequate or the patient's presentation is atypical, the authors recommend an endoscopic evaluation for mucosal integrity and to assess for other diagnoses.
- If there is no erosive reflux disease, the authors recommend ambulatory reflux monitoring to evaluate for reflux hypersensitivity. If the symptom profile is unclear, the authors then recommend esophageal function testing with high-resolution impedance manometry. These steps are to allow for best practices management and minimize risk and cost.

DOCUMENTATION GUIDELINES

- Discomfort: Timing, character, location, duration, precipitating factors
- Nutrition: Food and fluid intake; understanding of dietary restriction and weight reduction for each meal; daily weight measurement

- Medication management: Understanding drug therapy, response to medications
- Response to nighttime positioning: Progress of changing position of head of the bed at night, tolerance to position change

DISCHARGE AND HOME HEALTHCARE GUIDELINES

Teach the patient how to maintain adequate nutrition and hydration and to manage medications. Make sure the patient and family understand all aspects of the treatment regimen. Review dietary limitations, recommendations to reduce weight and cut out tobacco, and dosage and side effects of all medications. Make referrals for smoking cessation and alcohol management as needed. Make sure the patient understands the need to change position at nighttime and that the patient has the supplies required to do so.

Glaucoma

DRG Category:	117
Mean LOS:	2.7 days
Description:	SURGICAL: Intraocular Procedures Without Complication or Comorbidity or Major Complication or Comorbidity
DRG Category:	124
Mean LOS:	5.2 days
Description:	MEDICAL: Other Disorders of the Eye With Major Complication or Comorbidity

Glaucoma is the second leading cause of irreversible blindness behind macular degeneration. More than 2 million people in the United States over the age of 40 years are diagnosed with glaucoma, and estimates are that only half of the people who have glaucoma know it. Over half have significant visual impairment, and over 100,000 have bilateral blindness. While long defined as a problem with intraocular pressure (IOP), glaucoma is now defined as a problem with the integrity of optic nerve structure or function that causes specific visual field defects. It is an optic neuropathy that is chronic and progressive, leading to irreversible damage and loss of optic nerve fibers. The process of optic nerve damage can be stopped or slowed by lowering the IOP, but some patients can have optic nerve damage and visual field defects while having a normal IOP. In a healthy person, the IOP (10–21 mm Hg) exists as long as there is a balance between the production, circulation, and outflow of aqueous humor. Aqueous humor is produced in the posterior chamber ciliary processes and flows through the pupil into the anterior chamber. From the anterior chamber, it passes through the canal of Schlemm and out through the aqueous veins into the anterior ciliary veins.

Increased IOP compromises blood flow to the optic nerve and retina. Tissue damage occurs as a result of the deficient blood supply and progresses from the periphery toward the fovea centralis. If IOP is left untreated, the primary complication is blindness.

CAUSES

The cause of glaucoma is not certain, but risk factors are known. They include elevated IOP, family history, age older than 40 years, and myopia. Other risk factors may include obesity, smoking, alcohol misuse and abuse, history of stress, anxiety, and sleep apnea. Chronic open-angle glaucoma (primary open-angle glaucoma [POAG]) is the most common form of glaucoma, accounting for 90% of all glaucoma cases. It is caused by an overproduction of aqueous humor or obstruction to its flow through the trabecular meshwork or the canal of Schlemm. The chamber angles between the iris and the cornea remain open. IOP intensifies gradually because aqueous humor cannot leave the eye at the same rate that it is produced, leading to pressures that are incompatible with the health of the eye.

Acute glaucoma, also referred to as *closed-angle glaucoma* or *narrow-angle glaucoma*, is less common and, with its sudden onset, is treated as an emergency situation. Obstruction of the outflow of aqueous humor occurs by anterior displacement of the iris against the cornea, which narrows or obstructs the chamber angle. Attacks of acute glaucoma are caused by injury, pupil dilation, or stress. Secondary glaucoma occurs in other diseases of the eye when the circulation of aqueous humor is disrupted with either a decreased angle or an increased intraocular volume. Uveitis, iritis, trauma, tumors, and postsurgical procedures on the eye are common causes of secondary glaucoma. Congenital glaucoma is caused by an autosomal recessive trait that results in dysfunctional development of the trabecular meshwork through which aqueous humor flows.

GENETIC CONSIDERATIONS

Several genes have been associated with the occurrence of glaucoma. Genetic causes of both congenital glaucoma (Rieger syndrome) and adult-onset POAG have been identified. Hereditary factors are believed to account for between 13% and 25% of POAG cases. POAG has been reported to be caused by mutations in myocilin, optineurin, and *CYP1B1*. Autosomal dominant and recessive patterns of inheritance have been described, and there appear to be both wide variability in expression and incomplete penetrance.

SEX AND LIFE SPAN CONSIDERATIONS

Individuals over age 40 years are at a higher risk of developing glaucoma. Approximately 2% of the U.S. population over age 40 years and 10% of people over age 80 years have glaucoma. Glaucoma affects both men and women.

HEALTH DISPARITIES AND SEXUAL/GENDER MINORITY HEALTH

Glaucoma is the leading cause of blindness among Black persons, and is three to four times more common in Black Americans than in White Americans. Black persons are more likely to develop glaucoma early in life and often have rapidly progressing disease as compared to other groups. Medicaid recipients with OAG receive less glaucoma testing than other groups, and disparities are even more profound in Black Medicaid patients. Asian American and Native American persons seem to be at higher risk than other populations for angle-closure glaucoma. Experts note that glaucoma is significantly underdiagnosed in Hispanic persons in the United States. Sexual and gender minority status has no known effect on the risk for glaucoma.

GLOBAL HEALTH CONSIDERATIONS

The leading cause of blindness in the world is uncorrected cataracts, followed by glaucoma. Approximately 3.5 million people have bilateral POAG that has led to blindness, which is irreversible. Estimates are that each year, 2 million people will be newly diagnosed with POAG, which raises concerns that the number of people experiencing blindness will continue to increase globally. The health burden of glaucoma is increasing globally, and people of older age, lower socioeconomic level, higher amount of ultraviolet radiation, and higher level of pollution have a higher burden. Asian ancestry is associated with angle-closure glaucoma, whereas African or European ancestry is associated with POAG.

ASSESSMENT

HISTORY. Patients with POAG will often have no presenting symptoms until late in the disease. Acute glaucoma (narrow-/closed-angle glaucoma) is more likely to cause earlier symptoms. Question patients about any history of eye disease in their family. Establish a history of eye pain, headache, eye redness, or multicolored halos. Ask patients if they have had recent eye surgery, eye or head trauma, or infection, or if they have diabetic retinopathy. Use of antihistamines can precipitate closed-angle glaucoma because antihistamines cause pupils to dilate, and this may result in obstruction of fluid flow. Family visual history can help with a diagnosis of chronic POAG. Because POAG develops slowly, the visual history should focus on foggy vision, diminished accommodation, frequent changes in eyeglass prescription, mild eye pain, headache, visual field deficits, and halos around lights.

PHYSICAL EXAMINATION. Many patients do not have symptoms. Common symptoms include **eye redness or pain**, **headaches**, and **visual changes such as fogginess or multicolored halos**. Perform a standard eye examination as recommended by the American Academy of Ophthalmology. Compare current visual acuity to previous visual examinations if possible. Blind spots and peripheral field losses are confirmed by a visual field examination. Gentle palpation of the covered eyeball reveals a firmer globe, which has been caused by the increased IOP. Inspect the patient's eyes for reddened sclera, turbid aqueous humor, and moderately dilated nonreactive pupils. Other symptoms include extreme unilateral eye pain, blurred vision, and possibly nausea and vomiting. Symptoms of congenital glaucoma include photophobia, cloudy corneas, excessive tearing, and muscle spasms around the orbital ridge (blepharospasm).

PSYCHOSOCIAL. Validate observations of anxiety and explore coping strategies to deal with patient concerns. Grieving for the potential of vision loss or vision already lost follows the stages of denial, anger, bargaining, depression, and acceptance. Reassure the patient that early treatment can prevent irreversible damage.

Diagnostic Highlights

Test	Normal Result	Abnormality With Condition	Explanation
Tonometry	12–20 mm Hg	Elevated: 22–28 mm Hg warning level; > 38 mm Hg major concern	Measures IOP using a tonometer (instrument that is pressed directly against the anesthetized eye); if a recording device is used (tonography), recorded slope indicates adequacy of drainage
Gonioscopy	Normal drainage angle in eye	Presence of adhesions, aberrant blood vessels, signs of injury	Visualization of entire 360-degree circumference of iridocorneal angle

Other Tests: Tests include direct opthalmoscopic examination and visual field testing, perimetry, fundus photography, ultrasound biomicroscopy, and retinal nerve fiber imaging. Newly developed imaging studies include scanning laser techniques and optical coherence tomography.

PRIMARY NURSING DIAGNOSIS

DIAGNOSIS. Anxiety related to decreased visual acuity as evidenced by visual changes and/or headache

OUTCOMES. Body image; Anxiety level; Neurological status; Knowledge: Disease process; Self-care: Activities of daily living

INTERVENTIONS. Vision screening; Communication enhancement: Visual deficit; Environmental management; Fall prevention; Eye care; Medication management

✳ PLANNING AND IMPLEMENTATION

Collaborative

Patients should be screened for glaucoma every 3 to 5 years after the age of 40 years and more often if the person is Black. Blindness from glaucoma can frequently be prevented by early detection and lifelong treatment. Patients are informed that vision loss is permanent, but further vision loss may be prevented if IOP is controlled through medications or surgery. Glaucoma is often treated medically to lower the IOP (see Pharmacologic Highlights). Surgery is required when medications are ineffective in reducing IOP. Argon laser trabeculoplasty is preferred because it has an 80% success rate in reducing IOP. Surgical filtering treatment produces a permanent fistula from the anterior chamber and the subconjunctival space. Filtering procedures include trabeculectomy, cyclodialysis, peripheral iridectomy, sclerectomy, and ocular implantation devices such as the Molento implant.

After surgical filtering, postoperative care includes dilation and topical steroids to rest the pupil. Postoperative care after peripheral iridectomy includes cycloplegic eyedrops in only the affected eye to relax the ciliary muscle and to decrease inflammation, thus preventing adhesions. When other surgical procedures have failed, cyclocryotherapy may be performed. Parts of the ciliary body are destroyed by the freezing effect of the probe, which reduces aqueous humor production.

Pharmacologic Highlights

Medication or Drug Class	Dosage	Description	Rationale
Miotic eyedrops	Varies with drug	Pilocarpine hydrochloride, carbachol	Constrict pupil and contract ciliary muscle to promote outflow
Beta blockers	Varies with drug	Timolol, levobunolol, metipranolol, carteolol or betaxolol ophthalmic	Reduce the production of aqueous humor
Alpha-2 adrenergic agonists	Varies with drug	Brimonidine, apraclonidine	Lower intraocular pressure
Carbonic anhydrase inhibitors	Varies with drug	Acetazolamide, methazolamide, dorzolamide, brinzolamide	Reduce the production of aqueous humor

Other Drugs: Combination solutions may be used to increase utility and compliance. Epinephrine and dipivefrin hydrochloride reduce aqueous humor production (not for use in closed-angle glaucoma); osmotic agents such as oral glycerin or mannitol in emergencies to reduce IOP rapidly; prostaglandin analogs (latanoprost, bimatoprost)

Independent

Note that miotics, which cause pupillary constriction, blur vision for 1 to 2 hours after installation and reduce adaptation to darkness. To prevent injury related to reduced peripheral vision, arrange the environment to ensure safety. Place frequently used items where the patient can view them through central visual fields. If the patient has difficulty with balance and is fearful of falling, consider balance training to promote confidence in ambulating. Teach the patient to administer miotics, which are often given four times a day to fit the patient's schedule; the gel form (pilocarpine HS gel) can be given once a day at night. Some patients benefit by the use of Ocusert, a pilocarpine time-released wafer. The wafer is inserted weekly and is helpful to patients who cannot insert eyedrops.

To minimize self-care deficits, encourage independence with activities of daily living and assist the patient as necessary. Encourage the patient to express anxiety, grieving, and concerns about glaucoma or blindness. Listen supportively, and explore coping strategies. Reinforce compliance with the recommended treatment plan and follow-up care. If the patient has suffered significant loss of vision, arrange for consultation with a specialist who can assist the patient to achieve the highest possible quality of life.

Evidence-Based Practice and Health Policy

Rossetti, L., Lester, M., Tranchina, L., Ottobelli, L., Coco, G., Calcatelli, E., Ancona, C., Cirafici, P., & Manni, G. (2020). Can treatment with citicoline eyedrops reduce progression in glaucoma? The results of a randomized placebo-controlled clinical trial. *Journal of Glaucoma, 29*, 513–520.

- The authors wanted to test whether additional therapy with citicoline eyedrops along with other IOP-lowering treatments could slow glaucoma progression in patients with worsening of damage and IOP 18 mm Hg or less. The authors conducted a randomized, double-masked, placebo-controlled, multicenter 3-year study.
- Patients ($N = 80$) were randomized to receive citicoline eyedrops or placebo three times daily for 3 years, were followed every 3 months, and underwent visual field examinations. On average, patients receiving citicoline eyedrops lost 1.86 mcm of retinal nerve fiber layer in 3 years, versus 2.99 mcm in the placebo group. The addition of citicoline eyedrops to IOP-lowering treatment might reduce disease progression in patients with progressing glaucoma.

DOCUMENTATION GUIDELINES

- Cupping and atrophy of the optic disk, palpation of the eyeball, peripheral field losses, reddened sclera, nonreactive pupils, turbid aqueous humor, pain, and nausea or vomiting
- Presence of surgical complications: Pain, nausea, infection, hemorrhage, profuse sweating, change in vital signs
- Response to medication teaching
- Response to any limitations in quality of life because of visual changes

DISCHARGE AND HOME HEALTHCARE GUIDELINES

To prevent increased IOP, teach the patient to avoid the following: bending at the waist, lifting heavy objects, coughing, vomiting, and straining to have a bowel movement. Note that following the medication schedule and routinely seeing the eye doctor can prevent further visual loss. Glaucoma requires strict, consistent treatment to prevent blindness.

Validate the patient's understanding of all medications, including dosage, route, action, and side effects. Be sure the patient has the dexterity to instill eyedrops correctly. Suggest a daily calendar log to record medication use. Written guidelines may be helpful. Review the date and time of the return visit to the eye surgeon after surgery. Instruct the patient to wear an eye shield over the operated eye at night and eyeglasses during the day to prevent accidental injury. Explain the need for the patient to call the eye doctor right away if any of the following symptoms occurs: pain in the eye, shortness of breath, nausea or vomiting, loss of vision, nonreactive pupils, reddened sclera, bleeding, discharge, or tingling in the hands or feet. Visiting nurses for home healthcare or social services can assist with rehabilitation or finances. Refer the patient to a Web resource from the Glaucoma Research Foundation on living with glaucoma: https://www.glaucoma.org.

Glomerulonephritis, Acute

DRG Category: 699
Mean LOS: 4.2 days
Description: MEDICAL: Other Kidney and Urinary Tract Diagnoses With Complication or Comorbidity

Acute glomerulonephritis (AGN) is a specific set of renal inflammatory diseases of the specialized tuft of capillaries within the kidney called the *glomerulus*. It is defined by its sudden onset of hematuria, proteinuria, and red blood cell casts in the urine, and it may be accompanied by hypertension, edema (sodium and water retention), and decreased glomerular filtration. In its several forms, glomerulonephritis (GN) was the leading cause of chronic renal failure in the United States until the mid-1980s, but because of more aggressive treatment approaches, it is now third, after diabetes mellitus and hypertension. GN continues to be a fairly common disorder worldwide, however. The inflammatory changes occur because of deposits of antigen-antibody complexes lodged within the glomerular membrane. Antigen-antibody complexes are formed within the circulation in response to an antigen or foreign protein. The antigen may be of external origin, such as a portion of the *Streptococcus* bacterial cell wall, or of internal origin, such as the changes that occur in systemic diseases like systemic lupus erythematosus (SLE).

Acute poststreptococcal glomerulonephritis (APSGN) results from an infection with nephritogenic strains of group A beta-hemolytic streptococci (GABHS). These infections occur in the skin (impetigo) or throat (pharyngitis). If the source of the causative antigen is temporary, such as a transient infection, the inflammatory changes subside, and renal function usually returns to normal; if the source of antigen is long term or permanent, the AGN may become chronic. During the acute phase of the disease process, major complications include hypertension, hypertensive encephalopathy, acute renal failure, cardiac failure, and seizures. Chronic glomerular nephritis leads to contracted, granular kidneys and end-stage renal disease. Rapidly progressive glomerulonephritis (RPGN; also known as *crescentic nephritis*), an acute and severe form of kidney inflammation, can cause loss of kidney function within days. Inflammation at the sites of renal filtration (the glomerular basement membrane) causes leakage of blood proteins into the urinary space. The condition is caused by inflammation of cells in the urinary space that form crescents, hence the name crescentic nephritis. Complications of AGN include acute kidney failure, end-stage renal failure, hypertension, hypertensive retinopathy, hypertensive encephalopathy, and nephrotic syndrome.

CAUSES

Etiological factors are unclear, but most experts identify an immunological origin for the disease. The exact triggers for formation of immune complexes (primarily composed of immunoglobulins and complement) that are deposited in the glomerulus are unclear, but they cause swelling and inflammatory changes of the glomerular tufts. The basement membrane of the glomerulus is also thicker than normal, with deposits of dense material that can lead to irreversible injury. AGN may occur as an isolated (primary) disorder, as a disorder associated with an infectious disease, or as a secondary disorder. Primary AGN occurs in mesangiocapillary GN and in IgA nephropathy. Infection-associated AGN follows an infection such as a GABHS. Nonstreptococcal postinfectious GN may occur after an attack of infective endocarditis, sepsis, pneumococcal pneumonia, viral hepatitis, mumps, or measles, which are considered risk factors. RPGN is associated with vasculitis, SLE, Goodpasture syndrome, and IgA nephropathy, which are considered risk factors.

GENETIC CONSIDERATIONS

Single-gene disorders with GN as a feature include Fechtner syndrome (*MYH9* mutation) and Barraquer-Simons syndrome (possibly caused by *LMNB2* mutation). There is also a familial form of IgA nephropathy. Alport syndrome is a hereditary nephritis that includes X-linked Alport syndrome (80%), autosomal recessive Alport syndrome (15%), and autosomal dominant Alport syndrome (5%). Mutations in collagen genes (*COL4A3*, *COL4A4*, *COL4A5*) are also associated with GN.

SEX AND LIFE SPAN CONSIDERATIONS

AGN occurs primarily in the pediatric population, ages 2 to 15 years, after an infectious event; GABHS is most common in boys ages 3 to 7 years. About 95% of children and 70% of adults have a full recovery from APSGN. In adults, AGN may occur after an infection or with multisystem diseases such as SLE. Because adults may exhibit more signs of cardiovascular compromise than children, treatment of the adult may require more support of the cardiovascular system through medications. RPGN primarily affects adults in their sixth and seventh decades of life. As a whole, twice as many males as females are affected with GN.

HEALTH DISPARITIES AND SEXUAL/GENDER MINORITY HEALTH

Ethnicity, race, and sexual/gender minority status have no known effect on the risk for GN.

GLOBAL HEALTH CONSIDERATIONS

While APSGN has decreased in Western countries, it is common in developing regions of Africa, the Caribbean, and South America and in countries such as India, Pakistan, and Malaysia. Globally, the most common cause of AGN is IgA nephropathy (Berger disease), which likely has a genetic cause or is related to infections such as HIV or hepatitis.

ASSESSMENT

HISTORY. A typical person with AGN is a boy 2 to 15 years of age who develops facial swelling and puffiness of the eyelids following a streptococcal infection. Question the patient or parents about an untreated respiratory tract infection that has occurred in the last 1 to 3 weeks, as well as any other recent infections. The timing and duration of the infection are important. Some adult patients, particularly patients with diabetes mellitus, may describe a recent history of a skin abscess or skin infection. Ask the patient about the medical history to identify any multisystem diseases. Because patients often describe a history of weight gain and edema of the hands and face, ask them if their rings are tighter than usual. Some patients may also describe decreased urine volume, changes in urine color (dark, smoky), headache, increased fatigue and activity intolerance, muscle and joint achiness, shortness of breath, and orthopnea. Older patients' symptoms may be more vague and nonspecific, such as achiness and nausea.

PHYSICAL EXAMINATION. Symptoms generally have an abrupt onset. The most common symptoms are **hematuria, oliguria,** and **peripheral or periorbital edema**. Note any signs of fluid retention, such as edema in the face and hands. You may notice ascites. As you speak to the patient, you may notice dyspnea and labored breathing from a pleural effusion or pulmonary edema. Inspect the neck veins to determine if engorgement is present. The patient's urine output is usually decreased and is often dark or even coffee colored. When you auscultate the patient's heart and lungs, you may hear basilar crackles and an S_3 heart sound. Most patients have an elevated arterial pressure. Weigh the patient each day, and monitor abdominal girth. Some patients may have nausea, vomiting, and abdominal pain. Provide ongoing monitoring for visual changes, sinusitis, adventitious breath sounds, abdominal distention, and seizure activity.

These signs and symptoms indicate the potential onset of the complications and need to be reported to the physician.

PSYCHOSOCIAL. Patients and families may be anxious about changes in the patient's appearance, an uncertain prognosis, and the possibility of lifestyle changes. Assess the patient's and family's coping mechanisms, support systems, and stress levels.

Diagnostic Highlights

Test	Normal Result	Abnormality With Condition	Explanation
Creatinine clearance	100–140 mL/min	50 mL/min	Damaged glomerulus no longer able to clear or filter normal amounts of creatinine from blood
Serum creatinine	0.51–1.21 mg/dL	> 2 mg/dL	Decreased ability of glomerulus to filter creatinine leads to accumulation in the blood
Urinalysis	Minimal red blood cells; moderate clear protein casts; negative for protein	Red blood cells and red blood cell casts; elevated protein and urine specific gravity	May also have renal tubular cells, white blood cells, increased white blood cell casts

Other Tests: Supporting tests include cultures of the throat and skin lesions if streptococcus infection is suspected, serum electrolytes, serum potassium, serum blood urea nitrogen, complete blood count, erythrocyte sedimentation rate, C-reactive protein, complement levels, cryoglobulins, serum mucoprotein levels, antistreptolysin O titers, streptozyme test, and percutaneous renal biopsy. Blood cultures may be drawn if the patient is immunosuppressed, febrile, or has a history of using IV drugs. Computed tomography, ultrasonography, or echocardiography may be performed.

PRIMARY NURSING DIAGNOSIS

DIAGNOSIS. Excess fluid volume related to glomerular inflammation and decreased renal filtration as evidenced by oliguria, weight gain, and/or peripheral edema

OUTCOMES. Fluid balance; Hydration; Nutrition status: Food and fluid intake; Knowledge: Treatment regime; Knowledge: Acute illness management; Knowledge: Weight management

INTERVENTIONS. Fluid/electrolyte management; Fluid monitoring; Medication administration; Medication management; Weight management

PLANNING AND IMPLEMENTATION

Collaborative

Because most patients with AGN recover spontaneously, treatment is supportive. During the acute phase, when urine is grossly hematuric and blood pressure is elevated, the patient is placed on bedrest, and symptoms are managed pharmacologically. All infections need to be identified and treated. A dietary consultation is necessary to implement dietary restrictions that can manage increased blood pressure, decreased urine output, and the presence of nitrogenous products in the urine. Usually, sodium and fluid restriction is instituted to manage hypertension and edema. Depending on the course of their disease, some patients also need potassium and protein restrictions. If the patient is on fluid restriction, work with the patient and family to devise a schedule of fluid intake that maximizes patient preference and comfort. Pediatric patients may require hemodialysis, particularly in the setting of crescentic nephritis.

Pharmacologic Highlights

Medication or Drug Class	Dosage	Description	Rationale
Antihypertensive and diuretics	Varies with drug	Antihypertensives; hydralazine; diuretics: furosemide; nifedipine	Manage hypertension and fluid overload
Antibiotics	Varies with drug for a 10-day course of therapy	Penicillin, erythromycin, cephalexin	Kills streptococcal infection if the disease is believed to be APSGN

Other Drugs: Antibiotics may be administered for 7 to 10 days if the etiological factor was an infectious agent such as streptococcus. Corticosteroids are controversial and considered by many experts to be of no value. Labetalol may be used for hypertensive encephalopathy and malignant hypertension. Cyclophosphamide may be used for treatment of AGN due to Wegener granulomatosis.

Independent

Focus on decreasing discomfort, promoting rest, reducing complications, and providing patient education. Work with the patient to develop a schedule for daily hygiene that limits fatigue and overexertion. Cluster care to provide for rest periods and assist the patient with relaxation techniques. Assist children with the usual bedtime rituals. Increase activity gradually as symptoms subside.

While the patient is on bedrest, perform active or passive range-of-motion exercises each shift and assist the patient to a new position every 2 hours. Monitor the patient's skin for breakdown. If the patient is recovering from an infection, prevent secondary infection. Take time to answer the patient's and parents' questions fully. If you note that the family is coping ineffectively with the illness or prognosis, make a referral to a clinical nurse specialist.

Evidence-Based Practice and Health Policy

Moran, S., Barbour, S., Dipchand, C., Garland, C., Hladunewich, M., Jauhal, A., Kappel, J., Levin, A., Pandeya, S., Reich, H., Thanabalasingam, S., Thomas, D., Ma, J., & White, C. (2020). Management of patients with glomerulonephritis during the COVID-19 pandemic: Recommendations from the Canadian Society of Nephrology COVID-19 Rapid Response Team. *Canadian Journal of Kidney Health and Disease, 7*, 1–8.

- The authors aimed to provide guidance on how to manage patients with GN during the COVID-19 epidemic. They performed a literature review and collected surveys from nephrologists to identify practice patterns. They identified nine areas of management that may be affected by the pandemic.
- The identified areas were clinic visit scheduling, clinic visit type, provision of multidisciplinary care, blood and urine testing, home-base monitoring, immunosuppression, other medications, patient education and support, and employment. These recommendations were based on the best route to optimal care delivery during the COVID-19 pandemic.

DOCUMENTATION GUIDELINES

- Cardiovascular responses: Blood pressure, pulse, presence of abnormal heart sounds; presence, location, and severity of edema; daily weights
- Renal responses: Character, amount, odor of urine
- Respiratory responses: Respiratory rate and effort, breath sounds
- Presence of complications: Fever, food intolerance, pulmonary congestion, shortness of breath, increasing peripheral edema, weight gain, skin breakdown, anuria
- Comfort: Type of discomfort, location and intensity, character, response to attempts to provide relief

DISCHARGE AND HOME HEALTHCARE GUIDELINES

Inform patients and families about the disease process, prognosis, and treatment plan. Discuss with them the possibility that abnormal urinary findings may persist for years after AGN has been diagnosed. Demonstrate all home care techniques, such as medication administration. Discuss the dosage, action, route, and side effects of all medications. If the patient is placed on antibiotics, encourage the patient to complete the entire prescription. Teach the patient and family to seek professional assistance for all infectious processes (particularly respiratory infections with sore throat and fever); monitor body weight and blood pressure at home or through a clinic; and avoid contact with individuals with infectious processes. Discuss the need for ongoing laboratory monitoring of electrolytes and renal function tests during the months of convalescence, as recommended by the physician. Explain that after APSGN, any gross hematuria that occurs when the patient has a viral infection needs to be reported to the physician.

Goiter

DRG Category:	644
Mean LOS:	4.3 days
Description:	MEDICAL: Endocrine Disorders With Complication or Comorbidity

Goiter is the enlargement of the thyroid gland. It is usually a response to a thyroid hormone deficiency (primary hypothyroidism) that results in the hypersecretion of thyroid-stimulating hormone (TSH) from the anterior pituitary gland. Oversecretion leads to subsequent thyroid hypertrophy and hypervascularity. The body's response may compensate for thyroid hormone deficiency, leaving the patient asymptomatic. Goiter may also occur in conjunction with hyperthyroidism, known as Graves disease. Finally, goiter may occur with the growth of thyroid tumors. Secondary hypothyroidism occurs with TSH deficiency in the pituitary gland and is not associated with goiter.

Most goiters are classified as *nontoxic goiters* (simple goiters). They result from any enlargement of the thyroid gland that is not caused by an inflammation or a neoplasm. Simple goiters can be classified as sporadic or endemic and are not associated initially with either hyperthyroidism or hypothyroidism. Sporadic goiters occur after a person eats certain foods (peaches, strawberries, radishes, spinach, peas, cabbage, soybeans, or peanuts) or takes certain medications (iodides, lithium, propylthiouracil) that decrease thyroxine (T_4). Endemic goiters, in contrast, occur because of the patient's geographic location in areas where the soil is depleted of iodine. Endemic goiter that results from soil deficiencies is most likely to occur during autumn and winter. *Toxic goiters* are associated with hyperthyroidism and elevated thyroid hormones.

Goiter becomes a problem only when the enlargement exerts pressure on other neck structures, such as the trachea, or when the enlargement is unsightly, causing the patient to become concerned. If the goiter is related to hyperthyroidism, cardiovascular complications may occur, such as hypertension, cardiac dysrhythmias, myocardial infarction, and heart failure. If the goiter is related to hypothyroidism, complications include fatigue, cold sensitivity, heart failure, an enlarged heart, cardiac dysrhythmias, intestinal obstruction, obesity, anemia, deafness, psychiatric problems, carpal tunnel syndrome, and impaired fertility.

CAUSES

The causes of goiter include iodine deficiency, excess iodine ingestion, autoimmune processes, benign or malignant tumors, radiation exposure, infection, and inflammation of the thyroid gland. The use of iodine food additives has greatly reduced the incidence of endemic goiter.

Difficulty in determining the incidence of endemic goiter is complicated because many individuals with the condition experience no symptoms and are not diagnosed. Sporadic goiter, or goiter caused by interference with iodine metabolism, is affected by either hereditary factors or ingestion of foods or pharmacologic agents, such as lithium, that inhibit T_4 production.

Goiter caused by thyroid nodules, a common condition, may also cause no symptoms. Although thyroid nodules or tumors may be either benign or malignant, more than 75% of thyroid nodules are benign.

GENETIC CONSIDERATIONS

Among infants with hypothyroidism, 10% to 20% have an inherited form of the disorder, which is often associated with a visible enlargement of the thyroid gland. A mutation in the thyroid peroxidase gene on chromosome 2 is usually involved. Goiter may also appear in conjunction with deafness in the single-gene disorder Pendred syndrome, which is caused by mutations in the *SLC26A4* gene.

SEX AND LIFE SPAN CONSIDERATIONS

Endemic goiter may be experienced by adolescents during growth spurts, but most thyroid dysfunction is found in women in their second to fifth decades. Additional thyroid hormone is required by the body during pregnancy and lactation, conditions that may result in the need for a higher index of suspicion of endemic goiter during these life stages. Older individuals who have depressive symptoms should also be assessed for uncompensated hypothyroidism. Patients over the age of 80 years have a higher complication rate after thyroidectomy than those between 65 and 79 years of age.

HEALTH DISPARITIES AND SEXUAL/GENDER MINORITY HEALTH

Ethnicity, race, and sexual/gender minority status have no known effect on the risk for goiter.

GLOBAL HEALTH CONSIDERATIONS

Approximately 30% of the world's population lives in countries with low iodine content in the soil. Around the globe, endemic goiter from iodine deficiency is a leading cause of brain damage and mental retardation in children. Severe iodine deficiency impairs thyroid hormone synthesis and delays fetal brain growth and development. According to the World Health Organization, iodine deficiency is a particular problem for children living in developing countries in Asia, South America, and Africa.

ASSESSMENT

HISTORY. Patients with suspected goiter most often complain of visible enlargement of the neck or difficulty in activities such as buttoning shirts with no accompanying weight gain to account for the problem. In advanced stages, they may complain of pressure on the neck or chest, difficulty in swallowing, hoarseness, or respiratory distress. Other symptoms may reflect either hypothyroidism or hyperthyroidism.

Obtain a drug history to determine past use of iodine-containing medications (including recent contrast media or oral contraceptives), which may falsely elevate serum thyroid function tests. Similarly, a severe illness, malnutrition, or the use of aspirin, corticosteroids, or phenytoin sodium may falsely depress serum thyroid function tests.

PHYSICAL EXAMINATION. The patient with a significantly enlarged goiter may have a **visible thyroid gland on the anterior neck**. Note that the gland rises with swallowing. When you palpate the gland, stand behind the patient and palpate the gland for tender areas, areas of irregularity, firmness, or any nodules. A normal lateral lobe is approximately the size of the distal phalanx (most remote bony segment) of the thumb. Remember that excessive palpation of the thyroid gland can precipitate thyroid storm (acute thyrotoxic crisis from an oversecretion of the thyroid hormones); therefore, palpate the gland gently and only when necessary. You may also hear a bruit over an enlarged thyroid gland when you auscultate over the lateral lobes. Some patients also have respiratory stridor from compression of the trachea. The patient may also have Pemberton sign (dizziness, flushed face, fainting when the patient's arms are raised above the head) caused by compression from the goiter.

PSYCHOSOCIAL. While most types of thyroid dysfunction can be treated noninvasively, goiter that is caused by cancer will likely precipitate concern. Assess the patient's degree of anxiety about the illness and potential complications.

Diagnostic Highlights

Normal iodine levels can be determined by a urine sample. Median urine iodine is greater than 100 mg/dL; severe iodine deficiency is associated with median urine iodine 20 to 49 mg/dL.

Test	Normal Result	Abnormality With Condition	Explanation
Plasma TSH level	In most healthy patients, TSH values are 0.4–4.2 mU/L	> 4.2 mU/L	TSH is overproduced to stimulate the poorly functioning thyroid gland; increased levels indicate primary hypothyroidism and decreased levels indicate secondary hypothyroidism
TSH stimulation test	> 10% in radioactive iodine uptake	Primary hypothyroidism: no response; secondary hypothyroidism: normal response	Differentiates between primary and secondary hypothyroidism
Tri-iodothyronine (T_3) and thyroxine (T_4)	T_3: 80–210 ng/dL; T_4: 4.6–12 mcg/dL	Hyperthyroid: increased; hypothyroid: decreased	Results depend on underlying disease process

Other Tests: Supporting tests include thyroid antibodies, thyroid scan, plasma T_4 index, thyroid antibody tests, and urinary iodine excretion; ultrasound, computed tomography, and magnetic resonance imaging. Barium swallow documents esophageal obstruction for patients who are having difficulty swallowing.

PRIMARY NURSING DIAGNOSIS

DIAGNOSIS. Risk for ineffective airway clearance as evidenced by stridor, hoarseness, and/or dysphagia

OUTCOMES. Respiratory status: Airway patency; Respiratory status: Ventilation; Symptom severity; Medication response; Comfort status; Knowledge: Treatment regimen

INTERVENTIONS. Airway management; Anxiety reduction; Artificial airway management; Positioning; Respiratory monitoring; Surveillance; Ventilation assistance; Medication management

PLANNING AND IMPLEMENTATION
Collaborative

MEDICAL. The goal of medical management for the patient with a simple goiter is to reduce the size of the goiter by correcting the underlying cause. Both hyperthyroidism and hypothyroidism need to be treated. If the patient has decreased iodine stores, small doses of iodide (e.g., Lugol solution) may correct the problem. If the patient is ingesting a known substance that leads to goiter, avoidance of the food or drug is necessary. Commonly, no specific cause of the goiter is found, and the patient is placed on thyroid-replacement therapy.

If the patient is an older adult or has a longstanding goiter with many nodules, further testing is needed because levothyroxine may lead to thyrotoxic crisis; the patient may need radioiodine ablation therapy to destroy areas of hypersecretion. Surgical treatment is rarely indicated and is used only when symptoms of obstruction occur after a trial of medications. Patients with goiter and thyroid nodules may also need surgical exploration to determine if they have cancer.

Pharmacologic Highlights

Medication or Drug Class	Dosage	Description	Rationale
Levothyroxine sodium	1.5–2.5 mcg/kg PO daily; use lowest dose possible because overreplacement of thyroid can cause bone loss or cardiovascular complications	Synthetic thyroid hormone replacement	Suppresses TSH formation and allows the thyroid to rest

Independent

The first priority is to ensure an adequate airway and breathing. If you suspect that the patient's airway is compromised, keep an intubation tray and suction equipment at the bedside at all times. Pay particular attention to any sign of airway obstruction, such as stridor or dyspnea, and check on the patient frequently. Elevate the head of the patient's bed to high Fowler position during meals and for 30 minutes afterward to limit the risk of aspiration. If you suspect that the goiter is increasing in size, monitor the patient's neck circumference daily.

Care of the patient with goiter also focuses on the patient's anxiety and knowledge deficits. Whatever the cause of the goiter, the patient may be highly anxious about the medical diagnosis itself or the resulting symptoms. Make sure patients have the information they need to understand the disease. If the goiter is unsightly, recommend that the patient choose clothing that neither restricts activity nor draws attention to the neck. If the patient's appearance is extremely distressing, refer the patient for appropriate counseling.

If surgery for goiter removal is necessary, monitor the patient for acute airway obstruction and for thyrotoxic crisis, which is a potential complication of the surgery and leads to tachycardia, increased blood pressure, diaphoresis, and anxiety. Check both the incision and behind the neck for postoperative bleeding; notify the physician immediately if significant bleeding occurs. Each time you monitor the vital signs, assess the patient's vocal quality and compare it with the patient's preoperative speaking. Maintain the neck and head in good alignment and support them during position changes to prevent traction on the sutures and damage to the operative site.

Evidence-Based Practice and Health Policy

Zheng, R., Rios-Diaz, A., Thibault, D., Crispo, J., Willis, A., & Willis, A. (2020). A contemporary analysis of goiters undergoing surgery in the United States. *American Journal of Surgery*, *220*, 341–348.

- The authors identified disparities and at-risk populations among patients with goiters undergoing thyroidectomy. The authors queried the National Inpatient Sample (NIS) database to identify patients ($N = 103,678$) with goiter who underwent thyroidectomy between 2009 and 2013 and to determine factors associated with surgery.
- Only 7.4% of patients had simple goiter, 70.9% had nodular goiter, 13.5% had thyrotoxicosis, 1.2% had thyroiditis, and 7.0% had thyroid cancer. Factors associated with operation for simple goiter included age over 65 years, being Black, and being uninsured. Patients with cancerous goiters undergoing thyroidectomy were less likely to be Black or uninsured.

DOCUMENTATION GUIDELINES

• Physical findings: Respiratory status, postoperative wound healing, presence of dysphagia (difficulty swallowing), neck circumference
• Response to and understanding of medications

DISCHARGE AND HOME HEALTHCARE GUIDELINES

Teach the patient to avoid medications and foods that lead to endemic or sporadic goiter. Patients with endemic goiter should use iodized salt to supply at least 300 mcg of iodine daily to prevent goiter. Be sure the patient understands all medications, including the dosage, route, action, adverse effects, and the need for any laboratory monitoring of thyroid medications. Encourage the patient to take thyroid hormone supplements at the same time each day to maintain constant thyroid levels in the blood.

Have the patient immediately report to the physician any signs and symptoms of thyrotoxic crisis; these include rapid heart rate and palpitations, perspiration, shakiness and tremors, difficulty breathing, and nausea and vomiting. Teach the patient to report any increased neck swelling, difficulty in swallowing, or weight loss.

If the patient had surgery, teach the patient to change any dressings; to inspect the incision for redness, swelling, and discharge; and to notify the physician about changes that indicate infection.

Gonorrhea

DRG Category:	728
Mean LOS:	3.6 days
Description:	MEDICAL: Inflammation of the Male Reproductive System Without Major Complication or Comorbidity
DRG Category:	758
Mean LOS:	4.4 days
Description:	MEDICAL: Infections, Female Reproductive System With Complication or Comorbidity

Gonorrhea is one of the most common sexually transmitted infections (STIs) in the United States. It is an infection of mucous membranes caused by a gram-negative microorganism, *Neisseria gonorrhoeae*. The Centers for Disease Control and Prevention (CDC) estimate that 1.6 million new infections occur each year in the United States, and more than half occur in young people 15 to 24 years of age. Estimates are that only half of cases that occur are actually reported. In 2018, 583,405 cases were reported to the CDC. Rates are highest in the District of Columbia and Mississippi and lowest in Vermont. The risk of developing the infection from intercourse with an infected partner is between 50% and 90% for females and is 20% for males. The risk for males increases threefold to fourfold after four exposures. Two types of infection develop: local and systemic (disseminated). Local infection involves the mucosal surfaces of the genitourinary tract, rectum, pharynx, or eyes. Systemic infections occur because of bacteremia and can lead to multisystem involvement with connective tissues, the heart, and the brain.

If left untreated, gonorrhea will involve the fallopian tubes, ovaries, and peritoneum, resulting in gonococcal pelvic inflammatory disease (PID) in women. Systemic complications of untreated or undertreated infections are disseminated gonococcal infections that lead to acute arthritis, tenosynovitis, dermatitis, polyarthritis, endocarditis, and meningitis. With adequate treatment, most people recover fully, but reinfection is common. If gonorrhea is contracted during pregnancy, preterm premature rupture of membranes, preterm birth, and increased risk for neonatal morbidity and mortality exist.

CAUSES

Gonorrhea is an STI caused by the bacterium *N gonorrhoeae*, an aerobic, pyrogenic, gram-negative diplococcus that produces inflammatory reactions characterized by purulent exudates. It is commonly spread during sexual contact. The organism grows best in warm, mucus-secreting epithelia and can enter the body through the genitourinary tract, eyes, oropharynx, anorectum, or skin. An infant born to an infected pregnant person can contract gonorrhea when it passes through the birth canal. Self-inoculation to the eyes can also occur if a person with gonorrhea touches their eyes with a contaminated hand. Risk factors include having multiple sex partners, having an unknown sex partner, being a man who has sex with men, having low-income status, initiating sexual intercourse at an early age, doing sex work, and having unprotected sex.

GENETIC CONSIDERATIONS

Heritable immune responses could be protective or increase susceptibility.

SEX AND LIFE SPAN CONSIDERATIONS

Gonorrhea is particularly prevalent in the young adult population ages 15 to 24 years; the highest incidence of infection is in the 20- to 24-year-old age group. Slightly more females than males have gonorrhea, but females may be asymptomatic as compared to males, who are generally symptomatic. Infection in children is considered a marker for child sexual abuse and should be investigated and reported. Experts note that pregnant people and those who are menstruating may be particularly prone to infection.

HEALTH DISPARITIES AND SEXUAL/GENDER MINORITY HEALTH

The incidence of gonorrhea in the United States is increased among urban dwellers, people of lower socioeconomic status, and minority groups. Explanations for these disparities include decreased access to diagnosis and treatment and bias in data collection (data are often collected in urban emergency departments). In contrast, experts suggest that in recent years, gonorrhea infections have been climbing in rural areas, where adolescents and preadolescents have an earlier sexual debut than urban youth, with higher pregnancy rates. Men who have sex with men are at risk for sexual transmission of *N gonorrhoeae*. They may also experience multiresistant strains of organisms, which makes the illness more difficult to treat (Newman et al., 2020). A focus on prevention and condom use is important for this group of persons. While little research has been done studying gonorrhea in transgender persons, experts note that rates of gonorrhea among transgender women is approximately 10%.

GLOBAL HEALTH CONSIDERATIONS

Approximately 99 million new cases of gonorrhea occur each year around the world according to the World Health Organization. Prevalence data are not available from developing regions, but the highest numbers of new cases are in South and Southeast Asia, Latin America, and the Caribbean.

ASSESSMENT

HISTORY. Take a complete sexual history. To direct specimen collection, elicit information regarding sexual orientation and sexual practices (vaginal, oral, and anal). Explore the patient's birth control practices and determine if the patient and partner regularly use condoms. Explore the number of sex partners, the incidence of unprotected sexual contacts, frequency of sex with unknown partners, and any history of sexual assault. Determine the treatment history for STIs. Note that people may wish to have someone of the same sex take their sexual history.

Men usually develop symptoms of urethritis 2 to 5 days after exposure, but symptoms may not appear until 3 weeks later. Usually, they describe a purulent yellow or greenish-yellow penile discharge. In addition, dysuria, urinary frequency, and malaise may also be present. If the infection remains untreated after 10 to 14 days, it spreads from the anterior urethra to the posterior urethra, resulting in more intense dysuria, headaches, and lymphadenopathy. Untreated, the infection can result in prostatitis, epididymitis, and cystitis. With an anorectal infection, there is often a history of mucopurulent rectal discharge, rectal bleeding, rectal pain, and changes in bowel habits. Inspection will reveal erythema and discharge from the rectal and anal mucosa.

In women, the incubation takes at least 2 weeks, although women are often asymptomatic. The most common site (90%) of infection in women is the endocervix. Women may describe symptoms such as yellowish or greenish vaginal discharge, dysuria, urinary frequency, vaginal spotting between periods, heavy menses, backache, and abdominal and pelvic pain. In addition, there may be pruritus and burning of the vulva. If the infection is left untreated, it may ascend to the pelvic cavity, resulting in pelvic pain, fever, and pelvic inflammatory disease. Frequently, women have a gonococcal infection involving the rectum and anus, presumably from the spread of the exudate.

PHYSICAL EXAMINATION. The most common symptoms are **vaginal discharge, dysuria, intermenstrual bleeding,** and **dyspareunia** for women and **urethritis** and **penile discharge** for men. The patient may appear uncomfortable with symptoms of a local infection and may be mildly ill with a low-grade fever. When you inspect the female genitalia, you may note a greenish-yellow discharge from the Skene or Bartholin glands, along with a mucopurulent discharge at the cervical os. The vagina is engorged, red, and swollen. The cervix is usually friable and erythematic. Abdominal palpitation will reveal both lower quadrant and rebound tenderness. Pelvic examinations will be painful, especially with cervical movement. The male's urethral meatus usually has purulent discharge. An anal infection in either gender leads to purulent discharge and bleeding from the rectum.

In newborns, gonorrheal conjunctivitis appears 1 to 12 days after birth. If conjunctivitis is left untreated, blindness results from corneal ulcerations. Symptoms include bilateral edema of the lid, followed by a profuse purulent discharge from the eye.

PSYCHOSOCIAL. When taking a sexual history and counseling on sexual matters, be sensitive to the patient's need for privacy and yet be aware of the public health responsibility to report STIs. States hold the legal authority for notification of partners. Urge the patient to notify all sexual partners of the infection promptly so that they can receive treatment. Because gonorrhea is an STI, sexual abuse should be considered and reported when it is diagnosed in a child. Follow up immediately with appropriate referrals.

Diagnostic Highlights

General Comments: A simple tissue culture is the most accurate diagnostic method. Reculture 1 to 2 months later to detect both failures and reinfections; reinfection is more common than resistance to antibiotics. A Gram stain may also be used for diagnosis.

Test	Normal Result	Abnormality With Condition	Explanation
Gonococcal culture	Negative culture	Positive culture	Growth of the organism confirms the diagnosis

Other Tests: Pelvic ultrasonography; Gram stains; tests for other STIs, such as HIV infection, syphilis, herpes simplex, chlamydia; pregnancy test; nucleic acid amplification tests (DNA probe, polymerase chain reaction assay)

PRIMARY NURSING DIAGNOSIS

DIAGNOSIS. Risk for infection as evidenced by vaginal discharge, dysuria, and/or dyspareunia (females) and urethritis and/or penile discharge (males)

OUTCOMES. Risk control: Sexually transmitted diseases; Risk control: Infectious process; Knowledge: Infection management; Knowledge: Medication

INTERVENTIONS. Teaching: Safe sex; Medication management; Fertility preservation; Infection protection; Teaching: Prescribed medication

PLANNING AND IMPLEMENTATION

Collaborative

Treatment of gonorrhea is primarily pharmacologic, with antibiotic regimens. The CDC recommend that treatment for gonorrhea include concomitant therapy for chlamydia because it is found in 20% to 40% of all patients with gonorrhea. Both partners should be treated at the same time and instructed to avoid sexual activity until negative cultures are obtained. If the partners are heterosexual and the male partner is symptomatic, the female partner should have a pregnancy test to assist in the choice of therapy because some medications are not approved for use in pregnancy. Then the female partner should be treated even before culture results are obtained to prevent infertility.

Pharmacologic Highlights

Medication or Drug Class	Dosage	Description	Rationale
Ceftriaxone and azithromycin (for people with cephalosporin allergies, may consider gemifloxacin or gentamicin, both with azithromycin)	Ceftriaxone 250 mg IM single dose plus azithromycin 1 g PO single dose	Third-generation cephalosporin	Effective regimen recommended by the CDC; treats chlamydia also because both STIs often present simultaneously; should be administered on the same day
Erythromycin ointment (0.5%); tetracycline 1%	Apply to conjunctiva once at delivery	Macrolide antibiotic	Ophthalmic prophylaxis; prevents newborn blindness if maternal-newborn transmission occurred

Independent

Comfort measures are important. Loose, absorbent undergarments that the patient changes frequently will decrease discomfort from the genitourinary mucous discharge. Discuss the importance of perineal or penile cleansing and good hand-washing techniques. Sitz baths may help decrease lower abdominal discomfort.

In addition to explanations of all current treatments, teach patients strategies to prevent reinfection with gonorrhea because no natural immunity develops. Additional instruction focuses on transmission of gonorrhea and identification of symptoms of other STIs. Because of the confidential and private nature of the health history and health teaching, interact with the patient in a private location where you are unlikely to be interrupted. Many experts in STIs recommend that treatment be initiated before questioning the patient about all sexual contacts so that patients will not avoid treatment when they learn that STIs are reported to the Department of Public Health. Help the patient who has had multiple sexual partners compile a list so that the partners can be notified and treated. Note that this procedure is apt to be embarrassing and stressful for the patient, who will require support and a nonjudgmental approach from the nurse.

Instruct the patient about safe sexual practices. If the patient has several sexual partners, encourage the patient to receive regular checkups to screen for STIs. Remind patients that latex condoms are the only form of birth control known to decrease the chance of contracting an STI. Provide the patient and partner with the CDC STI hotline number: 1-800-232-4636.

High-risk populations are targeted for sexual health education and screening due to increased rates of STIs and include detained adults and juveniles, men who have sex with men, and adolescent girls who binge drink (five or more drinks). Once an adolescent is treated, the likelihood of reinfection within the next 2 years is more than 30%. College health centers are in a prime position to screen for gonorrhea.

Evidence-Based Practice and Health Policy

Williams, A., Kreisel, K., & Chesson, H. (2019). Impacts of federal prevention funding on reported gonorrhea and chlamydia rates. *American Journal of Preventative Medicine, 56,* 352–358.

- The authors assess the effectiveness of CDC STI prevention funding for reducing rates of reported STIs. They assessed the impact of STI prevention funding on reported chlamydia rates from 2000 to 2016 and reported gonorrhea rates from 1981 to 2016 while assessing the impact of funding over time. They also controlled for state-level socioeconomic factors, such as poverty rates.
- Increased annual funding led to decreased infection rates in general as well as when stratified by sex. The authors concluded that federally funded STI prevention activities have a discernible effect on reducing the burden of STIs. The funding rate in a given year depends more on prevention funding in previous years than on prevention funding in the current year.

DOCUMENTATION GUIDELINES

- History: Onset of symptoms, risk factors
- Physical response: General symptoms; discomfort; type, color, odor, amount of discharge
- Response to treatment, lessening of symptoms, willingness to implement prevention strategies

DISCHARGE AND HOME HEALTHCARE GUIDELINES

Explain that federal regulations require notification of all sexual partners so that they can seek treatment. Encourage the patient to refrain from all sexual activity (vaginal, anal, oral) until treatment is complete because of the high risk of reinfection. Explain that abstinence is the surest way to prevent STIs. If the partner's sexual history is unknown or the partner is suspected of having an STI, suggest the use of condoms. Encourage patients to wash the genitalia with soap and water before and after intercourse and to avoid sharing washcloths or douching equipment.

Guillain-Barré Syndrome

DRG Category:	98
Mean LOS:	7.1 days
Description:	MEDICAL: Non-Bacterial Infections of Nervous System Except Viral Meningitis With Complication or Comorbidity

Guillain-Barré syndrome (GBS; also known as *acute idiopathic demyelinating polyneuropathy*) is an acute, rapidly progressing form of polyneuritis that results in a temporary, flaccid paralysis lasting for 4 to 8 weeks. It is the most common cause of acute flaccid paralysis in the United States. Motor, sensory, and autonomic functions may be involved. GBS is actually a collection of syndromes that result from diffuse inflammation or demyelination (or both) of the ascending or descending peripheral nerves that leads to a viral illness and then paralysis.

Although the syndrome is considered to be a medical emergency, over 80% of persons who are affected with GBS recover their functional abilities completely. The remaining individuals have some degree of neurological deficit after recovery from the disease, which results in a chronic disability. Fewer than 5% of patients with GBS die, and usually, death is related to respiratory complications. Other complications include residual numbness, pain, thromboembolic phenomena, pressure sores, and relapse.

CAUSES

Although the exact cause of GBS is unknown, two-thirds of patients who develop it have had a viral or bacterial infection 1 to 3 weeks before the development of symptoms. It is considered a postinfectious, immune-mediated disease. The most typical site and cause of infections are a lung or intestinal infection caused by *Campylobacter jejuni* or cytomegalovirus (CMV). Infections with Epstein-Barr virus and *Mycoplasma pneumoniae* are also associated with GBS. Another 10% of patients have had recent surgical procedures during the 4 weeks before GBS developed. The immune response is directed against the lipopolysaccharide antigens of the bacteria; the antibodies react not only with the bacteria but also with the myelin of the nerves. When the myelin is stripped from the nerves, there is altered propagation of electrical impulses leading to flaccid paralysis. Other diseases that have been linked to the development of GBS are lymphoma, HIV disease, gastroenteritis, Hodgkin disease, and lupus erythematosus. Several cases of GBS have been linked to the novel coronavirus 2019 disease (COVID-19). In some cases, GBS develops after immunization for influenza.

There are two subtypes of GBS. Acute inflammatory demyelinating polyneuropathy (AIDP) is generally preceded by a bacterial or viral infection. Less than half of these patients are seropositive for *C jejuni*, and symptoms generally resolve with remyelination. Acute motor axonal neuropathy (AMAN) is more prevalent among pediatric age groups, and most of these patients are seropositive for *C jejuni*. AMAN is identified with rapidly progressive weakness, respiratory failure, and good recovery.

GENETIC CONSIDERATIONS

GBS is considered to be an autoimmune disorder, with some reports of familial inheritance. New evidence suggests that polymorphisms in the gene *TNFA* lead to increased susceptibility to GBS. Rare cases may also be caused by a mutation in the *PMP22* gene.

SEX AND LIFE SPAN CONSIDERATIONS

The incidence of GBS is 1.2 to 3 per 100,000 individuals, and it affects individuals of both sexes and of all ages but is rare in infants. Most commonly, it affects young (15–35 years) and older-aged adults (50–75 years) and men slightly more than women.

HEALTH DISPARITIES AND SEXUAL/GENDER MINORITY HEALTH

There are no known racial and ethnic considerations except that Asian American persons are most likely to have GBS after an infection with *C jejuni* as compared with other agents. For unknown reasons, active-duty U.S. military personnel have a slightly higher risk for GBS than other groups, particularly in the setting of gastroenteritis. Sexual and gender minority status has no known effect on the risk for GBS.

GLOBAL HEALTH CONSIDERATIONS

The underlying cause of GBS varies by country, but the syndrome has been reported in all regions of the world. AIDP occurs most often in Western Europe and North America, whereas people in China, Japan, and Mexico are more likely to have AMAN.

ASSESSMENT

HISTORY. Determine if the patient has had a recent viral illness or surgical procedure. Often, 2 to 4 weeks after the infection, the patient describes a minor upper respiratory or gastrointestinal febrile illness. Many, but not all, patients complain of finger paresthesia (numbness, prickling, tingling) early in the course of the illness, followed by muscle weakness of the legs. The patient or family generally seeks assistance when bilateral lower limb weakness begins to spread toward the trunk or has progressed to paralysis of the limbs. Urinary incontinence may be a problem initially, followed by difficulty in swallowing and speaking. Impairment of respiratory functions, the most life-threatening effect of GBS, does not occur until the paralysis has affected all of the peripheral areas and the trunk. Often the patient reaches the lowest point of functioning 4 weeks after the start of symptoms.

PHYSICAL EXAMINATION. The major neurological sign found in GBS is **muscle weakness**, but symmetrical **sensory loss, particularly in the legs and later in the arms,** often occurs. Most patients experience **pain** during their illness and at least half describe severe pain. Although the progression of symptoms is variable, the disease often progresses upward from the legs in 1 to 3 days. To follow the progression of symptoms, test for ascending sensory loss by gently using a pinprick upward from the level of T12 on the vertebral column (level of the iliac crests) to the midscapular point (about T6). Mark the patient's skin with a pen every 4 hours to document changes. Notify the physician immediately if the level reaches T8 or higher, because muscles at that level are needed for breathing. Patients may also have ocular muscle paralysis, loss of position sense, and diminished or absent reflexes.

The function of cranial nerve VII (facial nerve) may be affected, especially in the later stages of the paralysis. To test for facial nerve weakness, inspect the patient's face at rest and during conversation. Have the patient raise both eyebrows, smile, frown, puff out the cheeks, and show both upper and lower teeth. If the facial nerve is involved, the patient may have problems talking, chewing, and swallowing.

Patients often have changes in their vital signs. Rapid or slow heart rates and a labile blood pressure may occur because of the effects on the vagus nerve (cranial nerve X); profuse sweating and facial flushing may also occur. Patients require continuous cardiac monitoring to assess for dysrhythmias. Although respiratory function may be impaired in the later stages of paralysis, the nurse needs to assess the patency of the airway and adequacy of breathing in order to initiate prompt interventions when necessary. Weakness and paralysis usually last 2 to 4 weeks before symptoms begin to improve, and the average time to full recovery is 200 days.

PSYCHOSOCIAL. The patient is alert but paralyzed, and this leads to considerable fear and anxiety both during the initial stages and throughout the course of the disease. As the paralysis ascends, patients' level of anxiety will probably rise; their anxiety level can be reduced with antianxiety agents, and pain control helps manage the condition. The patient and significant others will need a great deal of emotional support to deal with the health crisis.

Diagnostic Highlights

Note that the diagnosis generally is made on the basis of clinical symptoms.

Test	Normal Result	Abnormality With Condition	Explanation
Cerebrospinal fluid (CSF) assay	Protein: 15–60 mg/dL; glucose: 40–70 mg/dL; erythrocytes: 0–5/mcL; leukocytes: 0–5/mcL	Increase in CSF protein without an increase in cell count; lymphocytes might be present but are usually < 20/mcL	High protein levels (as high as 500 mg/dL) are often noted 1–2 wk of illness; peak at 4–6 wk

Other Tests: Most laboratory values are not particularly helpful in the initial diagnosis of GBS. White blood cell counts may show mild leukocytosis; other tests include

Diagnostic Highlights (continued)

electromyography, pulmonary function tests, arterial and venous blood gases, and blood cultures. Electromyography and nerve conduction studies may be used to monitor neuromuscular changes.

PRIMARY NURSING DIAGNOSIS

DIAGNOSIS. Ineffective airway clearance related to weakness and respiratory muscle paralysis as evidenced by loss of gag reflex and/or dysphagia

OUTCOMES. Respiratory status: Airway patency; Respiratory status: Gas exchange; Respiratory status: Ventilation; Symptom control; Symptom severity; Knowledge: Disease process

INTERVENTIONS. Airway management; Oxygen therapy; Airway suctioning; Airway insertion and stabilization; Cough enhancement; Mechanical ventilation management: Invasive and noninvasive; Positioning; Respiratory monitoring

PLANNING AND IMPLEMENTATION

Collaborative

During the acute phase of the illness, the patient may be in the intensive care unit, particularly to support pulmonary function with oxygenation, endotracheal intubation, and mechanical ventilation. Sequential neurological, cardiopulmonary, and hemodynamic assessments are needed. Some patients have chest physiotherapy ordered, and all require aggressive pulmonary toileting to maintain a patent endotracheal or tracheostomy tube. Most patients need a Foley catheter to manage urinary function. Compression boots limit the risk of thromboembolic complications. Physical and occupational therapy consults should occur early in the illness.

IV immunoglobulin administration may hasten recovery. Plasmapheresis (plasma exchange) may be completed during the early stages (first few days) of the syndrome; research suggests that the procedure may reduce the circulating antibodies and shorten the period of paralysis. Care of the patient who is having plasmapheresis includes monitoring the amount of plasma removed and reinfused and monitoring for any reactions to the fluid replacement. Transfusion reactions should not occur because the patient's own blood is being returned. Complications such as infection and hypertension require pharmacologic management. Other patients may become hypotensive and require fluid boluses or vasopressors.

Pharmacologic Highlights

Medication or Drug Class	Dosage	Description	Rationale
Antihypertensives	Varies with drug	Nitroprusside (Nipride); propranolol (Inderal)	Control hypertensive episodes
Low-molecular-weight heparin (enoxaparin, dalteparin)	Varies with drug	Anticoagulant	Prevents thromboembolism during periods of immobility
Antibiotics	Varies with drug	Chosen on the basis of cultures and sensitivities	Combat urinary or pulmonary infection

Other Drugs: Tricyclic antidepressants are effective to relieve pain associated with paresthesias. Note that muscles are tender (particularly in the trunk, thighs, and shoulders) during range-of-motion and turning procedures. Analgesics may be needed for muscle stiffness, pain, and spasm. Antacids and histamine blockers may be used to reduce the risk of gastrointestinal bleeding. Corticosteroids may be given early in the course of the disease, but their usefulness is unproved, and they are generally considered ineffective by most experts.

Independent

The most important interventions center on maintaining a patent airway and adequate breathing. Teach deep-breathing and coughing techniques. Monitor the patient who is mechanically ventilated for airway obstruction. Use deep endotracheal suction to maintain a patent airway, but monitor the patient carefully for dysrhythmias and a dropping oxygen saturation. Because respiratory complications are seen in 35% to 40% of patients, preparation for intubation or eventually a tracheostomy is appropriate. A viable call system for the patient is vital, and the type will depend on the extent of the paralysis. Cardiac dysrhythmias also occur in GBS, so patients require continuous cardiac monitoring.

Provide passive range-of-motion exercises at least twice a day, turn the patient at least every 2 hours, and use splints and pillow supports to keep the limbs in functional positions. Control the environment to limit the risk of injury from falls. Inspect for integrity of the skin. Frequent eye care is necessary for the individual with cranial nerve VII involvement. Protect the cornea with eye shields (some eye specialists may recommend suturing the eyes closed) and provide eye lubricants. Give mouth care at least every 4 hours.

The patient's psychological state is most important. Use relaxation exercises, include the patient in decision making, and provide frequent explanations of care to decrease the patient's anxiety. Mood swings are to be expected. Encourage the patient to ventilate fears and anger related to the paralysis and the prognosis, and refer the patient for consultation if the patient's emotional needs are not being met. If the patient cannot speak because of endotracheal intubation or paralysis, try to establish communication by having the patient blink once for "yes" and twice for "no."

Evidence-Based Practice and Health Policy

Sedaghat, Z., & Karimi, N. (2020). Guillain-Barré syndrome associated with COVID-19 infection: A case report. *Journal of Clinical Neuroscience, 76*, 233–235.

- A novel coronavirus (COVID-19) outbreak has led to thousands of infections with many body systems involved. The authors report on one patient who developed acute progressive ascending quadriparesis following diagnosis with COVID-19.
- The authors theorized that the virus stimulated inflammatory cells, producing an immune-mediated process that resembled GBS. The authors also noted that it was unclear whether COVID-19 produced the antibodies against molecules in the nervous system that led to GBS or it was the result of the immune response. The authors concluded that it is important to pay attention to the neurological symptoms of COVID-19.

DOCUMENTATION GUIDELINES

- Respiratory and cardiovascular functions: Patency of airway, description of breathing, vital sign changes with rest or activity
- Neurological functions: Level of paralysis, level of motor and sensory function, level of consciousness
- Bowel and bladder functions: Frequency of voiding, consistency and number of stools
- Pain: Location, duration, precipitating factors, interventions that alleviate pain
- Activity: Strength and motion of extremities, presence of deformities or atrophy and strategies used to manage dysfunction, response to activity
- Skin: Areas of potential or actual breakdown, successful strategies to manage breakdown

DISCHARGE AND HOME HEALTHCARE GUIDELINES

Especially during the recovery period, teach the patient to avoid exposure to further upper respiratory infections. Encourage self-care, but stress the avoidance of fatigue and the importance of frequent planned rest periods. Continue ongoing rehabilitation with physical therapy sessions to teach walking with a cane or walker and to provide active and passive range-of-motion exercises. Teach strengthening exercises for the hands, such as modeling clay or squeezing balls. Work with physical therapy to teach the patient and family how to manage the transfer from the bed to a wheelchair and from a wheelchair to the toilet or bathtub.

Teach the patient to maintain a high-calorie, high-protein diet and to include at least 2,000 mL of fluid intake per day. Avoid constipation by increasing fluids and dietary fiber and using stool softeners as required. Teach the patient to use warm baths to manage muscle pain and diversional activities to decrease boredom during the slow recovery period.

Gunshot Wound

DRG Category:	205
Mean LOS:	5.5 days
Description:	MEDICAL: Other Respiratory System Diagnoses With Major Complication or Comorbidity
DRG Category:	228
Mean LOS:	9.2 days
Description:	SURGICAL: Other Cardiothoracic Procedures With Major Complication or Comorbidity
DRG Category:	405
Mean LOS:	12.6 days
Description:	SURGICAL: Pancreas, Liver, and Shunt Procedures With Major Complication or Comorbidity
DRG Category:	799
Mean LOS:	10.7 days
Description:	SURGICAL: Splenectomy With Major Complication or Comorbidity
DRG Category:	958
Mean LOS:	8.3 days
Description:	SURGICAL: Other Operating Room Procedures for Multiple Significant Trauma With Complication or Comorbidity

Penetrating trauma from a gunshot wound (GSW) or firearm injury can cause devastating injuries. The most commonly injured organs and tissues are the intestines, liver, vascular structures, spleen, and intrathoracic structures. Evaluating injuries is difficult; it is important to determine the type of weapon, energy dissipated from the weapon, firing range of the weapon at the time of injury, and characteristics of the injured tissue.

In the United States, 35,000 to 40,000 people are killed each year in gun-related events. The United States has 4% of the world's population but possesses 50% of the world's privately owned firearms. Firearm deaths are the highest in Alaska, Mississippi, New Mexico, Wyoming, and Alabama and lowest in Massachusetts, New York, New Jersey, and Hawaii. Approximately 63% of gun deaths are suicides, 36% are homicides, and the rest are from other causes, primarily unintentional death. GSWs can be perforating, when the bullet exits the body, or penetrating, when the bullet is retained in the body. GSWs can lead to the need for extensive débridement, resection, or amputation. Among the many complications are sepsis, organ dysfunction, exsanguination, and death.

CAUSES

The energy of the missile is dissipated into tissues of the body, causing destruction of vital and nonvital structures. When the missile enters the body, it creates a temporary cavity, which stretches, distorts, and compresses the surrounding anatomic structures. The cavity that is produced often has a greater diameter than the missile itself. In a situation called *blast effect* or *muzzle blast*, damage occurs in structures outside the direct path of the missile. High-velocity missiles (bullets from shotguns, rifles, or high-caliber handguns) cause extensive cavitation and significant tissue destruction, while low-velocity missiles (bullets from low-caliber handguns) have limited cavitation potential with less tissue destruction. Another characteristic of missiles is the yaw, which is the amount of tumbling and movement of the nose of the missile that occurs. The more yaw, the greater the tissue damage.

GENETIC CONSIDERATIONS

No clear genetic contributions to susceptibility have been defined.

SEX AND LIFE SPAN CONSIDERATIONS

Penetrating injuries from gunshot wounds and stab wounds, which are on the increase in U.S. preteens, teens, and young adults, are more common in males than females. In urban areas, drive-by shootings are increasing, and in some cities they are associated with half of all youth gunshot wounds. Males have different patterns of injury than females, and a higher injury severity. Analysis of trauma outcomes indicates that, following traumatic injury, males have higher rates of multiple organ failure, pneumonia, and sepsis than females, creating health disparities for men (Marcolini et al., 2019). Trauma is the third leading cause of death in people ages 45 to 65 years and the seventh leading cause of death in people older than 65 years.

HEALTH DISPARITIES AND SEXUAL/GENDER MINORITY HEALTH

In the United States, Black youth ages 15 to 24 years have the highest homicide rate from GSWs, followed by Hispanic youth. Suicide rates are highest among Native American males and non-Hispanic white males. Penetrating injuries from gunshot wounds and stab wounds are more common in non-Hispanic Black persons than in non-Hispanic White persons. Non-Hispanic Black males have adjusted firearm death rates from two to seven times higher than males of other groups. Healthy People 2020 reports that non-Hispanic Black persons have the highest injury death rate in the United States (79.9 injury deaths per 100,000 people), followed by non-Hispanic White people (79.2), Native American people (78.2), Hispanic people (45.5), and Asian/Pacific Islander people (25.6). Geographic information system mapping has shown that impoverished neighborhoods have a higher incidence of gunshot injury than other neighborhoods (Bayouth et al., 2019). Socioeconomic status and injury are linked, with people living with lower incomes having higher risk. Children under 14 years of age living in rural areas have higher rates of unintentional firearm injuries than urban children have. Recent work has shown evidence that rural populations have injury mortality rates that are more than twice as high as urban rates. Many factors contribute to these health disparities, including the distance from major trauma centers. Sexual and gender minority persons have high risk for dating and interpersonal violence, violence related to bullying, and intentional and unintentional injury (Healthy People 2020).

GLOBAL HEALTH CONSIDERATIONS

Countries with high levels of civil strife or political instability or are at war have a high prevalence of GSW death and disability. South Africa, Brazil, Colombia, El Salvador, Guatemala, Honduras, and Jamaica have high rates of gun-related deaths as compared to other countries. Mortality rates are lowest in Japan and highest in the United States.

ASSESSMENT

HISTORY. Establish a history of the weapon, including the type, caliber, and range at which it was fired. Determine if the GSW was self-inflicted as well as the patient's hand dominance and tetanus immunization history. Obtain a history from the patient or family using AMPLE: allergies, medications, prior illnesses and operations, last meal, events and environments surrounding injury. Because injuries are often associated with alcohol and substance use, determine if the patient ingested drugs and/or alcohol prior to the incident.

PHYSICAL EXAMINATION. The most common symptom is an **open puncture wound from the bullet with bleeding**. The initial evaluation is always focused on assessing the airway, breathing, circulation, disability (neurological status), and exposure (completely undressing the patient); these assessments are done simultaneously by the trauma resuscitation team. The secondary survey is a head-to-toe assessment, including vital signs.

After completing the primary survey, begin the secondary survey. Examine the patient's entire skin surface carefully for abrasions, open wounds, powder burns, and hematomas, paying special attention to skinfolds, groin, and axillae. Assess the patient's abdomen, back, and extremities for lacerations, wounds, abrasions, and deformities. Some high-velocity weapons may cause extensive tissue destruction and fractures. Inspect the patient for both entrance and exit wounds (Table 1).

• TABLE 1 Types and Descriptions of Gunshot Wounds

TYPE OF WOUND	DESCRIPTION	DESCRIPTION OF WOUND	EXPLANATION
Entrance: Soft contact	Gun is pressed against skin prior to shooting	Searing of edges of bullet hole, soot or smoke depositions around wound	Hot gases and flame when gun is shot burn edges of wound
Entrance: Hard contact	Gun barrel is pressed firmly into skin	Little or no soot on edges of bullet hole; smoke and soot in deep layers of wound	Soot, burning gun powder fragments, smoke, and hot gases are forced to penetrate deep into wound
Entrance: Blow back	Hard contact wound of head	Wound is very large, irregular, and gaping	The thin layer of skin and muscle over bones of skull causes a large amount of energy to be forced directly into the wound

(table continues on page 498)

• **TABLE 1** Types and Descriptions of Gunshot Wounds (continued)

TYPE OF WOUND	DESCRIPTION	DESCRIPTION OF WOUND	EXPLANATION
Entrance: Intermediate range	No contact but within 48 in.	Tattooing: Fragments of gunpowder strike surface of skin and become embedded; Stippling: Fragments of gunpowder strike with enough force to cause abrasions but do not penetrate skin	Pieces of burning gunpowder exit the gun barrel while firing and damage the skin; the closer the muzzle is to skin, the smaller the area of distribution and greater the concentration of fragments around the entrance wound
Entrance: Indeterminate range (unable to determine distance)	No contact but more than 48 in.	Bullet hole surrounded by area of abrasion	Size of hole depends on angle of entry, caliber of weapon, layers of clothing, other factors
Exit	Same general appearance regardless of range of fire	Configuration of wound varies widely: irregular, jagged, round, slitlike	Size of bullet does not determine size of wound; small, highly deformed bullet may produce a larger wound than a large bullet

Perform a thorough fluid volume assessment on at least an hourly basis until the patient is stabilized. This assessment includes hemodynamic, urinary, and central nervous system parameters. Notify the physician of overt bleeding and of any early indications that hemorrhage is continuing; this includes delayed capillary refill, tachycardia, urinary output less than 0.5 mL/kg per hour, and alterations in mental status, including restlessness, agitation, and confusion, as well as decreases in alertness. Body weights are helpful in indicating fluid volume status; note that many of the critical care beds have incorporated bed scales.

PSYCHOSOCIAL. The violent and often unexplained nature of this type of trauma can lead to ineffective coping for both the patient and the family. Determine if the patient is at risk from themself or others by questioning the patient, significant others, or police. If the patient is on police hold, determine the patient's and family's response to the pending legal charges. Injuries may be associated with alcohol or substance use. Determine if alcohol and substance abuse assessment and treatment are needed.

Diagnostic Highlights

Test	Normal Result	Abnormality With Condition	Explanation
Complete blood count	Red blood cells: 3.7–5.8 million/mcL; hemoglobin: 11.7–17.4 g/dL; hematocrit: 33%–52%; white blood cells: 4,500–11,100/mcL; platelets: 150,000–450,000/mcL	Decreased values reflective of the degree of hemorrhage	Determines the extent of blood loss; note that it takes 2 hr for hemorrhage to be reflected in a dropping hemoglobin and hematocrit after injury

Diagnostic Highlights (continued)

Test	Normal Result	Abnormality With Condition	Explanation
X-rays of areas near the GSW; if head or neck injury is suspected or patient is unconscious, x-rays of chest, pelvis, and lateral cervical spine are needed	No injury in bony structures	Damage to bones and joints in area of wound	If wound is near bony structures, entire surrounding area needs to be assessed for injury
Computed tomography scan	No injury to body structures	Damage to organ and supporting structures; collection of blood in tissues, location of foreign bodies (missiles)	May be used to identify abdominal, urological, chest, and head injuries (actual and suspected); injuries to bony structure; trajectory of penetrating missile

Other Tests: Blood chemistries, angiography, endoscopy, indirect laryngoscopy, arterial blood gases, pulse oximetry, urinalysis, excretory urography, ultrasound, magnetic resonance imaging, diagnostic peritoneal lavage, laparoscopy. Blood and urine toxic screen.

PRIMARY NURSING DIAGNOSIS

DIAGNOSIS. Ineffective airway clearance related to airway obstruction as evidenced by wheezing, dyspnea, and/or tachypnea

OUTCOMES. Respiratory status: Airway patency; Respiratory status: Ventilation; Respiratory status: Gas exchange; Symptom control; Symptom severity; Medication response; Knowledge: Treatment regimen

INTERVENTIONS. Airway insertion and stabilization; Airway management; Airway suctioning; Anxiety reduction; Artificial airway management; Mechanical ventilation management: Invasive and noninvasive; Oxygen therapy; Positioning; Respiratory monitoring; Ventilation monitoring; Vital signs monitoring

PLANNING AND IMPLEMENTATION

Collaborative

Maintaining a patent airway, maintaining oxygenation and ventilation, and supporting the circulation are the first priorities. Assist with endotracheal intubation and mechanical ventilation. Maintain the Pao_2 at greater than 100 mm Hg and the $Paco_2$ at 35 to 45 mm Hg. The patient may require placement of a tube thoracostomy to drain blood and relieve a pneumothorax.

The focus is on four broad components of care: control of bleeding, identification of injuries, control of contamination, and reconstruction of the injured area. Restoring fluid volume status is critical in maximizing tissue perfusion and oxygenation; the use of pressure infusers and rapid volume/warmer infusers for trauma patients requiring massive fluid replacement is essential. Administering warm blood products and crystalloids assists in maintaining normothermia. Be prepared to administer vasopressors after fluid volume status is stabilized. Patients who require massive fluid resuscitation are at risk for developing hypothermia, which exacerbates existing coagulopathy and compounds their hemodynamic instability. Paramount in managing patients is a rapid fluid resuscitation with blood, blood products, colloids, and crystalloids through a large-bore peripheral IV catheter or a large-bore trauma catheter.

Patients frequently require surgical exploration to identify specific injuries and control hemorrhage. After surgical exposure is obtained, any of the following may be required: assessment of structures, control of hemorrhage, débridement, resection, or amputation. If definitive surgical intervention is not possible because of the patient's instability, a temporizing method known as *damage control* may be instituted. Damage control consists of the placement of packing to achieve a temporary tamponade, correction of coagulopathy, and aggressive management of hypothermia. The patient is then transferred to the critical care unit for continued monitoring and stabilization. The "second look" surgical exploration is generally done in 24 hours for definitive surgical intervention.

Pharmacologic Highlights

Medication or Drug Class	Dosage	Description	Rationale
Antibiotics: Prophylactic antibiotic use is controversial; surgeons follow culture results and institute antibiotics sensitive to the organism that was cultured	Varies with drug	Second-generation cephalosporins or cephamycin	Prevent gram-negative infections when there is traumatic violation of the gastrointestinal tract
Low-molecular-weight heparin (enoxaparin, dalteparin)	Varies with drug	Anticoagulant	Prevents thromboembolism during periods of immobility after hemorrhage is controlled; not generally administered in patients with neural injuries

Other: Many trauma surgeons may choose to administer a tetanus booster to patients with chest trauma whose immunization history indicates a need or whose history is unavailable.

Independent

In the emergency phase of treatment, maintain the patient in a supine position unless it is contraindicated because of other injuries. Ensure adequate airway and breathing in this position. Avoid the Trendelenburg position because it may have negative hemodynamic consequences, increase the risk of aspiration, and interfere with pulmonary excursion. If the patient can tolerate the position, elevate the head of the bed to limit the risk of aspiration and to improve gas exchange.

Wound care varies, depending on the severity of wounds, whether an open fracture is present, and what type of fixation device is applied. Wounds and any exposed soft tissue and bone are covered with wet, sterile saline dressings. Standard Betadine-soaked dressings may not be used because of the need to limit iodine absorption and skin irritation. To decrease the risk of infection of the patient, use a gown, mask, gloves, and hair covers when caring for patients with extensive wounds. Document the size, description, and healing of the wound each day, and notify the surgeon if there are signs of wound infection. Use universal precautions in handling all bloody drainage.

If another person has initiated the violence toward the patient, consider assigning the patient a pseudonym for all hospital records to prevent another assault. Do not provide any information about the patient over the phone unless you are sure of the caller's name and relationship to the patient. If you fear for the patient's safety, talk to hospital security about strategies to ensure the patient's safety. If the patient has a self-inflicted injury, make a referral to a clinical nurse specialist or discuss a psychiatric consultation with the surgeon. If the patient is self-destructive, initiate suicide precautions according to unit protocol.

If the patient is being held by police, remember that the patient receives competent and compassionate care even when under arrest. Determine from hospital policy the regulations about visitors if the patient is held by the police. Provide a supportive atmosphere to promote healing of the injury, but use care to avoid being drawn into the legal aspects of the patient's arrest.

Evidence-Based Practice and Health Policy

Parker, S. (2020). Estimating nonfatal gunshot injury locations with natural language processing and machine learning models. *JAMA Network Open*. Advance online publication. https://doi .org/10.1001/jamanetworkopen.2020.20664

- The author aims to determine if natural language processing and machine learning methods can predict the locations of nonfatal shootings and improve the accuracy of national estimates of gunshot injuries. The authors used 59,025 gunshot wound cases from the National Electronic Injury Surveillance System Firearm Injury Surveillance Study.
- The primary outcomes were injury location and subsequent estimation of nonfatal gunshot injury location. Patients with these injuries were predominantly male, Black, and ages 15 to 24 years. The analysis was able to determine the most likely locations (street, highway) for gunshot injuries. The findings showed that machine learning models may be used to determine location, and that highways or streets were the most likely location rather than in the home.

DOCUMENTATION GUIDELINES

- Physical and emotional response: Location, size and appearance of wound; description of dressings and drainage on dressings; amount of bleeding from wound; description of accompanying injuries, breath sounds, heart sounds; emotional recovery; mental health status
- Response to treatment: Vital signs, pulse oximetry, urine output, mental status, patency of airway, adequacy of circulation
- Presence of complications: Infection, hemorrhage, organ dysfunction, poor wound healing
- Pain: Location, duration, precipitating factors, response to interventions
- Laboratory results: Electrolytes, measures of organ function, complete blood count, coagulation studies

DISCHARGE AND HOME HEALTHCARE GUIDELINES

PREVENTION. To prevent complications of wound infection and impaired wound healing, review wound care instructions with the patient and family. Verify that they can demonstrate proper care with understanding and accuracy.

MEDICATIONS. Verify that the patient understands all medications, including dosage, route, action, and adverse effects. Provide written instructions to the patient or family.

FOLLOW-UP. Review with the patient all follow-up appointments that are arranged. If home care is necessary, verify that appropriate arrangements have been completed. Make sure that patients with self-inflicted wounds have counseling and support before and after the discharge.

Heart Failure

DRG Category:	292
Mean LOS:	3.9 days
Description:	MEDICAL: Heart Failure and Shock With Complication or Comorbidity

Heart failure (HF) occurs when the heart is unable to pump sufficient blood to meet the metabolic needs of the body. It is the most common nonfatal consequence of cardiovascular disorders and is the only major heart disease that is increasing significantly throughout the world. The American Heart Association (AHA) estimates that as many as 6.5 million people in the United States have HF, and in the next 15 years, it anticipates an increase of 46% in HF prevalence. Almost 1 million hospital admissions occur each year for acute decompensated HF, and the rehospitalization rates during the 6 months following discharge are as much as 50%. In spite of recent advances in the treatment of HF, the 5-year estimated mortality rate is almost 50%.

In HF, the result of inadequate cardiac output (CO) is poor organ perfusion and vascular congestion in the pulmonary or systemic circulation. HF may be described as backward or forward failure, high- or low-output failure, or right- or left-sided failure. In backward failure, the ventricle fails to eject its contents, which results in pulmonary edema on the left side of the heart and systemic congestion on the right. In forward failure, an inadequate CO leads to decreased organ perfusion. High-output failure is the inability of the heart to meet the increased metabolic demands of the body despite a normal or high CO. Low-output failure occurs when the ventricle is unable to generate enough CO to meet the metabolic demands of the body. This type of failure consists of impaired peripheral circulation and compensatory vasoconstriction. Right-sided failure occurs when the right ventricle is unable to maintain an adequate CO, and systemic congestion occurs. When the left ventricle is unable to produce a CO sufficient to prevent pulmonary congestion, left-sided failure occurs.

Several pathophysiological mechanisms are involved in HF. Local angiotensin II production increases the heart's workload because of sodium and water retention, promotes progressive loss of myocardial function, and increases myocardial mass. As the heart fails, myocytes (heart muscle cells) enlarge, go through apoptosis (cellular death), and the heart muscle is remodeled and becomes maladaptive. Both systolic and diastolic failure occurs, and atrial natriuretic peptide and beta-type natriuretic peptide promote vasodilation and sodium loss. Complications of HF include pulmonary edema, renal failure, cerebral insufficiency, myocardial infarction, and cardiac dysrhythmias.

CAUSES

HF may result from a number of causes that affect preload (venous return), afterload (impedance the heart has to overcome to eject its volume), or contractility. Elevated preload can be caused by incompetent valves, renal failure, volume overload, or a congenital left-to-right shunt. Elevated afterload occurs when the ventricles have to generate higher pressures in order to overcome impedance and eject their volume. This disorder may also be referred to as an *abnormal pressure load*. An elevation in afterload also may be caused by hypertension, valvular stenosis, or hypertrophic cardiomyopathy. Abnormal muscle conditions may diminish contractility and cause a decrease in the ability of the heart muscle to act as a pump. Some common causes of diminished contractility include cardiomyopathy, coronary heart disease (CHD), acute myocardial infarction, myocarditis, amyloidosis, sarcoidosis, hypocalcemia, hypomagnesemia, or iatrogenic myocardial damage caused by drugs (doxorubicin or disopyramide) or radiation therapy for mediastinal tumors or Hodgkin disease. Some clinical experts classify the causes as underlying causes (acquired or congenital structural abnormalities), fundamental causes (biochemical or physiological mechanisms), precipitating causes (valvular conditions, medications, radiation), and genetic causes (see next section). Risk factors include myopathy, previous myocardial infarction, valvular heart disease, alcohol use, substance abuse, hypertension, diabetes mellitus, dyslipidemia, sleep disorders, thyroid disease, and chemotherapy/radiotherapy.

GENETIC CONSIDERATIONS

HF is a complex disease combining the actions of numerous genes with environmental factors. Many HF risk factors have genetic causes or are associated with genetic predispositions. These include hypertrophic cardiomyopathy (HCM) and dilated cardiomyopathy (DCM), CHD, myocardial infarction, and hypertension. Genetic polymorphisms of the renin-angiotensin-aldosterone system (RAAS) and sympathetic system have also been associated with susceptibility to and/or mitigation of HF. Gene variants in the *ADRA2C* adrenoceptor and the *ADRB1* adrenoceptor have been associated with a higher risk of HF among Black persons.

SEX AND LIFE SPAN CONSIDERATIONS

HF may occur at any age and in both sexes as a result of congenital defects, hypertension, valve disease, CHD, or autoimmune disorders. Older adults, however, are much more prone to the condition because of chronic hypertension, CHD, myocardial infarction, chronic ischemia, or valve disease, all of which occur more frequently in the older population. HF is the primary cause of hospitalizations in older people. Although men and women have similar rates of HF, women tend to have the condition later in life than men, and they survive longer with HF than their male counterparts. Women are less likely to have procedures such as cardiac catheterization as compared to men, which is an important health disparity for women because they may not have associated ischemic heart disease identified (Tandon et al., 2020 [see Evidence-Based Practice and Health Policy]).

HEALTH DISPARITIES AND SEXUAL/GENDER MINORITY HEALTH

Experts have found that people with HF who do not have private health insurance consistently receive hospital care that does not meet the quality standards that privately insured patients receive, such as the use of cardiac devices and the most current medication protocols. People without private health insurance also have poorer outcomes than insured people. Persons with Medicare and Medicaid are less likely to receive heart transplants than people with private health insurance. The same is true for people living in rural areas as compared to urban areas; rural patients are less likely to receive guideline-directed care. Regional differences occur in the use of medications such as beta blockers and mineralocorticoid receptor antagonists as well as technology such as the implantable cardioverter defibrillator, with rural patients receiving lower-quality care. Adults without housing, even when controlling for insurance, are less likely to undergo percutaneous coronary intervention and coronary artery bypass grating compared with people with a permanent residence. Thus, housing, income, geography, and insurance status all contribute to health disparities in the care of HF.

As compared with White persons, the incidence and prevalence of HF are higher in Black, Hispanic, and Native American persons. Black persons present with the condition at an average age of 63 years, as compared to 77 years in White persons. The Centers for Disease Control and Prevention report that 11.5% of White people, 9.5% of Black people, 7.4% of Hispanic people, and 6.0% of Asian people have heart disease. Black persons have higher morbidity and mortality rates of CHD, and the burden for Black individuals is higher than for White individuals because of the prevalence of hypertension, obesity, metabolic syndrome, and decreased physical activity. People from developing countries who immigrate to the United States have a higher prevalence of HF, possibly because of lack of preventive healthcare. Significant health disparities exist in the cardiac care of underrepresented groups as compared to White persons. Black, Indigenous, and other people of color are known to receive care less often guided by standard cardiac care guidelines than White persons. Unless patients have health insurance, White patients are more likely to receive coronary angiograms and other coronary interventions than Black, Indigenous, and other people of color, who are also less likely to be referred to cardiologists and cardiac surgeons than White persons (Batchelor et al., 2019). In the United States, Asian Indian persons have a higher prevalence of CHD than White persons.

Transgender is a term used to describe persons whose gender identity is different from their sex assigned at birth. Approximately 1% of the U.S. population identify themselves as transgender. Sexual and gender minority people have higher odds for multiple chronic conditions, cancer, and poor quality of life, and are more apt to have disabilities than cisgender males and females. (Cisgender is a term used to describe persons whose gender identity and gender expression are aligned with their assigned sex listed on their birth certificate.) Gender-affirming hormone therapy is the use of hormone therapy for gender transition or gender affirmation and can be masculinizing or feminizing. It may also affect cardiovascular health in transgender females. In a large sample, researchers have found that transgender men and women are more likely to be overweight than cisgender women. Compared to cisgender women, transgender women reported higher rates of diabetes, ischemic stroke, angina/coronary disease, and myocardial infarction. Gender-nonconforming men and women reported higher odds of myocardial infarction than cisgender women. Transgender women also had higher rates of any cardiovascular disease than cisgender men (Cacerese, Jackman, et al., 2020; Connelly et al., 2019). Although large-scale studies are not available, these factors may place some sexual and gender minority persons at risk for HF.

GLOBAL HEALTH CONSIDERATIONS

HF occurs in all regions of the globe, but the cause of HF varies. In developing countries, such as South and Central America, Chagas disease, an infection that generally occurs in the tropics by a protozoan parasite, plays an important role. Valvular cardiomyopathy is also more common in developing countries, and HF occurs at earlier ages than in developed countries. Outcomes in patients from developing countries are worse than in developed countries, likely because of a shortage of healthcare resources in developing countries. In developed parts of the world such as North America and Western Europe, HF is most often caused by ischemic heart disease and ischemic cardiomyopathy. Compared with people living in North American and Western European countries, recent immigrants from developing countries and the former Soviet republics have a higher prevalence of HF.

ASSESSMENT

HISTORY. Patients with HF typically have a history of a precipitating factor such as myocardial infarction, recent open heart surgery, dysrhythmias, alcohol/substance abuse, or hypertension. Symptoms vary depending on the type and severity of failure. Ask patients if they have experienced any of the following: anxiety, irritability, fatigue, weakness, lethargy, mild shortness of breath with exertion or at rest, orthopnea that requires two or more pillows to sleep, nocturnal dyspnea, cough with frothy sputum, nocturia, weight gain, anorexia, or nausea and vomiting. Take a complete medication history and determine if the patient has been on any dietary restrictions. Ask patients to describe their patterns of alcohol and drug use. Determine if the patient regularly participates in a planned exercise program.

The New York Heart Association has developed a commonly used classification system that links the relationship between symptoms and the amount of effort required to provoke the symptoms:

• Class I: No limitations. No symptoms (fatigue, dyspnea, or palpitations) with ordinary activity.
• Class II: Slight mild limitation of physical activity. Comfortable at rest or mild exertion but more than ordinary exertion leads to fatigue, palpitations, dyspnea, or angina.

• Class III: Marked limitation of physical activity. Comfortable at rest but less than ordinary activity leads to fatigue, dyspnea, palpitations, or angina.
• Class IV: Symptomatic at rest; discomfort increases with any physical activity; confined to bed or chair.

PHYSICAL EXAMINATION. The most common symptom of heart failure is **shortness of breath**, which may occur with exertion (exertional dyspnea) or at night (orthopnea and paroxysmal nocturnal dyspnea). Dyspnea at rest may occur. Observe the patient for mental confusion, anxiety, or irritability caused by hypoxia. Pale or cyanotic, cool, clammy skin is a result of poor perfusion. In right-sided HF, the jugular veins may become engorged and distended. If the pulsations in the jugular veins are visible 4.5 cm or more above the sternal notch with the patient at a 45-degree angle, jugular venous distention is present. The liver may also become engorged, and pressure on the abdomen increases pressure in the jugular veins, causing a rise in the top of the blood column. This positive finding for HF is known as *hepatojugular reflux* (HJR). The patient may also have peripheral edema in the ankles and feet, in the sacral area, or throughout the body. Ascites may occur as a result of passive liver congestion.

With auscultation, inspiratory crackles or expiratory wheezes (a result of pulmonary edema in left-sided failure) are heard in the patient's lungs. The patient's vital signs may demonstrate tachypnea or tachycardia, which occur in an attempt to compensate for the hypoxia and decreased CO. Gallop rhythms such as an S_3 or an S_4, while considered a normal finding in children and young adults, are considered pathological in the presence of HF and occur as a result of early rapid ventricular filling and increased resistance to ventricular filling after atrial contraction, respectively. Murmurs may also be present if the origin of the failure is a stenotic or incompetent valve.

PSYCHOSOCIAL. Note that experts have found that the physiological measures of HF (such as ejection fraction) do not always predict how active, vigorous, or positive patients feel about their health; rather, a person's view of health is based on many factors such as social support, level of activity, and outlook on life. HF is often accompanied by depression or anxiety because of physical limitations, concern over job or family responsibilities, or difficulty managing the burden of the illness.

Diagnostic Highlights

Test	Normal Result	Abnormality With Condition	Explanation
Echocardiography (ECHO)	Normal heart size, structure, and cardiac output	Depressed cardiac output, evidence of cardiomegaly	Measures chamber size, valvular structure and function, ventricular wall motion, and an estimated ejection fraction
Multigated blood pool imaging	Normal cardiac output and ejection fraction	Alterations in cardiac output and ejection fraction, often decreased	Assesses cardiac volume during both systole and diastole; data are used to determine ejection fraction; values are depressed in low-output failure
B-type natriuretic peptide (BNP) and pro-B-type natriuretic peptide (pro-BNP)	BNP: < 100 pg/mL; pro-BNP: < 125 pg/mL	100–300 pg/mL: HF is present; 300+: mild HF; 600+: moderate HF; 900+: severe HF	Naturally formed polypeptide; major source of plasma BNP in the cardiac ventricles; BNP level increases when HF symptoms worsen and decreases when the condition stabilizes

(highlight box continues on page 506)

Diagnostic Highlights (continued)

Cardiac Magnetic Resonance Imaging (cMRI): Has the ability to obtain information on structure and function with one noninvasive test. Electrocardiography: Reveals ventricular hypertrophy, ventricular dilatation, and axis deviation, although this test is not conclusive in itself and needs to be followed up with an ECHO. Chest X-ray: May show cardiomegaly, pulmonary vascular congestion, alveolar or interstitial edema, or pleural effusions. Other Tests: Tests include serum electrolytes, blood urea nitrogen, arterial blood gases, genetic testing, liver enzymes, prothrombin time, color flow mapping, and cardiac angiograms. Genetic testing.

PRIMARY NURSING DIAGNOSIS

DIAGNOSIS. Decreased cardiac output related to an ineffective ventricular pump as evidenced by dyspnea, tachycardia, and/or peripheral edema

OUTCOMES. Cardiac pump effectiveness; Circulation status; Tissue perfusion: Cardiac; Tissue perfusion: Cerebral; Tissue perfusion: Abdominal organs; Tissue perfusion: Peripheral; Vital signs; Electrolyte and acid-base balance; Knowledge: Heart failure management; Energy conservation; Fluid balance

INTERVENTIONS. Cardiac care; Circulatory care: Mechanical assist device; Fluid/ electrolyte management; Medication administration; Medication management; Oxygen therapy; Vital signs monitoring

PLANNING AND IMPLEMENTATION

Collaborative

MEDICAL. Initial management of the patient with HF depends on severity of HF, seriousness of symptoms, etiology, presence of other illnesses, and precipitating factors. Medication management is paramount in patients with HF. The general principles for management are treatment of any precipitating causes, control of fluid and sodium retention, increasing myocardial contractility, decreasing cardiac workload, and reducing pulmonary and systemic venous congestion. Nonpharmacologic therapy includes nutrition, weight loss, and exercise. The physician may also prescribe fluid and sodium restriction in an attempt to reduce volume and thereby reduce preload.

SURGICAL. If the elevated preload is caused by valvular regurgitation, the patient may require corrective surgery. Corrective surgery may also be warranted if the elevated afterload is caused by a stenotic valve. Another measure that may be taken to reduce afterload is an intra-aortic balloon pump (IABP). This is generally used as a bridge to surgery or in cardiogenic shock after acute myocardial infarction. It involves a balloon catheter placed in the descending aorta that inflates during diastole and deflates during systole. The balloon augments filling of the coronary arteries during diastole and decreases afterload during systole. IABP is used with caution because there are several possible complications, including dissection of the aortoiliac arteries, ischemic changes in the legs, and migration of the balloon up or down the aorta.

OTHER MEASURES. Other measures the physician may use include supplemental oxygen, thrombolytic therapy, percutaneous transluminal coronary interventions, directional coronary atherectomy, placement of a coronary stent, or coronary artery bypass surgery to improve oxygen flow to the myocardium. Circulatory devices such as ventricular assist devices and total artificial hearts can serve as a bridge to transplantation. Intra-aortic balloon counterpulsation or extracorporeal membrane oxygenation may be used for organ underperfusion in emergency situations. Finally, a cardiac transplant may be considered if other measures fail; if all other organ systems are viable; if there is no history of other pulmonary diseases; and if the patient does not smoke or use alcohol, is generally under 60 years of age, and is psychologically stable.

Pharmacologic Highlights

Medication or Drug Class	Dosage	Description	Rationale
Vasodilators	Varies by drug	Decrease arterial and venous vasoconstriction due to activation of adrenergic and renin-angiotensin systems; increase venous capacitance; drugs such as nitroglycerin and angiotensin-converting enzyme inhibitors (ACEIs) such as captopril, enalapril, and lisinopril; angiotensin receptor blockers (ARBs) such as losartan, valsartan, candesartan	Reduce vasoconstriction, thereby reducing afterload and enhancing myocardial performance and decreasing preload and ventricular filling pressures
Diuretics	Varies by drug	Increase excretion of sodium and water with drugs such as furosemide (Lasix) and metolazone (Zaroxalyn)	Used for patients with volume overload
Digoxin	0.125–0.375 mg PO daily	Cardiotonic	Increases cardiac contractility and helps manage some atrial dysrhythmias; may increase myocardial oxygen demand

Human B-Type Natriuretic Peptides: Dilates arteries and veins; used in case of serious HF. Dobutamine: Sympathomimetic, selective beta-1 stimulator that increases contractility, improves CO, decreases pulmonary capillary wedge pressure, and increases renal blood flow (as a result of improved CO). Dopamine: Low doses to stimulate dopaminergic receptors, causing renal vasodilation and improved renal function. Beta-Adrenergic Blocking Agents (Metoprolol, Carvedilol): Agents improve symptoms, exercise tolerance, cardiac hemodynamics, and left ventricular performance; they decrease mortality in HF patients, especially those with ischemic and idiopathic cardiomyopathy. Other Drugs: Antihypertensive agents (hydralazine, minoxidil) and, in severe cases of HF, nitroprusside may be used in an attempt to reduce afterload and improve CO. Norepinephrine is used for profound hypotension; phosphodiesterase inhibitors (milrinone, amrinone) cause increased contractility, decreased pulmonary vascular resistance, and decreased afterload. Anticoagulants may be used to decrease the risk of thromboembolism.

Independent

To conserve the patient's energy and to maximize the oxygen that is available for body processes, encourage the patient to rest. Elevation of the head of the bed to 30 to 45 degrees may alleviate some of the dyspnea by lowering the pressure on the diaphragm that is caused by the contents of the abdomen and by decreasing venous return, thereby decreasing preload. The patient may need assistance with activities of daily living, even eating, if the HF is at end stage and the least bit of activity causes fatigue and shortness of breath. To assess the patient's response to activity, check the blood pressure and heart rate, as well as the patient's subjective response both before and after any increase in activity level. Prolonged periods of little or no activity can be very difficult to reverse; therefore, maintaining some level of activity is highly encouraged.

To control symptoms, provide ongoing monitoring throughout the acute phases of the patient's disease. Monitor the patient for signs and symptoms of fluid overload, impaired gas exchange, and activity intolerance. Routine assessment of the cardiovascular and pulmonary systems is imperative in the early detection of exacerbation. Monitor daily intake and output, as well as daily weight, and conduct cardiopulmonary assessment.

Education of the patient and family is important for preventing exacerbations and frequent hospital visits. HF is clearly a condition that can be managed on an outpatient basis. A clear explanation of the disease process helps the patient understand the need for the prescribed medications, activity restrictions, diet, fluid restrictions, and lifestyle changes. Written material should be provided for the patient to take home and use as a reference.

Patients may no longer be able to live alone or support themselves. Fear, anxiety, and grief can all stimulate the sympathetic nervous system, leading to catecholamine release and additional stress on an already compromised heart. Helping the patient work through and verbalize these feelings may improve psychological well-being and CO. The patient and family may need end-of-life care and a referral to hospice.

Evidence-Based Practice and Health Policy

Tandon, V., Stringer, B., Conner, C., Gabriel, A., Tripathi, B., Balakumaran, K., & Chen, K. (2020). An observation of racial and gender disparities in congestive heart failure admissions using the national inpatient sample. *Cureus, 12*, 1–22.

- The authors analyzed the National Inpatient Sample database from 2009 to 2014 to determine that nature of sex and racial disparities that occur in congestive health failure (CHF) admissions to the hospital. They studied over 5 million admissions with a primary diagnosis of CHF. Females accounted for 49.7% of the admissions. Black people had the lowest mortality rate and the lowest average admission age of 63.5 years, indicating that they were getting sick earlier in their life span than other groups.
- Total charges for males were $42,920 and for females were $36,744. Males had significantly more procedures than females. The authors suggested that women may be less inclined to utilize hospital services during the early states of their disease. Other studies have shown that women have a less positive experience with hospitalization than men, which may explain the delay. They were also less likely to receive a cardiac catheterization than men when hospitalized with myocardial infarction, which is a significant health disparity for women.

DOCUMENTATION GUIDELINES

- Physical findings indicative of HF: Mental confusion; pale, cyanotic, clammy skin; presence of jugular vein distention and HJR; ascites; edema; pulmonary crackles or wheezes; adventitious heart sounds
- Fluid intake and output, daily weights
- Response to medications such as diuretics, nitrates, dopamine, dobutamine, and oxygen
- Psychosocial response to illness; evaluation of depression and anxiety, referral to end-of-life care if appropriate

DISCHARGE AND HOME HEALTHCARE GUIDELINES

PREVENTION. To prevent exacerbations, teach the patient and family to monitor for an increase in shortness of breath or edema. Tell the patient to restrict fluid intake to 2 to 2.5 L per day and restrict sodium intake as prescribed. Teach the patient to monitor daily weights and report weight gain of more than 4 pounds in 2 days.

MEDICATIONS. Be sure the patient and family understand all medications, including effect, dosage, route, adverse effects, and the need for routine laboratory monitoring for drugs such as digoxin.

COMPLICATIONS OF HF. Tell the patient to call for emergency assistance for acute shortness of breath or chest discomfort that is not alleviated with rest.

Hemophilia

DRG Category:	813
Mean LOS:	4.9 days
Description:	MEDICAL: Coagulation Disorders

Hemophilia refers to a group of congenital coagulation disorders characterized by a deficiency or malfunction of specific clotting factors. The Centers for Disease Control and Prevention estimate that approximately 20,000 people in the United States have hemophilia, and approximately 400 babies are born each year with the disease. Hemophilia A, or classic hemophilia, is caused by a defect in factor VIII (antihemophilic factor). Hemophilia B, or Christmas disease, is caused by a defect in factor IX (plasma thromboplastin component, or Christmas factor). Hemophilia A is more common, occurring once per 5,000 to 10,000 live male births, contrasted with hemophilia B, which occurs once per 30,000 live male births. Hemophilia C, or factor XI (plasma thromboplastin antecedent) deficiency, is even more rare, accounting for less than 5% of hereditary coagulopathies. The mortality rate for persons with hemophilia is twice that of the healthy male population, and for severe hemophilia, the rate is almost six times higher.

Of patients who have hemophilia, 85% have hemophilia A, which is classified by levels of factor VIII. Severe hemophiliacs have less than 1% activity and have bleeding episodes that require factor VIII therapy several times per month. Moderate hemophiliacs have 1% to 5% activity and have varying need for factor VIII therapy, whereas mild hemophiliacs have greater than 5% activity and require intervention only after trauma or surgery.

Persons with hemophilia are able to form a platelet plug but are unable to form a stable clot. Clinical manifestations and complications of hemophilia are usually secondary to recurrent bleeding. Complications from subcutaneous and intramuscular hematomas are caused by compression of nerves or other structures, resulting in peripheral neuropathies, pain, compromised airway, muscle atrophy, ischemia, and gangrene. Hemarthrosis, or bleeding into the joint or synovial cavity, is a common complication that often results in joint deformities. Life-threatening hemorrhage may result from minor injuries.

CAUSES

All forms of hemophilia are the result of an X-linked recessive trait disorder (see Genetic Considerations). Approximately one-third of all hemophiliacs have no family history of bleeding disorders, which indicates that there may be factors other than heredity involved and that the illness is a result of a new mutation.

GENETIC CONSIDERATIONS

Hemophilia is an X-linked recessive condition. Both factor VIII (hemophilia A) and factor IX (hemophilia B) genes are located on the X chromosome; therefore, hemophilia affects males almost exclusively. Daughters of men with hemophilia are obligate carriers, but sons of affected men are normal. When a carrier woman has a son, his risk of disease is 50% and each of her daughters has a 50% risk of also being a carrier. Female offspring have a 50% chance of being affected with hemophilia if an affected male has a child with a carrier female.

SEX AND LIFE SPAN CONSIDERATIONS

Males who inherit the genetic trait have hemophilia. Most females with the defective gene do not develop clinical manifestations because they usually inherit a normal X chromosome from the other parent. Hemophiliac males do not transmit the disease to their sons because the Y chromosome is not affected. However, all daughters of afflicted males become carriers of the trait because they inherit the defective X chromosome. Female carriers have a 50% chance of transmitting the trait to their offspring. Half of the daughters become carriers, and half of their sons have manifestations of hemophilia. Girls have a 50% chance of being affected with hemophilia if their father is an affected male and their mother is a carrier female.

Bleeding abnormalities associated with hemophilia are usually noticed when the child becomes active and learns to walk, but mild cases may go undetected until adulthood. Approximately 40% of children have their first bleeding during their first year of life, and by age 4 years, 90% of children with hemophilia have had episodes of persistent bleeding from minor injuries. Bleeding episodes seem to decrease at or after adolescence, which may be because of the decreased risk of trauma as well as stabilization of the disease process.

HEALTH DISPARITIES AND SEXUAL/GENDER MINORITY HEALTH

Hemophilia A and B are found in all ethnic and racial groups, although a lower prevalence may exist in the Chinese population. The prevalence in general follows the racial and ethnic distribution of the U.S. population. Sexual and gender minority status has no known effect on the risk for hemophilia.

GLOBAL HEALTH CONSIDERATIONS

The National Hemophilia Foundation estimates that approximately 400,000 people in the world have severe or moderate hemophilia A and B. Experts suggest that about 10,000 infants are born with hemophilia each year worldwide. Underdiagnosis of hemophilia in developing countries is a critical problem because of little access to care, no money for screening, lack of diagnostic tests to identify patients, and no factor replacement therapies. Estimates of nondiagnosis are as high as 75% in developing countries, and many infants born with hemophilia die during childhood.

ASSESSMENT

HISTORY. Question the patient, parents, or caregiver about any history of prolonged bleeding episodes, either spontaneous or following any injury in the patient or family. Determine the patient's age at diagnosis and the specific nature of the bleeding problem; in the case of a child, determine the family member's relationship to the patient. Ask if the patient has any signs of internal bleeding or excessive blood loss like weakness, lethargy, fast heart rate, or orthostasis. Pubertal females should be questioned about their menstrual cycles and blood flow as symptoms often do not present before that time.

PHYSICAL EXAMINATION. Note hematomas from **subcutaneous and intramuscular bleeding**. Tissue over the bleeding site is hard, raised, and dark purple. The hemorrhage extends from this center concentrically, with each successive outer circle becoming lighter in color. Intramuscular bleeding usually spreads within a single fascial space. Fever or pain may occur, with or without the skin discoloration. Signs of excessive blood loss are tachycardia, hypotension, shortness of breath, dizziness, and orthostatic changes in blood pressure.

Monitor the patient for frank or occult hematuria, melena, or hematemesis. Bleeding disproportionate to the extent of a traumatic injury is characteristic of hemophilia. Typically, the bleeding is an intermittent oozing type that develops over several hours or days after the injury or procedure. Wound healing is often delayed.

When the patient's extremities are moved, note joint pain and swelling caused by hemarthrosis or spontaneous or trauma-induced bleeding into the joint or synovial cavity. Acute hemarthrosis is often preceded by a warm tingling sensation in the affected joint. If absorption of the blood from around the periarticular structures is incomplete, the remaining blood can cause chronic inflammation of the synovial membranes. Other long-term clinical sequelae of hemarthrosis include impaired joint mobility, bone deformity and demineralization, and stunted growth. Approximately 40% of hemophilia patients have splenomegaly; there have been some reported cases of spontaneous splenic rupture.

PSYCHOSOCIAL. Patients with hemophilia and their families contend with the challenges of a rare chronic illness and the constant threat of life-threatening hemorrhage. Children often feel isolated from their peers because of the activity restrictions. Feelings of guilt are common among parents of hemophilic children. Research studies have shown a positive correlation between children's adaptation to hemophilia and parental acceptance of the disease. Also, children who have a greater understanding of hemophilia and its treatment are less likely to experience psychological distress.

Diagnostic Highlights

Test	Normal Result	Abnormality With Condition	Explanation
Genetic testing	Normal factors VIII, IX, or XI genes	Mutation on factors VIII, IX, or XI genes	Identifies genetic alterations from normal
Assay of factors VIII, IX, XI	VIII: 50%–150% of normal control activity; IX: 50%–150%; XI: 65%–135%	< 5% normal control activity	Determines level of activity of essential factors needed for blood clotting
Coagulation studies; activated partial thromboplastin time (APTT); prothrombin time (PT); bleeding time; platelet count	APTT: 25–35 sec; PT: 10–13 sec; bleeding time (Duke, varies by method): 1–5 min; platelets: 150,000–450,000/mm³	Hemophilia A and B: prolonged APTT; normal bleeding time, platelet count, PT	Determine clot formation; APTT measures the time for clot to form in a section of clotting cascade affected by factors VIII, IX, and XI

Other Tests: Thrombin time, x-rays of hemarthrotic joints, computed tomography scan, magnetic resonance imaging

PRIMARY NURSING DIAGNOSIS

DIAGNOSIS. Risk for bleeding as evidenced by bruising, swelling, joint pain, and/or muscle pain

OUTCOMES. Risk control; Safe home environment; Blood coagulation; Knowledge: Personal safety; Knowledge: Medication; Knowledge: Fall prevention; Medication response

INTERVENTIONS. Bleeding precautions; Bleeding reduction; Fall prevention; Environmental management; Health education; Surveillance; Medication administration; Medication management

PLANNING AND IMPLEMENTATION

Collaborative

Replacement therapy and drug therapy may be used prophylactically or to control mild or major bleeding episodes. Factor VIII, also found in fresh-frozen plasma (FFP), is usually reserved for patients with hemophilia A who are actively bleeding. Factor VIII concentrates replace deficient factor VIII, with the goal of achieving normal hemostasis. The current recommendation is to use recombinant (synthetic) products initially and thereafter in all newly diagnosed cases. Recombinant factor VIII contains less risk of viral transmission than pooled plasma products but has a relatively high cost. Purified plasma-derived factor VIII concentrates are derived from large pools of plasma donors. Recent methods of screening and heating of these concentrates have greatly diminished the risk of contamination with HIV but have little effect on the risk of hepatitis transmission. High-potency factor VIII preparations (those that are highly purified) are considered to be virtually virus free. A rule of thumb is that for every 1 unit/kg infused, factor VIII levels will increase 2%. In an emergency, a 50-unit/kg IV bolus will increase levels to 100%. Desmopressin will raise factor VIII levels twofold to threefold (see Pharmacologic Highlights).

Bleeding episodes in hemophilia B can be treated with FFP or purified factor IX. Hemophilia C rarely requires intervention. Factor VIII replacement therapy is indicated for active bleeding or preparation for multiple tooth extractions or major surgery. Cryoprecipitate contains high levels of factor VIII and fibrinogen and may be administered in emergencies. Prophylactic replacement therapy for factor VIII or factor IX deficiency has been found to be beneficial in preventing spontaneous bleeding episodes and in minimizing bleeding complications such as joint disease. Any incidence of head trauma should receive immediate therapy that raises the factor VIII or IX levels to 100% normal before any diagnostic tests are performed. Intracranial hemorrhage is the most common cause of death in people with hemophilia; approximately 50% of these are associated with acute head injury.

Pharmacologic Highlights

Medication or Drug Class	Dosage	Description	Rationale
Emicizumab (Hemlibra)	Loading dose of 3 mg/kg SQ once weekly for 4 weeks, the maintenance dosages of 1.5 mg/kg once per week, 3 mg/kg once every 2 weeks or 6 mg/kg once every 4 weeks	Nonfactor replacement therapy	Routine prophylaxis to prevent or minimize episodic bleeding with hemophilia A with or without factor VIII inhibitors; increases the ability for blood to clot
Desmopressin, 1-deamino-8-darginine vasopressin	0.3 mcg/kg IV diluted in 50 mL normal saline solution; intranasal: 300 mcg, one spray in each nostril	Antidiuretic	Stimulates rapid release of von Willebrand factor into the blood; treatment of choice in patients with hemophilia A who do not have life-threatening bleeding problems; avoided with infants; does not play a role in treatment for hemophilia B

Other Drugs: Analgesia for hemarthrosis; avoid products containing aspirin and NSAIDs; monoclonal antibodies (rituximab); antifibrinolytic agents: aminocaproic acid (Amicar) can be used in oral surgery or bleeding.

Independent

To prevent trauma that may precipitate bleeding episodes, avoid intramuscular injections and minimize the number of venipuncture attempts. Alert other health team members about the patient's high risk for bleeding. Avoid sources of mucosal irritation such as rectal temperatures, urinary catheters, and suppositories. Use only sponge sticks and nonalcoholic rinses for oral care. Ensure that tourniquets or blood pressure cuffs are applied no longer than necessary. Perform nasopharyngeal or oropharyngeal suctioning very gently and only when needed. Prevent skin breakdown through the use of frequent turning and preventive skin care.

When bleeding occurs, apply firm, direct pressure for at least 5 minutes or until bleeding has stopped completely to sites of subcutaneous injections and venipuncture sites. Use sandbags and pressure dressings to maintain pressure on large puncture sites after hemostasis has been established. Initially, provide rest and elevation to a bleeding joint. Initiate mobilization within a few days after the bleeding is controlled to facilitate restoration of normal joint range of motion. Apply ice packs to control epistaxis, hematoma formation, and hemarthrosis.

Evaluate the family's current coping mechanisms and the level of anxiety. Encourage the patient and family members to verbalize their feelings openly and clearly with staff and with each other. Encourage family members to discuss the needs of their child with child care centers, schools, babysitters, and persons overseeing sports or extracurricular activities.

Evidence-Based Practice and Health Policy

Shima, M., Nogami, K., Nagami, S., Yoshida, S., Yoneyama, K., Ishiguro, A., Suzuki, T., & Taki, M. (2019). A multicenter, open-label study of emicizumab given every 2 or 4 weeks in children with severe haemophilia A without inhibitors. *Haemophilia*, *25*, 979–987.

• The authors use a multicenter, open-label, nonrandomized study design to evaluate the efficacy, safety, and pharmokinetics of emicizumab on eligible children less than 12 years old weighing over 3 kg with severe congenital hemophilia A without factor VIII inhibitors. Children received a loading dose of emicizumab 3 mg/kg once a week for 4 weeks, followed by a maintenance dose of 3 mg/kg every 2 weeks or 6 mg/kg every 4 weeks. Those patients with sustained clinical benefit were permitted to continue prophylaxis treatment or offered to titrate up the dose in those with insufficient control of bleeding. Caregivers participated by recording physical activity level, preference of treatment, and influencing factors.

• While sample size was limited, the results indicated efficacy and safety of the biweekly or every 4 weeks drug regimens. Caregivers reported preference for this treatment due to less frequency of drug needed and less effect on other activities.

DOCUMENTATION GUIDELINES

• Bleeding episodes: Site, extent, duration, associated signs and symptoms, response to interventions
• Physical responses: Alteration in circulation, movement, or sensation; redness, warmth or swelling around joints; changes in vital signs, intake and output, cognition
• Pain: Location, precipitating factors, quality, intensity, associated signs and symptoms, factors that alleviate or exacerbate the pain
• Therapeutic and adverse effects of medical or surgical interventions

DISCHARGE AND HOME HEALTHCARE GUIDELINES

Teach the patient and family the early and late clinical manifestations of bleeding. Outline measures to prevent bleeding episodes, such as use of a soft-bristled toothbrush or sponge sticks, avoidance of activities that are likely to result in trauma, and avoidance of NSAIDs.

Emphasize the importance of carrying identifying medical information at all times. Teach the patient or caregiver to inform all healthcare providers about the patient's diagnosis. Describe immediate actions the patient or caregiver should take to control bleeding. List indicators of the need for medical assistance. Teach the patient or caregiver the purpose of each medication, the correct procedure for administration, and potential adverse effects. Provide the patient or family with a list of referrals for genetic counselors, social workers, vocational counselors, or psychologists to assist in the long-term adjustment as necessary.

Hemorrhoids

DRG Category:	394
Mean LOS:	3.8 days
Description:	MEDICAL: Other Digestive System Diagnoses With Complication or Comorbidity
DRG Category:	348
Mean LOS:	4.4 days
Description:	SURGICAL: Anal and Stomal Procedures With Complication or Comorbidity

Hemorrhoids are a common, generally insignificant swelling and distention of veins (hemorrhoidal venous cushions) in the anorectal region. They cause symptoms when they become enlarged or inflamed, bleed, or become prolapsed (enlarged internal hemorrhoids that actually protrude through the anus). In the United States, at least 10 million people have hemorrhoids, and up to one-third of these people seek treatment. Hemorrhoids are categorized as either internal or external. Internal hemorrhoids, produced by dilation and enlargement of the superior plexus, cannot be seen because they are above the anal sphincter, whereas external hemorrhoids, produced by dilation and enlargement of the inferior plexus, are below the anal sphincter and are apparent on inspection.

Experts suggest that hemorrhoids may develop when increased intra-abdominal pressure produces increased systemic and portal venous pressure, thus causing increased pressure in the anorectal veins. The arterioles in the anorectal area send blood directly to the swollen anorectal veins, further increasing the pressure. Recurrent and repeated increased pressure causes the distended veins to separate from the surrounding smooth muscle and leads to their prolapse. Complications include rectal bleeding, infection, thrombosis, fibrosis, abscess, necrosis, and strangulation.

CAUSES

There is little evidence to point to a direct cause of hemorrhoids, but most experts agree that low-fiber diets cause small, hard stools, which can lead to straining and increased pressure during defecation. Pressure leads to engorgement and swelling of the venous cushions. The link between pregnancy and hemorrhoids is also thought to be due to decreased venous return, engorgement, and hormone changes. Other related factors include obesity, elevated anal resting pressure, having an episiotomy, and anal intercourse. Conditions that are associated with hemorrhoids include chronic diarrhea, heart failure, colon malignancy, liver disease, spinal cord injury, and inflammatory bowel disease.

GENETIC CONSIDERATIONS

It is unclear whether familial occurrences of hemorrhoids are related to genetic or environmental factors or a combination of the two. A familial tendency toward weak rectal vein walls and/or valves and varicose veins would increase susceptibility. A recent genetic study identified variants in the myosin gene, *MYH9*, that are associated with hemorrhoids, providing evidence that there is a genetic component to hemorrhoids.

SEX AND LIFE SPAN CONSIDERATIONS

Hemorrhoids are more common in women during late pregnancy and immediately after delivery. Young people who are engaged in heavy weightlifting and exercise are prone to hemorrhoids, and college students who do not eat balanced diets or who eat low-fiber diets are also at risk. The greatest incidence occurs in adults from 45 to 65 years of age. Men and people with high socioeconomic status are more likely to pursue medical care for the treatment of hemorrhoids than women and people from underresourced communities. In later life, congestive heart failure and obesity contribute to the development of hemorrhoids.

HEALTH DISPARITIES AND SEXUAL/GENDER MINORITY HEALTH

There are no known racial or ethnic considerations with respect to prevalence, but people requesting treatment are most likely to be White with income in the middle or upper range. Women and men who have receptive anal intercourse may have a higher risk for hemorrhoids and may have pain and bleeding during sexual encounters.

GLOBAL HEALTH CONSIDERATIONS

In Western countries, approximately 4% to 5% of the population is affected with symptoms. This prevalence is likely comparable to most regions around the world.

ASSESSMENT

HISTORY. Establish a history of anal itching, blood on the toilet tissue or in the toilet bowl after a bowel movement, and anorectal pain or discomfort. The blood is usually bright red. Determine the onset and duration of symptoms. Ask if the patient has experienced any mucous discharge. Determine if the patient can feel the external hemorrhoids. Elicit a history of risk factors, activity patterns, and dietary patterns. Determine if the patient has a person or familial history of inflammatory bowel disease, coagulation problems, or immune suppression such as HIV disease or cancer.

PHYSICAL EXAMINATION. The most common symptoms are **anal itching**, **rectal bleeding after a bowel movement**, and **anorectal pain**. Inspect the patient's anorectal area, noting external or prolapsed hemorrhoids. The preferred position to complete the visual inspection and digital examination is the left lateral decubitus with the patient's knees flexed to the chest. Internal hemorrhoids are discovered through digital rectal examination or anoscopy. Note any subcutaneous large, firm lumps in the anal area.

PSYCHOSOCIAL. Patients with hemorrhoids may delay seeking treatment because of embarrassment relating to the anatomic location. Provide privacy and foster dignity when interacting with these patients. Inform the patient of every step of the procedure. Provide comfort during examination.

Diagnostic Highlights

Test	Normal Result	Abnormality With Condition	Explanation
Anoscopy: Endoscopic examination of rectum and anal canal (flexible sigmoidoscopy/colonoscopy may be included)	Normal rectal lining: Consistently reddish, free of lesions or inflammation	Visualization of external and internal hemorrhoids	Determines size and location of hemorrhoids
Other Tests: Barium enema, proctoscopic ultrasound, virtual colonoscopy, complete blood count			

PRIMARY NURSING DIAGNOSIS

DIAGNOSIS. Acute or chronic pain related to rectal swelling and prolapse as evidenced by self-reports of pain, swelling, and/or itching

OUTCOMES. Comfort status; Pain control; Pain level; Symptom severity; Knowledge: Pain management

INTERVENTIONS. Analgesic administration; Anxiety reduction; Pain management: Acute and chronic; Medication management; Heat/cold application; Bowel management; Coping enhancement

✳ PLANNING AND IMPLEMENTATION

Collaborative

Generally, hemorrhoids can be managed pharmacologically, with adequate fluid intake and dietary changes. Conservative treatments include application of cold packs to the anal region, sitz baths for 15 minutes twice a day, and local application of over-the-counter treatments such as witch hazel (Tucks) or dibucaine (Nupercainal) ointment. Increasing fiber intake in the diet, avoiding spicy and fatty foods, and increasing fluid intake are components of conservative treatment. If conservative treatment does not alleviate symptoms in 3 to 5 days, more invasive management may be needed.

Invasive treatment may be indicated for thrombosis or severe symptoms. Sclerotherapy obliterates the vessels when the physician injects a sclerosing agent into the tissues around the hemorrhoids. With rubber band ligation (RBL), rubber bands are put on the hemorrhoids in an outpatient setting. The banded tissue sloughs. Successive visits may be necessary for many hemorrhoids. Although RBL has a high success rate, it may temporarily increase local pain and cause hemorrhage. In cryosurgery, the physician freezes the hemorrhoid with a probe to produce necrosis. Cryosurgery and infrared coagulation are used primarily for first- and second-degree hemorrhoids. All nonoperative treatments have similar outcomes when implemented by an experienced clinician (Ma et al., 2020 [see Evidence-Based Practice and Health Policy]).

The most effective treatment is hemorrhoidectomy, the surgical removal of hemorrhoids, which is performed in an outpatient setting in 10% of patients. Because conservative treatment is often successful, however, hemorrhoidectomy is much less common than previously. Postoperative care includes checking the dressing for excessive bleeding or drainage. The patient needs to void within the first 24 hours. If prescribed, spread petroleum jelly on the wound site and apply a wet dressing. Complications include urinary retention and hemorrhage. The newest surgical technique for treating internal hemorrhoids is stapled hemorrhoidectomy. The surgery does not actually remove hemorrhoids but rather the supporting tissue that causes hemorrhoids to prolapse downward.

Pharmacologic Highlights

Medication or Drug Class	Dosage	Description	Rationale
Docusate sodium (Colace)	100 mg bid PO	Stool softener	Eases defecation
Anusol suppositories	1 bid PR	Analgesic, emollient	Relieve pain and itching
Hydrocortisone ointment or suppositories	Topical or PR as needed for brief courses of therapy	Corticosteroid	Relieve itching and swelling

Pharmacologic Highlights (continued)

Other Drugs: Over-the-counter analgesics such as acetaminophen or topical anesthetics such as lidocaine ointment. NSAIDS may decrease discomfort. Some people find that hamamelis water (witch hazel) effectively reduces anal itching. Note: Laxatives are prohibited. Supplements high in fiber such as psyllium seed and methylcellulose are commonly used.

Independent

Most patients can be treated on an outpatient basis. Teach patients and families about over-the-counter local applications for comfort. Explain the importance of promoting regular bowel habits and avoiding prolonged sitting on the toilet. Emphasize the need for increasing dietary fiber and fluid through a balanced diet high in whole grains, raw vegetables, and fresh fruit. Moderate exercise such as walking can also help regulate bowel function.

Postoperative actions include administering ice packs for pain control and positioning the patient for comfort. After the first 12-hour postoperative period, sitz baths three or four times a day may be instituted to prevent rectoanal spasms and reduce swelling. Explain that the first postoperative bowel movement is painful and may require suitable narcotic intervention for comfort.

Evidence-Based Practice and Health Policy

Ma, W., Guo, J., Yang, F., Dietrich, C., & Sun, S. (2020). Progress in endoscopic treatment of hemorrhoids. *Journal of Translational Internal Medicine, 8,* 237–244.

* This article discusses several endoscopic treatment techniques: RBL, sclerotherapy, and electrocoagulation. The development, efficacy, and advantages of these treatments are summarized and evaluated. The authors offer an overview of the three techniques, providing history, a description of the technique, and a table that reviews research studies on the technique.
* They note that current research shows that compared with traditional treatment methods, endoscopic hemorrhoid treatment techniques can also effectively treat hemorrhoids in a minimally invasive fashion. These procedures allow for a shortened procedure time, reduced intraprocedural bleeding, decreased pain, and shortened recovery time; other important colorectal pathologies can be detected at the same time. The authors expect that going forward, endoscopic technology will be applied in clinical practice and may become the first-line method for the treatment of hemorrhoids.

DOCUMENTATION GUIDELINES

* Physical findings: Rectal examination, urinary retention, bleeding, mucous drainage
* Wound healing: Drainage, color, swelling
* Pain management: Pain (location, duration, frequency), response to interventions
* Postoperative bowel movements: Tolerance for first bowel movement

DISCHARGE AND HOME HEALTHCARE GUIDELINES

Teach the patient the importance of a high-fiber diet, increased fluid intake, mild exercise, and regular bowel movements. Be sure the patient schedules a follow-up visit to the physician. Teach the patient which analgesic applications for local pain may be used. If the patient has had surgery, teach the patient to recognize signs of urinary retention, such as bladder distention and hemorrhage, and to contact the physician at their appearance.

Hemothorax

DRG Category:	165
Mean LOS:	3.3 days
Description:	SURGICAL: Major Chest Procedures Without Complication or Comorbidity or Major Complication or Comorbidity
DRG Category:	186
Mean LOS:	5.6 days
Description:	MEDICAL: Pleural Effusion With Major Complication or Comorbidity
DRG Category:	199
Mean LOS:	6.7 days
Description:	MEDICAL: Pneumothorax With Major Complication or Comorbidity

Hemothorax, an accumulation of blood in the pleural space, affects oxygenation, ventilation, and hemodynamic stability. Approximately 60% of people who experience multiple trauma have chest injuries, and experts estimate that approximately 300,000 cases of trauma-related hemothorax occur each year. Oxygenation is affected because the accumulation of blood exerts pressure on pulmonary structures, leading to alveolar collapse, a decreased surface area for gas exchange, and impaired diffusion of oxygen from the alveolus to the blood. Ventilation is likewise impaired as the accumulating blood takes the place of gas in the lungs. Hemodynamic instability occurs as bleeding increases in the pleural space and vascular volume is depleted. Pneumothorax, or air in the pleural cavity, often accompanies hemothorax.

The hemorrhage can occur from pulmonary parenchymal lacerations, intercostal artery lacerations, or disruptions of the pulmonary or bronchial vasculature. Low pulmonary pressures and thromboplastin in the lungs may aid in spontaneously tamponading parenchymal lacerations. Complications of hemothorax include hypovolemic shock, atelectasis, intrathoracic hematoma, wound infection, pneumonia, sepsis, exsanguination, organ failure, cardiopulmonary arrest, and death. Some experts define a hemothorax only when the hematocrit is greater than 50%, as compared to a bloody pleural effusion, but most do not differentiate between the two conditions.

CAUSES

Approximately 150,000 people die in the United States each year from trauma, and most are caused by blunt trauma from motor vehicle crashes (MVCs), assaults, and falls or by penetrating trauma from knives or gunshot wound. All of these injuries can cause a hemothorax. MVCs cause 70% of chest trauma, and one of every four patients with chest trauma has a hemothorax. Other causes of hemothorax include thoracic surgery, pulmonary infarction, dissecting thoracic aneurysms, tumors, tuberculosis, and anticoagulant therapy.

GENETIC CONSIDERATIONS

Hemothorax may occur more commonly in people with clotting or bleeding disorders.

SEX AND LIFE SPAN CONSIDERATIONS

Hemothorax from traumatic injury occurs in both pediatric and adult populations. Because trauma is the leading cause of death in the first four decades of life, hemothorax is most commonly seen in children and young adults. Penetrating injuries from gunshot wounds and stab wounds, which are on the increase in U.S. preteens, teens, and young adults, are more common in males than females. In urban areas, drive-by shootings are increasing, and in some cities, they are associated with half of all youth gunshot wounds. Males have different patterns of injury than females and a higher injury severity. Analysis of trauma outcomes indicates that, following traumatic injury, males have higher rates of multiple organ failure, pneumonia, and sepsis than females, creating health disparities for men (Marcolini et al., 2019). Trauma is the third leading cause of death in people 45 to 65 years old and the seventh leading cause of death in people older than age 65 years. Because they often have fewer compensatory mechanisms to respond to the injury, older adults with such an injury have higher rates of complications and death.

HEALTH DISPARITIES AND SEXUAL/GENDER MINORITY HEALTH

Many types of injuries lead to hemothorax, and injury rates vary by group. In the United States, Black youth ages 15 to 24 years have the highest homicide rate from gunshot wounds, followed by Hispanic youth. Suicide rates are highest among Native American males and non-Hispanic White males. Penetrating injuries from gunshot wounds and stab wounds are more common in non-Hispanic Black persons than in non-Hispanic White persons. Non-Hispanic Black males have adjusted firearm death rates from two to seven times higher than males of other groups. Healthy People 2020 reports that non-Hispanic Black persons have the highest injury death rate in the United States (79.9 injury deaths per 100,000 people), followed by non-Hispanic White people (79.2), Native American people (78.2), Hispanic people (45.5), and Asian/Pacific Islander people (25.6). Geographic information system mapping has shown that impoverished neighborhoods have a higher incidence of gunshot injury than other neighborhoods (Bayouth et al., 2019). Socioeconomic status and injury are linked, with people living with lower incomes having higher risk. Children under 14 years of age living in rural areas have higher rates of unintentional firearm injuries than urban children have. Recent work has shown evidence that rural populations have injury mortality rates that are more than twice as high as urban rates. Many factors contribute to these health disparities, including the distance from major trauma centers. Sexual and gender minority persons have high risk for dating and interpersonal violence, violence related to bullying, and intentional and unintentional injury (Healthy People 2020).

GLOBAL HEALTH CONSIDERATIONS

Specifically with respect to thoracic trauma, MVCs are the leading cause of injury, and they occur most commonly in males 14 to 30 years of age. According to the World Health Organization, injury accounts for 9% of global mortality. Falls from heights of less than 5 meters are the leading cause of injury globally, but estimates are that only a small percentage of those are related to thoracic trauma. In areas of civil and political strife and war, ballistic injuries and stab wounds to the chest also cause hemothorax.

ASSESSMENT

HISTORY. Establish a history of the injury. If the patient has been shot, ask the paramedics for ballistic information, including the caliber of the weapon and the range at which the person was shot. If the patient was in an MVC, determine the type of vehicle (truck, motorcycle, car); the speed of the vehicle; the victim's location in the car (driver or passenger); and the use, if any, of safety restraints. Determine if the patient has had recent tetanus immunization. If the patient can communicate, determine the location of chest pain and whether the patient is experiencing shortness of breath. If there is no chest trauma, establish a history of other risk factors. Determine if the patient has undergone thoracic surgery or anticoagulant therapy. Determine if the patient has a history of alcohol or substance use and abuse both at the time of injury and daily. Establish a history of pulmonary infarction, dissecting thoracic aneurysm, or tumor.

PHYSICAL EXAMINATION. The most common symptoms are **chest pain, tachypnea,** and **dyspnea,** but symptoms may be subtle or vary depending on the nature of the injury and the amount of bleeding. The initial evaluation focuses on assessing the adequacy of the patient's airway, breathing, and circulation (ABCs) as well as neurological status. The patient should be completely undressed for a thorough visual assessment. The initial evaluation, or primary survey, is completed by the trauma resuscitation team and may occur simultaneously with life-saving interventions as needed.

The secondary survey, completed after life-threatening conditions are stabilized, includes serial vital signs and a complete head-to-toe assessment. Assess the patient for a patent airway. Note respiratory rate, breathing pattern, and lung sounds on an hourly basis. Observe the patient's breathing; the affected side of the chest may expand and stiffen while the unaffected side rises. Auscultate for lung sounds; the loss of breath sounds is evidence of a collapsed lung. Percuss the lungs; blood in the pleural space yields a dullness. Physical findings are best determined when the patient is sitting upright if the patient's condition allows. Note signs of respiratory failure; the patient may appear anxious, restless, even stuporous, and cyanotic. If the patient has a chest tube, monitor its functioning, the amount of blood loss, the integrity of the system, and the presence of air leaks.

Examine the thorax area, including the anterior chest, posterior chest, and axillae, for contusions, abrasions, hematomas, and penetrating wounds. Note that even small penetrating wounds can be life threatening if vital structures are perforated. Observe carefully for pallor, blood pressure, and pulse rate, noting the early signs of shock or massive bleeding such as a falling pulse pressure, a rising pulse rate, and delayed capillary refill. Note that a delayed hemothorax may occur hours to days after the initial injury from a rupture of a chest wall hematoma or displacement of a fractured rib.

PSYCHOSOCIAL. The patient may be fearful or panic-stricken because of difficulties in breathing and intense pain. Ongoing assessment of coping strategies of patient and family assists in planning and evaluating interventions. Note that approximately half of all traumatic injuries are associated with alcohol and other drugs of abuse. Assess the patient's drinking and drug-taking patterns and refer for counseling if appropriate.

Diagnostic Highlights

Test	Normal Result	Abnormality With Condition	Explanation
Chest x-rays, upright	Air-filled lungs	Opacity at the area of bleeding and lung collapse; blunted costophrenic angle; may show widening of mediastinum and intercostal spaces with depressed diaphragm	Determines the location and extent of lung collapse and fluid accumulation
Complete blood count	Red blood cells: 3.6–5.8 million/mcL; hemoglobin: 11.7–17.4 g/dL; hematocrit: 33%–52%; white blood cells: 4,500–11,100/mcL; platelets: 150,000–450,000/mcL	Decreased values reflective of the degree of hemorrhage	Determines the extent of blood loss; note that it takes 2 hr for hemorrhage to be reflected in a dropping hemoglobin and hematocrit after injury

Diagnostic Highlights (continued)

Test	Normal Result	Abnormality With Condition	Explanation
Computed tomography (CT)	Air-filled lungs with normal lung structure	Localized collection of blood	Determines the location and extent of lung collapse and fluid accumulation if findings from chest x-rays are uncertain; helpful in identifying loculated (saclike) collection of blood
Arterial blood gases	Pao_2: 80–95 mm Hg; $Paco_2$: 35–45 mm Hg; SaO_2: 95%–100%; pH: 7.35–7.45	Hypoxemia; Pao_2 < 80 mm Hg; SaO_2 < 95%; $Paco_2$ > 45 mm Hg	Determine adequacy of oxygenation; accumulation of blood and air in functional tissue of lungs decreases gas exchange leading to hypoxemia and hypercapnea

Other Tests: Coagulation studies, ultrasonography, electrocardiogram, thoracentesis/needle aspiration, cervical spine x-rays

PRIMARY NURSING DIAGNOSIS

DIAGNOSIS. Ineffective airway clearance related to airway obstruction as evidenced by stridor, hoarseness, cough, air hunger, restlessness, confusion, and/or dyspnea

OUTCOMES. Respiratory status: Airway patency; Respiratory status: Ventilation; Respiratory status: Gas exchange; Vital signs; Symptom control; Medication response; Mechanical ventilation response: Adult

INTERVENTIONS. Airway management; Airway insertion and stabilization; Airway suctioning; Artificial airway management; Oxygen therapy; Respiratory monitoring; Ventilation assistance; Vital signs monitoring

PLANNING AND IMPLEMENTATION

Collaborative

Treatment of a hemothorax focuses on stabilizing the patient's condition by maintaining airway and breathing, stopping the bleeding, emptying blood from the pleural cavity, and re-expanding the underlying lung. Because pneumothorax also occurs with hemothorax, emergency care usually includes needle decompression if tension pneumothorax is suspected. Mild cases of hemothorax may resolve in 10 days to 2 weeks, requiring only observation for further bleeding. A tube thoracostomy is the treatment of choice for hemothorax; approximately 80% of penetrating and blunt trauma can be managed successfully with this procedure. A hemothorax with a volume of 500 to 1,000 mL that does not continue to bleed can be managed with a chest tube alone. Placement of more than one chest tube may be necessary to drain a hemothorax adequately. After the procedure is completed, a repeat chest x-ray helps identify chest tube position and determines results of hemothorax evacuation. If drainage is not complete, then placement of other drainage tubes may be necessary. The preferred procedure to accomplish the evacuation of the pleural space in this situation is video-assisted thoracic surgery operative procedure.

More severe cases of hemothorax (hemorrhaging that arises from arterial sites or major hilar vessels) generally require aggressive surgical intervention. A massive hemothorax with an initial volume of 1,000 to 2,000 mL or one that continues to bleed between 150 and 200 mL per hour after 2 to 4 hours is an indication for a formal thoracotomy. An emergency thoracotomy at the bedside may be necessary in the setting of a massive hemothorax with accompanying hemodynamic instability. The approach is a left anterolateral incision and is reserved for those patients who are in a life-threatening situation. A formal thoracotomy performed in the operating room is accomplished by a variety of incisions. Once exposure is obtained, lung parenchyma and vascular structures, including the great vessels, can be evaluated and repaired.

Pharmacologic Highlights

Medication or Drug Class	Dosage	Description	Rationale
Antibiotics	Varies with drug	Physicians may follow cultures of wounds, urine, blood, and sputum rather than use prophylactic antibiotics	Protect from or combat bacterial infections
Analgesics	Varies with drug	IV morphine sulfate provides pain control and can be reversed with naloxone if complications occur	Reduce pain and thereby increase mobility

Other Drugs: Some experts recommend intrapleural instillation of fibrinolytic agents such as streptokinase or urokinase to remove residual hemothorax if chest tube drainage is inadequate. Patients with significant chest trauma causing a hemothorax may benefit by the placement of an epidural catheter for pain management. A tetanus booster is administered to patients with chest trauma whose immunization history indicates a need or whose history is unavailable.

Independent

The most critical nursing intervention is maintaining the ABCs. Have an intubation tray available in case endotracheal intubation and mechanical ventilation are necessary. Maintain a working endotracheal suction at the bedside as well. If the patient is hemodynamically stable, position the patient for full lung expansion, using the semi-Fowler position with the arms elevated on pillows. Because the cervical spine is at risk after injury, maintain body alignment and prevent flexion and extension by a cervical collar or by other strategies dictated by trauma service protocols.

If the patient is hemodynamically unstable, consider alternate positions but never place the adequacy of the patient's airway and breathing at risk. When the patient has inadequate circulation, consider placing the patient flat with the legs raised if airway and breathing are adequate (usually when the patient is intubated and on mechanical ventilation). Trendelenburg position is not recommended because it may increase the systemic vascular resistance and decrease the cardiac output in some patients, interfere with chest excursion by pushing the abdominal contents upward, and increase the risk of aspiration.

Establish adequate communication. The patient is likely to be very anxious, even fearful, for several reasons. If the hemothorax is the result of a chest trauma, the injury itself is unexpected and possibly quite frightening. The patient is experiencing pain and may not be receiving sedatives or analgesics until the pulmonary status stabilizes. The patient may have low oxygen levels, which leads to restlessness and anxiety. Remain with the patient at all times and provide reassurance until the ABCs have been stabilized.

Evidence-Based Practice and Health Policy

Gonzalez, G., Robert, C., Petit, L., Biais, M., & Carrié, C. (2021). May the initial CT scan predict the occurrence of delayed hemothorax in blunt chest trauma patients? *European Journal of Trauma and Emergency Surgery, 47*, 71–78.

• The authors assessed the impact of delayed hemothorax on outcomes in patients with blunt chest trauma without life-threatening condition at admission. They aimed to characterize the predictive value of predefined anatomic factors to identify delayed hemothorax. The authors conducted a retrospective study, including all spontaneous breathing patients ($N = 109$) admitted to an intensive care unit for a blunt chest trauma.

• The patients with delayed hemothorax had higher rates of pulmonary infections. Other markers of hemothorax were a posterior location and a displaced rib fracture. At least one displaced rib fracture was more specific for delayed hemothorax than the commonly used threshold of three or more rib fractures. The authors concluded that posterior location and the displacement of at least one rib fracture in the initial CT scan were independent risk factors for predicting the occurrence of delayed hemothorax.

DOCUMENTATION GUIDELINES

• Physical findings: Patency of airway, presence of clear breath sounds, vital signs, level of consciousness, urinary output, capillary blanch, skin temperature
• Response to pain: Location, description, duration, response to interventions
• Response to treatment: Chest tube insertion—type and amount of drainage, presence of air leak, presence or absence of crepitus, amount of suction, presence of clots, response to fluid resuscitation; response to surgical management
• Complications: Hemorrhage (ongoing bleeding), infection (fever, wound drainage), inadequate gas exchange (restlessness, dropping SaO_2)

DISCHARGE AND HOME HEALTHCARE GUIDELINES

Be sure the patient and family understand any pain medication prescribed, including dosage, route, action, and side effects. Review with the patient all follow-up appointments that are arranged. Follow-up often involves chest x-rays and arterial blood gas analysis, as well as a physical examination. If the injury was alcohol related, explore the patient's drinking pattern. If the injury was binge related, explain the relationship between injury and alcohol by stating the facts without being judgmental. If you think the patient is either a problem or a dependent drinker, refer the patient to an advanced practice nurse or an alcohol counselor. Refer patients with a drug use or abuse problem to an appropriate counselor or program. Teach the patient when to notify the physician for complications such as signs of infection, an unhealed wound, or anxiety and inability to cope. Provide the patient with a phone number for a primary healthcare provider, trauma clinic, or advanced practice nurse.

Hepatitis

DRG Category:	441
Mean LOS:	6.3 days
Description:	MEDICAL: Disorders of Liver Except Malignancy, Cirrhosis, Alcoholic Hepatitis With Major Complication or Comorbidity

Hepatitis is a widespread inflammation of the liver that results in degeneration and necrosis of liver cells. While hepatitis can be caused by toxic substances, it is most commonly caused by viruses. Several forms of virus are involved, but each enters the bloodstream and spreads to the liver, where it infects and damages the hepatocytes (the functional cells of the liver). The resulting inflammation in the hepatocytes interferes with the normal function of the liver, which includes detoxifying substances, producing proteins and clotting factors, and metabolizing vitamins. Millions of people live with chronic viral hepatitis in the United States, although estimates range widely on the number of people with both the acute and chronic conditions. In most cases, the damage is reversible after the acute phase; in some cases, however, massive necrosis can lead to liver failure and death.

Acute viral hepatitis is a major public health concern because it is highly communicable and is transmitted before the onset of symptoms in the infected host. In general, the majority of cases of hepatitis are self-limiting and resolve without complications. Hepatitis A viral (HAV) infection has an incubation period averaging 4 weeks, is the most common type of hepatitis, and occurs when an acute infection spreads with close contact with infected persons. It does not lead to chronic hepatitis. Hepatitis B virus (HBV) has a longer incubation period averaging 12 weeks. Both the virus and the immune response to the virus can lead to liver cell damage. A large proportion of infants and children infected with the disease will develop a chronic infection. The Centers for Disease Control and Prevention estimate that from 820,000 to 2.2 million people in the United States have chronic HBV. Hepatitis C virus (HCV) has an average incubation period of 8 weeks, and more than half of people who acquire it will have chronic infection.

The most serious complication of hepatitis is fulminant hepatitis, which occurs in approximately 1% of all patients and leads to liver failure and hepatic encephalopathy and, in some, to death within 2 weeks of onset. Other complications include a syndrome that resembles serum sickness (muscle and joint pain, rash, angioedema), as well as cirrhosis, pancreatitis, myocarditis, aplastic anemia, or peripheral neuropathy.

CAUSES

Hepatitis can be caused by bacteria; by hepatotoxic agents (drugs, alcohol, industrial chemicals); or, most commonly, by a virus. Five agents are commonly recognized as the cause of acute viral hepatitis (Table 1): HAV, HBV, HCV, delta virus or hepatitis D virus (HDV), and hepatitis E virus (HEV).

• TABLE 1 Causative Agents of Hepatitis

VIRAL AGENT	ROUTE OF TRANSMISSION	CHARACTERISTICS AND RISK GROUPS	INCUBATION PERIOD	CARRIER/ CHRONIC HEPATITIS
HAV (infectious hepatitis) (acute)	Fecal-oral route (contaminated water or food); sexual contact	Military personnel, children in day care, international travelers. Incidence is rising in men who have sex with men and in those with HIV infections	2–7 wk (often 4 wk)	No/no
HBV (accounts for 5%–10% of posttrans-fusion hep-atitis) (acute and chronic)	Blood; sexual con-tact; perinatal contact	IV drug abusers; Native Asians; healthcare workers; transfusion recipients; incidence is rising in those with HIV infections	2–5 mo (often 12 wk)	Yes/yes

• **TABLE 1** Causative Agents of Hepatitis (continued)

VIRAL AGENT	ROUTE OF TRANSMISSION	CHARACTERISTICS AND RISK GROUPS	INCUBATION PERIOD	CARRIER/ CHRONIC HEPATITIS
HCV (acute and chronic)	Blood; sexual contact; perinatal contact; unknown factors	IV drug abusers; health-care workers; transfusion recipients	1 wk to several mo	Yes/yes
HDV (delta hepatitis) (acute)	Blood; sexual contact; perinatal contact	IV drug abusers; people with HBV	3 wk to 3 mo	Yes/yes
HEV (acute)	Fecal-oral (contaminated water or food)	Most common in people who travel to India, Asia, Africa, Central America	14–60 days	No/no

GENETIC CONSIDERATIONS

While viral hepatitis is considered an infectious disease, affected persons may have significantly varying courses. Certain APOE2 and APOE4 alleles contribute to HCV clearance, reducing the chance of chronic hepatitis. Several other genes have recently been reported to influence hepatitis infection severity. These include interleukin 10 (*IL10*) for HBV and the killer cell immunoglobulin-like receptor genes (*KIR2DS3, KIR2D*) for HCV.

Autoimmune hepatitis does not have a clear underlying cause, but individuals with another autoimmune condition or a family history of autoimmune disease are at increased risk of developing autoimmune hepatitis. It is likely that a combination of genetic and environmental factors plays a role in the development of this disease.

SEX AND LIFE SPAN CONSIDERATIONS

All age, sex, and socioeconomic groups can be affected by hepatitis. Children ages 5 to 14 years are most likely to acquire acute HAV infection. HDV infection is more common in adults than children. Experts have found in large studies that women with HCV have worse overall heath than men, whereas men were more likely to have comorbidities such as obesity or diabetes that put them at risk for developing life-threatening complications. People who acquire HCV at a younger age have a better prognosis than people who acquire it at an older age.

HEALTH DISPARITIES AND SEXUAL/GENDER MINORITY HEALTH

Significant health disparities occur with HCV. It is more common in Black and Hispanic persons than White persons, and Black, Indigenous, and other people of color have higher mortality rates from the disease. HCV is also more likely to occur in people with lower economic status. Although a safe and effective vaccine is available for HBV, Black and Hispanic persons have lower vaccine coverage than White persons. HBV and HCV have higher prevalence among Black and Hispanic persons as compared to other groups. Marginalized groups, and people living in poverty in particular, are disproportionately at risk for HAV, HBV, and HCV because of homelessness, mental illness, injection drug use, and lack of healthcare. Sexual minority men and women who have multiple sex partners, inject drugs, or are sex workers are at high risk for HBV. Gay, bisexual, and men who have sex with men have a higher chance of getting HAV,

HBV, and HCV than other groups. Approximately 10% of new cases of HAV and 20% of new cases of HBV infections in the United States are found in gay and bisexual men.

GLOBAL HEALTH CONSIDERATIONS

Viral hepatitis is the seventh leading cause of death in the world. Globally, approximately 257 million people are chronically infected with HBV and 71 million with HCV. The World Health Organization estimates that the highest rates of infection of HAV and HBV occur in sub-Saharan Africa, Eastern Asia, and South America. HCV is more common in Europe and the Eastern Mediterranean region.

ASSESSMENT

HISTORY. Note that the incubation period varies by virus (see Table 1) and that variation should be considered during history-taking. Question the patient about potential sources of transmission and risks: a history of blood dyscrasias, multiple blood or blood product transfusions, alcohol or drug abuse (sharing of needles), exposure to hepatotoxic chemicals or medications, and travel to developing countries or areas where the sanitation is poor. Because HAV transmission occurs in association with day-care centers, among male sexual minorities, and among household contacts of persons with acute cases, inquire into these areas. Take a sexual history to determine if sexual behaviors place the patient and others at risk. Also ask about recent meals because hepatitis A occasionally occurs from contaminated food or improper sewage treatment. Determine the patient's occupation; teratogen exposure may cause a nonviral hepatitis.

From the patient's history, determine the patient's phase in the disease. The first phase is the viral replication phase when patients are asymptomatic. Patients in the prodromal (second) phase may complain of nausea, vomiting, malaise, headache, fatigue, anorexia (a distaste for cigarettes in smokers is characteristic of early profound anorexia), and fever. Ask about any changes in the sense of taste or smell, recent weight loss, and the presence of urticaria or arthralgias, which can occur early in the disease process. Pruritus may be mild and transient and is caused by the accumulation of bile salt in the skin. During the icteric phase (3 to 10 days later), in addition to dark urine and yellowish (jaundice) skin, there may be right upper-quadrant pain and no flu-like symptoms. The final phase is the convalescent phase.

PHYSICAL EXAMINATION. Symptoms vary individually and by infectious virus, but common symptoms are **anorexia, nausea, vomiting, fever, fatigue**, and **pruritus**. In the prodromal phase (period of infection and appearance of early symptoms), inspect the skin for a rash. Fever is usually between 101°F (38.3°C) and 102°F (38.9°C). In the icteric phase, the urine often appears dark and concentrated. Observe stools for a pale, clay color. Inspect the skin, sclera, and mucous membranes for jaundice, which is caused by the poor ability of the damaged liver to remove bilirubin from the bloodstream. Jaundice peaks within 1 to 2 weeks and fades during the convalescent phase over the next 2 to 4 weeks.

On palpation, the liver is usually enlarged and sometimes tender. The edges remain soft and smooth. In 15% to 20% of cases, mild splenomegaly is present. In uncomplicated cases, signs of chronic liver disease are not seen. In alcoholic hepatitis, inspect the skin for spider nevi.

Potential complications include bleeding and the possibility of progressive liver degeneration. Assess for petechiae, bruising, bleeding gums or nose, prolonged bleeding from puncture sites, and obvious or occult blood in body secretions and fluids. Note that restlessness and confusion, decreasing blood pressure and pulse, abnormal complete blood count, and platelet and coagulation tests may indicate increased bleeding. Monitor for worsening symptoms, edema, ascites, and encephalopathy. Because an early sign of hepatic encephalopathy is deterioration of handwriting, have patients write their name each shift and monitor the signature for changes.

PSYCHOSOCIAL. The patient with hepatitis has a communicable disease. Assess for knowledge of possible sources of transmission, including behavioral risk factors. Ask about the patient's living conditions to assess the risk of spread of hepatitis to the family and significant others. Determine the patient's ability to cope with a communicable disease, anxiety level, and support mechanisms. Some families have a magnified fear of contracting a communicable disease and may respond to the diagnosis with irrational fears and concerns.

Diagnostic Highlights

Test	Normal Result	Abnormality With Condition	Explanation
Viral hepatitis serologies	Negative results	Acute HAV: Positive anti-HAV immunoglobulin M (IgM) Acute HBV: IgM hepatitis B core antigen (HBcAg), HB surface antigen Acute HCV: Anti-HCV antibody, HCV RNA HDV: Anti-HDV IgM, HDV antigen HEV: Not available HGV: All tests negative	Identify immune response to virus; leads to markers such as immunoglobulins (IgG and IgM), antigens, antibodies
Liver function tests	Alanine aminotransferase (ALT): 13–40 units/L; aspartate aminotransferase (AST): 15–40 units/L; alkaline phosphatase: 25–142 units/L	ALT elevated as high as or higher than 1,000 units/L; AST elevated ≥ 1,000 units/L; alkaline phosphatase mildly elevated	Determine the extent of inflammation

Other Tests: Bilirubin, gamma glutamyl transferase, lactate dehydrogenase, prothrombin time, complete blood count, albumin, liver biopsy

PRIMARY NURSING DIAGNOSIS

DIAGNOSIS. Imbalanced nutrition: less than body requirements related to decreased oral intake, nausea, vomiting, and/or anorexia as evidenced by weight loss, thirst, and/or fatigue

OUTCOMES. Nutritional status: Food and fluid intake; Nutritional status: Nutrient intake; Nutritional status: Energy; Weight: Body mass

INTERVENTIONS. Nutritional therapy; Fluid management; Nutritional counseling; Nutritional monitoring; Weight management; Medication management; Teaching: Prescribed diet

PLANNING AND IMPLEMENTATION
Collaborative

HAV is generally treated supportively by treating symptoms such as nausea, fatigue, and dehydration. HBV may be treated with antivirals or interferons. Vaccination against HAV and HBV is available and should be considered in high-risk groups, including medical and healthcare personnel and people traveling to high-risk locations. Immunoglobulin can provide protection against clinically apparent HAV. It should be given to household contacts of patients with HAV and to persons who plan to travel on prolonged visits to developing countries or other places where sanitation is poor. Passive immunization with immunoglobulin (Gammagard) reduces infection when administered within 2 weeks of exposure but has been replaced by immunization in many situations.

Dietary management usually includes a high-caloric, high-protein, high-carbohydrate, low-fat diet as tolerated. If oral intake is limited or compromised, parenteral or enteral nutrition may be implemented. With fluid retention or encephalopathy, sodium or protein restriction (because of the buildup of ammonia in the blood) may be indicated. Alcoholic beverages should not be taken at all during recovery.

Pharmacologic Highlights

Note: Much research is occurring around the pharmacologic management of hepatitis; drugs and dosages are changing frequently.

Medication or Drug Class	Dosage	Description	Rationale
Antivirals for HBV and HCV	Varies by drug	Amantadine (Symmetrel); tenofovir disoproxil fumarate (Viread), lamivudine (Epivir), adefovir dipivoxil (Hepsera); entecavir (Baraclude); telbivudine (Tyzeka); famciclovir (Famvir)	To reduce viral replication
Interferons: alpha, beta, and gamma for HBV and HCV	Varies by drug	Naturally produced proteins with antiviral, antitumor, and immunomodulatory actions that are manufactured by genetically engineering techniques; given through a variety of routes including topical, systemic, and directly into lesions	Binds with receptors to modulate host-immune response; produces remission in 25%–50% of people with chronic HBV and 40% with chronic HCV

Other Drugs: Hepatitis B vaccine (recombinant) and hepatitis A vaccine (inactivated) are available for active immunization. Antiemetics such as trimethobenzamide hydrochloride (Tigan) can be given 30 minutes before meals to decrease nausea and vomiting and to increase the likelihood of an adequate intake. Avoid prochlorperazine maleate (Compazine) because of the effects on the liver. In addition, analgesics and antipruritics may be administered to assist with comfort. Dosages may be decreased because of the altered ability of the liver to clear certain medications. Immune gamma globulin provides passive immunity to those exposed to HAV, HBV, and hepatitis B surface antigen. Vitamin K phytonadione (AquaMephyton) is a nutrition supplement to enhance formation of coagulation factors II, VII, IX, and X. A brief course of corticosteroids may improve the course of the disease.

Independent

Observe enteric precautions if the patient has HAV or HEV and universal precautions for HBV, HCV, or HDV. To maintain fluid and electrolyte balance, implement measures to reduce nausea and vomiting. Encourage the patient to eat, but avoid greasy foods. Avoid overmedication, which can decrease appetite. Encourage rest before meals. Assist in providing oral care and maintain a relaxed environment to enhance the palatability of the meal. Encourage fluids to at least 4,000 mL per day unless there are fluid restrictions for other accompanying illnesses. Supplement dietary fluids with soft drinks, ice chips, and ice pops. Determine if the patient is maintaining body weight.

Provide pain relief measures such as heat, back rubs, positioning, relaxation techniques, and age-appropriate diversion. Relieve pruritus with skin care. Implement measures to improve activity tolerance; facilitate adequate rest periods by organizing nursing and multidisciplinary care activities, adjusting visitation schedules, and reducing environmental stimulation. Institute measures to promote safety. Measures to prevent bleeding include using the smallest-gauge needle possible for venipunctures or injections; applying gentle, prolonged pressure to puncture sites; avoiding overinflation of the blood pressure cuff; and avoiding risk for trauma and falls by limiting clutter in the room.

Evidence-Based Practice and Health Policy

Flores, B., Fernandez, A., Wang, C., Bobadilla, R., Hernandez, L., Jain, M., & Turner, B. (2022). Educating primary care providers and associate care providers about hepatitis C screening of baby boomers: A multi-practice study. *Journal of Cancer Education, 37*(1), 217–223.

• Chronic HCV increases the risk for hepatocellular carcinoma. Despite higher prevalence of HCV in persons born from 1945 to 1965 (baby boomer years), screening has not been widely adopted. We aimed to determine knowledge and attitudes of primary and associate care providers about HCV. In five federally qualified health centers serving low-income Hispanic communities, staff attended a 50-minute training lecture about HCV epidemiology, screening methods, and evaluation.
• While a higher proportion of PCPs correctly answered knowledge questions as compared to associates, the associates had more favorable attitudes about linking patients to care. Engaging the entire primary care practice team in learning about HCV screening promotes knowledge and attitudes necessary for successful implementation.

DOCUMENTATION GUIDELINES

• Findings of physical examination and ongoing assessments: Nausea, vomiting, anorexia, diarrhea, color of stools and urine, daily weights, vital signs, jaundice, pruritus, edema, ascites, pain, level of consciousness
• Response to medical and nursing interventions: Medications, comfort measures, diet, hydration
• Pain: Location, duration, precipitating factors, response to interventions
• Presence of complications: Bleeding, progressive liver degeneration, changes in mental status
• Protection of household: Isolation procedures, family prophylaxis

DISCHARGE AND HOME HEALTHCARE GUIDELINES

Provide instruction on the prevention of the spread of hepatitis to others. With HAV, do the following for 1 to 2 weeks after the onset of jaundice: Use strict hand washing after bowel movements and before meals. Have separate toilet facilities if possible (if not, clean the seat with bleach after each use). Wash linens, towels, and undergarments separately from other items in hot, soapy water. Do not donate blood or work in food services until such work is cleared by a physician.

With HBV, HCV, or HDV, do the following, as directed by a physician, until antigen-antibody tests are negative: Maintain strict hand washing after urination and defecation; do not share personal items (toothbrush, razor, washcloth); use disposable eating utensils or wash utensils separately in hot, soapy water; do not share food or eating utensils; do not share needles and dispose of them properly after a single use; avoid intimate sexual contact (when sex can be resumed, use a condom and avoid intercourse during menstruation); and do not donate blood. Instruct the patient to inform household members and sexual partners of the fact that the patient has developed hepatitis and to encourage them to notify a primary healthcare provider immediately to assess the risk of the disease.

To prevent complications, teach the patient to avoid alcohol for 6 months to 1 year, avoid illicit drugs and toxic chemicals, and take acetaminophen only when necessary and not beyond the recommended dosage. Note that in viral hepatitis, the patient has immunity only to the type of hepatitis the patient has had.

Herniated Disk

DRG Category: 518
Mean LOS: 6.1 days
Description: SURGICAL: Back and Neck Procedures Except Spinal Fusion With Major Complication or Comorbidity or Disc Device or Neurostimulator

DRG Category: 552
Mean LOS: 3.5 days
Description: MEDICAL: Medical Back Problems Without Major Complication or Comorbidity

The intervertebral disk is a complex structure situated between vertebrae; it provides additional structural support to the spinal column and cushions the vertebrae. The outer layer of the disk contains numerous concentric rings of tough, fibrous connective tissue called the *annulus fibrosus*. The central portion of the disk consists of a softer, spongier material called the *nucleus pulposus*. If the annulus fibrosus weakens or tears, then the nucleus pulposus may "slip" or herniate outward, creating the condition known as a "slipped disk," or more precisely, *herniated nucleus pulposus*. When the disk material herniates, it can compress the spinal cord or the nerve roots that come from the spinal cord. Disk injury results in the release of inflammatory mediators such as tumor necrosis factor and interleukins. White blood cells enter the area to "clean up" the injury, scarring follows, and substance P is released, which leads to pain. Of herniations, 90% usually occur in the lumbar and lumbosacral regions, 8% occur in the cervical area, and 1% to 2% occur in the thoracic area. The disk between the fifth and the sixth cervical vertebrae is involved most frequently.

CAUSES

Disk deterioration causes the condition, but the exact reasons for the deterioration are not known. Injury and the loss of disk height may shift the balance of weight-bearing, furthering traumatic damage. The injury is followed by a degenerative cascade of inflammatory mediators in a sequence similar to that which occurs in aging. Experts understand a number of risk factors. Smoking is one of the most important risk factors because of chronic coughing. Disk herniation is often seen in individuals who have had previous episodes of back problems; however, a herniation may occur without such a history. Repeated episodes are thought to weaken the annulus fibrosus. Heavy physical labor, including repetitive bending, twisting, and lifting, is a risk factor for herniated disk, especially if combined with weak abdominal and back muscles or poor body mechanics. Advancing age produces desiccations of the disk and friability of the annulus, which can increase the likelihood of injury. Other risk factors include stress, long hours of driving vehicles (cab drivers, truck drivers), and sitting for long hours without lumbar support.

GENETIC CONSIDERATIONS

While disk herniations are the result of trauma, various genetic factors may increase a person's susceptibility to injury or progressive disc degeneration. Twin studies have supported the contribution of genetic factors to back and neck pain reporting in women. Associated factors include both genetic determinants of structural disk degeneration and genetic determinants of psychological distress. Some of the implicated genes in intervertebral disc degeneration include collagen genes (*COL1A1*, *COL1A2*, *COL9A1*, *COL9A2*, *COL9A3*), aggrecan (*ACAN*), interleukins (*IL1A*, *IL6*), and matrix metalloproteinase-3 (*MMP3*).

SEX AND LIFE SPAN CONSIDERATIONS

Disk herniations most often occur in adults, with a mean age at surgery of 40 years. Men are affected more often than women, and the highest incidence is in men ages 30 to 60 years. Experts have found that people over 65 years of age have similar surgical outcomes as people who are younger. The condition rarely occurs in people 80 years of age or older.

HEALTH DISPARITIES AND SEXUAL/GENDER MINORITY HEALTH

Patients who were self-paying or with private insurance or military-based insurance are more likely to have the most advanced disk replacement surgery as compared to people with Medicaid or Medicare, who are more apt to receive cervical fusion. Ethnicity, race, and sexual/gender minority status have no known effect on the risk for herniated disk.

GLOBAL HEALTH CONSIDERATIONS

While herniated disk occurs worldwide, no epidemiological data are available.

ASSESSMENT

HISTORY. Establish a history of back pain, including a description of the location and intensity of the pain. Determine if the patient has a history of smoking or tobacco use. Determine if the person has ever had a back injury. Ask patients about their work history, with particular attention to jobs involving sedentary work or heavy lifting. Obtain a history of activity intolerance or pain with activity. Often, the symptoms are of a gradually progressing nature over a period of days to weeks. The development and distribution of extremity pain help determine the level of the involved disk. Ask about weakness in the extremities, altered sensation, or muscle spasms; ask if pain intensifies during Valsalva maneuver, coughing, sneezing, or bending. Establish a history of sensory and motor loss in the area that has been innervated by the compressed spinal nerve root.

PHYSICAL EXAMINATION. The most common symptom is **back pain exacerbated by activity**. Document any gait abnormalities, such as a limp. Test the patient's deep tendon reflexes in the upper and lower extremities. Perform a sensory evaluation of the patient's sharp-dull and fine-touch discrimination. Motor strength testing of the involved extremities is also important, again to determine the extent of injury to the spinal cord or nerve roots. Perform range-of-motion studies of either the cervical, the thoracic, or the lumbar regions. Conduct stretch tests for nerve root irritation, including the straight leg-raise test; if the sciatic nerve is irritated, there will be pain in the involved leg. The Braggart test, passive stretching of the foot in dorsiflexion, is positive if it elicits pain along the sciatic nerve distribution. The "bow string" sign is performed with the patient sitting and the knees flexed just beyond a 90-degree angle and the body bent slightly forward to increase the stretch on the sciatic nerve. A positive response occurs when gentle pressure with the examiner's finger into the popliteal space further stretches the sciatic nerve, producing more pain. Check the patient's peripheral vascular status, including peripheral pulses and skin temperatures, to rule out ischemic disease, another possible cause of leg pain and numbness.

PSYCHOSOCIAL. The individual may be unexpectedly debilitated. The assessment should include an evaluation of the patient's ability to deal with unexpected changes in lifestyle, roles, and income. Along with severe pain, an employed person may be facing a prolonged period of disability and reduced income.

Diagnostic Highlights

Test	Normal Result	Abnormality With Condition	Explanation
Magnetic resonance imaging is the diagnostic test of choice; computed tomography scan	Normal bony skeleton and soft tissue	Changes in spinal structure and alignment, deterioration or herniation of soft tissues	Indicates the extent of bony and soft tissue injury and deterioration
X-rays	Normal bony skeleton	Changes in spinal structure and alignment	Indicate the extent of bony injury

Other Tests: Myelography, electromyography

PRIMARY NURSING DIAGNOSIS

DIAGNOSIS. Acute pain related to inflammation and compression as evidenced by self-reports of pain, facial grimacing, and/or protective behavior

OUTCOMES. Comfort status; Pain control; Pain level; Symptom severity; Knowledge: Pain management

INTERVENTIONS. Analgesic administration; Anxiety reduction; Pain management: Acute; Medication management

PLANNING AND IMPLEMENTATION
Collaborative

MEDICAL. Bedrest may be used for several days, followed by physical therapy. Physical therapy includes various passive modalities of treatment, such as heat, ice, massage, ultrasound, and electrogalvanic stimulation, often directed by a physical therapist, and exercises to stretch and strengthen the spine and supporting musculature. Pharmacologic measures are often used to manage pain. Spinal adjustments performed by osteopathic or chiropractic physicians can also relieve symptoms. Generally, if symptoms are not resolved with 6 weeks of therapy, other treatments may be considered.

SURGICAL. When the medical and pharmacologic treatments are not successful or if the symptoms become debilitating, then surgery is considered. Surgery involves removal of the disk using a microscope. A microdiskectomy removes fragments of the nucleus pulposus. During a laminectomy, the protruding disk and a portion of the lamina are removed. A spinal fusion (anterior cervical diskectomy and fusion [ACDF]) of the bony tissues may be performed if there is evidence that the disk herniation is accompanied by instability of the surrounding tissues. Cervical disk arthroplasty (CDA) is a newer procedure designed to preserve motion and reduce disease in adjacent segments. While controversial, some studies over the past 10 years since CDA has been available have shown that outcomes from CDA are improved as compared to ACDF.

Postoperatively, enforce bedrest and monitor dressings for excessive drainage. Position the patient depending on the type of surgery performed. Teach the patient who has undergone spinal fusion how to wear a brace. Teach the patient proper body mechanics. Encourage the patient to lie down when tired and to sleep on the side, using an extra firm mattress or bed board. Caution the patient to maintain proper weight because obesity can cause lordosis. Ongoing assessments are important if the patient requires surgery. Monitor the patient for signs of weakness, pain, changes in circulation, and numbness in the extremities. Assess the cardiovascular status of the patient's legs by observing for color, temperature, and motion. Assess the degree of pain in terms of intensity, location, and character.

Pharmacologic Highlights

Medication or Drug Class	Dosage	Description	Rationale
NSAIDs	Varies with drug	Ibuprofen (Ibuprin, Advil, Motrin); ketoprofen (Oruvail, Orudis, Actron); flurbiprofen (Ansaid); naproxen (Anaprox, Naprelan, Naprosyn)	Reduce acute inflammation
Muscle relaxants	Varies with drug	Cyclobenzaprine hydrochloride (Flexeril)	Relieve muscular irritation, recommended for use for a short period of time

Other Drugs: Narcotic analgesics such as codeine and meperidine may be used to control pain for a short period of time. Nonnarcotics (e.g., propoxyphene [Darvon]) may also be used. Acute inflammation is usually treated with either a corticosteroid or NSAIDs.

Independent

Place the patient in a semi-Fowler position or in a flat position with a pillow between the patient's legs for side-lying to help reduce the pain. Instruct the patient to roll to one side when sitting up to minimize pain during position changes. Perform active and passive range-of-motion exercises within the prescribed regimen. Keep a schedule of progress to encourage the patient when the patient becomes discouraged, and provide an estimate of when the patient will return to normal functioning. Allow the patient to direct or perform self-care. Provide meticulous skin care.

Evidence-Based Practice and Health Policy

Yang, X., Donk, R., Arts, M., Bartels, R., & Vieggeert-Lankamp, C. (2020). Prosthesis in anterior cervical herniated disc approach does not prevent radiologic adjacent segment degeneration. *Spine*, *45*, 1024–1029.

- The authors report on the incidence of radiological adjacent segment degeneration (ASD) in patients with cervical radiculopathy due to a herniated disc who were randomized to receive cervical arthroplasty or arthrodesis. Outcomes were measured at 1- and 2-year follow-ups.
- Adjacent segment degeneration was similar in both groups, 59% as compared to 56%. The authors noted that radiological ASD occurs in a similar manner in patients who were subjected to arthrodesis in cervical radiculopathy and in patients who received arthroplasty to maintain motion. The outcomes were similar in both groups.

DOCUMENTATION GUIDELINES

- Physical findings: Neural and musculoskeletal system assessments, degree of pain, tolerance to activity; presence of postoperative complications (infection, pain, immobility, poor wound healing)
- Response to physical therapy: Work status of the patient, ability to cope with both immobility and inability to return to work

DISCHARGE AND HOME HEALTHCARE GUIDELINES

Teach the patient the mechanics of disk function and how herniation occurs. Instruct the patient in proper body mechanics and advise avoiding high-torsion activities, such as twisting and heavy lifting. Discuss an exercise program with the patient as a maintenance program, following the 6-week physical therapy regimen. Be sure the patient understands any medication prescribed, including dosage, route, action, and side effects. Advise the patient against driving or operating heavy machinery if the medications are likely to impair judgment.

Herpes Simplex Virus

DRG Category: 606
Mean LOS: 5.9 days
Description: MEDICAL: Minor Skin Disorders With Major Complication or Comorbidity

There are two types of herpes simplex virus (HSV): type 1 and type 2. HSV-1 causes infection above the waist, such as "cold sores" that occur on the mouth. This type may occur in the genital area as a result of oral-genital sexual practices. After the initial infection, the virus is dormant, but the patient is a carrier and likely to have recurrent infections. Events that trigger recurrences are sun exposure, fever, menses, stress, and lack of sleep. The virus is inactivated at room temperature, and humans are the only carriers.

HSV-2 causes lesions in the genital area and is a common sexually transmitted infection (STI). In the primary episode, multiple blisterlike, painful vesicles erupt on the vulva, perineum, cervix, tip or shaft of the penis, or perianal area within 3 to 5 days after the initial exposure. The virus then becomes dormant and resides in the nerve ganglia of the affected area. Repeated outbreaks can happen at any time, but most patients have less severe regular recurrences that are more likely to occur during menses, pregnancy, or times of illness and stress. The more severe the primary outbreak, the more frequent the recurring infections. The Centers for Disease Control and Prevention estimates that one in six people in the United States ages 14 to 19 years have HSV-2 genital infection.

HSV-2 is associated with significant complications. Active HSV is associated with spontaneous abortion in the first trimester of pregnancy and an increased risk of preterm labor after 20 weeks' gestation. If a patient has active herpes around the time of the estimated date of delivery, cesarean section is the preferred method of delivery. Infected infants can develop the following signs and symptoms after an incubation period of 2 to 12 days: fever, hypothermia, jaundice, seizures, poor feeding, and vesicular skin lesions. When people have HSV-2 lesions, studies have shown that they are at risk for infection with HIV. Experts suggest that this risk occurs because the T cells that are part of the body's reaction to HSV-2 create an environment conducive to HIV proliferation. As a result, scientists note that HIV replicates three to five times faster in tissues that have healed from an HSV-2 infection as compared to normal tissue.

CAUSES

HSV infection occurs through attachment by receptors to human cells after close personal contact with an infected person, usually through a mucosal surface such as the oropharynx, cervix, or conjunctiva or through contact with cracks in the skin. The virus also attaches to sensory neurons, leading to latency (the infection can reappear during times of physiological stress). HSV-1 is particularly attracted to the oral mucosa, and HSV-2 is particularly attracted to the genital epithelium. Pregnant women can transmit the herpes virus to the fetus, especially during a primary outbreak. Transmission can occur when the membranes rupture or during a vaginal delivery, but transplacental transmission is extremely rare. Asymptomatic transmission is very uncommon.

GENETIC CONSIDERATIONS

Heritable immune responses could be protective or increase susceptibility.

SEX AND LIFE SPAN CONSIDERATIONS

HSV-1 is usually acquired during childhood when children come in contact with oral secretions of others with the infection. By age 30 years in the United States, 50% of people with higher socioeconomic status are seropositive for HSV-1, and 80% of people with lower socioeconomic status are positive. HSV-2 affects one in five men and one in four women. Because teenagers are engaging in sexual activity earlier than ever before, they have a higher risk today than in the past of contracting HSV-2; the number of adolescents with HSV-2 is therefore increasing. Because there is no cure for herpes, recurrent outbreaks of HSV occur over a lifetime.

HEALTH DISPARITIES AND SEXUAL/GENDER MINORITY HEALTH

HSV-2 is more prevalent in Black persons (seroprevalence of 45%) and Hispanic persons (seroprevalence of 22%) than in White persons (seroprevalence of 17%). Men who have sex with men are at higher risk for infection with HSV, with infections of both the oropharynx and genito-anal tract, than men who do not have sex with men.

GLOBAL HEALTH CONSIDERATIONS

HSV is present around the globe, and the global prevalence of HSV infections is increasing with more than 23 million new cases a year. Just as in the United States, around the globe there are increasing numbers of people who are seropositive for HSV-2.

⁂ ASSESSMENT

HISTORY. If the patient has an oral lesion, ask about a sore throat, increased salivation, anorexia, and mouth pain. During a primary episode, the patient may experience flu-like symptoms, such as fever, malaise, and enlarged lymph nodes. The patient may describe pain at the site of the lesion. If the lesion is not a primary one, the patient usually does not have any systemic complaints but may complain of a tingling, an itching, or a painful sensation at the site of the lesion. If patients have a genital lesion, obtain a description about when symptoms began and obtain a detailed summary of their sexual activity, including number of partners, use of barrier protection and birth control measures, participation in oral or anal intercourse, and previous (if any) history of STIs. Inquire about any burning with urination, dysuria, dyspareunia, pruritus, fever, chills, headache, and general malaise. On some occasions, the patient may be asymptomatic or have such mild symptoms that the outbreak goes unnoticed.

PHYSICAL EXAMINATION. The most common symptom is the **appearance of a herpetic lesion**. Inspect the lips and the oral and pharyngeal mucosa for lesions and inflammation. The lesion may appear as a red, swollen vesicle, or if it has ruptured, it is ulcerlike with yellow crusting. Palpation of the lymph nodes in the neck may reveal cervical adenopathy. Take the patient's temperature. Inspect the genitalia for fluid-filled vesicles, or if the vesicles have ruptured, note an edematous, erythematous oozing ulcer with a yellow center. Examine the cervix by using a speculum and inspect the walls of the vagina. Inspect the patient's perianal skin and the labia and vulva or penis and foreskin carefully to identify all lesions; note any abnormal discharge. Lesions can also appear in the perianal region, rectum, scrotum, thighs, and buttocks. If herpetic urethritis occurs in men, they will experience pain while urinating and a mucous discharge from the penis.

PSYCHOSOCIAL. Ask the patient about sexual practices, partners, and birth control methods. Assess the patient's knowledge of STIs and their implications. Assess the patient's ability to cope with having an STI. The diagnosis of an STI can be very upsetting to people who believe they were involved in a monogamous relationship. Tell patients that an outbreak of genital HSV may have had its origins even 20 to 30 years before the outbreak.

Diagnostic Highlights

Test	Normal Result	Abnormality With Condition	Explanation
Polymerase chain reaction (PCR)	Negative for HSV DNA	Positive for HSV DNA	Demonstrates presence of viruses
Viral culture	Negative	Positive for HSV; differentiates between HSV-1 and HSV-2	Demonstrates presence of viruses in an active lesion; cultures are most accurate in the first several days of ulceration

Other Tests: Serological tests for antibodies may also be done in the presence of symptoms and a negative culture. Tzanck preparation assists with diagnosis of cutaneous herpes simplex but does not differentiate between HSV-1 and HSV-2. It is performed by aspirating and analyzing fluid from the vesicle.

PRIMARY NURSING DIAGNOSIS

DIAGNOSIS. Anxiety related to a knowledge deficit (cause, treatment, and prevention of HSV) as evidenced by apprehension, distress, fear, and/or uncertainty

OUTCOMES. Anxiety level; Coping; Social interaction skills; Acceptance: Health status; Symptom control; Knowledge: Infection management; Knowledge: Sexual functioning

INTERVENTIONS. Anxiety reduction; Coping enhancement; Teaching: Individual; Counseling; Medication prescribing; Medication management

PLANNING AND IMPLEMENTATION

Collaborative

Because HSV is not curable, treatment focuses on relieving the symptoms. The drug of choice to treat a primary infection of HSV-1 or HSV-2 is acyclovir.

Pharmacologic Highlights

Medication or Drug Class	Dosage	Description	Rationale
Antiviral	Depends on the drug and whether the outbreak is primary or recurrent	Penciclovir (Denavir); acyclovir (Zovirax); valacyclovir (Valtrex); famciclovir (Famvir)	Relieves symptoms, decreases viral shedding (acyclovir is contraindicated during pregnancy); daily dosage for primary episodes is slightly lower than for recurrent infections; some physicians may order chronic suppressive drug therapy, where acyclovir is taken for up to 6 mo

Other Drugs: Antipyretics, analgesics, viscous lidocaine

Independent

Instruct the patient to take all medication ordered, even if symptoms recede before the medication is used up. For comfort during the outbreak, patients may take prescribed analgesics or use warm soaks with Epsom salts or sitz baths. Lesions can be cleaned with Betadine. Encourage patients to wear loose clothing and cotton underwear and to avoid ointments that contain cortisone and petroleum because they slow healing and promote the growth of the virus. Encourage exercise, good nutrition, and stress reduction to decrease the number of recurrent outbreaks (Box 1).

Inform patients that for persons with HSV-2, the risk of acquiring HIV is likely more than double than for persons without HSV-2. Help patients understand that this is a minor problem with which they will be inconvenienced from time to time. Adherence to strict guidelines when active lesions are present allows patients to have normal sexual relationships. Healthcare workers with active herpes are prohibited from working with immunosuppressed patients or in a nursery setting because of the complications that result in the neonate if HSV transmission occurs.

Evidence-Based Practice and Health Policy

Marcocci, M., Napoletani, G., Protto, V., Kolesova, O., Piacentini, R., Donatella, D., Lomonte, P., Grassi, C., Palamara, A., & De Chiara, G. (2020). Herpes simplex virus-1 in the brain: The dark side of a sneaky infection. *Trends in Microbiology, 28*, 808–820.

* After infection, HSV-1 remains alive but resting in sensory nerves, but a variety of stresses can induce reactivation of the virus, which spreads and replicates to the site of primary infection (usually the lips or eyes). Viral particles can also reach the brain, causing herpes simplex encephalitis. This infection is usually clinically asymptomatic but has recently been correlated with the production of biomarkers of Alzheimer disease.
* The authors highlight three issues that need to be studied: (1) identification of the biomarkers in people with recurrent infections; (2) understanding of the virus- and host-related factors determining the frequency and extent of virus spread to the brain; (3) identification of strategies to limit virus reactivation and diffusion to the brain; and (4) evaluation of their potential to prevent neurodegenerative damage.

DOCUMENTATION GUIDELINES

* Appearance, location, and number of lesions; drainage from lesions
* Presence of flu-like symptoms that accompany outbreaks
* Patient's knowledge of cause, treatment, and prevention of HSV
* Patient's reaction to the diagnosis of an STI

DISCHARGE AND HOME HEALTHCARE GUIDELINES

Be sure the patient understands the correct dosage, route, and time of the medication, as well as the importance of taking all prescribed medication even if the symptoms subside. Review events that trigger outbreaks; emphasize the importance of avoiding contact with the lesion in preventing transmission. Teach the female patient that a potential long-term complication is the development of cervical cancer; yearly Papanicolaou (Pap) tests are critical.

• BOX 1 Living With Genital Herpes: What Patients Need to Know

BACKGROUND	TRANSMISSION
• Each patient's symptoms are different; lesions can resemble blisters, cuts in the skin, or spider bites on the buttocks; flu-like symptoms that accompany lesions also vary, as do the frequency and duration of outbreaks.	• Patients are at the highest risk of transmitting HSV to a partner during the time an active lesion is present until complete healing takes place. • Condoms are not a safe barrier for transmission if an active lesion is present; they reduce but do not eliminate the risk for infection.

(box continues on page 538)

• BOX 1 Living With Genital Herpes: What Patients Need to Know (continued)

- During the time when active lesions are present, patients should engage in sexual activities that avoid contact with the lesions. Abstinence is encouraged if an active lesion is present.
- When lesions are active, extreme caution needs to be taken to avoid transmission by contact with articles such as towels, washcloths, and razors. Good hand washing with soap and water helps prevent the spread of the virus.
- Patients can prevent self-infection to other areas of the body by not touching the sores and by using good hand washing.
- It is a myth that if one person has herpes, so does their partner.

OUTBREAKS

- Patients should be aware of prodromal symptoms—tingling, itching, pain, numbness—and should begin pharmacologic treatment earlier to better alleviate symptoms.
- Patients should be aware of events that can trigger a repeated outbreak: pregnancy, menses, stress, fever, infectious illness.
- For more information, patients should contact the Herpes Resource Center at 800-230-6039 or the National Herpes Hotline at 919-361-8488.

Herpes Zoster (Shingles)

DRG Category:	595
Mean LOS:	7.5 days
Description:	MEDICAL: Major Skin Disorders With Major Complication or Comorbidity

Herpes zoster, also known as *shingles*, is a common viral skin eruption that is estimated to affect approximately 1 million persons each year in the United States. Approximately 95% of adults in the United States have antibodies to the varicella zoster virus (VZV), which means they have been exposed to it. The virus causes acute unilateral inflammation of a dorsal root ganglion. Each nerve innervates a particular skin area on the body called a dermatome, which bends around the body in a pattern that has been mapped corresponding to the vertebral source. Generally, herpes zoster eruptions occur in the thoracic region and, less commonly, affect a single cervical, facial (trigeminal nerve), lumbar, or sacral ganglion.

Most patients recover completely, but approximately 12% experience complications that include uveitis, motor deficits, infection, and systemic involvement such as meningoencephalitis, pneumonia, deafness, or widespread dissemination. In some patients, the scars are permanent. Another serious complication is postherpetic neuralgia (PHN), persistent pain lasting for 30 or more days after the acute infection has ended. The pain is generally at the same location as the original dermatome lesions and can be severe, long lasting, and incapacitating. Ophthalmic involvement (herpes infection of the trigeminal, or fifth, cranial nerve) is also a serious complication that threatens vision. Herpes zoster has been considered a foreshadow or harbinger of a possible diagnosis of other diseases such as malignancies in older patients. These conditions may have remained hidden but have led to immunocompromise, leading the patients to a shingles outbreak.

CAUSES

The VZV, which causes chickenpox, remains dormant in a nerve ganglion and may be reactivated later in life. A decrease in cellular immunity may allow the latent virus to become active and spread along the nerve, resulting in clinical zoster. Conditions associated with reactivation include acute systemic illness, HIV disease, lymphoma, Hodgkin disease, lupus erythematosus, and situations in conjunction with immunosuppressive therapy such as steroids or antineoplastic drugs. Herpes zoster is seen seven times more often in people with HIV disease than in other groups.

GENETIC CONSIDERATIONS

Genetic susceptibility has been identified as an important risk factor for herpes zoster. Postherpetic neuralgia (PHN) has been associated with certain human leukocyte antigen alleles.

SEX AND LIFE SPAN CONSIDERATIONS

Shingles can occur at any age and in both genders, although it is uncommon in children and young adults unless they are immunocompromised. Prevalence doubles in patients over the age of 50 years, and approximately 80% of all cases occur in people older than 20 years. It is hypothesized that 50% of all people who live to the age of 85 years will have an attack and that at least 10% may suffer from more than one occurrence. Older adults who are frail or immunocompromised are at particular risk for shingles.

HEALTH DISPARITIES AND SEXUAL/GENDER MINORITY HEALTH

Of those people who have been exposed to chickenpox, Black persons are 25% less likely than White persons to develop herpes zoster. Beginning in 2006, adults have the option to receive a shingles vaccine. By 2018, only 35% of people age 60 years and older were vaccinated. However, 19% of Black and Hispanic persons were vaccinated as compared to 39% of White persons (Singh et al., 2021). Possible reasons are lack of insurance and mistrust of vaccines. Sexual and gender minority status has no known effect on the risk for herpes zoster unless persons are immunocompromised with conditions such as lymphoma, organ transplant, or HIV infection.

GLOBAL HEALTH CONSIDERATIONS

Herpes zoster infection is present around the globe. Vaccinations may have the long-term effect of decreasing the global prevalence.

⬚ ASSESSMENT

HISTORY. Generally, patients describe a history of itching, numbness, tingling, tenderness, and pain in the affected area for 1 to 2 days before skin lesions develop. The rash begins as maculopapules (discolored patches on the skin mixed with elevated red pimples) that rapidly develop into crops of vesicles (blisters) on an erythematous (diffuse redness) base. New lesions continue to appear for 3 to 5 days as the older lesions ulcerate and crust. Malaise, low-grade fever, and adenopathy may accompany the rash. The patient will report a history of chickenpox.

PHYSICAL EXAMINATION. Often the earliest symptoms prior to the breakout of a rash are **fever, anorexia,** and **fatigue** followed by **pain and numbness in the affected area**. Observe the rash, noting the color, temperature, and appearance of lesions and their location and distribution over the body. Note lesion grouping and identify the type. The involved skin may reveal redness, warmth, swelling, vesicles, or crusted areas. This area is generally tender to touch. Determine if lesions are present in the patient's mouth.

The appearance of the lesions changes over time. The initial maculopapules and blisters may evolve in 10 days to scabbed dry blisters and in 2 weeks to small, red nodular skin lesions spread around the area of the dermatome. The patient usually experiences intermittent or continuous pain for up to 4 weeks, although, in rare situations, intractable neurological pain may persist for years.

PSYCHOSOCIAL. Assess the patient's ability to cope with a sudden, unexpected illness that is generally very painful. Assess the amount of pain and degree of relief obtained. Some patients with facial palsy or visible skin lesions may have an altered body image that may cause anxiety.

Diagnostic Highlights

Test	Normal Result	Abnormality With Condition	Explanation
Polymerase chain reaction	Negative for herpes zoster DNA	Positive for herpes zoster DNA	Demonstrates presence of viruses
Viral culture	Negative culture	Positive for herpes zoster	Demonstrates presence of viruses in an active lesion; cultures are most accurate in first several days of ulceration

Other Tests: Tzanck smear (obtained from lesions but cannot differentiate between herpes zoster and herpes simplex), direct immunofluorescence assay (can distinguish herpes zoster from herpes simplex), monoclonal antibody tests. Because herpes zoster infections are frequently seen in people who are HIV positive, the patient should be asked about having an HIV test.

PRIMARY NURSING DIAGNOSIS

DIAGNOSIS. Acute or chronic pain related to nerve root inflammation and skin lesions as evidenced by self-reports of pain, facial grimacing, and/or protective behavior

OUTCOMES. Comfort status; Pain control; Pain level; Symptom severity; Symptom control; Knowledge: Medication

INTERVENTIONS. Analgesic administration; Anxiety reduction; Pain management: Acute and chronic; Medication administration; Medication management

PLANNING AND IMPLEMENTATION

Collaborative

The goals of therapy are to dry the lesions, relieve pain, and prevent secondary complications (see Pharmacologic Highlights). These goals are met primarily through pharmacologic therapy. A wet-to-dry compress application of a Burow solution (aluminum acetate) three to four times a day will help dry the lesions. Isolation procedures are evolving, but recent evidence is that herpes zoster infections are more infectious than was previously thought. Some dermatologists are recommending as part of isolation procedures that all lesions be covered to prevent transmission to other immunocompromised patients.

Pharmacologic Highlights

General Comments: Antihistamines may help with itching. Pain relief may vary from the use of mild analgesics (e.g., aspirin or acetaminophen) to mild opiates (e.g., codeine) if the pain is excruciating. Nighttime sedation also may be helpful. Topical lidocaine sprays can be used to provide analgesia. The use of systemic corticosteroids appears to decrease the severity of PHN pain. Early corticosteroid therapy for 7 to 10 days can both shorten the duration of pain and prevent its chronic reoccurrence.

Pharmacologic Highlights (continued)

Medication or Drug Class	Dosage	Description	Rationale
Antiviral	Varies with drug	Valacyclovir (Valtrex); acyclovir (Zovirax); famciclovir (Famvir)	Treats herpes zoster; most effective if given in the first 48 hr of onset of rash
Capsaicin (Zostrix)	Topical cream applied directly to area of discomfort tid, qid	Topical analgesic	Treats neuralgia after shingles; avoid contact with broken skin
Zoster vaccine recombinant, adjuvanted (Shingrix) (Note: For people with allergies, live, attenuated VZV vaccine [Varivax, Zostavax] is given)	Single dose vial, 0.5 mL IM; given twice 2 to 6 mo apart	Antigen (glycoprotein E) and adjuvant system (AS01B)	Protects from VZV infection; Centers for Disease Control and Prevention (CDC) recommends vaccine be administered to all healthy adults 50 years and older

Other Drugs: Corticosteroids (use is controversial), analgesics (oxycodone, acetaminophen, ibuprofen, naproxen)

Independent

Normally, the only patients treated in the hospital for a herpes zoster infection are those with a primary disease that leads to immunosuppression and can place them at risk for shingles. The most important nursing intervention focuses on prevention of complications and transmission to other vulnerable patients. Monitor for signs and symptoms of infection. Because involvement of the ophthalmic branch of the trigeminal nerve may result in conjunctivitis and possible blindness, be alert for lesions in the eye, and refer the patient to an ophthalmologist. Patients with involvement of sacral dermatomes may have changes in patterns of urinary elimination from acute urinary retention. Monitor intake and output to identify this complication.

Pain may be reduced by splinting the affected area with a snug wrap of nonadherent dressings and covering with an elastic bandage. Manage malaise and elevated temperature with bedrest and a quiet environment. Encourage diversionary activities and teach relaxation techniques to help the patient manage pain without medication. If oral lesions are painful, encourage use of a soft toothbrush and swishing and rinsing every 2 hours with a mouthwash based on a normal saline solution. A soft diet may be necessary during periods of painful oral lesions.

Discuss communicability of the disease and check current guidelines from the CDC. Experts are considering that herpes zoster may be more infectious than was previously thought. In addition, the patient can transmit chickenpox to people who have not had it or who are immunocompromised.

Evidence-Based Practice and Health Policy

Liu, B., Yang, Y., Zhang, Z., Wang, H., Fan, B., & Sima, L. (2020). Clinical study of spinal cord stimulation and pulsed radiofrequency for management of herpes zoster-related pain persisting beyond acute phase in elderly patients. *Pain Physician, 23*, 263–270.

- This study aimed to investigate the effects of spinal cord stimulation (SCS) and pulsed radiofrequency (PRF) on the treatment of elderly patients with herpes zoster–related pain persisting beyond the acute phase. The authors employed a prospective, randomized-controlled trial ($N = 63$) and divided the subjects randomly into an SCS group and a PRF group.
- Outcomes included response and remission rates as well as the use of analgesics and calcium channel antagonists. There were no differences in the outcomes in both groups. Analyses showed that the operation method, age, gender, and course of disease did not affect surgical efficacy. Therefore, the authors concluded that SCS and PRF can both effectively relieve PHN.

DOCUMENTATION GUIDELINES

- Physical findings of rash: Vesicles, redness, and location; degree of healing
- Response to pain medications, rest, relaxation; response to antiviral medications
- Presence of complications: Infection, involvement of eyes, urinary retention, central nervous system symptoms

DISCHARGE AND HOME HEALTHCARE GUIDELINES

PREVENTION. Explain that there is no means for eliminating the varicella virus from the nerve ganglia. Encourage vaccinations when appropriate for children and adults older than age 60 years. The CDC recommends the shingles vaccine for all adults 50 years and older to prevent shingles.

MEDICATIONS. Be sure the patient understands all medications, including the dosage, route, action, and adverse effects.

COMPLICATIONS. Instruct the patient to report redness, swelling, or drainage of the rash to the primary healthcare provider.

Hodgkin Lymphoma

DRG Category:	824
Mean LOS:	7.1 days
Description:	SURGICAL: Lymphoma and Non-Acute Leukemia With Other Procedures With Complication or Comorbidity
DRG Category:	841
Mean LOS:	5.4 days
Description:	MEDICAL: Lymphoma and Non-Acute Leukemia With Complication or Comorbidity

Hodgkin lymphoma is a group of neoplastic disorders characterized by painless, progressive enlargement of the lymph nodes, spleen, and other lymphoid tissue. The enlargement is caused by a proliferation of lymphocytes, histiocytes, eosinophils, and Reed-Sternberg giant cells, the cells that characterize Hodgkin lymphoma; their absence classifies a lymphoma as non-Hodgkin. Generally, the disease tends to begin within a single lymph node region and spreads to nodes in close proximity. Only late in the disease will widespread dissemination occur. It is a progressive and fatal disease if not treated but is one of the most curable neoplastic diseases with treatment. The World Health Organization has classified Hodgkin lymphoma in five ways: nodular sclerosis, mixed cellularity, lymphocyte depleted, lymphocyte rich, and nodular lymphocyte-predominant Hodgkin lymphoma.

In the United States in 2021, the American Cancer Society estimated 8,830 new cases of Hodgkin lymphoma and 960 deaths from the disease. Depending on the stage when the diagnosis was made, the 1-year survival rate with treatment was 93%, and the 5-year survival rate was 87%. Poorer survival rates occur in older people, those with bulky disease, males, and those with lymphocyte and red blood cell depletion.

CAUSES

The cause of Hodgkin lymphoma is unknown. Researchers note that DNA changes in B lymphocytes that are infected with the Epstein-Barr virus lead to Reed-Sternberg cells, which are the cancer cells in Hodgkin lymphoma. Some of the early symptoms include fever, chills, and leukocytosis, as if a viral infection were present. Gene fragments similar to those of a murine leukemia virus have been found in tissue of people with the disease. In particular, higher-than-usual levels of Epstein-Barr antibodies have been found in many patients, and a small increase in incidence has been found in people who have had Epstein-Barr–induced infectious mononucleosis. In addition to Epstein-Barr and mononucleosis infections, other risk factors are older age, male sex, family history, affluent social background, and previous HIV infection.

GENETIC CONSIDERATIONS

Twin studies and ethnic distribution patterns and occurrences of several affected persons in a family support a genetic predisposition for Hodgkin lymphoma, and heritability is estimated at 35% to 40%. Variation at human leukocyte antigen-linked genes (*HLA-A*, *HLA-DRA*) and a major histocompatibility complex region gene (*MICB*) has been shown to influence risk.

SEX AND LIFE SPAN CONSIDERATIONS

Hodgkin lymphoma tends to strike in young adulthood from the ages of 15 to 38 years and is more common in males than in females. When children get the disease, approximately 85% of the patients are male. There is also a bimodal incidence, with the first major peak being in young adults and the second peak later in life after age 50 years. Older people tend to have a more advanced disease at diagnosis and a worse prognosis for cure.

HEALTH DISPARITIES AND SEXUAL/GENDER MINORITY HEALTH

The disease is more common among White persons than persons of other groups. However, in pediatric Hodgkin lymphoma patients, Black children have a lower survival rate at 5 years (91.5%) as compared to White children (95.9%). As with many cancers, patients without health insurance are more likely to have more advanced disease when they are diagnosed as compared to people with private insurance or managed care. In studies of older adults with Hodgkin lymphoma, experts have identified that older age, Medicaid insurance, being unmarried, being frail, having cardiac comorbidities, having prior cancer, and having advanced disease were associated with not receiving first-line (standard) treatment. These factors can lead to health disparities if people do not receive the accepted standard of care (Rodday et al., 2020). The Centers for Disease Control and Prevention reported in 2018 that 69% of new HIV diagnoses in the United States were in gay and bisexual men. People who are immunocompromised, such as those with HIV disease and organ transplantation, are at higher risk for Hodgkin lymphoma. Gender and sexual minority persons are a vulnerable group because people with low income, long travel distances to cancer screening sites, or who lack health insurance or paid medical leave are less likely to be treated according to cancer care guidelines (National Institutes of Health, 2021).

GLOBAL HEALTH CONSIDERATIONS

The global incidence of Hodgkin lymphoma is 1.2 per 100,000 males per year and 0.8 per 100,000 females per year. The incidence is two to four times higher in developed countries than in developing countries. Rates appear to be lower in Asian countries and the islands of the Pacific Ocean.

❄ ASSESSMENT

HISTORY. Many patients present with asymptomatic peripheral lymphadenopathy. Because there are numerous causes for enlarged lymph nodes, it is important to elicit information about recent infections, allergic reactions, and other events. In Hodgkin lymphoma, the nodes tend to be cervical, supraclavicular, and mediastinal. About 40% of patients report fever, night sweats, and recent weight loss, collectively called *B symptoms*. Some patients report cough, chest pain, or dyspnea. Pain at the lymph node site after drinking alcohol does not occur often but is specific to Hodgkin lymphoma. Less commonly, they may report pruritus during any stage (Table 1). Because the B symptoms are necessary for staging, it is important to elicit that information in the history.

• **TABLE 1** Staging for Hodgkin Lymphoma

STAGES AND SUBCLASSIFICATIONS	DESCRIPTION	5-YEAR SURVIVAL RATE BASED ON STAGE
Stage I	Localized to a single lymph node or nodal group	90%–95%
Stage II	More than one nodal group on the same side of the diaphragm	90%–95%
Stage III	More than one nodal group on both sides of the diaphragm	84%
Stage IV	Spread to organs other than lymph nodes or spleen	Approximately 65%
Subclassification	A: Asymptomatic	
	B: Fevers, weight loss, night sweats are present; symptoms suggest bulky disease and a poor prognosis (sometimes classified as "X" category)	
	E: Extralymphatic involvement such as stomach, small intestine	
	S: Spleen involvement	

PHYSICAL EXAMINATION. The most common presenting symptom is **asymptomatic swelling of the lymph nodes above the diaphragm**. During advanced phases of the disease, the patient may have edema of the face and neck, weight loss, and jaundice. Palpate all lymph node chains, including the submental, infraclavicular, epitrochlear, iliac, femoral, and popliteal nodes. Involved nodes are characteristically painless, firm, rubbery in consistency (unlike the rock-hard nodes of carcinoma), freely movable, and of varying size. Palpate the liver and spleen, which may be enlarged.

PSYCHOSOCIAL. The diagnosis of a neoplastic disorder in young adulthood is a devastating event for the patient and significant others. Rather than pursuing educational goals, job obligations, social interactions, or parenting responsibilities, the young adult is suddenly managing a potentially terminal disease. Although the disease is treatable in most cases, the patient needs to manage short- and long-term complications of therapy that may profoundly alter the patient's body image. Infertility in young adults after treatment may affect the patients' view of themselves and the long-term potential for the desired role of parenthood.

Diagnostic Highlights

Test	Normal Result	Abnormality With Condition	Explanation
Lymph node biopsy or bone marrow biopsy	Normal cells	Positive for Hodgkin lymphoma cells (Reed-Sternberg giant cells)	Determines extent of disease and allows for staging of disease; bone marrow biopsy is generally done only for patients with anemia or fever and night sweats
Computed tomography (CT) scan, positron emission tomography (PET), or magnetic resonance imaging of chest, abdomen, and pelvis	Normal structures	Spread of Hodgkin lymphoma into organs and body cavities	Assists with staging; common sites of extralymphatic involvement include spleen, stomach, small intestine; combined with lymphangiography, can predict nodal involvement in 90% of cases; CT and PET scanning are often performed together; PET can distinguish between tumor and necrosis/fibrosis

Other Tests: Complete blood cell count, chest x-ray, erythrocyte sedimentation rate; tests for liver and renal function, including lactate dehydrogenase, alkaline phosphatase, blood urea nitrogen, creatinine, HIV testing

PRIMARY NURSING DIAGNOSIS

DIAGNOSIS. Risk for infection as evidenced by fever and/or diaphoresis

OUTCOMES. Immune status; Knowledge: Infection management; Knowledge: Cancer management; Risk control: Infectious process; Risk detection; Nutritional status; Tissue integrity: Skin and mucous membranes

INTERVENTIONS. Infection control; Infection protection; Surveillance; Nutritional management; Medication management; Teaching: Disease process

PLANNING AND IMPLEMENTATION

Collaborative

Treatment begins with accurate classification and staging. Clinical staging is determined by initial biopsy, history, physical examination, and radiological findings. Pathological staging involves a more extensive surgical assessment of possible sites for spread. Owing to continued improvement in radiological staging, a staging laparotomy (thorough abdominal exploration, splenectomy, liver biopsy, bone marrow biopsy, and multiple lymph node samplings) is performed infrequently.

In general, radiation combined with chemotherapy is used for early, less extensive disease. PET is used to determine response to treatment before doses are adjusted. A combination of radiation and chemotherapy is used for stages I, IIB, IIIA, and B. Combination chemotherapy with drugs such as Adriamycin (doxorubicin), bleomycin, vinblastine, and dacarbazine (ABVD) is used for stage IV (see Pharmacologic Highlights). Involved-site radiation (ISRT) is a radiation field that includes both pre- and postchemotherapy node volumes and a margin of healthy tissue around the node. ISRT is recommended for Hodgkin lymphoma, and doses are set to maximize response and minimize complications. Surgery is not used as a treatment modality in Hodgkin lymphoma except in the role of staging. A dietary consultation may be needed to help the patient maintain weight and to help support healing.

If the disease does not respond to standard treatment, bone marrow transplantation may be offered, either as part of a clinical trial or outside of a clinical trial. The patient's own bone marrow is removed and stored. Then very high doses of chemotherapy, sometimes in combination with radiation therapy, are administered to eradicate the cancer. High doses also destroy bone marrow. The stored marrow is administered intravenously to the patient, and bone marrow cells enter the bloodstream and return to the bone. The transplanted marrow produces new red and white blood cells. In another type of transplant, peripheral blood stem cell transplant, only the stem cells (immature cells from which all blood cells develop) are removed and the rest of the blood is returned to the body. Stem cells are then frozen until they are returned to the patient after treatment is finished.

Pharmacologic Highlights

General Comments: Typically, chemotherapy is given in six or more cycles of treatment in combination with radiotherapy. Common side effects are alopecia, nausea, vomiting, fatigue, myelosuppression, and stomatitis. Patients who are receiving chemotherapy are administered antinausea drugs, antiemetics, and pain medicines as needed to help control adverse experiences. Note that older patients are at particular risk for developing toxicity from chemotherapy and need to be monitored carefully. Toxicities are associated with the treatment regimes and include hematological, pulmonary, and cardiac toxicity as well as infections, secondary cancers, and psychiatric difficulties such as depression and anxiety.

Medication or Drug Class	Dosage	Description	Rationale
Chemotherapy	Varies with drug	Common examples are MOPP (mechloreth-amine, vincristine, procarbazine, prednisone), ABVD, Stanford V (doxorubicin, vinblastine, mustard, bleomycin, vincristine, etoposide, prednisone), and BEACOPP (bleomycin, etoposide, doxorubicin, cyclophosphamide, vincristine, procarbazine, prednisone)	IV chemotherapy is used depending on early or advanced disease

Other Drugs: If chemotherapy fails or patients have relapse, "salvage" chemotherapy is given. These drugs include ICE (ifosfamide, carboplatin, etoposide), DHAP (cisplatin, cytarabine, prednisone).

Independent

The primary nursing roles are to maintain comfort, protect the patient from infection, provide teaching and support about the complications of the treatment, and give emotional support. Complications from radiation, such as dry mouth, loss of taste, dysphagia, nausea, and vomiting can be managed with frequent mouth care. Manage skin irritation and redness. Encourage the patient to avoid applying lotions, perfumes, deodorants, and powder to the treatment area. Explain that the skin must be protected from sunlight and extreme cold. Before starting treatments, arrange for the patient to have a wig, scarf, or hat to cover any hair loss, which occurs primarily at the nape of the neck. Explain to the patient that pneumonitis and hypothyroidism may occur; explain the signs and symptoms of each and when to notify the physician.

If the patient develops bone marrow suppression during hospitalization, make sure all staff and visitors use good hand-washing techniques. Do not assign a nurse who is caring for patients with infections. Encourage staff and visitors with infections to avoid all contact with the patient. If the patient receives chemotherapy, the side effects are equally uncomfortable. In addition to many of the symptoms that occur in response to radiation therapy (gastrointestinal symptoms, oral lesions, hair loss, bone marrow depression), the patient may develop joint pain, fever, fluid retention, and a labile emotional state (euphoria or depression) that need specific interventions based on their incidence and severity.

The disease presents severe emotional stressors to the patient and the patient's significant others. The complexity of the diagnostic and staging process may make the patient feel lost in a crowd of specialists. It is important for the nurse to provide supportive continuity. Patience and repeated explanations are needed. Provide the patient with information about support groups, and refer the patient to either a clinical nurse specialist, support groups associated with the American or Canadian Cancer Society, or counselors.

Evidence-Based Practice and Health Policy

Gupta, S., Baxter, N., Hodgson, D., Punnett, A., Sutradhar, R., Pole, J., Nagamuthu, C., Lau, C., & Nathan, P. (2020). Treatment patterns and outcomes in adolescents and young adults with Hodgkin lymphoma in pediatric versus adult centers: An IMPACT cohort study. *Cancer Medicine, 9,* 6933–6945.

• The authors aimed to compare population-based treatment patterns and outcomes in adolescent and young adults ($N = 954$) with Hodgkin lymphoma by locus of care (adult versus pediatric cancer centers). They examined locus of care–based differences in treatment, cumulative doses, event-free survival, overall survival, and late effects.

• Most of the adolescent and young adult patients received treatment at adult cancer centers (74.5%). Patients treated in pediatric centers received higher rates of radiation therapy but lower cumulative doses of chemotherapy. While pediatric and adult centers used different treatment strategies, the outcomes were similar. However, the authors note that differences in treatment might lead to different late-term effects.

DOCUMENTATION GUIDELINES

• Response to staging: Emotional and physical response to diagnostic testing, healing of incisions, signs of ineffective coping, response to diagnosis, ability to participate in planning treatment options, response of significant others
• Response to treatment: Effects of chemotherapy or radiation therapy, or both; response to treatment of symptoms, presence of complications (weight loss, infection, skin irritation)
• Emotional state: Effectiveness of coping, presence of depression, interest in group support or counseling, referrals made

DISCHARGE AND HOME HEALTHCARE GUIDELINES

Although they are cured of the disease, patients who survive Hodgkin lymphoma continue to have immune defects that persist throughout life. Defects include transiently depressed antibody production, decreased polymorphonuclear chemotaxis, decreased antigen-induced T-cell proliferation, and changes in delayed hypersensitivity. Coupled with the sometimes lingering aftereffects of radiation and chemotherapy, the patient needs to maintain infection vigilance even after remission is obtained. Teach the patient lifelong strategies to avoid infection.

Patients may have other complications for up to 25 years after some types of radiation therapy, including hypothyroidism, Graves disease, and thyroid cancer. Irradiation can also cause pulmonary and pericardial fibrosis and coronary artery changes, and it may increase the risk for the development of solid tumors such as lung cancer, breast cancer, and others. Explain the presenting symptoms of the disorder, provide written information for the patient, and encourage yearly physicals to maintain follow-up. Because infertility may be a complication of chemotherapy, men may want to think of sperm banking before treatments, although many have sperm dysfunction at diagnosis.

Human Immunodeficiency Virus Disease

DRG Category:	975
Mean LOS:	5.5 days
Description:	MEDICAL: HIV With Major Related Condition With Complication or Comorbidity
DRG Category:	977
Mean LOS:	4.8 days
Description:	MEDICAL: HIV With or Without Other Related Condition

HIV is a blood-borne retrovirus transmitted primarily through sexual intercourse, blood transfusions, and mother-to-child transmission during pregnancy and/or breastfeeding. *AIDS* was a term more appropriate in the early years of the AIDS epidemic, when healthcare providers were aware only of the late stages of the disease and did not fully understand its mechanisms. The more current name for the condition is *HIV disease*, which refers to the pathogen that causes symptoms and physiological derangements. HIV disease encompasses all the phases of the disease, from infection to the deterioration of the immune system. AIDS is still the name that most people use to refer to the immune deficiency caused by HIV disease.

The Centers for Disease Control and Prevention (CDC) first described AIDS in 1981, and since then, the disease has become one of the most widely publicized and feared diseases of our time. The CDC's most recent prevalence statistics indicate that there are approximately 1.2 million adults and adolescents living with HIV infection in the United States. Of those people, one in seven do not know that they are infected. Each year there are an estimated 37,000 new HIV infections in the United States.

The early, acute phase in an immunocompetent person occurs with widespread viral production and seeding of lymph tissues (acute retroviral syndrome). The symptoms are generally nonspecific, such as sore throat, myalgia, fever, weight loss, and fatigue; they occur 3 to 6 weeks after infection and resolve 2 to 4 weeks later. As the disease progresses, people may remain asymptomatic or may develop a persistent generalized lymphadenopathy. In either case, HIV replication occurs primarily in the lymphoid tissues. HIV infection of lymphocytes and other cells that bear specific protein markers leads to lymphopenia and impaired T-cell and B-cell function. There is a specific decline in CD4$^+$ helper T cells and a resultant change in the proportion of CD4:CD8 ratio. In addition, B-cell antibody production is dysregulated, reducing the immune response to certain antigens and increasing the risk of opportunistic nonbacterial infections such as cytomegalovirus and *Candida* species. HIV disease generally occurs when the CD4 count is below 200/mL, and it is characterized by the appearance of opportunistic infections.

The CDC classifies HIV infection into three categories. Category A includes people with an asymptomatic HIV infection. Category B includes people with symptoms that are directly attributable to an HIV infection. These symptoms include, among others, oral thrush (candidiasis), vulvovaginal thrush, pelvic inflammatory disease, fever, diarrhea, peripheral neuropathy, and shingles (herpes zoster). Category C is HIV infection with AIDS-defining opportunistic infections and conditions such as candidiasis, cervical cancer, cytomegalovirus disease, Kaposi sarcoma, and others. The three categories are further subdivided based on the CD4 T-cell counts.

CAUSES

Two HIV strains have been identified: HIV-1 and HIV-2. HIV-1 is the prototype virus and is responsible for most cases of HIV disease in the United States. HIV-2 is found chiefly in

Africa, appears to be less easily transmitted, and has a longer incubation period. Susceptibility to infection is unclear. The presence of sexually transmitted infections (STIs) with open lesions, such as herpes and syphilis, may increase the patient's susceptibility to viral entry. People with cytomegalovirus and Epstein-Barr virus infections may also be more susceptible because of an increased number of target cells. Routes of transmission are through sexual contact (male to male, male to female, female to male, and female to female); by blood to blood or transfusion contact (generally blood products given between 1977 and 1985); through the use of needles contaminated by an HIV-infected person; by blood or other HIV-infected fluids coming in contact with open lesions or mucous membranes; and by mother to child during the in utero period, during delivery, or by breastfeeding. Risk factors for HIV disease include needle sharing during drug use, blood transfusions, receptive anal intercourse, insertive anal intercourse, needle sticks, having multiple sex partners, and unprotected anal and vaginal sexual intercourse. Use of alcohol and drugs are associated with HIV transmission because these substances change people's judgment about safe practices.

GENETIC CONSIDERATIONS

Susceptibility to HIV disease varies among people. Investigators are finding genetic variants that increase or mitigate susceptibility to HIV infection. CCL3L1 is a protein that interacts with the *CCR5* coreceptor that is used by HIV to infect cells. Persons with more copies of the gene that codes for CCL3L1 are less likely to contract HIV infection than others of the same ethnicity with fewer copies. Polymorphisms in *CCR5* itself also affect viral entry, with one particular 32 base pair deletion in *CCR5* preventing viral infection and disease progression. Genetic variants for other coreceptors or coreceptor ligands, such as *CCR2*, *CCL5*, *CXCL12*, *CX3CR1*, *CXCR1*, and certain *HLA* alleles, also affect viral entry and/or progression of the disease.

SEX AND LIFE SPAN CONSIDERATIONS

The patterns of HIV-related deaths have changed during the past 20 years. In the late 1990s, HIV was the second leading cause of death in the United States in men ages 25 to 44 years and the third leading cause of death in women of the same age range. The most recent mortality statistics from the CDC (2021) indicate that in 2019, 15,815 deaths in the United States and U.S.-dependent areas were directly attributed to HIV disease, a much lower rate of death. Individuals can contract HIV at any time during their life span, including infancy. The average time between exposure and diagnosis in adults is from 8 to 10 years, although the incubation period varies among people. In children, the incubation period is approximately 18 months. Children are likely to have a history of repeated bacterial infections, such as middle ear infections and pneumonia. Most HIV disease in children is the result of maternal-child transmission.

The progression of HIV disease and response to seropositive status vary in men and women in several ways. Women seek healthcare interventions later than men and are at risk for gynecological complications, such as pelvic inflammatory disease and cervical dysplasia. Women make up 15% of new HIV infections. Approximately 86% of HIV infections among U.S. women occur through heterosexual contact and 14% through use of injected drugs.

HEALTH DISPARITIES AND SEXUAL/GENDER MINORITY HEALTH

Black and Hispanic persons bear a disproportionate burden of HIV disease compared with other populations. In addition, 65% of women with newly diagnosed HIV disease are Black, and many of those women live in the southern parts of the United States. In 2019, male to male sexual contact was the source for new HIV diagnoses in 65.4% of the cases, heterosexual contact in 23.4% of the cases, and injected drug use in 6.8% of the cases. Approximately 4% new HIV diagnoses were made in males who have had both male-to-male sexual contact and injected drug use. The CDC reported in 2021 that 69% of new HIV diagnoses in the United States were gay, bisexual, and other men who have sex with men. In young people ages 13 to 24 years, young gay and bisexual men and men/youth who have sex with men account for 83% of all new HIV diagnoses.

GLOBAL HEALTH CONSIDERATIONS

The most current statistics from the CDC indicate that there were 1.7 million new cases of HIV in 2019 worldwide. Approximately 38 million people are living with HIV around the world, and 24.5 million are receiving antiretroviral therapy. Sub-Saharan Africa is the region most affected by HIV disease and AIDS worldwide, but other regions that have a significant number of people with disease are Asia, Latin America, the Caribbean, and Eastern Europe.

ASSESSMENT

HISTORY. Note that patients may come to the healthcare system in any of the stages of HIV disease, and therefore, symptoms vary in their severity. If patients are in the asymptomatic phase, they may have generalized lymphadenopathy and may notice a "stiff" neck and pain. They may have gait disturbance and burning, numbness, and tingling in the extremities. Establish a history of night sweats, fever, weight loss, and fatigue. The patient may have flu-like symptoms, fever, and rash or gastrointestinal (GI) disturbances such as nausea, vomiting, diarrhea, and anorexia. The patient may describe neurological manifestations, including headache, lightheadedness, memory loss, word-finding difficulty, inability to concentrate, and mood swings. A history of infections such as tuberculosis, herpes, hepatitis B, fungal infections, or STIs is common in the HIV disease population. Discuss with patients possible exposure through unprotected sexual intercourse, a large number of sexual partners, a prior history of STIs, sharing of IV drug paraphernalia, transfusion of blood products (particularly prior to 1986), or maternal HIV infection.

PHYSICAL EXAMINATION. Common symptoms include **night sweats**, **lymphadenopathy**, **fever**, **weight loss**, **fatigue**, and **rash**. Patients with HIV disease are at risk for opportunistic infections that affect all systems and diseases common to their age group (Box 1). Wasting syndrome is common to patients with HIV disease and includes weight loss of at least 10% of body weight, diarrhea, weakness, and documented fever for at least 30 days. The patient's skin may have a generalized rash or lesions from herpes or Kaposi sarcoma (a metastasizing skin cancer). Ask the patient to walk during the examination to examine the patient's gait. Note ataxia, motor weakness, gait disturbance, and hemiparesis. Palpate the patient's lymph nodes to determine if lymphadenopathy is present, particularly in two or more extra-inguinal sites. Patients may or may not be febrile.

• BOX 1 Symptoms Requiring Medical Attention in Patients With HIV Disease

- New cough
- Shortness of breath or dyspnea on exertion
- Increased fatigue or malaise
- Fever
- Night sweats
- Headache or stiff neck
- Visual changes: Floaters, blurring, photophobia, changes in visual fields
- Mental status alteration: Change in level of consciousness, loss of memory, forgetfulness, loss of concentration, depression, mood swings
- New onset of diarrhea
- Sudden weight loss
- Increased size of or pain in lymph nodes
- Skin lesions
- Pain

PSYCHOSOCIAL. While HIV disease is now a treatable disease, diagnosis of HIV remains a crisis, and the crisis may exacerbate any underlying physical and psychiatric disorders. A person may be in a state of denial or have anxiety, psychological numbness, and depression. Remember that in this state, people cannot focus and do not hear what healthcare professionals tell them. The patient undergoes a fear of the loss of sex life, contaminating others, rejection, and stigma. While fears about loss of employment, financial independence, and insurance are realities, they are less likely than 25 years ago. As the disease progresses, grief over losses, hopelessness, suicidal ideation, and emotional exhaustion may occur. The patient deals with stress over the demands of treatment, embarrassment because of physical symptoms, and loneliness.

Diagnostic Highlights

Test	Normal Result	Abnormality With Condition	Explanation
HIV p24 antigen	Negative	Positive for HIV 24 antigen	Detects HIV in the blood; this test is followed by a test that can differentiate HIV-1 from HIV-2
HIV-1/2 Ag/Ab combo test (rapid HIV test)	Negative	Positive	Simultaneously detects HIV-1 p24 antigen as well as antibodies to both HIV-1 and HIV-2 (does not distinguish between HIV-1 and HIV-2)
Enzyme-linked immunosorbent assay (ELISA) and Western blot	Negative for HIV antibodies	Positive for HIV antibodies; 50% of people are positive within 22 days and 95% within 6 wk after HIV transmission	Positive ELISA test is confirmed by a Western blot; identifies HIV types including HIV-1 (M, N, O) and HIV-2
T-lymphocyte and B-lymphocyte subsets; CD4 counts, CD4 percentages	B cells: 65–4,785/mL; CD4 T cells: 527–2,846/mL (49%–81%); CD4 to CD8 T-cell ratio: 1:2.5	B-cell and T-cell values decreased. CD4 counts less than 500/mL are generally associated with symptoms; CD4 counts less than 200/mL are associated with severe immune suppression. Any HIV-infected person with a CD4 level less than 200/mL is considered to have HIV disease; CD4:CD8 ratio inverts to less than 1:1 (CD4 count may decrease and CD8 count may increase).	HIV infects cells with the CD4 protein marker
HIV viral load: Polymerase chain reaction, nucleic acid sequence-based amplification	Negative	Detects number of copies/mL; test depending on sensitivity has a lower limit of 20 copies/mL but levels in HIV disease can reach 30,000 copies/mL and higher; test correlates with disease progression and response to therapy	Quantitative assay that measures amount of HIV-1 RNA in plasma

Other Tests: Tests include complete blood count, viral culture, and indirect fluorescent antibody. The HIV rapid antibody test is a screening test that can be performed with limited training. A lymph node biopsy may help with diagnosis or staging. Results must be confirmed by ELISA and Western blot.

PRIMARY NURSING DIAGNOSIS

DIAGNOSIS. Risk for infection as evidenced by diaphoresis, weight loss, anorexia, lymphadenopathy, fever, and/or rash

OUTCOMES. Immune status; Knowledge: Infection management; Knowledge: Human immunodeficiency virus management; Risk control: Infectious process; Respiratory status: Gas exchange; Respiratory status: Ventilation; Thermoregulation

INTERVENTIONS. Infection control; Infection protection; Respiratory monitoring; Teaching: Disease process; Temperature regulation

⚕ PLANNING AND IMPLEMENTATION

Collaborative

Much of the collaborative management is based on pharmacologic therapy (see Pharmacologic Highlights). HIV-infected people should also be screened for diabetes, osteoporosis, and colon cancer, and their vaccinations for influenza, varicella, hepatitis, and pneumococcal infection should be current. They should also be assessed for cardiovascular risk and have STI screening. Supportive management consists of treatment of malignancies with chemotherapy and irradiation, treatment of infections as they develop, and the management of discomfort with analgesia. Surgical management may be needed to excise lesions from Kaposi sarcoma or to drain abscesses. If the patient becomes short of breath, oxygen is often prescribed to improve gas exchange. Dietary support is important in the treatment of HIV disease throughout the progression of the illness.

Pharmacologic Highlights

Antiretroviral therapies are grouped into four categories and should always be used in combination. Introduction of highly active antiretroviral therapy (HAART) is capable of maximally suppressing viral replication. The clinical benefits of HAART are significant and durable. Drugs have important interactions with other medication. Interactions need to be reviewed carefully.

Medication or Drug Class	Dosage	Description	Rationale
Antiretroviral therapy classification: Nucleotide reverse transcriptase inhibitors: tenofovir	300 mg PO daily	Nucleotide analog	Decreases HIV replication by incorporation into the strand of DNA, leading to chain termination
Antiretroviral therapy classification: protease inhibitors	Varies by drug	Protease inhibitor	Blocks the action of the viral protease required for protein processing near the end of the viral cycle
Antiretroviral therapy: non-nucleoside reverse transcriptase inhibitors	Varies by drug	Non-nucleoside reverse transcriptase inhibitors	Inhibits HIV by binding noncompetitively to reverse transcriptase
Antiretroviral therapy: HIV entry inhibitors (fusion inhibitor)	Varies by drug	New class of antiretroviral agents	Targets different stages of the HIV entry process
Antiretroviral therapy: Integrase inhibitor: raltegravir	400 mg PO daily	New class of antiretroviral agents	Slows HIV replication by blocking the HIV integrase enzyme needed for viral multiplication

Note: Drugs are usually used in combination. The monthly cost of antiretroviral agents ranges from $400 to $3,200 for each medication. The CDC estimates that the lifetime cost of treating HIV is $379,000.

Independent

Nursing interventions are complex because of the many physical, psychological, and social effects that occur from HIV disease. Because patients can live a full life using HAART, nursing care can focus on living healthily in the community by screening for risks, implementing safe sex strategies, maintaining nutrition, keeping vaccinations current, and living a healthy lifestyle without IV drugs. During the more acute and severe stages of the illness, focus on maximizing the patient's health and promoting comfort. Educate the patient and significant others regarding self-care by keeping any lesions and the skin clean and dry. Diarrhea can limit activities and also cause pain, both abdominal and perianal, if any lesions are present. Keep the perianal area clean and assist the patient with cleaning immediately. Instruct the patient about the food substances that are GI irritants. Explain that diarrhea can cause dehydration, electrolyte disturbances, and malabsorption; provide the patient with ways to maintain fluid and electrolyte balance. All patients need to be instructed to perform frequent and thorough oral care. Teach patients to avoid toothbrushes. Tell them to clean the teeth, gums, and membranes with a soft gauze pad; to use mouthwashes without alcohol; to lubricate the lips; and to avoid foods that are spicy, acidic, thermally hot, and hard to chew. Also explain the need to seek treatment for *Candida* and herpes and to use lidocaine (Xylocaine) for discomfort.

Explain the mechanisms for HIV transmission and teach the patient and significant others the precautions regarding transmission by both casual and sexual routes. Discuss safe sex behaviors. Explore mechanisms to assist with the large financial cost of retroviral therapy. Explain that if the patient has spills of blood or secretion, they should be cleaned up with a 1:10 solution of bleach and water to limit the risk of infection to others. Use universal precautions whenever you are exposed to blood, body fluids, or secretions, and teach the patient's significant others to do the same.

Note that the best outcomes result from early intervention. Many times, the patients' family members are unaware of their sexual practices, or spouses or partners may be unaware that their partner had high-risk behavior that exposed them to HIV infection. The diagnosis of HIV disease may increase the distance between friends and family members. Social isolation often occurs because others avoid the patient out of the fear of being infected. Allow the patient to talk about the diagnosis and isolation.

If the patient has severe immunodeficiency at the end of life, use touch and encourage others to touch, hug, hold hands, and give back rubs to the patient to help fulfill the patient's need for touch. Encourage the patient's participation in support groups and use of volunteer "friends." The patient may experience anger, denial, anxiety, hopelessness, and depression. Ensure that the needed support services are available for home healthcare; make sure the patient has support for meals, financial assistance, and hygienic care.

Evidence-Based Practice and Health Policy

Graham, L., & Makic, M. (2020). Nursing considerations for patients with HIV in critical care settings. *AACN Advanced Critical Care, 31*, 308–317.

- With the advent of antiretroviral therapy, people living with HIV have a life expectancy approaching that of the general population. However, they are also at increased risk for cardiovascular disease, renal disease, type 2 diabetes, neurologic conditions, and cancers, often with worse outcomes than in patients without HIV.
- The authors describe issues surrounding antiretroviral therapy, which is critical for successful management and should be continued when possible during intensive care unit stays. Antiretroviral regimens result in drug-drug interactions, adverse drug-related events, and secondary complications such as insulin resistance and prolonged QT intervals and must be monitored carefully by critical care nurses.

DOCUMENTATION GUIDELINES

- Physical changes: Weight, mental status, vital signs, skin integrity, bowel habits
- Tolerance to activity, fatigue, ability to sleep, ability to manage self-care; response to medications

- Understanding of safe sex behaviors
- Emotional response, coping, signs of ineffective coping, support from family and friends
- Presence of opportunistic infections, complications of infections, medications, resistance, recurrence
- Requests for management of living with a chronic disease, living with a critical disease, and pertinent information about the patient's wishes regarding the final stages of life

DISCHARGE AND HOME HEALTHCARE GUIDELINES

PREVENTION. Teach the patient or caregiver universal precautions at home; adequate nutritional strategies; the names and telephone numbers for support organizations; self-assessments daily for temperature elevations; signs of thrush (*Candida*), herpes, and other opportunistic infections; symptoms of complications such as cough, lesions, and fever; and strategies to limit situations with high infection potential (crowds, people with colds or flu).

TRANSMISSION. Teach the patient strategies to practice safe sex. Inform the patient that the disease can be transmitted during high-risk sexual practices that expose partners to body fluids. These practices include vaginal and anal intercourse without a condom and/or oral sex without protection. Encourage the patient to use safe sex practices such as hugging, petting, mutual masturbation, and protected anal and vaginal sex. Explore the patient's knowledge about male and female condom use.

Encourage patients to notify any sexual partners and healthcare providers that they have HIV infection. Explain that the patient should not donate blood, blood products, or organs, tissues, or sperm. If the patient continues to use IV drugs, make sure the patient knows never to share needles.

Explain to patients of childbearing age that any pregnancy may result in an infant with HIV infection. Explain that HIV may also infect an infant during delivery or during breastfeeding. Encourage the patient to notify the physician as soon as pregnancy occurs to allow preventive treatment to limit the risk to the fetus.

SUPPORT SYSTEMS. Inform patients about the possible physiological, emotional, and mental effects of the disease, along with the treatments and resources that are available to them. At the end of life, encourage patients to explore hospice care early in the treatment cycle to establish a possible long-term relationship as the disease progresses.

Human Papillomavirus

DRG Category:	760
Mean LOS:	3.4 days
Description:	MEDICAL: Menstrual and Other Female Reproductive System Disorders With Complication or Comorbidity or Major Complication or Comorbidity

Human papillomavirus (HPV) is a highly specific virus that affects only humans. It has an affinity for epidermal sites like mucous membranes and skin, and causes the most common sexually transmitted infection (STI) in the United States. There are more than 100 types of HPV viruses, but HPV types 16 and 18 seem to be high-risk types because they are linked to the high-grade epithelial lesions that often progress to carcinomas, particularly those in the anogenital area or in the mucosa. It is the primary cause of cervical cancer. HPV is associated with esophageal and anal epithelial tumors in both men and women and is associated with a threefold risk of developing esophageal cancer. HPV also causes anogenital warts, which are usually found near moist surfaces such as the perianal area, vaginal introitus, and vagina. They also may occur on dry surfaces, such as the shaft of the penis.

Women are infected with HPV most commonly through sexual contact, which can be male to female and, more uncommonly, female to female. It is important to note that most women infected with these viruses do not develop cervical cancer. A number of factors, however, seem to contribute to HPV infection progressing to cervical cancer. They include having sexual intercourse at an early age, having multiple sexual partners, decreased frequency of showering and bathing, oral contraception, and having unprotected sexual intercourse. Other factors that might be related to risk are tobacco use, ultraviolet radiation, pregnancy, folate deficiency, and immune suppression.

Men are infected with HPV most commonly by having sex with men. Anal cancer has been strongly associated with men having sex with men, and more specifically, with engaging in receptive anal intercourse. It is possible that circumcision reduces the risk of HPV transmission. For people living with HIV, HPV infection is detected more often and is more resistant to treatment than in HIV-negative individuals. Complications include cervical dysplasia, genital warts, skin tumors, cervical cancer, cancer of the vulva, esophageal cancer, anal cancer, and penile cancer.

CAUSES

Infection likely occurs via a disrupted epithelial barrier, such as a tear or abrasion that occurs during sexual intercourse or after minor skin injury such as a scrape. The virus infects the basal skin cells (keratinocytes) of the epidermis through the disruptions and spreads through the skin, not the bloodstream. People with immune deficiencies such as HIV disease are particularly susceptible to HPV infection because of decreases in cell-mediated immunity. HPV causes epithelial tumors of the skin and mucous membranes, most likely because of proliferation of infected basal keratinocytes.

GENETIC CONSIDERATIONS

More than 100 HPV types have been detected, and the genomes of more than 80 viruses have been sequenced. The current classification system is based on similarities in the viral genomic sequences and can be divided into anogenital and/or mucosal, nongenital cutaneous, and epidermodysplasia verruciformis.

Women have twice the risk of developing cervical cancer if they have a first-degree relative (mother, sister, or daughter) with carcinoma of the cervix. Various immune response genes have been suggested to modulate risk of developing cervical cancer, including *IL1B*, *TNFA*, *HLA*, *IL12A*, *IL12B*, *IFNG*, *IL10*, and *CTLA4*.

SEX AND LIFE SPAN CONSIDERATIONS

Young adults in the age range of 15 to 24 years account for approximately half of new HPV cases each year in the United States. Young, sexually active females have the highest rates of genital HPV infection; in the United States, 45% of young women ages 20 to 24 years screen positive for genital HPV. There are two explanations for the high rates of HPV in young women. First, the age range from 20 to 24 years is a time when many women have multiple sex partners. Second, it is possible that as women reach the age of 30 years, they have developed immunity to the virus. Both men and women can be infected without having any signs of infection, but asymptomatic disease is more typical in men.

Infants born of HPV-positive mothers and with HPV-positive nasopharyngeal aspirates are considered "contaminated" but not infected with HPV. Generally, these infants will eliminate the virus several months after birth.

HEALTH DISPARITIES AND SEXUAL/GENDER MINORITY HEALTH

The government does not keep statistics on HPV infections; therefore, the prevalence in various groups is uncertain. Some experts suggest that prevalence for Black women is 40% and for White and Hispanic women is 25%. In the United States, the cervical cancer death rate is 3.2/100,000 for Black women; 2.5/100,000 for Hispanic and Native American women; and 2.1/100,000 for White women (NIH, 2021). Because HPV is a cause of cervical cancer, Black women are at particular risk when they acquire an HPV infection. Men who have sex with men are at disproportionate risk for HPV infection. Commonly, men are infected with HPV by having sex with men, and uncommonly, women are infected with HPV by having sex with women. Sexual minority women (in this case, lesbian and bisexual women) are more likely to complete HPV vaccination protocols than heterosexual women (Boakye et al., 2021 [see Evidence-Based Practice and Health Policy]). Transgender is a term used to describe persons whose gender identity is different from their sex assigned at birth. Approximately 1% of the U.S. population identify themselves as transgender. Transgender men need to undergo cervical cancer screening if they have a cervix. For some transgender men, screening is needed even if gender-affirming surgery has occurred.

GLOBAL HEALTH CONSIDERATIONS

HPV is the most common STI in the world. More than 30 million people have genital warts. A significant health disparity exists for women in developed versus developing countries with respect to cervical cancer, which can be caused by HPV. Cervical cancer is the second leading cause of cancer-related death for women in developing countries and 10th leading cancer-related death for women in developed countries. Regions around the world that have a high prevalence of HIV-infected people have high rates of HPV infection. Estimates are that 70% to 80% of women who are HIV infected are also HPV positive.

ASSESSMENT

HISTORY. Take a complete sexual history. To direct specimen collection, elicit information regarding sexual orientation and sexual practices (vaginal, oral, and anal). Explore the patient's birth control practices and determine if the patient and partner regularly use condoms. Explore the number of sex partners, the incidence of unprotected sexual contacts, and the frequency of sex with unknown partners. Determine how often the patient receives the Papanicolaou (Pap) test. It is important that during this discussion the provider and the patient have privacy and the provider use sensitive communication skills to elicit specific information.

Many patients do not have symptoms from an HPV infection. Ask if the patient has a history of warts in the genital area or in the nares, mouth, larynx, and conjunctiva. Determine how long the warts have been present. Ask patients if they have noticed rectal bleeding or a sensation of a rectal mass. Ask patients if they have experienced vaginal bleeding between periods or after sexual intercourse, dyspareunia, and pelvic fullness. Note that genital warts can appear weeks or even months after sexual contact with a person infected with HPV virus; patients may not know they are infected or that they may be responsible for HPV transmission to other partners.

PHYSICAL EXAMINATION. Generally, an HPV infection will lead to a **lesion such as a wart at the infected location**. Inspect the skin, particularly the genitourinary area, for genital warts, which take on many different appearances and sizes. They are most typically found on the anus, cervix, scrotum, groin, thigh, or penis.

Warts may be raised, flat, pink, or the same color as the patient's skin. They are often described as being shaped like a cauliflower and may be a single wart or a cluster of warts. Perform a gynecological examination, including cervical inspection, on women.

PSYCHOSOCIAL. When taking a sexual history and counseling on sexual matters, be sensitive to the patient's need for privacy. As of 2021, HPV is not a national reportable disease, but some states have reporting requirements. Remember that the diagnosis of an STI is very upsetting to most people. Urge the patient to notify all sexual partners of the infection promptly so that they can receive treatment. Follow up immediately with appropriate referrals.

Diagnostic Highlights

General Comments: The Pap test is the standard screening procedure for cervical cancer. Current national recommendations include the following: Pap tests should be performed at age 21 years and then every 3 years until age 30 years. The interval can then be increased to every 5 years in patients receiving a Pap test and HIV screening. A Pap test can be discontinued at 65 years if the patient has had no abnormal Pap tests in the previous 20 years. Application of acetic acid can identify the presence of HPV by showing a foamy, white appearance ("acetowhite") but should not be used for regular screening when the Pap test is available. HPV DNA confirms HPV infection. Two types of testing are completed: hybrid capture II and the polymerase chain reaction enzyme immunosorbent assay. Tissue biopsy may also be used to confirm HPV infection.

PRIMARY NURSING DIAGNOSIS

DIAGNOSIS. Risk of infection as evidenced by warts, dyspareunia, and/or unexpected rectal or vaginal bleeding

OUTCOMES. Knowledge: Infection management; Knowledge: Medication; Risk control: Sexually transmitted infections; Infection severity; Immunization behavior; Knowledge: Sexual functioning

INTERVENTIONS. Teaching: Safe sex; Medication management; Fertility preservation; Infection control; Infection protection

⁂ PLANNING AND IMPLEMENTATION

Collaborative

While collaborative treatment focuses on elimination or reduction of symptoms, elimination of abnormal (dysplastic) lesions is the goal in treating intraepithelial lesions. Treatment likely does not eliminate HPV infection or decrease the ability of the infected person to infect others. Treatment options include surgical excision, chemical ablation, and cryotherapy, but each should be used carefully so as not to damage healthy tissue. Note that warts may recur after treatment because the virus is latent in healthy skin around the lesion. No single treatment is recommended; treatment depends on the size, shape, number, and location of lesions as well as on the cost and side effects of the treatment or the preference of the patient. Treatment generally occurs over weeks and months with medications that are applied topically to the area of infection.

Surgical treatment has the advantage over medical treatment because it may lead to complete elimination of the infection. Types of surgery include cryosurgery; electrodesiccation, loop electrosurgical excision procedure, or simple surgical excision.

Pharmacologic Highlights

Medication or Drug Class	Dosage	Description	Rationale
Immune-response modifiers	Varies by drug	Imiquimod, interferon alfa	Reduce or eliminate external anogenital warts or condylomata acuminatea; treatment continues until warts are completely cleared to a maximum of 16 wk

(highlight box continues on page 558)

Pharmacologic Highlights (continued)

Medication or Drug Class	Dosage	Description	Rationale
Cytotoxic agents	Varies by drug	Antiproliferative drugs: podofilox, podophyllin, 5-fluorouracil; chemodestructive or keratolytic agents: salicylic acid, trichloroacetic acid (TCA), bichloracetic acid (BCA)	Cause cell death or necrosis of warts; duration of treatment varies

Independent

Encourage the patient to have a healthy lifestyle. Folate deficiency may increase the risk of cervical carcinogenesis, as does smoking and secondhand smoke. Assess the need for a nutrition or smoking-cessation consultation. Make sure the patient understands the use of all medications and also understands surgical treatment choices.

In addition to explanations of all current treatments, teach patients strategies to prevent reinfection or infecting others. Provide additional instruction on transmission and identification of symptoms of other STIs. Because of the confidential and private nature of the health history and health teaching, interact with the patient in a private location where you are unlikely to be interrupted. While a list of partners for notification and treatment is not essential with HPV infection, it may be helpful so that the partners can be examined. Note that this procedure is apt to be embarrassing and stressful for the patient, who will require support and a nonjudgmental approach from the nurse. Teach the patient safe sex behaviors (see Discharge and Home Healthcare Guidelines).

An HPV vaccine available in North America prevents infection by HPV types 6, 11, 16, and 18 and is most effective when given before the onset of sexual activity. Current recommendation by the Centers for Disease Control and Prevention (CDC) is to vaccinate preadolescents beginning at age 11 or 12 years with a series of two injections 6 months apart. The CDC also recommends that adolescents and young adults ages 15 to 26 years receive three doses of the vaccination if they have not previously received it. Give patients and their families accurate information about the HPV vaccination. Skepticism, religious concerns, and fears that the vaccine will precipitate early sexual behavior in preadolescents have limited the numbers of teens receiving the preventative treatment. Provide the evidence to patients and their families about the importance of prevention.

Evidence-Based Practice and Health Policy

Boakye, E., Osazuwa-Peters, N., Lopez, J., Pham, V., Tobo, B., Wan, L., Schootman, M., & McElroy, J. (2021). Disparities in human papillomavirus (HPV) vaccine initiation and completion based on sexual orientation among women in the United States. *Human Vaccines & Immunotherapeutics*, *17*, 428–433.

- The authors aimed to compare HPV vaccine initiation of heterosexual women as compared to lesbian and bisexual women. They used the National Health and Nutrition Examination Survey data between 2009 and 2016 ($N = 3,017$) for females ages 18 to 34 years. HPV vaccination initiation was defined as reported receipt of at least one dose of the vaccine, and completion was defined as receipt of the three recommended doses. Approximately 12% of the sample identified as lesbian or bisexual.
- Compared to heterosexual women, lesbian/bisexual women were 60% more likely to initiate and 63% more likely to complete the HPV vaccine. However, both groups (heterosexual women and lesbian and bisexual women) had lower rates than the Healthy People 2020 target, which was 80%. Strategies need to be implemented to increase both initiation and completion of HPV vaccination in women.

DOCUMENTATION GUIDELINES

• History: Onset of symptoms, risk factors
• Physical response: General symptoms; changes in skin appearance
• Response to treatment, lessening of symptoms

DISCHARGE AND HOME HEALTHCARE GUIDELINES

Instruct the patient about safe sexual practices. If the patient has several sexual partners, encourage the patient to receive regular checkups to screen for STIs. Stress the following points:

• Remind patients that latex condoms are the only form of birth control known to decrease the chance of contracting an STI. Condom use may reduce the transmission of HPV, but use does not eliminate the risk of infection.
• Remind patients that treatment does not eliminate the possibility of HPV transmission; the latent virus still may be present in tissues near treated areas.
• Provide the patient and partner with the STI hotline number: 1-800-232-4636. High-risk populations are targeted for sexual health education, screening, and vaccination due to increased rates of STIs and include detained adults and juveniles, men who have sex with men, and adolescent girls who binge drink (five or more drinks).
• Explain that there is a direct correlation among anogenital HPV infection, age of first intercourse, and the lifetime number of sexual partners.
• Anal cancer is associated with male sexual practices for men who have sex with men, such as engaging in receptive anal intercourse.
• HPV vaccine is available for preadolescents; the recommended time for administration is at 11 to 12 years of age.

Hydronephrosis

DRG Category:	659
Mean LOS:	8.1 days
Description:	SURGICAL: Kidney and Ureter Procedures for Non-Neoplasm With Major Complication or Comorbidity
DRG Category:	693
Mean LOS:	5.1 days
Description:	MEDICAL: Urinary Stones With Major Complication or Comorbidity
DRG Category:	694
Mean LOS:	2.7 days
Description:	MEDICAL: Urinary Stones Without Major Complication or Comorbidity

Hydronephrosis is the distention of the pelvis and calyces of one or both kidneys, resulting in thinning of the renal tubules, because of obstructed urinary flow. The obstruction can be anatomic or pathological, acute or chronic, and/or in one kidney or both. When the obstruction is a stone or kink in one of the ureters, only one kidney is damaged. The obstruction causes backup, resulting in increased pressure in the kidneys. If the pressure is low to moderate, the kidney may dilate with no obvious loss of function.

Over time, intermittent or continuous high pressure causes irreversible nephron destruction, and the urinary stasis may lead to infection and ultimately to sepsis. If the patient has a chronic partial obstruction, the kidneys lose their ability to concentrate urine. The kidneys may lose renal mass and atrophy and have a lowered resistance to infection and pyelonephritis because of urinary stasis. If hydronephrosis is caused by an acute obstructive uropathy (any disease of the urinary tract), the patient may develop a paralytic ileus. If bilateral hydronephrosis is left untreated, renal failure can result. At the time of death, approximately 3% of the U.S. population has hydronephrosis. In addition to renal failure, other complications include fluid and electrolyte imbalances, urinary stasis, renal calculus formation, hypertension, infection, sepsis, and septic shock.

CAUSES

Any anatomic or functional process from the kidneys to the urethral meatus that interrupts the flow of urine can cause hydronephrosis. The most common types of obstruction are caused by prostate hypertrophy (enlargement), renal calculi that form in the renal pelvis or drop into the ureter, or urethral strictures. More unusual causes include structure of the ureter or bladder outlet, tumors pressing on the ureter, congenital abnormalities, pregnancy, cancer, blood clots, and a neurogenic bladder. Note that during pregnancy, hydronephrosis is normal because of hormonal changes and compression on the ureters. It generally resolves during the postpartum period.

GENETIC CONSIDERATIONS

Hereditary hydronephrosis is an autosomal dominant trait that causes pelviureteric junction obstruction and has been linked to mutations in the gene *TBX18*. There is evidence supporting possible contributions at several different loci resulting in genetic heterogeneity for this condition.

SEX AND LIFE SPAN CONSIDERATIONS

Hydronephrosis can occur in patients of either gender, regardless of age. Men age 60 years and older with prostate difficulties have a higher risk of hydronephrosis than women of the same age. The most common causes of hydronephrosis in women are gynecological cancers and pregnancy; because of the frequency of these conditions, rates of hydronephrosis are higher in women than men. When cervical cancer is complicated by hydronephrosis, experts suggest that women may have a higher mortality and morbidity than when it does not occur. Urinary tract obstruction is rare in children. In young adults, calculi are the most common causes of hydronephrosis, whereas in children, reflux and ureteropelvic junction obstruction are the most common causes.

HEALTH DISPARITIES AND SEXUAL/GENDER MINORITY HEALTH

Ethnicity, race, and sexual/gender minority status have no known effect on the risk for hydronephrosis.

GLOBAL HEALTH CONSIDERATIONS

While hydronephrosis occurs around the world, no global data are available.

ASSESSMENT

HISTORY. Ask the patient to describe any recent history of mild or severe renal or flank pain that radiates to the groin or a history of fever. Elicit a description of urinary patterns to determine if burning sensations or abnormal color have occurred. The patient may be completely anuric (no urine flow) or experience polyuria (large urine output) or nocturia (excessive urination at night) because of a partial urinary obstruction. Establish if women of childbearing years are pregnant. Determine if the patient has a history of any chronic conditions such as diabetes mellitus, genitourinary or gynecological cancer, or prostate problems. Ask about vomiting, nausea, or abdominal fullness. Establish any history of blood clots, bladder problems, or prior urinary difficulties. Some patients will report very mild or even no symptoms.

PHYSICAL EXAMINATION. The most common symptoms are **pain** and **changes in urinary pattern** (anuria, polyuria, or nocturia). In acute hydronephrosis, pain is more pronounced, whereas in chronic hydronephrosis, the pain may be minimal or absent. The location of pain may help identify the location of the obstruction. Upper ureteral or renal pelvic obstruction may lead to flank pain, whereas lower ureteral obstruction may cause pain radiating to the labia or scrotum. Inspect the flank area for asymmetry, which indicates the presence of a renal mass. Inspect the male urethra for stenosis, injury, or phimosis (narrowing so that the foreskin cannot be pushed back over the glans penis). A genitourinary (GU) examination is performed in the female patient to inspect and palpate for vaginal, uterine, and rectal lesions. When the flank area is palpated, a large fluctuating soft mass may be felt in the kidney area that represents the collection of urine in the renal pelvis. Palpate the abdomen to help identify tender areas. If the hydronephrosis is the result of bladder obstruction, markedly distended urinary bladder may be felt. Gentle pressure on the urinary bladder may result in leaking urine from the urethra because of bladder overflow. Rectal examination may reveal enlargement of the prostate or renal or pelvic masses.

PSYCHOSOCIAL. Although hydronephrosis is a treatable condition, the patient is likely to be upset and anxious. Many find GU examinations embarrassing. Urinary catheterization can also be a stressful event, particularly if it is not performed by someone of the same sex. If the patient's renal condition has been permanently affected, determine the patient's ability to cope with a serious chronic condition.

Diagnostic Highlights

Test	Normal Result	Abnormality With Condition	Explanation
Ultrasonography	Normal kidney and ureters	Distention of the renal pelvis and calyces	Obstruction of urine outflow
Serum creatinine	0.51–1.21 mg/dL	> 2 mg/dL if renal damage has occurred	Decreased ability of glomerulus to filter creatinine leads to accumulation in the blood
Blood urea nitrogen	8–21 mg/dL	May be elevated	Urinary tract obstruction with diffusion of urea nitrogen back into bloodstream through renal tubules may occur
Urinalysis and culture	Minimal numbers of red and white blood cells; no bacteria; clear urine with no occult blood and no protein	Urinary tract infection may occur with presence of bacteria and abnormally increased numbers of red and white blood cells; colony counts as low as 100–10,000 bacteria/mL may indicate infection; bacteriuria: more than one organism per oil-immersion field; pyuria: more than eight leukocytes per high-power field	Urinary retention may lead to infection

Other Tests: Serum electrolytes, computed tomography, magnetic resonance imaging, complete blood count, IV pyelogram (excretory urogram), retrograde pyelogram, renal ultrasound, radionuclide studies

PRIMARY NURSING DIAGNOSIS

DIAGNOSIS. Risk for infection as evidenced by dysuria, pain on urination, hematuria, and/ or fever

OUTCOMES. Knowledge: Infection control; Infection severity; Knowledge: Medications; Knowledge: Disease process

INTERVENTIONS. Infection control; Tube care: Urinary; Infection protection; Medication management; Teaching: Disease process

PLANNING AND IMPLEMENTATION

Collaborative

Temporary urinary drainage may be achieved by a nephrostomy or ureterostomy. Other options are ureteral, urethral, or suprapubic catheterization. When no infection is present, immediate surgery is not necessary even if there is complete obstruction and anuria. Urologists often place a ureteral stent, which is performed along with a cystoscopy and retrograde pyelography. Stents can bypass an obstruction and dilate the ureter for further evaluation and treatment such as a percutaneous nephrostomy tube, which may be placed when a retrograde stent cannot be passed because of an obstruction in the ureter. Advances in endoscopic and percutaneous instrumentation have reduced the surgical role, although some cases of hydronephrosis still require treatment with open surgery. Many surgeons will wait until acid-base, fluid, and electrolyte balances are restored before operating. Surgery includes options such as prostatectomy for benign prostatic hypertrophy, tumor removal, and dilation of urethral strictures.

When bilateral complete urinary obstruction is relieved, the patient usually has massive polyuria and excessive natriuresis (sodium loss in the urine). In general, the physician will prescribe the replacement of two-thirds of the loss of urinary volume per day to be replaced by salt-containing IV solutions. Further expansion of the extracellular volume may sustain the diuresis. With impaired renal function, a diet low in sodium, potassium, and protein is often prescribed. Preoperative diet restrictions are sometimes used to limit the progression of renal failure before surgical removal of the obstruction.

The urinary drainage system requires close monitoring. Check the color, consistency, odor, and amount of urine hourly and as needed. Inspect the tube insertion site for signs of infection (purulent drainage, swelling, redness) and bleeding. If the tube is obstructed, follow the appropriate protocol for either irrigation or physician notification. Clamp the drainage tube only after specific discussion with the physician.

Pharmacologic Highlights

Medication or Drug Class	Dosage	Description	Rationale
Antibiotics	Varies with drug	Anti-infectives to manage bacterial infections: Trimethoprim sulfamethoxazole (Bactrim, Septra), ciprofloxacin hydrochloride (Cipro)	Treatment based on bacterial sensitivity as well as the ability of the antibiotic to concentrate in the urinary system; course of treatment is at least 1–4 wk
Analgesics	Varies with drug	Acetaminophen; mild narcotics	Relieve pain

Independent

The patient requires careful fluid balance. Weigh the patient at the same time of day on the same scale with the same clothing. Elicit the patient's and family's support in maintaining an accurate record of fluid intake and output. Assess the patient for fluid and electrolyte imbalances, particularly at the time of removal of the obstruction.

Pay particular attention to the patient's response to the illness. Respect the patient's privacy by isolating the patient from others during urinary drainage system insertion and insertion site care. Provide an honest appraisal of the patient's condition and answer all questions. Note that patients link urinary functioning to sexual functioning. Be open to and supportive of the patient's fears of sexual dysfunction and provide accurate information.

Provide meticulous skin care. Request a consultation from the enterostomal nurse for unusual problems.

Evidence-Based Practice and Health Policy

Laquerre, J. (2020). Hydronephrosis: Diagnosis, grading, and treatment. *Radiologic Technology*, *92*, 135–151.

- The author described hydronephrosis as dilation of the renal collecting system. The aim was to explore the causes of hydronephrosis and its effects on the urinary system, presenting signs, symptoms, diagnostic techniques, and the role of various imaging specialists. In addition, there is an explanation of the grading scale for hydronephrosis and the common diagnostic tests used to diagnose the condition. Most commonly, sonography is performed initially to confirm suspected hydronephrosis. Other diagnostic tests included radiographic IV urography, computed tomography, magnetic resonance imaging, nuclear medicine radioisotope scanning techniques, excretory urography, and cystoscopy.
- The author noted that retroperitoneal sonography of the kidneys and bladder using color Doppler is a reliable modality for evaluating hydronephrosis in the emergency department. The author also described the Society for Fetal Urology score to indicate severity, ranging from stage 0 (no hydronephrosis) to 4 (severe hydronephrosis including dilation of the renal pelvis and all calyces plus thinning of the renal functional tissue).

DOCUMENTATION GUIDELINES

- Physical changes: Abdominal pain, abdominal distention, bladder distention, signs of infection (painful urination, cloudy urine, fever, fatigue)
- Fluid balance: Daily weights, intake and output, description and appearance of urine
- Emotional response: Anxiety, coping, depression, response to analgesia
- Presence of complications: Infection, urinary tract obstruction, electrolyte imbalance

DISCHARGE AND HOME HEALTHCARE GUIDELINES

PREVENTION. Teach the importance of adequate fluids. Explain the importance of notifying the physician at the first signs of inability to void or of urinary infection, such as burning or painful urination, cloudy urine, rusty or smoky urine, blood-tinged urine, foul odor, flank pain, or fever.

MEDICATIONS. Be sure the patient, family, or other caregiver understands all medications, including the dosage, route, action, and adverse effects. Encourage the patient to take the entire course of antibiotics as prescribed.

CARE OF INDWELLING CATHETERS. Teach the patient, family, or other caregiver how to drain a Foley catheter or nephrostomy tube and to examine the insertion site for infection. Encourage older patients with a family history of benign prostatic hypertrophy or prostatitis to have annual medical checkups.

Hypercalcemia

DRG Category:	640
Mean LOS:	4.5 days
Description:	MEDICAL: Miscellaneous Disorders of Nutrition, Metabolism, Fluids, and Electrolytes With Major Complication or Comorbidity

Hypercalcemia occurs with a serum calcium level above 10.5 mg/dL in the bloodstream, although clinical manifestations generally occur at concentrations exceeding 12 mg/dL. It develops when an influx of calcium into the circulation overwhelms the calcium regulatory hormones (parathyroid hormone [PTH] and metabolites of vitamin D) and renal calciuric mechanisms (calcium excretion in the urine) or when there is a primary abnormality of one or both of these hormones.

Calcium is vital to the body for the formation of bones and teeth, blood coagulation, nerve impulse transmission, cell permeability, and normal muscle contraction. Although 98% of the body's calcium is found in the bones, three forms of serum calcium exist: free or ionized calcium (50% of serum total), calcium bound to protein (primarily albumin, 45% of serum total), and calcium complexed with citrate or other organic ions (5% of serum total). Ionized calcium is resorbed into bone, absorbed from the gastrointestinal (GI) mucosa, and excreted in urine and feces as regulated by the parathyroid glands. Ionized calcium is the active, physiological component of total calcium fraction. When extracellular calcium levels rise, a sedative effect occurs within the body, causing the neuromuscular excitability of cardiac and smooth muscles to decrease and impairing renal function. The calcium precipitates to a salt, causing calculi to form, and this leads to diuresis and volume depletion.

Hypercalcemia occurs relatively often and is often mild, but may last weeks or months. It can also be serious and life threatening. At levels above 12 mg/dL, renal failure and soft tissue calcification may occur. Hypercalcemic crisis exists when the serum level reaches 14 mg/dL. Serious cardiac dysrhythmias and hypokalemia can result as the body wastes potassium in preference to calcium. Hypercalcemia at this level can cause coma and cardiac arrest. It is considered to be a serious electrolyte imbalance, with a mortality rate as high as 50% when not treated quickly. Hypercalcemia is a common metabolic emergency, and approximately 10% to 20% of patients with cancer develop it at some point during their disease. Alkalosis protects from hypercalcemia because it leads to increased calcium-protein binding and decreased ionized calcium; acidosis can induce hypercalcemia because it leads to decreased calcium-protein binding and increased ionized calcium. Prognosis of hypercalcemia associated with malignancy is also poor, with a 1-year survival rate of 10% to 30%. Complications include cardiac dysrhythmias, hypertension, kidney stones, renal failure, osteoporosis, confusion, coma, and cardiac arrest.

CAUSES

More than 90% of cases of hypercalcemia result from primary hyperparathyroidism or malignancy. Pituitary adenomas can lead to hyperparathyroidism and therefore hypercalcemia. Malignancies likely to cause hypercalcemia include squamous cell carcinoma of the lung; cancer of the breast, ovaries, prostate, bladder, kidney, neck, and head; leukemia; lymphoma; and multiple myeloma. These conditions raise serum calcium levels by destroying bone or by releasing PTH or a PTH-like substance (osteoclastic-activating factor), or prostaglandins. Other causes of hypercalcemia are vitamin D toxicity, the use of or abuse (in eating disorders) of thiazide diuretics or lithium, sarcoidosis, immobilization, renal failure, excessive administration of calcium during cardiopulmonary arrest, and metabolic acidosis.

GENETIC CONSIDERATIONS

Hypercalcemia can be heritable through a number of different mechanisms. Mutation in the gene encoding the calcium-sensing receptor (*CASR*) results in familial hypocalciuric hypercalcemia (HHC1) and neonatal severe hyperparathyroidism. Gain-of-function mutations in *CASR* result in autosomal dominant hypocalcemia. Multiple endocrine neoplasia type I is an inherited disease usually resulting in enlargement of the parathyroid, pancreas, and pituitary glands. This disorder results in an increased lifetime risk of hyperparathyroidism. Other mutations near 19q13 are also suspected, but no particular gene has yet been identified.

SEX AND LIFE SPAN CONSIDERATIONS

Hypercalcemia can occur in all people. In infants, it can be caused by ingestion of large amounts of chicken liver or vitamin D or vitamin A supplements. Children and adolescents who consume large amounts of calcium-rich foods and drinks may develop hypercalcemia. Paget disease, which causes increased bone turnover, leads to hypercalcemia in older people who are immobilized. Primary hyperparathyroidism, usually from an adenoma of a single parathyroid gland, causes most cases of hypercalcemia in people who are ambulatory and is more common in older women than in older men. Hypercalcemia related to cancer occurs equally in men and women.

HEALTH DISPARITIES AND SEXUAL/GENDER MINORITY HEALTH

Ethnicity, race, and sexual/gender minority status have no known effect on the risk for hypercalcemia.

GLOBAL HEALTH CONSIDERATIONS

Prevalence seems to vary by developed country, but differences may be related to index of suspicion by healthcare providers rather than true prevalence. No data are available in developing regions of the world.

ASSESSMENT

HISTORY. Determine a history of risk factors, with a particular focus on medications. Ask patients if they have a history of kidney stones, bone disease, endocrine/pituitary problems, or malignancies. Establish a history of lethargy, confusion, anorexia, nausea, vomiting, constipation, polyuria, or polydipsia. Ask about muscular weakness or digital and perioral paresthesia (tingling) and muscle cramps. Ask family members if the patient has manifested personality changes.

PHYSICAL EXAMINATION. The signs and symptoms are directly related to the serum calcium level and result from **reduced neuromuscular excitability** (lethargy, weakness, malaise, confusion). In some patients, hypercalcemia is discovered upon routine physical examination. Evaluate the patient's neuromuscular status for muscle weakness, hypoflexia, and decreased muscle tone. Observe for signs of confusion. Hypercalcemia slows GI transit time; therefore, assess the patient for abdominal distention, hypoactive bowel sounds, and paralytic ileus. Strain the urine for renal calculi. Assess for fluid volume deficit by checking skin turgor and mucous membranes. Auscultate the apical pulse to determine heart irregularities.

PSYCHOSOCIAL. Increased calcium in the cerebrospinal fluid may result in behavior changes. The symptoms can range from slight personality changes to the manifestations of psychosis. They may include mental confusion, impaired memory, slurred speech, or hallucinations. Assess the patient's mental status and the family's response to alterations in it.

Diagnostic Highlights

Test	Normal Result	Abnormality With Condition	Explanation
Serum calcium: Total calcium including free ionized calcium and calcium bound with protein or organic ions	8.4–10.2 mg/dL	> 10.5 mg/dL; critical value: > 14 mg/dL	Accumulation of calcium above normal levels in the extracellular fluid compartment; clinical manifestations generally occur when calcium levels are > 12 mg/dL and tend to be more severe if hypercalcemia develops rapidly; if ionized calcium cannot be measured, total serum calcium can be corrected by adding 0.8 mg/dL to the total calcium level for every 1 g/dL decrease of serum albumin below 4 g/dL; the corrected value determines whether true hypocalcemia is present. When calcium levels are reported as high or low, calculate the actual level of calcium by the following formula: Corrected total calcium (mg/dL) = (measured total calcium mg/dL) + 0.8 (4.4 measured albumin g/dL).
Serum ionized calcium: Unbound calcium; level unaffected by albumin level	4.6–5.3 mg/dL; critical value: > 6.5 mg/dL	> 5.5 mg/dL	Ionized calcium is approximately 46%–50% of circulating calcium and is the form of calcium available for enzymatic reactions and neuromuscular function; levels increase and decrease with blood pH levels; for every 0.1 pH decrease, ionized calcium increases 1.5%–2.5%
Serum parathyroid hormone level	10–65 pg/mL	Elevated in more than 90% of people with primary hyperparathyroidism	Determines presence of hyperparathyroidism

Other Tests: Because malignancy is a common cause of hypercalcemia, a search for malignancy is important. Therefore, radiographs or computed tomography are completed to rule out malignancies (breast, lung, kidney, multiple myeloma, lymphoma, leukemia), sarcoidosis, or Paget disease. Other tests include electrocardiogram (shortened ST and QT interval), urine calcium clearance, serum electrolytes, and immunoreactive parathyroid hormone.

PRIMARY NURSING DIAGNOSIS

DIAGNOSIS. Risk for injury as evidenced by bone demineralization and/or bone fracture

OUTCOMES. Hypercalcemia severity; Fluid balance; Electrolyte/acid-base balance; Risk control: Falls; Mobility; Knowledge: Personal safety; Knowledge: Medication; Neurological status: Consciousness

INTERVENTIONS. Electrolyte management: Hypercalcemia; Medication management; Medication administration; Fall prevention; Environmental management: Safety; Fluid/electrolyte management; Neurological monitoring; Exercise promotion

PLANNING AND IMPLEMENTATION

Collaborative

The goals of treatment are to reduce the serum calcium level and to identify and correct the underlying cause. Conservative measures include administering fluids to restore volume and enhance renal excretion of calcium; prescribing a low-calcium diet; eliminating calcium-containing medications (calcium supplements, calcium-containing antacids) or medications that impair calcium excretion (thiazide diuretics, lithium); and, when possible, keeping active.

In severe cases of hypercalcemia, administer large volumes of normal saline (0.9% NaCl) at a rate of 300 to 500 mL per hour until the extracellular volume is restored (usually 3 to 4 L in the first 24 hr), at which time the rate is slowed and the infusion is maintained to promote renal calcium excretion. The physician may prescribe furosemide with the saline infusion, which helps prevent fluid volume overload. Monitor for signs of congestive heart failure in patients who are receiving 0.9% NaCl solution diuresis therapy. If hypercalcemia is the result of a malignancy, then surgery, chemotherapy, or radiation may be used.

Pharmacologic Highlights

Medication or Drug Class	Dosage	Description	Rationale
Furosemide (Lasix)	20–40 mg IV bid–qid	Loop diuretic	Excretion of sodium also leads to calcium excretion; furosemide lowers serum calcium as natriuresis occurs; used with saline diuresis when clinical evidence of heart failure occurs
Calcitonin	4–8 units/kg IM or SC daily 6–12 hr	Calcium regulator	Inhibits bone resorption and increases renal calcium excretion; lowers calcium 1–3 mg/dL within several hours, but hypocalcemic effect wanes after several days
Biphosphonates	Varies by drug	Pamidronate, zole-dronic acid, etidro-nate, alendronate	Inhibits bone reabsorption and reduces serum calcium levels, particularly in hypercalcemia in malignancy and Paget disease

Other Drugs: Denosumab (monoclonal antibody that prevents osteoclast formation and decreased bone resorption). Bulk laxatives and stool softeners; loop rather than thiazide diuretics; glucocorticoids such as prednisone (inhibit serum calcium by inhibiting cytokine release, inhibiting intestinal calcium absorption, and increasing urinary calcium excretion).

Independent

Encourage sufficient fluid intake. Encourage ambulation as soon as possible to strengthen bones and prevent calcium loss; if patients are bedridden, use care to handle them to prevent fractures. Reposition bedridden patients frequently and encourage range-of-motion exercises to promote circulation and prevent urinary stasis as well as calcium loss from bone. Choose fluids containing sodium unless contraindicated. Discourage a high intake of calcium-rich foods and fluids and provide adequate bulk in the diet to help prevent constipation. If confusion or other mental symptoms occur, institute safety precautions as necessary. Orient the patient frequently and design a safe environment to prevent falls.

Evidence-Based Practice and Health Policy

Thongprayoon, C., Cheungpasitporn, W., Hansrivijit, P., Medaura, J., Api Chewcharat, A., Mao, M., Bathini, T., Vallabhajosyula, S., Thirunavukkarasu, S., & Erickson, S. (2020). Impact of changes in serum calcium levels on in-hospital mortality. *Medicina, 56,* 106–120.

- The authors aimed to assess the association between changes in calcium levels during hospitalization and mortality. They reviewed 9,868 cases of patients with at least two changes in serum calcium levels. They defined serum calcium changes as the absolute difference between the maximum and the minimum calcium levels.
- Hospital mortality progressively increased with higher calcium changes when adjusted for age, sex, race, principal diagnosis, comorbidity, kidney function, acute kidney injury, number of measurements of serum calcium, and hospital length of stay. The authors concluded that larger serum calcium changes in hospitalized patients were progressively associated with increased in-hospital mortality.

DOCUMENTATION GUIDELINES

- Current mental status and any recent changes
- Physical findings: Skin turgor and appearance of mucous membranes, presence or absence of bowel sounds, presence of any muscular changes, presence or absence of renal calculi
- Response to pain medications
- Tolerance of activity
- Vital signs, pulse rhythm

DISCHARGE AND HOME HEALTHCARE GUIDELINES

Encourage ambulation and a fluid intake of 3 to 4 L of fluid per day, including acid-ash juices (e.g., cranberry juice). Explain the importance of avoiding excessive amounts of calcium-rich foods and calcium-containing medications. Caution the patient against taking large doses of vitamin D. Be sure the patient understands any medication prescribed, including dosage, route, action, and side effects. Remind the patient to report to the physician the appearance of any symptoms of flank pain, hematuria, palpitations, or irregular pulse.

Hyperchloremia

DRG Category: 640
Mean LOS: 4.5 days
Description: MEDICAL: Miscellaneous Disorders of Nutrition, Metabolism, Fluids, and Electrolytes With Major Complication or Comorbidity

Serum chloride excess, hyperchloremia, occurs when the serum chloride level is greater than 112 mEq/L. Normal serum chloride level is 97 to 107 mEq/L. Chloride is the major anion in extracellular fluid (ECF). Chloride is regulated in the body primarily through its relationship with sodium, and primarily by the kidney. Serum levels of both sodium and chloride often parallel each other.

Chloride performs a number of essential physiological functions. One is to join with hydrogen to form hydrochloric acid (HCl), which aids in digestion and activates enzymes, such as salivary amylase. Chloride also plays a role in maintaining the serum osmolarity and the body's water balance. The normal serum osmolarity ranges from 275 to 295 mOsm/L. Hyperchloremia, like hypernatremia, causes an increase in the serum osmolarity (the proportion of sodium and chloride ions to water in ECF). Chloride influences the acid-base balance as well. To maintain acid-base balance, the kidneys excrete chloride or bicarbonate. Each sodium ion that is reabsorbed in the renal tubules reabsorbs either a chloride or a bicarbonate ion depending on the acid-base balance of the ECF. In metabolic acidosis, the kidney excretes chloride in exchange for bicarbonate. Complications of hyperchloremia include hypotension, cardiac dysrhythmias, kidney stones, kidney failure, and coma.

CAUSES

The most common cause of hyperchloremia is body fluid loss, or dehydration, which leads to renal retention of water, sodium, and chloride. Other causes are changes in hormones, trauma, kidney failure, liver failure, diabetes insipidus, diabetic coma, and acid-base imbalances (hyperchloremic acidosis). Excessive levels of adrenal cortical hormones (corticosteroids, estrogens, androgens) can cause excess sodium levels, and thereby chloride, in the body. In head-injured patients, sodium is frequently retained, and thus chloride is also retained. In addition, hyperchloremia can be caused by any condition that allows for excessive chloride intake or absorption.

GENETIC CONSIDERATIONS

Hyperchloremia may be a feature of various genetic diseases resulting in electrolyte imbalances. Type I renal tubular acidosis causes hyperchloremia and has been demonstrated to be caused by mutations in *ATP6V1B1*, *ATP6V0A4*, and *SLC4A1*.

SEX AND LIFE SPAN CONSIDERATIONS

Infants, young children, and older people of both sexes are at particular risk for hyperchloremia because they are prone to dehydration.

HEALTH DISPARITIES AND SEXUAL/GENDER MINORITY HEALTH

Ethnicity, race, and sexual/gender minority status have no known effect on the risk for hyperchloremia.

GLOBAL HEALTH CONSIDERATIONS

No data are available, but hyperchloremia occurs around the world.

ASSESSMENT

HISTORY. Ask the patient about factors or conditions that could cause hyperchloremia, such as severe dehydration, a recent head injury, renal disease, or use of adrenal corticosteroids. Ask if the patient has recently had any of the following conditions: diarrhea, ingestion of salt water, or ingestion of very high-salt foods. Be aware that thought processes may be affected, so self-reported information may not be totally accurate. Ask about all of the patient's medications (carbonic anhydrase inhibitors, bromide-containing drugs, or large quantities of laxatives), past illnesses and surgeries, and any recent signs and symptoms that deviate from past health patterns.

PHYSICAL EXAMINATION. Patients may have no symptoms, but for symptomatic patients, the most common signs are **dyspnea, fatigue, muscle weakness,** and **tachycardia.** Physical findings depend on the source of the chloride imbalance. Assess the patient's respiratory status. If the hyperchloremia is associated with metabolic acidosis, the patient may have rapid, deep respirations. Tachycardia and hypertension may also be noted. Perform a thorough neurological assessment and note that patients may experience weakness; cognitive changes; and, if the condition is severe, mental status deterioration and loss of consciousness. Because most patients who have hyperchloremia also have hypernatremia, assess for signs and symptoms associated with this imbalance, including excessive thirst, dry mucous membranes, restlessness, agitation, irritability, muscle twitching, hyperreflexia, and seizures.

PSYCHOSOCIAL. Assess the patient's and family's knowledge and understanding of dehydration to prevent future episodes. In the trauma patient, assess the patient's and family's ability to cope with a head injury and assist the patient with understanding the effects of head injury on fluid and electrolyte regulation. Patients on corticosteroids often have to deal with complications, such as fluid retention. Assess the patient's knowledge regarding steroid use.

Diagnostic Highlights

Test	Normal Result	Abnormality With Condition	Explanation
Serum chloride	97–107 mEq/L	> 112 mEq/L; critical value: 120 mEq/L	Reflects an excess of chloride
Serum osmolarity	275–295 mOsm/L	> 295 mOsm/L; critical value: > 335 mOsm/L	Reflects increased concentration of particles in ECF

Other Tests: Serum bicarbonate, serum electrolytes, urinary anion gap

PRIMARY NURSING DIAGNOSIS

DIAGNOSIS. Deficient fluid volume related to water loss and dehydration as evidenced by thirst, dry mouth, and/or tachycardia

OUTCOMES. Hyperchloremia severity; Fluid balance; Electrolyte and acid-base balance; Hydration; Nutritional status: Food and fluid intake; Knowledge: Treatment regimen

INTERVENTIONS. Fluid/electrolyte management; IV therapy; Electrolyte monitoring; Fluid monitoring; Medication management; Nutrition management

PLANNING AND IMPLEMENTATION
Collaborative
Report any serum chloride levels greater than 112 mEq/L and observe the patient for increases in serum potassium and sodium levels as well. Note any decrease in serum bicarbonate level, which may indicate metabolic acidosis.

Severe hyperchloremia secondary to hypernatremia because of dehydration may require an IV solution of hypotonic saline, such as 0.45% sodium chloride (one-half normal saline). Infuse the solution cautiously because rapid infusion can cause a rapid shift of water into the cerebral cells, creating cerebral edema and the risk of death. Patients with hyperchloremia from metabolic acidosis may receive IV sodium bicarbonate; monitor them closely for overcorrection (metabolic alkalosis and respiratory depression). Dietary changes are seldom necessary; however, for severe conditions, a low-sodium diet prevents further accumulation of chloride and sodium.

Pharmacologic Highlights

Medication or Drug Class	Dosage	Description	Rationale
Sodium bicarbonate	IV 2–5 mEq/kg over 4–8 hr	Alkalinizing agent	Corrects metabolic acidosis; dosage is guided by laboratory values

Independent

Maintain safety measures for patients who develop neuromuscular weakness or lethargy. If the patient's mental status is affected, initiate strategies to maintain adequate airway, breathing, and circulation. Guard patients' airways by positioning them on their side. Keep the patient's mouth free of secretions. If you suspect airway compromise, insert an oral or nasal airway; if airway compromise is accompanied by impaired breathing, notify the physician immediately and prepare for endotracheal intubation. If the patient is able to take fluids by mouth, avoid drinks containing caffeine and alcohol, which can worsen dehydration.

Evidence-Based Practice and Health Policy

Yeh, P., Pan, Y., Sanchez-Pinto, L., & Luo, Y. (2020). Hyperchloremia in critically ill patients: Association with outcomes and prediction using electronic health record data. *BMC Medical Informatics and Decision Making, 20,* 302–320.

- The authors aimed to examine if the increased chloride load in IV fluid and serum chloride levels (hyperchloremia) are associated with increased morbidity and mortality in critically ill patients with sepsis. They used the Medical Information Mart for Intensive Care database to assess chloride load and hyperchloremia in association with outcomes (mortality, new acute kidney injury by day 7, and multiple organ dysfunction syndrome on day 7).
- Hyperchloremia had an independent association with increased odds of mortality, new acute kidney injury by day 7, and multiple organ failure on day 7. High chloride load was also associated with increased odds of mortality. The authors concluded that monitoring chloride levels and chloride load has the potential to improve patient outcomes.

DOCUMENTATION GUIDELINES

- Laboratory findings: Serum electrolytes, serum osmolarity; daily flowsheet for easy day-to-day comparisons
- Physical responses: Respiratory status (rate, quality, depth, ease, breath sounds); vital signs with any tachycardia or hypertension; muscle strength, steadiness of gait, ability to perform activities of daily living; fluid balance, intake and output
- Nutrition: Tolerance for dietary restrictions, interest in and understanding of diet teaching

DISCHARGE AND HOME HEALTHCARE GUIDELINES

Educate about the effect of dehydration on chloride levels. Teach the patient to report any signs and symptoms of neuromuscular weakness or changes in body weight in 1 week to the primary healthcare provider. Teach the patient to maintain a healthy diet with all the components of adequate nutrition. Teach the patient the name, dosage, route, action, and side effects of all medications, particularly those that affect chloride and sodium balance in the body.

Hyperglycemia

DRG Category:	640
Mean LOS:	4.5 days
Description:	MEDICAL: Miscellaneous Disorders of Nutrition, Metabolism, Fluids, and Electrolytes With Major Complication or Comorbidity

Hyperglycemia exists when the fasting blood glucose level is greater than 110 mg/dL or the 2-hour postprandial level is above 140 mg/dL. Prediabetes occurs when blood glucose levels are higher than normal but not high enough for a diagnosis of diabetes. This condition is sometimes called impaired fasting glucose or impaired glucose tolerance. About one in three U.S. adults aged 20 years or older—or 88 million people—have prediabetes according to the Centers for Disease Control and Prevention.

Normal blood glucose levels can be maintained between 70 and 100 mg/dL when there is an adequate balance between insulin supply and demand. In acutely ill individuals, hyperglycemia is usually not diagnosed until a random test of serum glucose level shows an increase above the 150 to 200 mg/dL range. Glucose is the most important carbohydrate in body metabolism. It is formed from the breakdown of polysaccharides, especially starch and is absorbed from the intestines into the blood of the portal vein. As it passes through the liver, glucose is converted into glycogen for storage, but the body maintains a blood level for tissue needs.

Insulin is produced by the beta cells of the pancreas, which are stimulated to release it when the blood glucose level rises. Insulin transports glucose, amino acids, potassium, and phosphate across the cell membrane. Insufficient production or ineffective use of insulin causes an elevated blood glucose level (hyperglycemia), which promotes water movement into the bloodstream from the interstitial space and intracellular fluid compartments. As blood glucose levels increase, the renal threshold for glucose reabsorption is exceeded, and glycosuria (loss of glucose in the urine) occurs. Glucose in the urine acts as an osmotic diuretic, and the patient has an increased urinary output in response that can lead to a serious fluid volume deficit. As glucose levels climb, the blood becomes more viscous, and the patient is also at risk for thromboembolic phenomena.

Insulin resistance and hyperglycemia have been linked with any critical illness or traumatic injury, and the condition has been named the "diabetes of injury." Current research has found links between hyperglycemia and poor outcomes from acute illnesses and trauma. Current thinking is that with better control of hyperglycemia, patient outcomes may improve during an acute illness. Complications of hyperglycemia include neuropathy, nephropathy, vascular damage, dehydration, and coma.

CAUSES

The two primary causes of hyperglycemia are diabetes mellitus (DM) and hyperosmolar nonketotic syndrome (HNKS). Other conditions that can lead to hyperglycemia include glucocorticoid imbalances (Cushing syndrome), increased epinephrine levels during times of extreme stress (multiple trauma, surgery), excess growth hormone secretion, excessive ingestion or administration of glucose by total parenteral nutrition or enteral feedings, and pregnancy. In patients with extreme physiological stress, such as thermal injuries, multiple trauma, or shock, a serum glucose of approximately 200 to 250 mg/dL is expected, considering the release of epinephrine that accompanies the stress response.

GENETIC CONSIDERATIONS

Hyperglycemia is a prominent feature of DM, which has a significant genetic component. Polymorphisms in the adiponectin gene have also been associated with elevated blood sugar levels as well as increased body mass index, insulin sensitivity, and type 2 diabetes in some cross-sectional studies. Glucokinase mutations are also associated with hyperglycemia and non-insulin-dependent type 2 diabetes.

SEX AND LIFE SPAN CONSIDERATIONS

Children and young adults of both sexes who are at risk for type 1 DM are between the ages of 6 months and 30 years, whereas adults older than 35 years are more at risk for type 2 DM. Older people are at highest risk for HNKS.

HEALTH DISPARITIES AND SEXUAL/GENDER MINORITY HEALTH

While there are no racial or ethnic considerations or sexual and gender minority health issues for hyperglycemia itself, there are different patterns of types 1 and 2 DM across populations (see **Diabetes Mellitus**).

GLOBAL HEALTH CONSIDERATIONS

The prevalence of DM is increasing dramatically. DM is a global epidemic, with the number of people with DM exceeding 422 million. The International Diabetes Federation states that by 2045, the number will exceed 700 million, and the countries with the most cases include the most populous countries of the world as well as Western Europe. Some experts note that type 1 DM is increasing by up to 5% each year in the Middle East, Western Europe, and Australia. Scandinavian countries have the highest prevalence rates for type 1 DM, while China and Japan have the lowest prevalence.

Type 2 DM is more common in developed countries than in developing countries. Experts suggest that in developing countries, and particularly in Africa, people ingest fewer calories and have higher levels of activity (less sedentary) than in North America and Western Europe. As countries become more developed, however, the prevalence of weight gain and type 2 DM increases dramatically. Africa will likely be the location for the largest increase in people with type 2 DM in the next decade.

⬛ ASSESSMENT

HISTORY. Ascertain if the patient has any disorders that are risk factors for hyperglycemia. Elicit a complete medication history, focusing on whether the patient has ever taken insulin or oral antidiabetic medications. Ask about polyuria (excessive urination) and polydypsia (excessive thirst). Because it is common to have large amounts of dilute urine, ask if the patient has noted a larger urinary output than usual and if the color was light yellow or clear. Determine if the patient is pregnant or has experienced a recent traumatic event or illness. Determine if the patient has been prescribed corticosteroids, which may increase blood glucose levels.

PHYSICAL EXAMINATION. The patient may not have any symptoms unless the blood glucose level has increased high enough to cause **fluid volume deficit** and **dehydration**. Perform a complete head-to-toe assessment, including a neurological examination. Patients with severe hyperglycemia also have an increased serum osmolarity (higher concentration of particles than water in the blood); when it goes above 300 mOsm/L, osmolarity causes decreased mental status. Assess the patient's level of consciousness and the cough and gag reflexes.

Inspect for signs of dehydration: dry mucous membranes, poor skin turgor, and dry scaly skin. Press gently on the patient's eyeballs; they may feel soft rather than firm. The patient's vital signs may reveal hypotension from fluid loss and tachycardia. If the dehydration has occurred for several days, the patient may have warm skin and an elevated temperature. In spite of the state of dehydration, the urine may not appear concentrated.

PSYCHOSOCIAL. Ask about the home environment, occupation, knowledge level, financial situation, and support systems, which may provide information that can be used to prevent future episodes. Determine the patient's and significant other's social, economic, and interpersonal resources to help manage a potentially chronic condition such as DM.

Diagnostic Highlights

Test	Normal Result	Abnormality With Condition	Explanation
Serum glucose level (fasting)	70–100 mg/dL	> 110 mg/dL; critical value: > 400 mg/dL	Elevation of glucose resulting from insulin deficit, insulin resistance, or pancreatic disease; fasting serum glucose > 126 mg/dL is an indication of possible DM
Serum osmolarity	275–295 mOsm/L	> 295 mOsm/L; critical value: > 335 mOsm/L	Reflects increased concentration of particles in extracellular fluid

Other Tests: Complete blood count, blood chemistries, sodium bicarbonate, blood urea nitrogen and creatinine, urine glucose and acetone

PRIMARY NURSING DIAGNOSIS

DIAGNOSIS. Deficient fluid volume related to high levels of blood glucose and hyperosmolarity as evidenced by excess urinary output and/or thirst

OUTCOMES. Hyperglycemia severity; Fluid balance; Electrolyte balance; Nutritional status: Food and fluid intake; Circulation status; Hydration; Knowledge: Medication

INTERVENTIONS. Medication management; Hyperglycemia management; Nutrition management; Electrolyte management; Electrolyte monitoring; Fluid management; Fluid monitoring; Fluid resuscitation; IV therapy

PLANNING AND IMPLEMENTATION

Collaborative

If the serum glucose level is above 250 mg/dL and the fluid balance is adequate, insulin is usually prescribed either as a subcutaneous (SC) injection or as an IV push injection. Often patients are placed on a "sliding scale" of insulin every 6 hours. If a patient has an elevated serum glucose along with a fluid volume deficit, the fluid volume deficit is corrected first, often with normal saline solution (0.9% sodium chloride), before the glucose excess. If glucose is reduced on a fluid volume–depleted patient before volume resuscitation, the vascular volume decreases, and the patient can develop hypovolemic shock.

If the patient has hyperglycemia because of DM or HNKS, management is based on the severity of symptoms. Because HNKS is associated with extraordinarily high levels of glucose (some reports describe levels higher than 1,000 mg/dL), the patient usually requires volume resuscitation followed by an insulin infusion. Often patients receive intermittent SC or IV doses of insulin as well. This should be done cautiously, however, because if the serum glucose level is reduced too rapidly, fluid shifts into the central nervous system, leading to cerebral edema and death. No matter what the diagnosis, once the glucose level and the patient are stabilized, a full work-up to determine the cause and long-term treatment is needed to prevent recurrences of hyperglycemia.

Current thinking with acutely and critically ill patients, particularly surgical patients, is that patient outcomes can be improved with more stringent control of hyperglycemia than in the past. The goal of control during the critical illness is a glucose level in the range of 80 to 125 mg/dL. Serial glucose monitoring at the bedside as frequently as every 30 minutes with point-of-care technology may be necessary during the administration of insulin through continuous insulin infusions.

Pharmacologic Highlights

Medication or Drug Class	Dosage	Description	Rationale
Insulin	Varies with severity of disease; adjusted to maintain blood glucose of 80–125 mg/dL	Hormone; hypoglycemic	Replaces deficient or absent levels of insulin

Independent

The first priority is to maintain adequate fluid balance. The action of glucose as an osmotic diuretic places the patient at risk for severe fluid volume deficits. If the patient is awake, encourage the patient to drink water and sugar-free drinks without caffeine. Because patients are usually tachycardic, caffeinated beverages are contraindicated, and they also cause increased urine output. Because severe hyperglycemia is accompanied by increased serum osmolarity and accompanying decreases in mental status, fluid replacement is accomplished by the IV route in most cases. If rapid fluid resuscitation is needed, use a large-gauge peripheral IV site with a short length to provide for rapid fluid replacement. Keep the tubing as short as possible from the IV bag or bottle and avoid long loops of tubing at a level below the patient's heart. Monitor for signs of underhydration (mental status that remains depressed, dry mucous membranes, soft eyeballs) and overhydration (pulmonary congestion, neck vein distention, shortness of breath, frothy sputum, cough).

Patients with the most severe cases of hyperglycemia have a risk of ineffective airway clearance because of decreased mental status and airway obstruction by the tongue. Have airway equipment, including an oral and nasal airway, an endotracheal tube, and a laryngoscope, near the patient's bedside at all times. If the patient develops snoring, slow respirations, or apnea, maintain the patient's airway and breathing with a manual resuscitator bag and notify the physician immediately.

If the patient has hyperglycemia because of DM or HNKS, provide appropriate patient teaching. Discuss the administration of insulin; a consistent and appropriate technique of insulin administration is critical for optimal blood glucose control. Whenever possible, have patient self-administer insulin. Encourage exercise. Instruct the patient about self-monitoring to recognize the signs and symptoms of hyperglycemia and hypoglycemia. Teach the patient and significant others how to prevent skin and lower-extremity infection, ulcers, and poor wound healing.

Evidence-Based Practice and Health Policy

Chatzi, G., Mason, T., Chandola, T., Whittaker, W., Howarth, E., Cotterill, S., Ravindrarajah, R., McManus, E., Sutton, M., & Bower, P. (2020). Sociodemographic disparities in non-diabetic hyperglycaemia and the transition to type 2 diabetes: Evidence from the English Longitudinal Study of Ageing. *Diabetic Medicine, 37*, 1536–1544.

- The authors explored whether there are social inequalities in nondiabetic hyperglycemia (NDH) and in transitions to type 2 diabetes mellitus. The authors used the English Longitudinal Study of Ageing (ELSA) from 2004 to 2016 to study patients ($N = 9,143$) in three groupings: low risk, NDH, and type 2 diabetes.
- NDH was more prevalent in older participants, those reporting a disability, those living in deprived areas, and those with more disadvantaged social classes. Older participants with

NDH were less likely to progress to undiagnosed type 2 diabetes. Individuals with NDH with limiting long-standing illness who were from disadvantaged social classes were more likely to progress to type 2 diabetes. Disparities included the greater likelihood of disadvantaged social groups with NDH developing type 2 diabetes and greater likelihood of advantaged social groups with NDH becoming low risk.

DOCUMENTATION GUIDELINES

- Fluid balance and nutrition: Intake and output, color of urine, amount and type of volume resuscitation, "sliding scale" and response to insulin, signs of hypoglycemia or hyperglycemia, daily weights, signs of dehydration or rehydration
- Effectiveness of diet, medications, and activity on blood glucose
- Patient's understanding of teaching: Pathophysiology of underlying disorder, nutrition education, insulin and technique of administration, oral hypoglycemic medication, exercise program, self-monitoring of blood glucose (if appropriate), prevention of complications
- Complications such as skin lesions, hypoglycemic reactions

DISCHARGE AND HOME HEALTHCARE GUIDELINES

Teach the patient strategies for managing the disorder. Provide a written list of all medications, including dosage, route, time, and side effects. If appropriate, give the patient a phone number to call if the patient has any problems with self-administration of insulin or self-monitoring of blood glucose. Provide the patient with a list of referrals, such as an outpatient diabetic clinic or community contacts, for follow-up care and information. Provide a list of equipment and materials needed for home care. Give the patient any pamphlets or written materials about the management of hyperglycemia. Patients should also be taught "sick day" rules for managing their diabetes when ill. Examples of sick day rules are to continue insulin doses when nausea and vomiting occurs, check blood glucose more frequently, and call the healthcare provider if unable to drink fluids.

Hyperkalemia

DRG Category: 640
Mean LOS: 4.5 days
Description: MEDICAL: Miscellaneous Disorders of Nutrition, Metabolism, Fluids, and Electrolytes With Major Complication or Comorbidity

Normal serum levels of potassium range from 3.5 to 5.3 mEq/L. Hyperkalemia, defined as a potassium level greater than 5.5 mEq/L, is usually associated with impaired renal function, but it may also be produced by treatments for other disorders. Mild hyperkalemia is from 5 to 6 mEq/L, moderate hyperkalemia is from 6.1 to 7 mEq/L, and severe hyperkalemia is 7 mEq/L and greater. It is diagnosed in up to 10% of hospitalized patients. Increased potassium intake, reduction in potassium excretion, and shift of potassium out of the cells all may result in hyperkalemia. Because potassium plays a key role in cardiac function, a high serum potassium level is of great concern. It is sometimes the first symptom of cardiac arrest.

Potassium functions as the major intracellular cation and balances sodium in the extracellular fluid (ECF) to maintain electroneutrality in the body. It is excreted by the kidneys. The normal ratio is approximately 40 mEq of potassium in 1 L of urine. Potassium is not stored in the body and needs to be replenished daily through dietary sources. It is also exchanged for hydrogen when changes in the body's pH call for a need for cation exchange. This situation occurs in metabolic alkalosis or other alterations that lead to increased cellular uptake of potassium, including insulin excess and renal failure. Potassium is regulated by two stimuli, aldosterone and hyperkalemia. Aldosterone is secreted in response to high renin and angiotensin II or hyperkalemia. The plasma level of potassium, when high, also increases renal potassium loss. Complications of hyperkalemia include altered neuromuscular control, respiratory paralysis, cardiac dysrhythmias (ventricular flutter or ventricular fibrillation), and sudden cardiac death.

CAUSES

Factors that result in decreased potassium excretion include oliguric renal failure, potassium-sparing diuretics (e.g., spironolactone), multiple transfusions or transfusions of stored blood, decrease in adrenal steroids, and NSAIDs. Too much potassium is taken into the body by overuse of oral potassium supplements, inappropriate IV administration of potassium, or excessive use of potassium-based salt substitutes.

Transcellular shift of potassium from within the cells to the ECF can also lead to hyperkalemia. This situation occurs in tumor lysis syndrome, rhabdomyolysis, strenuous and prolonged exercise, massive tissue destruction (hemolysis, major burns), metabolic acidosis, and insulin deficiency with hyperglycemia. Other causes include severe digitalis toxicity and the use of beta-adrenergic blockers and the drugs heparin, captopril, and lithium. Hyperkalemia can also be produced by adrenocortical insufficiency and hypoaldosteronism, and it may occur in eating disorders for people with little sodium in their diet.

GENETIC CONSIDERATIONS

Several genetic disorders can result in hyperkalemia. Familial hyperkalemia and hypertension (pseudohypoaldosteronism type II) is an autosomal dominant disorder caused by overexpression of *WNK1* kinase or loss of function of *WNK4*. Symptoms include hyperkalemia, hypertension, and low renin, despite a normal glomerular filtration rate.

SEX AND LIFE SPAN CONSIDERATIONS

Hyperkalemia can occur at any age and in both sexes. Men seem to be more prone to hyperkalemia than women, although the reasons are unknown. It may be more common in older adults because renal failure and potassium replacement therapy are more common in this group. Infants and older adults are at most risk for adverse consequences.

HEALTH DISPARITIES AND SEXUAL/GENDER MINORITY HEALTH

Ethnicity, race, and sexual/gender minority status have no known effect on the risk for hyperkalemia.

GLOBAL HEALTH CONSIDERATIONS

Hospitalized patients around the globe experience hyperkalemia at rates that are likely similar to the United States and Western Europe.

ASSESSMENT

HISTORY. Take a thorough history of medications and dietary patterns to determine if excess potassium is a result of excess ingestion. Ask if patients have a history of eating disorders. Because hyperkalemia is a side effect of a disease process (as in renal failure) or a treatment (as in overuse of potassium supplements), a careful history of all past and present illnesses is important. Determine if the patient has diabetes mellitus. The symptoms of potassium excess include nausea and diarrhea because of hyperactivity of the gastrointestinal (GI) smooth muscle. Patients often experience muscle weakness, which may extend to paralysis if severe. A complaint of general weakness is an early sign of hyperkalemia. A history of heart irregularities, dizziness, and postural hypotension may be reported.

PHYSICAL EXAMINATION. Many individuals have no symptoms. The most common effects of hyperkalemia are **muscle weakness, fatigue,** and **nausea.** Cardiac symptoms are reflected in the electrocardiogram (ECG) tracings (see Diagnostic Highlights). Heart sounds may reveal a slowed overall rate with or without irregular or extra beats.

Neuromuscular effects are primarily on the peripheral nervous system, leading to significant muscular weakness that progresses upward from legs to trunk. The muscles of respiration may be affected, as well as those that produce voice. Paresthesia of the face, feet, hands, and tongue may occur. The patient may have signs of a paralytic ileus such as hypoactive or absent bowel sounds. General anxiety and irritability, or depression, may also be present, and the patient may have a low urinary output.

PSYCHOSOCIAL. Feelings of physical weakness can increase the sense of powerlessness. The patient may experience feelings of irritability, restlessness, depression, and confusion. In addition, if the condition is caused by nonadherence to a medication regimen, the patient may feel personally responsible for the problem.

Diagnostic Highlights

Test	Normal Result	Abnormality With Condition	Explanation
Serum potassium	3.5–5.3 mEq/L	> 5.5 mEq/L; critical value: > 6 mEq/L	Potassium excess is reflected in serum and ECF compartment
ECG and continuous cardiac monitoring	Normal PQRST pattern	Early: Increased T-wave amplitude or peaked T waves Middle: Prolonged PR interval and QRS duration, atrioventricular conduction delay, loss of P waves Late: Progressive widening on QRS complex and merging with T wave to produce sine wave pattern	Cardiac toxicity does not correlate well with degree of hyperkalemia; depolarization is prolonged, and bradycardia may occur along with atrioventricular block
Transtubular potassium gradient (TTKG): formula is (urine K × serum osmolarity) (serum K × urine osmolarity) (Note: K is potassium level)	Normal value: 8–9	In hyperkalemia, higher than normal levels of potassium are excreted in the urine; TTKG > 10	Index that reflects the conservation of potassium in the renal collecting ducts; estimates the ratio of potassium in the lumen of collecting ducts as compared to peritubular capillaries

Other Laboratory Tests: Blood chemistry and electrolyte levels, calcium, glucose, digitalis level (if patient is on digitalis), urinalysis, cortisol, aldosterone level

PRIMARY NURSING DIAGNOSIS

DIAGNOSIS. Decreased cardiac output related to ineffective cardiac pumping and cardiac arrest as evidenced by shortness of breath, apnea, and/or heart rate irregularities

OUTCOMES. Hyperkalemia severity; Electrolyte and acid-base balance; Cardiac pump effectiveness; Circulation status; Tissue perfusion; Fluid balance; Vital signs

INTERVENTIONS. Electrolyte management: Hyperkalemia; Medication management; Medication administration; Fluid management; Cardiac care: Acute; Code management; Dysrhythmia management; IV therapy; Electrolyte monitoring; Fluid monitoring

▓ PLANNING AND IMPLEMENTATION

Collaborative

If hyperkalemia is not severe, it can often be remedied by simply eliminating potassium supplements or potassium-sparing diuretics and drugs that lead to the disorder.

In more serious situations, pharmacologic therapy is important. Be aware of concerns related to sodium retention when using sodium polystyrene sulfonate (cation exchange resin), which is given orally or by enema. Monitor the patient's response to the medication; if no stools result, notify the physician. Emergency management of hyperkalemia is threefold with IV administration of bicarbonate, calcium, and insulin given together with 50% dextrose. A thorough search needs to be made for the cause, and cation exchange resins may be needed in addition to other treatments to maintain potassium at normal levels. Excess potassium can also be removed by dialysis. This approach is reserved for situations in which less aggressive techniques have proved ineffective. Hemodialysis takes longer to initiate but is more effective than peritoneal dialysis.

Pharmacologic Highlights

Medication or Drug Class	Dosage	Description	Rationale
Calcium gluconate	10 mg of a 10% solution IV over 2–3 min	Electrolyte replacement	Decreases membrane excitability; one dose lasts 30–60 min; dose may be repeated after 5–10 min if no change in ECG occurs
Insulin	10–20 units of regular insulin IV	Hormone	Lowers serum potassium by enabling more potassium to enter the cell
Glucose	25–50 g IV	Sugar	Protects the patient from a hypoglycemic reaction
Sodium polystyrene sulfonate (Kayexalate)	Orally or by enema: 15 g/60 mL in 20–100 mL sorbitol to facilitate passage of resin through intestinal tract	Cation exchange resin: 0.5–1 mEq/L of potassium is removed with each enema, but an equivalent amount of sodium is retained	Exchanges sodium for potassium in the GI tract, leading to the elimination of potassium

Other Drugs: As an emergency measure, sodium bicarbonate delivered IV (one ampule of a 7.5% $NaHCO_3$ solution) increases pH and causes potassium to shift into the cells; it is particularly effective in treating metabolic acidosis. Note that pseudohyperkalemia

(highlight box continues on page 580)

Pharmacologic Highlights (continued)

(false elevation of potassium) may occur from an improper blood-drawing technique with hemolysis, laboratory error, leukocytosis, and thrombocytosis. Other medications are albuterol (has additive effect with insulin and glucose), loop diuretics such as furosemide, and magnesium sulfate. Patiromer sorbitex calcium may also be used as a cation exchange polymer.

Independent

Provide clear explanations and allow the patient to express concerns throughout the treatment course. Involve family members and the support system in teaching. Patients who are experiencing hyperkalemia should avoid foods high in potassium. These include potatoes, beet greens, bananas, orange juice, dried fruit, coffee, tea, and chocolate. Draw blood samples to ensure accurate potassium-level measurement. Do not draw a sample from above an IV site where potassium is infusing, make certain the sample gets to the laboratory quickly, do not leave a tourniquet on for prolonged periods, and do not have the patient repeatedly clench and relax the fist.

Evidence-Based Practice and Health Policy

Desai, N., Rowan, C., Alvarez, P., Fogli, J., & Toto, R. (2020). Hyperkalemia treatment modalities: A descriptive observational study focused on medication and health care resource utilization. *PLOS One, 15*, 1–10.

- Renin-angiotensin-aldosterone system inhibitor (RAASi) therapy has been shown to improve outcomes in people with congestive heart failure, diabetes, or renal disease. Hyperkalemia is a complication of therapy, which may lead to discontinuation of RAASi therapy. Patiromer is a new, sodium-free, nonabsorbed potassium. The authors studied potassium binders (patiromer and sodium polystyrene sulfonate [SPS]) and RAASi on healthcare resource utilization using the Optum's Clinformatics Data Mart.
- Overall baseline patient characteristics were a mean age 75 years, female 49%, low-income subsidy 29%, chronic kidney disease 48%, and congestive heart failure 29%. Following the continuous use of patiromer, statistically significant reductions in hospital admissions and emergency department visits were observed, which did not occur with SPS treatment.

DOCUMENTATION GUIDELINES

- Cardiac and musculoskeletal assessment: Cardiac rhythm changes and resolution of changes, respiratory effort, neuromuscular responses
- Musculoskeletal response, degree of fatigue, level of anxiety or depression
- Patient's understanding of potassium use if the cause of hyperkalemia is related to mismanagement of medication

DISCHARGE AND HOME HEALTHCARE GUIDELINES

PREVENTION. Assess the patient's understanding of the relationship between dietary intake of potassium-containing foods and supplements and hyperkalemia. Discuss strategies to improve or eliminate those factors that are leading to elevated potassium levels. Have the patient describe the changes in diet or home care that are necessary to prevent recurrence. For example, what could be done to ensure that potassium supplements are taken as prescribed?

MEDICATIONS. Evaluate the patient's understanding of the appropriate use of potassium supplements and salt substitutes.

Hyperlipoproteinemia

DRG Category: 642
Mean LOS: 4.1 days
Description: MEDICAL: Inborn and Other Disorders of Metabolism

Hyperlipoproteinemia is a condition of increased lipoprotein particles (fats) in the blood caused by an increased rate of synthesis or a decreased rate of lipoprotein breakdown. Because lipoproteins transport triglycerides and cholesterol in the plasma, an increased level may cause complications such as pancreatitis and atherosclerosis leading to coronary heart disease, myocardial infarction, stroke, and sudden death.

Lipids are a mixed group of biochemical substances manufactured by the body or derived from metabolism of ingested substances. The plasma lipids (cholesterols, triglycerides, phospholipids, and free fatty acids) are derived from dietary sources and lipid synthesis. Cholesterol and triglycerides are implicated in atherogenesis. Hyperlipemia, also known as hyperlipidemia, occurs with elevated plasma cholesterol or triglyceride levels or both and is present in all hyperlipoproteinemias.

Hyperlipidemia, an elevation of serum cholesterol or triglycerides, can be primary or secondary to another underlying condition. Lipoprotein elevation, or hyperlipoproteinemia, is described by five specific types: types I, II, III, IV, and V (Table 1).

• TABLE 1 Types of Hyperlipoproteinemia

TYPE	DEFINITION AND CAUSE	ASSESSMENT	LIPID LEVEL
I	Fat-induced hyperlipidemia or idiopathic familial hyperlipidemia, which is a rare condition caused by deficient or abnormal lipase; rare genetic disorder that is present in infancy	Recurrent attacks of severe abdominal pain after fat intake; malaise; anorexia; may be associated with pancreatitis	Triglycerides 1,000–10,000+ mg/dL, normal cholesterol
II	Familial hyperbetalipoproteinemia and essential familial hypercholesterolemia (FH) because of deficient cell surface receptors	Chest pain from prematurely accelerated coronary artery disease; tendinous xanthomas (firm masses) on Achilles tendons, tendons of hands and feet; juvenile corneal arcus (grayish ring around the cornea of the eye)	Elevated cholesterol and triglycerides, elevated low-density lipoproteins (LDL) and very low-density lipoproteins (VLDL)
III	Familial broad-beta disease xanthoma tuberosum caused by a deficient LDL receptor	Chest pain from early progression of atherosclerosis; xanthomas over elbows, knees, palms, and fingertips	Elevated cholesterol and triglycerides; elevated intermediate-density lipoproteins

(table continues on page 582)

• TABLE 1 Types of Hyperlipoproteinemia (continued)

TYPE	DEFINITION AND CAUSE	ASSESSMENT	LIPID LEVEL
IV	Endogenous hypertriglycer-idemia and hyperbeta-lipoproteinemia with an idiopathic cause; often associated with obesity and diabetes	Chest pain from early pro-gression of coronary heart disease (CHD); obesity, hypertension	Triglycerides < 1,000 mg/dL, normal cholesterol, elevated VLDL
V	Mixed hypertriglyceridemia from defective triglyceride clearance; often second-ary to other disorders such as renal disease or obesity	Abdominal pain from pan-creatitis; visual changes; xanthomas on arms and legs; enlarged liver and spleen	Triglycerides > 1,000 mg/dL, elevated choles-terol, normal LDL

CAUSES

Primary hyperlipoproteinemia results from rare genetic disorders. Secondary hyperlipopro-teinemia occurs as a manifestation of other diseases, which include hypothyroidism, nephrotic syndrome, diabetes mellitus, alcoholism, glycogen storage disease (type I), Cushing syndrome, acromegaly, anorexia, renal disease, liver diseases, immunological disorders, stress, and the use of oral contraceptives or glucocorticoids.

GENETIC CONSIDERATIONS

Familial hypercholesterolemia (FH) is an autosomal disorder caused by mutations in the LDL receptor gene (*LDLR*), leading to increases in both total cholesterol and low-density lipoprotein levels. FH is associated with an increased risk of coronary artery disease. Mutations in the lipoprotein lipase (*LPL*) gene cause autosomal recessive hyperlipoproteinemia, whereas *APOE* mutations yield a dominant disorder with incomplete penetrance. A clinically identical pheno-type is produced by mutations in the apolipoprotein B-100 gene (*APOB*). Other genetic and environmental factors may contribute.

SEX AND LIFE SPAN CONSIDERATIONS

Type I disease is a rare disorder that is present at birth. Type II disease usually causes symptoms in young adults in their 20s, but symptoms may begin as early as age 10 years. Symptoms from type III disease usually occur during the teenage years or early 20s. Type IV disease, more common than the other forms of hyperlipoproteinemia, occurs primarily in middle-aged men. Type V disease occurs in late adolescence or in the early 20s.

While there are no differences in incidence and prevalence in males and females, women with familial hypercholesterolemia are underrepresented in research and have to interrupt ther-apy during childbearing. Women also are less likely to be on guideline-recommended statin medications and less likely to be on nonstatin agents such as PCSK9 inhibitors as compared to men. As a result, women are less likely than men to achieve target low-density lipoprotein cho-lesterol (LDL-C) goals (Balla et al., 2020). While the condition is found in children, adolescents, and young adults, type IV is seen most often in middle-aged and older adults.

HEALTH DISPARITIES AND SEXUAL/GENDER MINORITY HEALTH

In general, Black persons are more likely to have hyperlipoproteinemia than White per-sons. People of Asian and Indian-Asian descent have lower prevalence than other groups in developed countries. Sexual and gender minority status has no known effect on the risk for hyperlipoproteinemia.

GLOBAL HEALTH CONSIDERATIONS

Hyperlipoproteinemia has a high prevalence in developed countries. Little is known about the prevalence in developing countries, but if trends in hyperlipoproteinemia follow obesity trends, prevalence will increase as developing regions become more urbanized.

ASSESSMENT

HISTORY. Take a thorough history of existing illnesses because secondary hyperlipoproteinemia is related to a number of other conditions. Ask if the patient has a history of renal or liver disease, diabetes mellitus, other endocrine diseases, or immune disorders. Determine the patient's height and weight, and calculate the body mass index.

Ask if the patient is taking corticosteroids or oral contraceptives and determine the extent of the patient's alcohol use. Because hyperlipoproteinemia is sometimes treated with a range of bile acid sequestrant medications, which can affect the absorption of other medications, ask if the patient is taking any of the following: warfarin, thiazides, thyroxine, beta-adrenergic blockers, fat-soluble vitamins, folic acid, diuretics, or digitoxin.

Symptoms of hyperlipoproteinemia vary, depending on which of the five types the patient has. Ask about recurrent bouts of severe abdominal pain, usually preceded by fat intake, or if the patient has experienced malaise, anorexia, or fever.

PHYSICAL EXAMINATION. Observe general appearance for **signs of obesity**, which may be an exacerbating factor for hyperlipoproteinemia. Classic symptoms include opaque ring surrounding the corneal periphery (**corneal arcus**), **xanthelasma** (lipid deposit on the eyelid), and **lipemia retinalis** (creamy appearance of the retinal vessels). Inspection may reveal papular or eruptive deposits of fat (xanthomas) over pressure points and extensor surfaces; likely locations include the Achilles tendons, hand and foot tendons, elbows, knees, and hands and fingertips (where you may observe orange or yellow discolorations of the palmar and digital creases). Ophthalmoscopic examination typically reveals reddish-white retinal vessels. Palpate the abdomen for spasm, rigidity, rebound tenderness, liver or spleen tenderness, and hepatosplenomegaly. Check for signs of hypertension and hyperuricemia.

PSYCHOSOCIAL. Hyperlipoproteinemia is not an abrupt illness; it develops over years. The patient may have developed coping mechanisms during that time, but the patient may be anxious because of accelerated symptoms of atherosclerosis and CHD. Patients may have experienced the premature death of parents from this disorder and have long-lasting fears about their own early death. Body image disturbance may also occur because of obesity or the presence of unsightly xanthomas. Cigarette smoking and alcohol misuse and dependence are known to contribute to the condition. Assess patients' patterns of use and abuse, and assess their readiness and willingness to change.

Diagnostic Highlights

Test	Normal Result	Abnormality With Condition	Explanation
Total cholesterol	Varies with age, ethnicity, and gender; desirable: < 200 mg/dL	Borderline high: 200–239 mg/dL; high: > 239 mg/dL	Used for screening and initial classification of risk of CHD; elevations determine hyperlipidemia; lipid and lipoprotein levels are collected after a 12-hr fast
LDL cholesterol (LDL-C)	Optimal: < 100 mg/dL; desirable level: < 130 mg/dL	Borderline high risk: 130–159 mg/dL; high risk: > 159 mg/dL	Elevated levels are associated with increased risk for CHD; VLDL normal range: 10–31 mg/dL; lipid and lipoprotein levels are collected after a 12-hr fast

(highlight box continues on page 584)

Diagnostic Highlights (continued)

Test	Normal Result	Abnormality With Condition	Explanation
High-density lipoprotein cholesterol (HDL-C)	Desirable: > 60 mg/dL; acceptable: 40–60 mg/dL	Low: < 40 mg/dL	Considered a major risk factor for CHD; high HDL-C (> 60 mg/dL) is considered protective; lipid and lipoprotein levels are collected after a 12-hr fast
Triglycerides	< 150 mg/dL	Borderline high risk: 150–199 mg/dL; high risk: 200–499 mg/dL; very high risk: > 500 mg/dL	Used for screening and initial classification of risk of CHD; elevations determine hyperlipidemia

Other Tests: Electrocardiogram, genetic testing, ophthalmological examination

PRIMARY NURSING DIAGNOSIS

DIAGNOSIS. Readiness for enhanced nutrition related to concern over lipoprotein accumulation and accelerated blockage of the coronary arteries as evidenced by expressing a desire to change dietary patterns

OUTCOMES. Nutritional status: Food and fluid intake, Nutrient intake; Knowledge: Medication; Knowledge: Disease process

INTERVENTIONS. Teaching: Prescribed diet; Weight management; Medication management; Nutritional monitoring; Nutrition therapy; Nutritional counseling; Exercise promotion; Mutual goal setting; Teaching: Individual

PLANNING AND IMPLEMENTATION

Collaborative

The primary treatment is dietary management, weight reduction, increased physical activity, and the restriction of saturated animal fat and cholesterol intake. Adding polyunsaturated vegetable oils to the diet helps reduce LDL-C concentration. Secondary treatment is aimed at reducing or eliminating aggravating factors, such as alcoholism, diabetes mellitus, or hypothyroidism. To reduce risk factors that contribute to atherosclerosis, the regimen includes treating hypertension, implementing an exercise program, controlling blood sugar, and stopping tobacco use. For type V hyperlipoproteinemia, female patients are taken off oral contraceptives. Medications may also be prescribed to lower the plasma concentration of lipoproteins, either by decreasing their production or by increasing their removal from plasma.

Target levels for lipoprotein are shown in Table 2.

• TABLE 2 Target Levels for Lipoprotein

LEVEL OF RISK	DEFINITION	TARGET LIPOPROTEIN LEVEL RISK
Low risk	All must be present: Nonsmoker; total cholesterol < 200 mg/dL, HDL-C > 40 mg/dL; systolic blood pressure (BP) < 120, diastolic BP < 80; no evidence of diabetes; not overweight; no family history of premature vascular disease	LDL-C should be lowered to < 160 mg/dL

• TABLE 2 Target Levels for Lipoprotein (continued)

LEVEL OF RISK	DEFINITION	TARGET LIPOPROTEIN LEVEL RISK
Moderate risk	Does not fit in low-risk or high-risk categories	LDL-C should be lowered to < 130 mg/dL; consideration to lower LDL-C to < 100 mg/dL
High risk	Any of the following present: Known coronary artery disease or other vascular disease; type 2 diabetes; over age 65 years with multiple (more than one) risk factors	LDL-C should be lowered to < 100 mg/dL; consideration to lowering LDL-C to < 70 mg/dL

In rare instances, for patients who cannot tolerate medication therapy, surgical creation of an ileal bypass may be necessary to accelerate the loss of bile acids in the stool and lower plasma cholesterol levels. For children with severe disease, surgery to create a portacaval shunt may be performed as a last resort to decrease plasma cholesterol levels. Plasma exchanges may also be used to reduce cholesterol levels.

Pharmacologic Highlights

Medication or Drug Class	Dosage	Description	Rationale
Drugs that lower LDL-C	Varies with drug	Statins such as lovastatin, pravastatin, simvastatin, fluvastatin, and atorvastatin are the first line of therapy; bile acid sequestrant resins (cholestyramine, colestipol); nicotinic acid (niacin); 3-hydroxy-3-methylglutaryl coenzyme A reductase inhibitors; estrogen in postmenopausal women	Lower the plasma concentration of lipoproteins either by decreasing their production or by increasing their removal from plasma
Drugs that increase HDL-C	Varies with drug	Nicotinic acid (niacin), estrogen in postmenopausal women	Lower the plasma concentration of lipoproteins either by decreasing their production or by increasing their removal from plasma

Independent

Teach the patient about ways to manage diet to control the disorder. Urge the patient to adhere to a 1,000- to 1,500-calorie daily diet and avoid excess sugar intake. Explain the components of the lipid profile and their ramifications and discuss various means of lowering VLDL and LDL levels and increasing HDL levels. Several dietary additions are thought to reduce LDL cholesterol, such as 1.5 cups of oatmeal with fiber-containing fruit (soluble fiber reduces LDL), 1.5 ounces of nuts (walnuts, almonds, peanuts, pecans), olive oil, and fatty fish containing omega-3 fatty acids such as mackerel, lake trout, herring, sardines, albacore tuna, and salmon.

Explain the prescribed medication regimen and provide verbal and written information to the patient or significant others. Refer to effective programs or support groups for controlling cigarette and alcohol use. Teach alternative methods of contraception to the female patient who can no longer use oral contraceptives. Encourage strategies for weight loss and weight maintenance.

A patient faces significant health threats unless the patient makes permanent lifestyle changes. Encourage the patient to verbalize fears, such as those concerning CHD. Offer support and provide clear explanations for the patient's questions about the lifestyle changes and consequences.

Evidence-Based Practice and Health Policy

Sergei, N., Pokrovsky, S., Afanasieva, O., & Ezhov, M. (2020). Therapeutic apheresis for management of Lp(a) hyperlipoproteinemia. *Current Atherosclerosis, 22,* 1–11.

* High lipoprotein(a) (Lp[a]) level is an independent cardiovascular risk factor with higher prevalence among patients with atherosclerotic cardiovascular disease (ASCVD). Lipoprotein apheresis (LA) is an effective method for elimination of lipoproteins, but it is approved only in some countries for treatment of elevated Lp(a) in people with progressive ASCVD.
* The purpose of this review was to present the information on optimal management of Lp(a) hyperlipoproteinemia by LA. Most clinical studies suggest inflammatory and prothrombotic processes begin to reduce in a few months, and there is plaque regression in 1.5 years. Treatment with LA for 2 to 5 years shows ongoing reduction by 60% to 80%. Therapeutic Lp(a) apheresis is the only method that solely targets Lp(a).

DOCUMENTATION GUIDELINES

* Physical findings: Xanthelasma, corneal arcus, organ enlargement, abdominal pain or distention, chest pain
* Response to lifestyle recommendations, smoking cessation, diet and nutrition control, exercise maintenance

DISCHARGE AND HOME HEALTHCARE GUIDELINES

PREVENTION. Teach the patient the importance of dietary and lifestyle changes. Refer the patient to a dietitian if appropriate. Provide information on smoking cessation and sensible drinking if appropriate. Discuss an exercise plan.

MEDICATIONS. Be sure the patient understands all medications, including the dosage, route, action, adverse effects, and the need for routine laboratory monitoring for lipid profiles.

COMPLICATIONS. Teach the patient to report to the physician the occurrence of signs and symptoms of CHD, such as chest pain, shortness of breath, and changes in mental status. Teach the patient the need for follow-up serum cholesterol and serum triglyceride tests. Instruct the patient to maintain a stable body weight and to adhere to any dietary restrictions before undergoing cholesterol tests. Most tests require the patient to fast for 12 hours before the test.

Hypermagnesemia

DRG Category:	640
Mean LOS:	4.5 days
Description:	MEDICAL: Miscellaneous Disorders of Nutrition, Metabolism, Fluids, and Electrolytes With Major Complication or Comorbidity

Hypermagnesemia occurs when the serum magnesium concentration is greater than 2.5 mg/dL, but signs and symptoms do not occur until the magnesium reaches 4 mg/dL. The normal serum magnesium level is 1.6 to 2.2 mg/dL. Magnesium is found in the bones—just 1% is located in the extracellular compartment, and the remainder is found within the cells. Hypermagnesemia is fairly uncommon, and generally people do not have symptoms.

Magnesium plays an important role in neuromuscular function. It also has a role in several enzyme systems, particularly the metabolism of carbohydrates and proteins, as well as maintenance of normal ionic balance (it triggers the sodium-potassium pump), osmotic pressure, myocardial functioning, and bone metabolism. Because the kidneys are able to excrete large amounts of magnesium (> 5,000 mg/day), either the patient has to ingest extraordinary amounts of magnesium or the glomerular filtration of the kidneys needs to be very depressed for the patient to develop hypermagnesemia. Complications include complete heart block, cardiac arrest, and respiratory paralysis.

CAUSES

Hypermagnesemia, although rare, usually occurs in patients with chronic renal disease, and is exacerbated by patients with renal failure who consume excessive quantities of magnesium in the form of magnesium-containing laxatives or antacids. Obstetric patients who are treated with parenteral magnesium for preeclampsia or patients with acute adrenocortical insufficiency (Addison disease) may also develop hypermagnesemia. Both hypothermia and shock can also lead to a high serum magnesium level. Other causes include lithium therapy, hypothyroidism, and depression.

GENETIC CONSIDERATIONS

Familial hypocalciuric hypercalcemia may cause a mild hypermagnesemia due to an increase in the sensitivity of the loop of Henle to calcium and magnesium ions.

SEX AND LIFE SPAN CONSIDERATIONS

Hypermagnesemia may occur at any age and across all groups, but it is seen much more frequently in the older patient with chronic renal failure. Children may develop this condition if they have renal failure or consume significant quantities of medications that contain magnesium.

HEALTH DISPARITIES AND SEXUAL/GENDER MINORITY HEALTH

Ethnicity, race, and sexual/gender minority status have no known effect on the risk for hypermagnesemia.

GLOBAL HEALTH CONSIDERATIONS

Most experts suggest that hospitalized patients around the globe experience hypermagnesemia at rates that are likely similar to the United States and Western Europe.

ASSESSMENT

HISTORY. Question the patient about precipitating factors, which may include renal failure, laxative or antacid abuse, adrenal insufficiency, diabetes, or acidosis. Medication history may include magnesium-containing laxatives such as milk of magnesia, antacids that contain magnesium hydroxide, or parenteral administration of magnesium sulfate. Ask the patient to describe any symptoms, which may range from none to full cardiopulmonary arrest. The patient may experience muscle weakness, diminished reflexes, lethargy, depression, or even paralysis as well as nausea and vomiting, flushed skin, thirst, or diaphoresis. Patients may have changes in the cardiac rhythm that lead to palpitations or dizziness.

PHYSICAL EXAMINATION. Common symptoms are **muscle weakness** and **fatigue**. Generally, patients do not develop signs and symptoms until the serum magnesium reaches more than 4 mg/dL. Assess the vital signs, which may show tachycardia, bradycardia, heart block, or hypotension. Cardiopulmonary arrest may occur when the respiratory muscles are paralyzed as a result of a magnesium level in excess of 10 mg/dL or as a consequence of depressed myocardial contractility. The patient may be disoriented, confused, or even unresponsive. When strength and movement are assessed, you may find the patient has lost deep tendon reflexes, has muscle weakness, and may even have some paralysis. Smooth muscle paralysis may lead to paralytic ileus and gastrointestinal symptoms.

PSYCHOSOCIAL. The patient with hypermagnesemia usually has chronic renal failure. Assess the patient's ability to cope with a chronic disease as well as an acute complication. The patient may have had to cope with a change in lifestyle and roles that may be compromised by the sudden and potentially life-threatening complication of hypermagnesemia. The patient's degree of anxiety about the illness should also be assessed.

Diagnostic Highlights

Test	Normal Result	Abnormality With Condition	Explanation
Serum magnesium	1.6–2.2 mg/dL	> 2.5 mg/dL; critical value: > 4.9 mg/dL	Excess of magnesium ions
Electrocardiogram	PQRST pattern	Early: Bradycardia, prolonged PR, QRS, and QT intervals; late: complete heart block, asystole	Magnesium excess leads to alterations in generation and conduction of the action potential

Other Tests: Serum calcium, blood urea nitrogen, serum creatinine, serum electrolytes

PRIMARY NURSING DIAGNOSIS

DIAGNOSIS. Risk for injury as evidenced by muscle weakness and/or fatigue

OUTCOMES. Hypermagnesemia severity; Cardiac pump effectiveness; Circulation status; Electrolyte and acid-base balance; Knowledge: Medication; Respiratory status

INTERVENTIONS. Artificial airway management; Electrolyte management: Hypermagnesemia; Cardiac care: Acute; Code management; Emergency care; Oxygen therapy; Medication administration; Medication management

PLANNING AND IMPLEMENTATION

Collaborative

All medications that contain magnesium need to be discontinued. Loop diuretics may be used to promote excretion of magnesium. The patient may be given calcium gluconate in emergencies to antagonize the effects of magnesium. If the patient does not have severe renal failure, 1,000 mL of 0.9% saline with 2 g of calcium gluconate may be infused to increase magnesium excretion at a rate of 150 to 200 mL per hour. Calcium antagonizes the toxic effects of magnesium as calcium and magnesium electrically oppose each other at their sites of action. In patients with inadequate renal function, the physician may prescribe dialysis with magnesium-free dialysate. Prompt supportive therapy is essential, such as mechanical ventilation if the patient has respiratory failure or a temporary pacemaker if the patient has symptomatic bradycardia.

During treatment, monitor the serum magnesium in patients at risk for hypermagnesemia. Monitor vital signs, urine output, and the neuromuscular status, including level of consciousness, orientation, and muscle strength and function. Assess the patellar (knee-jerk) reflex in patients with a magnesium level above 5 mEq/L: With the patient lying flat or sitting on the side of the bed, support the knee and tap the patellar tendon firmly just below the patella. A normal response is extension of the knee. An absent reflex may indicate a magnesium level greater than 7 mEq/L and should be reported to the physician.

Pharmacologic Highlights

Medication or Drug Class	Dosage	Description	Rationale
Furosemide (Lasix)	20–80 mg/day PO/IV/IM	Loop diuretic	Promotes excretion of magnesium and water by interfering with chloride-binding transport system and inhibiting sodium and chloride reabsorption in kidney
Calcium gluconate 10%	1,000 mL of 0.9% saline with 2 g of calcium gluconate at a rate of 150–200 mL/hr; in emergency, 100–300 mg calcium IV diluted in 150 mL D5W over 10 min	Electrolyte replacement; nutritional supplement	Antagonizes the effects of magnesium and counter-acts neuromuscular effects; improves cardiac function; effect is temporary
Glucose and insulin	10 units insulin IV and 50 mL D50W bolus or 500 mL D10W over 1 hr	Hypoglycemic hormone and sugar supplement	Promotes magnesium entry into cells; to prevent hypoglycemia, glucose is administered

Independent

Maintain the patient's airway, breathing, and circulation until the magnesium levels return to normal. Have emergency airway equipment and a manual resuscitator bag at the patient's bedside at all times. Keep a working endotracheal suction present. Maintain patient safety measures. Reassure the patient and significant others that the patient's neuromuscular status will return to baseline with treatment.

Educate the patient with chronic renal failure to review all over-the-counter medications with the physician and pharmacist before use. These medications include vitamin supplements that contain minerals because these usually contain magnesium. Provide a list of common magnesium-containing medications that the patient should avoid.

Evidence-Based Practice and Health Policy

Tan, L., Xu, Q., Chan, L., Liu, J., & Shi, R. (2021). High-normal serum magnesium and hypermagnesemia are associated with increased 30-day in-hospital mortality: A retrospective cohort study. *Frontiers in Cardiovascular Medicine.* Advance online publication. https://doi .org/10.3389/fcvm.2021.625133

- The authors assessed the association of admission serum magnesium level with all-cause in-hospital mortality in critically ill patients with acute myocardial infarction (AMI). They performed a medical record review on patients in the intensive care unit ($N = 9,005$) within 24 hours after intensive care unit admission.
- They found that abnormally high serum magnesium levels were significant predictors of all-cause in-hospital mortality in patients with AMI. They concluded that high-normal serum magnesium levels may be a useful and early predictor for 30-day in-hospital mortality in critically ill patients with AMI.

DOCUMENTATION GUIDELINES

• Serum magnesium level
• Vital signs; oxygen saturation; cardiac rhythm, electrocardiogram strip and interpretation
• Mental and neuromuscular status, including patellar reflex if appropriate
• Response to treatment: IV fluids, diuretics, dialysis, calcium gluconate, glucose, and insulin

DISCHARGE AND HOME HEALTHCARE GUIDELINES

PREVENTION. To prevent a recurrence of hypermagnesemia, teach the patient to avoid sources of magnesium such as laxatives, antacids, and vitamin-mineral supplements and to consult with the pharmacist or physician before using any over-the-counter medications. The patient should also be taught the signs and symptoms of hypermagnesemia (changes in level of consciousness, neuromuscular weakness, nausea and vomiting) and instructed to notify the physician if these return.

COMPLICATIONS OF NEUROMUSCULAR WEAKNESS. If the patient suffered from prolonged neuromuscular symptoms, the patient may have developed muscle weakness as a result of disease. Teach safety measures to the patient and significant others, including the use of any assistive devices (cane or walker) and seeking assistance when ambulating. The patient should also be taught muscle-strengthening exercises and may need a home-care evaluation before being discharged.

Hypernatremia

DRG Category:	640
Mean LOS:	4.5 days
Description:	MEDICAL: Miscellaneous Disorders of Nutrition, Metabolism, Fluids, and Electrolytes With Major Complication or Comorbidity

Hypernatremia is a condition in which the serum sodium concentration is greater than 145 mEq/L (normal range is 135 to 145 mEq/L). Sodium is the most abundant cation in the body; a 70-kg person has approximately 4,200 mEq of sodium. About 30% of the total body sodium, called silent sodium, is bound with bone and other tissues; the remaining 70%, called the exchangeable sodium, is dissolved in the extracellular fluid (ECF) compartment or in the compartments in communication with the ECF compartment. Sodium has five essential functions: It maintains the osmolarity of the ECF; it maintains ECF volume and water distribution; it affects the concentration, excretion, and absorption of other electrolytes, particularly potassium and chloride; it combines with other ions to maintain acid-base balance; and it is essential for impulse transmission of nerve and muscle fibers.

Hypernatremia occurs in less than 1% of all hospital admissions and is unusual in patients who are awake, are alert, and have an intact thirst response. Most of the cases of hypernatremia are acquired in the hospital, particularly during critical illnesses, when mortality may be as high as 50%. Hypernatremia usually occurs when there is an excess of sodium in relation to water in the ECF compartment, resulting in hyperosmolarity of the ECF, which produces a shift in water from the cells to the ECF. The result is cellular dehydration. It is a water problem rather than a problem of sodium regulation. Complications include tachycardia, hypotension, nerve cell shrinkage, brain injury, and ultimately circulatory and neurological collapse. Three different manifestations of hypernatremia have been described on the basis of the ratio of total body water (TBW) to total body sodium: hypovolemic hypernatremia, hypervolemic hypernatremia, and euvolemic hypernatremia (Table 1).

• TABLE 1 Types and Causes of Hypernatremia

TYPE OF HYPERNATREMIA	FLUID VOLUME AND SODIUM (Na) STATUS	CAUSES
Hypovolemic (most common)	TBW decreases in a greater proportion than Na is lost	Nonrenal: Fever, vomiting, diarrhea, exercise, heat exposure, severe burns, insensible loss from mechanical ventilation, profuse diaphoresis Renal: Diuresis, severe hyperglycemia, increased production of urea (high-protein diet), IV administration of mannitol
Hypervolemic (least common)	TBW is normal with increased Na	Overadministration of saline solutions, particularly in patients with diabetes keto-acidosis and osmotic diuresis; overad-ministration of hypertonic salt solutions; overingestion of salt
Euvolemic	TBW is decreased rela-tive to a normal total body Na	Acute diabetes insipidus; hypodipsia in infants; older persons, incarcerated people, and debilitated adults because of lack of access to water; medications such as lith-ium, dopamine, amphotericin B, ethanol

CAUSES

The cause of hypernatremia is associated with the ratio of TBW to total body sodium. In hyper-natremia, there is often an excess of sodium relative to TBW. Causes of hypernatremia are explained in Table 1.

GENETIC CONSIDERATIONS

One genetic cause for hypernatremia is congenital nephrogenic diabetes insipidus, which is an X-linked disorder resulting in a reduction of the renal collecting duct's sensitivity to arginine vasopressin. Variants in a few recently identified genes, *NFAT5*, *SLC4A10*, and *FAM49A*, may also contribute to hypernatremia.

SEX AND LIFE SPAN CONSIDERATIONS

Hypernatremia is most likely to occur in infants, older adults (especially those institutionalized), incarcerated patients, restrained patients, or debilitated patients. In these people, hypernatremia occurs when they are confused or not cognitively intact, or had water withheld from them, and therefore are unable to respond to the thirst response. Babies cannot respond independently to the thirst response and are dependent on the people feeding them. Hypernatremia is often associated with an acute infection associated with water loss and decreased water intake. The total body sodium level does not vary significantly depending on the person's sex or age once childhood is over.

HEALTH DISPARITIES AND SEXUAL/GENDER MINORITY HEALTH

Ethnicity, race, and sexual/gender minority status have no known effect on the risk for hypernatremia.

GLOBAL HEALTH CONSIDERATIONS

Experts suggest that hypernatremia may occur in hospitalized and nonhospitalized patients more frequently in developing regions compared to developed regions. Children in developing regions are particularly at risk because of nutritional problems and problems with infant feeding such as lack of maternal breast milk and improperly prepared infant formula. Western countries have rates of hypernatremia in patients in the intensive care unit similar to those in the United States.

ASSESSMENT

HISTORY. Determine if the patient has risk factors for hypernatremia: old age, uncontrolled diabetes mellitus, diuretic therapy, sedative therapy, mental impairment, nursing home residence, or being restrained. In hospitalized patients, the following treatment modalities are associated with hypernatremia: enteral feedings, hypertonic IV solutions, mechanical ventilation, and osmotic diuresis. In nonhospitalized patients, inquire about the patient's daily fluid and salt intake. Patients with hypernatremia often report a decrease in fluid intake and possibly a high salt intake. Since polyuria moving to oliguria is an early sign of hypernatremia, ask about daily urine output and if the urine appears concentrated. Question the patient about fever, diarrhea, and vomiting, which might contribute to dehydration. If hypernatremia is severe, the patient may be confused. Ask the family if the patient has been lethargic, disoriented, or agitated. These changes in mental status, along with occurrence of a seizure, indicate severe hypernatremia.

PHYSICAL EXAMINATION. The patient may be asymptomatic or have nonspecific symptoms such as **agitation, lethargy, nausea, vomiting**, and **signs of dehydration**. Cognitive dysfunction with symptoms such as confusion, irritability, and abnormal speech patterns is typical. Assess the patient's vital signs; fever, tachycardia, decreased blood pressure, and orthostatic hypotension are characteristic of hypernatremia. Assess the skin and mucous membranes for signs of dehydration. With pronounced hypernatremia, expect general weakness and weight loss, poor skin turgor, flushed skin color, dry mucous membranes, and a dry tongue. With more severe hypernatremia, assess the patient for obtundation, muscle twitching, hyperreflexia, tremors, seizures, and rigid paralysis.

PSYCHOSOCIAL. Assess the patient's ability to obtain adequate fluid intake. The patient's lethargic state contributes to the poor fluid intake. Assess the quality and support of the caregivers regarding their ability to provide for the patient's fluid intake. Because the symptoms of severe hypernatremia are primarily neurological, assess the patient's level of orientation and the patient's ability to communicate needs. Assess the safety needs of the patient, especially for the disoriented older or debilitated patient. Note that central nervous system symptoms are particularly upsetting for the patient and family and may create anxiety over the patient's long-term prognosis.

Diagnostic Highlights

Test	Normal Result	Abnormality With Condition	Explanation
Serum sodium	135–145 mEq/L	> 145 mEq/L; critical value: > 160 mEq/L	Imbalance between sodium and water leads to excess sodium
Blood urea nitrogen (BUN)	8–21 mg/dL	Usually elevated	Conditions that lead to dehydration and fluid loss may elevate BUN because of decreased renal blood flow and abnormal absorption of urea back into the blood
Serum chloride	97–107 mEq/L	> 112 mEq/L	Reflects an excess of chloride

Diagnostic Highlights (continued)

Test	Normal Result	Abnormality With Condition	Explanation
Serum osmolarity	275–295 mOsm/L	> 295 mOsm/L	Water loss in the urine and hypernatremia lead to hemo-concentration; levels above 320 mOsm/L are considered "panic levels" and require immediate intervention
Urine osmolarity	200–1,200 mOsm/L	Varies depending on cause; often > 800 mOsm/L; note that older people lose the ability to concentrate the urine, so urine may not be concentrated	Used to diagnose nature of hypernatremia; osmolarity refers to a solution's concentration of solute particles per liter of water; usual renal response to hypernatremia is excretion of maximally concentrated urine (< 500 mL/day) with an osmolarity > 800 mOsm/L

Other Tests: Complete blood count, blood urea nitrogen, creatinine, serum and urine electrolytes, serum glucose and protein level, urine-specific gravity

PRIMARY NURSING DIAGNOSIS

DIAGNOSIS. Deficient fluid volume related to fluid loss, inadequate fluid intake, or fluid shifts to the extravascular space as evidenced by agitation, dehydration, dry mucous membranes, and/or thirst

OUTCOMES. Hypernatremia severity; Electrolyte and acid-base balance; Hydration; Fluid balance; Nutritional status: Food and fluid intake; Knowledge: Health behavior; Urinary elimination

INTERVENTIONS. Electrolyte management: Hypernatremia; Fluid management; Fluid monitoring; Electrolyte monitoring; IV insertion; IV therapy

PLANNING AND IMPLEMENTATION

Collaborative

Treatment is based on the cause and type of hypernatremia. Often estimates are made by a formula to determine the fluid replacement considering total body water deficits and sodium levels. The goal is to decrease the total body sodium and replace the fluid loss. Encourage liquids; if the patient cannot tolerate fluids, an IV hypotonic electrolyte solution (0.2% or 0.45% sodium chloride) or salt-free solution is usually ordered. Sometimes these two types of solutions are alternated to prevent hyponatremia. If 5% dextrose in water is ordered, monitor the urine output because this solution encourages diuresis, which can aggravate the hypernatremic condition. Use care with dextrose-containing solutions if the patient is diabetic. Maintain intake and output records, and weigh the patient each day to monitor the fluid volume status.

Monitor the patient's serum and urine sodium levels daily to determine the effectiveness of IV fluids. Administer the water replacement slowly as prescribed to reduce the serum sodium levels to no more than 2 mEq/L per hour in acutely ill patients. In people with chronic hypernatremia, sodium balance is corrected more slowly at a rate of 0.5 mEq/L per hour. If hypernatremia is corrected too quickly, the ECF shifts into the cells, resulting in cerebral edema and neurological problems. Monitor the patient for signs and symptoms of cerebral edema: headache, lethargy, nausea, vomiting, widening pulse pressure, and decreased pulse rate. Sometimes, diuretic therapy is indicated to increase sodium excretion, along with a decrease of oral sodium intake in the diet. Pharmacologic management other than IV therapy usually is not required, although patients may receive sodium-wasting diuretic therapy (hydrochlorothiazide, furosemide).

Pharmacologic Highlights

Independent
Offer fluids and water frequently to patients with hypernatremia. Avoid caffeinated fluids and alcohol because they can increase the serum sodium level by causing water diuresis. Monitor intake and output as fluid and electrolytes are replaced. Notify the physician of any changes in mental status, such as agitation, confusion, and disorientation. If the patient is at risk for seizures, initiate seizure precautions.

Give oral care every 2 hours; avoid using lemon glycerin swabs and alcoholic mouthwashes because they have a drying effect and can cause discomfort. Monitor the condition of the skin and assist with position changes frequently. Determine the patient's ability to ambulate safely. If the patient is confused and disoriented, maintain the bed in the lowest position and maintain safety measures.

Evidence-Based Practice and Health Policy
Overwyk, K., Pfeiffer, C., Storandt, R., Zhao, L., Zhang, Z., Campbell, N., Wiltz, J., Merritt, R., & Cogswell, M. (2021). Serum sodium and potassium distribution and characteristics in the U.S. population, National Health and Nutrition Examination Survey, 2009–2016. *Journal of Applied Laboratory Medicine, 6*, 63–78.

- The authors aimed to examine averages of serum sodium and potassium levels by sex and age groups in people 12 years and older ($N = 25,520$). They wanted to examine the age-adjusted prevalence of low serum sodium and high serum potassium and consider selected sociodemographic characteristics, health conditions, and medication use.
- They found that 2% of U.S. adults had low sodium, and 0.6% had high potassium. Prevalence of low serum sodium and high serum potassium occurred most often in adults 71 years of age or older and in people with chronic kidney disease, diabetes, or using antihypertensive medications. Maintaining low levels of sodium may make some persons at risk for hyperkalemia.

DOCUMENTATION GUIDELINES
- Intake and output, daily weights, serum and urine electrolyte levels, urine-specific gravity
- Vital signs: Presence of fever, tachycardia, low blood pressure, orthostatic changes
- Mental status: Orientation to person, place, and time; observations of confusion or agitation; ability to drink oral fluids; presence of gag reflex
- Condition of oral mucosa and skin
- Response to treatments: Oral and parenteral fluids, sodium restrictions, diuretics

DISCHARGE AND HOME HEALTHCARE GUIDELINES
Teach the patient and caregivers the importance of an adequate fluid intake and normal sodium intake. Discuss the foods that are appropriate for a low-sodium diet if indicated. Advise the patient or significant others to avoid over-the-counter medications that are high in sodium. Teach the patient about the early signs of hypernatremia: lethargy, confusion, irritability, polyuria, nausea, vomiting, and orthostatic hypotension. Explain that as hypernatremia becomes severe, the patient or family will note clear decreases in the patient's mental status. Encourage the patient or significant others to notify the primary healthcare provider if any of these signs and symptoms occur.

Hyperparathyroidism

DRG Category:	626
Mean LOS:	3.5 days
Description:	SURGICAL: Thyroid, Parathyroid, and Thyroglossal Procedures With Complication or Comorbidity
DRG Category:	644
Mean LOS:	4.3 days
Description:	MEDICAL: Endocrine Disorders With Complication or Comorbidity

Hyperparathyroidism refers to the clinical condition associated with oversecretion of the parathyroid hormone (PTH). Primary hyperparathyroidism, the most common form, is a gland dysfunction that originates in the parathyroid gland. Secondary hyperparathyroidism, in contrast, is a parathyroid gland dysfunction that is a response to a disorder elsewhere in the body, such as chronic renal failure. PTH is produced by the parathyroid glands, which are four small endocrine glands located on the posterior surface of the thyroid gland. The primary function of PTH is to regulate calcium and phosphorus balance by affecting gastrointestinal (GI) absorption of calcium, bone resorption (removal of bone tissue by absorption) of calcium, and renal regulation of both calcium and phosphorus. Calcium and phosphorus have a reciprocal relationship in the body; high levels of calcium lead to low levels of phosphorus.

Hypercalcemia, the identifiable result of hyperparathyroidism, also leads to the most important clinical complications. The body is able to compensate for slowly increasing calcium levels but eventually is overcome with calcium excess and phosphorus deficiency. Because the bones hold the majority of the body's calcium, extracellular hypercalcemia is a result of demineralization of the bones. The calcium in the bones is replaced by cysts and fibrous tissue, leading to severe osteoporosis (reduction of bone mass per volume) and osteopenia (diminished bone tissue). Increased levels of extracellular calcium may be deposited in the soft tissues of the body and the kidney and lead to renal calculi, renal insufficiency, urinary tract infections, and eventually, renal failure. Hypercalcemia can also trigger the increased secretion of gastrin, which leads to peptic ulcer disease. Other GI dysfunctions that may result include cholelithiasis and pancreatitis. In addition to osteoporosis, renal disease, and GI dysfunction, complications include bone fractures, high blood pressure, and heart disease.

CAUSES

Primary hyperparathyroidism, which leads to the enlargement of at least one of the parathyroid glands, occurs in more than 85% of the cases because of a single benign adenoma (neoplasm of glandular epithelium). Other causes include genetic disorders and endocrine cancers, such as pancreatic or pituitary cancers. Patients who have had head or neck radiation are also at increased risk. Secondary hyperparathyroidism occurs when a source for hypocalcemia occurs outside the parathyroid gland, stimulating the parathyroid glands to overproduce PTH to try to correct the calcium. These conditions include chronic renal failure, rickets, vitamin D deficiency, and laxative abuse.

GENETIC CONSIDERATIONS

Primary hyperparathyroidism is usually sporadic but also can run in families. Several genes, such as *MEN1* and *CDC73*, have been identified that cause or contribute to this disorder. Primary hyperparathyroidism may be a feature of familial syndromes, such as multiple endocrine neoplasia type I (MEN I), which causes hyperactivity of all four parathyroid glands. Most individuals who inherit a susceptibility to MEN I will develop hyperparathyroidism by age 50 years. MEN I is transmitted in an autosomal dominant pattern with widely variable penetrance.

SEX AND LIFE SPAN CONSIDERATIONS

Primary hyperparathyroidism affects women more than men, is more frequent in individuals older than 50 years, and is unusual in children. It is usually diagnosed when people are in their 50s. Postmenopausal women between the ages of 35 and 65 years and older women are especially at risk. Regular screening of calcium levels as part of an annual physical examination is very important for all people older than age 50 years.

HEALTH DISPARITIES AND SEXUAL/GENDER MINORITY HEALTH

The incidence of hyperparathyroidism is highest among Black persons, followed by White persons. A short time between the diagnosis of hyperparathyroidism and the surgical procedure is an indication of whether appropriate medical care was received. Among patients undergoing surgery, time from diagnosis to surgical treatment is longer for Black persons than White persons. These differences remained after adjusting for age, calcium levels, insurance, and comorbidities. Black persons face delays in access to parathyroidectomy that could impair quality of life and increase healthcare costs (Mallick et al., 2021 [see Evidence-Based Practice and Health Policy]). Black patients also have more severe disease and more comorbidities than White patients. Experts also note that patients who have parathyroidectomy, which is a complicated surgery, have better outcomes when operated on by experienced surgeons. Hispanic patients, men, and patients with Medicaid health coverage were more likely to be managed by less-experienced surgeons and had more postoperative complications (Al-Qurayshi et al., 2017). Sexual and gender minority status has no known effect on the risk for hyperparathyroidism.

GLOBAL HEALTH CONSIDERATIONS

Hyperparathyroidism occurs around the world but is relatively rare, and no global prevalence statistics are available.

☀ ASSESSMENT

HISTORY. Early symptoms are polyuria (large amounts of urine), anorexia, and constipation, as well as weakness, fatigue, drowsiness, and lethargy. As the hypercalcemia increases, abdominal pain (from peptic ulcer disease), nausea, and vomiting are typical. The patient may report generalized bone and joint pain and may have had recent fractures from minor situations that normally would not cause a fracture (also known as *pathological* or *fragility* fractures). They may report a history of kidney stones. Some patients may describe depression, inability to concentrate, and memory problems or subtle differences in mental acuity.

PHYSICAL EXAMINATION. Many patients do not have physical findings when examined until the late stages of the disease. Hypertension is common, and if the patient is on digitalis, there may be a significantly lowered pulse rate, which signals increased sensitivity to the drug. Muscle atrophy and depressed tendon reflexes are late signs of hypercalcemia. The patient may have marked muscle weakness and atrophy (particularly in the legs) and skeletal deformities. If the central nervous system is affected, there will be changes in mental status, such as confusion, disorientation, and even coma. Palpation of even grossly enlarged parathyroid glands is generally impossible because of their location.

PSYCHOSOCIAL. The hypercalcemic patient or significant others may note memory changes, confusion, irritability, and symptoms of depression or paranoia (or both). The psychological clinical manifestations may range from mild to acute psychosis or possibly paranoid hallucinations. The patient and significant others may be understandably upset or anxious about the changes in the patient's behavior.

Diagnostic Highlights

Test	Normal Result	Abnormality With Condition	Explanation
Serum calcium: Total calcium, including free ionized calcium and calcium bound with protein or organic ions	8.4–10.2 mg/dL	> 10.5 mg/dL; critical value: > 14 mg/dL in primary hyperparathyroidism (Note: In secondary hyperparathyroidism, a source for hypocalcemia exists outside the parathyroid glands)	Accumulation of calcium above normal levels in the extracellular fluid compartment; clinical manifestations generally occur when calcium levels are above 12 mg/dL and tend to be more severe if hypercalcemia develops rapidly; if ionized calcium cannot be measured, total serum calcium can be corrected by adding 0.8 mg/dL to the total calcium level for every 1 g/dL decrease of serum albumin below 4 g/dL; the corrected value determines whether true hypocalcemia is present. When calcium levels are reported as high or low, calculate the actual level of calcium by the following formula: Corrected total calcium (mg/dL) = (measured total calcium mg/dL) + 0.8 (4.4 measured albumin g/dL).
Serum ionized calcium: Unbound calcium; level unaffected by albumin level	4.6–5.3 mg/dL	> 5.5 mg/dL	Ionized calcium is approximately 46%–50% of circulating calcium and is the form of calcium available for enzymatic reactions and neuromuscular function; levels increase and decrease with blood pH levels; for every 0.1 pH decrease, ionized calcium increases 1.5%–2.5%.
Serum parathyroid hormone level	10–65 pg/mL	Elevated in more than 90% of people with primary hyperparathyroidism	Determines presence of hyperparathyroidism

Other Tests: Serum phosphorus level; 24-hour urine for calcium; vitamin D level; supporting tests include x-rays, electrocardiogram, technetium-99m sestamibi imaging, ultrasonography of the neck, computed tomography, and magnetic resonance imaging

PRIMARY NURSING DIAGNOSIS

DIAGNOSIS. Decreased activity tolerance related to electrolyte imbalance as evidenced by fatigue, muscle weakness, and/or bone pain

OUTCOMES. Hypercalcemia severity; Energy conservation; Knowledge: Disease process, Diet, Medication, and Prescribed activity; Nutritional status: Energy; Pain level; Symptom severity

INTERVENTIONS. Electrolyte management: Hypercalcemia; Electrolyte monitoring; Fluid management; Fluid monitoring; Medication management; Exercise promotion; Fall prevention

☀ PLANNING AND IMPLEMENTATION

Collaborative

Surgical removal of the parathyroid glands is the only definitive treatment and is the treatment of choice for symptomatic primary hyperparathyroidism. Indications for surgery include symptoms resulting from hypercalcemia, nephrolithiasis, reduced bone mass, serum calcium level in excess of 12 mg/dL, age younger than 50 years, and infeasibility of long-term follow-up. If hyperplasia (proliferation of normal cells) of the glands is excessive, all but one-half of one gland is removed because only a small amount of glandular tissue is necessary to maintain appropriate levels of PTH. The individual who has had all four glands removed will quickly become hypoparathyroid and must be treated accordingly. To prevent postoperative deficits of calcium, magnesium, and phosphorus, the patient may need either IV or oral supplements. Bone pain may subside as soon as 3 days after surgery, but renal dysfunction may be irreversible.

Nonsurgical management includes medications to assist in the excretion of calcium by the kidneys. Medical therapy, however, has not been shown to affect the clinical outcome of primary hyperparathyroidism. Patients are asked to maintain a moderate daily calcium intake and vitamin D intake appropriate for their age and sex. To increase calcium excretion, the patient needs a large fluid intake, at least 2 to 3 L per day, and 8 to 10 g of salt per day. Foods high in fiber will assist the patient to have normal bowel function.

Secondary hyperparathyroidism is managed by treating the underlying cause; either vitamin D therapy or non-calcium-based phosphate binders may be used, depending on the underlying cause of the disorder. The patient may receive etelcalcetide (see below) after each dialysis session.

Pharmacologic Highlights

Medication or Drug Class	Dosage	Description	Rationale
Etelcalcetide	Initial dose: 5 mg IV three times/wk; adjusted does 2.5–5 mg three times/wk until PTH levels reach target level; maintenance dose 2.5–5 mg IV three times/wk	Calcimimetics	For secondary hyperparathyroidism; binds to and activates calcium sensing receptor and decreases parathyroid hormone secretion
Furosemide (Lasix)	20–40 mg IV bid-qid	Loop diuretic	Used with normal saline to cause diuresis and to reduce calcium levels

Other Drugs: Cinacalcet (Sensipar) is used in parathyroid carcinoma, bisphosphonates in patients who cannot receive surgery for primary hyperparathyroidism.

Independent

Unless contraindicated, increase the patient's mobility, protect the patient from injury, monitor for possible complications, and provide patient education. Provide comfort measures for bone and joint pain. Increased activity limits further bone demineralization. Moderate weight-bearing activities are more beneficial to the patient than range-of-motion exercises in bedrest or chair rest. Patients with hyperparathyroidism may be weak and at risk for falls and trauma. If the patient is hospitalized, maintain safety measures.

If the patient is recovering from a parathyroidectomy, the most life-threatening complication is airway compromise, either from swelling or from acute hypocalcemia. Keep emergency intubation and tracheostomy equipment in a readily available location. Notify the surgeon immediately if the patient develops respiratory distress, stridor, neck swelling, or hoarseness because of laryngeal nerve damage. Maintain the patient in a semi-Fowler position to decrease postoperative edema. If the patient develops tingling in the hands and around the mouth, notify the surgeon and obtain serum calcium levels if prescribed to determine if tetany is beginning.

As with many endocrine disorders, the patient may be frustrated with the clinical manifestations of the disease and require frequent reassurance. Reassure the patient that most of the symptoms will reverse with the return of normal calcium levels. Assist the patient in identifying stressors and methods of coping with the stressors.

Evidence-Based Practice and Health Policy

Mallick, R., Xie, R., Kirklin, J., Chen, H., & Balentine, C. (2021). Race and gender disparities in access to parathyroidectomy: A need to change processes for diagnosis and referral to surgeons. *Annals of Surgical Oncology*, *28*, 476–483.

- The authors hypothesized that there would be race and gender disparities in the surgical treatment of hyperparathyroidism and studied the time from initial diagnosis to the time of treatment with parathyroidectomy. They performed a medical record review of 2,289 patients with hypercalcemia. The average age was 63 years; 57% were White, 41% Black, and 74% were female.
- Among patients undergoing surgery, time from index high calcium to surgical treatment was longer for Black men and women than White men and women. At 1 year after the index abnormal calcium, only 6% of Black men underwent surgery compared with 20% of White men. Similarly, 13% of Black women underwent surgery versus 20% of White women. These differences remained significant after adjusting for age, calcium levels, insurance, and comorbidities. The authors concluded that Black individuals face delays in access to parathyroidectomy that could impair quality of life and increase healthcare costs.

DOCUMENTATION GUIDELINES

- Physical findings: Signs and symptoms of calcium imbalance, bone deformity, patency of airway
- Prevention of complications: Postoperative swelling, postoperative wound healing
- Response to mobility: Level of activity tolerance, response to activity, energy level, pain level

DISCHARGE AND HOME HEALTHCARE GUIDELINES

Teach the patient about the disease process and the signs and symptoms of calcium imbalance. Stress that the symptoms require immediate medical attention. Describe any dietary considerations, including a diet low in calcium with limitation/avoidance of milk products. If the patient is on potassium-depleting diuretics, note that a diet high in potassium-rich foods (apricots, fresh vegetables, citrus fruits) is necessary if no potassium supplements are prescribed. In addition, a diet with adequate fiber and fluid will aid normal bowel function. Teach the action, dosage, route, and side effects of all medications.

If the patient has a surgical incision, describe incisional care and arrange for a follow-up visit with the surgeon. Instruct the patient regarding an appropriate activity level. Note that recalcification of the bones will take some time. If the patient maintains mobility, recalcification will be increased. Suggest that the patient avoid bedrest; encourage the patient to space activity throughout the day and use energy levels as a guide to activity. Remind the patient to avoid contact sports or other activities that place the patient at risk for falls or fractures.

Hyperphosphatemia

DRG Category:	642
Mean LOS:	4.1 days
Description:	MEDICAL: Inborn and Other Disorders of Metabolism

Phosphorus is one of the primary intracellular ions in the body. It is found as both organic phosphorus and inorganic phosphorus salts. Phosphorus plays a critical role in all of the body's tissues. It is an important structural element in the bones and is essential to the function of muscle, red blood cells, and the nervous system. It is responsible for bone growth and interacts with hemoglobin in the red blood cells, promoting oxygen release to the body's tissues. Phosphorus is responsible for promotion of white blood cell phagocytic action and is important in platelet structure and function. It also acts as a buffering agent for urine. In one of its most important roles, phosphorus is critical for the production of adenosine triphosphate, the chief energy source of the body. Approximately 85% of body phosphorus is in bone, and most of the remainder is intracellular; only 1% is in the extracellular fluid.

Normal serum phosphorus levels are 2.5 to 4.5 mg/dL, whereas intracellular phosphorus levels are as high as 300 mg/dL. Hyperphosphatemia occurs when serum phosphorus levels exceed 4.5 mg/dL. It is rare in the general population, but in patients with renal insufficiency or acute or chronic renal failure, the rate of hyperphosphatemia is approximately 70%. Phosphorus is absorbed primarily in the jejunum from foods such as red meats, fish, poultry, eggs, and milk products. Phosphorus is regulated by the kidneys; 90% of phosphorus excretion occurs by the renal route and 10% by the fecal route. Phosphorus is also regulated by vitamin D and by parathyroid hormone. Phosphorus levels are inversely related to calcium levels, and therefore complications of hyperphosphatemia include hypocalcemia and tetany as well as seizures, vascular calcification, arterial stiffness, myocardial infarction, peripheral vascular disease, and sudden death.

CAUSES

The primary cause of hyperphosphatemia is decreased phosphorus excretion because of renal insufficiency or renal failure (acute or chronic). Decreased phosphorus excretion also occurs with hypoparathyroidism. Decreased parathyroid activity leads to decreased calcium concentration and increased phosphorus concentration. Increased serum phosphorus absorption may also occur with increased intake of vitamin D or excessive quantities of milk. An increased intake of phosphorus or phosphorus-containing medications, such as enemas, laxatives, or antacids, can cause substantial absorption of phosphorus. Blood transfusions may also cause increased levels of phosphorus because it leaks from the blood cells during storage. Phosphorus may be released in excessive quantities in patients who are receiving chemotherapy for neoplastic diseases. Muscle necrosis because of trauma, viral infections, or heat stroke may also cause hyperphosphatemia because muscle tissues store the bulk of soft-tissue phosphorus.

GENETIC CONSIDERATIONS

Hyperphosphatemia can be seen as a feature of inherited endocrine abnormalities, such as hyperphosphatemic familial tumoral calcinosis (HFTC). Biallelic pathogenic mutations in *FGF23*, *GALNT3*, or *KL* are diagnostic of HFTC.

Other mutations in the *GALNT3* or *FGF23* genes cause hyperostosis with hyperphosphatemia (HHS). There is an autosomal dominantly transmitted form of hypoparathyroidism with variable expressivity that includes high phosphate with low calcium and magnesium levels.

SEX AND LIFE SPAN CONSIDERATIONS

Serum levels of phosphorus are normally higher (3.3–6.5 mg/dL) in children because of the increased rate of skeletal growth. Infants who are fed cow's milk or formula may develop hyperphosphatemia because cow's milk contains more phosphorus (940 mg/L) than human milk (150 mg/L). The most common cause, renal failure, occurs across the life span and in all people. Women have a slight but nonclinical elevation of serum phosphorus levels after menopause.

HEALTH DISPARITIES AND SEXUAL/GENDER MINORITY HEALTH

Black, Hispanic, and Native American persons have higher rates of renal failure than other groups, which can result in a higher prevalence of hyperphosphatemia. Sexual and gender minority status has no known effect on the risk for hyperphosphatemia.

GLOBAL HEALTH CONSIDERATIONS

Experts suggest that rates of hyperphosphatemia parallel those of renal failure around the world.

ASSESSMENT

HISTORY. Assess the patient's mental status, which may be affected by high levels of phosphorus. Determine if the patient has a history of end-stage renal disease. While most people will be asymptomatic, some patients with increased serum phosphorus levels exhibit signs and symptoms associated with renal failure and/or hypocalcemia. Ask about a recent history of frequent laxative or enema use, excess antacid use, and increased intake of foods containing large amounts of phosphorus (dried beans and peas, eggs, fish, meats, milk, nuts). Note if the patient has been admitted for massive burns or trauma, acute pancreatitis, acute or chronic renal failure, neoplastic disorders, or hypoparathyroidism. Because most hyperphosphatemia is associated with renal failure, query if patients experience nausea, vomiting, fatigue, and shortness of breath.

Tetany, a condition that leads to increased neural excitability due to calcium deficit, may develop. Determine if the patient has experienced tingling in the fingertips or around the mouth. As tetany progresses, tingling may progress up the limbs and around the face and increase in intensity from tingling to numbness followed by pain accompanied by muscle spasm. Tetany is more common in patients who have taken an increased phosphorus load by diet or through medication. It is less likely in the renal patient because calcium ionization is increased in the presence of acidosis.

PHYSICAL EXAMINATION. An elevated serum phosphorus level may cause **few signs or symptoms**. Central nervous systems may include altered mental status, delirium, coma, convulsions, and seizures. Some patients may have sleep disturbance. Patients may have symptoms of renal failure, such as dyspnea and vomiting. Long-term consequences may involve soft-tissue calcification for the patient with chronic renal failure resulting from precipitation of calcium phosphates in nonosseous sites, often the kidney, liver, and lungs. Other nonosseous sites may include arteries, joints, skin, or the corneas. Muscle cramps and tetany may account for the majority of signs and symptoms because of hypocalcemia. Check for Trousseau (development of carpal spasm when a blood pressure cuff is inflated above systolic pressure for 3 minutes) and Chvostek (twitching facial muscles when the facial nerve is tapped anterior to the ear) signs.

PSYCHOSOCIAL. Hyperphosphatemia is most often associated with other chronic problems, such as renal failure, hypoparathyroidism, or chemotherapy for neoplastic diseases. Assess the patient's ability to cope with a serious disease, and evaluate the patient's social network for available support and coping abilities. Changes in mental status are upsetting for both the patient and significant others.

Diagnostic Highlights

Test	Normal Result	Abnormality With Condition	Explanation
Serum phosphorus	2.5–4.5 mg/dL	> 4.5 mg/dL (adults); > 5.5 mg/dL (children); critical value: > 5 mg/dL in adults	Reflects phosphorus excess
Serum calcium	8.4–10.2 mg/dL	< 8.4 mg/dL	Reflects calcium deficit
Serum ionized calcium (free calcium)	4.6–5.3 mg/dL	< 4.5 mg/dL	Reflects ionized calcium (46%–50% of circulating calcium)

Other Tests: Electrocardiogram, blood urea nitrogen, creatinine, serum magnesium levels

PRIMARY NURSING DIAGNOSIS

DIAGNOSIS. Decreased activity tolerance related to electrolyte imbalance as evidenced by fatigue, muscle weakness, and/or bone pain

OUTCOMES. Hyperphosphatemia severity; Hypocalcemia severity; Knowledge: Energy conservation; Knowledge: Disease process; Nutritional status: Energy; Pain level; Symptom severity

INTERVENTIONS. Electrolyte management: Hyperphosphatemia; Electrolyte management: Hypocalcemia; Medication management; Exercise promotion; Fall prevention

PLANNING AND IMPLEMENTATION

Collaborative

Medical treatment is aimed at managing the underlying disease process. If the hyperphosphatemia is caused by excessive phosphate administration in medications, elimination or substitution of the products remedies the problem. In some cases, pharmacologic agents, such as calcium-containing phosphate binders or phosphate binders without calcium or aluminum, are used. Hemodialysis may be needed to control the excess phosphorus levels. Because hyperphosphatemia can impair kidney function, the physician monitors the patient's renal function carefully.

Adequate levels of phosphorus are easily maintained by a normal diet because phosphorus is abundant in many foods, including red meat, poultry, eggs, vegetables, hard cheese, cream, nuts, cereals such as bran and oatmeal, dried fruits, and desserts made with milk. These foods may need to be restricted in the diet when patients have increased levels of phosphorus because of chronic diseases. Because the most common dietary factor causing hyperphosphatemia is vitamin D, it is often temporarily eliminated from the diet. A referral to a dietitian can help the patient with menu alternatives.

Pharmacologic Highlights

Medication or Drug Class	Dosage	Description	Rationale
Acetazolamide (Diamox)	250–375 mg PO/IV daily	Diuretic carbonic anhydrase inhibitor	Increases renal excretion of phosphorus Note: Furosemide (Lasix) may also be used to increase renal excretion of phosphate

Pharmacologic Highlights (continued)

Medication or Drug Class	Dosage	Description	Rationale
Phosphate-binding agents (aluminum-containing binders are no longer prescribed because of the toxic effects of aluminum)	Varies with drug	Sevelamer hydrochloride (Renagel); lanthanum carbonate (Fosrenol); sucroferric osyhudroxide (Velphoro); calcium acetate, calcium carbonate	Cause phosphate binding in the gastrointestinal tract, thereby decreasing serum phosphate levels

Other Drugs: Calcium supplements to prevent tetany, normal saline infusion with a forced diuresis with a loop diuretic

Independent

Identify patients at risk for hyperphosphatemia. If those patients develop any signs of tetany (tingling sensations, numbness, or muscle spasms and cramps), notify the physician immediately because airway compromise from laryngospasm is a potential complication.

Teach patients at risk for phosphorus imbalances to use care in choosing over-the-counter medications such as antacids, laxatives, and enemas. Patients should learn to read medication ingredients and check with the healthcare provider about any questions regarding the phosphorus content of medications. Make sure the patient understands the mechanism of action of phosphate binders. Stress the need to take phosphate binders with or after meals to maximize their effectiveness. Explain that phosphate-binding medications may lead to constipation. Encourage the patient to use bulk-building supplements or stool softeners if constipation occurs.

Evidence-Based Practice and Health Policy

Bacchetta, J., Bernardor, J., Garnier, C., Naud, C., & Ranchin, B. (2021). Hyperphosphatemia and chronic kidney disease: A major daily concern both in adults and in children. *Calcified Tissue International, 108*, 116–127.

- The objective of this review is to explore the pathophysiology of hyperphosphatemia in chronic kidney disease (CKD), with a focus on its negative effects. The authors also provide a description of the clinical management of hyperphosphatemia considering the complex mineral and bone disorders associated with CKD. They note that hyperphosphatemia is common in CKD and is seen as the "silent killer" because of its dramatic effect on vascular calcifications.
- CKD along with bone abnormalities may be complicated by secondary hyperparathyroidism or delayed with poor growth, bone deformities, fractures, and vascular calcifications. The clinical management of hyperphosphatemia is a challenge, primarily because of the phosphate overload in diets that is mainly due to the phosphate "hidden" in food additives. The management begins with a dietary restriction of phosphate intake, the use of calcium-based and non-calcium-based phosphate binders, and increasing the frequency of dialysis.

DOCUMENTATION GUIDELINES

- Physical response: Signs of tetany (tingling sensations, numbness, muscle spasms, or cramps), neurological symptoms
- Phosphorus levels, calcium levels
- Emotional response to chronic illness, response to changes in management

DISCHARGE AND HOME HEALTHCARE GUIDELINES

Teach the patient to avoid the use of over-the-counter medications that contain phosphorus, such as certain enemas, antacids, or laxatives, and ensure that the patient understands the information.

Instruct the patient to avoid foods high in phosphorus (meats, poultry, fish, nuts, beans, and dairy products) and vitamin D. Teach the patient to recognize signs of low calcium. Notify the patient of the next appointment with the healthcare provider.

Hypertension

DRG Category:	305
Mean LOS:	2.7 days
Description:	MEDICAL: Hypertension Without Major Complication or Comorbidity

The American Heart Association (AHA) estimates that 47.3% of U.S. adults have hypertension. In 2018 (the most current data), there were 95,876 deaths primarily attributed by AHA to hypertension. AHA defines normal blood pressure as a systolic blood pressure of less than 120 mm Hg and a diastolic blood pressure less than 80 mm Hg. AHA guidelines define hypertension by three levels. People with elevated blood pressure have a systolic pressure between 120 and 129 mm Hg and diastolic pressure less than 80 mm Hg. People with stage 1 hypertension have a systolic blood presssure of 130 to 139 mm Hg or a diastolic pressure of 80 to 89 mm Hg. People with stage 2 hypertension have a systolic blood pressure of 140 mm Hg or more or a diastolic blood pressure of 90 mm Hg or more. Hypertension results in significant economic and personal costs, including disability and an increased mortality rate.

Hypertension is classified by three types: Primary (essential) accounts for over 90% of cases and is often referred to as *idiopathic* because the underlying cause is not known. This type has an insidious onset with few, if any, symptoms, so it is often not recognized until complications have occurred. Secondary hypertension results from a number of conditions that impair blood pressure regulation, and this type accounts for only 2% to 10% of all cases of hypertension. A severe or accelerating form of hypertension, malignant hypertension, results from either type and can cause blood pressures as high as 240/150 mm Hg, possibly leading to coma and death.

Approximately 16% of adults in the United States with hypertension are unaware that they have it. Untreated, hypertension can cause major complications. It contributes to the development of atherosclerosis and increases the workload of the heart, thereby reducing perfusion to major organs and possibly resulting in transient ischemic attacks, strokes, myocardial infarction, left ventricular hypertrophy, heart failure, and renal failure. Damage to small arteries in the eye can lead to blindness.

CAUSES

The cause of primary hypertension is not known; however, it is known that the disease is associated with risk factors such as genetic predisposition, stress, obesity, and a high-sodium diet. Secondary hypertension results from underlying disorders that impair blood pressure regulation, particularly renal, endocrine, vascular, and neurological disorders; hypertensive disease of pregnancy (formerly known as toxemia); and use of estrogen-containing oral contraceptives. It is associated with the use of alcohol, cocaine, NSAIDs, some herbal remedies containing ephedrine or licorice, and nicotine. Associated diseases and conditions include thyroid and parathyroid dysfunction, hypercalcemia, sleep apnea, and pregnancy.

The cause of malignant hypertension is also not known, but it may be associated with dilation of cerebral arteries and generalized arteriolar fibrinoid necrosis, which increases intracerebral blood flow, resulting in encephalopathy.

GENETIC CONSIDERATIONS

Hypertension is a complex disease combining the effects of multiple genes and environmental factors. Heritability varies from 15% to 70% depending on ethnicity and the contribution of environmental factors. Over 100 candidate genes have been suggested to increase susceptibility to hypertension, and there may be many more that have yet to be determined. Genetic mutations have been located for several syndromes that include hypertension as a feature (Liddle syndrome, glucocorticoid-remediable aldosteronism, the syndrome of apparent mineralocorticoid excess), but genetic causes of primary hypertension have been difficult to elucidate.

SEX AND LIFE SPAN CONSIDERATIONS

Approximately two-thirds of Americans over age 65 years have systolic hypertension, usually related to underlying atherosclerosis and stress. Younger individuals may also be affected, depending on the number of risk factors present. Malignant hypertension affects men more often than women, with an average age at diagnosis of 40 years. The age-related blood pressure rises for women and men are essentially the same from 45 to 60 years, and then women's blood pressure exceeds that of men after the age of 60 years.

HEALTH DISPARITIES AND SEXUAL/GENDER MINORITY HEALTH

The Centers for Disease Control and Prevention (CDC) report that the age-adjusted prevalence of hypertension in the United States for people 18 years of age and older is 57.1% for Black men, 56.7% for Black women, 50.2% for White men, 36.7% for White women, 50.1% for Hispanic men, and 36.8% for Hispanic women. Black persons and older people are most prone to hypertension and its complications, such as stroke and end-stage renal disease. Significant health disparities exist in cardiac care. Black, Indigenous, and other people of color are known to receive care less often guided by standard cardiac care guidelines than White persons. Unless patients have health insurance, White patients are more likely to receive coronary angiograms and other coronary interventions than Black and Hispanic patients, who are also less likely to be referred to cardiologists and cardiac surgeons than White persons (Batchelor et al., 2019).

Transgender is a term used to describe persons whose gender identity is different from their sex assigned at birth. Approximately 1% of the U.S. population identify themselves as transgender. Sexual and gender minority persons have higher odds for multiple chronic conditions, cancer, and poor quality of life, and are more apt to have disabilities than cisgender males and females (cisgender is a term used to describe persons whose gender identity and gender expression are aligned with their assigned sex listed on their birth certificate). Gender-affirming hormone therapy is the use of hormone therapy for gender transition or gender affirmation and can be masculinizing or feminizing. It may also affect cardiovascular health in transgender people. Authors of a recent study found that gender-affirming hormone therapy raised average systolic blood pressure in transgender men while lowering it in transgender women (Banks et al., 2021). In a large sample, researchers also found that transgender men and women are more likely to be overweight than cisgender women. Compared to cisgender women, transgender women reported higher rates of diabetes, ischemic stroke, angina/coronary disease, and myocardial infarction. Gender-nonconforming men and women reported higher odds of myocardial infarction than cisgender women. Transgender women also had higher rates of any cardiovascular disease than cisgender men (Cacerese, Jackman, et al., 2020; Connelly et al., 2019). While large-scale studies are not available, these factors likely place some sexual and gender minority people at risk for hypertension.

GLOBAL HEALTH CONSIDERATIONS

Hypertension is a critically important health condition globally. Approximately 26% of the world's adult population have hypertension. In some regions, more than half of the population over age 60 years has hypertension, and experts estimate that more than 1 billion people are hypertensive. High blood pressure is considered the leading modifiable risk factor for disability in the world and contributes to more than 7.5 million deaths per year around the globe. People of African descent have among the highest rates of hypertension, and global prevalence for this group of people is increasing. They have higher risks for nonfatal stroke, fatal stroke, heart disease, and end-stage renal disease than do most other groups.

ASSESSMENT

HISTORY. A diagnosis of hypertension is confirmed after an elevated blood pressure reading occurs on at least three separate occasions. Elicit a history of previously elevated blood pressure, elevated cholesterol counts, a family history of hypertension, and the presence of risk factors. Ask if the patient is experiencing stress at work or at home. Ask the patient about early signs and symptoms, such as malaise, fatigue, general weakness, or a vague sense of discomfort. Establish any history of headache, lightheadedness, dizziness, nosebleeds, ringing in the ears, or blurred vision. Ask about medications such as steroids, oral contraceptives, or cold medications. Ask if the patient has experienced any loss of vision, shortness of breath, chest pain, confusion, increased irritability, seizures, transient paralysis or stupor, sleepiness, visual disturbances, severe headaches, or vomiting. Because hypertension can exist for years without symptoms, assess the following organ systems, which may be affected by longstanding hypertension: heart (heart failure, myocardial infarction), eyes (retinopathy), peripheral circulation (peripheral arterial disease), kidney (end-stage renal disease), and brain (stroke, dementia).

PHYSICAL EXAMINATION. The patient may appear **symptom free** in early stages, although **flushing of the face** may be present. In later stages, a fundoscopic examination of the retina may reveal hemorrhage, fluid accumulation, and narrowed arterioles. Palpate peripheral pulses; note pulsus alternans (alternating strength of the pulse) and bounding arterial pulses. An atrial gallop (S_4 heart sound) on auscultation is suggestive of hypertension.

Have the patient rest quietly in a quiet room for 5 minutes before taking the blood pressure. Using a correctly sized blood pressure cuff, measure blood pressure in both arms three times, 2 to 3 minutes apart, while the patient is at rest in the sitting, standing, and lying positions. A systolic blood pressure of more than 160 mm Hg or a diastolic blood pressure of more than 100 mm Hg is associated with a risk for stroke.

PSYCHOSOCIAL. When symptoms are exacerbated, the patient may become anxious or fearful. Because hypertension can result in changes in lifestyle and perception of body image, assess the patient's coping mechanisms. Assess the patient's stress level and any mental health considerations, which may affect blood pressure control.

Diagnostic Highlights

Test	Normal Result	Abnormality With Condition	Explanation
Blood urea nitrogen	8–21 mg/dL	May be elevated	Determines if renal dysfunction or fluid imbalances are present as a complication of hypertension
Serum creatinine	0.5–1.2 mg/dL	May be elevated	Determines if renal dysfunction is present as a complication of hypertension
Total cholesterol	Individual variations; desirable: < 200 mg/dL	May be elevated	Used for screening to determine risk of coronary heart disease; assesses for hyperlipidemia
Triglycerides	< 150 mg/dL	May be elevated	Used for screening and initial classification of risk of coronary heart disease; elevations determine hyperlipidemia

Diagnostic Highlights (continued)

Test	Normal Result	Abnormality With Condition	Explanation
Electrocardiogram (ECG)	Normal PQRST pattern	ECG may be normal or show signs of left ventricular hypertrophy: conduction delays, ST-T changes	Electrical conduction system may be altered by hypertrophied left ventricle

Other Tests: Tests include urinalysis, chest x-ray, complete blood count, plasma glucose, hemoglobin A_{1C}, serum potassium and calcium, uric acid, plasma renin, and thyroid function tests. Head computed tomography or brain magnetic resonance imaging is indicated for people with hypertension and an abnormal neurological examination.

PRIMARY NURSING DIAGNOSIS

DIAGNOSIS. Deficient knowledge related to insufficient information as evidenced by inaccurate performance of medication and/or self-care management

OUTCOMES. Knowledge: Hypertension management; Knowledge: Medication; Anxiety self-control; Medication response; Health-promoting behaviors; Health-seeking behavior

INTERVENTIONS. Hypertension management; Teaching: Individual; Medication administration; Anxiety reduction; Health education

✴ PLANNING AND IMPLEMENTATION

Collaborative

The long-term goal of care is to limit organ damage. The primary goal is to reduce the blood pressure to less than 140/90 mm Hg, although in people with cardiovascular disease, blood pressure lowering medication may be prescribed for a blood pressure of 130/80 mm Hg. Hypertension in adults older than 60 years of age includes initiating treatment if they have persistent systolic blood pressure at or above 150 mm Hg. Conservative medical management includes diet, exercise, and changes in lifestyle. Because weight loss can result in a drop of 10 mm Hg in both systolic and diastolic blood pressure, patients are encouraged to reach a weight within 15% of their ideal body weight. Patients are encouraged to reduce sodium intake. Advise patients to cease smoking and to reduce alcohol intake to one glass of wine or beer per day. Recommend an aerobic exercise regimen that builds up to 20 to 30 minutes three times a week. When these changes are not effective, drug therapy, along with these recommendations, becomes necessary. Evidence-based recommendations are available through the AHA and other organizations.

If the blood pressure fails to respond to conservative management, the physician initiates pharmacologic management. In stages 1 and 2, pharmacologic therapy should be started along with lifestyle modifications and frequent follow-up. Note that calcium channel blockers and thiazide diuretics are recommended for Black patients (see Pharmacologic Highlights below). If hypertensive crisis occurs (accelerated malignant hypertension, intracranial hemorrhage, aortic dissection, progressive renal failure, or eclampsia), the physician prescribes IV antihypertensives to be given with an infusion device. Maintain continuous noninvasive blood pressure monitoring if the patient does not have an intra-arterial catheter for invasive blood pressure monitoring.

Pharmacologic Highlights

Medication or Drug Class	Dosage	Description	Rationale
Angiotensin-converting enzyme (ACE) inhibitors	Varies with drug	Captopril, enalapril, lisinopril, ramipril	Block production of angiotensin II by inhibiting ACE, leading to vasodilation
Angiotensin II receptor blocker	Varies with drug	Candesartan, irbesartan, losartan, telmisartan, valsartan	Block vasoconstricting and aldosterone-secreting effects of angiotensin II resulting in an antihypertensive effect
Diuretics	Varies with drug	Thiazides; loop; potassium sparing	Cause urinary sodium loss with subsequent intravascular volume loss; cause mild vasodilation
Calcium channel blockers	Varies with drug	Diltiazem, nifedipine, amlodipine, verapamil, isradipine, nicardipine	Cause arteriolar vasodilation by blocking calcium channels
Beta-adrenergic antagonists	Varies with drug	Commonly used: atenolol, metoprolol, nadolol, propranolol, timolol	Inhibit effects of catecholamines that decrease renin and cause resetting of baroreceptors to accept a lower level of blood pressure
Beta-adrenergic antagonists	Varies with drug	Commonly used: atenolol, metoprolol, nadolol, propranolol, timolol	Inhibit effects of catecholamines that decrease renin and cause resetting of baroreceptors to accept a lower level of blood pressure
IV antihypertensives	Varies with drug	Sodium nitroprusside, (IV infusion), diazoxide (IV bolus), labetalol (IV bolus), esmolol (IV bolus), nitroglycerin (IV infusion)	Manage hypertensive crisis with a variety of mechanisms of actions

Independent

Teach the patient the pathophysiology of hypertension. Explain the actions, dosages, and adverse effects of prescribed antihypertensive medications and discuss risk factors that can cause organ damage. Review dietary restrictions. Stress the importance of reading food labels and avoiding prepared foods with a high sodium content. Foods with sodium listed among the top five ingredients are not recommended. Recommend that canned meats and vegetables be rinsed for 1 minute to remove most of the sodium. Explain the need to decrease the intake of saturated fats and cholesterol. Encourage patients on potassium-losing medications to eat foods rich in potassium. Patients taking potassium-sparing diuretics should avoid excessive use of salt substitutes because they may be high in potassium.

Teach the patient the need for regular aerobic exercise and stress reduction. Refer patients to smoking cessation or substance abuse programs as appropriate. Demonstrate relaxation techniques. Teach the patient the correct use of a self-monitoring blood pressure cuff. Advise the patient to record the reading at least twice weekly in a journal and to bring the journal when visiting the physician. Explain the need to take the blood pressure at approximately the same time and following a similar type of activity. Also encourage the patient to keep a record of the medications prescribed and their efficacy. Suggest that the patient establish a daily routine for taking antihypertensive medications and remind the patient to avoid vasoconstricting over-the-counter cold and sinus medications.

Evidence-Based Practice and Health Policy

Hsieh, H-F., Heinze, J., Caruso, E., Scott, B., West, B., Mistry, R., Eisman, A., Assari, S., Buu, A., & Zimmerman, M. (2020). The protective effects of social support on hypertension among African American adolescents exposed to violence. *Journal of Interpersonal Violence.* Advance online publication. https://doi.org/10.1177/0886260520969390

- The authors note that African American individuals develop hypertension earlier in life than White individuals, and disparities occur as early as adolescence. They also note that violence victimization is a stressor that may be related to hypertension. They used eight waves of longitudinal data of African American youth ($N = 353$) that included youth in middle adolescence (mean 14.9 years) through emerging adulthood (mean 23.1 years).
- They found that higher levels of self-reported violence victimization during ages 14 to 18 years were associated with more reports of hypertension during ages 20 to 23 years. The authors adjusted the statistics for sex, socioeconomic status, substance abuse, and mental distress. The relationship between violence and hypertension was moderated by friends' support but not family support.

DOCUMENTATION GUIDELINES

- Physical findings: Blood pressure readings, presence of headache, mental status, daily weights
- Response to diet therapy and exercise
- Response to medications
- Presence of complications
- Side effects of medications, noncompliance
- Ability to deal with stress and a chronic condition

DISCHARGE AND HOME HEALTHCARE GUIDELINES

Make sure the patient understands the need to control risk factors through medication therapy, dietary modifications, exercise guidelines, stress-reduction methods, and follow-up care. Have the patient demonstrate an understanding of how to take medicine, how often, and the potential side effects. Emphasize the need for frequent monitoring of blood pressure and laboratory work. Explain which signs and symptoms indicate a need to contact the physician. These symptoms include headache, blurred vision, dizziness, sleepiness, confusion, and changes in sexual performance. If the patient experiences altered sexual performance after starting a medication, encourage the patient to notify the physician immediately to have the medication changed rather than just stopping it without consultation.

Hyperthyroidism

DRG Category: 644
Mean LOS: 4.3 days
Description: MEDICAL: Endocrine Disorders With Complication or Comorbidity

Hyperthyroidism is a condition caused by excessive overproduction of thyroid hormone by the thyroid gland. The thyroid hormones (triiodothyronine [T_3] and thyroxine [T_4]), produced in the thyroid gland under the control of thyroid-stimulating hormone (TSH), regulate the body's metabolism. Sustained thyroid hormone overproduction, therefore, causes a hypermetabolic state that affects most of the body organs, such as the heart, gastrointestinal tract, brain, muscles, eyes, and skin.

The seriousness of the disease depends on the degree of hypersecretion of the thyroid hormones. As the levels of thyroid hormones rise, the risk of life-threatening cardiac problems becomes progressively greater. The most common form of hyperthyroidism is called *Graves disease* or *thyrotoxicosis*. Graves disease is associated with hyperthyroidism, eye disorders, and skin disorders, and when uncontrolled, vital organs are stressed to their capacity. It is also associated with many autoimmune diseases such as diabetes mellitus, breast cancer, Addison disease, systemic lupus erythematosus, rheumatoid arthritis, myasthenia gravis, and pernicious anemia. Risk factors include tobacco use, high iodine intake, stress, and use of sex steroids.

Cardiac stress from increased myocardial oxygen requirements can lead to serious cardiovascular complications, such as systolic hypertension, life-threatening dysrhythmias, or heart failure. Large goiters can cause pressure on the neck and trachea, which can result in respiratory distress. Ophthalmopathy can result in corneal ulceration and loss of vision. Metabolic hyperactivity can cause high levels of anxiety, insomnia, and psychoses. The most severe form of hyperthyroidism is thyrotoxic crisis, known also as *thyroid storm* or *thyrotoxicosis*. This condition, which occurs when the body can no longer tolerate the hypermetabolic state, is a nursing and medical emergency and is fatal if not treated. Thyroid storm may be precipitated by a physiological stressor such as diabetic ketoacidosis, infection, trauma, or surgery.

CAUSES

Graves disease has an autoimmune derivation and is caused by circulating anti-TSH autoantibodies that displace TSH from the thyroid receptors and mimic TSH by activating the TSH receptor to release additional thyroid hormones. Graves disease is also associated with Hashimoto disease, a chronic inflammation of the thyroid gland that usually causes hypothyroidism but can also cause symptoms similar to those of Graves disease.

Thyrotoxicosis has several different pathophysiological causes, including autoimmune disease, functioning thyroid adenoma, and infection.

GENETIC CONSIDERATIONS

Hyperthyroidism has a strong genetic component, with heritability estimated at 40% to 60%. Mutations in the thyroid-stimulating hormone receptor gene (*TSHR*) cause a nonautoimmune form of hyperthyroidism that is inherited in an autosomal dominant manner. The autoimmune form of hyperthyroidism, Graves disease, is caused by mutations in several genes and follows either an autosomal recessive or X-linked inheritance pattern. Loci that have been linked with Graves disease include chromosome 6p11, CTKA4 on 2q33, AITD1, CTLA4, GRD1, GRD2, GRD3, HT1, and HT2. Other loci and the human leukocyte antigen (HLA) region types are also linked with Graves disease.

SEX AND LIFE SPAN CONSIDERATIONS

Hyperthyroidism is more frequently found in women than in men, and some experts suggest that the hormone cycles of women may in some way affect the incidence of thyroid disease. Although it can affect all ages, it is most typically diagnosed in 20- to 40-year-olds and is unusual in children, teenagers, and people over age 65 years. When hyperthyroidism occurs in older adults, their symptoms may be more subtle than those of younger persons, and the classic signs may even be absent. Occasionally, an older person with hyperthyroidism has apathy or withdrawal instead of the more typical hypermetabolic state.

HEALTH DISPARITIES AND SEXUAL/GENDER MINORITY HEALTH

White, Asian, and Hispanic persons have a slightly higher prevalence of hyperthyroidism than do Black persons. Sexual and gender minority status has no known effect on the risk of hyperthyroidism.

GLOBAL HEALTH CONSIDERATIONS

Hyperthyroidism is present in people of all countries. Areas of the world that have iodine deficiency place people at risk for both hyperthyroidism and hypothyroidism. Countries with insufficient iodine include Eastern Europe, Russia, and parts of Africa. Highest prevalence occurs in Brazil, China, India, Great Britain, and Northern Africa.

☀ ASSESSMENT

HISTORY. Ask patients about their medical history and if they have experienced nervousness, anxiety, or hyperactivity. Often, patients report intolerance to heat, excessive perspiration, and increased appetite accompanied by weight loss. Complaints of abdominal cramping and frequent bowel movements are customary. Patients may also describe discomfort when wearing clothing or jewelry that is close fitting at the neckline as well as generalized muscular weakness and increased fatigue. Physical exertion may cause chest pain, shortness of breath, or both. They may have a history of heart failure or cardiac dysrhythmias. A female patient may report oligomenorrhea (scanty or infrequent menses), and all patients might experience decreased libido. Ask patients if they use tobacco products or have high levels of stress in their life.

Determine if there is a family history of autoimmune disease or thyroid disease. Take a drug history to determine the use of iodides (oral contraceptives, contrast media) that may cause falsely elevated serum thyroid hormone levels. Determine if they lived in an area of the world that is iodine deficient. Similarly, severe illness, malnutrition, or the use of aspirin, corticosteroids, and phenytoin sodium may cause a false decrease in serum thyroid hormone levels.

PHYSICAL EXAMINATION. The most common symptoms are due to hypermetabolism, such as **anxiety**, **diaphoresis**, **nervousness**, and **palpitations**. The patient may have a short attention span and fine hand tremors or shaky handwriting. Note an increased resting pulse, a widened pulse pressure, or hypertension. The skin may have a sheen of perspiration or be salmon colored.

Stand behind the patient and palpate the thyroid gland at rest and during swallowing to note the size, tenderness, and nodularity. Remember that excessive palpation of the thyroid gland can precipitate thyroid storm; therefore, palpate gently and only when necessary. You may also hear a bruit when you auscultate the thyroid gland over the lateral lobes. Exophthalmos, bulging of the eye resulting in larger amounts of visible sclera, is often quite noticeable; a fixed stare because of the presence of fluid behind the eyeball and periorbital edema are also common. In patients who have had Graves disease for several years, there may be changes in the skin, such as raised and thickened areas over the legs or feet and hyperpigmentation and itchiness. Patients often exhibit fine, thin hair and fragile nails. Patients with thyroid storm have a racing heart, high fever, profound diaphoresis, diarrhea, severe dehydration, shaking, agitation, confusion, and coma.

PSYCHOSOCIAL. Well before a formal diagnosis, the patient may be aware that something is seriously wrong and report increased anxiety or nervousness, insomnia, and early awakening from sleep. The anxiety is often heightened by symptoms of the disease such as angina and the sense of loss of control over one's body.

Diagnostic Highlights

Test	Normal Result	Abnormality With Condition	Explanation
TSH assay	In most healthy patients, TSH values are 0.4–4.2 mU/L	Decreased so that values may be unmeasurable	Elevation of thyroid hormones; decreased TSH secretion by negative feedback

(highlight box continues on page 612)

Diagnostic Highlights (continued)

Test	Normal Result	Abnormality With Condition	Explanation
T₄ radioimmunoassay	5.5–12.5 mcg/dL	Elevated	Reflects overproduction of thyroid hormones; monitors response to therapy
T₃ radioimmunoassay	70–204 ng/dL	Elevated	Reflects overproduction of thyroid hormones

Other Tests: Tests include 24-hour radioactive iodine uptake, thyroid autoantibodies, antithyroglobulin, nuclear thyroid scan, and electrocardiogram.

PRIMARY NURSING DIAGNOSIS

DIAGNOSIS. Decreased activity tolerance related to increased metabolism as evidenced by exhaustion, palpitations, and/or fatigue

OUTCOMES. Activity tolerance; Energy conservation; Knowledge: Disease process; Knowledge: Medication; Endurance; Nutritional status; Symptom severity

INTERVENTIONS. Energy management; Exercise promotion; Nutrition management; Medication management; Vital signs monitoring

PLANNING AND IMPLEMENTATION

Collaborative

Most patients are diagnosed and treated on an outpatient basis. Symptoms are managed with oral hydration and beta-blockers for relief of neurological and cardiovascular symptoms. The goal of treatment is to return the patient to the euthyroid (normal) state and to prevent complications. Graves disease is treated pharmacologically (see Pharmacologic Highlights). Radioactive iodine (^{131}I) is given for two purposes: for diagnosing imaging in low doses and for therapeutic destruction of the thyroid gland in larger doses. Radioactive iodine is considered the definitive and most common treatment, but it is not without risks. The principal disadvantage is the potential for hypothyroidism because 40% to 70% of patients treated with ^{131}I develop hypothyroidism within 10 years after treatment. Other complications include parathyroid damage and exacerbation of hyperthyroidism. Surgical treatment with thyroidectomy is no longer the preferred choice of therapy for Graves disease but is an alternative therapeutic approach in some situations. In particular, it is used for patients who cannot tolerate antithyroid drugs, have significant ophthalmopathy, have large goiters, or cannot undergo radioiodine therapy.

If thyroid storm is suspected, emergency treatment needs to be instituted immediately. Patients may need cardiac monitoring, intubation and mechanical ventilation with supplemental oxygen, and IV fluids. The patient requires antithyroid medications and may receive IV corticosteroids and beta-adrenergic medications.

Pharmacologic Highlights

Medication or Drug Class	Dosage	Description	Rationale
Propylthiouracil (PTU)	Initial PTU: 300–400 mg/day PO divided tid; not to exceed 1,200 mg/day; maintenance: 100–300 mg/day PO	Antithyroid agent	Returns the patient to the euthyroid (normal) state; inhibits use of iodine by thyroid gland; blocks oxidation of iodine and inhibits thyroid hormone synthesis

Pharmacologic Highlights (continued)

Medication or Drug Class	Dosage	Description	Rationale
Methimazole (Tapazole)	Initial: 15 mg/day for mild hyperthyroidism; 30–40 mg/day for moderately severe hyperthyroidism; 60 mg/day for severe hyperthyroidism	Antithyroid agent	Returns the patient to the euthyroid (normal) state; inhibits use of iodine by thyroid gland

Other Drugs: Beta-adrenergic blockers, corticosteroids for vision threatening opthalmopathy, radioactive iodine

Independent

Nursing interventions center on ongoing monitoring, protecting the patient from injury, reducing stress, and initiating teaching. Patients with exophthalmos or other visual problems might be more comfortable wearing sunglasses or eye patches to protect the eyes from light. Report any changes in visual acuity to the physician and use artificial tears to lubricate the eyes.

Encourage patients to follow the medication regimen and reassure them while waiting for it to take effect. To determine the response to treatment and to prevent thyroid storm, assess the cardiovascular status, fluid and diet intake and output, daily weights, bowel elimination, and the ability of the patient to perform activities of daily living without excessive fatigue. Reassure the patient's family that the patient's mood swings, nervousness, or anxiety will diminish as treatment continues. If the patient or family requires additional support, ask a clinical nurse specialist or mental health counselor to see the patient or family. Note that extreme anxiety of the undiagnosed or uncontrolled patient makes patient education difficult for all concerned. If you recognize the patient's inability to maintain long cognitive or physical attention spans, you will have better success at patient education. One useful strategy is to ensure that significant others are present during all teaching sessions.

Evidence-Based Practice and Health Policy

Pan, Y., Xie, Q., Zhang, Z., Dai, Y., Lin, L., Quan, M., Guo, X., Shen, M., & Zhao, S. (2020). Association between overt hyperthyroidism and risk of sexual dysfunction in both sexes: A systematic review and meta-analysis. *Journal of Sexual Medicine, 17*, 2198–2207.

- The authors conducted a systematic review and meta-analysis using electronic databases to explain the association between overt hyperthyroidism and the risk of sexual dysfunction. They located seven relevant studies.
- Overt hyperthyroidism led to significant sexual dysfunction in both sexes. Men and women with overt hyperthyroidism were at over twofold higher risk of sexual dysfunction than the general population. Women had issues with arousal, lubrication, orgasm, and sexual satisfaction, whereas men had issues with ejaculation, erectile dysfunction, and desire. The authors concluded that sexual health consequences may occur as a result of hyperthyroidism.

DOCUMENTATION GUIDELINES

- Physical findings: Cardiovascular status (resting pulse, blood pressure, presence of angina or palpitations), bowel activity, edema, condition of skin, activity tolerance
- Physical findings: Hypermetabolism, eye status, heat intolerance, level of hydration, activity level
- Response to medications, skin care regimen, nutrition, body weight, comfort
- Psychosocial response to changes in bodily function, including mental acuity, behavioral patterns, emotional stability

DISCHARGE AND HOME HEALTHCARE GUIDELINES

DISEASE PROCESS. Provide a clear explanation of the role of the thyroid gland, the disease process, and the treatment plan. Explain possible side effects of the treatment. Ensure that the patient understands eye care.

MEDICATIONS. Be sure the patient understands all medications, including the dosage, route, action, adverse effects, and need for any laboratory monitoring of thyroid medications. If the patient is taking propylthiouracil or methimazole, encourage the patient to take the medications with meals to limit gastric irritation. If the patient is taking an iodine solution, mix it with milk or juice to limit gastric irritation and have the patient use a straw to limit the risk of teeth discoloration.

COMPLICATIONS. Have the patient report any signs and symptoms of thyrotoxicosis immediately: rapid heart rate, palpitations, perspiration, shakiness, tremors, difficulty breathing, nausea, and vomiting. Teach the patient to report increased neck swelling, difficulty swallowing, or weight loss.

Hypocalcemia

DRG Category: 640
Mean LOS: 4.5 days
Description: MEDICAL: Miscellaneous Disorders of Nutrition, Metabolism, Fluids, and Electrolytes With Major Complication or Comorbidity

Hypocalcemia is a diminished calcium level, below 8.2 mg/dL, in the bloodstream. Calcium is vital to the body for the formation of bones and teeth, blood coagulation, nerve impulse transmission, cell permeability, and normal muscle contraction. Although 98% of the body's calcium is found in the bones, three forms of calcium exist in the serum: free or ionized calcium (50% of serum total), calcium bound to protein (45% of serum total), and calcium complexed with citrate or other organic ions (5% of serum total). Ionized calcium is reabsorbed into bone, absorbed from the gastrointestinal mucosa, and excreted in urine and feces as regulated by the parathyroid glands. Ionized calcium is the active, physiological component of total calcium fraction. Parathyroid hormone (PTH) is necessary for calcium absorption and normal serum calcium levels.

Hypocalcemia is a more common clinical problem than hypercalcemia and may occur as frequently as 15% to 50% in acutely ill patients. Some experts estimate that over half of critically ill patients in intensive care units have hypocalcemia. Alkalosis can induce hypocalcemia because it leads to increased calcium-protein binding and decreased ionized calcium; acidosis protects from hypocalcemia because it leads to decreased calcium-protein binding and increased ionized calcium. When calcium levels drop, neuromuscular excitability occurs in smooth, skeletal, and cardiac muscle, causing the muscles to twitch. The result can lead to cardiac dysrhythmias. Hypocalcemia can also cause increased capillary permeability, pathological fractures, and decreased blood coagulation. Most severe cases result in tetany (condition of prolonged, painful spasms of the voluntary muscles of the fingers and toes [carpopedal spasm] as well as the facial muscles), which, if left untreated, leads to carpopedal and laryngeal spasm, seizures, and respiratory arrest.

CAUSES

The most frequent cause of hypocalcemia is a low albumin level, but if serum ionized (free) calcium is normal, then no disorder of calcium metabolism is present and no treatment is needed. In the clinical setting, the most common cause of hypocalcemia is acute/chronic kidney failure followed by vitamin D deficiency (vitamin D is needed for calcium absorption). Causes of low ionized calcium, which is needed for enzymatic reactions and neuromuscular function, also include hypoparathyroidism, severe hypomagnesemia, hypermagnesemia, and acute pancreatitis. It is also associated with thyroidectomy and radical neck dissection when there is postoperative ischemia to the parathyroid glands.

Low serum calcium levels can also occur after small bowel resection, partial gastrectomy with gastrojejunostomy, and Crohn disease. Severe diarrhea or laxative abuse may also cause hypocalcemia; when intestinal surfaces are lost, less calcium is absorbed. A transient low calcium level can result from massive administration of citrated blood. Some drugs that can result in hypocalcemia include loop diuretics, phenytoin, phosphates, caffeine, alcohol, antimicrobials (pentamidine, ketoconazole, aminoglycosides), antineoplastic agents (cisplatin, cytosine arabinoside), and corticosteroids.

GENETIC CONSIDERATIONS

Gain of function mutations in the calcium-sensing receptor (*CASR*) are associated with type 1 autosomal dominant familial hypocalcemia with hypercalciuria. Type 2 familial hypocalcemia with hypercalciuria is rarer and occurs from mutations in the *GNA11* gene.

Persistent low blood calcium levels are also seen in DiGeorge syndrome, which results from a deletion of several genes on chromosome 22 (22q deletion). Other features of 22q deletion include cleft palate, cardiac defects, characteristic facial features, and underdevelopment of the thymus.

SEX AND LIFE SPAN CONSIDERATIONS

Hypocalcemia can occur in all people at any age, but infants, children, and older adults are at high risk. In infants, it occurs with the use of cow's milk formula with a high concentration of phosphate. The large bone turnover during growth spurts accounts for hypocalcemia in children, especially if their calcium intake is deficient. Osteoporosis in older adults is associated with a lifetime low intake of calcium, which leads to a total body calcium deficit. Those older adults with osteoporosis who spend prolonged time on bedrest also have a risk for hypocalcemia.

HEALTH DISPARITIES AND SEXUAL/GENDER MINORITY HEALTH

Ethnicity, race, and sexual/gender minority status have no known effect on the risk for hypocalcemia.

GLOBAL HEALTH CONSIDERATIONS

Hypocalcemia occurs in all global regions from acute and chronic renal failure, nutritional deficiencies (vitamin D, calcium, and magnesium), parathyroid disease, and pancreatitis.

ASSESSMENT

HISTORY. Ask about a prior diagnosis of hypoparathyroidism, renal failure, pancreatic insufficiency, or hypomagnesemia. Elicit a history of severe infections or burns. Ask if the patient has been under treatment for acidosis, which might lead to alkalosis. Determine if the patient has an inadequate intake of calcium, vitamin D, or both. Investigate causes of vitamin D or magnesium deficiency, such as a gastrointestinal disease associated with malabsorption, poor diet, gastrectomy, intestinal resection or bypass, or hepatobiliary disease. Ask about medication use associated with disordered calcium metabolism, such as phenytoin, estrogen, loop diuretics, or plicamycin.

Inquire about anxiety, irritability, twitching around the mouth, laryngospasm, or convulsions, all central nervous system signs and symptoms of hypocalcemia. Establish a history of tingling or numbness in the fingers (paresthesia) or around the mouth, tetany or painful tonic muscle spasms, abdominal cramps, muscle cramps, or spasmodic contractions. Determine if the patient has experienced mental status changes. Ask the patient about gastrointestinal symptoms such as diarrhea.

PHYSICAL EXAMINATION. The most common symptoms of severe hypocalcemia include **neuromuscular excitability with muscle cramps, twitching and irritability**, and **laryngospasm**. Assess airway, breathing, and circulation. Hypocalcemia can lead to wheezing, laryngospasm, dyspnea, and difficulty swallowing. Central nervous system signs include confusion, disorientation, hallucinations, dementia, and seizures. Auscultate for heart sounds. The patient may have heart failure and/or dysrhythmias, especially heart block and ventricular fibrillation. Tetany, increased neural excitability, accounts for the majority of signs and symptoms of hypocalcemia. Check for Trousseau sign (development of carpal spasm when a blood pressure cuff is inflated above systolic pressure for 3 minutes) and Chvostek sign (twitching facial muscles when the facial nerve is tapped anterior to the ear).

Inspect the patient's skin to see if it is dry, coarse, or scaly, which are signs of hypocalcemia. Note any exacerbation of eczema or psoriasis along with hair loss or brittle nails. Check for dental abnormalities. Inspect the patient's eyes for cataracts of the cortical portion of the lens, which may develop within a year after the onset of hypocalcemia.

PSYCHOSOCIAL. Severe hypocalcemia may produce mental changes, which is frightening for the patient and the family. Assess for depression, impaired memory, and confusion. As the condition continues, delirium and hallucinations may be present. In severe cases of hypocalcemia, psychosis or dementia may develop. Electrolyte disturbances that affect a patient's personality often increase the patient's and family's anxiety. Assess the patient's and family's coping mechanisms.

Diagnostic Highlights

Test	Normal Result	Abnormality With Condition	Explanation
Serum calcium: Total calcium, including free ionized calcium and calcium bound with protein or organic ions	8.4–10.2 mg/dL	< 8.2 mg/dL; critical value: < 6.5 mg/dL	Deficit of calcium below normal levels in the extracellular fluid compartment; if ionized calcium cannot be measured, total serum calcium can be corrected by adding 0.8 mg/dL to the total calcium level for every 1 g/dL decrease of serum albumin below 4 g/dL; the corrected value determines whether true hypocalcemia is present. When calcium levels are reported as high or low, calculate the actual level of calcium by the following formula: Corrected total calcium (mg/dL) = (measured total calcium mg/dL) + 0.8 (4.4 measured albumin g/dL).

Diagnostic Highlights (continued)

Test	Normal Result	Abnormality With Condition	Explanation
Serum ionized calcium: Unbound calcium; level unaffected by albumin level	4.6–5.3 mg/dL	< 4.5 mg/dL; critical value: < 3.5 mg/dL	Ionized calcium is approximately 50% of circulating calcium and is the form of calcium available for enzymatic reactions and neuromuscular function; levels increase and decrease with blood pH levels; for every 0.1 pH decrease, ionized calcium increases 1.5%–2.5%
Serum PTH	10–65 mg/ mL pg	Elevated in disorders other than hypoparathyroidism and magnesium deficiency	Determines presence or absence of hypoparathyroidism; determines the cause of hypocalcemia

Other Tests: Tests include electrocardiogram (prolonged ST segment and QT interval; in patients taking digitalis preparations, hypocalcemia potentiates digitalis toxicity), phosphorus (elevated in hypocalcemia resulting from most causes, although in hypocalcemia from vitamin D deficiency, it is usually low), magnesium, creatinine, and urine calcium. Note that alkalosis augments calcium binding to albumin and increases the severity of symptoms of hypocalcemia.

PRIMARY NURSING DIAGNOSIS

DIAGNOSIS. Risk for ineffective airway clearance as evidenced by wheezing, laryngospasm, and/or dyspnea

OUTCOMES. Hypocalcemia severity; Respiratory status: Airway patency; Respiratory status: Gas exchange; Respiratory status: Ventilation; Electrolyte & acid/base balance; Fluid balance

INTERVENTIONS. Electrolyte management: Hypocalcemia; Fluid management; Airway management; Airway insertion and stabilization; Airway suctioning; Anxiety reduction; Oxygen therapy; Mechanical ventilation management: Invasive or noninvasive; Respiratory monitoring

▓ PLANNING AND IMPLEMENTATION

Collaborative

If the patient has an airway obstruction, endotracheal intubation and mechanical ventilation may be needed to manage laryngospasm. Hypocalcemia is treated pharmacologically. Acute hypocalcemia with tetany is a medical emergency that requires parenteral calcium supplements. Be aware of factors related to the administration of calcium replacement. A too-rapid infusion rate can lead to bradycardia and cardiac arrest; therefore, place patients who are receiving a continuous calcium infusion on a cardiac monitor and place the infusion on a controlled infusion device. The infusion rate should be adjusted to avoid recurrent symptomatic hypocalcemia and to maintain serum calcium levels between 8 and 9 mg/dL. Monitor the patient's serum calcium levels every 12 to 24 hours and immediately report a calcium deficit less than 8.5 mg/dL. When giving calcium supplements, frequently check pH levels because an alkaline state (pH < 7.45) inhibits calcium ionization and decreases the free calcium available for physiological reactions.

Chronic hypocalcemia can be treated in part by a high dietary intake of calcium. If the deficiency is caused by hypoparathyroidism, however, teach the patient to avoid foods high in phosphate. Vitamin D supplements are prescribed to facilitate gastrointestinal calcium absorption.

Pharmacologic Highlights

Medication or Drug Class	Dosage	Description	Rationale
Calcium supplements	Varies by drug	Electrolyte supplement; emergency supplementation: Calcium gluconate 2 g IV over 10 min followed by an infusion of 6 g in 500 mL D5W over 4–6 hr; oral calcium gluconate, calcium lactate, or calcium chloride; asymptomatic hypocalcemia can be alleviated with oral calcium citrate, acetate, or carbonate and vitamin D supplementation	Correct deficiency
Magnesium sulfate	1 g in 50 mL over 1 hr IV	Electrolyte supplement	Corrects magnesium deficiency; magnesium deficiency needs to be corrected in order to correct calcium deficiency; magnesium is needed to transport calcium across cell membrane

Independent

Monitor calcium supplements carefully. If calcium is given intravenously, the patient should have continuous cardiac monitoring attached and have calcium supplements on an infusion device to regulate dosage. If the patient has an altered mental status, institute the appropriate safety measures. Provide a quiet, stress-free environment for patients with tetany. Institute seizure precautions for patients with severe hypocalcemia. If tetany is a possibility, maintain an oral or a nasal airway and intubation equipment at the bedside. Initiate patient teaching to prevent future episodes of hypocalcemia.

Evidence-Based Practice and Health Policy

Lapointe, A., Moreau, N., Simonyan, D., Rousseau, F., Mallette, V., Préfontaine-Racine, F., Paquette, C., Mallet, M., St-Pierre, A., & Berthelot, S. (2021). Identification of predictors of abnormal calcium, magnesium and phosphorus blood levels in the emergency department: A retrospective cohort study. *Open Access Emergency Medicine, 13*, 13–21.

- Because rising healthcare costs require judicious use of diagnostic tests, the authors sought to determine risk factors that could predict abnormal calcium, magnesium, and phosphorus serum levels, as well as to identify patients who may need corrective interventions. They conducted a retrospective cohort study evaluating variables in 1,008 cases with serum calcium and/or magnesium and/or phosphorus levels drawn in the emergency department.
- The most significant risk factors for a hypocalcemia electrolytic abnormality were as follows: respiratory distress, diuretics (excluding loop and thiazide), antineoplastic medication, long QTc (cardiac dysrhythmia), and chronic kidney disease. Predictors of patients who needed an intervention included poor peripheral perfusion, nausea, and chronic obstructive pulmonary disease. Emergency physicians can possibly reduce unnecessary testing of calcium, magnesium, and phosphorus blood levels by targeting patients with high-acuity conditions or chronic comorbidities such as renal and pulmonary disease.

DOCUMENTATION GUIDELINES

• Maintenance of a patent airway, normal breathing, and adequate circulation; vital signs
• Presence or absence of increased neuromuscular activity: Seizures, Trousseau sign, Chvostek sign, numbness, tingling
• Response to calcium therapy

DISCHARGE AND HOME HEALTHCARE GUIDELINES

Instruct the patient about foods rich in calcium, vitamin D, and protein. Emphasize the effect of drugs on serum calcium levels. High intakes of alcohol and caffeine decrease calcium absorption, as does moderate cigarette smoking. Patients with a tendency to develop renal calculi should be told to consult their physician before increasing their calcium intake. When hypocalcemia is caused by hypoparathyroidism, milk and milk products are omitted from the patient's diet to decrease phosphorus intake.

Be sure the patient understands any calcium supplements prescribed, including dosages, route, action, and side effects. Advise the patient that calcium may cause constipation and review methods to maintain bowel elimination. Hypercalcemia may develop as a consequence of the treatment for hypocalcemia. Teach the patient the signs and symptoms of increased serum calcium levels and the need to call the physician if they develop.

Hypochloremia

DRG Category: 640
Mean LOS: 4.5 days
Description: MEDICAL: Miscellaneous Disorders of Nutrition, Metabolism, Fluids, and Electrolytes With Major Complication or Comorbidity

Hypochloremia is a serum chloride level below 95 mEq/L. Normal serum chloride level is 97 to 107 mEq/L. Chloride is the major anion in the extracellular fluid (ECF). The intracellular level of chloride is only about 2 to 4 mEq/L. Chloride is regulated in the body primarily through its relationship with sodium. Serum levels of both sodium and chloride often parallel each other.

A main function of chloride in the body is to join with hydrogen to form hydrochloric acid (HCl). HCl aids in digestion and activates enzymes, such as salivary amylase. Chloride plays a role in maintaining the serum osmolarity and body water balance. The normal serum osmolarity ranges between 275 and 295 mOsm/L.

Chloride deficit leads to a number of physiological alterations such as ECF volume contraction, potassium depletion, intracellular acidosis, and increased bicarbonate generation. Hypochloremia, similar to hyponatremia, also causes a decrease in the serum osmolarity. This decrease means that there is a decrease in sodium and chloride ions in proportion to water in the ECF. When there is a body water excess, chloride also may be decreased along with sodium, preventing reabsorption of body water by the kidneys. Complications of hypochloremia include dehydration, hypotension, muscle twitching, tetany, and seizure activity.

CAUSES

The most common cause of hypochloremia is gastrointestinal (GI) abnormalities, including prolonged vomiting or nasogastric suctioning leading to metabolic alkalosis, loss of potassium, and diarrhea. Loss of potassium, which occurs as a result of gastric suctioning and vomiting, further leads to hypochloremia because potassium frequently combines with chloride to form potassium chloride (KCl). Chloride is also lost through diarrhea, which has a high chloride content.

Other causes of hypochloremia are dietary changes, renal abnormalities, acid-base imbalances (particularly respiratory acidosis and metabolic alkalosis), and skin losses due to burn injury. Diets low in sodium can contribute to hypochloremia, as can medications such as thiazide and loop diuretics, corticosteroids, and bicarbonate. Another common cause in hospitalized patients is the combination of stopping all oral intake during an illness and placing patients on IV fluid.

GENETIC CONSIDERATIONS

Several genetic diseases can result in low blood chloride levels. These include cystic fibrosis and Bartter syndrome. Bartter syndrome is a group of several disorders of impaired salt reabsorption in the thick ascending loop of Henle: hypochloremia, hypokalemic metabolic alkalosis, and hypercalciuria. Several genes have been associated with Bartter syndrome (bumetanide-sensitive Na-K-2Cl cotransporter *SLC12A1*, the *BSND* gene, simultaneous mutation in both the *CLCNKA* and the *CLCNKB* genes, and the thiazide-sensitive sodium-chloride cotransporter *SLC12A3*). Another cause of hypochloremia is congenital adrenal hyperplasia, which is a heritable disorder of adrenal corticosteroid synthesis that is transmitted in an autosomal recessive pattern.

SEX AND LIFE SPAN CONSIDERATIONS

Infants, children, and adults of both sexes are at risk for developing hypochloremia. Older patients are particularly at risk when they are placed on multiple medications or if they have persistent bouts of vomiting and diarrhea. Identify high-risk groups, such as those with GI abnormalities. Note that hospitalized patients across the life span are often at risk because of the treatments, such as nasogastric suction, used to manage their illnesses.

HEALTH DISPARITIES AND SEXUAL/GENDER MINORITY HEALTH

Ethnicity, race, and sexual/gender minority status have no known effect on the risk for hypochloremia.

GLOBAL HEALTH CONSIDERATIONS

No data are available, but hypochloremia exists around the world in people with fluid and electrolyte imbalances.

⚒ ASSESSMENT

HISTORY. Ask about any recent signs and symptoms that deviate from past health patterns that could cause hypochloremia, such as vomiting and diarrhea. Ask the patient to list all medications, especially diuretics, which contribute to chloride loss. Obtain a history of past illnesses and surgeries. If the patient is already hospitalized, review the records for prolonged dextrose administration and a history of gastric suctioning or IV fluid therapy.

PHYSICAL EXAMINATION. Physical findings depend on the cause of the chloride deficit, but the patient can be asymptomatic. Inspect the patient for tetany-like symptoms, such as tremors and twitching; these neuromuscular symptoms are present with hypochloremia associated with hyponatremia. Assess if the patient has signs of dehydration such as thirst, dizziness, fatigue, confusion, or low urine output. If hypochloremia is caused by metabolic alkalosis secondary to the loss of gastric secretions, respiratory and neuromuscular symptoms appear. Other symptoms include muscular weakness, diaphoresis, and fever. Assess the patient's respirations and note the depth and rate; the patient's breathing may become shallow and depressed with severe hypochloremia. If the chloride deficit is not corrected, eventually a decrease in blood pressure occurs.

PSYCHOSOCIAL. In most cases, hypochloremia is a result of GI abnormalities or the use of loop diuretics. Assess the patient's tolerance and coping ability to handle the discomfort of GI symptoms. If the patient is upset about changes in nerves and muscles, explain that the symptoms disappear when chloride is supplemented.

Diagnostic Highlights

Test	Normal Result	Abnormality With Condition	Explanation
Serum chloride	97–107 mEq/L	< 95 mEq/L; critical value: < 90 mEq/L	Reflects a deficit in chloride
Serum osmolarity	275–295 mOsm/L	< 275 mOsm/L; critical value: < 250 mOsm/L	Reflects decrease in concentration of particles in ECF

Other Tests: Serum bicarbonate, serum electrolytes, urine electrolytes, urine osmolarity

PRIMARY NURSING DIAGNOSIS

DIAGNOSIS. Ineffective protection related to neuromuscular changes as evidenced by tremors and/or twitching

OUTCOMES. Hypochloremia severity; Electrolyte and acid-base balance; Hydration; Neurological status: Consciousness; Nutritional status; Fluid balance

INTERVENTIONS. Fluid/electrolyte management; Electrolyte monitoring; Fluid management; Fluid monitoring; Nutrition management; Medication management

PLANNING AND IMPLEMENTATION

Collaborative

Treatment of hypochloremia involves treating the underlying cause and replacing the chloride. Careful monitoring of fluid and electrolyte status is critical. Monitor serum chloride levels and report any levels less than 95 mEq/L. Observe for decreases in serum potassium and sodium and note any increase in serum bicarbonate, which indicates metabolic alkalosis. Maintain strict intake and output records, noting any excessive gastric secretion loss, emesis, and diarrhea. Weigh the patient at the same time each day.

In mild hypochloremia, replacement of chloride can be accomplished orally with salty broth. If the condition is severe, IV fluid replacement is necessary. If the patient is hypovolemic, administration of 0.9% sodium chloride increases fluid volume as well as serum chloride levels. Ammonium chloride can also be given for replacement, and if metabolic alkalosis is present, KCl is administered. Dietary changes are seldom necessary.

Pharmacologic Highlights

Medication or Drug Class	Dosage	Description	Rationale
KCl	Oral or IV: 10–40 mEq PO depending on severity of deficit; IV dosages should not exceed 20 mEq/hr except in unusual situations	Electrolyte replacement	Replaces needed electrolytes, particularly in metabolic alkalosis
Ammonium chloride	IV dose is dependent on patient's weight and serum chloride	Electrolyte replacement	Replaces needed electrolytes, particularly in metabolic alkalosis

Independent

Institute safety measures for patients who develop neuromuscular symptoms, with particular attention to changes in level of consciousness and risks to airway patency. Have emergency equipment for airway and breathing maintenance available at all times. Educate those at risk in preventive measures. Teach patients the complications of medication therapy and how to maintain fluid and electrolyte balance nutritionally.

Evidence-Based Practice and Health Policy

Oh, T., Do, S., Jeon, Y., Kim, J., Na, H., & Hwang, J. (2019). Association of preoperative serum chloride levels with mortality and morbidity after noncardiac surgery: A retrospective cohort study. *Anesthesia-Analgesia, 129,* 1494–1501.

- The authors aimed to evaluate the relationship between preoperative hyperchloremia or hypochloremia, using preoperative serum chloride levels, and 90-day mortality and morbidity after noncardiac surgery. They reviewed the medical records of adult patients (*N* = 103,505) who underwent noncardiac surgery and categorized their baseline chloride levels into three groups: normochloremia, hyperchloremia, and hypochloremia.
- Analysis revealed significantly increased 90-day mortality in the hypochloremia and hyperchloremia groups and increased odds of acute kidney injury in the preoperative hypochloremia group when compared with the normochloremia group. The authors concluded that preoperative serum chloride level could help predict mortality and acute kidney injury postoperatively.

DOCUMENTATION GUIDELINES

- Laboratory findings: Serum electrolytes, osmolarity; daily flow sheet for easy day-to-day comparisons
- Physical responses: Respiratory status (rate, quality, depth, ease, breath sounds); vital signs; GI symptoms (nausea, vomiting, diarrhea); muscle strength, signs of muscle twitching, steadiness of gait, ability to perform activities of daily living; fluid balance, intake and output
- Condition of IV site, complications of IV therapy (infection, infiltration phlebitis)

DISCHARGE AND HOME HEALTHCARE GUIDELINES

Caregivers of older adults and infants should be alerted to the effect of vomiting and diarrhea on chloride levels. Teach the patient to report any signs and symptoms of neuromuscular hyperactivity. Teach the patient to maintain a healthy diet with all the components of adequate nutrition. Teach the patient the name, dosage, route, action, and side effects of all medications, particularly those that affect chloride and sodium balance in the body.

Hypoglycemia

DRG Category:	640
Mean LOS:	4.5 days
Description:	MEDICAL: Miscellaneous Disorders of Nutrition, Metabolism, Fluids, and Electrolytes With Major Complication or Comorbidity

Hypoglycemia occurs when the blood glucose falls below 50 mg/dL. Normal blood glucose values range between 70 and 100 mg/dL. A series of complex physiological responses is set off when a patient develops a low level of blood glucose. The most dramatic is the sympathetic nervous system (SNS) or adrenergic response, which is primarily the result of epinephrine. Epinephrine stimulates the liver to convert glycogen into glucose to support the falling serum glucose. In addition, the reticular activating system creates a state of alertness and wakefulness (fight-or-flight reaction).

Cerebral dysfunction occurs when the central nervous system (CNS) is deprived of glucose for cellular needs. In contrast to muscle and fat cells in the body that can break down amino and fatty acids for energy, the brain cells depend on glucose for energy. When the liver's supply of glycogen is depleted and no replacement is available, brain damage results. Prolonged periods of hypoglycemia can lead to complications such as coma, permanent brain damage, and death.

CAUSES

Causes can best be understood by breaking them into the nondiabetic and diabetic categories. In the nondiabetic patient, there are four classifications of hypoglycemia: organic, iatrogenic, reactive, and gestational. Organic hypoglycemia is caused by liver diseases such as hepatitis, cirrhosis, liver cancer, and insulin-secreting tumors. Iatrogenic hypoglycemia is associated with consumption of alcohol and reactions to drugs such as beta-adrenergic blockers and sulfonylureas, the two most common for this problem. Reactive hypoglycemia is caused by an adrenergic response that is triggered within 5 minutes of meal consumption in susceptible individuals. Symptoms are transient. Reactive hypoglycemia occurs in approximately 75% of all spontaneous hypoglycemic reactions. Gestational hypoglycemia occurs during pregnancy and occurs most often in people with preexisting conditions.

Hypoglycemia occurs more often in diabetic patients who are receiving insulin or oral hypoglycemic agents. Usually, this reaction is the result of an imbalance between insulin/hypoglycemic agent intake and exercise or food intake. In the patient with diabetes mellitus (DM), hypoglycemia occurs usually for the following reasons: medication errors (too much insulin or hypoglycemic agent), diet changes (too little food intake or omission), and activity level (increase in activity in relation to medication and food intake). Other causes in the diabetic patient include alcohol consumption, drugs, emotional stress, and infections.

GENETIC CONSIDERATIONS

There are several familial forms of hyperinsulinemic hypoglycemia, inherited in autosomal dominant and recessive patterns. Mutations in nine genes have so far been shown to cause congenital hyperinsulinism: *ABCC8, KCNJ11, HADH, GLUD1, GCK, HNF1A, HNF4A, SLC16A1*, and *UCP2*. One form has been linked to a mutation in the human insulin receptor gene. Persistent hyperinsulinemic hypoglycemia of infancy is a rare disorder that often follows an autosomal recessive inheritance pattern. It is usually due to dysregulation of negative feedback of insulin secretion by low glucose levels.

SEX AND LIFE SPAN CONSIDERATIONS

People with diabetes and older adults are at higher risk for hypoglycemia than other people. Older adults may have fewer symptoms of hypoglycemia, and the symptoms may appear at a lower threshold of blood glucose. Reactive hypoglycemia, recurrent episodes of symptomatic hypoglycemia occurring within 4 hours after a high-carbohydrate meal, is more common in females than males. It is also more common in overweight and obese persons who are insulin resistant. Reactive hypoglycemia occurs in people with and without diabetes.

HEALTH DISPARITIES AND SEXUAL/GENDER MINORITY HEALTH

Ethnicity, race, and sexual/gender minority status have no known effect on the risk for hypoglycemia.

GLOBAL HEALTH CONSIDERATIONS

Hypoglycemia can result because of the treatment for DM or from other conditions. The prevalence of DM is increasing dramatically. The World Health Organization considers DM as a global epidemic with the number of people with DM exceeding 422 million. The International Diabetes Federation states that by 2030 the number will exceed 500 million, and the countries with the most cases include the most populous countries of the world, such as China and India as well as Western Europe. Experts estimate that in the developing world, large increases will occur in sub-Saharan Africa, Latin America, and the Middle East.

ASSESSMENT

HISTORY. Determine if the patient has DM, renal insuffiency or failure, alcoholism, liver failure, endocrine disease, or recent surgery. General complaints include headaches, tiredness, palpitations, hunger, tremulousness, irritability, diaphoresis, nervousness, dizziness, mental confusion, and blurred vision. Question the patient or significant others about the patient's current medications. Ask about the possibility of medication errors and changes in diet and activity. Determine if the patient has been on a weight loss regime. Find out when the patient last ate and the content of the meal.

PHYSICAL EXAMINATION. The most common symptoms are **dizziness, difficulty concentrating, headache, shakiness, tachycardia**, and **diaphoresis**. The patient may be apprehensive, stare into space, and have trouble with speech or train of thought. Skin changes include pallor and diaphoresis. Trembling of the hands and seizures are possible. If the hypoglycemia has persisted, the patient may be unresponsive. Infants and children with hypoglycemia tend to have vague signs and symptoms, such as refusing to eat or nurse or a weak, high-pitched cry. As hypoglycemia progresses, children may appear to have poor muscle tone or have twitching, seizures, or coma.

PSYCHOSOCIAL. Ask about the home environment, occupation, knowledge level, financial situation, and support systems, which may provide information that can be used to prevent future episodes. Determine the patient's and significant others' social, economic, and interpersonal resources to help manage a potentially chronic condition such as reactive hypoglycemia or DM.

Diagnostic Highlights

Test	Normal Result	Abnormality With Condition	Explanation
Serum glucose level	70–100 mg/dL (fasting)	< 70 mg/dL in adults; < 60 mg/dL in children; critical value: < 40 mg/dL	Deficiency of glucose

Other Tests: Oral glucose tolerance test, 72-hour fasting plasma glucose level, insulin levels. C-peptide measurement (elevated in insulinoma, normal or low with exogenous insulin, elevated with oral sulfonylureas), liver function tests, thyroid levels, cortisol levels

PRIMARY NURSING DIAGNOSIS

DIAGNOSIS. Imbalanced nutrition: less than body requirements related to glucose deficit or insulin excess as evidenced by dizziness, difficulty concentrating, headache, shakiness, diaphoresis, and/or tachycardia

OUTCOMES. Hypoglycemia severity; Nutritional status: Food and fluid intake; Nutritional status: Nutrient intake; Nutritional status: Energy; Fluid balance; Electrolyte and acid/base balance

INTERVENTIONS. Nutrition management; Nutritional counseling; Energy management; Hypoglycemia management; Fluid/electrolyte balance; IV therapy; Medication management; Teaching: Individual

▓ PLANNING AND IMPLEMENTATION
Collaborative

The immediate management is to maintain a patent airway, regular breathing, and adequate circulation and to replace the glucose to restore the energy source for cells. If the patient is alert, has a patent airway, and can safely ingest oral carbohydrates, you may provide a cup of milk, fruit juice without additives, a granola bar, or cheese and crackers. Approximately 15 to 20 g of carbohydrates can be found in each of the following foods: 4 ounces of orange or grapefruit juice or regular soda; 8 ounces of milk; three graham crackers; 2 to 3 teaspoons of honey; or 6 to 10 hard candies. Oral glucose and sugar-containing fluids are effective but may lead to hyperglycemia. The blood glucose should be tested again after 15 minutes and treated again if it is less than 70 to 75 mg/dL.

The unconscious, hospitalized patient with severe hypoglycemia or the patient with suspected medication overdose needs a source of IV glucose immediately. Occurring simultaneously with glucose administration, if needed, is management of the airway and breathing with endotracheal intubation and breathing with a manual resuscitator bag. Usually, with restoration of airway, breathing, and serum glucose, the patient does not have circulatory instability, but the patient may receive IV fluid hydration and inotropic drugs to maintain circulation. If the patient is receiving insulin by continuous infusion either in a crystalloid or in total parenteral nutrition, the infusion is tapered or turned off, and the physician reevaluates the dose.

Once the patient regains consciousness, the oral intake of carbohydrates is increased to maintain the serum glucose. Whether in the hospital or at home, the healthcare provider needs to conduct an aggressive search to identify the precipitating cause of the hypoglycemic episode and to institute preventive strategies.

Pharmacologic Highlights

Medication or Drug Class	Dosage	Description	Rationale
50% dextrose	IV 25–50 mL, followed by an infusion of D₅W or D₁₀W to maintain a blood glucose of 100 mg/dL	Sugar; antihypoglycemic	Supplies a source of carbohydrate that can be immediately converted to glucose
Glucagon	1 mg IM or SC	Antihypoglycemic; promotes hepatic glycogenolysis and gluconeogenesis, stimulates production of cyclic adenosine monophosphate	Treats hypoglycemia if the person cannot maintain oral intake and if IV access is not available; note that the drug may cause vomiting

(highlight box continues on page 626)

> ### Pharmacologic Highlights (continued)
>
> Note: Diazoxide (Hyperstat), an inhibitor of insulin secretion, may be used rarely as an adjunct to a glucose infusion because it increases hepatic glucose output and decreases cellular glucose uptake.

Independent

Assessment and management of airway, breathing, and circulation is the highest priority. Never force an unconscious or semiconscious patient to drink liquids because of the risk of aspiration into the lungs. Continue to repeat the oral intake of carbohydrates until the blood glucose rises above 100 mg/dL and administer the next meal as soon as possible. If the next scheduled meal is not ready for more than 30 minutes or longer, provide the patient with a combination of carbohydrates and protein, such as ½ cup milk, 1 ounce of cheese, and three saltine crackers.

Teach the patient and family prevention, detection, and treatment of hypoglycemia. Encourage a daily exercise, diet, and medication regimen on a consistent basis. Remind the patient to consume extra foods before increased exercise and to carry a rapid-absorbing carbohydrate at all times. Teach the patient and significant others to keep glucagon available in the home or at work or school. Instruct coworkers, teachers, and neighbors how to treat hypoglycemia.

Evidence-Based Practice and Health Policy

Chalew, S., Kamps, J., Jurgen, B., Gomez, R., & Hempe, J. (2020). The relationship of glycemic control, insulin dose, and race with hypoglycemia in youth with type 1 diabetes. *Journal of Diabetes and Its Complications, 34,* 1–6.

- The authors aimed to study whether Black pediatric patients with type I diabetes may be prescribed higher daily doses of insulin than White pediatric patients, putting them at greater risk for hypoglycemia. They performed a retrospective analysis of 88 cases studying social and environmental factors, changes of insulin dose, hemoglobin (Hb)A$_{1c}$ levels, and episodes of hypoglycemia.
- Age, duration of diabetes, and body mass index were similar in both groups. Black patients had higher levels of HbA$_{1c}$, and insulin dose increased with increasing HbA$_{1c}$ and mean blood glucose. The authors found no differences in Black and White patients with respect to the occurrence of hypoglycemia and insulin dosing.

DOCUMENTATION GUIDELINES

- Physical response: Patency of airway, regularity of breathing, adequacy of circulation; assessment of the CNS (level of consciousness, signs and symptoms of hypoglycemia; strength and motion of extremities; pupillary response; SNS response); response to therapeutic interventions
- Blood glucose level; trend of levels after interventions

DISCHARGE AND HOME HEALTHCARE GUIDELINES

Teach the patient and significant others about the signs and symptoms of hypoglycemia and how to manage them at home. Include written materials to reinforce the assessment and management of hypoglycemia and instructions to the patient to carry a diabetic identification card or bracelet.

Discuss with the patient and family the reason for the hypoglycemic episode and explore ways to prevent its recurrence. If appropriate, assess the patient's understanding of DM and the medications used to manage the disorder. Refer the patient to a dietitian if you note the need for more in-depth dietary consultation than you are able to provide.

Hypokalemia

DRG Category: 640
Mean LOS: 4.5 days
Description: MEDICAL: Miscellaneous Disorders of Nutrition, Metabolism, Fluids, and Electrolytes With Major Complication or Comorbidity

Hypokalemia is a serum potassium ion level below 3.5 mEq/L, although symptoms do not usually occur until the potassium is below 3 mEq/L. Mild hypokalemia is between 3 and 3.5 mEq/L, moderate hypokalemia is between 2.5 and 3 mEq/L, and severe hypokalemia (critical value) is less than 2.8 mEq/L. As many as 21% of hospitalized patients are hypokalemic, but the condition is clinically significant in only 5% of patients.

It typically occurs when there is an increase in the potassium concentration gradient between the intracellular fluid (ICF) and extracellular fluid (ECF). Potassium functions as the major intracellular cation and balances sodium in the ECF to maintain electroneutrality in the body. It is excreted by the kidneys: approximately 40 mEq of potassium in 1 L of urine. Potassium is not stored in the body and needs to be replenished daily through dietary sources. It is also exchanged for hydrogen when changes in the body's pH call for a need for cation exchange. This situation occurs in metabolic alkalosis or other alterations that lead to increased cellular uptake of potassium, including insulin excess and renal failure. Potassium is regulated by two stimuli, aldosterone and hyperkalemia. Aldosterone is secreted in response to high renin and angiotensin II or hyperkalemia. The plasma level of potassium, when high, also increases renal potassium loss.

Because 98% of the body's potassium is intracellular, small variations in the potassium concentration gradient can cause major changes in cell membrane excitability. Hypokalemia is a relatively common electrolyte imbalance with potentially life-threatening consequences because symptoms can affect virtually all body systems. Complications of hypokalemia include paralytic ileus, cardiac dysrhythmias, shock, and sudden cardiac death.

CAUSES

Decreased potassium intake can be caused by decreased intake, transcellular shifts, nonrenal loss, and renal loss. Situations that lead to decreased intake include anorexia, poverty, fad diets, prolonged periods without oral intake (NPO), and prolonged IV therapy without potassium. Abnormal movement of potassium from ECF to ICF can be caused by alkalosis, hyperalimentation, hyperinsulinism, and transfusion of frozen red blood cells, which are low in potassium.

Increased nonrenal loss occurs from prolonged use of digitalis or corticosteroids, laxative abuse, excessive vomiting or diarrhea, excessive diaphoresis, excessive wound drainage (especially gastrointestinal), and prolonged nasogastric suctioning. Renal excretion can be caused by inappropriate or prolonged use of potassium-wasting diuretics, such as acetazolamide, ethacrynic acid, furosemide, bumetanide, and thiazides; diuresis phase after severe bodily burns; increased secretion of aldosterone as in Cushing syndrome; and renal disease that has impaired reabsorption of potassium.

GENETIC CONSIDERATIONS

Hypokalemia is a feature of various disorders that can have genetic etiology. These include Bartter syndrome, a group of several disorders of impaired salt reabsorption in the thick ascending loop of Henle, which causes hypochloremia, hypokalemic metabolic alkalosis, and hypercalciuria. Mutations in the Na-K-2Cl cotransporter gene (*SLC12A1*) are often involved. The disorder hypokalemic periodic paralysis is inherited as an autosomal dominant pattern, caused by mutations in *CACNA1S*, *SCN4A*, or *KCNJ2*. It features intermittent episodes of muscle weakness or paralysis that can last from several hours to days. Gitelman syndrome (GS) is caused by mutations in *SLC12A3* and is characterized by hypokalemic alkalosis, low urinary calcium, and hypomagnesemia. GS is transmitted in an autosomal dominant pattern.

SEX AND LIFE SPAN CONSIDERATIONS

Potassium imbalance may occur at any age and in both sexes. Older patients are at a particularly high risk because the concentrating ability of the kidney diminishes with age, and excessive urinary potassium loss may occur. They also are more likely to take medications that place them at higher risk for potassium deficit.

HEALTH DISPARITIES AND SEXUAL/GENDER MINORITY HEALTH

Ethnicity, race, and sexual/gender minority status have no known effect on the risk for hypokalemia.

GLOBAL HEALTH CONSIDERATIONS

Hospitalized patients around the globe experience hypokalemia at rates that are likely similar to the United States and Western Europe.

ASSESSMENT

HISTORY. Question the patient about dietary habits, recent illnesses, recent medical or surgical interventions, and medication use (prescribed or over-the-counter), especially the use of digitalis, diuretics, and corticosteroids. Ask if the patient has diabetes mellitus. Patients with hypokalemia may complain of anorexia, nausea and vomiting, fatigue, drowsiness, constipation, lethargy, muscle weakness, and leg cramps. They may describe exercise intolerance. Knowledge of the patient's usual mental status and mood is helpful. Changes in cognitive ability, behavior, and level of consciousness are not uncommon in hypokalemic patients.

PHYSICAL EXAMINATION. Symptoms vary greatly from patient to patient but usually do not occur unless the potassium drops below 3 mEq/L. Common symptoms include **anorexia, nausea and vomiting, lethargy, muscle weakness,** and **leg cramps.** Assess the patient's level of consciousness and orientation. Hypokalemic patients may be confused; apathetic; anxious; irritable; or, in severe cases, even comatose. Assess the rate and depth of respirations and the color of nailbeds and mucous membranes. Note cardiovascular changes, such as weak and thready peripheral pulses and heart rate variability. The apical pulse may be excessively slow or excessively rapid depending on the type of dysrhythmia present. Check the patient's blood pressure when lying, sitting, and standing to assess for postural hypotension. These changes occur in early stages, and the patient's symptoms deteriorate to a generalized hypotensive state in advanced stages of hypokalemia. Note the presence of skeletal muscle weakness, as evidenced by bilateral weak hand grasps, inability to stand, hyporeflexia, and profound flaccid paralysis in severe hypokalemic states. Gastrointestinal function is altered during hypokalemia, and the patient may have abdominal distention and hypoactive bowel sounds.

PSYCHOSOCIAL. Although it is seldom long term and can be easily corrected, hypokalemia can lead to life-threatening complications. Typically, the patient is dealing not only with the hypokalemic state but also with the underlying cause of the hypokalemia. Assess the patient's ability to cope.

Diagnostic Highlights

Test	Normal Result	Abnormality With Condition	Explanation
Serum potassium	3.5–5.3 mEq/L	< 3.5 mEq/L; critical value: < 2.8 mEq/L	Potassium deficit is reflected in serum and ECF compartment
Electrocardiogram	Normal PQRST pattern	Early: Flat or inverted T wave, prominent U wave, ST segment depression, prolonged QU interval Late: Prolonged PR interval, decreased voltage and widening of QRS interval, increased risk of ventricular dysrhythmias	Potassium deficit leads to changes in the generation and conduction of action potential

Other Tests: Blood urea nitrogen, creatinine, calcium, glucose, digitalis level (if patient is on digitalis), urinalysis and urine electrolytes, cortisol, aldosterone level

PRIMARY NURSING DIAGNOSIS

DIAGNOSIS. Imbalanced nutrition: less than body requirements related to decreased potassium intake and/or vomiting as evidenced by leg cramps, muscle weakness, anorexia, and/or lethargy

OUTCOMES. Hypokalemia severity; Nutritional status: Nutrient intake; Electrolyte and acid-base balance; Fluid balance; Cardiac pump effectiveness; Circulation status; Knowledge: Medication

INTERVENTIONS. Electrolyte management: Hypokalemia; Electrolyte monitoring; Fluid management; Fluid monitoring; IV therapy; Nutrition management; Nutrition monitoring; Vital signs monitoring; Medication management; Medication administration

PLANNING AND IMPLEMENTATION

Collaborative

To prevent hypokalemia, most physicians closely monitor serum potassium levels and prescribe supplements to patients who are in the high-risk categories. Most patients who develop hypokalemia are placed on either oral or parenteral potassium supplements. Potassium is not administered intramuscularly or subcutaneously because potassium is a profound tissue irritant. Parenteral potassium should be administered with extreme caution. Potassium solutions irritate veins and can cause a chemical phlebitis.

Foods high in potassium can help restore potassium levels as well as prevent further potassium loss. Collaboration between the nurse and a registered dietitian can ensure accurate teaching on dietary maintenance of potassium levels. Common foods high in potassium are bananas, cantaloupe, raisins, skim milk, avocados, mushrooms, potatoes, spinach, and tomatoes.

Pharmacologic Highlights

General Comments: Administer IV solutions that contain potassium through a controller or pump device to regulate the rate. Mix oral potassium supplements in at least 4 ounces of fluid or food to prevent gastric irritation. Angiotensin-converting enzyme inhibitors may be used to reduce some of the symptoms that occur but must be used with caution in patients with poor renal function.

(highlight box continues on page 630)

Pharmacologic Highlights (continued)

Medication or Drug Class	Dosage	Description	Rationale
Potassium chloride	Oral or IV: 10–40 mEq PO, depending on severity of deficit; IV dosages should not exceed 20 mEq/hr IV except in unusual situations, when 40 m/Eq/hr IV may be administered for critical levels	Electrolyte replacement	Replaces needed electrolytes; dilute IV potassium solutions because rapid IV administration can be dangerous as rapid increases of serum potassium levels depress cardiac muscle contractility and can lead to life-threatening dysrhythmias

Independent

Interventions are focused on the prevention of potassium imbalances, restoration of normal potassium balance, and supportive care for altered body functions until the hypokalemia is resolved. Teach all patients who are placed on potassium-depleting medications to increase their dietary intake of potassium. Encourage the patient to eat bulk-forming foods and drink at least 2 L of fluid a day unless fluids are restricted because of other patient conditions. Evaluate the patient's knowledge of dietary sources of potassium and teach the patient and family members the needed information. Institute safety measures to prevent falls because of confusion, muscle weakness, or fatigue.

Evidence-Based Practice and Health Policy

Shen, A., Lin, H-L., Lin, H-C., Tseng, Y., Hsu, C., & Chou, C. (2020). Urinary tract infection is associated with hypokalemia: A case control study. *BMC Urology, 20*(1), 108.

- The aim of the study was to determine if urinary tract infection (UTI) is associated with hypokalemia. The authors performed a record review of patients hospitalized with UTI ($N = 43,719$) from the Longitudinal Health Insurance Database. They identified UTI patients with hypokalemia ($n = 4,540$) and selected a control group ($n = 1,842$) composed of patients hospitalized for other reasons.
- The percentage of patients with hypokalemia was higher in patients with UTI. Several conditions (stroke, chronic obstructive pulmonary disease, hypertension, congestive heart failure, diarrhea, and selected medications) were independently associated with hypokalemia. They concluded that UTI was associated with hypokalemia among hospitalized inpatients. The association is independent of patients' comorbidities and medications.

DOCUMENTATION GUIDELINES

- Physical findings associated with hypokalemia, including the current cardiac rate and rhythm on electrocardiogram, bowel function, and degree of muscle weakness
- Detailed description of the potassium ion (K^+) supplement route and dosage administration
- Detailed description of the IV site and date of insertion
- Dietary intake, especially as related to foods high in potassium
- Presence of complications related to hypokalemia

DISCHARGE AND HOME HEALTHCARE GUIDELINES

Teach patients at risk, especially those on diuretics, measures to increase potassium in their diet. Teach signs and symptoms that may indicate the presence of hypokalemia: muscle weakness, leg cramps, slow or irregular heart rate, slight confusion or forgetfulness, inability to concentrate, abdominal distention, and nausea. These symptoms should be reported to the physician. Teach patients how to take their pulse each morning and how to keep a daily record of the pulse rate. Remind patients and family members to give oral K⁺ supplements in at least 4 ounces of fluid or food and not to take the supplement on an empty stomach. Instruct patients to report any dizziness, extreme anxiousness or irritability, confusion, extreme muscle weakness, heart palpitations or irregularities, or difficulties in breathing to the primary healthcare provider.

Hypomagnesemia

DRG Category: 640
Mean LOS: 4.5 days
Description: MEDICAL: Miscellaneous Disorders of Nutrition, Metabolism, Fluids, and Electrolytes With Major Complication or Comorbidity

Hypomagnesemia occurs when the serum magnesium concentration is less than 1.5 mg/dL. The normal serum magnesium level is 1.6 to 2.2 mg/dL. An average-sized adult has approximately 25 g of magnesium in the body. About 50% of the body's total magnesium is found in the bones, 1% is located in the extracellular compartment, and the remainder is found within the cells. The body's requirement is met by ingesting foods such as meat, milk, and chlorophyll-containing vegetables and fruits. The risk of hypomagnesemia is 2% in the general population, 20% in hospitalized patients, 60% in critically ill patients, 30% to 80% in alcohol-dependent patients, and 25% in diabetic patients.

Magnesium, the second most abundant cation inside the cell, is controlled by vitamin D–regulated gastrointestinal (GI) absorption and renal excretion. Magnesium plays an important role in neuromuscular function. It also has a role in several enzyme systems, particularly the metabolism of carbohydrates and proteins, as well as maintenance of normal ionic balance (it triggers the sodium-potassium pump), osmotic pressure, myocardial functioning, and bone metabolism. Deficits of magnesium lead to deficits in calcium, and the two electrolyte imbalances are difficult to differentiate. The hypocalcemia that accompanies hypomagnesemia cannot be corrected unless the magnesium is replaced. Hypomagnesemia is also a stimulus for renin release, which leads to aldosterone production, potassium wasting, and hypokalemia. Because magnesium regulates calcium entry into cells, consequences of magnesium deficiency include ventricular dysrhythmias, an enhanced digitalis toxicity, and sudden cardiac death. Deficits in potassium and calcium potentiate the dysrhythmogenic effect of low magnesium. In addition to cardiac dysrhythmias, complications include hypertension, neuromuscular disturbances, osteoporosis, and nephrolithiasis. People with diabetes mellitus and coronary heart disease often are magnesium deficient.

CAUSES

The primary sources of magnesium deficit are reduced intestinal absorption, redistribution of magnesium from the extracellular to intracellular space, and increased renal excretion. Sources of reduced GI absorption include losses from intestinal or biliary fistulae, prolonged nasogastric suction, diarrhea, malabsorption syndrome, and laxative abuse. Decreased oral intake of magnesium also decreases absorption and is caused by malnutrition, chronic alcoholism, starvation, and prolonged administration of magnesium-free parenteral fluids. Redistribution of magnesium occurs during the treatment of diabetic ketoacidosis, in acute pancreatitis, and in alcohol withdrawal. Increased renal excretion of magnesium occurs because of prolonged diuretic use; the diuretic phase of acute renal failure; acute alcohol intoxication; hyperaldosteronism; syndrome of inappropriate antidiuretic hormone; or medications such as cisplatin, digoxin, tobramycin, gentamicin, cyclosporine, and amphotericin. Other conditions associated with low magnesium include malignancies, hypocalcemia, hypoparathyroidism, burns, multiple transfusions of stored blood, and toxemia of pregnancy.

GENETIC CONSIDERATIONS

There are several heritable syndromes that include hypomagnesemia as a primary feature. Primary hypomagnesemia can be transmitted in an autosomal recessive or dominant pattern and is due to either poor intestinal absorption of magnesium or a defect in renal reabsorption of magnesium. Gitelman syndrome results in hypokalemic alkalosis, low urinary calcium, and hypomagnesemia. It is caused by mutations in *SLC12A3* and transmitted in an autosomal recessive pattern.

SEX AND LIFE SPAN CONSIDERATIONS

Anyone with a chronic illness that causes malabsorption or renal loss of magnesium is susceptible. Infants seem to be the age group most prone to hypomagnesemia. Pregnant persons with toxemia are particularly at risk, as are older adults who are placed on diuretic therapy and people with cancer who are taking chemotherapy. There are no known sex differences in prevalence and incidence.

HEALTH DISPARITIES AND SEXUAL/GENDER MINORITY HEALTH

Ethnicity, race, and sexual/gender minority status have no known effect on the risk for hypomagnesemia.

GLOBAL HEALTH CONSIDERATIONS

Most experts suggest that hospitalized patients around the globe experience hypomagnesemia at rates that are likely similar to the United States and Western Europe.

ASSESSMENT

HISTORY. As noted earlier, many diseases and disorders are associated with hypomagnesemia; a complete medical history of all preexisting conditions is important including diabetes mellitus, pancreatitis, and renal disease. The following conditions put a patient at risk: poor nutrition, diuretics or chemotherapy, pregnancy, old age, or a history of alcohol abuse. Ask about the patient's diet and drinking history, including the amount of alcohol intake on a usual day and an unusual day. Ask the patient to describe bowel patterns and note if the patient has diarrhea or a history of an eating disorder with laxative abuse. Determine if the patient has experienced irregular heartbeats, lethargy, muscle weakness, tremors, mood alterations, anorexia, nausea, or dizziness.

PHYSICAL EXAMINATION. Observe any signs of muscular changes, such as **tetany, spasticity**, or **tremors**. Note the person's affect and mental status because hypomagnesemia can lead to seizures, mood changes, irritability, confusion, hallucinations, psychosis, and depression. The patient's vital signs may reflect hypotension and tachycardia. Assess the patient for muscular weakness and numbness of the fingers (paresthesias). When you examine the patient's eyes, you may note nystagmus (involuntary cyclical movement of the eyeball) and positive Trousseau and Chvostek signs. Trousseau sign is the development of carpal spasm when a blood pressure cuff is inflated above systolic pressure for 3 minutes; Chvostek sign is twitching facial muscles when the facial nerve is tapped anterior to the ear.

PSYCHOSOCIAL. The patient may be confused, psychotic, or depressed, which can be relieved with magnesium replacement. If the patient has chronic alcoholism, symptoms may persist beyond treatment of the hypomagnesemia and should be addressed with appropriate consultation and possible rehabilitation. Assess the patient's and significant others' abilities to cope with this sudden illness and any changes in roles that may result. Determine if a referral is needed for alcohol treatment.

Diagnostic Highlights

Test	Normal Result	Abnormality With Condition	Explanation
Serum magnesium	1.6–2.2 mg/dL	< 1.5 mg/dL; critical value: < 1 mg/dL	Deficit of magnesium ions
Serum calcium: Total calcium, including free ionized calcium and bound calcium	8.4–10.2 mg/dL	< 8.2 mg/dL; critical value: < 6.5 mg/dL	Deficit of calcium below normal levels in the extracellular fluid compartment
Serum ionized calcium: Unbound calcium; level unaffected by albumin level	4.6–5.3 mg/dL	< 4.5 mg/dL; critical value: < 3.5 mg/dL	Ionized calcium is approximately 46%–50% of circulating calcium; calcium available for enzymatic reactions and neuromuscular function
Electrocardiogram (ECG)	Normal PQRST pattern	Prolonged PR and QT intervals; patients on digitalis may have atrial and ventricular dysrhythmias	Magnesium deficit leads to alterations in generation and conduction of the action potential

Other Tests: Serum potassium level, blood urea nitrogen, creatinine, glucose

PRIMARY NURSING DIAGNOSIS

DIAGNOSIS. Risk for injury as evidenced by muscle weakness, unstable gait, tremors, and/or spasticity

OUTCOMES. Hypomagnesemia severity; Cardiac pump effectiveness; Circulation status; Electrolyte and acid-base balance; Knowledge: Medication; Respiratory status

INTERVENTIONS. Electrolyte management: Hypomagnesemia; Cardiac care: Acute; Code management; Emergency care; Medication administration; Medication management

PLANNING AND IMPLEMENTATION

Collaborative

If the levels are severely low, the patient needs IV or intramuscular magnesium replacement with magnesium sulfate ($MgSO_4$). Calcium gluconate may be administered with IV magnesium replacement therapy to reduce the risk of sudden reversal to hypermagnesemia. If the patient does not suffer from chronic malabsorption requiring total parenteral nutrition, an increase in dietary intake of magnesium is prescribed. Foods high in magnesium include bananas, chocolate, green leafy vegetables, grapefruit, oranges, nuts, seafood, soy flour, and wheat bran.

Monitor for signs of hypermagnesemia during IV infusions. These symptoms include hypotension, labored respirations, and diminished or absent patellar reflex (knee jerk). If any of these symptoms occurs, stop the infusion and notify the physician immediately. If hypokalemia occurs simultaneously with hypomagnesemia, the magnesium level should be corrected first because magnesium is necessary for the movement of potassium into the cell. Be aware that hypomagnesemia may precipitate digitalis toxicity by enhancing the effects of digitalis, which places the patient at increased risk for digitalis-induced atrial and ventricular dysrhythmias and Mobitz type I atrioventricular (AV) block (Wenckebach). Alkalosis should be avoided or corrected because this condition may precipitate tetany.

Pharmacologic Highlights

Medication or Drug Class	Dosage	Description	Rationale
MgSO$_4$	1–2 g MgSO$_4$ IV over 15 min followed by an infusion of 6 g in 1 L over 24 hr	Electrolyte replacement	Replace magnesium
Magnesium gluconate (Almora, Mag-Ox)	500 mg/day (27 mg elemental magnesium) PO; oral preparations for mild/chronic hypomagnesemia: 240 mg elemental magnesium PO qd to bid; other preparations: Mag-Ox 400 and Uro-Mag; magnesium-containing antacids containing aluminum hydroxide and magnesium hydroxide (Mylanta or Maalox) if problem was not caused by chronic GI loss (e.g., diarrhea)	Electrolyte replacement	Given when patient is mildly depleted (magnesium >1 mEq/L and patient is asymptomatic)

Independent

The patient's safety is of primary concern. Reorient the patient as necessary and reassure both the patient and the family that mood changes and the altered level of consciousness are temporary and improve when magnesium levels return to normal. If neurological and muscle status places the patient at risk for injury, evaluate the patient's environment to limit risks for trauma. Symptoms of hypomagnesemia are similar to those of delirium tremens (DT) in chronic alcoholism; if you suspect the patient of developing either DT or hypomagnesemia, discuss the symptoms with the physician and monitor the magnesium levels to determine the cause of the symptoms.

Maintain seizure precautions for patients with symptoms and keep environmental stimuli to a minimum. Encourage active range-of-motion (ROM) exercises or perform passive ROM exercises several times a day to help prevent complications of inactivity. Dysphagia may also occur in these patients, and their ability to swallow should be assessed before giving them food or liquids. Encourage the intake of magnesium-enriched foods in small, frequent meals if the patient is suffering from inadequate nutrition. Keep the environment as pleasant as possible. Include the patient and family in meal planning and request a nutritional consultation if necessary.

Evidence-Based Practice and Health Policy

van Dijk, P., Waanders, F., Qiu, J., de Boer, H., van Goor, H., & Bilo, H. (2020). Hypomagnesemia in persons with type 1 diabetes: Associations with clinical parameters and oxidative stress. *Therapeutic Advances in Endocrinology and Metabolism, 11.* Advance online publication. https://doi.org/10.1177/2042018820980240

- Among persons with type 1 diabetes mellitus (T1DM), low concentrations of magnesium have been reported. Previous studies suggested a relationship of hypomagnesemia with poor glycemic control and complications. The authors aimed to investigate the magnitude of

hypomagnesemia and the associations between magnesium with parameters of routine T1DM care in outpatients (*N* = 207).
• Hypomagnesemia was defined as a concentration below < 0.7 mmol/L. Magnesium deficiency was present in 4.3% of participants. There was no correlation between magnesium and HbA$_{1c}$ at baseline. In this group of outpatients, the presence of hypomagnesemia was infrequent and, if present, relatively mild, and not associated with glycemic control or with presence complications.

DOCUMENTATION GUIDELINES

• Serum magnesium, potassium, and calcium levels; patency of the IV line
• Vital signs, cardiac rhythm, and ECG strip and interpretation
• Neurological assessment findings: Level of consciousness, orientation, muscle strength and sensation, presence of Chvostek and Trousseau signs
• Presence of complications: Respiratory distress, tetany, IV infiltration
• Response to treatment: MgSO$_4$ or magnesium-containing antacids, calcium gluconate

DISCHARGE AND HOME HEALTHCARE GUIDELINES

Teach the patient to eat foods high in magnesium and to eat several small meals. Tell the patient to use any prescribed antiemetics before eating if nausea, vomiting, or diarrhea is a problem. Teach the signs and symptoms of hypomagnesemia (changes in level of consciousness, neuromuscular weakness), and instruct the patient to notify the physician if these return.

Explain any oral magnesium supplements, including the dosage, action, adverse effects, and need for routine laboratory monitoring if hypomagnesemia is a chronic problem. Explain that many of the magnesium-containing antacids may cause diarrhea, and instruct the patient to notify the physician if this occurs. Teach the use of assistive devices (cane or walker). The patient should also be taught muscle-strengthening exercises and may need a home-care evaluation before discharge.

Hyponatremia

DRG Category: 640
Mean LOS: 4.5 days
Description: MEDICAL: Miscellaneous Disorders of Nutrition, Metabolism, Fluids, and Electrolytes With Major Complication or Comorbidity

Hyponatremia is a serum sodium concentration less than 135 mEq/L (normal range is 135 to 145 mEq/L). Among hospitalized patients, 20% to 30% have hyponatremia, but only 1% to 4% have serious hyponatremia with levels lower than 130 mEq/L. Sodium is the most abundant cation in the body; a 70-kg person has approximately 4,200 mEq of sodium in the body. Sodium has five essential functions: It maintains the osmolarity of the extracellular fluid (ECF); regulates ECF volume and water distribution; affects the concentration, excretion, and absorption of other electrolytes, particularly potassium and chloride; combines with other ions to maintain acid-base balance; and is essential for impulse transmission of nerve and muscle fibers.

Hyponatremia is the most common of all electrolyte disorders. As serum sodium decreases, water in the ECF moves into the cells. There is less sodium available to move across an excitable membrane, which results in delayed membrane depolarization. Central nervous system cells are most likely to be affected by these changes. Four different manifestations of hyponatremia have been described on the basis of the ratio of total body water (TBW) to total body sodium: hypovolemic hyponatremia, hypervolemic hyponatremia, euvolemic hyponatremia, and redistributive hyponatremia (Table 1).

• TABLE 1 Types and Causes of Hyponatremia

TYPES OF HYPONATREMIA	FLUID VOLUME AND SODIUM (Na) STATUS	CAUSATIVE CLINICAL CONDITIONS
Hypovolemic	Na loss > TBW loss	Diuretic usage (especially thiazides), diabetic glycosuria, aldosterone deficiency, intrinsic renal disease, vomiting, diarrhea, excessive perspiration (found in exercise-associated hyponatremia), hemorrhage, burns, fever
Hypervolemic	TBW increases at a greater rate than Na	Edematous disorders, congestive heart failure, hepatic cirrhosis, nephrotic syndrome, renal failure
Euvolemic	TBW is moderately increased; Na is normal	Syndrome of inappropriate secretion of antidiuretic hormone (SIADH); continuous antidiuretic hormone secretion because of pain, emotion, medication
Redistributive	No change in TBW or Na; water shifts between extracellular and intracellular compartments, relative to Na concentrations	Pseudohyponatremia, hyperglycemia, hyperlipidemia

Important differences occur in patients with acute versus chronic hyponatremia. Acute hyponatremia develops over 48 hours or less, and patients are subject to more severe cerebral edema than those with chronic hyponatremia, which develops over more than 48 hours. If the serum sodium decreases slowly, or if it is greater than 125 mEq/L, the patient may be symptom free. If the serum sodium level drops below 115 mEq/L, cerebral edema and increased brain cell volume occur that could result in death. Serum sodium of less than 105 mEq/L is particularly life threatening in people who are alcohol dependent. If it is left untreated, hyponatremia can lead to potassium, calcium, chloride, and bicarbonate electrolyte imbalances; shock; convulsions; coma; and death.

CAUSES

The cause of hyponatremia is associated with the ratio of TBW to total body sodium. In many cases of hyponatremia, there is an excess of TBW relative to sodium. Causes are listed in Table 1.

GENETIC CONSIDERATIONS

Low blood sodium is a feature of several heritable endocrine imbalances. Pseudohypoaldosteronism type 1 is a salt-wasting disorder that can be transmitted in either an autosomal dominant or an autosomal recessive pattern. The autosomal dominant form is caused by mutations in a mineralocorticoid receptor (*NR3C2*) and is characterized primarily by renal resistance to aldosterone. The recessive form is caused by mutations in the epithelial sodium channel genes (*SCNN1A*, *SCNN1B*, *SCNN1G*) and features kidney, colon, and sweat/salivary gland resistance to aldosterone.

SEX AND LIFE SPAN CONSIDERATIONS

Hyponatremia can occur in any age group, and there are no differences by sex. It is more common in infants, young children, older adults, and debilitated patients because these groups are more likely to experience variation in the TBW. It is most common in the very young and in the very old because these individuals may be less able than other individuals to regulate fluid intake. Symptoms are more likely to occur in young women than in young men; premenopausal women's sex hormones may affect their ability to balance sodium levels. Hyponatremia can occur in healthy individuals, such as athletes or outdoor laborers, as a result of sodium loss through excessive perspiration.

HEALTH DISPARITIES AND SEXUAL/GENDER MINORITY HEALTH

Ethnicity, race, and sexual/gender minority status have no known effect on the risk for hyponatremia.

GLOBAL HEALTH CONSIDERATIONS

Hyponatremia is common in hospitalized and nursing home patients around the globe. Some experts note that it is the most common electrolyte disturbance and occurs in all regions of the world with rates as high as 30% in acutely and critically ill hospitalized patients.

ASSESSMENT

HISTORY. Obtain a medical history of any of the disorders that might predispose the patient to hyponatremia, such as heart failure, liver failure, renal failure, nephrotic syndrome, SIADH, or pneumonia. Inquire if the patient is taking any prescribed or over-the-counter medications because some drug interactions may alter sodium balance, particularly the thiazide diuretics, antipsychotic medications, and antidepressants. Determine if the patient drinks alcohol, and assess the pattern and amount of drinking. Ask if the patient does regular, strenuous exercise. Obtain a diet history to determine the normal sodium and fluid consumption patterns. Ask about nausea, vomiting, diarrhea, abdominal cramps, headache, or dizziness. Inquire about weight loss; mild hyponatremia can cause anorexia. Ask the patient and family if they have noted any change in mental status or behavior. Often, the patient with hyponatremia experiences confusion, a flat affect, and personality changes.

PHYSICAL EXAMINATION. Symptoms vary depending on the extent of the electrolyte imbalance and the speed that it develops. Slowly developing hyponatremia may be asymptomatic, whereas more rapidly progressing imbalances may be accompanied by **headache, muscle cramps, confusion, reduced mental awareness,** and **coma.** Assess the patient's vital signs. In hyponatremia, a low diastolic blood pressure, tachycardia, orthostatic hypotension, and a weak pulse may be noted. Inspect the skin and mucous membranes for dryness and a pale color. Note the skin turgor and peripheral vein refilling time. Assess the patient for decreased muscle strength and decreased deep tendon reflexes. Auscultate the lung fields bilaterally and note that you may hear adventitious breath sounds with congestive heart failure. Auscultate the bowel sounds and note any hyperactivity that may accompany hyponatremia.

PSYCHOSOCIAL. Assess the patient for anxiety, hostility, and the level of orientation to reality. Discuss the family's ability to cope with changes in the patient's mental status and their ability to provide dietary supervision and care for the patient at home. The patient may progress rapidly from confusion and agitation to seizure activity or coma. Because symptoms are primarily neurological in severe hyponatremia, assess the patient's level of orientation and ability to communicate needs.

Diagnostic Highlights

Test	Normal Result	Abnormality With Condition	Explanation
Serum sodium	135–145 mEq/L	< 135 mEq/L; critical value: < 120 mEq/L	Imbalance between sodium and water leads to deficits in sodium
Serum osmolarity	275–295 mOsm/L	< 275 mOsm/L; critical value: < 250 mOsm/L	Hyponatremia leads to hemodilution, showing a decrease in the ratio of water to particles
Urine osmolality and specific gravity (SG) 8.5 mg/dL	200–1,200 mOsm/L; SG = 1.016–1.022	Varies depending on cause; often < 100 mOsm/L with SG < 1.003	Show that urine is very diluted as kidneys excrete free water and retain as much sodium as possible

Other Tests: Complete blood count, urine and serum electrolytes, serum uric acid

PRIMARY NURSING DIAGNOSIS

DIAGNOSIS. Acute confusion related to neurological dysfunction and/or electrolyte imbalance as evidenced by altered cognitive function, headache, and/or coma

OUTCOMES. Hyponatremia severity; Electrolyte and acid-base balance; Cognition; Neurological status: Consciousness; Fluid balance; Respiratory status: Gas exchange

INTERVENTIONS. Electrolyte management: Hyponatremia; Electrolyte monitoring; Cerebral perfusion promotion; IV therapy; Fluid management; Fluid monitoring; Seizure precautions

PLANNING AND IMPLEMENTATION
Collaborative

The course of treatment depends on the cause; the goal is to correct the TBW-to-sodium ratio. Hypovolemic hyponatremic patients should be treated with isotonic saline to correct the volume deficit. If hyponatremia is severe (serum sodium > 115 mEq/L), an infusion of 3% to 5% sodium chloride solution may be administered slowly in small volumes via an infusion device. Monitor the patient carefully for signs and symptoms of circulatory overload (dyspnea, crackles, engorged veins). Fluid administration should be regulated with an IV controller to decrease the possibility of fluid overload. A diuretic may be given concurrently to avoid the occurrence of circulatory overload. Because IV hypertonic solutions are irritating to the vein, monitor the IV site closely. Monitor the effectiveness of fluid administration by following the serum sodium and osmolality levels, as well as daily weights and intake and output. Because osmolality of the brain takes longer to adjust than osmolality of the ECF, correction of hyponatremia should be done carefully to prevent rapid fluid shifts.

Hypervolemic or edematous patients are treated with a fluid restriction: 800 to 1,000 mL of fluid is allowed per day. Euvolemic patients need only a water restriction without a sodium restriction. Endocrine abnormalities (e.g., SIADH) should be specifically addressed and treated.

Pharmacologic Highlights

Medication or Drug Class	Dosage	Description	Rationale
3%–5% saline IV solutions	3% saline administered at a rate of 1–2 mL/kg per hr for the first 3–4 hr to target 120–125 mEq/L over 24–48 hr	Hypertonic saline	Correct the sodium deficit

Independent

If the patient is on a fluid restriction, offer cold liquids because they satisfy thirst better than hot liquids. If indicated, encourage the patient to drink liquids high in sodium, such as broth. Report the signs and symptoms of water intoxication (increased irritability, change in sensorium, headache, hyperreflexia) to the physician immediately. If the patient is confused, provide frequent orientation to person, place, and time. Because seizures are a possible consequence of hyponatremia, institute seizure precautions. Keep the side rails padded and raised, if that is appropriate for the patient, and the bed in the low position.

Maintain a stable, safe environment. Avoid sensory overload and confusing stimuli that may contribute to the patient's confused or agitated state. Explain to family members the rationales for disturbances in the patient's thought processes, for the fluid restriction, and for the measurement of intake and output.

Evidence-Based Practice and Health Policy

Potasso, L., Sailer, C., Blum, C., Cesana-Nigro, N., Schuetz, P., Mueller, B., & Christ-Crain, M. (2020). Mild to moderate hyponatremia at discharge is associated with increased risk of recurrence in patients with community-acquired pneumonia. *European Journal of Internal Medicine*, *75*, 44–49.

* The authors wanted to determine the impact of hyponatremia at discharge related to patients' mortality, rehospitalization, and recurrence rate at 180 days in patients with pneumonia. The authors analyzed data collected from hospital records ($N = 708$) from a double-blind, randomized, placebo-controlled trial of hospitalized patients with community-acquired pneumonia and prednisone treatment.
* The authors found that mild to moderate hyponatremia at discharge was associated with an increased risk of recurrence in hospitalized patients with pneumonia. This finding is particularly important for patients who are hyponatremic both on admission and at discharge.

DOCUMENTATION GUIDELINES

* Fluid intake and output, daily weights, urine SG, serum sodium level
* Vital signs: Presence of fever, tachycardia, low blood pressure, orthostatic changes
* Mental status: Orientation to person, place, and time; observations of confusion or agitation, ability to drink oral fluids, presence of gag reflex
* Response to treatments: Oral and parenteral fluids, dietary and fluid restrictions

DISCHARGE AND HOME HEALTHCARE GUIDELINES

Teach the patient and caregivers the importance of an adequate fluid intake and normal sodium intake and the food appropriate for a balanced sodium diet. If fluid restriction is indicated, tell the patient that using ice chips, iced pops, or lemon drops may reduce thirst. Teach the family that hyponatremia can recur with persistent vomiting or diarrhea because sodium is abundant in the gastrointestinal tract; this fact is especially important for infants, children, and older adults, and debilitated patients.

Hypoparathyroidism

DRG Category:	644
Mean LOS:	4.3 days
Description:	MEDICAL: Endocrine Disorders With Complication or Comorbidity

The parathyroid glands—four small endocrine glands located on the posterior surface of the thyroid gland—produce the parathyroid hormone (PTH), which regulates calcium and phosphorus balance by affecting gastrointestinal (GI) absorption of calcium, bone resorption (removal of bone tissue by absorption) of calcium, and renal regulation of both calcium and phosphorus. Calcium and phosphorus have a reciprocal relationship in the body; high levels of calcium lead to low levels of phosphorus. Hypoparathyroidism is a rare clinical syndrome and is associated with a deficiency or absence of PTH or a decreased peripheral action of PTH.

Although both hypocalcemia and hyperphosphatemia result from hypoparathyroidism, hypocalcemia accounts for the majority of clinical manifestations. The human body is able to compensate for low or moderate hypocalcemia. The seriousness of the disease is variable with the degree of hypocalcemia and the speed with which it develops. Acute hypoparathyroidism follows swiftly after trauma or removal of the parathyroid glands. The acute form, as with most hormone deficiencies, can result in life-threatening complications such as tetany, hypocalcemic seizures, cardiac dysrhythmias, and respiratory obstruction caused by laryngospasm. Autoimmune hypoparathyroidism develops more slowly. Most clinical manifestations are reversible with treatment; those caused by calcification deposits associated with chronic hypoparathyroidism (such as cataracts, malformed teeth) and parkinsonian symptoms are not reversible.

CAUSES

Hypoparathyroidism can be classified as idiopathic, acquired, or reversible. Idiopathic hypoparathyroidism has an unknown cause with an unspecified origin. Acquired hypoparathyroidism is irreversible and is most commonly caused by damage to or removal of the parathyroid gland therapeutically (parathyroidectomy) to treat hyperparathyroidism. Some patients receive an autotransplantation of a segment of a parathyroid gland in the forearm or neck to prevent hypoparathyroidism after a parathyroidectomy. Acquired hypoparathyroidism may also occur as an iatrogenic complication during thyroid or other neck surgery in about 1% to 3% of all patients postoperatively, but with repeated neck explorations, the incidence increases to 10%.

Reversible hypoparathyroidism occurs in children before age 16 years as a result of a rare autoimmune disease. It has also been known to occur as a rare side effect of ^{131}I treatment for Graves disease or with metastases of malignant tumors. Other causes of reversible hypoparathyroidism include hypomagnesemia (which impairs PTH synthesis) and delayed maturation of the parathyroid glands.

GENETIC CONSIDERATIONS

Hypoparathyroidism is characterized by hypocalcemia and hyperphosphatemia. Many genetic disorders are associated with hypoparathyroidism and have varied patterns of inheritance (autosomal recessive, autosomal dominant, and X-linked recessive). Some examples include DiGeorge syndrome (*TBX1* or *NEBL*), Charge syndrome (*CHD7* or *SEMA3E*), and Kenny-Caffey syndrome (*TBCE*). Other genes associated with hypoparathyroidism are *CASR*, *GNA11*, and *PTH*, which are involved in parathyroid development.

SEX AND LIFE SPAN CONSIDERATIONS

The disease may occur at any age. In several epidemiological studies in the United States and Europe, 75% of the people with hypoparathyroidism were female and 25% were male.

No specific life span considerations exist, although most people living with hypoparathyroidism are over the age of 45 years.

HEALTH DISPARITIES AND SEXUAL/GENDER MINORITY HEALTH

Ethnicity, race, and sexual/gender minority status have no known effect on the risk for hypoparathyroidism.

GLOBAL HEALTH CONSIDERATIONS

Hypoparathyroidism occurs around the world but is relatively rare, and no global prevalence statistics are available.

ASSESSMENT

HISTORY. History may reveal damage to the parathyroid glands during some form of neck surgery. The patient may report many GI symptoms, including abdominal pain, nausea and vomiting, diarrhea, and anorexia. Signs of hypocalcemia—such as paresthesia (numbness and tingling in the extremities), increased anxiety, headaches, irritability, and sometimes depression—may be reported. Muscle cramps, particularly involving the lower back, legs, and feet, are common. Some patients complain of difficulty swallowing, hoarseness, wheezing, or throat tightness. Others report difficulty with balancing and a history of falls or injuries.

PHYSICAL EXAMINATION. Most common symptoms are **numbness and tingling of the extremities and around the mouth, anxiety and irritability, muscle cramps, seizures, hoarseness**, and **wheezing**. Note dry skin, thin hair with patchy areas of hair loss, ridged fingernails, and teeth in poor condition. The patient may speak with a hoarse voice or have unexplained wheezing. The patient may have neuromuscular irritability with involuntary tremors and muscle spasms. Check for Trousseau sign (development of a carpal spasm when a blood pressure cuff is inflated above systolic pressure for 3 minutes) and Chvostek sign (twitching facial muscles when the facial nerve is tapped anterior to the ear). Increasing neuromuscular irritability and tetany can be life threatening.

PSYCHOSOCIAL. Patients may have altered behavior, exhibiting irritability, depression, and anxiety. The patient and significant others may describe an inability to cope with the physical manifestations of the disease and the stressors of daily life. These symptoms will create a great deal of anxiety for patients and families.

Diagnostic Highlights

Test	Normal Result	Abnormality With Condition	Explanation
Serum PTH level	10–65 pg/mL	< 10 pg/dL	Determines presence of hypoparathyroidism
Serum calcium: Total calcium, including free ionized calcium and calcium bound with protein or organic ions	8.4–10.2 mg/dL	< 8.4 mg/dL	Deficit of calcium below normal levels in the extracellular fluid compartment; if ionized calcium cannot be measured, total serum calcium can be corrected by adding 0.8 mg/dL to the total calcium level for every 1 g/dL decrease of serum albumin below 4 g/dL; the corrected value determines whether true hypocalcemia is present. When calcium levels are reported as high or low, calculate the actual level of calcium by the following formula: Corrected total calcium (mg/dL) = (measured total calcium mg/dL) + 0.8 (4.4-measured albumin g/dL).

(highlight box continues on page 642)

Diagnostic Highlights (continued)

Test	Normal Result	Abnormality With Condition	Explanation
Serum ion-ized calcium: Unbound calcium; level unaffected by albumin level	4.6–5.3 mg/dL	< 4.5 mg/dL	Ionized calcium is approximately 46%–50% of circulating calcium and is the form of calcium available for enzymatic reactions and neuromuscular function; levels increase and decrease with blood pH levels; for every 0.1 pH decrease, ionized calcium increases 1.5%–2.5%

Other Tests: Electrocardiogram (ECG; prolonged QT interval; in patients taking dig-italis preparations, hypocalcemia potentiates digitalis toxicity), phosphorus (elevated in hypocalcemia resulting from most causes, although in hypocalcemia from vitamin D deficiency, it is usually low), magnesium, creatinine, urine calcium. Bone x-rays and computed tomography to determine increased bone density. Note that alkalosis augments calcium binding to albumin and increases the severity of symptoms of hypocalcemia.

PRIMARY NURSING DIAGNOSIS

DIAGNOSIS. Risk for ineffective airway clearance as evidenced by laryngospasm, hoarseness, and/or wheezing

OUTCOMES. Hypocalcemia severity; Respiratory status: Airway patency; Respiratory status: Gas exchange; Respiratory status: Ventilation; Symptom control; Vital signsl

INTERVENTIONS. Electrolyte management: Hypocalcemia; Airway insertion and stabili-zation; Airway management; Airway suctioning; Oxygen therapy; Anxiety reduction; Cough enhancement; Mechanical ventilation: Invasive and noninvasive; Positioning; Respiratory monitoring

PLANNING AND IMPLEMENTATION

Collaborative

The treatment is to increase the ingestion and absorption of calcium. When the patient is acutely hypocalcemic, generally calcium chloride or gluconate is rapidly administered intravenously. Give oral calcium supplements with meals but not with foods that interfere with calcium absorp-tion, such as chocolate. Vitamin D supplements are usually given to increase the absorption of calcium. The individual with hypoparathyroidism needs a diet that is rich in calcium, low in phosphorus, and includes a high fluid and fiber content.

During the acute phase of hypocalcemia, monitor the ECG patterns for conduction block, the patient's respiratory status for dyspnea and stridor, and the central nervous system for seizure activity. Alkalosis worsens the symptoms of hypocalcemia because more free calcium binds with proteins when the blood pH increases. Strategies that increase carbon dioxide retention, such as breathing into a paper bag or sedating the patient, can control muscle spasm and other symptoms of tetany until the calcium level is corrected.

Pharmacologic Highlights

Medication or Drug Class	Dosage	Description	Rationale
Calcium supplements	Varies by drug	Electrolyte supplement; emergency supplementation: Calcium gluconate 2 g IV over 10 min followed by an infusion of 6 g in 500 mL D_5W over 4–6 hr; oral calcium gluconate, calcium lactate, or calcium chloride; asymptomatic hypocalcemia can be alleviated with oral calcium citrate, acetate, or carbonate	Correct deficiency: IV calcium is given cautiously to patients who are receiving epinephrine or digitalis; note that calcium can be irritating to veins when given by the IV route
Vitamin D	Ergocalciferol (Calciferol, Drisdol) 50,000–100,000 units/day PO/IM	Vitamin supplement	Stimulates absorption of calcium and phosphate from small intestine; promotes release of calcium from bone
Human parathyroid hormone, recombinant	Individualized dosage, 25–100 mcg/dose SC	Parathyroid hormone analog	Raises serum calcium by increasing renal tubular reabsorption, increasing calcium absorption, and increasing bone turnover

Independent

The primary nursing goals are to maintain a patent airway and prevent hypocalcemia in the high-risk population: patients with recent neck surgery. In addition to a careful, ongoing assessment for the symptoms of hypocalcemia, the patient should have a calm environment. Tell the patient to notify you immediately if experiencing difficulty swallowing or tightness in the throat. Listen to the patient's speech for hoarseness. To prepare for emergency airway obstruction from tetany, have intubation or tracheostomy equipment available, as well as IV calcium supplements.

Once the acute phase is over and the patient has been switched to oral medications and foods, begin patient teaching about a diet high in calcium and medications. The neuromuscular irritability and weakness place the patient at increased risk for falls. Evaluate the patient's ability to ambulate, and remove any obstructions in the patient's room. Assist the patient to identify both stressors and coping mechanisms to deal with the stressors. In particular, the patient needs to learn to avoid stressors such as fatigue and infection. Encourage the patient to ventilate feelings of anger or fear.

Evidence-Based Practice and Health Policy

Sardella, A., Bellone, F., Morabito, N., Minisola, S., Basile, G., Corica, F., & Catalano, A. (2021). The association between hypoparathyroidism and cognitive impairment: A systematic review. *Journal of Endocrinological Investigation, 44*, 905–919.

• The authors noted that hypocalcemia and low parathyroid hormone levels may induce central nervous system disturbances. Evidence of cognitive impairment is possibly underestimated. The authors performed a systematic review of the available literature using online databases to summarize the evidence of cognitive impairment in patients with idiopathic and secondary hypoparathyroidism.

• The authors found only 16 case report studies and one cross-sectional controlled study. Five case reports discussed the occurrence of cognitive impairment. The case-controlled study found a significant presence of reduced control over inhibitions, visual-spatial impairment, and slowed psychomotor ability among patients with hypoparathyroidism compared to controls. They concluded that neurological and psychological dysfunctions occur consistently in hypoparathyroid patients.

DOCUMENTATION GUIDELINES

• Physical findings: Signs and symptoms of calcium imbalance, bone deformity, patency of airway, ability to swallow and speak, assessment for signs of hypocalcemia
• Response to mobility: Level of activity tolerance, response to activity, ability to maintain a safe environment
• Psychological and neurological findings: Mood, cognition, coordination, cooperation

DISCHARGE AND HOME HEALTHCARE GUIDELINES

Encourage the patient to maintain a balance between dietary and pharmacologic calcium. Dietary calcium should be increased, and phosphorus should be decreased. Fluid and fiber should be increased. Milk, milk products, meat, poultry, fish, egg yolks, and cereals, although high in calcium, should be limited because of their phosphorus content. Chocolate is known to interfere with calcium absorption.

Remind the patient to take medications exactly as prescribed and not to substitute over-the-counter medications for prescribed calcium. Vitamin D supplements are frequently prescribed as well, sometimes in large doses. The patient may take a phosphate binder before or after meals. Some patients may also be placed on thiazide diuretics to control serum calcium. Remind women of childbearing age that pregnancy will significantly alter their calcium needs. Teach the patient about the disease process and the signs and symptoms of calcium imbalance. Stress which symptoms require immediate medical attention, and teach the patient the necessity of ongoing medical follow-up and the need to wear a Medic Alert bracelet.

Hypophosphatemia

DRG Category: 642
Mean LOS: 4.1 days
Description: MEDICAL: Inborn and Other Disorders of Metabolism

Phosphorus is a major anion in the intracellular fluid that is measured in the serum; normal serum phosphorus levels range between 1.7 and 2.6 mEq/L (2.5 and 4.5 mg/dL). In children, the serum phosphorus level is higher, at 4 to 7 mg/dL. Hypophosphatemia occurs when the serum phosphorus levels fall below 1.7 mEq/L (2.5 mg/dL). Patients with moderate hypophosphatemia (1 to 2.5 mg/dL) are usually asymptomatic and require no treatment except to manage the underlying cause; patients with severe hypophosphatemia (< 1 mg/dL) need more aggressive treatment to prevent complications. Hypophosphatemia occurs in approximately 5% of all hospitalized patients, 30% of patients admitted to critical care units, and 40% to 80% of patients with alcohol dependence, diabetic ketoacidosis, sepsis, or septic shock. Severe hypophosphatemia is rare and occurs in less than 1% of all hospitalized patients.

Approximately 85% of body phosphorus is in bone, and most of the remainder is intracellular. Only 1% is in the extracellular fluid. Phosphorus serves many functions in the body, such as maintenance of the normal nerve and muscle activity; formation and strength of bones and teeth; maintenance of cell membrane structure and function; metabolism of carbohydrates, proteins, and fats; maintenance of oxygen delivery to the tissue; maintenance of acid-base balance; and activation of the B complex vitamins. Phosphorus is excreted by the kidneys (90%) and gastrointestinal (GI) tract (10%). Regulation of phosphorus is controlled by parathyroid hormone (PTH). PTH stimulates a vitamin D derivative (calcitriol) to increase phosphorus absorption by the GI tract. PTH acts on the renal tubules to increase phosphate excretion. The possible complications of hypophosphatemia are grave and include dysrhythmias, heart failure, shock, destruction of striated muscles, seizures, and coma.

CAUSES

Hypophosphatemia occurs because of inadequate intake of phosphorus, increased excretion, and extracellular shifts of phosphorus to the intracellular space. Inadequate intake can occur because of changes in the diet as a result of malnutrition or alcoholism. Inadequate amounts of phosphorus in total parenteral nutrition may also lead to hypophosphatemia. GI problems that result in a phosphorus deficit include vomiting, chronic diarrhea, and intestinal malabsorption because of vitamin D deficiency. Increased excretion occurs in a number of ways. Two types of medications that most commonly decrease serum phosphorus are aluminum-containing antacids and diuretics. Aluminum binds with phosphorus in the GI tract, and most diuretics promote urinary excretion of phosphorus. Other phosphate binding agents include sevelamer hydrochloride and lanthanum carbonate. Increased levels of PTH, which increase the urinary excretion of phosphorus, occur with hyperparathyroidism. Extracellular shifts occur with infusion of glucose, which also leads to phosphate depletion. Cellular changes in several disorders, such as diabetic ketoacidosis, burns, and acid-base disorders, lead to hypophosphatemia. Liver and kidney transplantation may also lead to hypophosphatemia.

GENETIC CONSIDERATIONS

Familial hypophosphatemia (formerly called vitamin D–resistant rickets) results in the inability of the kidney to effectively reabsorb phosphate. Low blood levels of phosphate can be seen beginning between 6 and 10 months. In most cases, transmission of the trait follows an X-linked dominant (from *PHEX* mutations) pattern, although autosomal recessive (via *DMP1* mutations), autosomal dominant (from *FGF23* mutations), and X-linked recessive transmissions have been reported. About one-third of cases involve a de novo mutation.

SEX AND LIFE SPAN CONSIDERATIONS

Hypophosphatemia can occur at any age and in all people. Identifying high-risk groups—such as individuals with alcoholism, diabetes, malnourishment, or parathyroid disease—is critical. Children begin to show signs of hypophosphatemia from the genetic syndromes in infancy or childhood, whereas acquired hypophosphatemia occurs in late adolescence or adulthood. Adolescents who develop the condition may have eating disorders, whereas with aging, hypophosphatemia is usually associated with alcohol dependence, cancerous tumors, malabsorption syndrome, or vitamin D deficiency.

HEALTH DISPARITIES AND SEXUAL/GENDER MINORITY HEALTH

Ethnicity, race, and sexual/gender minority status have no known effect on the risk for hypophosphatemia.

GLOBAL HEALTH CONSIDERATIONS

While no international data are available, hypophosphatemia is known to occur around the world.

ASSESSMENT

HISTORY. Although most patients are asymptomatic or have nonspecific symptoms, a careful history will help to determine possible causes. Ask patients about their diet and if they have had any nausea, vomiting, diarrhea, muscle pain or weakness, or loss of appetite. Inquire about medications, especially aluminum-containing antacids and diuretics. Determine if the patient is diabetic or has a history of alcoholism, hyperparathyroidism, or a serious recent burn. Inquire about their alcohol drinking patterns. Ask if they have had a liver or kidney transplant. Look for signs of contributing conditions such as poor nutrition, malabsorption, eating disorders, or diabetes mellitus.

PHYSICAL EXAMINATION. Symptoms do not usually occur unless there is total body depletion of phosphorus or the serum level drops below 1 mg/dL. With acute hypophosphatemia, the patient appears **apprehensive and/or confused.** Ask if the patient has any **chest pain, muscle pain, weakness,** or **paresthesia.** With chronic hypophosphatemia, an accurate history may be difficult to obtain because often there is memory loss. The patient may report a history of anorexia, muscle and bone pain, double vision, or difficulty with speech.

Hypophosphatemia generally creates neuromuscular, cardiopulmonary, hematological, and GI abnormalities. Perform a thorough neuromuscular assessment; assess the patient's hand grasp and leg strength and note tremors of the extremities. Assess the deep tendon reflexes; often hyporeflexia is found. Neurological deficits include paresthesia, dysarthria, confusion, stupor, seizures, and coma. The patient's voice may be weak and shaky. Assess the patient's ability to swallow and the gag reflex. Auscultate the heart; the pulse may be weak and irregular. Assess the respiratory status, and note if the respirations are rapid and shallow because of impaired diaphragmatic function. Weigh the patient and assess for signs and symptoms of malnutrition, such as pallor, dull hair, poor skin turgor, weight loss, and fatigue.

PSYCHOSOCIAL. The patient with hypophosphatemia may be anxious and concerned about the muscular weakness, paresthesia, and ability to perform activities of daily living. Assess coping skills and family support and ability to assist with care.

Diagnostic Highlights

Test	Normal Result	Abnormality With Condition	Explanation
Serum phosphorus	2.5–4.5 mg/dL	Moderate: 1–2.5 mg/dL; severe: < 1 mg/dL; critical value: < 1.1 mg/dL	Reflects phosphorus deficit
Urine phosphorus	400–1,300 mg/day	100 mg/day when patient is hypophosphatemic	Reflects excessive renal loss of phosphorus

Other Tests: Electrocardiogram, serum total calcium, serum ionized calcium, serum magnesium, parathyroid hormone level, serum albumin level, urine amino acids, blood urea nitrogen, creatinine, serum vitamin D assays, bone radiographs

PRIMARY NURSING DIAGNOSIS

DIAGNOSIS. Imbalanced nutrition: less than body requirements related to alcoholism, dietary changes, GI abnormalities as evidenced by confusion, apprehension, weakness, and/or paresthesia

OUTCOMES. Hypophosphatemia severity; Nutritional status: Nutrient intake; Electrolyte & acid/base balance; Neurological status; Cardiac pump effectiveness; Knowledge: Medication

INTERVENTIONS. Electrolyte management: Hypophosphatemia; Nutrition management; Nutrition monitoring; Vital signs monitoring; Medication management

PLANNING AND IMPLEMENTATION

Collaborative

The most important goals are to replace the phosphorus and to correct the underlying cause of the phosphorus deficit. The average person requires 1,000 to 2,000 mg of phosphate daily. Phosphorus is replaced either by dietary intake or by oral administration of phosphate salt tablets or capsules. If hyperphosphatemia inadvertently occurs, hypocalcemia is also likely. Assess for tetany and be sure the patient has an open airway, adequate breathing, normal circulation, and an adequate urine output. Routine serum phosphate and calcium levels are ordered to determine the effectiveness of the replacement. Monitor the IV site for infiltration because potassium phosphate can cause tissue sloughing and necrosis.

Pharmacologic Highlights

Medication or Drug Class	Dosage	Description	Rationale
Phosphate supplements	Oral: 0.5–1 g elemental phosphorus PO bid-tid IV: Phosphate infusion IV over 6 hr	Oral: Neutra-Phos (250 mg phosphorus and 7 mEq each of sodium and potassium); Neutra-Phos K (250 mg phosphorus and 14 mEq sodium) IV: Potassium phosphate and sodium phosphate, 2.5–5 mg/kg in 500 mL 0.45% saline solution	Replace phosphorus; often capsules are preferred because the tablet form may cause nausea; if the deficit is severe, IV infusion of potassium phosphate is needed

Note: The response to IV phosphorus supplementation is variable and may lead to hyperphosphatemia and hypocalcemia. When using potassium phosphate as a supplement, monitor the potassium level and note that hyperkalemia may limit the amount of phosphate that can be given safely. Other Drugs: Analgesics may be ordered for bone pain. Monitor the effectiveness of the pain medications. Avoid administering antacids that contain aluminum. Vitamin D supplements may be given for vitamin D deficiency. If the patient develops alcohol withdrawal, the treatment of choice is the benzodiazepine class of medications.

Independent

Many organ systems may be affected by low phosphorus levels, and serial monitoring is important. Maintain an open airway and adequate breathing. Keep an artificial airway, manual resuscitator bag, and suction at the bedside at all times. If you hear stridor or see respiratory distress, notify the physician immediately, insert an oral or nasal airway if appropriate, and keep the airway clear with oral or nasal suction. If the patient is unresponsive, use the jaw lift or chin thrust to maintain the airway until a decision is made whether to intubate the patient. If the patient is disoriented, explain procedures carefully and simply.

Maintain a safe environment. The patient may need assistance with ambulation and activities of daily living. Orient the patient as needed. Encourage patient involvement in self-care as much as possible. If the patient develops signs of alcohol withdrawal (restlessness, insomnia, thirst, and tremors progressing to fever, hallucinations, and combative and irrational behavior), notify the physician and decrease stimulation as much as possible. Place the patient in a quiet, darkened room with a cool temperature. Provide frequent sips of water and fruit juices, but avoid fluids with caffeine. Place the patient in a room where frequent monitoring is easily accomplished.

Evidence-Based Practice and Health Policy

Glaspy, J., Lim-Watson, M., Libre, M., Karkare, S., Hadker, N., Bajic-Lucas, A., Strauss, W., & Dahl, N. (2020). Hypophosphatemia associated with intravenous iron therapies for iron deficiency anemia: A systematic literature review. *Therapeutics and Clinical Risk Management, 16*, 245–259.

- Administration of IV iron (IVI) preparations are associated with hypophosphatemia. The authors systematically assessed the prevalence, clinical consequences, and reporting of hypophosphatemia within literature IVI therapies marketed in the United States. They used electronic databases of the scientific literature.
- Most studies ($N = 40$) did not report phosphate monitoring methodology or an explicit definition of hypophosphatemia and discussed a variety of iron therapies. Eleven case reports detailed hypophosphatemia in patients treated with ferric carboxymaltose. Patients with acute hypophosphatemia primarily developed severe fatigue, and those with chronic hypophosphatemia developed osteomalacia (softening of bones) and bone deformities.

DOCUMENTATION GUIDELINES

- Laboratory: Maintain a flowsheet of serum electrolytes for easy day-to-day comparisons
- Physical responses: Adequacy of airway, breathing, and circulation; vital signs, noting any respiratory difficulties such as rapid, shallow breathing patterns; cardiac rhythm; intake and output; presence of any neuromuscular twitching, tetany, or seizure activity; ability to swallow; presence or absence of gag reflex
- Any signs of alcohol withdrawal; management of the symptoms; response to treatment
- Duration, intensity, location, and frequency of pain; effectiveness of analgesics

DISCHARGE AND HOME HEALTHCARE GUIDELINES

Instruct the patient on all medications regarding dosage, route, action, and adverse effects. Instruct the patient to avoid antacids that contain aluminum and about the higher risk for recurrence if taking diuretics. Instruct the patient to eat foods high in phosphorus, such as meats (kidney, liver, and turkey), milk, whole-grain cereals, dried fruits, seeds, and nuts. Many carbonated drinks are high in phosphate as well. Discuss with the patient how to prevent recurrence of hypophosphatemia.

Hypothyroidism

DRG Category:	644
Mean LOS:	4.3 days
Description:	MEDICAL: Endocrine Disorders With Complication or Comorbidity

Hypothyroidism occurs when the thyroid gland produces a deficient amount of the thyroid hormones, resulting in a lowered basal metabolism. Many individuals with mild hypothyroidism are frequently undiagnosed, but the hormone disturbance may contribute to an acceleration of atherosclerosis or complications of medical treatment, such as intraoperative hypotension and cardiac complications after surgery. In severe hypothyroidism, a hydrophilic ("water-loving") mucopolysaccharide is deposited throughout the body, causing nonpitting edema (myxedema) and thickening of the facial features. The most severe level of the disease is myxedema coma, a life-threatening state characterized by cardiovascular collapse, severe electrolyte imbalances, respiratory depression, and cerebral hypoxia. Risks for hypothyroidism include a family history of thyroid disease or autoimmune diseases, a personal history of rheumatoid arthritis, type 1 diabetes, treatment with radioactive iodine, thyroid surgery, or radiation exposure to the neck.

Hypothyroidism is generally classified as cretinism, juvenile hypothyroidism, and adult hypothyroidism. Cretinism is a state of severe hypothyroidism found in infants. When infants do not produce normal amounts of thyroid hormones, their skeletal maturation and central nervous system development are altered, resulting in retardation of physical growth or mental growth, or both. Juvenile hypothyroidism is most often caused by chronic autoimmune thyroiditis and affects the growth and sexual maturation of the child. Signs and symptoms are similar to adult hypothyroidism, and the treatment reverses most of the clinical manifestations of the disease. The majority of people with hypothyroidism have the adult form, in which the thyroid gland is unable to produce sufficient amounts of thyroid hormone to support body processes.

Complications of the disease affect every organ system. Cardiovascular depression can lead to poor peripheral perfusion, congestive heart failure, and an enlarged heart. Intestinal obstruction, obesity, anemia, deafness, psychiatric problems, carpal tunnel syndrome, and impaired fertility are a few of the systemic complications.

CAUSES

Hypothyroidism can be a primary disorder that results from disease in the thyroid gland itself or a secondary or tertiary disorder. In most cases, hypothyroidism occurs as a primary disorder and results from the loss of thyroid tissue, which leads to inadequate production of thyroid hormones (primary hypothyroidism). It is most frequently autoimmune in origin but can also be related to iodine deficiency. Secondary hypothyroidism, which occurs in only 5% of cases, is caused by a failure of the pituitary gland to stimulate the thyroid gland or a failure of the target tissues to respond to the thyroid hormones. Tertiary hypothyroidism is caused by failure of the hypothalamus to produce thyroid-releasing factor.

The most common cause of goitrous hypothyroidism in North America is Hashimoto disease, which causes defective iodine binding and defective thyroid hormone production. Hashimoto disease is common in the same family and is considered an autoimmune disorder leading to chronic inflammation of the thyroid gland and hypothyroidism but can also lead to hyperthyroidism.

GENETIC CONSIDERATIONS

Mutations in over a dozen genes (e.g., *PAX8*, *NKX2-8*, *SLC5A5*, *TG*, *TPO*, *TSHB*, and *TSHR*) can lead to congenital hypothyroidism. Mutations in two of these genes (*TSHR* and *PAX8*) prevent or interrupt thyroid development in the fetus, while the exact mechanism of the others is not as clear. Approximately 15% to 20% of cases are thought to be inherited, with almost all following an autosomal recessive pattern. Alleles associated with autoimmune hypothyroidism are also being investigated as genetic etiologies.

SEX AND LIFE SPAN CONSIDERATIONS

Hypothyroidism is more frequently found in women between ages 30 and 50 years as compared to men, although it may also affect infants and older adults. It is more common in females with small body size at birth and low body mass index (BMI) throughout childhood years. Some women experience transient hypothyroidism with pregnancy; generally, they may experience it again with subsequent pregnancies. Women with hypothyroidism have elevated mortality risks of diabetes mellitus, cardiovascular disease, and cerebrovascular disease, and older adults with hypothyroidism have an elevated mortality risk of cardiovascular disease.

Approximately 10% of all adults have laboratory evidence of Hashimoto disease. Aging makes a difference. Experts suggest that approximately 20% of older people have some form of hypothyroidism. Because patients with myxedema may have confusing signs and symptoms that mimic the aging process, it is often undiagnosed in older patients. Lack of a timely diagnosis can lead to serious side effects from medications such as sedatives, opiates, and anesthetics.

HEALTH DISPARITIES AND SEXUAL/GENDER MINORITY HEALTH

Hypothyroidism likely has a higher prevalence in White females than in other groups. White and Hispanic persons have a higher prevalence than Black persons. Sexual and gender minority status has no known effect on the risk of hypothyroidism.

GLOBAL HEALTH CONSIDERATIONS

In developed regions of the world, the incidence of hypothyroidism is approximately 8% in women and 3% in men. In regions such as North America and Western Europe, the most common cause is due to autoimmune processes, whereas in developing regions, iodine deficiency is the most common cause. Experts suggest that approximately 30% of the world's population is iodine deficient, including people in China, India, Northern Africa, and Great Britain. In these areas, women are 5 to 10 times more likely to have hypothyroidism than men. Recent attention on nutritional deficiencies with iodine supplementation in salt and flour has decreased prevalence of hypothyroidism in low-resource areas, but the problem of iodine deficiency persists.

☀ ASSESSMENT

HISTORY. The patient's history may be vague with subtle changes in mental acuity or physical stamina, or the patient may be asymptomatic. The patient may describe a history of cold intolerance, constipation, fatigue even with little activity, weight gain with decreased food intake, aches and stiffness, generalized weakness, slowing of intellectual functions, impaired memory, and loss of initiative. Some patients seek healthcare for obstructive sleep apnea, carpal tunnel syndrome, or menstrual disturbances. Patients with more severe or untreated disease, if hypothyroidism is accompanied by goiter, may describe discomfort with clothes or jewelry that is close fitting around the neck. The patient may complain of hair loss or slow growing of hair and nails. Women may note heavy, irregular menstrual periods, and men may describe impotence. Both may experience decreased libido.

Determine if the patient's diet is deficient in iodine. Some foods (cabbage, spinach, radishes) and medications (antithyroids, lithium carbonate) can cause hypothyroidism in a person predisposed to the disease. In addition, medications such as digoxin and insulin are potentiated by the hypothyroid state.

PHYSICAL EXAMINATION. The most common early symptoms are **sensitivity to cold, weight gain, joint achiness,** and **fatigue.** The patient has signs of a slowed metabolism and a slow tendon-reflex relaxation, with hypotension and bradycardia. Note a slow speech pattern, flat affect, and difficulty in forming replies to interview questions. The patient may have a dry, thick tongue and hoarseness; dry, flaky skin with a pale or yellowish tint; and edema of the hands and feet. Fingernails and toenails may appear thick, grooved, and brittle. The patient's face may have a distinctive appearance, with thick features, a masklike appearance, edema around the eyes, drooping eyelids, and abbreviated eyebrows. The patient's hair is often thin and dry; patchy hair loss is common.

If the condition has existed for some time, the skin feels cool, rough, and "doughy" on palpation. You may not be able to feel the thyroid tissue unless the patient has a goiter. Weak peripheral pulses, distant heart sounds, bradycardia, and hypotension are common findings. The patient has either decreased or absent bowel sounds and may have abdominal distention. Other findings include hypothermia, shortness of breath, and either depressive or agitated mood states. Rare findings include hypoventilation, pericardial or pleural effusions, deafness, and carpal tunnel syndrome.

PSYCHOSOCIAL. The patient's behavior may be depressed, agitated, disoriented, or even paranoid with severe, untreated disease. You may notice intellectual slowing and impaired interactions with others; the patient and family members may be upset about the change in behavior.

Diagnostic Highlights

Test	Normal Result	Abnormality With Condition	Explanation
Thyroid-stimulating hormone (TSH) assay	In most healthy patients, TSH values are 0.4–4.2 mU/L	> 4.2 mU/L	Normal value excludes primary hypothyroidism, and a markedly elevated value confirms the diagnosis
Thyroxine (T$_4$) radioimmunoassay	5.5–12.5 mcg/dL	Decreased	Reflects underproduction of thyroid hormones; monitors response to therapy
Triiodothyronine (T$_3$) radioimmunoassay	70–204 ng/dL for adults	Decreased	Reflects underproduction of thyroid hormones
Electrocardiogram	Normal PQRST pattern	Low-voltage T-wave abnormalities, bradycardia	Determines electrical impulse generation and conduction

Other Tests: Tests include 24-hour radioactive iodine uptake, thyroid autoantibodies, and antithyroglobulin.

PRIMARY NURSING DIAGNOSIS

DIAGNOSIS. Decreased activity tolerance related to hormonal deficiency as evidenced by joint achiness, fatigue, and/or weakness

OUTCOMES. Activity tolerance; Energy conservation; Knowledge: Disease process; Knowledge: Medication; Nutritional status; Endurance; Symptom severity

INTERVENTIONS. Energy management; Exercise promotion; Nutrition management; Medication management; Vital signs monitoring

PLANNING AND IMPLEMENTATION

Collaborative

Most patients are diagnosed and treated on an outpatient basis. The goal of treatment is to return the patient to the euthyroid (normal) state and to prevent complications; patients generally have no changes to quality of life when they are treated adequately. The treatment of choice is to provide thyroid hormone supplements to correct hormonal deficiencies. Treatment of the older patient is approached more cautiously because of higher risk for cardiac complications and toxic effects. The medication should not be given if the pulse rate is greater than 100. The treatment is considered to be lifelong, requiring ongoing medical assessment of thyroid function. Polypharmacy is a significant concern for the hypothyroid patient. Several classifications of drugs are affected by the addition of thyroid supplements, including beta blockers, oral anticoagulants, bronchodilators, digitalis preparations, tricyclic antidepressants, and cholesterol-lowering agents.

Because significant cardiovascular disease often accompanies hypothyroidism, the patient is at risk for cardiac complications if the metabolic rate is increased too quickly. Therefore, the patient needs to be monitored for cardiovascular compromise (palpitations, chest pain, shortness of breath, rapid heart rate) during early thyroid therapy. The diet for the hypothyroid patient is generally low in calories, high in fiber, and high in protein. As the metabolic rate rises, the caloric content can be increased. The patient's intolerance to cold may extend to cold foods, making meal planning more difficult.

Pharmacologic Highlights

Treatment consists of replacing the deficient hormone with a synthetic thyroid hormone; low doses are initially used, and the dose is increased every 1 to 2 months on the basis of clinical response and serial laboratory measurements that show normalization of TSH levels in primary hypothyroidism. The patient begins to experience clinical benefits in 3 to 5 days, which level off after approximately 4 to 6 weeks. After the dose is stabilized, patients can be monitored with laboratory measurement of TSH annually.

Medication or Drug Class	Dosage	Description	Rationale
Levothyroxine sodium	1.5–2.5 mcg/kg PO daily; use lowest dose possible because overreplacement of thyroid can cause bone loss or cardiovascular complications	Synthetic thyroid hormone replacement	Returns the patient to the euthyroid (normal) state

Independent

Monitor the patient carefully for cardiac complications (chest pain, shortness of breath, palpitations, rapid pulse), check vital signs frequently, and monitor the patient's intake and output. Monitor the patient's weight at least twice a week.

The patient with myxedema is generally weak and therefore progressively immobile. One goal is to increase the patient's mobility while accommodating the patient's extreme weakness with frequent rest periods and safety measures. Hypothyroidism exposes the patient to the risk of skin breakdown. Provide meticulous skin care.

Another patient concern is intolerance to cold. Caution the patient against using electric blankets or other electric heating devices because the combination of vasodilation, decreased sensation, and decreased alertness may result in unrecognized burns. Use of layered clothing and extra bedclothes is helpful to increase comfort. Patients tolerate warm liquids better than cold. Decreased mental acuity, significant weakness, and slower reflexes make the individual at risk for many injuries.

Patients may have difficulty interacting with significant others who have not understood or accepted the changes in their loved one. As their condition improves, patients and families may feel guilty that they did not notice the changes until they were severe. The return to the euthyroid state takes some time. Patients need frequent reassurance that the treatment is appropriate. Patient learning may be difficult for the hypometabolic patient; you can facilitate understanding that most of the physical manifestations are abnormal and reversible.

Evidence-Based Practice and Health Policy

Thavaraputta, S., Dennis, J., Laoveeravat, P., Nugent, K., & Rivas, A. (2019). Hypothyroidism and its association with sleep apnea among adults in the United States: NHANES 2007–2008. *Journal of Clinical Endocrinology and Metabolism, 104*, 4990–4997.

• The authors aimed to assess whether there is a positive association between hypothyroidism and sleep apnea in the U.S. population. The authors performed a cross-sectional study and included all subjects age 18 years and older who met inclusion criteria ($N = 5,515$). Participants were classified as hypothyroid, hyperthyroid, and euthyroid (normal thyroid). The diagnosis of sleep apnea was based on participants' response when asked whether they had been diagnosed by their doctors.
• The prevalence of hypothyroidism and hyperthyroidism was calculated at 9.47% and 1.19%, respectively. After controlling for demographics, healthcare access, body mass index, socioeconomic factors, alcohol use, smoking, and other comorbidities, the authors found a significant association between hypothyroidism and sleep apnea.

DOCUMENTATION GUIDELINES

• Physical findings: Cardiovascular status, bowel activity, edema, condition of hair, nails, and skin, fatigue level, and activity tolerance
• Response to medications, skin care regimen, nutrition, safety precautions
• Psychosocial response to changes in bodily function, including mental acuity

DISCHARGE AND HOME HEALTHCARE GUIDELINES

Explain all medications, including dosage, potential side effects, and drug interactions. Instruct the patient to check the pulse at least twice a week and to stop the thyroid supplement and notify the physician if the pulse is greater than 100. Explain that the healthcare professional should be notified about the condition. Explain that ongoing medical assessment is required to check thyroid function and that the medications may lead to hyperthyroidism despite the patient's underlying hypothyroidism.

Teach the patient about the thyroid gland and hypothyroidism, as well as complications such as heart disease and edema. Teach the patient that new cardiac or hyperthyroidism symptoms need to be reported immediately. Explain that the caloric and fiber requirements vary. The patient should report any abnormal weight gain or loss or change in bowel elimination.

Hypovolemic/ Hemorrhagic Shock

DRG Category:	640
Mean LOS:	4.5 days
Description:	MEDICAL: Miscellaneous Disorders of Nutrition, Metabolism, Fluids and Electrolytes With Major Complication or Comorbidity

Hypovolemic shock results from a decreased effective circulating volume of water, plasma, or whole blood and is the most common type of shock in adults and children. Rapid fluid loss leads to inadequate tissue perfusion and, if not reversed, ultimately, to organ failure. External, sudden blood loss resulting from penetrating trauma and severe gastrointestinal (GI) bleeding are common causes of hemorrhagic shock. A significant loss of greater than 30% of circulating volume results in a decrease in venous return, which in turn diminishes cardiac output, decreases perfusion to vital organs, and causes the symptoms associated with shock. When there is insufficient oxygen available to the cells, metabolism shifts from aerobic to anaerobic pathways. In this process, lactic acid accumulates in the tissues, and the patient develops metabolic acidosis. In addition, the tissues do not receive adequate glucose, and they cannot accomplish the removal of carbon dioxide. This disruption in normal tissue metabolism results initially in cellular destruction and, if left uncorrected, multiple organ failure and death. Significant hypovolemic shock (< 40% loss of circulating volume) lasting several hours or more is associated with a fatal outcome.

The American College of Surgeons separates hypovolemic/hemorrhagic shock into four classifications: Stage I occurs when up to 15% of the circulating volume, or approximately 750 mL of blood, is lost. These patients often exhibit few symptoms except perhaps anxiety and a slight increase in heart rate because compensatory mechanisms support bodily functions. Stage II occurs when 15% to 30%, or up to 1,500 mL of blood, of the circulating volume is lost. These patients have subtle signs of shock, but vital signs usually remain normal except for tachycardia and mild tachypnea. Patients may be slightly confused or irritable, and their skin may feel cool. Urine output will likely be reduced. Stage III occurs when 30% to 40% of the circulating volume, or from 1,500 to 2,000 mL of blood, is lost. This patient looks acutely ill, with significant tachycardia, thready pulses, hypotension, tachypnea, cold and clammy skin, lethargy, oliguria, and metabolic acidosis. The most severe form of hypovolemic/hemorrhagic shock is stage IV. The patient has severe tachycardia, weak or absent pulses, significant hypotension, hypothermia, acidosis, severe tachypnea, coma, cyanosis, and anuria. This patient has lost more than 40% of circulating volume, or least 2,000 mL of blood, and is at risk for exsanguination. Complications of hypovolemic shock include adult respiratory distress syndrome, sepsis, acute renal failure, disseminated intravascular coagulation, cerebrovascular accident, multiple organ dysfunction syndrome, and death.

CAUSES

The loss of circulating volume can result from a number of conditions. Hemorrhage caused by active blood loss that results from trauma is a frequent source of hypovolemia. Both motor vehicle crashes (MVCs) and penetrating injuries from guns or knives can lead to hypovolemic shock. Active bleeding or rupture of internal organs, such as the bowel or the fallopian tube when caused by an ectopic pregnancy, can quickly result in hypovolemia even without obvious bleeding. Ruptured aortic aneurysm leads to hypovolemic shock due to rapid internal hemorrhage. Profound decreases in circulating fluid volume can be caused by the plasma shifts seen in burns and ascites. Other sources of hypovolemia include decreases in fluid intake (dehydration) and increases in fluid output (vomiting, diarrhea, excessive nasogastric drainage, draining wounds, and diaphoresis). Excessive diuresis from diuretic overuse, diabetic ketoacidosis, and diabetes insipidus can also cause hypovolemia. Pregnancy-related disorders that can lead to hypovolemic shock include ruptured ectopic pregnancy, placenta previa, and abruption of the placenta.

GENETIC CONSIDERATIONS

No clear genetic contributions to susceptibility have been defined.

SEX AND LIFE SPAN CONSIDERATIONS

Hypovolemic shock can occur at any age and in all people. The most common cause of hypovolemic shock in children and older adults is dehydration. In comparison, although trauma can occur at any age, in young adults the major cause of hypovolemic shock is hemorrhage from multiple trauma. Most blunt trauma is associated with MVCs, which are two to three times more common in males than in females in the 15- to 24-year-old age group. Penetrating injuries from gunshot wounds and stab wounds, which are on the increase in U.S. preteens, teens, and young adults, are also more common in males than females. Chronic illness can alter an individual's compensatory abilities in the setting of hypovolemia. Hypovolemic shock related to an ectopic pregnancy occurs in females of childbearing age, and GI bleeding disorders are common in adults.

HEALTH DISPARITIES AND SEXUAL/GENDER MINORITY HEALTH

Trauma leading to hypovolemic shock may occur after traffic crashes and penetrating injury. In recent years, Black persons have been killed in traffic crashes at a rate almost 25% higher than that for White persons (National Highway Traffic Safety Administration [NHTSA], 2021). Native American persons have the highest rate of MVC injury in the United States, more than twice the rate of Black persons (NHTSA, 2021). Experts have noted that Black and Native American communities tend to be crisscrossed by more dangerous roads than other communities. Non-Hispanic Black males have adjusted firearm death rates from two to seven times higher than males of other groups. Healthy People 2020 reports that non-Hispanic Black persons have the highest injury death rate in the United States (79.9 injury deaths per 100,000 people), followed by non-Hispanic White persons (79.2), Native American persons (78.2), Hispanic persons (45.5), and Asian/Pacific Islander persons (25.6). Recent work has shown evidence that rural populations have injury mortality rates that are more than twice as high as urban rates. Many factors contribute to these health disparities, including the risk of traffic injury in narrow rural roads, the lack of graded curves and lighted traffic signals on rural highways, and the distance from major trauma centers. Many of the most dangerous occupations, such as mining and agriculture, are found in rural areas and can result in injury, disability, and death. Sexual and gender minority persons have high risk for dating and interpersonal violence, violence related to bullying, and intentional and unintentional injury (Healthy People 2020). All of these situations may lead to hypovolemic shock.

GLOBAL HEALTH CONSIDERATIONS

The World Health Organization has identified MVCs as a growing epidemic in developing regions of the world. Both blunt and penetrating traumatic injury resulting in excessive bleeding can result from MVCs. In regions at war or with civil or political strife, traumatic injuries also lead to hemorrhagic shock. GI bleeding is a source of hypovolemic/hemorrhagic shock around the world.

ASSESSMENT

HISTORY. If the patient is actively bleeding or is severely compromised, the history, assessment, and early management merge together into the primary survey. The primary survey is a rapid (30- to 60-second) head-to-toe assessment that encompasses the emergency management of threats to airway, breathing, and circulation (ABCs) or life. If the patient's condition is stable enough to warrant a separate history, ask questions about allergies, current medications, preexisting medical conditions, and the factors that surround the hypovolemic/hemorrhagic condition.

Generally, patients who are experiencing hypovolemia because of trauma have either obvious bleeding or a history of injury to a vascularized area. Elicit information from the patient, emergency medical personnel, or the family as to how much blood was lost or how long the bleeding has continued. In the case of traumatic blood loss, it is important to remember that the most obvious injury site may not be the cause of the evolving hypovolemic shock.

Explore the possibility of a mechanism of injury, such as a burn or crush injury, leading to plasma fluid shifts extravascularly. Likewise, a history of either recent alterations in fluid volume intake or excessive loss—as in vomiting, diarrhea, excessive diaphoresis, or diuresis—is a potential indicator. In addition, obtain a subjective history of thirst, lethargy, and decreased urinary output.

PHYSICAL EXAMINATION. Early signs include **restlessness, anxiety, agitation, confusion, weakness, lightheadedness,** and **tachycardia.** The patient may appear either stable and alert or critically ill depending on the phase of hypovolemic shock. If the patient can maintain the ABCs, assess the patient's level of consciousness. Mental status changes may be indicators of diminished cerebral perfusion and are among the early signs of hypovolemic shock. Other early indicators include a decreased urinary output of less than 30 mL/hour, delayed capillary blanching, and signs of sympathetic nervous system stimulation (tachycardia, piloerection [gooseflesh]). Monitor vital signs, including heart and respiratory rate, blood pressure, and temperature. Changes in blood pressure (particularly hypotension) are a late rather than an early sign; pulse pressure, however, does initially widen and then narrow in the first two stages of shock. Orthostatic blood pressure changes also indicate hypovolemia. Inspect the patient's neck veins and palpate them for the quality of carotid pulse and neck vein appearance.

Four areas of the body where life-threatening hemorrhage may occur include the chest, abdomen, thighs (from a femoral fracture), and on the body's surface. Percuss the chest and lung fields for the presence of fluid. Auscultate the patient's bilateral breathing to check for decreased breath sounds and note the patient's respiratory effort. Auscultate the patient's heart and note any new murmurs or other adventitious heart sounds. Inspect the patient's abdomen for possible sites of fluid loss or compartmentalization. When you auscultate the patient's abdomen, note the absence of bowel sounds, which may indicate a paralytic ileus, internal GI bleeding, or peritonitis. If bowel sounds are hypoactive, bleeding may be causing blood to shunt to other more vital organs. Check the abdomen for tenderness or enlargement. If the thighs have deformities or are enlarged, those may be signs of femoral fracture and bleeding into the thigh. Palpate the patient's peripheral pulses and note signs of decreased blood flow and inadequate tissue perfusion (cold, clammy skin; weak, rapid pulses; delayed capillary refill), but remember that these signs are late indicators of hypovolemic shock and may not be present until the patient reaches stage III. Check all parts of the body for external bleeding.

PSYCHOSOCIAL. If the patient has a decreased level of consciousness, attempt to identify a family member or significant other to discuss the patient's psychosocial history. Expect family members to be frightened, anxious, and in need of support. Of particular concern are the parents of young trauma patients who have to deal with a sudden, life-threatening event that may lead to the death of a child. Spouses of critically injured patients deal with role reversals, economic crises, and the fear of loss. Expect the family and partner of critically injured patients to express a range of emotions from fear and anxiety to grief and guilt.

Diagnostic Highlights

General Comments: No one specific diagnostic test identifies the degree of hypovolemic/hemorrhagic shock state. Several laboratory indicators provide valuable information on the status of the patient, however. These include arterial blood gases, hemodynamic parameters (cardiac output and cardiac index, oxygen delivery, oxygen consumption, central venous pressure, pulmonary capillary wedge pressure, and systemic vascular resistance), blood lactate level, electrolyte levels, hemoglobin, and hematocrit. The shock index (SI), which is the heart rate divided by the systolic blood pressure, is an indication of a patient's hypovolemic state. If the SI is less than 0.6, there is no shock. Mild shock is indicated by a value of 0.6 to less than 1.0. Moderate shock is from 1.0 to less than 1.4. Severe shock is a value of 1.4 or more. Radiographic, ultrasound, and imaging studies are important depending on the location of interest and might include chest and abdominal x-rays, transesophageal echocardiography, aortography,

Diagnostic Highlights (continued)

computed tomography, magnetic resonance imaging, or focused abdominal sonography for trauma. A pregnancy test should be completed for females of childbearing years, and if positive, followed by pelvic sonography.

PRIMARY NURSING DIAGNOSIS

DIAGNOSIS. Risk for bleeding as evidenced by hypotension, tachycardia, restlessness, frank hemorrhage, occult hemorrhage, and/or dyspnea

OUTCOMES. Blood loss severity; Fluid balance; Circulation status; Shock severity: Hypovolemic; Hydration; Vital signs

INTERVENTIONS. Bleeding reduction; Fluid resuscitation; Fluid monitoring; Blood product administration; IV therapy; Shock prevention; Shock management: Volume

PLANNING AND IMPLEMENTATION

Collaborative

The initial care of the patient with hypovolemic shock follows the ABCs of resuscitation. Measures to ensure adequate oxygenation and tissue perfusion include establishing an effective airway and a supplemental oxygen source, controlling the source of blood loss, and replacing intravascular volume. The American College of Surgeons recommends crystalloid fluids such as normal saline solution or lactated Ringer solution for stages I and II and crystalloids plus blood products for stages III and IV. Although vasopressors, such as norepinephrine or dopamine, do increase blood pressure in the setting of hypovolemic shock, they should never be started if there is insufficient intravascular fluid or if tissues remain underperfused despite an adequate blood pressure.

The objective of fluid replacement is to provide for adequate cardiac output to perfuse the tissues. Generally, any fluid transiently improves perfusion, but only red blood cells (RBCs) can carry enough oxygen to maintain cellular function. Three milliliters of crystalloid solutions should be infused for every 1 mL of blood loss. It is currently recommended to use caution in replacing fluids after trauma because the low flow state may protect the patient from further bleeding until the traumatic injury is repaired. After repair, fluid resuscitation can be used aggressively. RBCs or whole blood should be considered when fluid resuscitation with crystalloids is not successful. RBCs are preferred because they contain an increased percentage of hemoglobin per volume. Type-specific blood is preferred, although O-negative blood can be used if type-specific blood is not immediately available.

Pharmacologic Highlights

Medication or Drug Class	Dosage	Description	Rationale
Somatostatin (Zecnil)	250 mcg IV bolus, followed by a 250–500 mcg/hr continuous infusion; maintain for 2–5 days	Naturally occurring peptide from hypothalamus, GI tract, and pancreas	Increases reabsorption of water from the kidney tubules
Other Drugs: Octreotide (Sandostatin)			

Independent

After initial stabilization of airway and breathing, the most important nursing intervention is to ensure timely fluid replacement. Fluid resuscitation is most efficient through a short, large-bore peripheral IV catheter in a large peripheral vein. The IV line should have a short length of tubing from the bag or bottle to the IV site. If pressure is applied to the bag, fluid resuscitation occurs more rapidly. If fluids can be warmed before infusion, the patient has a lower risk of hypothermia.

Positioning the patient can also increase perfusion throughout the body; place the patient in a modified Trendelenburg position to facilitate venous return and to prevent excessive abdominal viscera shift and restriction of the diaphragm that occurs with the head-down position. Fluid balance is of high importance; ongoing monitoring of intake and output is essential for care and decision making. Patients with hypovolemic shock require critical surveillance and monitoring at all times with serial vital signs.

Patients and their families are often frightened and anxious. If the patient is awake, provide a running explanation of the procedures to provide reassurance. Touch the patient's hand or arm to offer reassurance when possible. Explain the treatment alternatives to the family and keep them updated as to the patient's response to therapy. If blood component therapy is essential, answer the patient's and family's questions about the risks involved.

Evidence-Based Practice and Health Policy

Ozakin, E., Yazlamaz, N., Kaya, F., Karakilic, E., & Bilgin, M. (2020). Perfusion index measurement in predicting hypovolemic shock in trauma patients. *Journal of Emergency Medicine, 59,* 238–245.

- The aim of this study was to investigate the relationship between perfusion index (PI) and blood transfusion necessity in multitrauma patients ($N = 338$). PI is derived from a pulse oximeter and shows the ratio of the pulsatile blood flow to the nonpulsatile blood flow (static blood) in peripheral tissue, and is an indirect and noninvasive measure of peripheral perfusion. They also investigated the risk of hemorrhage and recorded laboratory and clinical parameters.
- The PI was less than 1 in 39 (11.5%) patients. They found positive correlations between PI and hemoglobin, hematocrit, base deficit, systolic blood pressure, SpO_2, and negative correlations with lactate, respiratory rate, and shock index. Thirty-one patients with PI less than 1 had blood transfusion within 24 hours. The main risk factors to predict blood transfusions were PI, pulse rate, and SpO_2. PI was more significant than lactate, base deficit, revised trauma score, and shock index measurements.

DOCUMENTATION GUIDELINES

- Adequacy of airway: Patency of airway, ease of respiration, chest expansion, respiratory rate, presence of stridor or wheezes
- Cardiovascular assessment: Capillary blanch, quality of peripheral pulses, presence of gooseflesh, changes in vital signs (blood pressure and heart rate), skin color, cardiac rhythm, signs of uncorrected bleeding
- Body temperature
- Fluid balance: Intake and output, patency of IV lines, speed of fluid resuscitation

DISCHARGE AND HOME HEALTHCARE GUIDELINES

Provide a complete explanation of all emergency treatments and answer the patient's and family's questions. Explain the possibility of complications to recovery, such as poor wound healing, infection, and anemia. Explain the risks of blood transfusion and answer any questions about exposure to blood-borne infections. As required, provide information about any follow-up laboratory procedures that might be needed after the patient is discharged.

Idiopathic Thrombocytopenic Purpura

DRG Category:	813
Mean LOS:	4.9 days
Description:	MEDICAL: Coagulation Disorders

Idiopathic thrombocytopenic purpura (ITP), also known as *primary immune thrombocytopenic purpura*, is an acquired hemorrhagic disorder characterized by an increased destruction of platelets because of antiplatelet antibodies. The antibodies attach to the platelets, reduce their life span, and lead to a platelet count below $100,000/mm^3$ and occasionally as low as $5,000/mm^3$. ITP can be divided into two categories: acute and chronic. Acute ITP is generally a self-limiting childhood disorder, whereas chronic ITP predominantly affects adults and is characterized by thrombocytopenia of more than 6 months.

The most life-threatening complication of ITP is intracerebral hemorrhage, which is most likely to occur if the platelet count falls below $1,000/mm^3$. Hemorrhage into the kidneys, abdominal cavity, or retroperitoneal space is also possible. Prognosis for acute ITP is excellent, with nearly 80% of patients recovering without treatment. The mortality rate from hemorrhage is 1% in children and 5% in adults. Older age and a previous history of hemorrhage increase the risk of severe bleeding in adults. Prognosis for chronic ITP is good, with remissions lasting weeks or even years. Complications include cerebral hemorrhage and hemorrhagic shock.

CAUSES

Acute ITP is thought to be a response to a viral infection; platelets are destroyed by antibodies (immunoglobulin G autoantibodies) to a platelet membrane glycoprotein. Generally, a viral infection, such as rubella or chickenpox, occurs 2 to 21 days before the onset of the disease. Acute ITP may occur after live vaccine immunizations and is most prevalent during the winter and spring months when the incidence of infection is high. It is also associated with HIV infection. Chronic ITP generally has no underlying viral association and is often linked to immunological disorders, such as lupus erythematosus, or to drug reactions. Immune thrombocytopenia occurs rarely during pregnancy.

GENETIC CONSIDERATIONS

There seems to be both a genetic and environmental component to ITP. ITP has been seen in monozygotic twins, and a predisposition to autoantibody production can run in families. Variants in the genes *FCGR3A* and *KIR2DS2* have been identified that increase susceptibility to ITP.

SEX AND LIFE SPAN CONSIDERATIONS

Approximately 40% of the cases of ITP occur in children under the age of 10 years. Up to age 10 years, acute ITP affects children of both sexes and is most common between ages 2 and 4 years. After age 10 years, more girls than boys have the condition. About half of the children recover in 1 month, and 93% recover completely by 1 year. More than 80% of patients with acute ITP recover, regardless of treatment, but 10% to 20% progress to chronic ITP. ITP can also occur during pregnancy, and 5% to 20% of the neonates born to these patients will have severe thrombocytopenia and are at risk of intracranial hemorrhage during vaginal birth. Chronic ITP occurs mainly between the ages of 20 and 50 years and affects women almost three times as often as men. ITP related to drug reactions can occur at any age.

HEALTH DISPARITIES AND SEXUAL/GENDER MINORITY HEALTH

Some experts have reported that the prevalence of ITP in Black children is lower than that of White children, although Black children are more likely than White children to have chronic conditions such as systemic lupus erythematosus in conjunction with ITP. Immune thrombocytopenia in pregnancy is more common in White pregnant people as compared to pregnant people of other groups. Sexual and gender minority status has no known effect on the risk for ITP.

GLOBAL HEALTH CONSIDERATIONS

Global incidence of ITP varies greatly depending on the country and ranges from 10 to 125 cases per 1 million per year in developed regions of the world such as North America, Western Europe, and the Middle East. Few data are available in developing regions.

ASSESSMENT

HISTORY. Ask if the patient has recently had rubella or chickenpox or a viral infection with symptoms such as upper respiratory or gastrointestinal (GI). Ask if the patient was recently immunized with a live vaccine. Check for a history of systemic lupus erythematosus; easy bruising; or bleeding from the nose, gums, or GI or urinary tract. Ask about the onset of bruising and bleeding. Usually, children have an abrupt onset and adults have a more general onset. Because the symptoms of chronic ITP are usually insidious, patients may not have noticed an increase in symptoms. Ask the patient for the date of the last menstrual period, whether recent menses lasted longer and were heavier than usual, or whether the patient is pregnant. Ask if the patient has had HIV testing.

PHYSICAL EXAMINATION. Physical examination of patients with acute ITP reveals **diffuse petechiae** (red to purple dots on the skin 1 to 3 mm in size) or **bruises on the skin and in the oral mucosa**. Patients with chronic ITP may have no obvious petechiae. Other clinical features of ITP include ecchymoses (areas of purple to purplish-blue fading to green, yellow, and brown with time), which can occur anywhere on the body from even minor trauma. You may note bleeding from the gums and/or nose. In both types of ITP, the spleen and liver are often slightly palpable with lymph node swelling. Ongoing assessment throughout patient management is essential to evaluate for signs of life-threatening bleeding.

PSYCHOSOCIAL. Children with acute ITP are usually brought to the pediatrician by highly anxious parents who are concerned with the sudden appearance of easy bruising, petechiae, and occasionally bleeding gums and nosebleeds. Because these symptoms are so commonly associated with leukemia, parents and children need swift diagnosis and reassurance. Pregnant people are concerned about their own health as well as the health of the fetus.

Diagnostic Highlights

Test	Normal Result	Abnormality With Condition	Explanation
Platelet count	150,000–450,000/ mm³	> 100,000/mm³	Platelets are consumed during clot formation; degree of platelet suppression predicts the severity of symptoms: 30,000–50,000/mm³, bruising with minor trauma; 15,000–30,000/mm³, spontaneous bruising, petechiae, particularly on the arms and legs; > 15,000/mm³, spontaneous bruising, mucosal bleeding, nosebleeds, bloody urine or stool, intracranial bleeding

Other Tests: Tests include complete blood count and coagulation profiles, blood smear studies, bone marrow aspiration, HIV testing, and computed tomography of the head if intracerebral hemorrhage is suspected.

PRIMARY NURSING DIAGNOSIS

DIAGNOSIS. Risk for injury as evidenced by petechiae, bruising, and/or bleeding from the gums, nose, or mucous membranes

OUTCOMES. Risk control; Safe home environment; Blood coagulation; Knowledge: Personal safety; Knowledge: Medication

INTERVENTIONS. Bleeding precautions; Bleeding reduction; Fall prevention; Environmental management; Health education; Surveillance; Medication management

PLANNING AND IMPLEMENTATION

Collaborative

Treatment for ITP is primarily pharmacologic. Because the risk of hemorrhage occurs early in the course of acute ITP, therapy is focused on a rapid, sustained elevation in platelet counts. Children with active bleeding or a risk of cerebral hemorrhage may be treated with platelet transfusion, high-dose steroids, and IV immunoglobulin infusion. Children with non-life-threatening disease are not generally given transfused platelets because the antiplatelet antibody found in their serum is directed against both autologous and transfused platelets. They are likely monitored at home, observed for changes, and followed up frequently.

Adults with platelet counts above 50,000/mm^3 do not need treatment. If the patient fails to respond within 1 to 4 months or needs a high steroid dosage, splenectomy is usually considered. Splenectomy is effective because the spleen is a major site of antibody production and platelet destruction; research suggests that splenectomy is successful 85% of the time. In the face of life-threatening bleeding, such as intracranial or massive GI hemorrhages, a splenectomy is indicated.

Pharmacologic Highlights

Medication or Drug Class	Dosage	Description	Rationale
IV immune globulin; IV anti-(Rh)D (IV RhIG)	1 g/kg IV qd for 2 days	Immune serum	Increases antibody titer and antigen-antibody reaction; provides passive immunity against infection and induces rapid but short-term increases in platelet count
Glucocorticoids	Varies with drug	Prednisone 1–2 mg/kg PO daily; methyl-prednisolone 1–2 g IV for 3 days	Decrease inflammatory response; glucocorticoids are highly controversial therapy for children. Chronic ITP requires a slow steroid taper over several months.

Other Therapy: Alternative treatments include immunosuppression agents such as cyclophosphamide (Cytoxan) and vincristine sulfate. Plasmapheresis has been attempted with limited success. Eltrombopag (Promacta; a molecular agonist of a thrombopoietin receptor) and romiplostim (Nplate; fusion protein analogue of thrombopoietin) have been used in children older than 1 year of age with low blood platelets associated with chronic ITP when other medications have failed to work. Serious side effects have been reported, and the child should be monitored closely.

Independent

Many children are managed as outpatients with frequent outpatient visits for therapeutics and platelet counts. If the platelet count is less than 15,000/mm^3 and the child has bleeding symptoms, the condition may be considered serious enough to warrant hospitalization. Institute safety precautions to prevent injury and the resultant bleeding and to assist with ambulation. Protect areas of hematoma, petechiae, and ecchymoses from further injury. Avoid intramuscular injections, but if they are essential, apply pressure for at least 10 minutes after the intramuscular injection and for 20 minutes after venipuncture. Avoid nasotracheal suctioning, if possible, to prevent bleeding. If a child is being managed as an outpatient, discuss the home environment with the parents or caregivers. Encourage the parents to set up one or two rooms at home (e.g., the child's bedroom and the family room) as a protected environment. Pad all hard surfaces and corners with pillows and blankets and remove obstructions, furniture, and loose rugs.

Teach the patient and significant others about the nature of this disorder and necessary self-assessments and self-care activities. Teach the patient to report any signs of petechiae and ecchymoses formation, bruising, bleeding gums, and other signs of frank bleeding. Encourage the patient to stand unclothed in front of a mirror once a day to check for areas of bruising. Headaches and any change in level of consciousness may indicate cerebral bleeding and need to be reported to the healthcare worker immediately. Teach the signs and symptoms of blood loss, such as pallor or fatigue. Demonstrate correct mouth care for the patient and significant others by using a soft toothbrush to avoid mouth injury. Recommend electric shavers. Teach the patient to use care when taking a rectal temperature to prevent rectal perforation. Recommend care when clipping fingernails or toenails. If any bleeding does occur, instruct the patient to apply pressure to the area for up to 15 minutes or to seek help. Teach the patient to avoid aspirin, ibuprofen in any form, and other drugs that impair coagulation, with particular attention to over-the-counter remedies.

Provide a private, quiet environment to discuss the patient's or parents' concerns. The period of diagnosis is an anxious one, and parents need a great deal of emotional support. If the child is managed at home, parents need an opportunity to express their fears.

Evidence-Based Practice and Health Policy

Grace, R., Shimano, K., Bhat, R., Neunert, C., Bussel, J., Klaassen, R., Lambert, M., Rothman, J., Breakey, V., Hege, K., Bennett, C., Rose, M., Haley, K., Buchanan, G., Geddis, A., Lorenzana, A., Jeng, M., Pastore, Y., Crary, S., . . . Despotovic, J. (2019). Second-line in children with immune thrombocytopenia: Effect on platelet count and patient-centered outcomes. *American Journal of Hematology*, 94, 741–750.

- This longitudinal observational cohort study included 120 children, 1 to 17 years of age, with ITP who required second-line treatments including IV immunoglobulin (rituximab), romiplostim (fusion protein analog of thrombopoietin), corticosteroids, or anti-D immunoglobulin as a result of any of the following variables: bleeding risk, fatigue, activity restrictions, and poor quality of life. The outcomes measured included bleeding response, rescue medication, and platelet response.
- Only patients on romiplostim and rituximab had a significant reduction in both skin-related and non-skin-related bleeding symptoms after 1 month of treatment. The authors recommended that healthcare providers should take a patient-centered approach when considering treatment plans to select the best optimal second-line treatment for the child with recurrent bleeding.

DOCUMENTATION GUIDELINES

- Physical findings of skin and mucous membranes: Presence of petechiae, ecchymoses, blood blisters, hematoma, bleeding from the gums or nose
- Reaction to rest and activity, parents' response to the diagnosis and their child's well-being
- Presence of complications: Bleeding, petechiae, ecchymoses, headache, increased bruising

DISCHARGE AND HOME HEALTHCARE GUIDELINES

To prevent bleeding episodes, the patient should avoid both physical activity that may lead to injury and medications that have anticoagulant properties. Instruct the patient or caregiver when to notify the physician and how to monitor for bleeding in the stool, urine, and sputum. Remind the patient or caregiver to notify any medical personnel of bleeding tendencies. If the patient is a school-age child, encourage the parents to notify the school of the diagnosis, treatment, and complications. Check with the medical staff about the child's activities, including playground play and sports activities. These activities will likely be curtailed.

Explain all discharge medications, including dosage, route, action, adverse effects, and need for routine laboratory monitoring. If the patient is being discharged on a tapering corticosteroid dosage, be sure the patient or caregiver understands the schedule. If the patient had a central line placed for IV therapy, be sure the patient or caregiver has been properly trained in care, dressing changes, and sterile techniques. Teach the patient that antacids and oral drugs taken with meals can reduce gastric irritation. Weight gain, anxiety, and mood alterations are frequent side effects of steroid therapy. Parents and families need to be encouraged to lift activity restrictions when the child's platelet count returns to a safe range.

Infective Endocarditis

DRG Category:	216
Mean LOS:	15.9 days
Description:	SURGICAL: Cardiac Valve and Other Major Cardiothoracic Procedures With Cardiac Catheterization With Major Complication or Comorbidity
DRG Category:	218
Mean LOS:	6.7 days
Description:	SURGICAL: Cardiac Valve and Other Major Cardiothoracic Procedures With Cardiac Catheterization Without Complication or Comorbidity or Major Complication or Comorbidity
DRG Category:	219
Mean LOS:	10.9 days
Description:	SURGICAL: Cardiac Valve and Other Major Cardiothoracic Procedures Without Cardiac Catheterization With Major Complication or Comorbidity
DRG Category:	221
Mean LOS:	4.7 days
Description:	SURGICAL: Cardiac Valve and Other Major Cardiothoracic Procedures Without Cardiac Catheterization Without Complication or Comorbidity or Major Complication or Comorbidity
DRG Category:	307
Mean LOS:	3.1 days
Description:	MEDICAL: Cardiac Congenital and Valvular Disorders Without Major Complication or Comorbidity

Infective endocarditis (IE) is an inflammatory process of the endocardial lining of the heart. It typically affects a deformed or previously damaged valve, which is usually the focus of the infection, or a septal defect. Typically, endocarditis occurs when an invading organism enters the bloodstream and attaches to a sterile fibrin clot already present on the leaflets of the valves or the endocardium. The bacteria "innoculate" the clot, multiply, and form a projection of tissue that includes bacteria, fibrin, red blood cells, and white blood cells on the valves of the heart including the valve leaflets. This clump of material, called *vegetation*, may eventually cover the entire valve surface, leading to ulceration and tissue necrosis. Vegetation may even extend to the chordae tendineae, causing them to rupture and the valve to become incompetent. Approximately 10% to 20% of the infections occur with prosthetic valves. Most commonly, the mitral or aortic valve is involved. The tricuspid valve is mainly involved in IV drug abusers but is otherwise rarely infected. Infections of the pulmonary valve are rare.

IE can occur as an acute or a subacute condition. Generally, acute IE is a rapidly progressing infection, whereas subacute IE progresses more slowly. Acute endocarditis usually occurs on a normal heart valve and is rapidly destructive and fatal in 6 weeks if it is left untreated. Subacute endocarditis usually occurs in a heart already damaged by congenital or acquired heart disease on damaged valves and takes up to a year to cause death if it is left untreated. Complications include thromboembolic phenomenon such as stroke, myocardial infarction, cardiac valvular insufficiency, heart failure, sepsis, myocardial abscesses, arthritis, and myositis.

CAUSES

Since the 1960s, the most common causes of IE have been nosocomial infections from IV catheters, IV drug abuse, and prosthetic valve endocarditis. IVs become infected at the insertion site, on the catheter itself, from another site in the body, or from the IV infusate. IE can result from injected drug use and abuse as well.

The etiology of acute IE is predominantly bacterial. The two most common causes of bacterial endocarditis are staphylococcal and streptococcal infections (Box 1), and *Staphylococcus aureus* is the primary pathogen of endocarditis. Subacute IE occurs in people with acquired cardiac lesions. Possible ports of entry for the infecting organism include lesions or abscesses of the skin and genitourinary (GU) or gastrointestinal (GI) infections. Surgical or invasive procedures such as tooth extraction, tonsillectomy, bronchoscopy, endoscopy, colonoscopy, cystoscopy, transesophageal echocardiography, and prosthetic valve replacement also place the patient at risk.

• BOX 1 Conditions Predisposing to Endocarditis

- Rheumatic heart disease
- Congenital heart disease (CHD; patent ductus arteriosus, ventricular septal defect, bicuspid aortic valve, Fallot tetralogy)
- Prosthetic valve surgery
- Parenteral drug abuse
- Placement of intravascular foreign bodies (IV catheters, dialysis shunts, pacemakers, hyperalimentation catheters)
- Mitral valve prolapse
- Asymmetric septal hypertrophy
- Marfan syndrome
- Previous episodes of endocarditis
- Skin, bone, and pulmonary infections

GENETIC CONSIDERATIONS

Heritable immune responses could be protective or increase susceptibility.

SEX AND LIFE SPAN CONSIDERATIONS

The incidence of IE in infancy and childhood is low. Nearly all children infected have an identifiable predisposing lesion. Men over age 45 years are at highest risk, as males are affected three times more than females. More than half the cases occur in people older than age 60 years.

HEALTH DISPARITIES AND SEXUAL/GENDER MINORITY HEALTH

Ethnicity, race, and sexual/gender minority status have no known effect on the risk for IE.

GLOBAL HEALTH CONSIDERATIONS

The incidence of IE in the United States, Western Europe, and other developed regions is approximately 13 cases per 100,000 persons per year. Less is known about the incidence in developing countries, but because many of their healthcare systems are underresourced and medical procedures are less frequent, rates of IE are likely lower than in developed countries.

☀ ASSESSMENT

HISTORY. Discuss with the patient symptoms, such as anorexia and weight loss, fever and chills, malaise, headache, muscle and joint aches, shortness of breath, and cough. Ask the patient for a history of medical, surgical, and dental procedures during the past 5 years. A common finding of patients with preexisting cardiac abnormalities is a recent history (3 to 6 months) of dental procedures. Question the patient about the type of procedure performed and whether bleeding of the gums occurred. Ask the patient for a history of alcohol and drug use, particularly IV drug use.

Patients with IE may have complaints of continuous fever (103°F to 104°F [39.3°C to 40°C]) in acute IE, whereas in the subacute form, temperatures are generally in the range of 99°F to 102°F (37.2°C to 38.9°C). Patients with subacute IE may describe variable and vague symptoms, such as anorexia, weight loss, malaise, and headache.

PHYSICAL EXAMINATION. The patient appears **acutely ill**. Observe for signs of **temperature elevation**, such as **warm skin, dry mucous membranes,** and **alternating chills and diaphoresis**. Determine if the patient has symptoms of heart failure such as lung congestion and peripheral swelling. Inspect the conjunctivae, upper extremities, and mucous membranes of the mouth for the presence of petechiae, splinter hemorrhages in nailbeds, Osler nodes (painful red nodes on pads of fingers and toes), and joint tenderness. Some patients may have neurological symptoms from an embolic stroke due to clots from the valvular vegetation. Check whether drug track marks are apparent on the patient's skin. Palpate the abdomen for splenomegaly, which is present in approximately 30% of patients with IE. Auscultate the heart for the presence of tachycardia and murmurs. Approximately 95% of those with subacute IE have a heart murmur (most commonly mitral and aortic regurgitation murmurs), which is typically absent in patients with acute IE.

PSYCHOSOCIAL. Lengthy interventions, such as prophylactic antibiotic treatment, are generally required. Therefore, determine the patient's ability to understand the disease, as well as to comply with prescribed long-term treatments. If the patient acknowledges IV drug abuse, refer the patient to a substance use counselor or program.

Diagnostic Highlights

General Comments: There are no specific serum laboratory tests or diagnostic procedures that conclusively identify IE, although some are highly suggestive of its presence. Special cultures or serologic tests may detect nonbacterial IE.

(highlight box continues on page 666)

Diagnostic Highlights (continued)

Test	Normal Result	Abnormality With Condition	Explanation
Blood cultures and sensitivities (three to five sets of cultures over a 24-hr period)	Negative	Positive for microorganisms in 90% of patients but a high (50%) false-positive rate; continuous bacteremia for more than 30 min documented on blood cultures	If patients have been on antibiotics, they are less likely to have positive cultures; three sets of blood culture should be taken from separate sites over at least a 1-hr period before antibiotics are begun

Other Tests: Tests include complete blood count, computed tomography, M-mode and two-dimensional echocardiography, transesophageal echocardiogram, transthoracic echocardiogram, two-dimensional cardiac ultrasound Doppler, electrocardiogram, and rheumatoid factor.

PRIMARY NURSING DIAGNOSIS

DIAGNOSIS. Risk for infection as evidenced by fever, tachycardia, chills, and/or diaphoresis

OUTCOMES. Infection severity; Immune status; Knowledge: Infection management; Risk control; Risk detection; Knowledge: Medication

INTERVENTIONS. Infection control; Infection protection; Medication management; Teaching: Prescribed medication

PLANNING AND IMPLEMENTATION

Collaborative

Antibiotics are the mainstay of the treatment for IE. Antibiotics are chosen depending on the infecting organisms and are traditionally given intravenously for 4 to 6 weeks. Some physicians are prescribing oral step-down antibiotics after 3 weeks of IV antibiotics rather than the longer IV course (Spellberg et al., 2020 [see Evidence-Based Practice and Health Policy]). For persons at high risk for contracting IE, most physicians prescribe antibiotic therapy to prevent episodes of bacteremia before, during, and after invasive procedures. Procedures that are particularly associated with endocarditis are manipulation of the teeth and gums or GU and GI systems and surgical procedures or biopsies that involve respiratory mucosa.

Supportive treatment with oxygen, treatment of congestive heart failure, or management of acute renal failure with dialysis may be necessary. If the patient has developed endocarditis as a result of IV drug abuse, an addiction consultation is essential, with a possible referral to an appropriate treatment program. Surgical replacement of the infected valve is needed in those patients who have an infecting microorganism that does not respond to available antibiotic therapy and for patients who have developed infectious endocarditis in a prosthetic heart valve. (See **Coronary Heart Disease** for a full discussion of the collaborative and independent management of a patient following open heart surgery.)

Pharmacologic Highlights

Medication or Drug Class	Dosage	Description	Rationale
Penicillin G	2 million units IV daily 4 hr for 4 wk	Antibiotic	Treats penicillin-susceptible streptococcal infections in subacute bacterial endocarditis; patients who are allergic to penicillin may receive vancomycin

Pharmacologic Highlights (continued)

Medication or Drug Class	Dosage	Description	Rationale
Oxacillin; ceftriaxone, gentamicin, vancomycin, or tobramycin; cefazolin	Varies with drug	Antibiotic	Treats acute bacterial endocarditis; S aureus and gram-negative bacilli are the most likely bacteria
Acetaminophen (Tylenol)	650 mg as needed daily 4–6 hr	Nonnarcotic analgesic; antipyretic	Relieves joint and muscle achiness; controls fever

Other Drugs: Ceftriaxone at 2 g/day IV for 4 weeks; may also be given intramuscularly if problems occur with venous access and can be given once a day as an outpatient if the patient is stable. Other antibiotics are cefepime and nafcillin.

Independent

During the acute phase of the disease, provide adequate rest by assisting the patient with daily hygiene. Use strategies to increase the patient's comfort during the acute phase of the illness, during which symptoms such as fever, diaphoresis, and shortness of breath are uncomfortable. Space all nursing care activities and diagnostic tests to provide the patient with adequate rest. During the first few days of hospital admission, encourage the family to limit visitation.

Emphasize patient education. Individualize a standardized plan of care and adapt it to meet the patient's needs. Areas for discussion include the cause of the disease and its course, medication regimens, technique for administering IV antibiotics, and practices that help avoid and identify future infections.

If the patient is to continue parenteral antibiotic therapy at home, make sure that before the patient is discharged from the hospital, the patient has all the appropriate equipment and supplies that will be needed. Make a referral to a home health nurse as needed, and provide the patient and family with a list of information that describes when to notify the primary healthcare provider about complications.

Evidence-Based Practice and Health Policy

Spellberg, B., Chambers, H., Musher, D., Walsh, T., & Bayer, A. (2020). Evaluation of a paradigm shift from intravenous antibiotics to oral step-down therapy for the treatment of infective endocarditis: A narrative review. *JAMA Internal Medicine, 180,* 769–777.

- While prolonged IV antibiotic courses have long been used to treat IE, they are associated with high rates of adverse events. Recent studies have shown that oral step-down antibiotic treatment may be an alternative. The authors reviewed electronic databases to determine whether evidence supports the notion that oral step-down antibiotic therapy for IE is associated with inferior outcomes compared with IV-only therapy. They found 21 observational studies evaluating oral antibiotics for treating IE, typically after an initial course of IV therapy.
- None of the observational studies found oral step-down therapy to be inferior to IV-only therapy. Three randomized clinical trials also demonstrated that oral step-down antibiotic therapy is at least as effective as IV-only therapy in IE. In the largest trial, patients who received oral step-down antibiotic therapy had a significantly improved cure rate and reduced mortality rate compared with those who received only IV antibiotic therapy.

DOCUMENTATION GUIDELINES

- Observations and physical findings regarding level of consciousness, degree of abdominal or chest pain, skin temperature, and color; presence of petechiae, splinter hemorrhages, Osler nodes, joint tenderness, abnormal vital signs, dyspnea, cough, and crackles or wheezing
- Presence and characteristics of heart murmurs, vital signs

• Response to antibiotic therapy and antipyretics
• Presence of complications: Signs of right- or left-sided heart failure, arterial embolization

DISCHARGE AND HOME HEALTHCARE GUIDELINES

To prevent IE, provide patients in the high-risk category with the needed information for early detection and prevention of the disease. Instruct recovering patients to inform their healthcare providers, including dentists, of their endocarditis history because they may need future prophylactic antibiotic therapy to prevent subsequent episodes.

Be sure the patient understands all medications, including the dosage, route, action, and adverse effects. Make sure the patient understands the need to complete the course of antibiotic therapy. Explain the side effects that may occur during antibiotic administration (GI distress, yeast infection, sun sensitivity, skin rash). Encourage the patient to seek prompt medical attention if side effects occur. Make sure the patient or significant others can demonstrate the appropriate method of antibiotic administration. Instruct the patient on proper IV catheter site care as well as the signs of infiltration. Encourage good oral hygiene and advise the patient to use a soft toothbrush and to brush at least twice a day. Teach patients to avoid irrigation devices and flossing. Teach the patient to monitor and record temperature daily at the same time. Encourage the patient to take antipyretics according to physician orders. Instruct the patient to report signs of heart failure and embolization as well as continued fever, chills, fatigue, malaise, or weight loss.

Influenza

DRG Category:	152
Mean LOS:	4.0 days
Description:	MEDICAL: Otitis Media and Upper Respiratory Infection With Major Complication or Comorbidity

Influenza (flu) is an acute, highly contagious viral respiratory infection caused by one of three types of myxovirus influenzae. Influenza occurs all over the world and in the Northern Hemisphere begins in early fall, peaks in February, and ends in the late spring. The incubation period is 24 to 48 hours. Symptoms appear approximately 72 hours after contact with the virus, and the infected person remains contagious for 3 days.

Influenza is usually a self-limited disease that lasts from 2 to 7 days. The disease also spreads rapidly through populations, creating epidemics and pandemics. In the United States, the Centers for Disease Control and Prevention (CDC) estimate deaths associated with seasonal influenza. However, because individual states have a variety of reporting mechanisms and some do not report seasonal influenza in adults, the exact figure is unknown. In 2018 the CDC reported that in the past 8 years, the range of deaths per year was a low of 12,000 and a high of 56,000. Complications of influenza include pneumonia, myositis, exacerbation of chronic obstructive pulmonary disease, and Reye syndrome. In rare cases, influenza can lead to encephalitis, transverse myelitis, myocarditis, or pericarditis.

CAUSES

Influenzavirus A causes the most serious epidemics. Influenzavirus B produces milder respiratory infections. Influenzavirus C causes mild respiratory infections like the common cold. Infection with a specific strain of virus produces immunity only to that specific virus strain.

Therefore, each year an influenza vaccine is developed to provide immunity against influenza virus strains that are projected to be prevalent for that season. Older persons, those with chronic diseases, and healthcare workers are advised to get influenza vaccinations annually in October or November in the Northern Hemisphere. In tropical areas of the world, influenza occurs year-round, whereas in the Northern Hemisphere, it peaks in February. Influenzavirus A strains are classified by two proteins found on the surface of all influenzavirus A strains: hemagglutinin (H) and neuraminidase (N). The structures of these proteins vary from strain to strain.

GENETIC CONSIDERATIONS

Heritable immune responses could be protective or increase susceptibility.

SEX AND LIFE SPAN CONSIDERATIONS

All people are susceptible to influenza. The incidence of influenza cases is highest in school-age children and generally decreases with age, probably because of immunity established by repeated infections as people age. During an outbreak of the disease, however, older persons and those disabled by chronic illnesses are most likely to develop severe complications. During the third trimester of pregnancy, women are at high risk for complications of influenza A and B.

HEALTH DISPARITIES AND SEXUAL/GENDER MINORITY HEALTH

Ethnicity, race, and sexual/gender minority status have no known effect on the risk for influenza.

GLOBAL HEALTH CONSIDERATIONS

Influenza occurs around the world and during all seasons depending on the location and season. Globally it causes up to 5 million cases of severe illness and 500,000 deaths. In addition to the novel coronavirus 2019 disease (COVID-19), recent global epidemics included avian influenza (H5N1; H7N2) and swine flu (H1N1). Cases of avian influenza occur most commonly in eastern Asia, Eastern Europe, the Middle East, and Northern Africa.

ASSESSMENT

HISTORY. Determine if the patient has had contact with an infected person within the past 72 hours. Ask whether vaccination occurred in the current year. Establish a history of fever and chills, hoarseness, laryngitis, sore throat, rhinitis, or rhinorrhea. Elicit a history of myalgia (particularly in the back and limbs), fatigue, anorexia, malaise, headache, or photophobia. Ask if the patient has a nonproductive cough; in children, the cough is likely to be croupy. Determine if the patient has experienced gastrointestinal symptoms, such as vomiting and diarrhea.

PHYSICAL EXAMINATION. Common symptoms include **cough, fever, sore throat, headache,** and **muscle ache**. The patient usually appears ill and fatigued. Observe the patient for a flushed face and conjunctivitis. When you inspect the patient's throat, you may note redness of the soft palate, tonsils, and pharynx. Palpate for enlargement of the anterior cervical lymph nodes. The patient's temperature usually ranges from 102°F to 103°F (38.9°C to 39.4°C) and often rises suddenly on the first day before falling and rising again on the third day of illness. Patients are often tachycardic, and their skin is warm. Auscultate the lungs if influenza has produced respiratory complications such as tachypnea, rhonchi, rales, or focal wheezing. Some patients will experience nausea, vomiting, and diarrhea.

PSYCHOSOCIAL. Patients who feel very ill and are unable to continue with normal activities should be assured that the illness is self-limiting and that improvement occurs with rest and time. They may describe weakness and the need for additional sleep. Arrangements need to be made for time off from work while the patient is contagious and recovers.

Diagnostic Highlights

General Comments: No specific diagnostic tests are used because diagnosis is made by the history of symptoms and onset. If the patient has symptoms of a bacterial infection that complicates influenza, cultures and sensitivities, and complete blood count may be required. Rapid influenza diagnostic tests have better sensitivity in children (67%) than adults (54%) and may be used in primary care providers' offices to detect the virus with a result in 30 minutes. Viral culture and reverse transcription-polymerase chain reaction testing may be used in some situations. Chest radiography may be used for people with pulmonary complications.

PRIMARY NURSING DIAGNOSIS

DIAGNOSIS. Risk for infection as evidenced by fever, sore throat, headache, and/or muscle ache

OUTCOMES. Infection severity; Immune status; Symptom severity; Knowledge: Infection management; Fluid balance; Risk control; Risk detection; Knowledge: Medication

INTERVENTIONS. Infection control; Infection protection; Fluid management; Medication management; Temperature regulation

PLANNING AND IMPLEMENTATION

Collaborative

Prevention with annual influenza vaccination is the most effective collaborative strategy for influenza. Medical treatment does not cure influenza but is aimed at controlling the symptoms and preventing complications. Bedrest and increased intake of fluids are prescribed for patients in the acute stage of infection. Hospitalization occurs most often when influenza exacerbates an underlying chronic condition. For seriously ill people, supplemental oxygen, mechanical ventilation, and IV replacement of fluid and electrolytes may be necessary. For persons who are not immunized but are exposed to the virus, amantadine may prevent active infection. Amantadine or other antiviral medications may be used for outbreaks of influenza A within a closed population, such as a nursing home.

Pharmacologic Highlights

General Comments: Phenylephrine and antitussive agents such as terpin hydrate with codeine are often prescribed to relieve nasal congestion and coughing. In patients with influenza that is complicated by pneumonia, antibiotics may be administered to treat a bacterial superinfection.

Medication or Drug Class	Dosage	Description	Rationale
Oseltamivir (Tamiflu)	75 mg PO for at least 10 days	Antiviral	Initiate within 48 hr of exposure, for prophylaxis and treatment of flu
Acetaminophen	500–1,000 mg PO	Antipyretics	Control fever and discomfort
Amantadine	100–200 mg PO daily, bid for several days	Antiviral infective	Provides antiviral action against influenza (prophylaxis and symptomatic); usually prescribed for outbreaks of influenza A within a closed population, such as a nursing home

> **Pharmacologic Highlights** (continued)
>
> Other Drugs: Neuraminidase inhibitors (oseltamivir and zanamivir) for use in treatment and prophylaxis of influenza A and B; rimantadine for treatment and prophylaxis of influenza A only; other antivirals include peramivir, baloxavir marboxil; antiviral treatment should be initiated within 48 hours of the onset of symptoms to be effective.

Independent

The most important nursing intervention is prevention. Encourage all patients over age 65 years or those with chronic conditions to receive annual influenza vaccinations. The vaccination becomes effective approximately 2 weeks after it is given. Teach the patient about potential side effects of vaccination, such as fever; malaise; discomfort at the injection site; and, in rare instances, Guillain-Barré syndrome. Note that influenza vaccine is not recommended for pregnant women unless they are highly susceptible to influenza.

Instruct patients and families to cover their mouths and noses when coughing, to dispose of used tissues appropriately, and to wash their hands after patient contact to prevent the virus from spreading. Teach people to cough and sneeze into their sleeves rather than their hands. Limit visitors when necessary. Encourage a fluid intake of 3,000 mL/day for adults. Explain that warm baths or the use of a heating pad may relieve myalgia. Provide cool, humidified air; maintain bedrest; and monitor vital signs to detect any change in the rhythm or quality of respirations. Encourage patients to get as much rest and sleep as possible.

Evidence-Based Practice and Health Policy

Ward, B., Makarkov, A., Séguin, A., Pillet, S., Trépanier, S., Dhaliwall, J., Libman, M., Vesikari, T., & Landry, N. (2020). Efficacy, immunogenicity, and safety of a plant-derived, quadrivalent, virus-like particle influenza vaccine in adults (18–64 years) and older adults (≥65 years): Two multicentre, randomised phase 3 trials. *The Lancet*, 396, 1491–1503.

- The authors aimed to explore plant-based manufacturing of influenza vaccines to determine if they might address the limitations of current egg-derived and other vaccines. They conducted two randomized studies with people age 8 to 64 years old and people 65 years and older. In the younger group, healthy subjects received either recombinant quadrivalent virus-like particle (QVLP) vaccine or placebo. In the older group, healthy subjects received either QVLP vaccine or quadrivalent inactivated vaccine (QIV).
- The study did not meet its primary endpoint of 70% absolute vaccine efficacy for the QVLP vaccine against respiratory illness caused by matched strains. The efficacy studies showed that the plant-derived vaccine can provide substantial (approximately 40% efficacy) protection against influenza illnesses in adults. The plant-derived vaccine was tolerated well by the participants, and no safety concerns were raised by the side effects.

DOCUMENTATION GUIDELINES

- Physical findings: Elevated temperature; erythema of pharynx; enlarged lymph nodes; change in skin color, amount and characteristics of sputum, fluid intake and output; level of hydration
- Presence of chest pain or difficulty in breathing
- Response to bedrest; complications of bedrest; tolerance to activity
- Response to patient teaching regarding immunization, hand washing, and disposal of infected articles

DISCHARGE AND HOME HEALTHCARE GUIDELINES

PREVENTION. To prevent complications, emphasize to the patient the need to maintain bedrest and high fluid intake for 2 to 3 days after the temperature returns to normal.

MEDICATIONS. Instruct the patient and family about the dosage, route, action, and side effects of all medications.

COMPLICATIONS. Instruct the patient and family to report any chest pain, ear pain, or change in respirations to the physician.

Inguinal Hernia

DRG Category:	394
Mean LOS:	3.8 days
Description:	MEDICAL: Other Digestive System Diagnoses With Complication or Comorbidity
DRG Category:	352
Mean LOS:	2.5 days
Description:	SURGICAL: Inguinal and Femoral Hernia Procedures Without Complication or Comorbidity or Major Complication or Comorbidity

A hernia is a protrusion or projection of an organ or organ part through the wall of the cavity that normally contains it. An inguinal hernia occurs when either the omentum, the large or small intestine, or the bladder protrudes into the inguinal canal, passages in the anterior abdominal wall on each side of the midline. In an indirect inguinal hernia, the sac protrudes through the internal inguinal ring into the inguinal canal and, in males, may descend into the scrotum. In a direct inguinal hernia, the hernial sac projects through a weakness in the abdominal wall in the area of the rectus abdominal muscle and inguinal ligament.

Inguinal hernias make up approximately 80% of all hernias, and they occur in approximately 15% of the adult population. Repair of this defect is one of the most frequently performed procedures by both pediatric and adult surgeons. Hernias are classified into three types: reducible, which can be easily manipulated back into place manually; irreducible or incarcerated, which usually cannot be reduced manually because adhesions form in the hernial sac; and strangulated, in which part of the herniated intestine becomes twisted or edematous. Complications include pressure on surrounding tissues leading to pain and swelling, obstruction, necrosis, and sepsis.

CAUSES

An inguinal hernia is the result of either a congenital weakening of the abdominal wall (when the processus vaginalis fails to atrophy and close) or weakened abdominal muscles because of pregnancy, excess weight, or previous abdominal surgeries. In addition, if intra-abdominal pressure builds up, such as related to heavy lifting or straining to defecate, a hernia may occur. Other causes include aging and trauma. Risk factors include being male, White, and older; family history; previous hernia repair; chronic cough or constipation; pregnancy; and prematurity.

GENETIC CONSIDERATIONS

There may be a genetic contribution to inguinal hernia development and reoccurrence. While patterns of transmission are unclear, autosomal dominant inheritance with incomplete penetrance and sex influence has been suggested.

SEX AND LIFE SPAN CONSIDERATIONS

A hernia may be detected in both children and adults. Low-birth-weight infants and male infants are at higher risk (8:1) for this defect than female infants or full-term infants. Indirect hernias can develop at any age and are 25 times more common in males than in females. Nearly 90% of all inguinal hernia repairs are performed on males. Approximately 2% of females have an inguinal hernia in their lifetime.

HEALTH DISPARITIES AND SEXUAL/GENDER MINORITY HEALTH

Umbilical hernias are more common in Black infants than in infants of other groups. Disparities exist with the availability of inguinal repair because they are less likely to occur for Medicaid patients as compared to people with private insurance or Medicare. Patients older than 65 years and women are less likely to receive minimally invasive inguinal hernia repair than younger patients. Black patients are more likely to receive emergency surgery than elective surgery and have poorer outcomes than other groups, possibly indicating that routine healthcare and follow-up are less available to Black patients. Sexual and gender minority status has no known effect on the risk for inguinal hernia.

GLOBAL HEALTH CONSIDERATIONS

While little is known about the prevalence of inguinal hernias in developing countries, most experts suspect that factors related to anatomy and sex are similar in developing and developed regions of the world.

ASSESSMENT

HISTORY. Infants or children may be relatively symptom free until they cry, cough, or strain to defecate, at which time the parents note painless swelling in the inguinal area. The adult patient may complain of pain or a sense of fullness, or may report bruising in the area of a hernia after a period of exercise. More commonly, the patient complains of a slight bulge along the inguinal area, which is especially apparent when the patient coughs or strains. The swelling may subside on its own when the patient assumes a recumbent position or if slight manual pressure is applied externally to the area. Some patients describe a steady, aching pain that worsens with tension and improves with hernia reduction. People with an incarcerated hernia may describe more severe pain, nausea, vomiting, inability to defecate, and inability to manipulate the hernia.

PHYSICAL EXAMINATION. On inspection, the patient has a **visible swelling or bulge when asked to cough or bear down**. Another common symptom is **achiness radiating into the area of the hernia** but no pain or tenderness. If the hernia disappears when the patient lies down, the hernia is usually reducible. In addition, have the patient perform a Valsalva maneuver to inspect the hernia's size. Before palpation, auscultate the patient's bowel; absent bowel sounds suggest incarceration or strangulation.

You may be able to palpate a slight bulge or mass during this time and when the examiner slides the little finger 4 to 5 cm into the external canal located at the base of the scrotum. If you feel pressure against your fingertip when you have the patient cough, an indirect hernia may exist; if you feel pressure against the side of your finger, a direct hernia may exist. Palpate the scrotum to determine if either a hydrocele or cryptorchidism (undescended testes) is present. Signs of an incarcerated (irreducible hernia that cannot be returned to the abdominal cavity when pushed) hernia include painful engorgement, nausea, vomiting, and abdominal distention.

PSYCHOSOCIAL. A delay in seeking healthcare may result in strangulation of the intestines and require emergency surgery. In the adult population, surgical intervention to correct the defect takes the patient away from home and the work setting and causes anxiety. Parents of infants requiring surgery will be upset and worried about their child.

Diagnostic Highlights

> **General Comments:** No specific laboratory tests are useful for the diagnosis of an inguinal hernia. Diagnosis is made on the basis of a physical examination. On rare occasions, computed tomography or ultrasound may be used in diagnosis depending on the patient's body build.

PRIMARY NURSING DIAGNOSIS

DIAGNOSIS. Acute pain related to swelling and pressure as evidenced by self-reports of pain, facial grimacing, and/or protective behavior

OUTCOMES. Pain: Disruptive effects; Pain control; Knowledge: Pain management; Symptom severity; Knowledge: Disease process; Anxiety level

INTERVENTIONS. Analgesic administration; Pain management: Acute; Teaching: Disease process; Anxiety reduction

PLANNING AND IMPLEMENTATION

Collaborative

If the patient has a reducible hernia, the protrusion may be moved back into place and a truss for temporary relief can be applied. A truss is a thick pad with an attached belt that is placed over the hernia to keep it in place. Although a truss is palliative rather than curative, it can be used successfully in older or debilitated adult patients who are poor surgical risks or who do not desire surgery.

Collaboration with the surgical team is necessary to prepare the patient and family for surgery. A herniotomy is the removal of the hernial sac only. A herniorrhaphy is a herniotomy plus repair of the posterior wall of the inguinal canal. A hernioplasty is a herniotomy plus reinforcement of the posterior wall with a synthetic mesh. While open hernia repair is the most common approach, laparoscopic techniques are being used more frequently. These techniques reduce postoperative pain, time to recovery, and return to work, but the procedures are more expensive and take longer than other approaches. If the hernia is incarcerated, manual reduction may be attempted by putting the patient in Trendelenburg position with ice applied to the affected side. Manual pressure is applied to reduce the hernia. Surgery then may occur within 24 to 48 hours. The surgeon replaces hernial contents into the abdominal cavity and seals the opening in a herniorrhaphy procedure. A strangulated bowel requires immediate surgery to prevent peritonitis, bowel necrosis, sepsis, and shock.

IV fluids are administered to prevent dehydration, especially for the newborn who is prone to fluid shifts. The patient should be able to tolerate small oral feedings before discharge and should be able to urinate spontaneously. Postoperatively, inspect for signs and symptoms of possible peritonitis, manage nasogastric suction, and monitor the patient for the return of bowel sounds. As with any postoperative patient, monitor the patient for respiratory complications such as atelectasis or pneumonia; encourage the patient to use an incentive spirometer or assist the patient to turn, cough, and deep breathe every 2 hours.

Pharmacologic Highlights

Medication or Drug Class	Dosage	Description	Rationale
Antibiotics	Varies with drug	Broad-spectrum	Prevent infection postoperatively
Analgesics	Varies with drug	NSAIDs; narcotics	Relieve discomfort caused by hernial pressure or postoperatively

Independent

The nurse explains what to expect before, during, and after the surgery. Parents, especially those of a newborn, are anxious because their child requires general anesthesia for the procedure. If possible, use preoperative teaching tools such as pamphlets and videotapes to reinforce the information. Allow as much time as is needed to answer questions and explain procedures.

Instruct patients and parents on the care of the incision. Often, the incision is simply covered with collodion (a viscous liquid that, when applied, dries to form a thin transparent film) and should be kept clean and dry. Encourage patients to defer bathing and showering and instead to use sponge baths until they are seen by the surgeon at a follow-up visit. Explain how to monitor the incision for signs of infection. Infants or young children who are wearing diapers should have frequent diaper changes, or the diapers should be turned down from the incision so as not to contaminate the incision with urine. Teach the patient or parents about the possibility of some scrotal swelling or hematoma; both should subside over time.

If the patient does not have surgery, teach the signs of a strangulated or incarcerated hernia: severe pain, nausea, vomiting, diarrhea, high fever, and bloody stools. Explain that if these symptoms occur, the patient must notify the primary healthcare provider immediately. If patients use a truss, they should use it only after a hernia has been reduced. Assist the patient with the truss, preferably in the morning before the patient arises. Encourage the patient to bathe daily and to apply a thin film of powder or cornstarch to prevent skin irritation.

Evidence-Based Practice and Health Policy

Prabhu, A., Carbonell, A., Hope, W., Warren, J., Higgins, R., Jacob, B., Blatnik, J., Haskins, I., Alkhatib, H., Tastaldi, L., Fafaj, A., Tu, C., & Rosen, M. (2020). Robotic inguinal vs transabdominal laparoscopic inguinal hernia repair: The RIVAL randomized clinical trial. *JAMA Surgery, 155*, 1–8.

- The authors aimed to determine whether the robotic approach to inguinal hernia repair results in improved postoperative outcomes compared with traditional laparoscopic inguinal hernia repairs. They conducted a 3-year, multicenter prospective randomized clinical pilot study with a follow-up duration of 30 days ($N = 102$). Main outcomes included postoperative pain, health-related quality of life, mobility, and wound status. Two groups were formed (54 in the laparoscopic group, 48 in the robotic group).
- There were no differences at the preoperative, 1-week, or 30-day points between the groups in terms of wound events, readmissions, pain as measured by the Visual Analog Scale, or quality of life. Compared with traditional laparoscopic inguinal hernia repair, robotic transabdominal preperitoneal repair was associated with longer median operative times, higher cost, and higher frustration levels. Results of this study showed no clinical benefit to the robotic approach as compared to inguinal hernia repair with the laparoscopic approach.

DOCUMENTATION GUIDELINES

- Physical responses: Description of the hernia or incisional site, vital signs, gastrointestinal functioning, breath sounds
- Response to pain management; location, type, and duration of pain

DISCHARGE AND HOME HEALTHCARE GUIDELINES

Teach the patient signs and symptoms of infection: poor wound healing, wound drainage, continued incisional pain, incisional swelling and redness, cough, fever, and mucus production. Explain the importance of completion of all antibiotics. Explain the mechanism of action, side effects, and dosage recommendations of all analgesics. Caution the patient against lifting and straining. Explain that the patient can resume normal activities 2 to 4 weeks after surgery.

Intestinal Obstruction

DRG Category:	329
Mean LOS:	13.1 days
Description:	SURGICAL: Major Small and Large Bowel Procedures With Major Complication or Comorbidity
DRG Category:	389
Mean LOS:	4.0 days
Description:	MEDICAL: Gastrointestinal Obstruction With Complication or Comorbidity

Intestinal obstruction occurs when a blockage obstructs the normal flow of contents through the intestinal tract. Obstruction of the intestine causes the bowel to become vulnerable to ischemia. The intestinal mucosal barrier can be damaged, allowing intestinal bacteria to invade the intestinal wall and causing fluid exudation, which leads to hypovolemia and dehydration. About 7 L of fluid per day is secreted into the small intestine and stomach and is usually reabsorbed. During obstruction, however, fluid accumulates, causing abdominal distention and pressure on the mucosal wall, which can lead to peritonitis and perforation. Obstructions can be partial or complete. The most common type of intestinal obstruction is one of the small intestine from fibrous adhesions.

The patient's mortality risk depends on the type of lesion causing the small bowel obstruction (closed-loop or strangulated) and the time until diagnosis and treatment; when an early diagnosis is made, mortality is low, but if more than 75% of the small bowel is necrotic at the time of surgery, the mortality rate is 65%. Complications of intestinal obstruction include intestinal perforation, bacteremia, sepsis, intra-abdominal abscess, pneumonia from aspiration, dehydration, electrolyte disturbance, secondary infection, and metabolic alkalosis or acidosis. If it is left untreated, a complete intestinal obstruction can cause death within a few hours from hypovolemic or septic shock and vascular collapse.

CAUSES

The two major types of intestinal obstruction are mechanical and neurogenic (or nonmechanical). Mechanical obstruction of the bowel is caused by physical blockage of the intestine. Examples of mechanical obstruction include adhesions and strangulated hernias (usually associated with the small intestine), volvulus (twisting of the intestine) of the cecum or sigmoid, intussusception (telescoping of the bowel), strictures, fecal or barium impaction, carcinomas (usually associated with the large intestine), and foreign bodies such as gallstones and fruit pits. Neurogenic obstruction occurs primarily after manipulation of the bowel during surgery or with peritoneal irritation, pain of thoracolumbar origin, or intestinal ischemia. It is also caused by the effect of trauma or toxins on the nerves that regulate peristalsis, electrolyte imbalances, and neurogenic abnormalities such as spinal cord lesions.

GENETIC CONSIDERATIONS

No clear genetic contributions to susceptibility have been defined.

SEX AND LIFE SPAN CONSIDERATIONS

Intestinal obstructions can occur at any age and in all people, but they are more common in patients who have undergone major abdominal surgery or have congenital abnormalities of the bowel. When it occurs in a child, the obstruction is most likely to be an intussusception. Although small bowel obstructions in children are uncommon, the diagnosis should be considered for any child with persistent vomiting, abdominal distention, and abdominal pain; early diagnosis is critical because delayed diagnosis and treatment are associated with significant complications.

HEALTH DISPARITIES AND SEXUAL/GENDER MINORITY HEALTH

In a study using a national database of almost 600,000 cases of intestinal obstruction, Black, Medicaid, and Medicare patients who were managed operatively were more likely to have an operative delay of 5 or more days than other groups, indicating that health disparities in care likely exist (Jean et al., 2018). Ethnicity, race, and sexual/gender minority status have no known effect on the risk for intestinal obstruction.

GLOBAL HEALTH CONSIDERATIONS

While intestinal obstruction occurs around the world, no global data are available.

ASSESSMENT

HISTORY. Establish any predisposing factors: surgery, especially abdominal surgery; radiation therapy; gallstones; Crohn disease; diverticular disease; ulcerative colitis; or a family history of colorectal cancer. Ask if the patient has had hiccups, which is often a symptom of intestinal obstruction.

To establish the diagnosis of small bowel obstruction, ask about vomiting fecal contents, wavelike abdominal pain, or abdominal distention. Elicit a history of intense thirst, generalized malaise, or aching. A paralytic ileus usually causes a distended abdomen, with or without pain, but usually without cramping. To establish the diagnosis of large bowel obstruction, which has a slower onset of symptoms, ask about recent constipation with a history of spasmodic abdominal pain several days afterward. Establish a history of hypogastric pain and nausea. Ask if the patient has been vomiting. To establish neurogenic obstruction, ask about abdominal pain. Neurogenic obstruction characteristically produces diffuse abdominal discomfort rather than colicky pain. Establish a history of vomiting; ask the patient to describe the vomitus, which may consist of gastric and bile contents but rarely fecal contents.

PHYSICAL EXAMINATION. The most common symptoms are **abdominal pain and distention** and **vomiting**. Inspect the patient's abdomen for distention. Observe the patient's abdomen for signs of visible peristalsis or loops of large bowel. Measure the patient's abdominal girth every 4 hours to observe the progress of an obstruction. Auscultate the patient's abdomen for bowel sounds in all four quadrants; you may hear rushes or borborygmus (rumbling noises in the bowels). Always auscultate the abdomen for up to 5 minutes for bowel sounds before palpation. Lack of bowel sounds can indicate a paralytic ileus. High-pitched tingling sounds with rushes can indicate a mechanical obstruction. Palpate all four quadrants of the abdomen to determine areas of localized tenderness, guarding, and rebound tenderness.

Assess the patient for tachycardia, a narrowed pulse pressure, urine output less than 30 mL per hour, and delayed capillary blanching—all indicators of severe hypovolemia and impending shock. Assess for fever, which may indicate peritonitis. Inspect the patient's skin for loss of turgor and mucous membranes for dryness.

PSYCHOSOCIAL. The patient with an intestinal obstruction is acutely ill and may need emergency intervention. Assess the patient's level of anxiety and fear. Assess the patient's coping skills, support system, and the significant other's response to the illness. If the patient is a child, the family will have significant concerns about the emergency and surgical outcomes.

Diagnostic Highlights

Test	Normal Result	Abnormality With Condition	Explanation
Chest and abdominal x-ray, computed tomography (CT)	Normal abdominal structures	Distended loops of bowel; may have a ladder-like pattern with air-fluid levels	Identifies free air under the diaphragm if perforation has occurred or blockage of lumen of bowel with distal passage of fluid and air (partial) or complete obstruction; note that CT provides a more accurate and detailed image as compared to chest and abdominal x-rays

Other Tests: Complete blood count, serum electrolytes, blood urea nitrogen, coagulation studies, colonoscopy, sigmoidoscopy, abdominal ultrasound

PRIMARY NURSING DIAGNOSIS

DIAGNOSIS. Deficient fluid volume related to abnormal loss of gastrointestinal fluids as evidenced by thirst, dehydration, tachycardia, oliguria, and/or hypotension

OUTCOMES. Fluid balance; Hydration; Risk control: Dehydration; Vital signs; Knowledge: Disease process

INTERVENTIONS. Fluid management; Fluid monitoring; IV insertion and therapy; Venous access devices maintenance; Vital signs monitoring

☀ PLANNING AND IMPLEMENTATION

Collaborative

SURGICAL. Surgery is often indicated for a complete mechanical obstruction. The operative procedure varies with the location and type of obstruction. A strangulated bowel constitutes a surgical emergency as well as closed loop obstruction, volvulus, and bowel ischemia. A bowel resection may be necessary in some obstructions. A growing number of procedures can be handled with laparoscopic surgery, which may have shorter recovery time and reduced number of needed diagnostic procedures prior to laparoscopy.

Postoperative care includes monitoring the patient's cardiopulmonary response and identifying surgical complications. The highest priority is maintaining airway, breathing, and circulation. The patient may require temporary endotracheal intubation and mechanical ventilation to manage airway and breathing. The circulation usually needs support from parenteral fluids, and total parenteral nutrition may be prescribed if the patient has protein deficits. Electrolytes also need to be replaced. Care for the surgical site and notify the physician if you observe any signs of poor wound healing, bleeding, or infection. Antibiotics are generally given to cover both gram-negative aerobic and gram-negative anaerobic organisms.

MEDICAL. Medical management with IV fluids, electrolytes, and administration of blood or plasma may be required for patients whose obstruction is caused by infection or inflammation or by a partial obstruction. Insertion of a nasogastric (NG) tube, often ordered by the physician to rest and decompress the bowel, greatly decreases abdominal distention and patient discomfort.

Analgesic medication may be ordered after the cause of the obstruction is known, but it may be withheld until the diagnosis of intestinal obstruction is confirmed so as to not mask pain, which is an important clinical indicator. Explore nonpharmacologic methods of pain relief. The physician may order oxygen. Usually, until the patient is stabilized, the patient's condition precludes any oral intake.

Pharmacologic Highlights

Medication or Drug Class	Dosage	Description	Rationale
Antibiotics	Varies with drug	Broad-spectrum antibiotic coverage (clindamycin, metronidazole, cefoxitin, cefotetan, imipenem, and cilastatin)	May be prescribed when the obstruction is caused by an infectious process

Other Drugs: Analgesics

Independent

Patients with an intestinal obstruction are seriously ill and may require an emergency procedure to relieve the obstruction. They become hypovolemic very easily due to fluid shifts. Constant monitoring of vital signs, level of pain, and resulting symptoms is important. Focus on serial assessments and increasing the patient's comfort and monitoring for complications. Elevate the head of the bed to assist with patient ventilation. Position the patient in the Fowler or semi-Fowler position to ease respiratory discomfort from a distended abdomen. Reposition the patient frequently.

Instruct the patient about the need to take nothing by mouth. Frequent mouth care and lubrication of the mucous membranes can assist with patient comfort. Patient teaching should include the indications and function of the NG tube. Discuss care planning with the patient and the family.

Teach the causes, types, signs, and symptoms of intestinal obstruction. Explain the diagnostic tests and treatments, preparing the patient for the possibility of surgery. Explain surgical and postoperative procedures. Note the patient's and significant others' responses to emergency surgery if needed and provide additional support if the family or patient copes ineffectively.

Evidence-Based Practice and Health Policy

Sandy, N., Massabki, L., Goncalves, A., Ribeiro, A., Ribeiro, J., Servidoni, M., & Lomazi, E. (2020). Distal intestinal obstruction syndrome: A diagnostic and therapeutic challenge in cystic fibrosis. *Jornal de Pediatria, 96,* 732–740.

- The authors want to evaluate the demographics, genotype, and clinical presentation of pediatric patients with cystic fibrosis presenting with distal intestinal obstruction syndrome (DIOS) and factors associated with DIOS recurrence. They reviewed a series of 10 patients (median age 13.2 years) and analyzed age, gender, cystic fibrosis genotype, meconium ileus at birth, hydration status, pulmonary exacerbation, *Pseudomonas aeruginosa* colonization, pancreatic insufficiency (PI), body mass index, and clinical manifestations.
- All of the patients had two positive sweat chloride tests for cystic fibrosis, and nine of ten also had genotype study. In seven cases, a previous history of meconium ileus was reported. All patients had PI. Of the total number of episodes of DIOS, 85% were successfully managed with oral osmotic laxatives and/or rectal therapy (glycerin enema or saline irrigation). Ten patients had recurrence.

DOCUMENTATION GUIDELINES

- Physical findings: Vital signs, abdominal assessments, pulmonary assessment, fluid volume status, electrolyte status, presence of symptoms (vomiting, pain, distention, fever)
- Response to pain medications, antibiotics, NG intubation, and suctioning
- Presence of complications (preoperative): Peritonitis, sepsis, perforation, respiratory insufficiency, hypovolemia, shock
- Presence of complications (postoperative): Poor wound healing, hemorrhage, or infection

DISCHARGE AND HOME HEALTHCARE GUIDELINES

Teach postoperative care to patients who have had surgery. Explain the care of the surgical site. Teach the patient how to plan a paced progression of activities. Teach the patient the dosages, routes, and side effects for all medications. Review drug and food interactions with the patient. Instruct the patient to report bowel elimination problems to the physician. Emphasize that in the case of recurrent abdominal pain, fever, or vomiting, the patient should go to the emergency department for evaluation.

Intracerebral Hematoma

DRG Category:	70
Mean LOS:	6.2 days
Description:	MEDICAL: Nonspecific Cerebrovascular Disorders With Major Complication or Comorbidity
DRG Category:	955
Mean LOS:	11.0 days
Description:	SURGICAL: Craniotomy for Multiple Significant Trauma

An intracerebral hematoma (ICH) is a well-defined collection of blood within the brain parenchyma (functional tissue). Most ICHs are related to stroke or cerebral contusions; they account for approximately 10% of all strokes and are more likely than ischemic strokes to result in death or disability. Nontraumatic ICH commonly results from hypertensive damage to blood vessels but could also result from a ruptured aneurysm or other conditions. ICHs also complicate traumatic brain injury (TBI) in 2% to 3% of all head-injured patients. Although they are more frequently associated with closed-head injuries, they can also occur as a result of an open or penetrating injury or a depressed skull fracture. Similar to cerebral contusions, injury-related ICHs tend to occur most commonly in the frontal and temporal lobes and are uncommon in the cerebellum. They can also occur deep within the hemispheres in the paraventricular, medial, or paracentral areas in association with the shearing strain on small vessels that occurs with diffuse axonal injuries.

The patient can experience deterioration in cerebral functioning at the time of injury or in the first 48 to 72 hours after injury. Late hemorrhage into a contused area is possible for as long as 7 to 10 days after injury. ICHs result in a mortality rate between 25% and 72%. Complications include intracranial hypertension, brain herniation, and death.

CAUSES

In cases in which there is no apparent cause for spontaneous ICH, hypertension is the most frequently associated disease. Other potential causes of ICH include hemorrhage at the site of a brain tumor and stroke. Stroke results from hypertensive damage to the blood vessel wall, rupture of an aneurysm, or bleeding from an arteriovenous malformation. Traumatic causes of ICH include depressed skull fractures, penetrating missile injuries (gunshot wounds or stab wounds), or a sudden acceleration-deceleration motion. Depressed skull fractures cause penetration of bone into cerebral tissue. A high-velocity penetration (bullet) can produce shock waves that are transmitted throughout the brain in addition to the injury caused by the bullet directly. A low-velocity penetrating injury (knife) may involve only focal damage and no loss of consciousness. Motor vehicle crashes (MVCs) cause rapid acceleration-deceleration injuries.

GENETIC CONSIDERATIONS

Spontaneous ICH has been seen in familial congenital coagulation disorders such as factor XI deficiency.

SEX AND LIFE SPAN CONSIDERATIONS

About 20,000 people die from ICH in the United States each year. The peak incidence occurs in childhood (ages 3 to 12 years) and in older adults (ages 50 to 70 years). ICH can occur as a result of TBI, the leading cause of all trauma-related deaths. Many of these deaths are associated with MVCs. Males ages 15 to 24 years are three times more likely than females to be injured in a crash. Falls are the most common cause of TBI in adults over age 65 years. ICH can also occur from nontraumatic causes such as stroke, the third leading cause of death in the United States. Although a stroke can occur at any age, 72% occur in people over 65 years of age.

HEALTH DISPARITIES AND SEXUAL/GENDER MINORITY HEALTH

Hypertension and trauma may lead to ICH. Black persons have higher rates of intracerebral hemorrhage and ICH as compared to White persons, likely due to the higher prevalence of hypertension in Black persons. Asian Americans also have higher rates of ICH, perhaps related to the fish oil content in their diet.

In recent years, Black persons have been killed in traffic crashes at a rate almost 25% higher than White persons (National Highway Traffic Safety Administration [NHTSA], 2021). Native American persons have the highest rate of MVC injury in the United States, more than twice the rate of Black persons (NHTSA, 2021). Experts have noted that Black and Native American communities tend to be crisscrossed by more dangerous roads than other locations, placing people from those communities at risk for injury. Black youth ages 15 to 24 years have the highest homicide rate from gunshot wounds in the United States, followed by Hispanic youth. Penetrating injuries from gunshot wounds and stab wounds are more common in non-Hispanic Black persons than in non-Hispanic White persons, making Black youth at risk for ICH related to penetrating injuries. Stark disparities exist with the incidence, management, and rehabilitation of TBI. The Centers for Disease Control and Prevention (CDC) report that Native American children and adults have the highest TBI-related hospitalizations and deaths in the United States. Important health disparities exist in treatment, follow-up, and rehabilitation of TBI. Non-Hispanic Black and Hispanic patients are less likely to receive follow-up care and rehabilitation following TBI and more likely to have poor psychosocial, functional, and employment-related outcomes as compared to non-Hispanic White patients (CDC, 2021).

The CDC report that in the 20 years since the year 2000, more than 400,000 U.S. service members were diagnosed with TBI, including active military service members and Veterans. Approximately 80% of these injuries occurred when the service members were not deployed. These injuries may result in ongoing symptoms, posttraumatic distress syndrome, and suicidal thoughts. People in correctional or detention facilities, people who experience homelessness, and survivors of intimate partner violence may have long-term consequences from TBI. People with lower incomes and those without health insurance have less access to TBI care, are less likely to receive surgical procedures and cranial monitoring when indicated, less likely to receive rehabilitation, and more likely to die in the hospital. Recent work has shown that rural populations have injury mortality rates that are more than twice as high as urban rates. Many factors contribute to these health disparities, including the risk of traffic injury in narrow rural roads, the lack of graded curves and lighted traffic signals on rural highways, and the distance from major trauma centers. Many of the most dangerous occupations, such as mining and agriculture, are found in rural areas and can result in injury, disability, and death. People living in rural areas who experience a TBI have more time to travel to get emergency care, less access to high-level trauma care, and more difficulty accessing TBI services. Sexual and gender minority persons have high risk for dating and interpersonal violence, violence related to bullying, and intentional and unintentional injury, and therefore are at risk for TBI and ICH (Healthy People 2020).

GLOBAL HEALTH CONSIDERATIONS

While there are few data available about global trends, people who live in Asia have a higher incidence of intracerebral hemorrhage than people living in other regions of the world, as do people with Asian ancestry living in the United States.

ASSESSMENT

HISTORY. If the patient has a suspected stroke, determine the onset of symptoms and whether the patient has a history of hypertension. Elicit a history of headache, drowsiness, confusion, seizures, focal neurological deficits, dizziness, irritability, giddiness, visual disturbances (seeing stars), and gait disturbances. Determine if the patient experienced nausea or vomiting. In addition, others may describe symptoms related to increased intracranial pressure (ICP), such as increased drowsiness or irritability and pupillary dilation on the ipsilateral (same as injury) side. Generally, patients suspected of ICH have a history of traumatic injury to the head or an alteration in level of consciousness from a stroke. In trauma patients, if the patient is not able to report a history, question the prehospital care provider, significant others, or witnesses about the situation and timing of the injury. If the patient was in an MVC, determine the speed and type of the vehicle, the patient's position in the vehicle, whether the patient was restrained, and whether the patient was thrown from the vehicle on impact. If the patient was injured in a motorcycle crash, determine whether the patient was wearing a helmet. Determine if the patient experienced momentary loss of reflexes, momentary arrest of respirations, and possible retrograde or antegrade amnesia (loss of memory for events immediately before the injury or loss of memory for events after the injury). Ask about the patient's drinking history prior to the event.

PHYSICAL EXAMINATION. The most common symptoms are **alterations in level of consciousness, headache, nausea,** and **vomiting.** Seizures and focal neurological deficits may occur. When you examine the patient, note that, just as in cerebral contusions, small frontal lesions may be asymptomatic, whereas larger bilateral lesions may result in a frontal lobe syndrome of inappropriate behavior and cognitive deficits. Dominant hemispheric lesions are often associated with speech and motor deficits. Because many of the symptoms of alcohol intoxication mimic those of TBI, never assume that a decreased level of consciousness is caused by alcohol intoxication alone (even if you can smell the alcohol on the patient's breath or clothing) rather than a head injury (see **Stroke** for physical examination and treatment of stroke).

First evaluate and stabilize the patient's airway, breathing, and circulation with particular attention to the intactness of the patient's cervical spine (do not flex or extend the neck until you know the patient has no cervical spine injury). Next, perform a neurological assessment, watching for early signs of increased ICP: decreased level of consciousness, decreased strength and motion of extremities, reduced visual acuity, headache, and pupillary changes.

During the complete head-to-toe assessment, be sure to evaluate the patient's head for external signs of injury. Check carefully for scalp lacerations. Check the patient for cerebrospinal fluid (CSF) leakage from the nose (rhinorrhea) or ear (otorrhea), which is a sign of a basilar skull fracture (a linear fracture at the base of the brain). Other signs of basilar skull fracture include raccoon eyes (periorbital ecchymosis or bruising around the eyes) and Battle sign (bleeding and swelling behind the ear).

Be sure to evaluate the patient's pupillary light reflexes. An abnormal pupil reflex may result from increasing cerebral edema, which may indicate a life-threatening increase in ICP. Pupil size is normally 1.5 to 6 mm. Several signs to look for include ipsilateral miosis (Horner syndrome), in which one pupil is smaller than the other with a drooping eyelid; bilateral miosis, in which both pupils are pinpoint in size; ipsilateral mydriasis (Hutchinson pupil), in which one of the pupils is much larger than the other and is unreactive to light; bilateral midposition, in which both pupils are 4 to 5 mm and remain dilated and nonreactive to light; and bilateral mydriasis, in which both pupils are larger than 6 mm and nonreactive to light. Note the shape of the pupil as well because an oval pupil may indicate increased ICP and possible brain herniation. In more seriously injured patients, invasive ICP monitoring with an intraventricular catheter may be initiated for serial assessment of the ICP. Normally, ICP is 4 to 10 mm Hg, with an upper limit of 15 mm Hg. ICP is considered moderately elevated at levels of 15 to 30 mm Hg and severely elevated at levels above 30 mm Hg.

PSYCHOSOCIAL. Assess the patient's and family's ability to cope with a sudden illness and the change in roles that a sudden illness demands. Expect parents of children who are injured to be anxious, fearful, and sometimes guilt-ridden. Note if the injury was related to alcohol (approximately 40% to 60% of TBIs occur when the patient has been drinking), and elicit a drinking history from the patient or significant others.

Note that during the patient's recovery, subtle neurological deficits (such as subtle personality changes or inability to perform mathematical calculations) may exist long after hospital discharge and may interfere with the resumption of parenting, spousal, or occupational roles.

Diagnostic Highlights

Test	Normal Result	Abnormality With Condition	Explanation
Computed tomography (CT) scan	Intact cerebral anatomy	Identification of size and location of site of injury or bleeding	Shows anterior to posterior slices of the brain to highlight abnormalities

Other Tests: Skull x-rays, magnetic resonance imaging, cervical spine x-rays, electrocardiogram, complete blood count, coagulation studies, serum chemistries, glucose test of any drainage suspected to be CSF using a reagent strip, alcohol and drug screening, lumbar puncture

PRIMARY NURSING DIAGNOSIS

DIAGNOSIS. Acute confusion related to cerebral tissue injury and swelling as evidenced by agitation, restlessness, changes in cognition, and/or misperception

OUTCOMES. Cognition; Concentration; Decision making; Information processing; Memory; Neurological status: Consciousness; Neurological status: Central motor control

INTERVENTIONS. Cerebral perfusion promotion; Environmental management; Cerebral edema management; Medication management

PLANNING AND IMPLEMENTATION

Collaborative

Management of airway, breathing, and circulation is important, and endotracheal intubation is necessary if the patient develops increased intracranial pressure. If a lesion identified by CT scan is causing a shift of intracranial contents or increased ICP, immediate surgical intervention is necessary. Endoscopic evacuation is being attempted as a very early stage treatment for intracerebral hemorrhage. A craniotomy may be performed to evacuate the ICH and ischemic tissue if the site is operable or to release ICP if viable tissue will be preserved. A ventriculostomy (creation of a hole within a cerebral ventricle for drainage) allows for external drainage for patients experiencing ventricular bleeding.

Ongoing monitoring and serial assessments are essential. ICP monitoring and sequential CT scanning may be needed in critically ill patients, and serial neurological assessments are needed on all patients to determine if ICP is increasing. Because bleeding and swelling can progress over several days after injury, the patient is monitored for deterioration even up to 10 days after injury. During periods of frequent assessment, the patient should not be sedated for longer than 30 minutes at a time; longer-acting sedation may mask neurological changes and place the patient at risk for lack of detection. Blood pressure needs to be regulated carefully, keeping the mean arterial pressure less than 130 mm Hg but avoiding hypotension so that the brain is adequately perfused. Fluid and electrolytes need careful adjustment to maintain brain perfusion but reduce the potential for cerebral edema. Hyperthermia contributes to stress on the brain and needs to be corrected as soon as possible.

Pharmacologic Highlights

Medication or Drug Class	Dosage	Description	Rationale
Fentanyl (Sublimaze)	0.05 mg IV as needed	Short-acting opioid analgesic	Provides short-term (30 min) pain control and sedation without long-lasting effects that may mask neurological changes
Antihypertensives	Varies with drug	Labetalol, nicardipine	Reduce blood pressure to prevent worsening of ICH

Other Drugs: Some patients develop seizures as a complication and need anticonvulsants such as fosphenytoin. Drugs to reduce ICP, such as mannitol, may be used. Acetaminophen may be used to control fever. Phytonadione and protamine may be used to reverse coagulopathies, and famotidine may be used to prevent gastric ulcers.

Independent

After making sure the patient has adequate airway, breathing, and circulation, ongoing serial assessments of the patient's neurological responses are of highest priority. Timely notification of the trauma surgeon or neurosurgeon when a patient's assessment changes can save a patient's life. If the patient is intubated, make sure the endotracheal tube is anchored well. If the patient is at risk for self-extubation, maintain the patient in soft restraints. Notify the physician if the patient's Pao_2 drops below 80 mm Hg, if $Paco_2$ exceeds 40 mm Hg, or if severe hypocapnia ($Paco_2 < 25$ mm Hg) occurs. Aspiration pneumonia is a risk and can occur even with endotracheal intubation. Elevate the head of the bed at 30 degrees to help prevent this complication.

Help control the patient's ICP. Maintain normothermia by avoiding body temperature elevations. Avoid flexing, extending, or rotating the patient's neck because these maneuvers limit venous drainage of the brain and thus raise ICP. Avoid hip flexion by maintaining the patient in a normal body alignment, limiting venous drainage. Maintain a quiet, restful environment with minimal stimulation; limit visitors as appropriate. Time nursing care activities carefully to limit prolonged ICP elevations. Use caution when suctioning the patient. Hyperventilate the patient beforehand and suction only as long as necessary. When turning the patient, prevent Valsalva maneuver by using a draw sheet to pull the patient up in bed. Instruct the patient not to hold on to the side rails. Monitor the blood pressure carefully to avoid hypertension and hypotension. Regulate fluids to maintain euvolemia (normal fluid balance) to support brain perfusion but to reduce the chance of elevated ICP.

Strategies to maximize the coping mechanisms of the patient and family are directed toward providing support and encouragement. Provide educational tools about TBIs. Teach the patient and family appropriate rehabilitative exercises, as appropriate. Help the patient cope with long stretches of immobility by providing diversionary activities that are appropriate to the patient's mental and physical abilities. TBI support groups may be helpful. Referrals to clinical nurse specialists, pastoral care staff, and social workers are helpful in developing strategies for support and education.

Help the significant others and family face the fear of death, disability, and dependency; involve the patient and the family in all aspects of care.

Evidence-Based Practice and Health Policy

Xue, M., & Yong, V. (2020). Neuroinflammation in intracerebral haemorrhage: Immunotherapies with potential for translation. *The Lancet, 19*, 1013–1032.

- The authors suggest that current treatments for intracerebral hemorrhage are inadequate, and they aim to investigate literature on drugs that can reduce inflammation that can be neurotoxic. While the primary injury is serious and primarily mechanical, the secondary injury (occurs with swelling and biological changes in response to the primary injury) can lead to poor outcomes. The authors identified articles in electronic databases that discussed intracerebral hemorrhage and many terms associated with inflammation. They reviewed 10 clinical trials investigating drugs that reduced inflammation without interfering with the parts of inflammation that help with brain healing.
- The studies were conducted in both humans and animals. The articles supported the use of minocycline, sphingosine-1-phosphate receptor modulators, and statins after a brain hemorrhage. They note that quick initiation of these drugs in high systemic doses might counteract the evolving secondary injury in people with intracerebral hemorrhage. The studies provide a promising way to improve outcomes.

DOCUMENTATION GUIDELINES

- Descriptions of symptoms at time of stroke or trauma history, description of the event, time elapsed since the event, whether the patient had a loss of consciousness and, if so, for how long
- Adequacy of airway, breathing, circulation; serial vital signs
- Appearance: Bruising or lacerations, drainage from the nose or ears
- Physical findings related to the site of head injury: Neurological assessment, presence of accompanying symptoms, presence of complications
- Signs of complications: Seizure activity, infection (fever, purulent discharge from any wounds), aspiration pneumonia (shortness of breath, pulmonary congestion, fever, productive cough), increased ICP
- Response to medications used to control pain and increased ICP

DISCHARGE AND HOME HEALTHCARE GUIDELINES

Be sure the patient understands all medications, including the dosage, route, action, adverse effects, and the need for routine laboratory monitoring for convulsants. Teach the patient and caregiver the signs and symptoms that necessitate a return to the hospital. Teach the patient to recognize the symptoms and signs of postinjury syndrome, which may last for several weeks. Explain that mild cognitive changes do not always resolve immediately. Provide the patient and significant others with information about the trauma clinic and the phone number of a clinical nurse specialist in case referrals are needed. Stress the importance of follow-up visits to the physician's office. If alcohol counseling is needed, provide a phone number and the name of a counselor. Prepare the patient and family for the possible need for rehabilitation after the acute care phase of hospitalization.

Intrauterine Fetal Demise

DRG Category:	805
Mean LOS:	4.0 days
Description:	MEDICAL: Vaginal Delivery Without Sterilization or Dilation & Curettage With Major Complication or Comorbidity
DRG Category:	806
Mean LOS:	2.7 days
Description:	MEDICAL: Vaginal Delivery Without Sterilization or Dilation & Curettage With Complication or Comorbidity
DRG Category:	807
Mean LOS:	2.2 days
Description:	MEDICAL: Vaginal Delivery Without Sterilization or Dilation & Curettage Without Complication or Comorbidity or Major Complication or Comorbidity

An intrauterine fetal demise (IUFD), or stillbirth, is defined by the World Health Organization as death of the fetus prior to its complete expulsion, regardless of the duration of the pregnancy. The term *stillbirth* is used only for fetal deaths in pregnancies after 28 weeks' gestation. IUFD is more common with decreasing gestational age; 80% of all stillbirths occur before term, and more than half occur before 28 weeks. The specific gestational age and weight that classify the fetus as an IUFD vary among states in the United States. Labor and delivery of the dead fetus usually occur spontaneously within 2 weeks. Patients are under tremendous psychological stress and are at a higher risk for postpartum depression. Disseminated intravascular coagulation (DIC) is the main complication that can result. Thromboplastin released from the dead fetus is thought to mediate DIC.

CAUSES

Approximately 1%, or 30,000, pregnancies per year end in an IUFD. While 25% to 35% of fetal deaths are unexplainable, many potential causes have been identified via autopsy: genetic anomalies that are incompatible with life, uteroplacental insufficiency, umbilical cord prolapse or other cord problems, twin-to-twin transfusion, maternal disease (hypertension, diabetes mellitus, and gestational diabetes insipidus [GDI], advanced maternal age, sepsis, acidosis, hypoxia, infection, anaphylaxis), trauma, placenta previa, abruptio placentae, uterine rupture, pseudoamniotic band syndrome, premature rupture of membranes, and postterm pregnancy. New research is suggesting that IUFD may also be caused by various perinatal infections, including TORCH (toxoplasmosis, other, rubella, cytomegalovirus, herpes) infections, and some case reports have included positive fetal cultures for erythrovirus B19, *Haemophilus influenzae*, hepatitis E, group B streptococci, and even *Rothia dentocariosa*, a normal bacteria found in the oral cavity of humans. Also, intimate partner violence should be ruled out. Patients have the option of requesting an autopsy to determine the cause of death. If an autopsy is not performed, it may not be possible to determine the exact cause of fetal death. Risk factors include maternal disease, advanced maternal age, infections, trauma, abruptio placentae, previous stillbirths, intimate partner violence, hospitalization during pregnancy, anemia, and postterm pregnancy.

GENETIC CONSIDERATIONS

Genetic abnormalities of the fetus are a significant cause of pregnancy loss, including chromosomal abnormalities such as trisomies.

SEX AND LIFE SPAN CONSIDERATIONS

The likelihood of the occurrence of an IUFD decreases with good prenatal care. IUFD occurs more often in pregnant persons of advanced parental age (35 years and older) and is thought to be the reason for the increase in perinatal mortality in this age group. IUFD accounts for 50% of all perinatal deaths.

HEALTH DISPARITIES AND SEXUAL/GENDER MINORITY HEALTH

Factors associated with IUFD prior to 32 weeks of pregnancy include persons who are Black, persons with chronic hypertension, and fetal growth restriction as evidenced by small for gestational age (Brackett et al., 2020). Patients with intellectual disabilities likely have higher rates of adverse perinatal outcomes such as stillbirths. Pregnant persons who experience intimate partner violence are three times more likely to have a fetal or neonatal death than their counterparts not involved in violent relationships. Women who have sex with women, bisexual women, and lesbian women are more likely to report a pregnancy ending in stillbirth than heterosexual women (Everett et al., 2020).

GLOBAL HEALTH CONSIDERATIONS

IUFD rates globally vary significantly depending on the quality of healthcare in each region and the definition used for classifying fetal deaths.

ASSESSMENT

HISTORY. Obtain a thorough obstetric and medical history. Determine the gestational age of the fetus by asking the patient the date of the last menstrual period and using the Nagele rule. Inquire about any contractions, bleeding, or leakage of fluid. Ask about exposure to environmental teratogens or the use of recreational or prescription drugs. Ask when the patient last felt the baby move. Also inquire about any cultural and religious preferences related to labor, delivery, postpartum care, autopsy, and receiving a blood transfusion.

PHYSICAL EXAMINATION. Common symptoms are **cessation of fetal movement** and **loss of fetal heart tones**. Attempt to auscultate a fetal heart rate with a Doppler or electronic fetal monitor. If no heartbeat is heard, perform an ultrasound to be sure no heart rate is present. Determine the McDonald measurement, the measurement from the top of the uterus (fundus) to the top of the pubic symphysis, and compare it with previous data; the measurement is usually less than that expected for the gestational age if an IUFD has occurred. Palpate the abdomen for rigidity, which is often present with abruptio placentae, or for change in shape, which is often present with uterine rupture. Inspect the perineum for bleeding and note any foul odors. If there is no vaginal bleeding, perform a vaginal examination to check for a prolapsed cord and note any cervical dilation and effacement. If possible, determine the fetal presenting part and the station. Check the patient's vital signs. A temperature higher than 100.4°F (38°C) may indicate the presence of infection. Weigh the patient; some may experience a weight loss. Because DIC is a potential complication of IUFD, monitor the patient for the following signs and symptoms of DIC: bleeding from puncture sites, episiotomy, abdominal incision, or gums; hematuria; epistaxis; increased vaginal bleeding, bruising, and petechiae.

A thorough physical examination is done of the fetus, umbilical cord, amniotic fluid, placenta, and membranes to determine the cause of death. Knowing the cause may be therapeutic for the parents and helps relieve guilt feelings.

PSYCHOSOCIAL. Assess the patient's reaction and ability to cope with the fetal death and the patient's anxiety about going through the labor process. Determine the meaning of the pregnancy for the patient. Observe the interaction between the patient and significant other to assess potential support.

Diagnostic Highlights

General Comments: Abdominal ultrasound easily and accurately confirms the diagnosis of IUFD. Placental abnormalities at 19 to 23 weeks' gestation may be indicative of poor outcomes assessed by uterine artery Doppler.

Test	Normal Result	Abnormality With Condition	Explanation
Ultrasound (abdominal)	Heartbeat seen; fetal growth appropriate for gestational age	No heartbeat seen; "fetal collapse" noted; gestational age smaller than expected	Absence of heartbeat and shriveled fetal appearance indicative of IUFD

Other Tests: If sepsis or DIC is a potential threat, coagulation studies (fibrinogen, fibrin split products, prothrombin time, partial thromboplastin time, D-dimer) are done serially. Plasma cell-free DNA is a combination of both maternal and fetal DNA. Fetal fraction is the proportion of cell-free DNA derived from the fetus that is present in the mother's blood.

PRIMARY NURSING DIAGNOSIS

DIAGNOSIS. Risk for maladaptive grieving as evidenced by anger, blaming, despair, detachment, distress, personal growth, and/or finding meaning in a loss

OUTCOMES. Grief resolution; Guilt resolution; Personal resiliency

INTERVENTIONS. Grief work facilitation: Perinatal death; Active listening; Presence; Truth telling; Support group

☀ PLANNING AND IMPLEMENTATION

Collaborative

The treatment involves inducing labor to deliver the fetus. The timing of the delivery varies. A 48-hour wait is recommended to give the patient time to gather support from the family and to fathom the reality of the situation. Other patients may prefer to let the labor start on its own, but this could take weeks. The danger with this conservative treatment is that the necrotic fetus can lead to DIC or infection, or both, in the pregnant person. A cesarean section is rarely done unless the parental condition necessitates an immediate delivery.

Induction of labor is often a 2-day process. Insertion of a laminaria tent into the endocervical canal dilates the cervix. If necessary, the laminaria can be held in place by a tampon. The risk of infection in the presence of a dead fetus needs to be considered. Prostaglandin E_2 gel or 20-mg suppositories are alternatives to laminaria. By the second day, the cervix is usually ripe, and an oxytocic induction of labor can begin. When infusing oxytocin, assess often for resting tone, as uterine rupture caused by hyperstimulation can occur. Labor contractions are very uncomfortable for the patient. Liberal dosages of analgesia or anesthesia may be given if the patient desires because their effects on the fetus do not need to be considered. IV narcotics, an epidural, and sedatives may be ordered for relief of pain and anxiety.

If the patient has an epidural, turn the patient from side to side hourly to ensure an adequate distribution of anesthesia. Patients have limited mobility and require assistance in turning and positioning comfortably. Use pillows to support the back and abdomen and between the knees to maintain alignment. Check the blood pressure and pulse every 30 minutes. Most patients are unable to void and require a straight catheterization every 2 to 3 hours to keep the bladder empty. Maintain the infusion of IV fluids to prevent hypotension, which can result from regional anesthesia. Monitor the patient's pain relief and notify the nurse anesthetist or physician if the patient is uncomfortable.

Pharmacologic Highlights

Medication or Drug Class	Dosage	Description	Rationale
Dinoprostone (Prostaglandin, Cervidil, Prepidil gel)	20-mg suppository; 0.5-mg gel; 10-mg inserts	Prostaglandins	Ripens, softens, and begins to dilate the cervix and prepare it for labor
Oxytocin (Pitocin)	0.5–1 milliunits/min IV, titrate 1–2 milliunits/min every 15–60 min	Oxytocic	Induces labor contractions
Analgesia/ anesthesia	Varies by drug; medication given via either IV push or epidural catheter	Narcotic analgesics; anesthetics	Labor contractions are very uncomfortable and especially difficult to tolerate with a demise of the fetus
RhoD immunoglobulin (RhoGAM)	1,500 International Unit IM within 72 hr, prepared by blood bank	Immune serum	Prevents Rh isoimmunizations in future pregnancies; given if mother is Rh-negative and infant is Rh-positive

Independent

If possible, admit the patient to a room that is isolated from the nursery, patients in labor, and crying of newborns. Often, units have some small symbol (a small bear, a heart, a leaf with a raindrop representing a tear) to hang on the door that denotes the patient has an IUFD to alert any healthcare workers who encounter the patient to be sensitive. It is important to be available and not avoid the patient because the situation is uncomfortable.

The nurse is present through the entire labor and delivery and plays a key role in assisting the patient and family through the initial grieving process. Allow the patient to have more than one support person during labor. During this shocking event, encourage the patient and significant others to verbalize their feelings. Discuss the grieving process and expected feelings; use therapeutic communication skills and be empathic. Be aware of the content of your messages to the patient.

Involve the patient and significant other in all decisions and discussions related to the labor, delivery, and aftercare. Do not rush the patient and support group to make decisions regarding aftercare. Before the delivery, educate them about the labor process. Prepare them for the appearance of a dead fetus (maceration of the skin, discolorations, specific anomalies, and trauma that can occur during delivery). During delivery, have only the minimum number of staff needed to provide safe care. Keep the room quiet and dim to promote a calm and peaceful atmosphere. Honor the parents' desires for seeing, holding, and touching the newborn. Prepare a "memory box" that contains tangible items, such as footprints, handprints, pictures, a lock of hair, identification bands, and any other items used for the baby. After the patient delivers, monitor the patient's vital signs, location and firmness of fundus, amount of vaginal bleeding, ability to void, presence of edema and hemorrhoids, comfort level, and ability to cope. Provide time for the patient and significant other to be alone with the infant.

Provide reading material for the parents on coping with a neonatal loss. Offer to notify clergy if the patient desires and respect any religious requests. Although it may be difficult to discuss, offer information regarding funeral arrangements. Discuss an autopsy and explain the advantages of determining the exact cause of death. Refer the patient to a bereavement support group, such as SHARE. Often, follow-up counseling is done by a hospital grief counselor or by the nurse who was present at the delivery.

Evidence-Based Practice and Health Policy

Everett, B., Kominiarek, M., Mollborn, S., Adkins, D., & Hughes, T. (2019). Sexual orientation disparities in pregnancy and infant outcomes. *Maternal Child Health Journal, 23*, 72–81.

- The authors aimed to use a national data set to investigate sexual orientation inequities in pregnancy and birth outcomes, including miscarriage, stillbirth, preterm birth, and birth weight. They analyzed data on 19,955 eligible pregnancies and 15,996 singleton live births. Sexual orientation was measured using self-reported identity and histories of same-sex sexual experiences.
- Compared to heterosexual women, women who have sex with women, bisexual women, and lesbian women were more likely to report miscarriage. Bisexual women and lesbian women were more likely to report a pregnancy ending in stillbirth and preterm birth. Lesbian women were more likely to report low birth weight infants. The authors concluded that sexual orientation may lead to inequities in pregnancy and birth outcomes.

DOCUMENTATION GUIDELINES

- Progress of cervical dilation, progress of labor; response to pain of contractions; time of delivery; condition of fetus; vital signs
- Signs of abnormal bleeding; amount and character of lochia
- Patient's and significant other's expressions of grief
- Patient's ability to cope with the fetal loss

DISCHARGE AND HOME HEALTHCARE GUIDELINES

Teach the patient to be aware of the signs and symptoms that could indicate postpartum complications: pain in the calf of the leg; increase in vaginal bleeding; foul odor of vaginal discharge; fever; burning with urination; persistent mood change; or a hard, reddened area on the breast. A postpartum visit should be scheduled for 10 days to 2 weeks following birth so that the healthcare provider can monitor the emotional and physical state of the patient. Explain that the patient should not have intercourse or drive a car until after the postpartum check. Encourage participation in a bereavement support group, even if the patient and significant other seem to be coping with the loss. They may be able to help other couples cope.

Intussusception

DRG Category:	390
Mean LOS:	2.9 days
Description:	MEDICAL: Gastrointestinal Obstruction Without Complication or Comorbidity or Major Complication or Comorbidity

Intussusception occurs when a bowel segment invaginates or telescopes into an adjoining portion of bowel. As peristalsis continues, the segment is propelled farther into the bowel, blood supply is restricted, and bowel obstruction occurs. Tissue ischemia leads to an edematous and friable bowel, causing bleeding and, if the condition is not corrected, complications such as tissue necrosis, intestinal gangrene, shock, intestinal perforation, intestinal hemorrhage, and peritonitis. Intussusception is considered a pediatric emergency because it is one of the most common causes of bowel obstruction in children and can be fatal if it is not treated within 2 to 5 days.

Children with cystic fibrosis, gastroenteritis, polyps, lymphosarcoma, and celiac disease are particularly susceptible. Intussusception is classified according to the portion of the bowel involved. The most common location for intussusception is at or near the ileocecal valve, which usually occurs in infants and toddlers, but enteroenteral intussusception (jejunum and ilium) also occurs with older children. Intussusception can occur in both the small and the large bowels. Experts suggest that the recurrence rate is 10% to 15%.

CAUSES

In 90% of patients, the cause of intussusception is unknown. Some experts suggest that it develops because of an imbalance in the forces along the intestinal wall and a disorganized pattern of peristalsis. The result of this imbalance causes a portion of the intestine to telescope into the receiving portion of the intestine. In infants over 1 year, a "lead point" on the intestine may indicate the focal problem. Lead points may be Meckel diverticulum, a polyp, a foreign body, an enlarged lymph node, a hematoma, hypertrophy of lymphatic tissue of the bowel associated with infection (Peyer patch), or bowel tumors. When intussusception occurs in adults, it is most commonly associated with benign or malignant tumors or polyps. Current theories also suggest that intussusception may be associated with viral infections, such as an upper respiratory infection. Risk factors include congenital abnormalities in the intestine, celiac disease, cystic fibrosis, family history, male sex, and infancy.

GENETIC CONSIDERATIONS

A genetic predisposition to intussusception has been suggested in cases of multiple occurrences within families. However, the majority of cases of intussusception arise from an unknown cause. In addition, the jejunal polyps of Peutz-Jeghers syndrome (PJS; hereditary polyposis of the gastrointestinal tract) can lead to intussusception. PJS is due to a deletion in the *LKB1* gene, and it is transmitted in an autosomal dominant pattern with incomplete penetrance. PJS is also considered a cancer susceptibility syndrome.

SEX AND LIFE SPAN CONSIDERATIONS

About half the cases occur in children in their first year of life, particularly between the ages of 3 and 12 months. The majority of the rest of the cases occur before the age of 2 years. Intussusception occurs two to three times more frequently in males than in females. Once corrected, there are no lifetime complications of the condition that are known to occur. Intussusception is rare in adults, is often accompanied by a bowel obstruction, and in 90% of the cases is associated with a malignancy.

HEALTH DISPARITIES AND SEXUAL/GENDER MINORITY HEALTH

Ethnicity, race, and sexual/gender minority status have no known effect on the risk for intussusception.

GLOBAL HEALTH CONSIDERATIONS

In developed regions such as the United States, Canada, and Western Europe, intussusception occurs in approximately one to four cases per 1,000 live births. No data are available from developing regions of the world.

ASSESSMENT

HISTORY. The parents are likely to describe an infant or toddler, usually a healthy male with no previous illness, who experiences severe, intermittent abdominal pain, vomiting, and bloody stools; children often draw their legs up to the abdomen, turn pale and clammy, and cry sharply. The pain is intense, intermittent, and colicky. The attack is followed by a period of normal behavior and then developing symptoms occur (see below). Determine if this is a first episode or recurrence and if the child has had any gastrointestinal problems in the past. Adults may report general, chronic, intermittent symptoms such as abdominal tenderness; vomiting; and changes in bowel habits such as diarrhea, bloody stools, or constipation. Determine the child's past medical history and any medications.

PHYSICAL EXAMINATION. Usually the child looks well nourished and in good health. Common symptoms in children include **abdominal pain, vomiting,** and **changes in stool patterns** that last for a few minutes, followed by a period of lethargy. The cycle repeats every 15 to 30 minutes. The child may have bile-stained or fecal vomiting and may pass bloody stools. The stool is often called "currant jelly stool" because of the mucus and blood from the injured bowel. The child may show some guarding of the abdomen, and a sausagelike mass may be palpable in the abdomen. Location of the mass and the guarding vary depending on the location of the intussusception. Bloody mucus may be found on rectal examination. Hyperperistaltic rushes may be heard on auscultation.

Adult patients may have a distended abdomen and often pain in the right lower quadrant of the abdomen. Extremely severe pain, abdominal distention, rapid heart rate, and diaphoresis may indicate that intussusception has led to strangulation of the bowel.

PSYCHOSOCIAL. The sudden onset of intussusception and the severity of the pain and symptoms can provoke anxiety in the parents and the child. Assess the parents' coping ability and their support systems. Note that because the child experiences an emergency condition, the child has not been prepared for hospitalization, separation from the parents and the home environment, and possible surgery.

Diagnostic Highlights

Test	Normal Result	Abnormality With Condition	Explanation
Abdominal ultrasound	Normal abdominal structures	Distended loops of bowel	> 80% of children have positive ultrasound results in both ileocolic and jejunointestinal intussusception
Abdominal x-ray	Normal abdominal structures	Distended loops of bowel; may have a ladderlike pattern with air-fluid levels	Identifies blockage of lumen of bowel with distal passage of fluid and air (partial) or complete obstruction

Other Tests: Complete blood count, barium enema (for children under 3 years of age), abdominal computed tomography, colonoscopy, sigmoidoscopy

PRIMARY NURSING DIAGNOSIS

DIAGNOSIS. Acute pain related to inflammation as evidenced by self-reports of pain, facial grimacing, crying, and/or protective behavior

OUTCOMES. Pain level; Comfort status; Pain control; Symptom severity; Pain: Disruptive effects

INTERVENTIONS. Analgesic administration; Anxiety reduction; Pain management: Acute; Medication management

PLANNING AND IMPLEMENTATION

Collaborative

Reduction of the intussusception is accomplished by hydrostatic pressure or pneumatic reduction (barium enema), surgical manipulation, or surgical resection. Patients are often divided into groups by age with respect to treatment. Children ages 5 months to 3 years usually do not have a lead point and can be managed with nonoperative reduction. If the symptoms are less than 24 hours old and there is no evidence of complete obstruction, peritonitis, or shock, a therapeutic barium enema using fluoroscopic or ultrasonographic guidance can be used to reduce the high intestinal pressure. This technique has a 90% success rate. Other practitioners use a saline or air enema. The maximum safe intraluminal air pressure for young infants is 80 mm Hg and for older children is 110 to 120 mm Hg. If the procedure does not result in a change in the intussusception, the procedure is terminated, and the patient is evaluated for surgery. Adults and children ages 5 years and older often have a lead point and therefore require operative reduction.

Surgical resection of the affected bowel segment is performed in several situations: if the manipulation is unsuccessful, if the bowel is strangulated, or if it has necrotic areas. Laparoscopy, performed to reduce the intussusception and confirmed by radiological evidence, is becoming more common. It is associated with faster recovery time, decreased length of stay, lower pain medication requirements, and decreased time without eating. However, when used to treat adults, it is associated with complications such as paralytic ileus and wound infection. Recurrence, usually within the first 36 to 48 hours after treatment, can occur with the barium enema method, laparoscopy, or bowel manipulation in approximately 10% of patients who are treated nonoperatively. Parents need to understand that when the barium enema or laparoscopy is attempted, the child is also prepared for the possibility of surgery. Preoperatively, the child may have a nasogastric (NG) tube and IV lines for fluid replacement; the child also needs medications administered as needed for pain relief. Postoperative management contains the same three components: management of NG drainage and decompression, fluid replacement, and pain relief. Also monitor the child for signs of bleeding and infection. If the child had a successful reduction using the hydrostatic barium enema, the parents need to understand that feedings will be in small amounts and that stools will be grayish-white until the barium is passed. Children are usually kept in the hospital until they have normal stools.

Pharmacologic Highlights

Medication or Drug Class	Dosage	Description	Rationale
Antibiotics	Varies with drug	Broad spectrum	May be used to prevent peritonitis or postoperative infection

Other: Patient-controlled analgesia in adults, ibuprofen for pain relief, opioid analgesics for pain relief

Independent

Because intussusception occurs in otherwise healthy infants and is an emergency situation, the nurse's role is to provide comfort for the child and the parents, provide explanations to the parents, and evaluate the success of the treatment. Explain to the parents the differences in the various treatments, including nonoperative reduction, laparoscopy, and surgery. Because the child appears normal between attacks, you may sometimes have difficulty convincing parents of the potential severity of the condition. Make sure to explain the condition carefully. Early intervention is crucial to prevent complications. When you suspect intussusception, carefully elicit information from the parents about the progression of the symptoms and the type, location, and duration of pain. Comfort measures are needed for the child both before and after surgery, but do not mask abdominal pain with analgesia until a firm diagnosis is made.

If the child has surgery, check the incision for signs of infection (swelling, drainage, separation) or bleeding. Splint the wound with pillows and encourage coughing and deep breathing. If the child is old enough to follow directions, encourage deep breathing every hour. Elicit the parents' help in maintaining good pulmonary function after surgery.

Evidence-Based Practice and Health Policy

Zhang, M., Zhou, X., Hu, Q., & Jin, L. (2020). Accurately distinguishing pediatric ileocolic intussusception from small-bowel intussusception using ultrasonography. *Journal of Pediatric Surgery, 56*, 721–726.

- The clinical treatment of ileocolic intussusception as compared to small bowel intussusception (SBI) is different. The authors conducted a retrospective study of intussusception in patients aged 0 to 18 years and compared the clinical and ultrasonoscopy data to determine the differences between them. They studied 123 children with SBI and 60 children with ileocolic intussusception.
- Ultrasonoscopy features that were significantly different between the two groups included the lesion diameter, fat core thickness, outer wall thickness, lymph nodes inside intussusception, and lesion length. The author recommended using sonograms to distinguish SBI from ileocolic intussusception.

DOCUMENTATION GUIDELINES

- Location of pain, its duration, its patterns, time between episodes, and response to interventions
- Physical appearance and frequency of stool and vomitus
- If patient has surgery, appearance of wound or presence or absence of drainage; response to treatment and pain relief strategies
- Amount and type of food or formula eaten; tolerance to food and fluids
- Presence of complications: Infection, dehydration, poor wound healing

DISCHARGE AND HOME HEALTHCARE GUIDELINES

Parents should know the chance of recurrence, the time frame of the highest risk after the reduction, signs, and the action to take. If the child had surgery, parents should be prepared to care for the surgical incision. Parents should be informed of possible complications, such as infection and poor wound healing. Make sure the parents know how to monitor the infant or child's bowel function at home and when to return the infant or child to the hospital. Monitoring and follow-up are particularly important because of the chance of recurrence.

Provide a list of diet restrictions or recommendations. If the patient is discharged on antibiotics, make sure the parents know to complete the entire prescription before discontinuing the medication.

Iron Deficiency Anemia

DRG Category:	812
Mean LOS:	3.4 days
Description:	MEDICAL: Red Blood Cell Disorders Without Major Complication or Comorbidity

Iron deficiency anemia (IDA), the most common form of anemia, is a condition in which there is a decrease in normal body stores of iron and hemoglobin levels. IDA is caused by inadequate intake of iron, inadequate storage of iron, excessive loss of iron, or some combination of these conditions. The red blood cells (RBCs), which become pale (hypochromic) and small (microcytic), have a decreased ability to transport oxygen in sufficient quantities to meet body needs. Anemia is defined as a decrease in circulating RBC mass; the usual criteria for anemia are hemoglobin of less than 12 g/dL with a hematocrit less than 36% in women and hemoglobin less than 14 g/dL with a hematocrit less than 41% in men.

Generally, IDA is more common in people who are economically disadvantaged because of the high cost of a well-balanced diet with iron-rich foods. Complications from IDA include infection and pneumonia. It may lead to hypoxemia and exacerbation of coronary artery insufficiency. For patients suffering from pica (the urge to eat clay and other inappropriate items), lead poisoning may result from increased intestinal absorption of lead. Although it is a rare condition, Plummer-Vinson syndrome (IDA associated with difficulty swallowing, enlarged spleen, and spooning of the nails) may occur in severe cases of IDA, especially in middle-aged women who have recently had their teeth extracted.

CAUSES

The most common causes of IDA are menstrual blood loss and the increased iron requirements of pregnancy. Pathological bleeding, particularly gastrointestinal (GI) bleeding, is a common cause of iron depletion in men. Iron malabsorption can lead to IDA. Pathological causes include GI ulcers, hiatal hernias, malabsorption syndromes such as celiac disease, chronic diverticulosis, varices, and tumors. Other causes include surgeries such as partial gastrectomy and the use of prosthetic heart valves or vena cava filters. People at risk include those with heart failure (reduced iron stores) or renal transplant (kidneys regulate erythropoietin, which is necessary for red blood cell formation), people following bariatric surgery, and elite athletes (iron is lost in perspiration).

GENETIC CONSIDERATIONS

IDA has many possible etiologies, including blood loss, medications, or nutritional deficiency. One subtype of IDA, iron refractory iron deficiency anemia (IRIDA), is an autosomal recessive disease caused by mutations in *TMPRSS6*, which encodes the protein matriptase-2 (MT-2). MT-2 plays a role in the downregulation of hepcidin, which is crucial for iron homeostasis. When hepcidin levels are high, serum iron levels fall due to iron trapping within macrophages and hepatocytes.

SEX AND LIFE SPAN CONSIDERATIONS

Infants under age 2 years may develop IDA in situations of prolonged unsupplemented breastfeeding or bottle feeding; breast milk has some iron, but cow's milk has none. During periods of rapid growth in childhood, adolescence, and pregnancy, patients may ingest inadequate supplies of iron. Young women, in particular, are at risk as a result of heavy menses or unwise weight-reduction plans, and in the United States, females have a higher incidence of IDA than males. During childbearing years, adult females lose an average of 2 mg of iron daily that must be replaced nutritionally, whereas men lose only 1 mg of iron per day. Older patients with a poor diet and people who are alcohol dependent who fail to eat a well-balanced diet may also ingest inadequate supplies of iron.

HEALTH DISPARITIES AND SEXUAL/GENDER MINORITY HEALTH

IDA is associated with low-income households. Women at highest risk for IDA are women who live in urban poverty. Experts suggest that people who are uninsured and Black persons are less likely to receive colonoscopies and iron therapy than other groups when diagnosed with anemia

(Mirza et al., 2019). The lack of standardized care leads to health disparities for these groups. Sexual and gender minority status has no known effect on the risk for IDA.

GLOBAL HEALTH CONSIDERATIONS

In areas of the globe where meat is not a routine part of the diet, IDA is eight times more prevalent than in developed countries where meat is plentiful and culturally part of dietary patterns. Experts have reported that in Nepal and Sudan, IDA was present in two-thirds of the population. In certain underresourced regions of the world, intestinal parasites make iron deficiency worse because of GI blood loss.

ASSESSMENT

HISTORY. Inquire about recent weight loss, fatigue, weakness, dizziness, irritability, inability to concentrate, or sensitivity to cold. Ask about GI symptoms such as heartburn, loss of appetite, diarrhea, flatulence, bloody stools, or GI bleeding. Establish a history of difficulty in swallowing, which is a sign of long-term oxygen deficit, as esophageal webbing ensues. Elicit any history of neuromuscular effects, including vasomotor disturbances, tingling or numbness of the extremities, or pain along a nerve. Ask if the patient has experienced difficulty in breathing on exertion, rapid breathing, or palpitations. With infants and children, ask the parents to establish a history of growth patterns. With premenopausal women, ask about heavy bleeding during menses. Ask female patients for a pregnancy history.

Take a complete diet and illness history. Ask if the patient is following a strict vegetarian diet. Ask if the patient regularly eats foods that are rich in iron, such as whole grains, seafood, egg yolks, legumes, green leafy vegetables, dried fruits, red meats, and nuts; ask if the patient takes iron in vitamin supplements. Elicit the patient's history of alcohol use. Establish if the patient is a frequent blood donor. With infants, ask if breastfeeding or bottle feeding has been used and if any iron supplements have been added to the diet. Establish any history of frequent nosebleeds. With older patients, elicit a history of food preparation and diet planning to find out who takes responsibility for the patient's diet. Older patients in difficult economic circumstances may be hesitant to share their diet history if they are short of funds for food. Ask if the patient has had recent cravings for strange food (especially clay, laundry starch, or ice). Pagophagia is a form of pica involving compulsive eating or sucking of ice.

PHYSICAL EXAMINATION. While the condition may be asymptomatic, common symptoms include **leg cramps, fatigue, exercise intolerance,** and **craving for ice or cold foods (pagophagia).** Inspect the patient's mouth for pale mucous membranes and signs of inflammation (stomatitis) or eroded, tender, and swollen corners (angular stomatitis). Observe the tongue to see if it is inflamed and smooth because of atrophy of the papillae (glossitis). Note the color of the patient's skin to see if it is pale with poor turgor. Note the color of the patient's sclera, which may be pearly white to bluish. Inspect the patient's fingernails to check for brittleness; note the shape of the fingernails, which may be spoon-shaped with central depressions and raised borders. Check the patient's hair to see if it is brittle and easily broken. In later stages, ankle edema may be present. Note any breathlessness or rapid breathing. Auscultate for heart sounds, noting rapid heart rate or a functional systolic murmur.

PSYCHOSOCIAL. Patients may be anxious or fearful about symptoms that have made it difficult for them to function at their usual level of energy. Discomfort from oral mucosa symptoms may prove upsetting. A pregnant patient may have additional stress over the well-being of the baby. Some patients may be resistant to proposed changes that would disrupt long-held eating patterns or anxious about finding funds to eat the proscribed diet. Patients may also be upset about body changes such as pallor and weight loss. Children may have behavioral disturbances, difficulty in school, growth impairment, and psychiatric disorders such as bipolar disorders or anxiety disorder.

Diagnostic Highlights

Test	Normal Result	Abnormality With Condition	Explanation
Bone marrow biopsy	Normal cells	Cells show absent staining for iron	Cells are iron deficient
Complete blood count	RBCs 3.6–5.8 million/mcL	Decreased; normal unless infection is present	Cells are iron deficient; as hematocrit falls below 30%, hypochromic microcytic cells appear, followed by a decrease in MCV
	White blood cells (WBCs) 4,500–11,100/mcL		Usually the WBC count is normal unless other conditions, such as infection, occur
	Hemoglobin 11.7–17.3 g/dL	Decreased	Cells are iron deficient
	Hematocrit 36%–52%	Decreased	Cells are iron deficient
	Mean corpuscular volume (MCV) 77–103/mm^3	Decreased	Cells are iron deficient
Serum ferritin	10–263 ng/dL	< 10 ng/dL in women; < 20 ng/dL in men	Cells are iron deficient

Other Tests: Serum iron, total iron-binding capacity, reticulocyte hemoglobin content, hemoglobin electrophoresis, peripheral smear, hemoglobin A$_2$, fetal hemoglobin; urine tests for hemosiderinuria and hemoglobinuria

PRIMARY NURSING DIAGNOSIS

DIAGNOSIS. Decreased activity tolerance related to imbalance between oxygen supply and demand as evidenced by leg cramps, fatigue, and/or shortness of breath on exertion

OUTCOMES. Energy conservation; Self-care: Activities of daily living; Ambulation; Circulation status; Immobility consequences: Physiological; Mobility; Nutritional status: Energy; Symptom severity

INTERVENTIONS. Nutrition management; Medication management; Energy management; Exercise promotion; Exercise therapy: Ambulation; Vital signs monitoring

PLANNING AND IMPLEMENTATION

Collaborative

The two primary goals of treatment are to diagnose and correct the underlying cause of the iron deficiency and to correct the iron deficit. Medication therapy involves administering supplemental iron, which often shows results in the form of increased patient energy within 48 hours. Blood transfusions are not recommended for iron supplementation and should not be used to treat IDA unless there is cerebrovascular or cardiopulmonary compromise. Dietary supplementation of iron-rich food is needed to complement therapy and serve as a preventive model against future recurrence of the anemia. Pregnant persons may also need to take prenatal vitamins and iron supplements.

Pharmacologic Highlights

Medication or Drug Class	Dosage	Description	Rationale
Supplemental iron	Varies with drug	Oral therapy: Ferrous sulfate (Feratab ferrous citrate (Auryxia); carbonyl iron (Feosol)	Increases iron stores
Supplemental iron	25–100 mg IV or deep IM daily	Parenteral therapy: Iron dextran complex	Iron dextran complex (INFeD) is the preferred medication for IM injections; pregnant and older patients with severe IDA; drug may be given as total-dose IV infusion of iron dextran complex in a sodium chloride solution after a small test dose is given to check for allergic reaction

Independent

Nursing interventions focus on preventing infections, promoting comfort, and teaching the patient. Patients with IDA are apt to have other nutritional deficiencies that place them at risk for infection. Use good hand-washing techniques and encourage the patient to avoid contact with people with known upper respiratory infections. If the patient experiences discomfort from oral lesions, provide mouth care. To limit activity intolerance, allow rest periods between all activities. Before the patient's discharge, arrange for home health follow-up if needed.

Teach the patient and significant others the causal relationships between bleeding tendencies and poor diet in relation to this anemia. Discuss the need to pace activities and allow for periods of rest. Emphasize to the patient the need for a well-balanced diet rich in iron; provide a list of iron-rich foods. Consider a dietary consultation to discuss ways to eat nutritionally and still consider the patient's budget. Explain that any excess in iron stores may cause toxicity. Teach the patient that certain foods and medications—such as milk and antacids—interfere with the absorption of iron. Explain that stools normally turn greenish to black in color with iron therapy and that constipation may occur. Iron-rich foods, such as fresh vegetables and red meat, tend to be expensive, so budget planning activities or help with food assistance programs may be essential. A social service referral or arranging of home care needs may be necessary. Parents of infants may need follow-up home visits to ensure that the growth and development of the child are progressing normally.

Evidence-Based Practice and Health Policy

Li, N., Zhao, G., Wu, W., Zhang, M., Liu, W., Chen, Q., & Wang, X. (2020). The efficacy and safety of vitamin C for iron supplementation in adult patients with iron deficiency anemia: A randomized clinical trial. *JAMA Network Open, 3,* 1–9.

- The authors sought to determine whether the effects of oral iron supplements alone are equivalent to a regimen of oral iron supplements plus vitamin C in the treatment of IDA. Adult patients ($N = 440$) with newly diagnosed IDA were enrolled. Patients were randomized to receive a 100-mg oral iron tablet plus 200 mg of vitamin C or a 100-mg iron tablet alone every 8 hours daily for 3 months. The primary outcome was the change in hemoglobin level from baseline to 2 weeks of treatment.
- The authors found that among patients with IDA, oral iron supplements alone were equivalent to oral iron supplements plus vitamin C in improving hemoglobin recovery and iron absorption. These findings suggest that on-demand vitamin C supplements are not essential to take along with oral iron supplements for patients with IDA.

DOCUMENTATION GUIDELINES

• Physical findings: Oral mucosa alterations; weight loss; skin turgor
• Response to activity; ability to maintain activities of daily living
• Laboratory results: Reduced level of hemoglobin, RBCs, hematocrit, MCV
• Response to iron supplement therapy, side effects

DISCHARGE AND HOME HEALTHCARE GUIDELINES

Teach the patient that a well-balanced diet rich in both iron and iron supplements is necessary to prevent a recurrence of the anemia and provide a list of iron-rich foods. Advise continuation of iron supplementation therapy even after the patient begins to feel better. Teach the route, dosage, side effects, and indications for use of iron supplements. Infection is a possibility because of the patient's weakened condition. Therefore, stress the importance of meticulous wound care, good hand-washing techniques, and periodic dental checkups. Emphasize the need for the patient to immediately report any signs of infection to the physician, such as fever or chills.

Irritable Bowel Syndrome

DRG Category: 391
Mean LOS: 4.9 days
Description: MEDICAL: Esophagitis, Gastroenteritis, and Miscellaneous Digestive Disorders With Major Complication or Comorbidity

Irritable bowel syndrome (IBS), sometimes called *spastic colon*, is the most common digestive disorder in the United States with a prevalence as high as 10% to 20% of the population. It is a poorly understood syndrome of diarrhea, constipation, flatus, and abdominal pain that causes a great deal of stress and embarrassment to its victims. People often suffer with it for years before seeking medical attention.

Although people with IBS have a gastrointestinal (GI) tract that appears normal, colonic smooth muscle function is often abnormal. The autonomic nervous system, which innervates the large bowel, fails to provide the normal contractions interspaced with relaxations that propel stool smoothly forward. Excessive spasm and peristalsis lead to constipation or diarrhea, or both. Generally, patients with IBS have either diarrhea- or constipation-predominant syndrome. Although complications are unusual, they include diverticulitis, colon cancer, and chronic inflammatory bowel disease; IBS, however, does not increase mortality or the risk of inflammatory bowel disease or cancer.

CAUSES

IBS is a disorder of GI motility. Its exact cause remains unknown, although there is a familial link in about one-third of cases. Theories of IBS include alterations in the intestinal biome (fecal microflora and small bowel bacterial overgrowth), microscopic inflammation, dietary intolerance, and enhanced perception of motility and visceral pain. It is not caused by nerves or poor diet. Both stress and intolerance for some foods, however, can precipitate attacks. Other triggers include some types of abdominal surgery, acute illness that has disrupted bowel function, prolonged use of antibiotics, exposure to toxins, and emotional trauma. Ingestion of caffeine, alcohol, and other gastric stimulants and lactose intolerance seem to play roles for many individuals. The course of the disease is usually specific to the patient, who can identify the individual precipitating factors for exacerbations. Risk factors include smoking, frequent alcohol consumption, younger age (late 20s), being female, family history, depression, migraine headaches, and fibromyalgia.

GENETIC CONSIDERATIONS

There is some evidence that IBS runs in families, but it is likely a complex disorder with contributions from several genetic and environmental factors. Relatives of an individual with IBS are two to three times more likely to develop IBS. Numerous candidate genes have been proposed that may increase susceptibility. These include serotonin transporter and receptor gene polymorphisms (*SLC6A4*, 5-HT2A, 5-HT3A, and 5-HT3E), among others.

SEX AND LIFE SPAN CONSIDERATIONS

Most newly diagnosed patients are young women in their 20s or early 30s. Some recall at the time of diagnosis that as children they experienced abdominal pain or changes in bowel habits. The incidence of newly diagnosed IBS is rare over age 50 years. Fewer than one-third of the cases of IBS are in men.

HEALTH DISPARITIES AND SEXUAL/GENDER MINORITY HEALTH

IBS affects people in all groups, but there is some evidence that it is more common in White persons and Jewish persons than other groups. Sexual and gender minority status has no known effect on the risk for IBS.

GLOBAL HEALTH CONSIDERATIONS

Western Europe and the United States have similar prevalence statistics. The prevalence of IBS in developed countries is likely higher than in developing countries. These differences are likely because of sociocultural issues, eating patterns, and strategies of healthcare management.

ASSESSMENT

HISTORY. The 2016 Rome IV criteria are used to diagnose IBS: Patients must have recurrent abdominal pain on average of at least 1 day per week during the previous 3 months and associated with two or more of the following: (1) defecation that is increased or unchanged by defecation; (2) a change in stool frequency; (3) a change in stool form or appearance. The Rome IV criteria also include supporting symptoms: altered stool frequency, altered stool form, altered stool passage, mucorrhea, and abdominal bloating or distention.

Patients describe a variety of symptoms and a range of manifestations. Ask the patient to describe the usual bowel habits and have the patient detail patterns when there is no discomfort and when discomfort occurs. Determine if GI symptoms increase after meals and if pain occurs. Pain is often cramping in nature and may be accompanied by nausea, belching, flatus, bloating, and sometimes anorexia. As the disease progresses, the patient may suffer fatigue and anxiety related to the many attempts to control the symptoms and lead a normal life. For some individuals with this disorder, lifestyle is dictated by the need to remain close to a bathroom, which limits both occupation and social life.

PHYSICAL EXAMINATION. Symptoms that are reported most often are **pain in the left lower quadrant, abdominal distention, diarrhea,** and **constipation,** especially alternating bouts of the latter two. The pain may increase after eating and be relieved after a bowel movement. They may experience clear or whitish mucoid diarrhea. The patient often has a healthy appearance without weight loss or discomfort. With auscultation of the abdomen, normal bowel sounds may be heard, although they may be quiet during constipation. Tympanic sounds may be heard over loops of filled bowel. Although palpation often discloses a relaxed abdomen, it may reveal diffuse tenderness, which becomes worse if the sigmoid colon is palpable. The patient may have pain on rectal examination but does not usually experience rectal bleeding.

PSYCHOSOCIAL. Many patients have consulted physicians who fail to take IBS seriously, telling them to eat a high-fiber diet and relax. Unfortunately, a high-fiber diet, which is good for ordinary constipation, often makes the irritable bowel worse. As the person suffers more frequent bouts of diarrhea and constipation, any attempts to relax become futile. Anxiety over control of symptoms makes the symptoms of IBS worse, creating a vicious circle that becomes hard to break. Depression over the inability to control one's bodily functions or lead a normal life sometimes becomes a serious problem.

Diagnostic Highlights

Test	Normal Result	Abnormality With Condition	Explanation
Flexible sigmoidoscopy or colonoscopy	Visualization of normal sigmoid and colon	Intense spastic contractions; mucosa appears normal (smooth and pink)	Flexible sigmoidoscopy in adults younger than 40 yr; colonoscopy in adults older than 40 yr
Computed tomography, magnetic resonance imaging	Normal abdominal structures	May have a normal examination; checks for enteritis or tumor	Rules out other pathology

Other Tests: Often diagnostic testing will not occur unless the patient has weight loss, iron deficiency anemia, or a family history of GI illness. Investigation may include stool sample for ova and parasites, enteric pathogens, leukocytes, and *Clostridium difficile* toxin. Additional tests are complete blood count, serological tests, serum albumin, stool for guaiac (occult blood), and abdominal x-ray.

PRIMARY NURSING DIAGNOSIS

DIAGNOSIS. Acute pain related to abdominal cramping as evidenced by self-reports of pain, facial grimacing, and/or protective behavior

OUTCOMES. Comfort status; Pain control; Pain level; Symptom severity; Knowledge: Pain management

INTERVENTIONS. Comfort; Medication management; Analgesic administration; Anxiety reduction; Pain management: Acute

PLANNING AND IMPLEMENTATION

Collaborative

As the symptoms worsen during the stress of other physical illnesses or trauma, fluid volume deficit may become a serious problem. It is usually treated by hypotonic IV solutions such as half-strength normal saline, sometimes with a potassium supplement. If the diarrhea continues to be severe, antidiarrheal and antianxiety agents may be prescribed for a short period. Diarrhea, constipation, and abdominal pain are treated by a combination of drugs, diet, and attempts to establish an exercise routine that promotes normal bowel function.

For many years, diet recommendations included the addition of fiber and bulk. Recent reviews of evidence have not found that fiber or bulking agents are beneficial. Current recommendations are adequate water intake, avoidance of caffeine, avoidance of legumes (to decrease bloating), and limiting lactose and fructose. Generally, a gluten-free diet is not recommended, but experts believe that a subset of people with IBS have a gluten allergy, because their symptoms improve when they restrict gluten. Several diets under consideration are increasing probiotics, decreasing fermentable oligosaccharides, disaccharides, monosaccharides, and polyols (FODMAPs). Some specialists suggest that probiotics may be helpful for treating symptoms, but the appropriate treatment protocol and target population are unclear. Whether or not psychological treatment improves IBS is controversial. Possible choices are cognitive behavioral therapy and hypnotherapy.

Pharmacologic Highlights

Medication or Drug Class	Dosage	Description	Rationale
IBS agents	Varies with drugs	Lubiprostone, alosetron, linaclotide, eluxadoline	Enhances chloride-rich intestinal fluid secretions to treat constipation
Antidiarrheal agents	Varies with drug	Diphenoxylate hydrochloride with atropine sulfate (Lomotil); loperamide (Imodium)	Decrease cramping and diarrhea; used only during an acute episode because they have a narcotic base and could easily lead to dependency
Antispasmodic agents	Varies with drug	Dicyclomine hydrochloride (Bentyl); hyoscyamine (Anaspaz); propantheline bromide (Pro-Banthine); hyoscyamine (Levsin, Levbid)	Relieve abdominal cramping and spasms

Independent

The patient with IBS needs encouragement to eat meals at regular intervals, to chew the food slowly to help promote normal bowel function, and to drink eight glasses of water daily. Most of the fluid intake should be at times other than mealtime. Foods to avoid include alcohol, caffeine, and anything that may irritate the GI tract. For example, if milk or milk products or wheat or wheat products cause cramping or discomfort, they should be avoided. During acute episodes, it is important to monitor fluid balance and the patient's state of hydration.

Incorporating regular exercise in the daily routine may be helpful in controlling GI motility, but strenuous exercise is not desirable. Reassure the patient that stress does not cause the illness, even though it may be a major factor in its severity. Refer patients to a counselor if anxiety and stress management might help manage the condition.

Evidence-Based Practice and Health Policy

Staudacher, H., Ralph, F., Irving, P., Whelan, K., & Lomer, M. (2020). Nutrient intake, diet quality, and diet diversity in irritable bowel syndrome and the impact of the low FODMAP diet. *Journal of the Academy of Nutrition and Dietetics, 120,* 535–547.

- The authors' aim was to evaluate habitual nutrient intake, diet quality, and diversity in IBS and the effect of a 4-week diet low in fermentable oligosaccharides, disaccharides, monosaccharides, and polyols (FODMAP). Data from two randomized controlled trials were included for this secondary analysis. Participants were randomized to low FODMAP diet or control diet. Habitual (usual) dietary intake at baseline and after a 4-week intervention period was measured using 7-day food records.
- When examining habitual intake of individuals with IBS, fiber intake was low, with only six (5%) achieving the target (30 g/day). In those receiving low FODMAP advice, there was no

difference in intake of most nutrients compared with controls. This study demonstrates many individuals with IBS fail to meet dietary reference values for multiple nutrients.

DOCUMENTATION GUIDELINES

- Physical response: Hydration, GI assessment, frequency and consistency of bowel movements, level of discomfort
- Emotional response: Level of stress, mood and affect, coping ability
- Response to medications
- Nutritional status: Tolerance to food, body weight, appetite

DISCHARGE AND HOME HEALTHCARE GUIDELINES

Help the patient set a long-term goal to regain control of elimination patterns with manageable short-term goals to reduce stress. Progressive muscle relaxation helps relieve the tension that often stimulates stress-related diarrhea. Explain that as the patient experiences less frequent diarrhea, the patient begins to relax even more. Teach the patient about the disease, the treatment, and how to control the symptoms. Explain that the prognosis for control of the disease depends largely on the establishment of normal bowel habits and a plan for stress management. Explain all medications, including the dosage, action, route, and possible side effects. Explore the patient's dietary patterns and provide a dietary consultation if it is appropriate.

Junctional Dysrhythmias

DRG Category:	309
Mean LOS:	2.9 days
Description:	MEDICAL: Cardiac Arrhythmias and Conduction Disorders With Complication or Comorbidity

Cardiac rhythms that are generated from the area around the atrioventricular (AV) junction node are termed *junctional dysrhythmias*. They occur either as an automatic tachycardia or as an escape mechanism when a bradycardic rhythm drops below the intrinsic rate of the junctional pacemaker, which is 40 to 60 beats a minute. Impulses produced in the junction do not necessarily result in an atrial contraction that precedes the ventricular contraction. On the electrocardiogram, atrial contraction may be seen as retrograde P waves. This lack of coordination leads to a loss of ventricular filling during the last part of diastole; this loss of what is termed the *atrial kick* may reduce cardiac output by about 20% to 25%.

When the junctional pacemaker paces at its inherent rate, it produces what is called a *passive junctional rhythm* or a *junctional escape rhythm*. When it paces between 60 and 100 beats per minute, the term *accelerated junctional rhythm* is used. Junctional tachycardia occurs when the junctional pacemaker paces the heart at a rate between 100 and 160 beats per minute. Isolated complexes that arise from the junctional tissue are called *premature junctional complexes* (PJCs) if they come earlier than the expected sinus beat or *junctional escape beats* if they come later.

CAUSES

Junctional tissue may take over as the heart's pacemaker if the sinus node fails to produce an impulse or if that impulse is blocked in its conduction through the AV node. Junctional escape rhythms may be caused by digitalis toxicity, acute infections, oxygen deficiency, inferior wall myocardial infarction, or stimulation of the vagus nerve.

If the junctional tissue becomes irritable or increasingly automatic, it may override the sinus node and pace at a faster rate. Nonparoxysmal junctional tachycardia is often the result of enhanced automaticity, usually called irritability, which can be the result of digitalis toxicity, damage to the AV junction after an inferior myocardial infarction or rheumatic fever, open heart surgery, or excessive administration of catecholamines or caffeine. Paroxysmal junctional tachycardia (a rapid rhythm that starts and stops suddenly) is usually the result of a reentry mechanism.

PJCs may be found in healthy individuals or they may be the result of excessive intake of stimulants such as caffeine, tobacco, or sympathomimetic drugs. Digitalis toxicity or use of alcohol may also cause PJCs. Junctional escape beats occur after pauses in the heart's rhythm. When the sinus node fails to fire, the junctional pacemaker should take over impulse initiation. They may occur normally in people during periods of increased vagal tone (increased activity of the vagus nerve, which slows the firing of the sinoatrial node) such as during sleep.

GENETIC CONSIDERATIONS

Studies are ongoing into the inheritable origins of cardiac rhythm. Mutations in the gene encoding the gap junction protein connexin 40 (*GJA5*) are associated with atrial fibrillation. AV conduction block has been associated with various mutations in ion channels, including the sodium channel *SCN5A*, and transcription factors *NKX2-5* and *TBX5*.

SEX AND LIFE SPAN CONSIDERATIONS

Because of the common causes of junctional dysrhythmias, they occur more often in older patients with cardiac disease. They can occur in all people. In children and adolescents, and in young adult athletes, junctional escape rhythms may occur during times of increased vagal tone, particularly during sleep. They occur in males and females with equal prevalence.

HEALTH DISPARITIES AND SEXUAL/GENDER MINORITY HEALTH

The Centers for Disease Control and Prevention report that 11.5% of White persons, 9.5% of Black persons, 7.4% of Hispanic persons, and 6.0% of Asian persons have heart disease. Black, Indigenous, and other people of color are known to receive care less often guided by standard cardiac care guidelines than White persons. Unless patients have health insurance, White patients are more likely to receive coronary angiograms and other coronary interventions than Black and Hispanic patients. Black, Indigenous, and other people of color are also less likely to be referred to cardiologists and cardiac surgeons than White persons (Batchelor et al., 2019).

Transgender is a term used to describe persons whose gender identity is different from their sex assigned at birth. Approximately 1% of the U.S. population identify themselves as transgender. Sexual and gender minority persons have higher odds for multiple chronic conditions, cancer, and poor quality of life, and are more apt to have disabilities than cisgender males and females. (Cisgender is a term used to describe persons whose gender identity and gender expression are aligned with their assigned sex listed on their birth certificate.) Gender-affirming hormone therapy is the use of hormone therapy for gender transition or gender affirmation and can be masculinizing or feminizing. It may also affect cardiovascular health in transgender females. In a large sample, researchers have found that transgender men and women are more likely to be overweight than cisgender women. Compared to cisgender women, transgender women reported higher rates of diabetes, angina/coronary disease, and myocardial infarction. Gender-nonconforming men and women reported higher odds of myocardial infarction than cisgender women. Transgender women also had higher rates of any cardiovascular disease than cisgender men (Cacerese, Jackman, et al., 2020).

GLOBAL HEALTH CONSIDERATIONS

No global data are available, but it is reasonable to expect that junctional dysrhythmias exist in all populations around the world.

☀ ASSESSMENT

HISTORY. Many patients with suspected cardiac dysrhythmias describe a history of symptoms that indicate periods of decreased cardiac output, although it can occur without symptoms. Although some junctional dysrhythmias are asymptomatic, some patients report a history of dizziness, fatigue, activity intolerance, a "fluttering" in their chest, shortness of breath, and chest pain. In particular, question the patient about the onset, duration, and characteristics of the symptoms and the events that precipitated them. Obtain a complete history of all illnesses, dietary restrictions, and activity restrictions and a current medication history.

PHYSICAL EXAMINATION. Symptoms are usually rate dependent and may include **palpitations, dizziness, fatigue, activity intolerance**, and **bradycardia**. A passive junctional rhythm (junctional escape rhythm) is a bradycardia. Rates between 40 and 60 beats per minute with a loss of the atrial component to ventricular filling can produce signs of low cardiac output, such as syncope or lightheadedness. A patient who is experiencing accelerated junctional rhythm with a rate between 60 and 100 beats per minute is asymptomatic if cardiac status can accommodate the 20% to 25% reduction in cardiac output from loss of atrial kick. Otherwise, symptoms such as syncope and dizziness may occur.

Isolated PJCs usually produce no symptoms other than some palpitations and the sensation of a "skipped beat." Junctional tachycardia produces symptoms common to other supraventricular tachycardias. A junctional tachycardia may produce signs of low cardiac output and poor coronary perfusion. Common symptoms include labored breathing, shortness of breath, chest pain, feeling lightheaded, lowered blood pressure, and fainting.

PSYCHOSOCIAL. Patient response may vary depending on the origin of the dysrhythmia. Certainly, when the heart is beating unusually fast or slow or when palpitations are noticed, the patient may become distressed. Any disturbance in the brain's sensory apparatus as produced by low cardiac output can intensify fear or anxiety.

Diagnostic Highlights

Test	Normal Result	Abnormality With Condition	Explanation
12-lead electrocardiogram	Regular sinus rhythm	• Junctional escape: Heart rate of 40–60 beats/ min with regular R to R interval; P wave may be inverted and precedes the QRS with a short PR interval • Premature junctional beats: Early beat disrupts rhythm; P wave may be inverted and precedes the QRS with a short PR interval • Junctional tachycardia: Ventricular rate is 100–160 beats/min and regular; P wave may be inverted and precedes the QRS with a short PR interval	Detects specific conduction defects and monitors the patient's cardiac response to electrolyte imbalances, drug effects, and toxicities

Other Tests: Pulse oximetry, ambulatory or Holter monitoring: to provide a 12- to 24-hour continuous recording of myocardial electrical activity as the patient performs normal daily activities. Two-dimensional echocardiography, stress echocardiography, electrophysiological studies.

PRIMARY NURSING DIAGNOSIS

DIAGNOSIS. Risk for decreased cardiac tissue perfusion and ineffective cerebral tissue perfusion as evidenced by palpitations, bradycardia, dizziness, fatigue, and/or activity intolerance

OUTCOMES. Circulation status; Cardiac pump effectiveness; Knowledge: Cardiac disease management; Tissue perfusion: Cardiopulmonary, Cerebral, Peripheral; Vital signs; Medication response

INTERVENTIONS. Dysrhythmia management; Emergency care; Vital signs monitoring; Cardiac care; Oxygen therapy; Fluid/electrolyte management; Medication administration

PLANNING AND IMPLEMENTATION

Collaborative

People who are asymptomatic may need no therapy, particularly if the rhythm is due to increased vagal tone. Treatment of junctional dysrhythmias usually depends on the heart rate. Infrequent PJCs may also be tolerated as benign or by attempting to alleviate the cause. Stimulants such as caffeine, tobacco, and sympathomimetic drugs may be discontinued to improve symptoms. If digitalis toxicity is the cause, digitalis may be withheld, or the patient may receive digoxin immune FAB (Digibind). If PJCs are frequent, they may be suppressed by administration of an antidysrhythmic such as phenytoin. In contrast, junctional escape rhythm is a marked bradycardia that may be treated with IV atropine sulfate to increase the rate. In rare circumstances, a cardiac pacemaker is necessary if the bradycardia does not respond to treatment or if it is due to sick sinus syndrome or heart block.

An accelerated junctional rhythm, with a rate between 60 and 100 beats per minute, rarely compromises the cardiac output. In that situation, the patient is usually just observed. In contrast, if the ventricular rate is faster than 150 beats per minute such as in paroxysmal junctional tachycardia, a vagal maneuver, medications such as adenosine, or cardioversion may be indicated.

Pharmacologic Highlights

Medication or Drug Class	Dosage	Description	Rationale
Atropine sulfate	0.5–1 mg or 0.04 mg/kg IV daily 5 min, up to 3 mg total	Anticholinergic	Accelerates heart rate if patient has symptomatic bradycardia
Antidysrhythmics	Varies with drug	Phenytoin, amiodarone, flecanide	Suppress frequent PJCs or manages narrow complex tachycardia
Adenosine	6 mg IV over 1–3 sec; may repeat in 1–2 min	Antiarrhythmic	Suppresses junctional ectopic tachycardia

Other Drugs: Other drugs used for continuing significant bradycardias no matter what the origin, particularly when accompanied by hypotension, are dopamine (5–20 mcg/kg/min of IV infusion) and epinephrine (2–10 mcg/kg/min of IV infusion). If the patient is digitalis toxic, digoxin immune FAB may be used to prevent binding of digitalis molecules to tissues.

Independent

The nurse's role is one of monitoring and support. Support the patient who is experiencing symptoms from any rhythm disturbance. Maintain the patient's airway, breathing, and circulation.

To maximize oxygen available to the myocardium, encourage the patient to rest in bed until the symptoms are treated and subside. Remain with the patient to ensure rest and to allay anxiety. Discuss any potential precipitating factors with the patient. For some patients, strategies to reduce stress or lifestyle changes help limit the incidence of dysrhythmias. Teach the patient to reduce the amount of caffeine intake in the diet. If appropriate, encourage the patient to become involved in an exercise program or a smoking-cessation group. Provide emotional support and information about the dysrhythmia, the precipitating factors, and mechanisms to limit the dysrhythmia. If the patient is at risk for electrolyte imbalance, teach the patient any dietary considerations to prevent electrolyte depletion.

Evidence-Based Practice and Health Policy

Chen, Y., Nasrawi, D., Massey, D., Johnston, A., Keller, K., & Kunst, E. (2021). Final-year nursing students' foundational knowledge and self-assessed confidence in interpreting cardiac arrhythmias: A cross-sectional study. *Nurse Education Today*. Advance online publication. https://doi.org/10.1016/j.nedt.2020.104699

- The authors wanted to examine final-year nursing students' foundational knowledge and self-assessed confidence in interpreting cardiac dysrhythmias including junctional dysrhythmias. The authors developed an online survey to examine final-year nursing students' foundational knowledge and their self-assessed confidence when interpreting cardiac rhythms. A total of 114 participants at two Australian universities completed surveys, representing a response rate of 22%.
- More than 70% of the participants were able to interpret asystole, sinus rhythm, and sinus bradycardia. Over 50% correctly identified ventricular tachycardia, atrial flutter, sinus tachycardia, atrial fibrillation, and ventricular fibrillation. Less than 15% of the participants were able to interpret junctional rhythm, paced rhythm, and unifocal/multifocal premature ventricular contractions. Nursing curricula need to be supported and strategies need to be implemented to standardize educational electrocardiogram interpretation programs, which are critical to improving final-year nursing students' foundational knowledge.

DOCUMENTATION GUIDELINES

- Rhythm strips: Record and analyze according to hospital protocol, note the monitoring lead and document any change in leads
- Patient symptoms and vital signs with any change or new onset of dysrhythmia
- Patient's response to symptoms
- Patient's response to management

DISCHARGE AND HOME HEALTHCARE GUIDELINES

Make sure the patient understands the role of stimulants in generating dysrhythmias. Explain the importance of taking all medications before discharge. Explain the ordered dosage, route, action, and possible adverse effects. If the patient has required a pacemaker, make sure that the patient understands the type of pacemaker and the steps to take to make sure the pacemaker is functioning appropriately. Explain the hazards and limitations; provide written materials on follow-up after insertion. Teach the patient to monitor the pulse and to report to the physician any significant changes in rate or regularity.

Kidney Cancer

DRG Category:	656
Mean LOS:	7.5 days
Description:	SURGICAL: Kidney and Ureter Procedures for Neoplasm With Major Complication or Comorbidity
DRG Category:	687
Mean LOS:	4.3 days
Description:	MEDICAL: Kidney and Urinary Tract Neoplasms With Complication or Comorbidity

Kidney cancer is rare, accounting for about 3% of all adult cancers. The American Cancer Society estimates that 76,080 people will be newly diagnosed with kidney cancer in 2021, and approximately 13,780 people will die from the disease. For unknown reasons, the incidence of kidney cancers is increasing in the United States, where it is the 10th most common cancer. Kidney cancers are classified by cell type. The three most commonly seen in adults are renal cell carcinoma, transitional cell carcinoma, and sarcoma. Renal cell carcinoma arises in the renal tubules and accounts for more than 90% of kidney cancers. The other types of kidney cancer, transitional cell carcinoma and sarcomas, make up the remaining 10%. Most kidney cancers occur in one kidney only (unilateral) and are large and nodular. Renal metastases from other sites are unusual.

Renal cell tumors usually grow as a single mass; however, several tumors can form in one kidney. Because even large tumors may not cause pain, often the tumor is found only after it has become significant in size. Most are found before metastasis occurs, and often they are discovered incidentally during screening procedures that involve computed tomography (CT) scans. There are five main types of renal cell carcinoma, all diagnosed by microscopic examination: clear cell, pupillary, chromophobe, collecting duct, and unclassified. Renal cell cancer is also graded on a scale of 1 (have a cell nuclei that is similar to a normal kidney cell nuclei) to 4 (have a cell nuclei that looks very different from a normal kidney cell nuclei). Staging is a far better predictor of prognosis than grading.

The 5-year survival rate is as high as 90% if the cancer is confined to the kidneys and as low as 13% if metastasis has occurred. Complications from kidney cancer include renal hemorrhage and metastases to the lungs, central nervous system, and gastrointestinal tract. If it is left untreated, kidney cancer causes death.

CAUSES

Although the exact cause remains unknown, several factors seem to predispose a person to kidney cancer. Smokers increase their risk of developing kidney cancer by 40%. A link also exists between kidney cancer and occupational exposure to cadmium (found in batteries), asbestos, some herbicides, benzene, and organic solvents, particularly trichloroethylene. Family history, obesity, hypertension, certain medications (NSAIDs, diuretics), end-stage renal disease, and sedentary lifestyles are also risk factors for developing renal cell cancer.

GENETIC CONSIDERATIONS

Mutations in several genes can lead to kidney cancer as part of genetic syndromes, including von Hippel-Lindau (VHL). Renal cell carcinoma is a leading cause of mortality in VHL and occurs in about 25% to 40% of affected persons. About 80% of VHL is transmitted in an autosomal dominant pattern; the remaining 20% is due to new mutations. There is a hereditary form of papillary renal cell carcinoma associated with mutations in several genes, most notably *MET*, and there have been documented cases of familial renal cell carcinoma.

SEX AND LIFE SPAN CONSIDERATIONS

Kidney cancer occurs twice as frequently in men (who are more likely to be smokers and exposed to cancer-causing chemicals in the workplace) than women, commonly after age 45 years with a peak incidence between the ages of 65 and 74 years. The average age at diagnosis is 64 years. Men also have more aggressive, larger tumors, and worse outcomes than women, perhaps because of men's smoking patterns and the presence of male hormones. Diabetes mellitus is a risk factor for kidney cancer in nonobese postmenopausal women. Children and infants diagnosed with kidney cancer usually have Wilms tumors or a tumor of the renal pelvis and, with prompt treatment, usually have a good prognosis.

HEALTH DISPARITIES AND SEXUAL/GENDER MINORITY HEALTH

People who are overweight or obese have better kidney cancer outcomes than normal and underweight people. Renal cell carcinoma is more common in Black and Native American/Alaskan Native persons than in other groups. Some sexual and gender minority persons, gay and lesbian persons in particular, have higher rates of smoking than the general population (Centers for Disease Control and Prevention, 2021), which may place them at risk for kidney cancer. Gender and sexual minority persons are a vulnerable group because people with low income, long travel distances to cancer screening sites, or who lack health insurance or paid medical leave are less likely to be treated according to cancer care guidelines (National Institutes of Health, 2021).

GLOBAL HEALTH CONSIDERATIONS

The global incidence of kidney cancer is approximately 4 per 100,000 males per year and 3 per 100,000 females per year, but it varies by region. Males may have higher rates because of higher rates of tobacco use and occupational exposure. People living in developed countries have an incidence approximately eight times higher than those in developing countries.

ASSESSMENT

HISTORY. Question the patient about the classic triad of symptoms: hematuria, pain, and an abdominal mass. The most common single symptom is painless hematuria, whereas an abdominal mass is usually a late finding. Establish the presence or absence of signs and symptoms, such as a dull aching pain in the flank area. One-third of all patients diagnosed have these symptoms. One-third of patients have no symptoms at all, and the diagnosis is made during a routine physical examination or scanning procedure for other health-related issues. The other third of patients are diagnosed after the cancer has produced symptoms related to distant metastases. Ask about the patient's smoking history, and if weight loss, fever, hypertension, or malaise has occurred.

PHYSICAL EXAMINATION. It is not unusual for the patient to have a **normal physical examination**. Occasionally, the patient appears **weak** and has an **unintentional weight loss** since the last examination. The patient may have hypertension, edema, malaise, or persistent fever unrelated to cold or flu. A small number may have manifestations of hypercalcemia such as nausea, vomiting, changes in mental status, constipation, and lethargy. The placement of the kidneys, deep within the abdomen and protected by layers of fat, makes palpation of renal masses difficult. On occasion, palpation may reveal a smooth, firm abdominal mass.

PSYCHOSOCIAL. The patient may be preparing to retire or be retired when the diagnosis is made given the average age at the time of diagnosis. Consider the patient's and significant others' ability to cope with a life-threatening illness at this life stage. The diagnosis may be met with anger. The patient diagnosed with late kidney cancer is facing a possibly terminal diagnosis. Assess support systems and consider making appropriate referrals if needed.

Diagnostic Highlights

Test	Normal Result	Abnormality With Condition	Explanation
Kidney sonogram (ultrasound)	Bilateral kidneys are properly located and of normal size with smooth outer contours	Usually a unilateral tumor in one kidney	Serves as alternative to renal dye imaging tests for people with allergies; creates oscilloscopic picture from echoes of high-frequency sound waves that pass over the flank area
Abdominal CT scan; helical or spiral CT	Bilateral kidneys are properly located and of normal size with smooth outer contours	Usually a unilateral tumor in one kidney	Produces pictures of peritoneal and retroperitoneal cavity, based on differing densities and composition of body tissues; helical or spiral CT is a new rapid CT scan that immediately shows the passage of dye through the kidney; even very small tumors are evident

Other Tests: Magnetic resonance imaging, arteriography, blood urea nitrogen, creatinine, urinalysis, and IV pyelogram. To determine if metastasis has occurred: bone scan, chest x-ray, positron emission tomography scan.

PRIMARY NURSING DIAGNOSIS

DIAGNOSIS. Impaired urinary elimination related to renal tissue destruction as evidenced by hematuria, oliguria, and/or anuria

OUTCOMES. Urinary continence; Urinary elimination; Knowledge: Medication; Knowledge: Disease process; Knowledge: Treatment regimen; Symptom severity

INTERVENTIONS. Urinary elimination management; Fluid management; Medication prescribing; Urinary catheterization; Anxiety reduction; Pain management: Acute

PLANNING AND IMPLEMENTATION

Collaborative

Depending on the stage, surgical intervention and further staging is the primary treatment for renal cell cancer. A partial nephrectomy is reserved for those patients with very small renal cell tumors, those who have cancer in both kidneys, or those who only have one kidney. In the early stages, some experts are considering molecular approaches such as sunitinib or sorafenib as adjuvant therapy. A radical nephrectomy (removing the whole kidney, the attached adrenal gland, and fatty tissue that surrounds the kidney), sometimes with lymph node removal, offers the patient the best chance for cure. The procedure is the treatment of choice for localized cancer or in patients with tumor extension into the renal vein and vena cava. Surgical intervention is not curative for disseminated disease. Because of the proximity of the kidney to the diaphragm, the surgeon may explore the pleura on the surgical side. If that occurs, the patient could return from surgery with a chest tube placed to remove blood and air from the pleural space.

Nephrectomies involve large blood vessels and place the patient at risk for postoperative hemorrhage. Frequent assessment and serial vital signs to monitor for shock are part of postoperative management. Patients undergoing a nephrectomy experience moderate to severe pain; for this reason, the anesthesiologist may place an epidural catheter during surgery for pain management with morphine sulfate or other appropriate analgesia. Monitor the patient's urinary output through the Foley catheter for adequate volume and color and consistency of urine; if the patient's urine output decreases below 40 mL per hour, notify the physician.

Depending on the final stage of the kidney cancer, the surgeon may refer the patient to an oncologist for follow-up care. Kidney cancer is resistant to radiation therapy, which is used in high doses only when metastases have occurred into areas such as the perinephric region and the lymph nodes. Chemotherapy and hormonal therapy do not affect tumor growth. Although several experimental or alternative medications are being tested, they usually have many side effects or are of limited usefulness. Cytokines, proteins that activate the immune system, are currently being investigated as an approach to treat renal cell cancer by boosting the immune system to destroy cancer cells. Immunomodulatory agents (interferon, nivolumab, interleukin-2) may be used for patients with metastatic disease. Also being investigated are "targeted therapies," which include antiangiogenesis drugs, which kill cancer cells by cutting off their blood supply. Research on treatment of kidney cancer has shown that kidney-sparing treatment may prolong life. Cryoablative therapies with laparoscopic technique or radiofrequency ablation are now being used when the tumor is small and contained.

Pharmacologic Highlights

Medication or Drug Class	Dosage	Description	Rationale
Narcotics	Varies with drug and situation; should be taken on a regular basis to be effective	Patient-controlled analgesia; patient is placed on patient-controlled analgesia pump attached to the peripheral IV site	Manage pain

Independent

Two of the most important postoperative priorities are to enhance gas exchange and to maintain the patient's comfort. Institute pulmonary care on a routine basis. Patients with a smoking history may take longer to recover normal lung function after surgery. Encourage the patient to turn, cough, and breathe deeply at least every 2 hours. Show the patient how to use diaphragmatic breathing techniques and how to splint the incision. Teach the patient how to use an incentive spirometer to improve gas exchange. Ask the patient to describe the degree of pain on a scale of 1 to 10. Instruct the patient on nonpharmacologic methods for pain relief. If the patient is receiving analgesia that is insufficient to relieve the pain, notify the physician.

Patients and their significant others are dealing with stressors that cause anxiety and fear. Spend time each day discussing their concerns, being honest about the patient's chances for recovery. If the patient experiences an unusual degree of spiritual distress, refer to a chaplain or clinical nurse specialist. The diagnosis of kidney cancer is life threatening, and the patient may need to work through the issues associated with a serious disease.

Evidence-Based Practice and Health Policy

Harrison, H., Thompson, R., Lin, Z., Rossi, S., Stewart, G., Griffin, S., & Usher-Smith, J. (2021). Risk prediction models for kidney cancer: A systematic review. *European Urology Focus, 7*(6), 1380–1390.

- The authors identify and compare published models that predict the risk of developing kidney cancer in the general population. A search identified primary research reporting or validating models predicting the risk of kidney cancer in Medline and EMBASE. The risk models

were classified using the Transparent Reporting of a multivariable prediction model for Individual Prognosis Or Diagnosis (TRIPOD) guidelines and evaluated using an accepted assessment tool.
- The search identified 62 articles that satisfied the inclusion criteria. Six of the models had been validated, two using external populations. The most commonly included risk factors were age, smoking status, and body mass index. The highest performance was seen for the models using only biomarkers to detect kidney cancer.

DOCUMENTATION GUIDELINES

- Respiratory response: Patency of airway; adequacy of ventilation (rate, quality, and presence of adventitious breath sounds); maintenance of chest tube system (suction, presence of air leaks, amount and quality of drainage)
- Incisional care: Description of dressing; appearance of wound
- Degree of pain; response to interventions to lessen pain
- Presence of complications related to the surgical procedure
- Amount of urinary output, color of urine, and patency of Foley catheter

DISCHARGE AND HOME HEALTHCARE GUIDELINES

Be sure the patient understands what medications are to be taken at home, their effects, and dosages. Explain follow-up information, such as when the physician would like to see the patient. Provide a phone number and written discharge information and arrange for a home visit from nurses if appropriate. Refer the patient and family to hospital and community services such as support groups and the American Cancer Society. Reinforce any postoperative restrictions. Explain when normal activity can be resumed. Make sure the patient understands the need to have ongoing monitoring of the disease. Annual chest x-rays and CT are recommended to check for other tumors. Emphasize lifestyle choices that can aid in recovery: quit smoking; limit alcohol to one to two drinks per day; eat more fruits, vegetables, and whole grains and less animal fat; and exercise once the patient is able.

Kidney Disease, Chronic

DRG Category:	674
Mean LOS:	7.4 days
Description:	SURGICAL: Other Kidney and Urinary Tract Procedures With Complication or Comorbidity
DRG Category:	683
Mean LOS:	3.9 days
Description:	MEDICAL: Renal Failure With Complication or Comorbidity

Chronic kidney disease (CKD), formerly known as chronic renal failure, refers to decreased renal function across a continuum of severity from mild to moderate to severe chronic kidney failure. The Centers for Disease Control and Prevention (CDC, 2021) note that more than 7 in 10 Americans have CKD, and as many as 90% of those with CKD do not know that they have the condition. It is the eighth leading cause of death in the United States. Severe CKD is fatal if it is not treated. One classification of renal failure from the Kidney Disease Outcomes Quality

Initiative, based on glomerular filtration rate (GFR; the flow rate of filtered fluid through the kidney), is as follows:

- Stage 1: Kidney damage with normal or increased GFR (> 90 mL/min/1.73 m^2)
- Stage 2: Mild reduction in GFR (60–89 mL/min/1.73 m^2)
- Stage 3: Moderate reduction in GFR (30–59 mL/min/1.73 m^2)
- Stage 4: Severe reduction in GFR (15–29 mL/min/1.73 m^2)
- Stage 5: Kidney failure (GFR < 15 mL/min/1.73 m^2 or dialysis)

The kidney has many compensatory mechanisms to support its function as it becomes diseased. Each kidney contains approximately 1 million nephrons, the functional unit of the kidney that is responsible for glomerular filtration and reabsorption of solutes and solvents. When nephrons are injured, the kidneys maintain GFR by increasing filtration and reabsorption by hypertrophy of the healthy nephrons. Waste products such as urea and creatinine begin to accumulate in the body only when the GFR drops by 50%. The ability of the kidney to compensate for early disease gives rise to the continuum of severity; many patients can maintain borderline renal function with a mild or moderate reduction in GFR for years.

All individuals with stage 5 kidney failure experience similar physiological changes, regardless of the initial cause of the disease. The kidneys are unable to perform their normal functions of excretion of wastes, concentration of urine, regulation of blood pressure, regulation of acid-base balance, and production of erythropoietin (the hormone needed for red blood cell [RBC] production and survival). Complications of CKD include uremia (accumulation of metabolic waste products in the blood and body tissues), anemia, peripheral neuropathy, sexual dysfunction, osteopenia (reduction of bone tissue), pathological fractures, fluid overload, congestive heart failure, hypertension, pericarditis, electrolyte imbalances (hypocalcemia, hyperkalemia, hyperphosphatemia), metabolic acidosis, esophagitis, and gastritis.

CAUSES

CKD may be caused by either kidney disease or diseases of other systems (Table 1).

• TABLE 1 Causes of Chronic Kidney Disease

CATEGORY	DISEASES
Congenital/hereditary disorders	Polycystic kidney disease, renal tubular acidosis
Connective tissue disorders	Progressive systemic sclerosis, systemic lupus erythematosus
Infections/inflammatory conditions	Chronic pyelonephritis, glomerulonephritis, tuberculosis
Vascular disease	Hypertension, renal nephrosclerosis, renal artery stenosis
Metabolic/endocrine diseases	Diabetes mellitus, gout, amyloidosis, hyperparathyroidism
Obstructive diseases	Renal calculi
Nephrotoxic conditions	Medication therapy, drug overdose

Risk factors for CKD include diabetes mellitus, hypertension, medications that are toxic to the kidney (NSAIDs, some antibiotics, contrast media), smoking, hyperlipidemia, hyperphosphatemia, infections, and shock.

GENETIC CONSIDERATIONS

Several heritable diseases can lead to CKD, including the autosomal recessive condition Alport syndrome, which causes nephropathy that is often associated with sensorineural deafness and can be transmitted as X-linked recessive, autosomal recessive, and autosomal dominant forms. Mutations in atrial natriuretic peptide receptor-1 (*NPR1*) may also contribute to nephropathy and renal failure.

SEX AND LIFE SPAN CONSIDERATIONS

Both males and females are at risk for CKD. Because of anatomical differences in urethral valves, CKD is more common in boys than girls. Experts suggest that men progress to end-stage kidney disease (ESKD) more rapidly than women. Older patients are more susceptible to some of the causes of acute kidney injury (AKI) and may therefore experience CKD more frequently. CKD as a result of other diseases (diabetes mellitus or uncontrolled hypertension) is more common in older adults simply because they have had the disease longer. It is most typically diagnosed in people who are older than 60 years.

HEALTH DISPARITIES AND SEXUAL/GENDER MINORITY HEALTH

CKD affects all groups of people, and the prevalence in various populations depends on predisposing conditions such as diabetes and hypertension. The CDC (2021) report in the United States that 16.3% of Black adults over the age of 18 years have CKD, as well as 13.6% of Hispanic persons, 12.9% of Asian persons, and 12.7% of White persons. Early stage CKD is distributed evenly across racial and ethnic groups, but the burden of ESKD is highest in Black and Hispanic persons, possibly because of high rates of diabetes mellitus and hypertension in those groups. People with low incomes have an increased risk of progressive CKD as compared to people with middle- or upper-level incomes (Nelson et al., 2020). Transgender is a term used to describe persons whose gender identity is different from their sex assigned at birth. Approximately 1% of the U.S. population identify themselves as transgender. Sexual and gender minority persons have higher odds for multiple chronic conditions, cancer, and poor quality of life, and are more apt to have disabilities than cisgender males and females. (Cisgender is a term used to describe persons whose gender identity and gender expression are aligned with their assigned sex listed on their birth certificate.) Gender-affirming hormone therapy is the use of hormone therapy for gender transition or gender affirmation and can be masculinizing or feminizing. It may also affect cardiovascular health in transgender females. Current thinking is that kidney transplantation is safe and effective for transgender patients who are on gender-affirming treatments if drug interactions and calculation of renal function are managed carefully with consideration of hormone treatments (Jue et al., 2020). Recent research suggests that transgender people have an increased incidence of hypertension (Connelly et al., 2019), placing them at risk for CKD.

GLOBAL HEALTH CONSIDERATIONS

The global incidence of CKD is increasing, with rates highest in the United States and Japan. Worldwide, CKD is a critical public health problem that is acknowledged as a common condition associated with an increased risk of cardiovascular disease. Experts estimate that the global prevalence is 9.1%. Generally, treatments for ESKD are very expensive; developing countries may not have the economic resources to treat patients with renal failure. Few patients with CKD survive in developing countries where treatment is not government sponsored.

ASSESSMENT

HISTORY. Patients with CKD in stages 1, 2, and 3 are usually asymptomatic because their kidneys are able to compensate for decreasing GFR. Patients may report a history of AKI, which has progressed to a more chronic condition, although usually patients do not become symptomatic until they have a GFR less than 35% of normal. Ask the patient about the color of the urine, whether it is clear or cloudy, and whether it is frothy. The patient may also complain of a metallic taste in the mouth, anorexia, and stomatitis. Determine if the patient experienced weight loss and muscle weakness. Elicit a gastrointestinal (GI) history with particular attention to nausea, vomiting, hematemesis, diarrhea, and constipation.

Elicit the patient's description of any central nervous system (CNS) symptoms. In stages 4 and 5, blurred vision may occur. Patients may have impaired decision making and judgment, irritability, decreased alertness, insomnia, increased extremity weakness, and signs of increasing peripheral neuropathy (decreased sensation in the extremities, hands, and feet; pain; and burning sensations).

Patients often report changes in other body systems as well. Some have idiopathic bone and joint pain in the absence of a diagnosis of arthritis. Others suffer from loss of muscle mass and nocturnal leg cramping. Men may be impotent or notice gynecomastia, and women may mention amenorrhea (absence of menses). Both may have decreased libido.

PHYSICAL EXAMINATION. All body systems of patients with stage 5 CKD are affected, with significant cardiovascular involvement. Hypertension is usually noted and may indeed be the cause of CKD. Patients often have **rapid, irregular heart rates; distended jugular veins**; and, if pericarditis is present, a **pericardial friction rub** and **distant heart sounds** that may be accompanied by cardiac tamponade. Respiratory symptoms include hyperventilation, Kussmaul breathing, dyspnea, orthopnea, and pulmonary congestion. Rales may signify fluid overload. Frothy sputum combined with shortness of breath may indicate some degree of pulmonary edema.

The renal effects of CKD are pronounced. You may smell a urine-like odor on the breath and notice a yellow-gray cast to the skin. If the patient is producing any urine at all, it may be dilute, with casts or crystals present. The skin is fragile and dry, and there may be uremic frost on the skin or open areas owing to severe scratching (pruritus) by the patient. The patient may have bruising; petechiae; brittle nails; dry, brittle hair; gum ulcerations; or bleeding. The patient may appear malnourished with muscle wasting. If the patient has been followed for CKD, there may already be access sites created in preparation for dialysis. Assess the sites for patency (an arteriovenous fistula should have a palpable thrill and audible bruit) and signs of infection.

When you assess the CNS, you may find that the patient has difficulty with ambulation because of altered motor function, gait abnormalities, bone and joint pain, and peripheral neuropathy. The patient's mental status may range from mild behavioral changes to profound loss of consciousness and seizures. Electrolyte imbalances may result in signs of hypocalcemia (see **Hypocalcemia**), muscle cramps, and twitching.

PSYCHOSOCIAL. Patients with CKD present complex and difficult challenges to caregivers. Many have personality and cognitive changes. Apathy, irritability, and fatigue, which are part of the disease process, are common and interfere with interpersonal relationships. Sexual dysfunction is common. A careful assessment of the patient's capabilities, home situation, available support systems, financial resources, and coping abilities is important before any nursing interventions can be planned.

Diagnostic Highlights

Test	Normal Result	Abnormality With Condition	Explanation
Blood urea nitrogen	8–21 mg/dL	Elevated	Kidneys cannot excrete wastes
Serum creatinine	0.5–1.2 mg/dL	> 3 mg/dL	Kidneys cannot excrete wastes
Creatine clearance	Females: 75–115 mL/min/1.73 m²; males: 85–125 mL/min/1.73 m²	< 95% decrease	Acute damage to the kidney limits ability to clear creatinine

(highlight box continues on page 716)

> **Diagnostic Highlights (continued)**
>
> Other Tests: Urinalysis; complete blood count; erythrocyte sedimentation rate; hemodynamic monitoring; renal ultrasound; radionuclide scanning; magnetic resonance angiography; renal biopsy; serum levels of sodium, potassium, magnesium, and phosphorus; arterial blood gases

PRIMARY NURSING DIAGNOSIS

DIAGNOSIS. Excess fluid volume related to compromised regulatory mechanisms as evidenced by elevated heart rate, distended jugular veins, and/or hyperventilation

OUTCOMES. Fluid balance; Hydration; Circulation status; Cardiac pump effectiveness; Urinary elimination; Vital signs

INTERVENTIONS. Fluid monitoring; Fluid/electrolyte management; IV therapy; Medication management; Hemodialysis therapy; Vital signs monitoring

✺ PLANNING AND IMPLEMENTATION

Collaborative

Aggressive blood pressure control is important through all the stages of CKD to promote kidney function and slow the progression to CKD. In the early stages of CKD, the goals are to delay or halt the progression of the disease, treat the manifestations of CKD, and plan for renal replacement therapy. Patients who have progressed to stage 5 CKD, or ESKD, require either dialysis or renal transplantation. Renal transplantation is the treatment of choice for many patients; more than 375,000 kidney transplants have been performed in the United States, with 110,000 people on the kidney transplant waiting list. The transplanted kidney may come from a living donor or a cadaver. One-year survival rates are currently 90% to 95%. The new organ is placed in the iliac fossa. The original kidneys are not generally removed unless there is an indication, such as infection, for removing them. The greatest postoperative problem is transplant rejection. If kidney transplantation is not chosen, the patient will need lifelong dialysis. The three basic types of dialysis are peritoneal dialysis, hemodialysis, and continuous hemofiltration. Peritoneal dialysis uses the peritoneum as the semipermeable membrane. Access is achieved with the surgical placement of a catheter into the peritoneal cavity. Approximately 2 L of sterile dialysate is infused into the cavity and left for a variable period of time (usually 4 to 8 hr). At the end of the cycle, the dialysate is removed and discarded. A fresh amount of sterile dialysate is infused, and the cycle is continued.

Hemodialysis uses a surgically inserted vascular access, such as a shunt, or vascular access into an arterialized vein that was created by an arteriovenous fistula. In emergencies, vascular access through a large artery may be used. The blood is removed through one end of the vascular access and is passed through a machine (dialyzer). The dialyzer contains areas for the dialysate and the blood, separated by a semipermeable membrane. The fluid and waste products move quickly through the membrane because the pressure on the blood side is higher than that on the dialysate side. The blood is returned to a venous access site.

Continuous hemofiltration uses vascular access in the same manner as hemodialysis. The patient's heparinized blood goes from an arterial access, through the hemofilter (the semipermeable membrane), and back to the patient through venous access. No dialysate is used. The hemofilter uses the patient's own blood pressure as the source of pressure. One disadvantage is that frequently too much fluid is filtered, resulting in the need for IV fluid replacement. Other procedures, such as venovenous dialysis, are also used in some institutions. Glycemic control, control of blood pressure, dietary protein restrictions, smoking cessation, calcium supplementation, management of anemia, and control of hyperlipidemia are all components of collaborative management.

The diet for the CKD patient on dialysis is generally restricted in fluids, protein, sodium, and potassium. It is usually high in calories, particularly carbohydrates. The fluid restriction is generally the amount of the previous day's urine plus 500 to 600 mL. The patient with CKD is frequently taking many medications. A significant concern is that the patient's altered renal function also alters the action and the excretion of medications; toxicity, therefore, is always considered a possibility, and dosages are altered accordingly. Manifestations of CKD, such as anemia, electrolyte imbalances (hyperphosphatemia, hypocalcemia, hyperkalemia), hyperparathyroidism, fluid overload, and metabolic acidosis need treatment as well.

Pharmacologic Highlights

Medication or Drug Class	Dosage	Description	Rationale
Antihypertensives	Varies by drug	Angiotensin-converting enzyme (ACE) inhibitors; beta-adrenergic antagonists	Treat the underlying hypertension
Diuretics	Varies by drug	Loop and thiazide diuretics	Control fluid overload early in the disease if the patient is not anuric (total absence of urinary output)
Hematopoietic growth factors	Varies by drug	Epoetin alfa, darbepoetin	Stimulates RBC production to treat anemia
Sodium polystyrene sulfonate (Kayexalate)	Orally or by enema: 15 g/60 mL in 20–100 mL sorbitol to facilitate passage of resin through the intestinal tract	Cation exchange resin; 0.5–1 mEq/L of potassium is removed with each enema, but an equivalent amount of sodium is retained	Exchanges sodium for potassium in the GI tract, leading to the elimination of potassium

Other Drugs: Hypocalcemia and hyperphosphatemia may be treated with lanthanum carbonate; sevelamer; and sucroferric oxyhydroxide or phosphorus-lowering agents such as calcium acetate, calcium carbonate, calcitriol, or doxercalciferol. If long-term effects of aluminum hydroxide are a concern, an oral calcium (with vitamin D) preparation may be given. Anemia may be treated with iron salts such as ferrous sulfate. If the patient undergoes renal transplantations, immunosuppressives such as tacrolimus, azathioprine, mycophenolate mofetil, or cyclosporine are prescribed. Corticosteroids may also be given at this time to decrease antibody formation.

Independent

To help the patient deal with fluid restrictions, use creative strategies to increase the patient's comfort and compliance. Use ice chips, frozen lemon swabs, hard candy, and diversionary activities. Give medications with meals or with minimal fluids to maximize the amount of fluid that is available for patient use. Skin care is important because of the effects of uremia. Uremia results in itching and dryness of the skin. If the patient experiences pruritus, help the patient clip the fingernails short and keep the nail tips smooth. Teach the patient to use skin emollients liberally, to avoid harsh soaps, and to bathe only when necessary. You may need to speak to the physician to request an as-needed dose of an oral antihistamine such as diphen-hydramine (Benadryl). If the patient is hospitalized, frequent turning and range-of-motion exercises assist in preventing skin breakdown. If the patient is taking medications that cause frequent stools, teach the patient to clean the perineum and buttocks frequently to maintain skin integrity.

The patient needs to plan the week's activities to incorporate the level of fatigue, the dialysis routine, and any desired activities. The patient may also find that cognitive activities are more easily accomplished on certain days in relationship to dialysis treatments. Reassure the patient that this is not unusual but is caused by the shift of fluid and waste products. Counseling relative to role function, family processes, and changes in body image is important. Sexuality counseling may be required. Reassure the patient that adaptation to a chronic illness with an uncertain future is not easy for either the patient or the significant others. Participate when asked in discussions related to feasibility of home dialysis, placement on the transplant list, and decisions related to acceptance or refusal of dialysis treatment. Encourage decisions that increase feelings of control for the patient.

If the patient undergoes a kidney transplantation, provide preoperative and postoperative care as for any patient with abdominal surgery. Monitoring of fluids is more important for these patients than for other surgical patients because a decrease in output may be an early sign of rejection. Other signs include weight gain, edema, fever, pain over the site, hypertension, and increased white blood cell count. Emotional support is important for the patient and family, both preoperatively and postoperatively, because both positive and negative outcomes produce emotional turmoil. Teaching about immunosuppressive drugs is essential before discharge.

Evidence-Based Practice and Health Policy
Novick, T., Rizzolo, K., & Cervantes, L. (2020). COVID-19 and kidney disease disparities in the United States. *Advances in Chronic Kidney Disease, 27*, 427–433.

- The authors note that the coronavirus disease 2019 (COVID-19) disproportionately affected older adults, people who were not housed, underrepresented minorities, and immigrants. Not only were these groups affected by the societal aspects of the pandemic, but they were at an increased risk for infection and may have experienced more severe complications than other groups. Many people in those groups with underlying kidney disease had difficulties managing their kidney disease and had progression of their illness.
- For older adults, worsening of frailty and depression due to sheltering in place increased the risk of hospitalization for renal complications. For people without housing, limited computer and Internet access led to less healthcare contact, worsened chronic conditions, and more dependence on acute care settings and hospitalization. They also noted that minorities were disproportionately affected by COVID-19 which may have worsened kidney disease. They conclude that the pandemic may have exacerbated existing disparities in kidney disease.

DOCUMENTATION GUIDELINES
- Physical findings: Urinary output (if any) and description of urine, fluid balance, vital signs, findings related to complications of CKD, presence of pain or pruritus, mental status, GI status, skin integrity
- Condition of peritoneal or vascular access sites
- Nutrition: Response to dietary or fluid restrictions, tolerance to food, maintenance of body weight
- Complications: Cardiovascular, integumentary, infection
- Activity tolerance: Level of fatigue, ability to perform activities of daily living, mobility

DISCHARGE AND HOME HEALTHCARE GUIDELINES

CKD and ESKD are disorders that affect the patient's total lifestyle and the whole family. Patient teaching is essential and should be understood by the patient and significant others. Note that you may need to work collaboratively with social services to arrange for the patient's dialysis treatments. Issues such as the location for outpatient dialysis and follow-up, home health referrals, and the purchasing of home equipment are important. All teaching should be reinforced at intervals during the patient's lifetime.

CARE OF PERITONEAL CATHETER FOR DIALYSIS. The access site is a sterile area that requires a sterile dressing except when the site is being accessed. Teach the patient or significant others the dressing technique recommended by your institution. In addition, the patient needs to learn the signs of an infected access site, such as swelling, redness, drainage, and odor. In addition, teach the patient to avoid restrictive clothing around the waist and to avoid external abdominal pressure.

CARE OF EXTERNAL ARTERIOVENOUS DIALYSIS ACCESS (SHUNT). A shunt can be surgically inserted on any limb, but the dominant arm is usually avoided. The access site is considered sterile and is covered with a sterile dressing at all times. Teach the patient to cover the access site between dialysis treatments with a dressing and further support, such as a nonelastic tensor bandage. Because one end of the shunt is inserted directly into an artery, care must be taken to ensure that the shunt does not accidentally come apart, which would lead to immediate hemorrhage. Teach the patient to carry a clamp to use if the shunt becomes disconnected. Teach the patient to feel for the "thrill" of blood moving through the shunt when it is touched (except during dialysis). The presence of darker blood within the shunt may indicate clotting; if this condition occurs, the patient needs to notify the dialysis staff or physician immediately. Any pressure on that limb—such as blood pressure readings, sleeping with the affected limb under the body, carrying boxes or groceries with that arm, or tight clothing—is contraindicated. Tell the patient not to use creams or lotions on the access site and to protect the site during bathing.

CARE OF THE ARTERIOVENOUS FISTULA. The increased pressure in the arterialized vein creates a large and sometimes unsightly vessel but also creates an access site with enough pressure to complete hemodialysis. Teach the patient to palpate a thrill over the anastomosis or graft site every day. Postoperatively, the patient may be asked to do strengthening exercises (grasping ball) to increase the size of the arterialized vein. After hemodialysis, the nursing staff applies pressure for a lengthy period of time to ensure clotting of the patient's blood. If the patient notices excessive bleeding after a dialysis treatment, the patient must notify the dialysis unit. Teach the patient that the site does not need to be protected during bathing. Tell the patient to remind all healthcare personnel that the involved arm should not be used for blood pressure measurements and phlebotomy.

POSTTRANSPLANTATION TEACHING. Discharge teaching for the patient with a renal transplant includes information about medications and the signs of rejection. The immunosuppressive drugs place the patient at greater risk for infection and skin cancer. Teach the patient to avoid large groups of people in the first 3 to 4 months and strong sunlight for the duration of the transplant. Although most forms of daily activity are restricted only by how the patient is feeling, contact sports and heavy lifting are contraindicated because of the placement of the transplant. Teach the patient to report signs of infection, rejection, and skin changes immediately to the physician. Teach the patient or significant others about all medications, including dosage, potential side effects, and drug interactions.

Kidney Injury, Acute

DRG Category:	674
Mean LOS:	7.4 days
Description:	SURGICAL: Other Kidney and Urinary Tract Procedures With Complication or Comorbidity
DRG Category:	683
Mean LOS:	3.9 days
Description:	MEDICAL: Renal Failure With Complication or Comorbidity

Acute kidney injury (AKI), formerly termed acute renal failure, is the abrupt deterioration of renal filtration that results in the accumulation of fluids, electrolytes, and metabolic waste products. AKI is a common event in hospitalized patients. Approximately 1% of patients admitted to hospitals have AKI at the time of admission, and 2% to 5% develop AKI during hospitalization. One classification system that is helpful to establish a uniform definition of AKI is the RIFLE (Risk, Injury, Failure, Loss of function, and End-stage kidney disease) Classification (see Table 1, adapted from Lopes & Jorge, 2013).

● **TABLE 1** RIFLE Classification System

CLASS	SERUM CREATININE (SCr) AND GLOMERULAR FILTRATION RATE (GFR)	URINE OUTPUT
Risk	SCr increased 1.5–2 times or decrease in GFR > 25%	< 0.5 mL/kg/hr for 6 hr
Injury	SCr increased 2–3 times or decrease in GFR > 50%	< 0.5 mL/kg/hr for 12 hr
Failure	SCr increased > 3 times or decrease in GFR > 75% or baseline SCr ≥ 4 mg/dL	< 0.3 mL/kg/hr for 24 hr or anuria for 12 hr
Loss of function	Complete loss of kidney function for more than 4 wk	None
End-stage kidney disease	Complete loss of kidney function for more than 3 mo	None

Although AKI is often reversible, if it is ignored or inappropriately treated, it can lead to irreversible kidney damage and chronic renal failure. Two types of AKI occur: community acquired and hospital acquired. Community-acquired AKI is diagnosed in about 1% of hospital admissions at the time of initial assessment. In comparison, hospital-acquired AKI occurs in up to 4% of hospital admissions and 20% of critical care admissions. There are many reasons for a higher incidence of hospital-acquired AKI as compared to community-acquired AKI, and they include an aging population, the use of nephrotoxic medications, and higher acuity than previous decades in hospitalized patients.

Approximately 40% to 50% of patients develop oliguric (low output) AKI with a urine output of less than 400 mL/day. The other 50% to 60% of patients never develop oliguria and have what is considered nonoliguric renal failure. Oliguric AKI generally has three stages. During the initial phase (often called the *oliguric phase*), when trauma or insult affects the kidney tissue, the patient becomes oliguric. This stage may last a week or more. The second stage of AKI is the diuretic phase, which is heralded by a doubling of the urinary output from the previous 24 hours. During the diuretic phase, patients may produce as much as 5 L of urine in 24 hours but lack the ability to concentrate urine and regulate waste products. This phase can last from 1 to several weeks. The final stage, the recovery phase, is characterized by a return to a normal urinary output (about 1,500 to 1,800 mL/24 hr), with a gradual improvement in metabolic waste removal. Some patients take up to a year to recover full renal function after the initial insult.

Complications of AKI include severe electrolyte imbalances such as hyperkalemia and hypocalcemia. The patient is also at risk for secondary infections, congestive heart failure, myocarditis, cardiac dysrhythmias, and pericarditis. More than half of patients with AKI have pulmonary complications such as lung infections and alveolar hypoventilation. AKI that does not respond to treatment of the underlying cause can progress to chronic kidney disease (see **Kidney Disease, Chronic**).

CAUSES

The causes of AKI can be classified as prerenal, intrinsic (intrarenal), and obstructive (postrenal). Prerenal AKI results from conditions that cause diminished blood flow to the kidneys. Disorders that can lead to prerenal failure include cardiovascular disorders (dysrhythmias, cardiogenic shock, heart failure, myocardial infarction), disorders that cause hypovolemia (burns, trauma, dehydration, hemorrhage), maldistribution of blood (septic shock, anaphylactic shock), renal artery obstruction, and severe vasoconstriction.

Intrinsic AKI involves the actual destruction of the kidney parenchyma (functional cells). The most common cause of intrinsic failure is acute tubular necrosis (ATN), or damage to the renal tubules because of either a nephrotoxic or an ischemic injury. Nephrotoxic injuries occur when the renal tubules are exposed to a high concentration of a toxic chemical. Common sources of nephrotoxic injuries include antibiotics (aminoglycosides, sulfonamides), diuretics, NSAIDs (ibuprofen), and contrast media from diagnostic tests. Ischemic injuries occur when the mean arterial blood pressure is less than 60 mm Hg for 40 to 60 minutes. Situations that can lead to ischemic injuries include cardiopulmonary arrest, hypovolemic or hemorrhagic shock, cardiogenic shock, or severe hypotension.

Obstructive AKI is caused by a blockage to urine outflow. One of the most common causes of AKI in hospitalized patients is an obstructed Foley catheter. Other conditions that can lead to obstructive failure include ureteral inflammation or obstruction, accidental ligation of the ureters, bladder obstruction (infection, anticholinergic drug use, tumors, trauma leading to bladder rupture), or urethral obstruction (prostate enlargement, urethral trauma, urethral strictures).

GENETIC CONSIDERATIONS

Several heritable diseases that can lead to AKI include the autosomal recessive condition Alport syndrome, which causes nephropathy that is often associated with sensorineural deafness and can be transmitted as X-linked recessive, autosomal recessive, and autosomal dominant forms. Renal hypouricemia, which is caused by mutations in the genes *SLC2A9* or *SLC22A12*, can lead to exercise-induced AKI in about 10% of patients.

SEX AND LIFE SPAN CONSIDERATIONS

Persons across the life span develop AKI. Some experts report that the concentrating ability of the kidneys decreases with advancing age. Oliguria in the older patient, therefore, may be diagnosed with urine production of as much as 600 mL/day. Older patients may have a decreased blood flow, decreased kidney mass, decreased filtering surface, and decreased glomerular filtration rate. Older adults, therefore, are more susceptible to insults that result in AKI, and their mortality rates tend to be higher. Older men have an added risk of preexisting renal damage because of the presence of benign prostatic hypertrophy.

HEALTH DISPARITIES AND SEXUAL/GENDER MINORITY HEALTH

Growing evidence exists that AKI occurs more frequently in underrepresented groups and people who are uninsured. Sexual and gender minority status has no known effect on the risk for AKI.

GLOBAL HEALTH CONSIDERATIONS

AKI occurs around the globe, but no data are available on the international prevalence and incidence.

▓ ASSESSMENT

HISTORY. When you elicit the patient's history, look for a disorder that can lead to prerenal, intrinsic, or obstructive AKI. Question the patient about recent illnesses, infections, or injuries, and take a careful medication history with attention to maximum daily doses and self-medication patterns. Ask patients if they have had diagnostic procedures with contrast, were exposed to heavy metals like mercury or lead, had blood loss, or received a blood transfusion. Determine the patient's urinary patterns and document information such as frequency of voiding, approximate voiding volume, and pattern of daily fluid intake. Evaluate the patient for a recent history of gastrointestinal (GI) problems, such as anorexia, nausea, and changes in bowel patterns. Some patients have a recent history of weight gain, edema, headache, confusion, and sleepiness. People with the following conditions are at higher risk for AKI: heart failure or hypertension, preexisting renal disease, diabetes, obesity, cancer, autoimmune and connective tissue diseases, and liver disease.

PHYSICAL EXAMINATION. The symptoms reflect the underlying disease process and may be nonspecific. The patient **appears seriously ill and often drowsy, irritable, confused, and combative** because of the accumulation of metabolic wastes. In the oliguric phase, the patient may show signs of fluid overload such as **hypertension, rapid heart rate, peripheral edema,** and **crackles** when you listen to the lungs. Patients in the diuretic phase appear dehydrated, with dry mucous membranes, poor skin turgor, flat neck veins, and orthostatic hypotension. The patient may have increased bleeding tendencies, such as petechiae, ecchymosis of the skin, and bloody vomitus (hematemesis).

PSYCHOSOCIAL. The patient with AKI may be highly anxious because of the uncertain outcomes of the diagnosis. Because AKI may occur as an iatrogenic problem (a problem caused by the treatment of a disease), explain to the patient or significant others that some iatrogenic problems are not avoidable and are potential complications of the underlying disorder.

Diagnostic Highlights

Test	Normal Result	Abnormality With Condition	Explanation
Urinalysis	Clear, hazy, colorless; straw, yellow, or amber colored	Granular muddy-brown casts suggest tubular necrosis; tubular cells or tubular cell casts suggest ATN; reddish-brown urine and proteinuria suggest acute glomerular nephritis; presence of red blood cells may indicate glomerular nephritis; and white blood cells may indicate pyelonephritis	Acute damage to kidneys causes loss of red and white blood cells, casts (fibrous material or coagulated protein), or protein in the urine
Blood urea nitrogen	8–21 mg/dL	Elevated	Kidneys cannot excrete wastes
Serum creatinine	0.5–1.2 mg/dL	Elevated	Kidneys cannot excrete wastes

Diagnostic Highlights (continued)

Test	Normal Result	Abnormality With Condition	Explanation
24-hr urine creatinine	Females: 75–115 mL/min/1.73 m²; males: 85–125 mL/min/1.73 m²	50% decrease	Acute damage to the kidney limits ability to clear creatinine
Urine sodium	20–40 mEq/L	Prerenal: < 20 mEq/L; intrinsic: < 20 mEq/L; obstructive: > 40 mEq/L	Prerenal and sometimes inrinsic AKI leads to sodium retention, whereas obstructive AKI leads to sodium loss in urine; fractional excretion of sodium (FENa) is calculated as: urine Na/plasma Na/urine creatinine/plasma creatinine; FENa < 1% is likely prerenal AKI; FENa > 1% is likely ATN

Other Tests: Complete blood count; cystatin C; erythrocyte sedimentation rate; hemodynamic monitoring; renal ultrasound; radionuclide scanning; magnetic resonance angiography; renal biopsy; serum levels of sodium, potassium, magnesium, and phosphorus; arterial blood gases

PRIMARY NURSING DIAGNOSIS

DIAGNOSIS. Deficient fluid volume related to damage to kidney cells as evidenced by excessive urinary output and/or hypotension during the diuretic phase

OUTCOMES. Urinary elimination; Kidney function; Fluid balance; Electrolyte balance; Circulation status; Hydration

INTERVENTIONS. Fluid management, monitoring, and resuscitation; Urinary elimination management; Electrolyte management; IV therapy

PLANNING AND IMPLEMENTATION
Collaborative

Treatment is mainly supportive, with the focus on treating the underlying cause of AKI. No specific treatments have been found to correct kidney function. Any nephrotoxic medications should be discontinued. During the oliguric-anuric stage, diuretic therapy with furosemide (Lasix) or ethacrynic acid (Edecrin) may be attempted to convert oliguric AKI to nonoliguric AKI, which has a better renal recovery rate. During the diuretic phase, fluid volume replacement may be ordered to compensate for the fluid loss and to maintain adequate arterial blood flow to the kidneys. A daily record of intake, output, and weights assists the physician in making treatment decisions. During fluid replacement, monitoring with central venous pressures or pulmonary artery catheters helps track the patient's response to interventions. The physician should be notified if the patient's urine output drops below 0.5 mL/kg per hour or if the daily weight changes by more than 2 kg (4.4 lb).

Electrolyte replacement is based on the patient's serum electrolyte values. The physician attempts to limit hyperkalemia because of its potentially lethal effects on cardiac function. Note the excretory route for medications so that the already damaged kidneys are not further damaged by nephrotoxins. The patient's response to medications is important; drug dosages may need to be decreased because of decreased renal excretion. In addition, timing of medications may need to be changed because of increased excretion during dialysis.

Renal replacement therapy includes intermittent hemodialysis (IHD), continuous renal replacement therapy (CRRT), and peritoneal dialysis (PD). IHD is the most common and efficient way of removing extra volume from the blood but is associated with complications such as hypotension. CRRT is a better choice when hypotension is a problem, such as in hemodynamically unstable patients who have critical illness. CRRT has increased risks of bleeding but leads to better control of uremia and cerebral perfusion. PD, while less expensive, does not remove the volume as efficiently as other methods and is used infrequently. Indications for dialysis include fluid overload, hyperkalemia, metabolic acidosis, uremic intoxication, and the need to remove nephrotoxic substances such as metabolites or drugs. The diet for the patient with AKI is usually high in carbohydrates to prevent protein breakdown and low in protein to provide essential amino acids but to limit increases in azotemia (increased urea in the body). For patients who lose sodium in the urine, the diet is high in sodium; for patients with sodium and water retention, the diet is low in sodium and may also contain a fluid restriction. Potassium restrictions are frequently ordered based on laboratory values.

Pharmacologic Highlights

Medication or Drug Class	Dosage	Description	Rationale
Diuretics	Varies by drug	Furosemide (Lasix); bumetanide, ethacrynic acid (Edecrin); mannitol	Convert oliguric AKI to nonoliguric
Dopamine	0.5–3 mcg/kg/min IV	Vasodilator	Low-dose dopamine is a potent vasodilator, increasing renal blood flow and urine output

Other Drugs: Sodium polystyrene sulfonate (Kayexalate) can be administered orally or rectally to reduce potassium. Fenoldopam is a vasodilator that increases blood flow to the kidney in patients with hypertension. Sodium bicarbonate may be ordered to correct metabolic acidosis. If the patient is receiving hemodialysis, supplements of water-soluble vitamins are needed because they are removed during dialysis. Other medications include antihypertensives to control blood pressure, antibiotics to manage secondary infections, diphenhydramine (Benadryl) to manage itching, and recombinant human erythropoietin to increase red blood cell production.

Independent

Rest and recovery are important nursing goals. By limiting an increased metabolic rate, the nurse limits tissue breakdown and decreases nitrogenous waste production. A quiet, well-organized environment at a temperature comfortable for the patient ensures rest and recovery. To help the patient deal with fluid restrictions, use creative strategies to increase the patient's comfort and compliance. Give medications with meals or in minimal IV volumes to maximize the amount of fluid available for patient use.

Several factors place the patient with AKI at risk for impaired skin integrity. Uremia results in itching and dryness of the skin. If the patient experiences pruritus, help the patient clip the fingernails short and keep the nail tips smooth. Use skin emollients liberally, avoid harsh soaps, and bathe the patient only when necessary. Frequent turning and range-of-motion exercises assist in preventing skin breakdown. If the patient is taking medications that cause frequent stools, clean the perineum and buttocks frequently to maintain skin integrity.

Note that one of the most common sources of AKI is an obstructed urinary catheter drainage system. Before contacting the physician about a decreasing urinary output in an acutely or critically ill patient, make sure that the catheter is patent. If institutional policy permits, irrigate the Foley catheter using sterile technique with 30 mL of normal saline to check for obstruction. Note any kinks in the collecting system. If institutional policy permits, replace the indwelling Foley catheter with a new catheter and urinary drainage system to ensure it is functioning adequately. Signs that AKI is caused by obstruction in the urinary catheter include a sudden cessation of urinary output in a patient whose urinary output has previously been high or average and a urinary output with normal specific gravity and normal urinary sodium.

The patient with AKI is often irritable and confused. Recognize that the irritability is part of the disease process. Keep the environment free of unnecessary clutter to reduce the chance of falls. If the patient is on bedrest, maintain the bed in the low position and keep the side rails up. Keep the patient's call light within easy reach and the patient's belongings on a bedside table close to the bed. The patient with AKI is anxious not only because of the ambiguity of the prognosis but also because the patient may be in an acute care environment for treatment. Provide the patient with ongoing, repeated information about what is happening and why. Ongoing reassurance for both the patient and the significant others is essential.

Evidence-Based Practice and Health Policy

Gaudry, S., Hajage, D., Benichou, N., Chaibi, K., Barbar, S., Zarbock, A., Lumlertgul, N., Wald, R., Bagshaw, S., Srisawat, N., Combes, A., Geri, G., Jamale, T., Dechartres, A., Quenot, J., & Dreyfuss, D. (2020). Delayed versus early initiation of renal replacement therapy for severe acute kidney injury: A systematic review and individual patient data meta-analysis of randomised clinical trials. *The Lancet, 395*, 1506–1515.

• There is a debate about the best time to institute renal replacement therapy (hemodialysis, CRRT, or peritoneal dialysis) for severe kidney injury. The authors assessed delayed versus early treatment to determine if 28-day survival rates differed with early and late treatment. They reviewed nine studies with 2,083 individual patients.

• Early initiation was not associated with reduced mortality unless there were urgent indications for renal replacement therapy. Delaying therapy may save healthcare resources.

DOCUMENTATION GUIDELINES

• Physical findings: Urinary output and description of urine, fluid balance, vital signs, findings related to original disease process or insult, presence of pain or pruritus, mental status, GI status, and skin integrity
• Condition of peritoneal or vascular access sites
• Nutrition: Response to dietary or fluid restrictions, tolerance to food, maintenance of body weight
• Complications: Cardiovascular, integumentary infection

DISCHARGE AND HOME HEALTHCARE GUIDELINES

All patients with AKI need an understanding of renal function, signs and symptoms of renal failure, and how to monitor their own renal function. Patients who have recovered viable renal function still need to be monitored by a nephrologist for at least a year. Teach patients that they may be more susceptible to infection than previously. Advise daily weight checks. Emphasize rest to prevent overexertion. Teach the patient or significant others about all medications, including dosage, potential side effects, and drug interactions. Explain that the patient should tell the healthcare professional about the medications if the patient needs treatment such as dental work or if a new medication is added. Explain that ongoing medical assessment is required to check renal function.

Explain all dietary and fluid restrictions. Note if the restrictions are lifelong or temporary. Patients who have not recovered viable renal function need to understand that their condition may persist and even become chronic. If chronic renal failure is suspected, further outpatient treatment and monitoring are needed. Discuss with significant others the lifestyle changes that may be required with chronic renal failure.

Laryngeal Cancer

DRG Category:	12
Mean LOS:	9.8 days
Description:	SURGICAL: Tracheostomy for Face, Mouth, and Neck Diagnoses With Complication or Comorbidity
DRG Category:	148
Mean LOS:	2.9 days
Description:	MEDICAL: Ear, Nose, Mouth, and Throat Malignancy Without Complication or Comorbidity or Major Complication or Comorbidity

Cancer of the larynx is the most common malignancy of the upper respiratory tract. About 95% of all laryngeal cancers are squamous cell carcinomas; adenocarcinomas and sarcomas account for the other 5%. In 2021, the American Cancer Society reported that there will be 12,620 new cases of laryngeal cancer, and 3,770 people will die from the disease in the United States. Global rates of the disease in countries with high tobacco and alcohol use are high.

Most cases of laryngeal cancer are diagnosed before metastasis occurs. Most laryngeal cancer begins in the glottis (the true vocal cords), 35% begins in the supraglottis (false vocal cords), and 5% begins in the subglottis (downward extension from the vocal cords). If it is confined to the glottis, laryngeal cancer usually grows slowly and metastasizes late because of the limited lymphatic drainage of the cords. Laryngeal cancer that involves the supraglottis and subglottis tends to metastasize early to the lymph nodes in the neck because of the rich lymphatic drainage of this area. In early stages, the 5-year survival rates are approximately 60% to 80%, and in later stages, they are 30% to 40% depending on the location of the cancer. Complications include airway obstruction, disfigurement, dysphagia, and metastatic cancer.

CAUSES

The cause of laryngeal cancer is unknown, but the two major predisposing factors are prolonged use of tobacco and alcohol. Each substance poses an independent risk, but their combined use causes a synergistic effect. Experts view tobacco use as the foremost risk factor for the development of laryngeal cancer, because the risk for cancer increases during use and decreases when a person stops using. Other risk factors include a familial tendency, a history of frequent laryngitis or vocal straining, chronic inhalation of noxious fumes, poor nutrition (diets low in green leafy vegetables and high in preserved meats), human papillomavirus, and a weakened immune system.

GENETIC CONSIDERATIONS

Ongoing studies indicate a role for genetics in the susceptibility and course of laryngeal cancer. Several gene mutations (e.g., *PTEN* and *TP53*) have been associated with risk, especially in the presence of alcohol and tobacco intake. Other genes and pathways have been implicated to confer genetic susceptibility to laryngeal cancer, including variants in *CYP1A1*, *ADH1B*, *ALDH2*, *BCL11A*, and various nucleotide excision repair genes. Future studies are necessary to more completely elucidate their roles in the development of laryngeal cancer.

SEX AND LIFE SPAN CONSIDERATIONS

Cancer of the larynx is more common in men than in women (5:1 ratio). The increased incidence likely occurs because men have higher rates of cigarette and alcohol use, although the incidence in women is rising as more women smoke and drink. Cancer of the larynx occurs most frequently between the ages of 50 and 70 years. The average age at diagnosis is 66 years. Women are more likely to get laryngeal cancer between the ages of 50 and 60 years and men between the ages of 60 and 70 years.

HEALTH DISPARITIES AND SEXUAL/GENDER MINORITY HEALTH

Laryngeal cancer is 50% more common in Black persons than in White persons, and Black persons are diagnosed at a later stage of the disease than White persons, leading to poorer outcomes. In addition, low income, lack of health insurance, and unmarried status are associated with poorer outcomes in laryngeal cancer, creating health disparities among people associated with those factors (Chen et al., 2020 [see Evidence-Based Practice and Health Policy]). Sexual and gender minority persons have higher rates of smoking and alcohol consumption than the general population (Centers for Disease Control and Prevention, 2021), which may place them at risk for laryngeal cancer. Gender and sexual minority persons are a vulnerable group because people with low income, long travel distances to cancer screening sites, or who lack health insurance or paid medical leave are less likely to be treated according to cancer care guidelines (National Institutes of Health, 2021).

GLOBAL HEALTH CONSIDERATIONS

The global incidence of laryngeal cancer is approximately 5 per 100,000 for males per year and 1 per 100,000 females per year. The incidence is twice as high in developed regions of the world as compared to developing regions, likely because of the patterns of risk behaviors in developed countries.

ASSESSMENT

HISTORY. Be aware as you interview the patient that hoarseness, shortness of breath, and pain may occur as the patient speaks. Most patients describe hoarseness or throat irritation that lasts longer than 2 weeks and may report a change in voice quality. Ask about dysphagia, persistent cough, hemoptysis, weight loss, dyspnea, or pain that radiates to the ear, which are late symptoms of laryngeal cancer.

Obtain a history of risk factors: alcohol or tobacco usage, voice abuse, frequent laryngitis, and family history of laryngeal cancer. Obtain detailed information about the patient's alcohol intake; ask about drinks per day, days of abstinence, and patterns of drinking. Ask how many packs of cigarettes the patient has smoked per day for how many years, as well as the use of other tobacco products. Because of potential problems with alcohol and weight loss, inquire about the patient's nutritional intake and dietary habits.

PHYSICAL EXAMINATION. **A change in the quality of people's voices is often the first symptom.** Inspect and palpate the neck for lumps and involved lymph nodes. A node may be tender before it is palpable. Inspect the mouth for sores and lumps. Note if the patient has halitosis. Palpate the base of the tongue to detect any nodules. Perform a cranial nerve assessment because some tumors spread along these nerves.

PSYCHOSOCIAL. The patient with laryngeal cancer is faced with a potentially terminal illness. The patient may experience anger, guilt, denial, or shame because of the association with cigarette smoking and alcohol consumption. Efforts to cure patients of this disease often result in a loss of normal speech and permanent lifestyle changes. Patients may experience radical changes in both body image and role relationships (interpersonal, social, and work). Assess both the patient's and the significant others' coping mechanisms and support system because extensive follow-up at home is necessary.

Diagnostic Highlights

Test	Normal Result	Abnormality With Condition	Explanation
Nasopharyngoscopy/ laryngoscopy	Normal structures with no evidence of cancer	Visible cancers of the oral cavity and nasopharynx	Special fiberoptic scopes and mirrors allow for visual inspection of the mouth and behind the nose and biopsy of nodes
Panendoscopy	Normal structures with no evidence of cancer	Visible cancers of larynx, hypopharynx, esophagus, trachea, and bronchi	Special fiberoptic scopes and mirrors allow for visual inspection of larynx, hypopharynx, esophagus, trachea, and bronchi and biopsy of nodes
Barium swallow	Normal structures with no evidence of cancer	Locations and extent of cancers evident	X-rays performed while the patient swallows a liquid that contains barium

Other Tests: Magnetic resonance imaging, computed tomography scan, chest x-rays, arterial blood gases, thyroid hormone levels, pulmonary function tests, positron emission tomography, endoscopic biopsy, fine-needle aspiration

PRIMARY NURSING DIAGNOSIS

DIAGNOSIS. Ineffective airway clearance related to obstruction, swelling, and accumulation of secretions as evidenced by vocal changes, hoarseness, choking, and/or shortness of breath

OUTCOMES. Respiratory status: Airway patency; Respiratory status: Gas exchange; Respiratory status: Ventilation; Comfort status; Knowledge: Cancer treatment; Knowledge: Treatment regimen; Oral health

INTERVENTIONS. Airway insertion and stabilization; Airway management; Airway suctioning; Oxygen therapy; Oral health promotion; Respiratory monitoring; Ventilation assistance

PLANNING AND IMPLEMENTATION

Collaborative

The goals of treatment are to remove the tumor, prevent recurrence, and maintain laryngeal function if possible. Depending on the type and extent of cancer, endoscopic surgery, transoral laser microsurgery, chemoradiation, and laryngeal surgery may be used. A multidisciplinary team of speech pathologists, social workers, dietitians, respiratory therapists, occupational therapists, and physical therapists provides preoperative evaluation and postoperative care. The goal is to eliminate the cancer and preserve the ability to speak and swallow. Radiation therapy may be used if the cancer is small, particularly if preserving the voice quality is a priority. It is also used to treat patients who are too medically fragile to have surgery. To prevent recurrence after surgery, radiation therapy is used to kill any small areas of cancer that might remain. Chemotherapy has not been found to be beneficial in treating this type of cancer and, if used, is always employed in conjunction with surgery or radiation. Chemotherapy may be useful in treating cancer that has metastasized beyond the head and neck, however, and it may be useful as a palliative treatment for cancers that are too large to be surgically removed or for cancer that is not controlled by radiation therapy.

Treatment choice depends on cancer staging and the location of the tumor. Stage 0 cancer is treated either by surgical removal of the abnormal lining layer of the larynx or by laser beam vaporizing of the abnormal cell layer. Stages I and II are treated either surgically or with radiation therapy. A common course of radiation therapy consists of daily fractions or doses administered 5 days a week for 7 weeks. Radiation therapy is frequently used as the primary treatment of laryngeal cancer, especially for patients with small cancers. A partial laryngectomy is an alternative treatment; however, voice results are generally better with radiation.

Stages III and IV laryngeal cancer are generally treated with a combination of surgery and radiation, radiation and chemotherapy, or all three treatments. A total or partial laryngectomy may be performed. The patients lose their voice and sense of smell; the patient breathes through a permanent tracheostomy stoma. A radical neck dissection is done, in conjunction with a partial or a total laryngectomy, to remove carcinoma that has metastasized to adjacent areas of the neck.

Preoperatively, the physician and speech therapist should discuss the anticipated effect of the surgical procedure on the patient's voice. Postoperatively, the most immediate concern is maintaining a patent airway, and aspiration is a high risk. Suctioning needs to be done gently so as not to penetrate the suture line. Suction the patient's laryngectomy tube and nose because the patient can no longer blow air through the nose. Observe the suture lines for intactness, hematoma, and signs of infection. Assess the skin flap for any signs of infection or necrosis and notify the physician of any problems.

Restoring speech after a laryngectomy is a concern. Patients can use an electrolarynx, an electrical device that is pressed against the neck to produce a "mechanical voice." A new advance in restoring speech is a procedure called *tracheoesophageal puncture*, which is performed either at the time of the initial surgery or at a later date. Through the use of a small one-way shunt valve that is placed into a small puncture at the stoma site, patients can produce speech by covering the stoma with a finger and forcing air out of the mouth.

Pharmacologic Highlights

Medication or Drug Class	Dosage	Description	Rationale
Analgesics	Varies with drug	Morphine sulfate, fentanyl	Relieve pain

Other Drugs: Chemotherapy (usually 5-fluorouracil, carboplatin, cisplatin, docetaxel, paclitaxel, epirubicin) may be used in certain circumstances; however, no improvement in overall survival rate has been demonstrated. Targeted therapies (monoclonal antibodies such as cetuximab) may be used in larynx preservation.

Independent

Treatment for cancer is difficult for patients and families. Clear explanations about treatment are important. Because of the position of the larynx relative to the patient's airway, regardless of the treatment, make sure the patient has a patent airway and have emergency equipment available at all times. If the patient is scheduled for a partial or total laryngectomy, spend time with the patient preoperatively exploring changes in the patient's body, such as the loss of smell and the inability to whistle, gargle, sip, use a straw, or blow the nose. Explain that the patient may need to breathe through a stoma in the neck, learn esophageal speech, or learn to use mechanical devices to speak. Encourage the expression of feelings about a diagnosis of cancer and offer to contact the appropriate clergy or clinical nurse specialist to counsel the patient.

Postoperatively, assess the patient's level of comfort. Reposition the patient carefully; after a total laryngectomy, support the back of the neck when moving the patient to prevent trauma. Provide frequent mouth care, cleansing the mouth with a soft toothbrush, toothette, or washcloth. After a partial laryngectomy, the patient should not use the voice for at least 2 days. The patient should have an alternative means of communication available at all times, and the nurse should encourage its use. After 2 to 3 days, encourage the patient to use a whisper until complete healing takes place. Because the functional impairments and disfigurement that result from this surgery are traumatic, close attention should be paid to the patient's emotional status.

As soon as possible after surgery, the patient with a total laryngectomy should start learning to care for the stoma, suction the airway, care for the incision, and self-administer the tube feedings (if the patient is to have tube feedings after discharge). Assist the patient in obtaining the equipment and supplies for home use. Discuss safety precautions for patients with a permanent stoma. If appropriate, refer the patient to smoking and alcohol cessation counseling.

Evidence-Based Practice and Health Policy

Chen, S., Dee, E., Muralidhar, V., Nguyen, P., Amin, M., & Givi, B. (2020). Disparities in mortality from larynx cancer: Implications for reducing racial differences. *Laryngoscope, 131,* E1147–E1155.

- The authors used a national cancer database to determine if racial disparities affect laryngeal squamous cell carcinoma mortality in the United States. They identified 14,506 patients with a median age of 63 years. More than 80% were male and White, and 16% were Black. Most patients had early stage cancer (52%) and received radiotherapy only (28%), followed by chemoradiation (26%).
- Black patients had a higher overall mortality than White patients, but the cancer-specific mortality did not differ between groups. Black patients were diagnosed at a later cancer stage. Income and unmarried status were associated with poorer outcomes.

DOCUMENTATION GUIDELINES

- Preoperative health and social history, physical assessment, drinking and smoking history
- Postoperative physical status: Incisions and drains, patency of airway, pulmonary secretions, nasogastric feedings, oral intake, integrity of the skin
- Pain: Location, duration, frequency, precipitating factors, response to analgesia
- Preoperative, postoperative, and discharge teaching
- Patient's ability to perform self-care: Secretion removal, laryngectomy tube and stoma care, incision care, tube feedings

DISCHARGE AND HOME HEALTHCARE GUIDELINES

Teach the patient the name, purpose, dosage, schedule, common side effects, and importance of taking all medications. Teach the patient signs and symptoms of potential complications and the appropriate actions to be taken. Complications include infection (symptoms: wound drainage, poor wound healing, fever, achiness, chills); airway obstruction and tracheostomy stenosis (symptoms: noisy respirations, difficulty breathing, restlessness, confusion, increased respiratory rate); vocal straining; fistula formation (symptoms: redness, swelling, secretions along a suture line); and ruptured carotid artery (symptoms: bleeding, hypotension).

Teach patients the appropriate devices and techniques to ensure a patent airway and prevent complications. Explore methods of communication that work effectively. Encourage patients to wear a Medic Alert bracelet or necklace that identifies them as a mouth breather. Provide patients with a list of referrals and support groups, such as visiting nurses, American Cancer Society, American Speech-Language-Hearing Association, International Association of Laryngectomees, and the Lost Chord Club.

Laryngotracheobronchitis (Croup)

DRG Category:	153
Mean LOS:	2.9 days
Description:	MEDICAL: Otitis Media and Upper Respiratory Infection Without Major Complication or Comorbidity

Laryngotracheobronchitis (LTB) is an inflammation and obstruction of the larynx, trachea, and major bronchi of children. In small children, the air passages in the lungs are smaller than those of adults, making them more susceptible to obstruction by edema and spasm. Because of the respiratory distress it causes, LTB is one of the most frightening acute diseases of childhood and is responsible for over 250,000 emergency department visits each year.

LTB is sometimes called *croup*, although croup can be more specifically described as one of three entities: LTB, laryngitis (inflammation of the larynx), or acute spasmodic laryngitis (obstructive narrowing of the larynx because of viral infection, genetic factors, or emotional distress). Croup is the most common pediatric illness and causes 15% of all clinic and emergency department visits for child-related respiratory infections. Acute spasmodic laryngitis is particularly common in children with allergies and those with a family history of croup. Acute LTB usually occurs in the fall or winter in North America and is often mild, self-limiting, and followed by complete recovery. Complications include secondary bacterial infections such as pneumonia, pulmonary edema, pneumothorax, dehydration, and otitis media. Factors that are related to asthma later in life include recurrent episodes of croup.

CAUSES

More than 85% of LTB cases are caused by a virus. Parainfluenza 1, 2, and 3 viruses; respiratory syncytial virus; *Mycoplasma pneumoniae*; and rhinoviruses are the most common causes. The measles virus or bacterial infections such as pertussis and diphtheria are occasionally the cause. Epiglottitis, a life-threatening emergency caused by acute inflammation of the epiglottis and surrounding area, differs from LTB because it usually results from infection with the bacteria *Haemophilus influenzae* type B. Another rare occurrence is subglottic hemangioma, which can initially produce symptoms of croup. Recurrent croup may be associated with gastroesophageal reflux disease (GERD). Risk factors include prematurity, children with narrow upper airways, and asthma.

GENETIC CONSIDERATIONS

Although some anatomical structural anomalies have been associated with an increased incidence of croup, no direct genetic link has been made.

SEX AND LIFE SPAN CONSIDERATIONS

Children susceptible to LTB are generally between the ages of 3 months and 4 years, with peak incidence from 6 months to 3 years. The susceptibility decreases with age, although some children seem more prone to repeat episodes of LTB. Acute spasmodic laryngitis occurs in the same age group and peaks at age 18 months. As with many respiratory diseases, boys younger than 6 months are affected more often than girls, but in older children, the male-to-female ratio is equal.

HEALTH DISPARITIES AND SEXUAL/GENDER MINORITY HEALTH

Croup is more common in White as compared to Black children, but Black children are more likely to undergo diagnostic bronchoscopy or require intubation than other children. Experts suggest that this difference is related to a higher prevalence of subglottic stenosis in Black children. Sexual and gender minority status has no known effect on the risk for croup.

GLOBAL HEALTH CONSIDERATIONS

Epiglottitis usually results from infection with the bacteria *H influenzae* type B. This condition is more prevalent in developing countries that do not vaccinate for influenza B. Generally, children contract the illness during the cool months in their climate.

ASSESSMENT

HISTORY. The family usually reports that the child has a history of an upper respiratory infection and a runny nose (rhinorrhea) and fever. Parents may report that the child has dysphonia (impairment in the ability to make vocal sounds) and a sore throat. The symptoms tend to occur in the late evening and improve during the day, which may be due to the lower cortisol levels at night. The course of the infection lasts several days to several weeks, although 60% resolve within 48 hours. Some children may have a lingering, barking cough. A child may have LTB more than once but will outgrow it as the size of the airway increases.

PHYSICAL EXAMINATION. Symptoms can widely vary, with some children having a cough and hoarse cry and others having audible stridor at rest and significant respiratory distress. After 12 to 48 hours of respiratory symptoms, parents may describe symptoms such as **cough and increased respiratory rate.** The child may develop a **barking, seal-like cough**; a **hoarse cry**; and **inspiratory stridor.** Symptoms seem to worsen during the night hours. The child may develop flaring of the nares, a prolonged expiratory phase, and use of accessory muscles. When you auscultate the child's lungs, the breath sounds may be diminished and you may hear inspiratory stridor. The child may have a mild fever. Increasing respiratory obstruction is indicated by any of the following: increasing stridor, suprasternal and intercostal retractions, respiratory rate above 60, tachycardia, cyanosis, pallor, and restlessness. Assessment is done using the Westley scale, which evaluates the severity of symptoms on the basis of five factors: (1) stridor, (2) retractions, (3) air entry, (4) cyanosis, and (5) level of consciousness. In addition, each type of croup can have particular symptoms, as shown in Table 1.

• TABLE 1 Forms of Laryngotracheobronchitis

FORMS OF CROUP	SYMPTOMS
LTB	Fever, breathing problems at night, inability to breathe out because of bronchial edema, decreased breath sounds, expiratory rhonchi, scattered crackles
Laryngitis	Mild respiratory distress in children, increased respiratory distress in infants; sore throat and cough, inspiratory stridor, dyspnea; late phases: severe dyspnea, fatigue, exhaustion
Acute spasmodic laryngitis	Hoarseness, rhinorrhea, cough, noisy inspiratory phase that worsens at night, anxiety, labored breathing, cyanosis, rapid pulse; the most severe symptoms may occur on the first night, with lessening symptoms on each of the following nights

PSYCHOSOCIAL. The parents and child will be apprehensive. Assess the parents' ability to cope with the emergency situation, and intervene as appropriate. Note that many children are treated at home rather than in the hospital; your teaching plan may need to consider home rather than hospital management.

Diagnostic Highlights

General Comments: Most children require no diagnostic testing and can be diagnosed by the history and physical examination. If diagnostic testing is needed, it involves identifying the causative organism, determining oxygenation status, and ruling out masses as a cause of obstruction.

Test	Normal Result	Abnormality With Condition	Explanation
Blood culture; throat culture	No growth; no organism identified	Causative organism identified	Distinguishes between bacterial and viral infections
Laryngoscopy, bronchoscopy	Normal larynx and clear bronchial tree	Narrowing, inflamed, or blocked airways	Inflammatory response to invading organisms; used only during an atypical illness
Pulse oximetry	≥ 95%	< 95%	Low oxygen saturation is present if there is obstruction in the lung passages
X-rays	Normal structure	Narrowing of the upper airway and edema in epiglottal and laryngeal areas	Narrowing and/or blocked airway is characteristic of LTB

PRIMARY NURSING DIAGNOSIS

DIAGNOSIS. Ineffective airway clearance related to tracheobronchial infection and/or obstruction as evidenced by dysphonia, barking cough, dyspnea, inspiratory stridor, and/or fever

OUTCOMES. Respiratory status: Airway patency; Respiratory status: Gas exchange; Respiratory status: Ventilation; Comfort status; Symptom severity; Symptom control

INTERVENTIONS. Airway management; Airway suctioning; Respiratory monitoring; Vital signs monitoring; Anxiety reduction; Oxygen therapy

PLANNING AND IMPLEMENTATION

Collaborative

The aim of treatment is to maintain a patent airway and provide adequate gas exchange. Medical management includes bronchodilating medications, corticosteroids, nebulized adrenaline, and IV hydration if oral intake is inadequate. The role of cool mist or humidification therapy is controversial. Oxygen may be used, but it masks cyanosis, which signals impending airway obstruction. Sedation is contraindicated because it may depress respirations or mask restlessness, which indicates a worsening condition. Sponge baths and antipyretic medications may be needed to control temperatures above 102°F (38.9°C). You may need to isolate the child if the physician suspects syncytial virus or parainfluenza infections.

Laryngoscopy may be necessary if complete airway obstruction is imminent. A flexible nasopharyngoscopy can be used; an intubation or a tracheostomy is performed only if no other method of airway maintenance is available. Keep intubation and tracheostomy trays near the bedside at all times for use in case of emergencies.

Pharmacologic Highlights

Medication or Drug Class	Dosage	Description	Rationale
Racemic epinephrine	Per nebulizer, varies depending on size of child	Sympathomimetic	Dilates the bronchioles, opening up respiratory passages
Corticosteroids	Varies with drug	Dexamethasone, prednisone, prednisolone, budesonide inhaler	Decrease airway inflammation if epinephrine is not effective
Antipyretics	Varies with drug	Acetaminophen, NSAIDs	Reduce fever, often present in LTB
Antibiotics	Varies with drug	Type of antibiotic depends on the causative organism	Fight bacterial infections

Independent

Ongoing, continuous observation of the patency of the child's airway is essential to identify impending obstruction. Prop infants up on pillows or place them in an infant seat; older children should have the head of the bed elevated so that they are in the Fowler position. Sore throat pain can be decreased by soothing preparations such as iced pops or fruit sherbet. If the child has difficulty swallowing, avoid thick milkshakes.

Children should be allowed to rest as much as possible to conserve their energy; organize your interventions to limit disturbances. Provide age-appropriate activities. Crying increases the child's difficulty in breathing and should be limited if possible by comfort measures and the presence of the parents; parents should be allowed to hold and comfort the child as much as possible. Children sense anxiety from their parents; if you support the parents in dealing with their anxiety and fear, the children are less fearful. A child's anxiety and agitation will most likely exacerbate the symptoms and need to be avoided if possible. Carefully explaining all procedures and allowing the parents to participate in the care of the child as much as possible help relieve the anxieties of both child and parents.

Provide adequate hydration to liquefy secretions and to replace fluid loss from increased sensible loss (increased respirations and fever). The child also might have a decreased fluid intake during the illness. Clear liquids should be offered frequently. Apply lubricant or ointment around the child's mouth and lips to decrease the irritation from secretions and mouth breathing.

Evidence-Based Practice and Health Policy

Coughran, A., Balakrishnan, K., Ma, Y., Vaezeafshar, R., Capdarest-Arest, N., Hamdi, O., & Sidell, D. (2021). The relationship between croup and gastroesophageal reflux: A systematic review and meta-analysis. *Laryngoscope, 131*, 209–217.

- The authors conducted a systematic review with a meta-analysis component to evaluate the relationship between recurrent croup and GERD. They aimed to assess for evidence of improvement in croup symptoms when GERD is treated. The authors searched five separate databases according to prespecified criteria.
- Thirteen of 15 articles support an association between recurrent croup and GERD. Most studies lacked a control group, and all carried a moderate-to-high risk of bias. Further research is needed to assess for causality as most studies were retrospective, lacked a control group, and had a study design exposing them to bias. Patients treated with reflux medication appeared to demonstrate a reduced incidence of croup symptoms.

DOCUMENTATION GUIDELINES

- Respiratory status: Rate, quality, depth, ease, breath sounds
- Response to treatment: Cool mist tent, bronchodilators, racemic epinephrine, fluid, and diet
- Child's and parents' emotional responses
- Child's response to rest and activity

DISCHARGE AND HOME HEALTHCARE GUIDELINES

PREVENTION. Children may have recurring episodes of LTB; parental instruction on mechanisms to prevent airway obstruction is therefore important. Despite their continued widespread use, there is little evidence to support the effectiveness of cool mist humidifiers. Some parents may take the child into a closed bathroom with the shower or tub running to create an environment that has high humidity.

MEDICATIONS. If antibiotics have been prescribed, tell the parents to make sure the child finishes the entire prescription.

COMPLICATIONS. Instruct the parents to recognize the signs of increasing respiratory obstruction and advise them when to take the child to an emergency department. Remind the parents that ear infections or pneumonia may follow croup in 4 to 6 days. Immediate medical attention is needed if the child has an earache, productive cough, fever, or dyspnea.

HOME CARE. If the child is cared for at home, provide the following home care instructions: (1) Keep the child in bed or playing quietly to conserve energy; (2) prop the child in a sitting position to ease breathing; do not let the child stay in a flat position; (3) do not use aspirin products because of the chance of Reye syndrome; and (4) give plenty of fluids, such as sherbet, ginger ale left to stand so there are no bubbles, gelatin dissolved in water, and ice pops; withhold solid food until the child can breathe easily.

Legionnaires' Disease

DRG Category:	177
Mean LOS:	6.9 days
Description:	MEDICAL: Respiratory Infections and Inflammations With Major Complication or Comorbidity
DRG Category:	207
Mean LOS:	13.9 days
Description:	MEDICAL: Respiratory System Diagnosis With Ventilator Support > 96 Hours
DRG Category:	208
Mean LOS:	6.7 days
Description:	MEDICAL: Respiratory System Diagnosis With Ventilator Support ≤ 96 Hours
DRG Category:	3
Mean LOS:	30.3 days
Description:	SURGICAL: ECMO or Tracheostomy With Mechanical Ventilation > 96 Hours or Primary Diagnosis Except Face, Mouth, and Neck With Major Operating Room Procedures

Legionnaires' disease (LD) is an acute bronchopneumonia that was named because of a major outbreak at the 1976 American Legion Convention in Philadelphia, Pennsylvania, in which 182 American Legionnaires contracted the disease, and 29 persons died. It is now known as the most common type of atypical pneumonia in hospitalized patients and the second-most common cause of community-acquired bacterial pneumonia. Approximately 20% of cases occur in late summer and early fall; the rest are spaced throughout the year, and they may be epidemic or confined to a small number of sporadic cases. The Centers for Disease Control and Prevention (CDC) report that approximately 10,000 cases occur each year in the United States.

LD has an incubation period of 2 to 10 days and is characterized by patchy pulmonary infiltrates, lung consolidation, and flu-like symptoms. Pneumonia is the presenting clinical syndrome in more than 95% of cases. LD is spread by direct alveolar infection with the gram-negative bacterium *Legionella pneumophila*. The bacteria multiply in the alveolar cells of the lungs where, in the macrophages, the bacteria undergo phagocytosis. The bacteria are not destroyed in this process, however, but are released into the surrounding areas and multiply. The infection spreads through the bronchi, blood, and lymphatic systems. Bacteremia occurs in about 30% of the patients and is the source of nonrespiratory infections in most patients.

Complications are extensive and serious with LD. Hypoxemia and acute respiratory failure can result from the severe case of pneumonia. The disease can also cause hypotension and hyponatremia as a result of salt and water loss. Central nervous system involvement is seen in almost 30% of patients. Renal involvement, which ranges from interstitial nephritis to renal failure, may occur. Untreated immunosuppressed patients have a mortality rate of 80%; untreated patients with no immune system compromise have a mortality rate of 25%.

CAUSES

L pneumophila is an aerobic, gram-negative bacillus that seems to be transmitted by air. It is usually classified as a saprophytic water bacterium because it is natural to bodies of water such as rivers, lakes, streams, and thermally polluted waters. Optimal temperature for growth of the bacterium is 98.6°F (37°C). *L pneumophila* is also found in habitats such as cooling towers, evaporative condensers, humidifiers, respiratory therapy equipment, whirlpool spas, and water distribution centers, and it has been found in soil samples and at excavation sites. Pathogenic microorganisms can enter the lung by aspiration, direct inhalation, or dissemination from another focus of infection. Risk factors include older age, smoking or alcohol abuse, diabetes mellitus, chronic heart or lung disease, and immune diseases.

GENETIC CONSIDERATIONS

Although LD is the result of infection by *L pneumophila*, susceptibility has been associated with variants in the toll-like receptor-5 (*TLR5*) gene.

SEX AND LIFE SPAN CONSIDERATIONS

LD is two to three times more common in men than in women; it is uncommon in children, but when children acquire it, they are usually less than a year old. At-risk groups include middle-aged or older people; patients with a chronic underlying disease such as chronic obstructive pulmonary disease, diabetes mellitus, or chronic renal failure; patients with immunosuppressive disorders such as lymphoma or rheumatoid arthritis or those who receive corticosteroids after organ transplantation; people with alcohol dependence; and cigarette smokers.

HEALTH DISPARITIES AND SEXUAL/GENDER MINORITY HEALTH

Approximately 80% of the deaths from LD occur in White persons, with the most common comorbid conditions including leukemia and rheumatoid arthritis. Age-adjusted mortality rates for White and Black persons are similar. Sexual and gender minority status has no known effect on the risk for LD.

GLOBAL HEALTH CONSIDERATIONS

LD has been reported throughout the globe and on all populated continents.

⬛ ASSESSMENT

HISTORY. Ask about malaise, aching muscles, anorexia, headache, high fever, or recurrent chills. Often these symptoms occur over 1 to 2 days before other symptoms occur. Establish a history of chest pain or coughing, which begins as a nonproductive cough but eventually becomes productive. Ask the patient about gastrointestinal symptoms such as diarrhea, nausea, abdominal pain, and vomiting. Because the central nervous system is involved in about 30% of cases, ask the family or significant others if the patient has experienced recent confusion or decreased level of consciousness.

Determine if the patient has been close to a river, lake, or stream, which might have resulted in possible exposure to the bacteria. Establish a work history of employment at an excavation site or water distribution center, in a cooling tower, or near an evaporative condenser. Ask if the patient has had overnight stays away from home. Determine if the patient uses respiratory equipment or humidifiers, or if the patient works or lives in a facility with central air conditioning.

PHYSICAL EXAMINATION. Common symptoms include **mild headache, cough, muscle aches, high fever**, and **chills**. Note the respiratory rate, which may be rapid and accompanied by dyspnea. Auscultate the lungs to determine the presence of fine or coarse crackles. Percuss the chest for dullness over areas of secretions and consolidation or pleural effusions. Perform a neurological assessment to note altered level of consciousness, confusion, or coma. Inspect the patient's sputum, which may be grayish or rust colored, nonpurulent, and occasionally blood streaked. Auscultate the blood pressure and heart rate; note that some patients develop severe hypotension and bradycardia. Palpate the peripheral pulses to determine strength.

PSYCHOSOCIAL. A previously healthy person with a possible minor upper respiratory infection is at risk for life-threatening complications, such as multiple organ failure. Assess the patient's ability to cope with a sudden illness. Assess the patient's level of anxiety and fear.

Diagnostic Highlights

Test	Normal Result	Abnormality With Condition	Explanation
Sputum culture and sensitivity; direct fluorescent antibody staining	Negative	Presence of *L pneumophila*	Identify infecting organisms; bacteria is slow growing and may take 3–4 days for visible colonies
Chest x-ray	Air-filled lungs	Area of increased density of a lung segment, lobe, or entire lung; findings vary and may be non-specific; disease is often unilateral	Identifies the location and extent of infection

Other Tests: Urinalysis, serology for *Legionella* (urine antigen testing, indirect fluorescent antibody studies), arterial blood gases, pulse oximetry, complete blood count, erythrocyte sedimentation rate, blood urea nitrogen, creatinine, serum electrolytes

PRIMARY NURSING DIAGNOSIS

DIAGNOSIS. Risk for infection as evidenced by fever, chill, cough, muscle ache, and/or headache

OUTCOMES. Infection severity; Immune status; Knowledge: Infection management; Fluid balance; Risk control; Risk detection; Knowledge: Medication

INTERVENTIONS. Infection control; Infection protection; Fluid/electrolyte management; Medication management; Medication administration; Temperature regulation

☀ PLANNING AND IMPLEMENTATION

Collaborative

PHARMACOLOGIC. Antibiotics can be administered before test results are available. Generally, primary therapy is either levofloxacin or azithromycin. Erythromycin, sometimes in combination with rifampin, is also used, but the gastrointestinal effects of both the disease and drug can be cumulative and problematic. IV fluids and electrolyte therapy may be considered when the patient has fluid volume deficit. Careful monitoring of fluid balance is required because of the possible renal complications from interstitial nephritis or renal failure. If renal failure does ensue, the patient may require temporary renal dialysis.

Oxygen per cannula at 2 to 4 L/minute is effective with many patients, although in some patients with respiratory insufficiency, it is necessary to proceed with intubation and assisted ventilation. Atelectasis may occur at any stage of the pneumonia. Pleural effusion may occur, which may require a diagnostic thoracentesis and a chest tube. The patient may need continuous pulse oximetry to monitor the response to mechanical ventilation and suctioning. Continuous cardiac monitoring and hourly urine outputs may be necessary to assess the patient's response to the disease.

Pharmacologic Highlights

Medication or Drug Class	Dosage	Description	Rationale
Antibiotics	Varies with drug	Levofloxacin (Levaquin), azithromycin (Zithromax), erythromycin, doxycycline, ciprofloxacin, trimethoprim/sulfamethoxazole	Halt division of bacteria, thereby limiting infection
Other Treatment: Antipyretics			

Independent

The most important intervention is maintenance and improvement of airway patency. Retained secretions interfere with gas exchange and may cause slow resolution of the disease. Encourage a high level of fluid intake up to 3 L/day to assist in loosening pulmonary secretions and to replace fluid lost via fever and diaphoresis unless the patient has renal compromise. Provide meticulous sterile technique during endotracheal suctioning of the patient. Chest physiotherapy may be prescribed to assist with loosening and mobilizing secretions.

To maintain the patient's comfort, keep the patient protected from drafts. Institute fever-reducing measures if necessary. To ease the patient's breathing, raise the head of the bed at least 45 degrees and support the patient's arms with pillows. Provide mouth and skin care and emotional support. Include the patient and family in planning care and allow them to make choices.

Evidence-Based Practice and Health Policy

Mudali, G., Kilgore, P., Salim, A., McElmurry, S., & Zervos, M. (2020). Trends in Legionnaires' disease–associated hospitalizations, United States, 2006–2010. *Open Forum Infectious Diseases, 7*, 1–4.

- The authors aimed to offer an estimate of the annual incidence of LD-associated hospitalizations in the United States, identifying demographic, temporal, and regional characteristics of individuals hospitalized for LD. They conducted a retrospective study using the National

Hospital Discharge Survey (NHDS) data from 2006 to 2010. All discharges assigned with the LD diagnostic code (482.84) were included in this study.
• Over the 5-year period, 14,574 individuals were admitted with LD. A summer peak of LD-associated hospitalizations occurred June through September in 2006, 2007, 2008, and 2010. Peak age for infection was in the 60 to 69 years of age group. LD-associated hospitalizations significantly increased over the 5-year study period.

DOCUMENTATION GUIDELINES

• Physical findings: Vital signs, head-to-toe assessment, rate of breathing, breath sounds, description of sputum
• Response to treatments such as antibiotics, chest physiotherapy, oxygen, antipyretics, and fluid therapy
• Presence of complications: Hypotension, dehydration, chest pain, changes in patterns of urination, laboratory findings

DISCHARGE AND HOME HEALTHCARE GUIDELINES

Explain the medications to the patient, including the route, dosage, side effects, and need for taking all antibiotics until they are gone. Explain food and drug interactions. Provide information on smoking-cessation programs. Note the source of the patient's LD; if the cause was from within a patient's home or workplace, recommend appropriate action to prevent recurrence and decrease chances of further outbreaks. Instruct the patient to contact the physician if the patient has a fever or worsening pleuritic pain. Stress the need to go immediately to the nearest emergency department if the patient becomes acutely short of breath.

Leukemia, Acute

DRG Category:	835
Mean LOS:	6.8 days
Description:	MEDICAL: Acute Leukemia Without Major Operating Room Procedures With Complication or Comorbidity

Leukemias account for approximately 8% of all human cancers, and approximately half of these cases are classified as acute leukemia. Acute leukemia, a malignant disease of the blood-forming organs, results when white blood cell (WBC) precursors proliferate in the bone marrow and lymphatic tissues. The cells eventually spread to the peripheral blood and all body tissues. Leukemia is considered acute when it has a rapid onset and progression and when, if left untreated, it leads to 100% mortality within days or months.

There are two major forms of acute leukemia: lymphocytic leukemia and nonlymphocytic leukemia. Lymphocytic leukemia involves the lymphocytes (cells derived from the stem cells and that circulate among the blood, lymph nodes, and lymphatic organs) and lymphoid organs; nonlymphocytic leukemia involves hematopoietic stem cells that differentiate into monocytes, granulocytes, red blood cells (RBCs), and platelets. Up to 90% of acute leukemias are a form of lymphocytic leukemia, acute lymphoblastic leukemia (ALL), which is characterized by the abnormal growth of lymphocyte precursors called *lymphoblasts*. In ALL, the lymphoblasts have arrested development and also proliferate in the liver, spleen, and lymph nodes. Acute myelogenous leukemia (AML) (also known as *acute nonlymphocytic leukemia*, or ANLL) causes the rapid accumulation of megakaryocytes (precursors to platelets), monocytes, granulocytes, and RBCs. The physiology of AML is based on the maturational arrest of bone marrow cells; the cells never really develop, leaving the body with a deficit of mature RBCs, platelets, and WBCs. As the disease progresses, the patient may have central nervous system (CNS) dysfunction with seizures, decreased mental status, or coma and renal insufficiency. Death occurs when the abnormal cells encroach on vital tissues and cause complications and organ dysfunction.

Approximately 62,000 new cases of leukemia occur each year. AML is the most common adult leukemia, and three out of four children who develop leukemia develop ALL. Approximately 23,000 adults and children die of all forms of leukemia each year. Patients with AML or ALL can be kept in long-term remission or cured in approximately 20% to 40% of adult cases. Five-year survival rates for children with ALL are close to 90% and for children with AML are 65% to 70%.

CAUSES

The exact cause of acute leukemia is unknown, and most patients never have an identifiable cause. This is particularly true for adults with ALL. However, there are several risk factors for AML. Overexposure to radiation even years before the development of the disease, particularly if the exposure is prolonged, is a major risk factor. Other risk factors include exposure to certain chemicals (benzene), medications (alkylating agents used to treat other cancers in particular), and viruses. Other related factors in children include genetic abnormalities such as Down syndrome, albinism, and congenital immunodeficiency syndrome. People who have been treated with chemotherapeutic agents for other forms of cancer have an increased risk for developing AML. Such cases generally develop within 9 years of chemotherapy.

GENETIC CONSIDERATIONS

Several genetic disorders increase the risk of leukemia. Persons with Down syndrome have a lifetime leukemia risk that is 15 times greater than that of the general population. The heritable disorders Fanconi anemia, Bloom syndrome, and ataxia-telangiectasia also increase the likelihood of acute myeloid and acute lymphocytic leukemias. AML can be caused by mutations in *CEBPA* and *NPM1*. Familial platelet disorder also predisposes individuals to AML through autosomal dominant mutations in *RUNX1*. Familial myelodysplastic syndrome is caused by mutations in *GATA2*.

SEX AND LIFE SPAN CONSIDERATIONS

ALL is the most common type of childhood leukemia and accounts for 75% of pediatric leukemia; the majority of patients are under age 10 years, with the peak age for children to develop ALL between ages 2 and 3 years. Slightly more males than females develop ALL. In children, AML is more common in the first 2 years of life and again increases in the teen years. The disease is most common in older people; the average age of a patient with AML is 65 years, and the median age of onset is 70 years. Males are more susceptible to AML than are females.

HEALTH DISPARITIES AND SEXUAL/GENDER MINORITY HEALTH

More than twice as many White persons as compared to Black persons develop ALL. However, despite major advances in ALL treatment, poorer overall survival persists for Black children compared to White children. The factors most associated with disparities are age at diagnosis (younger than 1 year of age and older than 10 years of age), differences in laboratory test results, and lower socioeconomic status. AML is more common in White persons than other groups. There are likely poorer survival rates among people living in rural areas, particularly if patients live more than 50 miles from a cancer treatment center. Poorer AML survival is also related to smoking, lack of health insurance at the time of diagnosis, and socioeconomic deprivation.

A high body mass index (BMI) places a person at higher risk for leukemia than a normal BMI. Sexual and gender minority status has no known effect on the risk for ALL and AML. However, gender and sexual minority persons are a vulnerable group because people with low income, long travel distances to cancer screening sites, or who lack health insurance or paid medical leave are less likely to be treated according to cancer care guidelines (National Institutes of Health, 2021).

GLOBAL HEALTH CONSIDERATIONS

Leukemia comprises 2.5% of all cancers in the world. The global incidence of leukemia is approximately 6 per 100,000 males per year and 4 per 100,000 females per year. The incidence of diagnosed acute leukemia is three times higher in developed than in developing countries.

ASSESSMENT

HISTORY. Question the patient (or the parents of the patient, as appropriate) about any exposure to radiation, chemicals, viruses, and medications, including chemotherapy for cancer. Determine the adult patient's occupation and pay particular attention to radiation exposure of healthcare workers, workers in a power plant, or those serving in the military. Often, the patient describes a sudden onset of high fever and signs of abnormal bleeding (increased bruising, bleeding after minor trauma, nosebleeds, bleeding gums, petechiae, and prolonged menses). Fever is one of the most common symptoms of patients with ALL and AML. Some patients report increased fatigue and malaise, weight loss, palpitations, night sweats, and chills. Parents of children with leukemia often report a series of recurrent pulmonary, urinary tract, and perirectal infections. Patients may also complain of abdominal or bone pain.

PHYSICAL EXAMINATION. The patient appears **acutely ill, short of breath**, and **pale**, symptoms that occur because of anemia. Children are often **febrile**. When you inspect the lips and mouth, you may note **bleeding gums** and **ulcerated areas of the mouth and throat**. On palpation, you may feel lymph node swelling and enlargement of the liver and spleen. When you auscultate the patient's lungs, you may hear decreased breath sounds, shallow and rapid respirations, a rapid heart rate, and a systolic ejection murmur. Patients may have altered mental status from brain infiltration with leukemic cells.

PSYCHOSOCIAL. When the diagnosis of acute leukemia is made, patients, parents, and significant others are shocked and fearful. If the patient is a child, determine the patient's stage of development and relationship with parents, caregivers, or grandparents. If the patient is an adult, determine the patient's job, childcare, and financial responsibilities. Assess the patient's home situation to determine the possibility of home healthcare. Determine the support systems available to the patient, including emotional, religious, financial, and social support.

Diagnostic Highlights

Test	Normal Result	Abnormality With Condition	Explanation
Complete blood count and differential	RBCs: 3.6–5.8 million/mcL; hemoglobin: 11.7–17.3 g/dL; hematocrit: 36%–52%; WBCs: 4,500–11,100/mcL; platelets: 150,000–450,000/mcL	Increased WBC counts (notably blast cells), lowered RBC count, insufficient platelets	Changes in numbers of different blood cell types and how the cells look under a microscope can suggest leukemia; overproduction of WBCs halts production of RBCs and platelets

(highlight box continues on page 742)

Diagnostic Highlights (continued)

Test	Normal Result	Abnormality With Condition	Explanation
Bone marrow aspiration/ bone marrow biopsy	No leukemia cells present	Leukemia cells present; 30% blast cells required for diagnosis of acute leukemia; < 5% blast cells for diagnosis of remission; more advanced testing is done with flow cytometry, cytogenic analysis, and molecular marrow evaluation	A thin needle is used to draw a small amount of liquid bone marrow; a small cylinder of bone and marrow (about 1/2 in. long) is removed with a slightly larger needle; the site of both samples is usually at the back of the hipbone

Other Tests: Other supporting tests include x-rays, lymph node biopsy, computed tomography scan, magnetic resonance imaging, ultrasound, cytochemistry, flow cytometry, immunocytochemistry, cytogenetic analysis, lumbar puncture, blood chemistries, lactate dehydrogenase, uric acid, liver function tests, blood urea nitrogen, creatinine

PRIMARY NURSING DIAGNOSIS

DIAGNOSIS. Risk for infection as evidenced by fever, tachypnea, and/or chills

OUTCOMES. Infection severity; Immune status; Knowledge: Infection management; Risk control; Risk detection; Fluid balance; Symptom severity; Symptom control; Knowledge: Medication

INTERVENTIONS. Infection control; Infection protection; Fluid/electrolyte management; Medication management; Temperature regulation

PLANNING AND IMPLEMENTATION

Collaborative

The treatment for acute leukemia occurs in four phases: induction, consolidation, continuation, and treatment of (CNS) leukemia. During the induction phase, the patient receives an intense course of chemotherapy that is meant to cause a complete remission of the disease. Complete remission occurs when the patient has less than 5% of the bone marrow cells as blast cells and the peripheral blood counts are normal. Once remission has been sustained for 1 month, the patient enters the consolidation phase, during which the patient receives a modified course of chemotherapy to eradicate any remaining disease. The continuation, or maintenance, phase may continue for more than a year, during which time the patient receives small doses of chemotherapy every 3 to 4 weeks. Treatment of CNS leukemia has changed from irradiation, which leads to significant CNS complications, to intensive intrathecal and systemic chemotherapy for most patients.

Some patients also need transfusions with blood component therapy to control infection and prevent bleeding and anemia. Bone marrow transplantation (BMT) is an option for some patients. Early BMTs were allogenic transplants using stem cells that had been harvested from bone marrow from siblings or matched from other relatives or people listed in a donor registry. In autologous BMTs in the 1980s, physicians began using frozen cells harvested from the donor's own marrow during remission. More recently, a newer form of BMT has been developed that uses peripheral blood stem cell transplant (SCT) or peripheral blood progenitor cell transplant. Multiple pheresis, or removal of cells from the blood, provides the stem cells from the patient for transplantation. SCT permits the use of doses of chemotherapy and radiation therapy high enough to destroy the patient's bone marrow; after the treatment is completed, SCT restores blood-producing bone marrow stem cells. Radiation treatment is sometimes used to treat leukemic cells in the brain, spinal cord, or testicles.

Pharmacologic Highlights

Medication or Drug Class	Dosage	Description	Rationale
Chemotherapeutic agents: Note that chemotherapy regimes are continually changing with advances	Varies with drug; treatment for AML generally uses higher doses over a shorter period of time, whereas treatment for ALL uses lower doses over a longer period of time; treatment varies for children and adults and with phases of treatment	*Adult* AML remission induction: Anthracycline drug (idarubicin or daunorubicin) and cytarabine (araC); cladribine may be added For ALL, fludarabine and cyclophosphamide and rituximab (FCR) is commonly used *Child* AML induction: Daunomycin or idarubicin, cytosine arabinoside, and etoposide along with oral 6-thioguanine and dexamethasone. ALL induction: Prednisone, asparaginase, vincristine, and anthracycline	Decrease replication of leukemia cells and kill them

Other Drugs: Supportive care and management of complications from chemotherapy are handled with blood products and pharmacologically with antibiotics, antifungals, and antiviral drugs. Growth factors (colony-stimulating factors) may be given to elevate blood counts.

Independent

Focus on providing comfort and support, managing complications, and providing patient education. Determine how the patient is coping with the disease and where you can best provide support. For some patients, improving their comfort is the highest priority, either physically, such as with a bed bath or back rub, or emotionally, such as by listening to fears and concerns and providing interesting distractions. Teach the patient stress- and pain-reduction techniques. Provide mouth care to lessen the discomfort from oral lesions. Support the patient's efforts to maintain grooming and a positive body image. If the patient is a child, provide age-appropriate diversions, and work with the parents or caregivers to keep the significant others present and involved in the child's care.

Protect the patient from injury and infection. To limit the risk of bleeding, hold firm pressure on all puncture wounds for at least 10 minutes or until they stop oozing. Limit the use of intramuscular injections and IV catheter placement when the patient is pancytopenic. Avoid taking rectal temperatures, using rectal suppositories, or performing a rectal examination. If the patient does not respond to treatment, be honest about the patient's prognosis. Determine from parents how much information they want to share with the child about a terminal disease. Work with the patient, significant others, and chaplain to help the patient plan for a terminal illness and achieve a compassionate death.

Evidence-Based Practice and Health Policy

Liao, W., & Liu, Y. (2020). Treatment outcomes in children with acute lymphoblastic leukemia with versus without coexisting Down's syndrome: A systematic review and meta-analysis. *Medicine, 99*, e221015.

- The authors aimed to analyze the treatment outcomes for children with and without Down syndrome who have ALL. They used electronic databases to search for publications reporting treatment-related outcomes in children with ALL with follow-ups from 5 to 10 years. They reviewed studies with a total of 31,476 children.
- The authors found that event-free survival was similar for both groups of children, as were overall mortality and clinical remission. Treatment-related mortality, induction failure, and relapses of certain types were significantly higher in those with Down syndrome. Although these findings are important to the provider, it is important to note the number of children with Down syndrome was relatively low in comparison to the number without Down syndrome.

DOCUMENTATION GUIDELINES

- Physical response: Vital signs, physical assessment, signs of infection, signs of bleeding, ability to tolerate activity
- Response to chemotherapy or radiation treatments
- Emotional response to the diagnosis of cancer or the use of reverse isolation
- Comprehension of treatment plan, including care: Purpose and potential side effects of radiation and chemotherapy; bone marrow transplant
- Presence of complications: Infection, bleeding, poor wound healing, ineffective coping by the patient or significant others

DISCHARGE AND HOME HEALTHCARE GUIDELINES

Teach the patient and significant others about the course of the disease, the treatment options, and how to recognize complications. Explain that the patient or parents need to notify the physician if any of the following occur: fever, chills, cough, sore throat, increased bleeding or bruising, or new onset of bone or abdominal pain. Discuss the patient's home environment to limit the risk of exposure to infections. Encourage the patient to avoid close contact with family pets because dogs, cats, and birds carry infections. Animal licks, bites, and scratches are sources of infection. The patient should not clean birdcages, litter boxes, or fish tanks. Additional sources of bacteria in the home include water in humidifiers and standing water in flower vases. Encourage the patient to have air filters in furnaces and air conditioners changed weekly. Explain that raw fruits, vegetables, and uncooked meat carry bacteria and should be avoided. If the patient becomes injured, encourage the patient or significant others to apply pressure, use ice, and report excessive bleeding. Teach the patient to avoid blowing or picking the nose or straining at bowel movements to limit the risk of bleeding.

Explain the proper administration and potential side effects of any medications. Teach the patient how to manage pain with the prescribed analgesics and how to manage other side effects specific to each chemotherapeutic agent. Explain that the chemotherapy may cause weight loss, even anorexia. Encourage the patient to eat a diet high in calories and protein and to drink at least 2,000 mL of fluids per day. If the chemotherapy leads to anorexia, encourage the patient to eat frequent, small meals several times a day. Arrange for a dietary consultation if needed before discharge. If the patient has oral lesions, teach the patient to use a soft toothbrush or cloth and to avoid hot, spicy foods and commercial mouthwashes, which can irritate mouth ulcers. Encourage the patient to take frequent rest periods during the day and to space activities with rest.

Urge the patient to maintain a realistic but positive attitude. The return to an independent lifestyle is possible with the efforts of a competent healthcare team and the patient's cooperation. Provide a list of referral agencies as appropriate, such as the American Cancer Society, Leukemia & Lymphoma Society, hospice, and support groups.

Leukemia, Chronic

DRG Category:	841
Mean LOS:	5.5 days
Description:	MEDICAL: Lymphoma and Non-Acute Leukemia With Complication or Comorbidity

Leukemia is a malignant disease of the blood-forming organs that leads to a transformation of stem cells or early committed precursor cells and thus to an abnormal overproduction of certain leukocytes. Two types of chronic leukemia commonly occur: chronic lymphocytic leukemia (CLL) and chronic myelogenous leukemia (CML). The American Cancer Society predicted that approximately 60,530 new cases of all types of leukemia will occur in 2021; an estimated 21,250 of those cases will be CLL and 9,110 will be CML.

CLL, the most common form of leukemia in adults in the United States, involves lymphocytes (B cells), which derive from stem cells and circulate among blood, lymph nodes, and lymphatic organs. In CLL, an uncontrollable spread of abnormal, small lymphocytes occurs in the bone marrow, lymphoid tissues, and blood. The cells often build up slowly over time, and patients may be without symptoms for a number of years. In CLL, an underproduction of immunoglobulins (antibodies) leads to increased susceptibility to infections. Some patients also develop antibodies to red blood cells (RBCs) and platelets, which then leads to anemia and thrombocytopenia. Many patients live for years with CLL as a chronic disease requiring intermittent treatment. The 5-year survival rate of CLL is 87%, depending on the patient's stage of disease.

CML is characterized by the abnormal overgrowth of myeloblasts, promyelocytes, metamyelocytes, and myelocytes (all granulocytic precursors) in body tissues, peripheral blood, and bone marrow. In CML, the bone marrow becomes 100% cellular (rather than 50% cellular and 50% fat, the normal composition). The spleen enlarges with a greatly expanded red pulp area. CML has three phases: an insidious chronic phase, an accelerated phase, and an acute (or blast crisis) phase. In the insidious chronic phase, chronic leukemia originates in the pluripotent stem cell, with an initial finding of hypercellular marrow with a majority of normal cells. After a relatively slow course for a median of 4 years, the patient with chronic leukemia invariably enters an accelerated phase (increased white blood cell [WBC] counts, fever, weight loss, poor appetite), followed by a blast crisis, or acute phase (increasing blasts and more aggressive symptoms). The 5-year survival rate of CML is 70%, depending on the patient's stage of disease.

Both CLL and CML may metastasize to the blood, lymph nodes, spleen, liver, central nervous system, and other organs. Other complications include infection, anemia, lymphoma, and second cancers such as melanoma, colorectal cancer, lung cancer, or skin cancer.

CAUSES

The cause of chronic leukemia is uncertain. CLL appears to be an acquired disease because reports of cases with a familial history are rare. Long-term contact with herbicides and pesticides may increase the risk of CLL. CML appears to be acquired as well, but in most patients, there is the presence of a genetic mutation, the abnormal Philadelphia (Ph[1]) chromosome (see Genetic Considerations). Environmental factors such as exposure to high-dose radiation may increase the risk of CML.

GENETIC CONSIDERATIONS

Family members of individuals with CLL have an increased risk of developing CLL, and nine susceptibility loci have been implicated to increase risk. Approximately 90% of cases of CML result from the Ph^1 chromosome, a chromosomal translocation in which part of chromosome 9 is transferred to chromosome 22. This can be induced by radiation or carcinogenic chemicals. Several genetic disorders also increase the risk of leukemia. Persons with Down syndrome have a lifetime leukemia risk that is 15 times greater than that of the general population. The heritable disorders Fanconi anemia, Bloom syndrome, and ataxia telangiectasia also increase the likelihood of leukemia. Somatic mutations creating fusions between *BCR* and *ABL* genes cause chronic myeloid leukemia.

SEX AND LIFE SPAN CONSIDERATIONS

Chronic leukemia affects mostly older adults over age 50 years. Only about 2% of patients with chronic leukemia are children. CLL affects adults, and CML affects mostly adults in the fourth and fifth decades of life; uncommonly, CML affects children and older adults. The average age for the diagnosis of CLL is 72 years and for CML is 64 years. Twice as many males as females develop chronic leukemia.

HEALTH DISPARITIES AND SEXUAL/GENDER MINORITY HEALTH

The incidence of CLL is higher in White persons as compared to Black, Asian, or Hispanic persons. CML has no known racial or ethnic trends. A high body mass index (BMI) places a person at higher risk for leukemia than a normal BMI. Sexual and gender minority status has no known effect on the risk for CLL and CML. However, gender and sexual minority persons are a vulnerable group because people with low income, long travel distances to cancer screening sites, or who lack health insurance or paid medical leave are less likely to be treated according to cancer care guidelines (National Institutes of Health, 2021).

GLOBAL HEALTH CONSIDERATIONS

The global incidence of leukemia is approximately 6 per 100,000 males per year and 4 per 100,000 females per year. The incidence of a leukemia diagnosis is three times higher in developed regions than in developing regions. Chronic leukemia, and CLL in particular, is uncommon in people living in Asian countries.

◾ ASSESSMENT

HISTORY. Often, symptoms of chronic leukemia are nonspecific and vague. In CLL, swollen lymph nodes or enlarged liver and spleen may cause discomfort. The patient may report susceptibility to infections such as pneumonia, herpes simplex, and herpes zoster. They may report easy bruising, bleeding gums, or petechiae. In CML, sometimes the first symptom the patient reports is a dragging sensation caused by extreme splenomegaly, or it may be left upper quadrant pain that is caused by a splenic infarct. Assess the patient's activity tolerance to determine if the following occur: fatigue, loss of energy, or decreased exercise tolerance.

Question the patient about recent weight loss or appetite loss; blood in the urine; or black, tarry stools. Bone and joint tenderness may occur from marrow involvement. Determine if the patient has been running a low-grade fever. Take an occupational history to determine possible exposure to radiation or carcinogenic chemicals and determine a family history for leukemia and cancer.

PHYSICAL EXAMINATION. The patient may have a normal appearance because of the insidious onset of CLL and CML. Observe the patient's general appearance for **pallor** and inspect for **ecchymoses and bruises**. Examine the patient's eyes for **retinal hemorrhage**. Palpate the lymph nodes to determine the presence of lymphadenopathy and palpate the abdomen for enlargement of the spleen or liver. Palpate the patient's thorax for signs of sternal or rib tenderness, which may be indications of infiltration of the periosteum. Obtain the patient's weight and ask the patient to describe any recent weight loss. Inspect the ankles for edema. Note a low-grade fever. Examine the skin for macular to nodular eruptions, signs of skin infiltrations, bruising, and opportunistic fungal infections. Pulmonary infiltrates may appear when lung parenchyma is involved. Assess the patient's breathing for dyspnea. Auscultate the heart for signs of tachycardia and palpitation.

PSYCHOSOCIAL. Despite advances in treatment and cure, the diagnosis of cancer is an emotionally laden one. Determine the past coping mechanisms used to manage situations of severe stress. Assess the patient's home situation to determine the possibility of home healthcare. Assess the support systems available, including emotional, religious, financial, and social.

Diagnostic Highlights

Test	Normal Result	Abnormality With Condition	Explanation
Complete blood count and differential	RBCs: 3.6–5.8 million/mcL; hemoglobin: 11.7–17.3 g/dL; hematocrit: 36%–52%; WBCs: 4,500–11,100/mcL; platelets: 150,000–450,000/mcL; differential: neutrophils: 2.7–6.5/mcL (40%–75%); lymphocytes: 2.5–3.7/mcL (12%–44%); monocytes: 0.2–0.4/mcL (4%–9%); eosinophils: 0.05–0.5/mcL (0%–5.5%); basophils: 0–0.1/mcL (0%–1%)	Increased WBC counts; may be only slightly increased or > 200,000/mcL; RBCs, decreased; platelets, increased (early in CML) or decreased (CLL and late CML); CLL elevated lymphocytes	Overproduction of WBCs halts production of RBCs and platelets
Bone marrow aspiration/bone marrow biopsy	No leukemia cells present	Leukemic blast phase cells present; leukemic surface markers on cells	Thin needle used to draw up small amount of liquid bone marrow. In biopsy, small cylinder of bone and marrow (about 1/2 in. long) is removed; the site of both samples is usually at back of the hipbone

Other Tests: Coagulation studies (prothrombin time, activated partial thromboplastin time), peripheral blood smear, blood flow cytometry, chromosomal analysis, x-rays, computed tomography scan, magnetic resonance imaging, ultrasound

PRIMARY NURSING DIAGNOSIS

DIAGNOSIS. Risk for infection as evidenced by fever, chills, and/or tachypnea

OUTCOMES. Infection severity; Immune status; Knowledge: Infection management; Risk control; Risk detection; Fluid balance; Knowledge: Medication

INTERVENTIONS. Infection control; Infection protection; Fluid/electrolyte management; Medication management; Temperature regulation

PLANNING AND IMPLEMENTATION

Collaborative

Patients with CLL do not need drug therapy until they have evidence of progressive disease or have complications. In CLL, because treatments destroy normal cells along with malignant ones, therapy focuses on the prevention and resolution of complications from induced pancytopenia (anemia, bleeding, and infection in particular). When diagnosed, most patients do not require chemotherapy unless they have weight loss of more than 10%, extreme fatigue, fever related to leukemia, or night sweats. Other signs that warrant chemotherapy are progressive bone marrow failure; anemia or thrombocytopenia that does not respond to corticosteroid treatment; or progressive splenomegaly, lymphadenopathy, or lymphocytosis (> 50% in 2 months or doubling of count in less than 6 months). Chemotherapy is therefore employed to reduce symptoms.

Total body irradiation or local radiation to the spleen may also be given as a palliative treatment to reduce complications. Two complications during later stages of CLL are hemolytic anemia (caused by autoimmune disorder) and hypogammaglobulinemia, which further increases the patient's susceptibility to infection. Antibiotics, transfusions of RBCs, and injections of gamma globulin concentrates may be required for patients with these problems.

Therapy in the chronic phase of CML focuses on (1) achieving hematologic remission with a normal complete blood cell count and a physical examination without enlargement of organs (organomegaly), (2) achieving cytogenetic remission (normal chromosomes), and (3) achieving molecular remission (negative polymerase chain reaction result for mutated RNA). Allogeneic (belonging to same species) bone marrow transplantation (BMT) before blast crisis offers the best treatment option and can cure the condition. Best outcomes occur if the BMT is performed during the chronic phase of the disease. Chemotherapy is used in treating CML, but at this time, it has not proven satisfactory in producing long-term remission. Supportive care and management of complications from chemotherapy are handled pharmacologically with antibiotics, antifungals, and antiviral drugs.

Some patients also need transfusions with blood component therapy to control infection and prevent bleeding and anemia. To relieve the pain of splenomegaly, irradiation or removal may be used. As supportive treatment, leukapheresis (separating leukocytes from blood and then returning remaining blood to patient) may be performed to lower an extremely high peripheral leukocyte count quickly and to prevent acute tumor lysis syndrome, but the results are temporary. Platelet pheresis (separating platelets from blood and then returning remaining blood to patient) may be required for thrombocytosis as high as 2 million. Apheresis (separating blood into components) is usually performed with the use of automated blood cell separators that are designed to remove the selected blood element and return the remaining cells and plasma to the patient.

Pharmacologic Highlights

Medication or Drug Class	Dosage	Description	Rationale
Prednisone	20–60 mg daily initially, with gradual dose reduction	Corticosteroid	Decreases auto-immune response; manages immune hemolytic anemia or immune thrombocytopenia
Chemotherapy	Varies with drug	CLL: Fludarabine, cyclophosphamide, and rituximab (FCR); pentostatin, cyclophosphamide, and rituximab (PCR); fludarabine, cyclophosphamide, and mitoxantrone (FCM); cyclophosphamide, vincristine, and prednisone (CVP); cyclophosphamide, doxorubicin, vincristine, and prednisone (CHOP)	CLL: Controls symptoms and prevents proliferation of WBCs; patient is generally on chemotherapy for 2 wk and off for 2 wk

Pharmacologic Highlights (continued)

Medication or Drug Class	Dosage	Description	Rationale
Chemotherapy		CML: Tyrosine kinase inhibitors such as imatinib, dasatinib, nilotinib; in addition, busulfan (Myleran) and hydroxyurea; when a blast crisis occurs, other drugs are used: cytosine arabinoside, omacetaxine, daunorubicin, methotrexate, prednisone, vincristine	CML: Can destroy blast cells, prevent leukemic cells from inhibiting formation of normal granulocytes, or transform the blast cells into normal granulocytes
Other Drugs: Interferon therapy, monoclonal antibodies			

Independent

Management focuses on providing comfort, support, and patient education and managing complications. Determine how the patient is coping with the disease and where you can best provide support. For some patients, improving their comfort is the highest priority, either physically, such as with a bed bath or back rub, or emotionally, such as by listening to fears and concerns and providing interesting distractions. Teach stress- and pain-reduction techniques. Provide mouth care to lessen the discomfort from oral lesions. Support the patient's efforts to maintain grooming and a positive body image.

Institute measures to control infection and maintain a safe environment. To limit the risk of bleeding, hold firm pressure on all puncture wounds for at least 10 minutes or until they stop oozing. Limit the use of intramuscular injections and IV catheter placement when the patient is pancytopenic. Avoid taking rectal temperatures, using rectal suppositories, or performing a rectal examination.

Assist the patient in minimizing the discomfort of splenomegaly. Provide small, frequent meals. Maintain adequate fluid intake and a high-bulk diet. Prevent constipation. Encourage the patient to cough and perform deep-breathing exercises as a prophylactic for atelectasis.

For patients who are undergoing outpatient chemotherapy, teach about side effects, emphasizing dangerous ones such as bone marrow suppression. Emphasize that the physician should be called in case of a fever over 100°F (37.8°C), chills, redness or swelling, a sore throat, or a cough. Explain the signs of thrombocytopenia. Emphasize that the patient needs to avoid aspirin and aspirin-containing compounds that might exacerbate bleeding. Emphasize the need for adequate rest and the importance of a high-calorie, high-protein diet.

If the patient does not respond to treatment, be honest about prognosis. Implement strategies to manage pain, fever, and infection to ensure the patient's comfort. Work with the patient, significant others, and chaplain to help the patient plan for a terminal illness and achieve a compassionate death.

Evidence-Based Practice and Health Policy

Farooqui, A., Ashraf, A., Farooq, T., Anjum, A., Rehman, S., Akbar, A., Kanate, A., Dean, R., Ahmed, M., Tariq, M., Nabeel, S., Faisal, M., & Anwer, F. (2020). Novel targeted therapies for chronic lymphocytic leukemia in elderly patients: A systematic review. *Clinical Lymphoma, Myeloma & Leukemia, 20,* e414–426.

* CLL typically affects older patients. The administration of chemotherapies in older patients has modest benefits without improvement in survival. Trends are shifting toward the use of targeted therapies. The authors review the safety and efficacy of novel agents that specifically target the dysregulated pathways, with particular attention to older patients.
* They performed a comprehensive literature review of electronic databases and selected 36 studies using specific criteria for inclusion. New agents, including B-cell receptor (BCR)

inhibitors, spleen tyrosine kinase inhibitors, Bcl-2 inhibitors, immunomodulators, and mono-clonal antibodies have shown activity in CLL without toxicity. They concluded that newer agents have improved clinical outcomes and have tolerable toxicity profiles in older patients.

DOCUMENTATION GUIDELINES

- Physical response: Vital signs, physical assessment, signs of infection, signs of bleeding, ability to tolerate activity
- Response to chemotherapy or radiation treatments
- Comprehension of treatment plan, including care: Purpose and potential side effects of radiation and chemotherapy; bone marrow transplant
- Presence of complications: Infection, bleeding, poor wound healing, ineffective coping by the patient or significant others

DISCHARGE AND HOME HEALTHCARE GUIDELINES

Teach the patient and significant others about the course of the disease, the treatment options, and how to recognize complications. Explain that the patient or family needs to notify the physician if any of the following occur: fever, chills, cough, sore throat, increased bleeding or bruising, new onset of bone or abdominal pain. Urge the patient to maintain a realistic but positive attitude. The return to an independent lifestyle is possible with the efforts of a competent healthcare team and the patient's cooperation. Provide a list of referral agencies as appropriate, such as the American Cancer Society, the Leukemia & Lymphoma Society, hospice, and support groups.

Discuss the patient's home environment to limit the risk of exposure to infections. Encourage the patient to avoid close contact with family pets because they carry infections. The patient should not clean birdcages, litter boxes, or fish tanks. Additional sources of bacteria in the home include water in humidifiers and standing water in flower vases. Encourage the patient to have air filters in furnaces and air conditioners changed weekly. Explain that raw fruits, vegetables, and uncooked meat carry bacteria and should be avoided. If the patient is injured, encourage the patient to apply pressure, use ice to the area, and report excessive bleeding. Teach the patient to avoid blowing or picking the nose or straining at bowel movements to limit the risk of bleeding.

Explain the proper administration and potential side effects of any medications. Teach the patient how to manage pain with the prescribed analgesics and how to manage other side effects specific to each chemotherapeutic agent. Explain that the chemotherapy may cause weight loss and anorexia. Encourage the patient to eat a diet high in calories and protein and to drink at least 2,000 mL of fluids per day. If the chemotherapy leads to anorexia, encourage the patient to eat frequent, small meals several times a day. Arrange for a dietary consultation if needed before discharge. If the patient has oral lesions, teach the patient to use a soft toothbrush or cloth and to avoid hot, spicy foods and commercial mouthwashes, which can irritate mouth ulcers.

Liver Failure

DRG Category: 441
Mean LOS: 6.3 days
Description: MEDICAL: Disorders of Liver Except Malignancy, Cirrhosis, Alcoholic Hepatitis With Major Complication or Comorbidity

Liver (hepatic) failure is a loss of liver function because of the death of many hepatocytes. The damage can occur suddenly, as with a viral infection, or slowly over time, as with cirrhosis. Acute liver failure (ALF) refers to both fulminant hepatic failure (FHF) and subfulminant hepatic failure. FHF occurs when sudden (within 8 weeks from onset) severe liver decompensation caused by massive necrosis of the liver leads to coagulopathies and encephalopathy. Approximately 2,000 people in the United States develop FHF each year. Subfulminant hepatic failure, also known as *late-onset hepatic failure*, can take up to 26 weeks before hepatic encephalopathy develops. Hepatic encephalopathy occurs with neurological changes such as personality changes, changes in cognition and intellect, and reduced level of consciousness.

Because of the complex functions of the liver, liver failure leads to multiple system complications. When ammonia and other metabolic by-products are not metabolized, they accumulate in the blood and cause neurological deterioration. Cerebral edema likely results from impaired regulation of osmosis, resulting in swelling of brain cells and accumulation of toxic products of metabolism, particularly glutamine. Without normal vitamin K activation and the production of clotting factors, the patient has coagulation problems. Patients are at risk for infections because of general malnutrition, debilitation, impairment of phagocytosis, and decreased liver production of immune-related proteins. Fluid retention occurs because of decreased albumin production, leading to decreased colloidal osmotic pressure with failure to retain fluid in the bloodstream. Renin and aldosterone production cause sodium and water retention. Ascites occurs because of intrahepatic vascular obstruction with fluid movement into the peritoneum.

Complications of liver failure include bleeding esophageal varices (Box 1), hemorrhagic shock, hepatic encephalopathy, seizures, hepatorenal syndrome, coma, and even death.

• BOX 1 Bleeding Esophageal Varices

Esophageal varices (fragile, distended, and thin-walled veins in the esophagus) occur in patients with liver failure because of portal hypertension. Obstructed blood circulates to low-resistance alternate vessels around the portal circulation in the liver, which is a high-pressure system. One of these routes is through the esophageal veins, which become distended with blood, irritated from pressure, and susceptible to rupture. Treatment of esophageal varices includes the following:

Surgery. Procedures include placing a portal caval shunt or distal splenorenal shunt, esophageal repair, or devascularization.

Endoscopic Sclerotherapy. To cause fibrosis of the varices, patients are injected with solutions during an endoscopy procedure. Sodium tetradecyl sulfate or sodium morrhuate are commonly used sclerosants in the United States.

Esophageal Balloon Tamponade. Endoscopic therapy has replaced balloon tamponade in almost all situations. If balloon therapy is used, it is essential that it is initiated by an experienced clinician. In balloon tamponade, a multilumen gastrointestinal tube with an esophageal and gastric balloon is passed into the upper gastrointestinal tract through the patient's mouth. The gastric balloon, which is filled with 250 to 300 mL of air, acts as an anchor; the esophageal balloon, which is filled with enough air to cause 20 to 75 mm Hg pressure, compresses the esophageal varices to decrease bleeding. Traction may be inserted by taping the outer portions of the multilumen tube to the face mask of a football helmet.

Parenteral Therapy. Maintain a large-bore IV line and keep several units of packed cells on call from the blood bank at all times.

Vasopressin (Pitressin) Therapy. A continuous infusion of this vasoconstrictor causes constriction of the mesenteric circulation and decreased blood flow to the portal circulation.

CAUSES

The leading causes of FHF are viral hepatitis and hepatotoxic drug reactions. The most common drug associated with liver failure is acetaminophen (42%), but idiosyncratic drug reactions (12%) also can lead to ALF. Although viral hepatitis can lead to liver failure, fewer than 5% of patients with viral hepatitis actually develop it. Other causes include chronic alcohol abuse, acute infection or hemorrhage that leads to shock, fatty liver of pregnancy, prolonged cholestasis (arrest of bile excretion), and metabolic disorders. Many of these lead to cirrhosis, a chronic liver disease that results in widespread tissue fibrosis, nodule formation, and necrosis of the liver tissue. Risk factors for liver failure include chronic alcohol abuse, poor nutrition, pregnancy, chronic hepatitis B and C, use of untested alternative/complementary medications, and narcotic abuse.

GENETIC CONSIDERATIONS

Autosomal dominant polycystic kidney disease is mainly caused by mutations in two genes (*PKD1* and *PKD2*) that also increase susceptibility to liver cysts. Isolated liver cysts (the polycystic liver disease) have been linked to multiple genes (*PRKCSH*, *SEC63*, *LRP5*, and *ALG8*). Some affected persons develop massive hepatic cystic disease that results in liver failure. Wilson disease is an autosomal recessive genetic disorder caused by mutations in *ATP7B*, leading to a large liver accumulation of copper. About 5% of patients with Wilson disease suffer from acute liver failure or fulminant hepatitis.

SEX AND LIFE SPAN CONSIDERATIONS

Although acute liver failure can occur at any age, infants and children are more likely to have an inherited disease, whereas adult men are more likely to have alcohol-related disease. The poorest outcomes and mortality rates are found in children under 10 years or adults older than 40 years. Cirrhosis is the 12th leading cause of death in the United States and occurs most commonly between the ages of 35 and 55 years. Women develop acute liver failure at a later age than men and are more likely than men to have failure related to viral hepatitis E or autoimmune liver disease. Women are also more severely affected by alcohol- and drug-induced liver injury than men. Women are more likely to die while waiting for a liver transplant as compared to men.

HEALTH DISPARITIES AND SEXUAL/GENDER MINORITY HEALTH

White persons have the highest rates of ALF (74%), followed by Hispanic (10%), Asian (5%), and Black (3%) persons. Sexual and gender minority people have higher rates of alcohol consumption than the general population (Centers for Disease Control and Prevention, 2021), which may place them at risk for liver failure.

GLOBAL HEALTH CONSIDERATIONS

The cause of liver failure varies across different countries. Worldwide statistics indicate that postnecrotic cirrhosis is more common in women than men and is the most common type of liver failure worldwide. Acetaminophen overdose is a common cause of liver failure in Western Europe, whereas hepatitis B and hepatitis D viral infections are a major cause in developing countries. Hepatitis E virus is associated with liver failure in pregnant persons, particularly those living or traveling in developing regions in Mexico, India, China, and Northern Africa.

ASSESSMENT

HISTORY. Determine the patient's family history for liver disease. Take a detailed medication history with particular attention to hepatotoxic medications, such as anesthesia agents, analgesics, antiseizure medications, cocaine, alcohol, isoniazid, herbal medications, and oral contraceptives. Ask about any recent travel to China, southeast Asia, sub-Saharan Africa, the Pacific Islands, and areas around the Amazon River, which may have exposed the patient to hepatitis B. Explore the patient's occupational history for hepatitis exposure; patients who are day-care workers, dental workers, physicians, nurses, or hospital laboratory workers are particularly at risk. Ask if the patient has experienced previous liver or biliary disease. Elicit a history of IV drug use and/or men having sex with men, because these activities expose people to the risk for hepatitis and therefore liver failure. Those who eat raw shellfish are at similar risk.

Patients or families may describe early symptoms such as personality changes (agitation, forgetfulness, disorientation), fatigue, anorexia, drowsiness, and mild tremors. Some patients experience sleep disturbance and low-grade fevers. As larger areas of the liver are destroyed, patients have increasing fatigue, confusion, and lethargy. If patients have longstanding liver failure, they experience jaundice, dry skin, early morning nausea, vomiting, anorexia, weight loss, altered bowel habits, and epigastric discomfort. If sudden FHF occurs, patients may develop encephalopathy (decreased mental status, fixed facial expression), peripheral swelling, ascites, and bleeding tendencies. Urine is often dark from bilirubin, and stools are often light colored because of the absence of bilirubin.

PHYSICAL EXAMINATION. The patient with acute liver failure usually has **jaundiced skin and sclera**. Fluid retention results in **ascites and peripheral edema**. The patient's facial expression appears fixed, movements are hesitant, and speech is slow. Usually, the patient's mental status is markedly decreased, and you may smell fetor hepaticus, a sweet fecal odor, on the patient's breath. The patient may have multiple bruises, a bloody nose, or bleeding gums.

The patient's peripheral pulses are bounding and rapid, indicating fluid overload and a hyperdynamic circulation. You may also palpate peripheral edema, an enlarged firm liver in acute failure and a small hard liver in chronic failure, an enlarged spleen, a distended abdomen, and an abdomen with shifting dullness to percussion and a positive fluid wave because of ascites. As ascites worsens, the patient develops hernias, an everted umbilicus, and an elevated and displaced heart because of a raised diaphragm. Usually, the patient with late disease has neck vein distention, and men develop gynecomastia (enlarged breasts), testicular atrophy, and scant body hair. When you monitor the patient's vital signs, you may find an elevated temperature and a low-to-normal blood pressure; if the physician initiates hemodynamic monitoring, the cardiac output may be low if ascites is decreasing the right ventricular filling pressure and if the systemic vascular resistance is low.

PSYCHOSOCIAL. The patient may feel upset or guilty if the patient contracted the disease while traveling. Use a nonjudgmental approach to elicit the patient's feelings if the condition is related to alcohol or drug abuse. If the patient is a candidate for a liver transplant, determine the patient's emotional stability, ability to cope with a complex medical regimen, and ability to rely on significant others.

Diagnostic Highlights

Test	Normal Result	Abnormality With Condition	Explanation
Prothrombin time	Varies by laboratory; generally 10–13 sec	Prolonged > 15 sec	Prothrombin is formed in the liver and is a vitamin K–dependent glycoprotein necessary for firm clot formation
Viral hepatitis serologies: Hepatitis A virus (HAV); hepatitis B virus (HBV); hepatitis C virus (HCV); hepatitis D virus (HDV); hepatitis E virus (HEV) (see **Hepatitis**)	Negative results	If patient has hepatitis: acute HAV: positive anti-HAV IgM; acute HBV: anti-HBV IgM; HB surface antigen; acute HCV: anti-HCV antibody, HCV RNA; HDV: anti-HDV IgM, HDV antigen; HEV: not available; non-A, non-B: all tests negative	Identify patients with hepatitis; virus leads to markers such as immunoglobulins (IgG and IgM), antigens, antibodies

(highlight box continues on page 754)

Diagnostic Highlights (continued)

Test	Normal Result	Abnormality With Condition	Explanation
Liver function tests	Alanine amino-transferase (ALT): 19–36 units/L; aspartate amino-transferase (AST): 15–40 units/L; alkaline phosphatase: 25–142 units/L	ALT elevated as high as or higher than 1,000 units/L; AST elevated as high as or higher than 1,000 units/L; alkaline phosphatase mildly elevated	Determine the extent of liver damage

Other Tests: The most important aspect of the diagnostic work-up is to determine the underlying cause of liver failure. Tests include liver ultrasound, computed tomography, magnetic resonance imaging, drug and alcohol screening, bilirubin, lactate dehydrogenase, complete blood count, serum glucose, serum lactate, serum sodium and potassium, ammonia, albumin, and liver biopsy.

PRIMARY NURSING DIAGNOSIS

DIAGNOSIS. Excess fluid volume related to water and sodium retention as evidenced by rapid and bounding peripheral pulses, ascites, and/or peripheral edema

OUTCOMES. Fluid balance; Electrolyte balance; Fluid overload severity; Hydration; Nutrition status; Knowledge: Disease process; Knowledge: Treatment regimen

INTERVENTIONS. Fluid/electrolyte management; Fluid monitoring; Medication administration; Nutrition management

PLANNING AND IMPLEMENTATION

Collaborative

Liver transplantation is the definitive treatment for ALF. More than 17,000 people are waiting for liver transplantation in the United States, and approximately 6,000 transplants are done each year. A liver transplant is indicated for patients with irreversible progressive liver disease who have no alternatives to transplantation, have life-threatening complications, or have the inability to sustain a normal quality of life. Patients with ALF who meet specific criteria can increase their transplant waitlist priority ahead of patients with liver failure caused by chronic liver disease.

While waiting for transplantation, if indicated, patients are managed with supportive therapy depending on their symptoms. Maintenance of airway, breathing, and circulation is the highest priority. Fluid and electrolyte imbalances, malnutrition, ascites, respiratory failure, cerebral edema, and bleeding esophageal varices can all occur with liver failure. Unless the patient has clinically significant hyponatremia, the patient usually receives limited IV fluids and food that contains sodium because increased sodium intake makes peripheral edema and ascites worse. Patients with ascites are usually restricted to 500 mg of sodium per day. A paracentesis may be used to remove 4 to 6 L of fluid. If the ascites is refractory, surgical placement of a peritoneal-venous shunt may be needed. Hypokalemia usually needs to be corrected with IV replacements. If the patient has serious fluid imbalances, a pulmonary artery catheter may be inserted for hemodynamic monitoring. If problems occur with coagulation, the patient may receive fresh frozen plasma.

Encephalopathy and cerebral edema are managed with hospitalization. Patients need serial neurological assessments. They should be positioned with the head of their bed elevated, and they may have continuous intracranial pressure (ICP) monitoring instituted. Because ammonia levels are increased due to liver failure, and since accumulation of ammonia and glutamine increase ICP, medications such as lactulose may be administered to reduce ammonia levels. Increased ICP may be managed with osmotic diuretics and hyperventilation. Other strategies may be the administration of hypertonic saline and/or barbiturate agents.

If respiratory failure is present, the patient may need endotracheal intubation and mechanical ventilation with supplemental oxygen. To manage nutrition in patients without evidence of hepatic encephalopathy, a high-calorie, 80- to 100-g protein diet is prescribed to allow for cellular repair. Some patients may need enteral or total parenteral nutrition to maintain calorie and protein levels. Hepatorenal failure is treated by fluid restriction, maintenance of fluid and electrolyte balance, and withdrawal of nephrotoxic drugs. Renal dialysis is generally not used because it does not improve survival and can lead to additional complications.

Pharmacologic Highlights

Medication or Drug Class	Dosage	Description	Rationale
Histamine receptor (H₂) antagonists	Varies with drug	Famotidine, cimetidine	Decrease gastric secretion; used as prophylaxis for ulcers
Thiamine	100 mg qd for several days or longer, depending on nutritional deficiencies	Vitamin supplement	Reduces risk for neuropathies
Vitamin K	Up to 10 mg IV as needed	Vitamin supplement	Needed for prothrombin production

Other Drugs: Sedatives and acetaminophen are avoided because poor metabolism can precipitate encephalopathy. Aspirin is usually avoided because of the action on platelets, which can lead to increased bleeding. If ascites is present, diuretics, particularly aldosterone antagonists such as spironolactone (Aldactone), may be prescribed and, if ineffective, more potent loop diuretics may be added. Mannitol may be used as an osmotic diuretic to reduce cerebral edema. Barbiturates such as pentobarbital and thiopental may be used for intracranial hypertension. Silibinin is a derivative of silymarin, an active ingredient in herbal preparations that possesses antioxidant properties; its use may benefit liver disease management.

Independent

The most common problem for patients with liver failure is fluid volume excess. Measure the patient's abdominal girth at the same location daily and mark the location as a reference point for future measurements. Notify the physician if the girth increases by 2 inches in 24 hours. Provide the required fluid allotment over the three meals and at night. If the patient desires, reserve some fluids to be used as ice chips. Provide mouth care every 2 hours. Because areas of edema are likely to be fragile and prone to skin breakdown, provide skin care.

One of the most life-threatening complications of liver failure is airway compromise because of neurological or respiratory deterioration. Keep endotracheal intubation equipment and an oral airway at the bedside at all times. Elevate the head of the patient's bed to 30 degrees to ease respirations and support the patient's arms on pillows to decrease the work of breathing. It is essential to be at the bedside and to perform serial assessments of all critical systems. Space all activities and limit visitors as needed so that the patient gets adequate rest. To encourage rest, consider nonpharmacologic methods such as diversionary activities and relaxation techniques.

The patient may be anxious, depressed, angry, or emotionally labile. Allow the patient to verbalize anxieties and fears. If needed, refer the patient to a counselor. Evaluate thoroughly anyone who is a candidate for a liver transplant to ensure that they have the ability to cope with a complex situation. Answer all questions, and explain the risks and benefits. Refer to an alcohol counselor if appropriate.

Depending on the patient's condition, discussion of end-of-life care might be appropriate. Opening discussion of the patient's desires for hospice care may be appropriate, as may discussion about the patient's preferences for a funeral. The patient and family will need privacy for these discussions.

Evidence-Based Practice and Health Policy

Patterson, J., Hussey, H., Silal, S., Goddard, L., Setshedi, M., Spearman, W., Hussey, G., Kagina, B., & Muloiwa, R. (2020). Systematic review of the global epidemiology of viral-induced acute liver failure. *BMJ Open.* Advance online publication. http://doi.org/10.1136/bmjopen-2020-037473

- The authors conducted a systematic review to explain the epidemiology of viral-induced ALF to facilitate clinical case management and case prevention. They searched electronic databases and located 25 eligible studies. They estimated the burden of ALF after infection with HBV, HAV, HCV, HEV, herpes simplex virus/human herpesvirus, cytomegalovirus, Epstein-Barr virus, and parvovirus B19.
- The prevalence of hepatitis A–induced ALF was markedly lower in countries with routine hepatitis A immunization versus no routine hepatitis A immunization. HEV was the most common cause of viral-induced ALF. Viral-induced ALF had poor outcomes as indicated by high fatality rates, which appear to increase with poor economic status of the studied countries.

DOCUMENTATION GUIDELINES

- Physical responses: Vital signs, ease of respirations, breath sounds, heart sounds, level of consciousness, gastrointestinal distress, abdominal girth, daily weights, color of skin and sclera
- Nutrition: Tolerance of diet, appetite, ability to maintain body weight or to decrease fluid retention, presence of muscle wasting or signs of malnutrition, albumin level
- Response to therapy: Clearing of mental status, improvement in infection, decreased or stable blood ammonia level

DISCHARGE AND HOME HEALTHCARE GUIDELINES

Teach the patient to follow prescribed sodium and fluid restrictions. Assist the patient to individualize a diet plan to maximize personal choices, including a dietitian if necessary. Encourage sodium-restricted patients to read labels on all canned soups, sauces, and vegetables and on all over-the-counter medications. Be sure the patient understands any pain medication prescribed, including dosage, route, action, and side effects. Teach the patient and family the need to limit the rise of infections by good hand washing, avoidance of others with colds, and prompt treatment by a healthcare provider when an infection occurs. Refer the patient to an alcohol support group.

Lung Cancer

DRG Category:	165
Mean LOS:	3.3 days
Description:	SURGICAL: Major Chest Procedures Without Complication or Comorbidity or Major Complication or Comorbidity
DRG Category:	181
Mean LOS:	4.2 days
Description:	MEDICAL: Respiratory Neoplasms With Complication or Comorbidity

Lung cancer is the leading cause of cancer death in the United States. The Centers for Disease Control and Prevention also reported that it is the second-most common cancer diagnosis after breast cancer for women and prostate cancer for men. It accounts for 25% of all cancer deaths and accounts for more deaths than prostate, breast, and colon cancer combined. The American Cancer Society (ACS) estimates that 235,760 new cases of lung cancer will occur in 2021, and 131,880 people will die. About 14% of all new cancers are lung cancer.

There are two major types of lung cancer: small cell lung cancer (SCLC) and non–small cell lung cancer (NSCLC). Sometimes a lung cancer shows characteristics of both types and is labeled small cell/large cell carcinoma. Both types have the capacity to synthesize bioactive products and produce paraneoplastic syndromes such as syndrome of inappropriate secretion of antidiuretic hormone (SIADH), Cushing syndrome, and Eaton-Lambert syndrome of neuromuscular disorder.

SCLC accounts for 15% of all lung cancers and is almost always caused by smoking. SCLC is characterized by small, round to oval cells generally beginning in the neuroendocrine cells of the bronchoepithelium of the lungs. They start multiplying quickly into large tumors and can spread to the lymph nodes and other organs. At the time of diagnosis, approximately 70% have already metastasized, often to the brain. SCLC is sometimes called *small cell undifferentiated carcinoma* and *oat cell carcinoma*. The 5-year survival rate of SCLC that is localized is 27%, and if cancer has spread to distant parts of the body, the 5-year survival rate is 3%.

NSCLC accounts for approximately 85% of all lung cancers and includes three subtypes: squamous cell carcinoma, adenocarcinoma, and large cell undifferentiated carcinoma. Squamous cell carcinoma, also associated with smoking, tends to be located centrally, near a bronchus, and accounts for approximately 25% to 30% of all lung cancers. Adenocarcinoma, accounting for 40% of all large cell carcinoma, is usually found in the outer region of the lung. One type of adenocarcinoma, bronchioloalveolar carcinoma, tends to produce a better prognosis than other types of lung cancer and is sometimes associated with areas of scarring. Large cell undifferentiated carcinoma starts in any part of the lung, grows quickly, and results in a poor prognosis owing to early metastasis; approximately 10% to 15% of lung cancers are large cell undifferentiated carcinoma. The 5-year survival rate for localized NSCLC is 63%, and if cancer has spread to distant parts of the body, the 5-year survival rate is 7%.

The hilus of the lung, close to the larger divisions of the bronchi, is the most frequent site of lung cancer. Abnormal cells divide and accumulate over time. As the cells grow into a carcinoma, they make the bronchial lining irregular and uneven. The tumor may penetrate the lung wall and surrounding tissue or grow into the opening (lumen) of the bronchus. In more than 50% of patients, the tumor spreads into the lymph nodes and then into other organs.

Systemic effects of the lung tumor that are unrelated to metastasis may affect the endocrine, hematological, neuromuscular, and dermatological systems. These changes may cause connective tissue and vascular abnormalities, referred to as paraneoplastic syndromes. In lung cancer, the most common endocrine syndromes are SIADH, Cushing syndrome, and gynecomastia. Complications of lung cancer include emphysema, bronchial obstruction, atelectasis, pulmonary abscesses, pleuritis, bronchitis, and compression on the vena cava.

CAUSES

Approximately 80% of lung cancers are related to cigarette, pipe, and cigar smoking. Lung cancer is 10 times more common in smokers than in nonsmokers. In particular, squamous cell and small cell carcinoma are associated with smoking. Other risk factors include exposure to carcinogenic industrial and air pollutants (e.g., asbestos, coal dust, radon, and arsenic) and family history.

GENETIC CONSIDERATIONS

Lung cancer is predominately caused by environmental factors, with approximately 85% of all cases linked to smoking. However, there are some genetic factors that increase susceptibility. Both somatic and germline mutations in several genes, including *SLC22A18*, *TP53*, *KRAS2*, *BRAF*, *ERBB2*, *MET*, *STK11*, *PIK3CA*, and *EGFR*, have been implicated in pathogenesis of lung cancer. Recently, a locus for a lung cancer susceptibility gene has been linked to a site on chromosome 6 (6q23-25).

SEX AND LIFE SPAN CONSIDERATIONS

The average age of people diagnosed with lung cancer is 70 years, and it is an unusual diagnosis for people younger than 45 years. Of the total number of deaths from lung cancer each year, 57% are men and 43% are women. The chance of men developing lung cancer is 1 in 13 and women 1 in 18. There has been an observable decline in deaths among younger men, and this is probably related to the diminishing number of young men who smoke, while rates in younger women are climbing. This increase may be related to increased rates of smoking among young women; experts also suggest that women may be more susceptible to the toxins in smoke than young men. Squamous cell carcinoma is most common in male smokers. Adenocarcinoma is equally common in men and women.

HEALTH DISPARITIES AND SEXUAL/GENDER MINORITY HEALTH

The ACS reports that Black men are 15% more likely to develop lung cancer than White men. Conversely, White women are 14% more likely to develop lung cancer than Black women. Health disparities exist because the 5-year survival rate for White people is 16% and non-White people is 13%. In areas of the United States experiencing persistent poverty, mortality rates for lung cancer are higher than in areas with low poverty rates. Sexual and gender minority people have higher rates of tobacco consumption than the general population (Centers for Disease Control and Prevention, 2021), which may place them at risk for lung cancer.

GLOBAL HEALTH CONSIDERATIONS

Cancer is the second leading cause of death globally, with 14 million new cases each year. The World Health Organization expects the number of new cases to rise by 70% over the next two decades. Tobacco use is the most important causal agent for cancer worldwide and is estimated to cause 22% of all cancer deaths. The global incidence of lung cancer is approximately 13 per 100,000 females per year and 31 per 100,000 males per year. Worldwide, lung cancer causes 1.8 million deaths each year and is the most commonly diagnosed cancer. The incidence is four to five times higher in developed than in developing countries, with the highest incidence in Hungary, Serbia, Poland, and Korea. As smoking rates increase in developing countries such as India and China, experts expect rates of lung cancer to increase.

ASSESSMENT

HISTORY. While most patients will have a history of tobacco use, many will not report symptoms of lung cancer until they have advanced disease. Establish a history of persistent cough, chest pain, wheezing, dyspnea, weight loss, or hemoptysis. Ask if the patient has experienced a change in normal respiratory patterns or hoarseness. Some patients initially report pneumonia, bronchitis, epigastric pain, symptoms of brain metastasis, arm or shoulder pain, or swelling of the upper body. Ask if the sputum has changed color, especially to a bloody, rusty, or purulent hue. Obtain a smoking history with the type of tobacco use and the quantity and frequency of use. Elicit a history of exposure to risk factors by determining if the patient has been exposed to industrial or air pollutants. Check the patient's family history for incidence of lung cancer.

PHYSICAL EXAMINATION. **Many people are asymptomatic.** As the disease progresses, symptoms are **cough, dyspnea, wheezing,** and **hemoptysis.** The clinical manifestations of lung cancer depend on the type and location of the tumor. Because the early stages of this disease usually produce no symptoms, it is most often diagnosed when the disease is at an advanced stage. In 10% to 20% of patients, lung cancer is diagnosed without any symptoms, usually from an abnormal finding on a routine chest x-ray. Approximately 25% have regional metastasis, and 40% have distant metastasis with symptoms that reflect the organ affected (brain, spinal cord, bone, liver).

Auscultation may reveal a wheeze if partial bronchial obstruction has occurred. Auscultate for decreased breath sounds, rales, or rhonchi. Note rapid, shallow breathing and signs of an airway obstruction, such as extreme shortness of breath, the use of accessory muscles, abnormal retractions, and stridor. Tumor involvement of the pleura and chest wall may cause pleural effusion. Typically, pleural effusion causes dullness on percussion and breath sounds that are decreased below the effusion and increased above it. Monitor the patient for oxygenation problems, such as increased heart rate, decreased blood pressure, or an increased duskiness of the oral mucous membranes. Metastases to the mediastinal lymph nodes may involve the laryngeal nerve and may lead to hoarseness and vocal cord paralysis. The superior vena cava may become occluded with enlarged lymph nodes and cause superior vena cava syndrome; note edema of the face, neck, upper extremities, and thorax.

PSYCHOSOCIAL. The patient undergoes major lifestyle changes as a result of the physical side effects of cancer and its treatment. Interpersonal, social, and work role relationships change. The patient is faced with a psychological adjustment to the diagnosis of a chronic illness that frequently results in death. Evaluate the patient for evidence of altered moods such as depression or anxiety, and assess the patient's coping mechanisms and support system.

Diagnostic Highlights

Test	Normal Result	Abnormality With Condition	Explanation
Chest x-ray	Clear lung fields; patent bronchi	Presence of tumors; compression of vital structures	Air-filled lungs are radiolucent (x-rays pass through tissue, which appears as a dark area), but tumors or masses may appear denser
Computed tomography scan	Normal organ and tissues	Presence and size of tumor; enlarged lymph nodes; compression of pulmonary structures	Sequential x-rays combined by computer to produce a detailed cross-sectional image of lungs
Cytological sputum analysis	No cancer cells present in sputum	Presence of cancer cells in sputum	Microscopic examination of sputum sample to determine presence of cancer cells; even with large tumors, cells may not be obtained in sputum

(highlight box continues on page 760)

Diagnostic Highlights (continued)

Test	Normal Result	Abnormality With Condition	Explanation
Bronchos-copy	No tumors or lung blockages	Visualization of tumors or blockages	Visual examination of the lungs through the use of a flexible fiber-optic lighted tube; microscopic examination of cells taken by biopsy and bronchial brushings

Other Tests: Magnetic resonance imaging, thoracentesis, thoracoscopy, closed-check needle biopsy, fluoroscopy, positron emission tomography, bone scan, mediastinos-copy, bone marrow biopsy, complete blood count, arterial blood gas

PRIMARY NURSING DIAGNOSIS

DIAGNOSIS. Ineffective airway clearance related to obstruction caused by secretions or tumor as evidenced by cough, dyspnea, wheezing, and/or hemoptysis

OUTCOMES. Respiratory status: Airway patency; Respiratory status: Gas exchange; Respiratory status: Ventilation; Symptom severity; Comfort status

INTERVENTIONS. Airway management; Oxygen therapy; Airway suctioning; Airway insertion and stabilization; Cough enhancement; Mechanical ventilation management: Invasive and noninvasive; Positioning; Respiratory monitoring; Anxiety reduction

PLANNING AND IMPLEMENTATION
Collaborative

The treatment of lung cancer depends on the type of cancer and the stage of the disease. Surgery, radiation therapy, and chemotherapy are all used. Unless the tumor is small without metastasis or nodes when discovered, it is often not curable. As experts have understood the molecular changes that occur in lung cancer, molecular-targeted therapy has led to testing for mutations to determine if specific targeted agents might be successful.

Surgical treatment ranges from segmentectomy or wedge resection (removal of a part of a lobe) to lobectomy (removal of a section of the lung) to pneumonectomy (removal of an entire lung). These procedures all require general anesthesia and a thoracotomy (surgical incision in the chest). Video-assisted thoracoscopic surgery is a minimally invasive procedure used for both diagnosis and treatment. It involves a shorter hospital stay, less pain, and a lower perioperative mortality. Outcome measures along with recurrence rates are currently being followed and compared with those from more invasive procedures. If patients are unable to undergo a thoracotomy because of other serious medical problems or widespread cancer, laser surgery may be performed to relieve blocked airways and diminish the threat of pneumonia or shortness of breath. Chemotherapy is used for cancer that has metastasized beyond the lungs. It is used both as a primary treatment and an adjuvant treatment to surgery. Combined treatment with radiation therapy and chemotherapy is the standard of care for SCLC. The chemotherapy most often uses a combination of anticancer drugs; different combinations are used to treat NSCLC and SCLC.

Radiation therapy is sometimes the primary treatment for lung cancer, particularly in patients who are unable to undergo surgery. It is also used palliatively to alleviate symptoms of lung cancer. In conjunction with surgery, radiation is sometimes used to kill deposits of cancer that are too small to be seen and thus to be surgically removed. Radiation therapy takes two forms: External beam therapy delivers radiation from outside the body and focuses on the cancer and is most frequently used to treat a primary lung cancer or its metastases to other organs; brachytherapy uses a small pellet of radioactive material that is placed directly into the cancer or into the nearby airway.

Pharmacologic Highlights

Medication or Drug Class	Dosage	Description	Rationale
Chemotherapy	Varies with drug	Cisplatin or carboplatin in combination with gemcitabine, paclitaxel, pemetrexed, docetaxel, etoposide, or vinorelbine	More effective in treating NSCLC
		Etoposide and cisplatin or etoposide and carboplatin, ifosfamide, carboplatin, and etoposide, or cyclophosphamide, doxorubicin, and vincristine, topotecan, irinotecan	More effective in treating SCLC

Independent

Maintain a patent airway. Position the head of the bed at 30 to 45 degrees. Increase the patient's fluid intake, if possible, to assist in liquefying lung secretions. Provide humidified air. Suction the patient's airway if necessary. Assist the patient in controlling pain and managing dyspnea. Assist the patient with positioning and pursed-lip breathing. Allow extra time to accomplish the activities of daily living. Teach the patient to use guided imagery, diversional activities, and relaxation techniques. Provide periods of rest between activities.

Discuss the expected preoperative and postoperative procedures with patients who are undergoing surgical intervention. Emphasize the importance of coughing and deep breathing after surgery. Splinting the patient's incision may decrease the amount of discomfort the patient feels during these activities. Monitor closely the patency of the chest tubes and the amount of chest tube drainage. Notify the physician if the chest tube drainage is greater than 200 mL/hour for more than 2 to 3 hours, which may indicate a postoperative hemorrhage. Early in the postoperative period, begin increasing the patient's activity. Help the patient sit up in the bedside chair and assist the patient to ambulate as soon as possible.

Explain the possible side effects of radiation or chemotherapy. Secretions may become thick and difficult to expectorate when the patient is having radiation therapy. Encourage the patient to drink fluids to stay hydrated. Percussion, postural drainage, and vibration can be used to aid in clearing secretions.

The patient may experience less anxiety if allowed as much control as possible over their daily schedule. Explaining procedures and keeping the patient informed about the treatment plan and condition may also decrease anxiety. If the patient enters the final phases of lung cancer, provide emotional support. Refer the patient and family to the hospice staff or the hospital chaplain. Encourage them to verbalize their feelings surrounding impending death. Allow for the time needed to adjust while helping the patient and family begin the grieving process. Assist in the identification of tasks to be completed before death, such as making a will; seeing specific relatives and friends; or attending an approaching wedding, birthday, or anniversary celebration. Urge the patient to verbalize specific funeral requests to family members.

Evidence-Based Practice and Health Policy

Becker, N., Motsch, E., Trotter, A., Heussel, C., Dienemann, H., Schnabel, P., Kauczor, H., Maldonaldo, S., Miller, A., Kaaks, R., & Delorme, S. (2020). Lung cancer mortality reduction by LDCT screening—Results from the randomized German LUSI trial. *International Journal of Cancer, 146,* 1503–1513.

• In 2011, the U.S. National Lung Cancer Screening Trial reported a 20% reduction of lung cancer mortality after regular screening by low-dose computed tomography (LDCT), as compared to x-ray screening. A lung cancer screening program in Europe, the German Lung Cancer Screening Intervention, is a randomized trial among 4,052 long-term smokers, 50 to 69 years of age, with a screening arm ($n = 2,029$ participants) and a control arm ($n = 2,023$).

• They followed both groups for an average of 8.8 years. They found that women showed a significant reduction in lung cancer mortality as compared to men when screened by LDCT. Regular screening by LDCT shows promise in decreasing cancer mortality when compared to screening with x-ray screening.

DOCUMENTATION GUIDELINES

• Physical findings: Adequacy of airway and breathing; vital signs; heart and lung sounds; pain (nature, location, duration, and intensity); intake and output
• Complications: Pneumonia, hypoxia, infection, dehydration, poor wound healing
• Response to interventions and counseling: Response to pain medication, discussions about end-of-life care
• Response to treatment: Chest tube drainage; wound healing; condition of skin following radiation; side effects from chemotherapy

DISCHARGE AND HOME HEALTHCARE GUIDELINES

Teach the patient to recognize the signs and symptoms of infection at the incision site, including redness, warmth, swelling, and drainage. Explain the need to contact the physician immediately. Be sure the patient understands any medication prescribed, including dosage, route, action, and side effects. Provide the patient with the names, addresses, and phone numbers of support groups, such as the American Cancer Society, the National Cancer Institute, the local hospice, the Lung Cancer Alliance, and the Visiting Nurse Association. Teach the patient how to maximize their respiratory effort.

Lupus Erythematosus

DRG Category:	546
Mean LOS:	4.4 days
Description:	MEDICAL: Connective Tissue Disorders With Complication or Comorbidity
DRG Category:	595
Mean LOS:	7.5 days
Description:	MEDICAL: Major Skin Disorders With Major Complication or Comorbidity

Lupus erythematosus is an autoimmune disease that affects the connective tissue of the body as well as the kidney, blood cells, and nervous system. The Lupus Foundation of America (2021) reports that 1.5 million people have lupus in the United States, with more than 16,000 new cases reported each year. The course of disease is variable and unpredictable, with episodes of remission and relapse. Only a small percentage of patients (< 10%) have long-lasting remissions.

Lupus takes two forms. Systemic lupus erythematosus (SLE) is a multisystem inflammatory disease that affects any body system but primarily the musculoskeletal, cutaneous, renal, nervous, and cardiovascular systems. People with SLE develop an autoantibody response to proteins (antigens) in the nucleus and cytoplasm of body cells leading to inflammation and the formation of circulating immune complexes in the capillaries. These complexes are deposited in the basement membranes of the skin and kidneys, disrupting the function of these organs. Discoid lupus erythematosus (DLE) is a less serious form of the disease that primarily affects the skin. DLE is characterized by skin lesions of the face, scalp, and ears. Longstanding lesions can cause scarring, hypopigmentation, and redness. Only 5% to 10% of patients with DLE develop SLE. The multisystem nature of SLE places the patient at risk for multiple complications, and the disease is ultimately fatal. The survival rates of patients with SLE are about 90% at 10 years, and 80% at 15 years. Because of recent advances in treatment, many people are living 25 or 30 years after diagnosis. The most common causes of death are renal failure and infections, followed by neurological and cardiovascular disorders.

CAUSES

The cause of lupus erythematosus is not known. A familial association has been noted that suggests a genetic predisposition, but a genetic link has not been identified. Approximately 8% of patients with SLE have at least one first-degree family member (parent, sibling, child) with the disease. Environmental factors, susceptibility to certain viruses, and an immune system dysfunction with production of autoantibodies are possible causes. Hormonal abnormality and ultraviolet radiation are considered possible risk factors for the development of SLE. Some drugs have been implicated as initiating the onset of lupus-like symptoms and aggravating existing disease; they include hydralazine hydrochloride, procainamide hydrochloride, penicillin, isonicotinic acid hydrazide, chlorpromazine, phenytoin, and quinidine. Possible childhood risk factors include low birth weight, preterm birth, and exposure to farming pesticides.

GENETIC CONSIDERATIONS

While familial clustering of lupus erythematosus is relatively rare, twin studies have shown concordance in 24% to 59% of identical twins and in only 2% to 5% of nonidentical twins, which suggests a significant genetic predisposition. Heritability is estimated at 43%, and there are now over 80 loci that are associated with lupus erythematosus. Genes encoding proteins of the complement system appear to have the strongest association with lupus erythematosus. Polymorphisms in the toll-like receptor-5 (*TLR5*) gene are also associated with SLE.

SEX AND LIFE SPAN CONSIDERATIONS

SLE occurs most frequently in females between the ages of 15 and 44 years, with the average age of onset at 30 years. Approximately 90% of people with SLE are women. DLE is more common in women than in men, and approximately 60% of cases are female patients in their late 20s or older.

HEALTH DISPARITIES AND SEXUAL/GENDER MINORITY HEALTH

Lupus erythematosus is more prominent in Black, Native American, Asian, and Hispanic persons as compared to White persons. Native American and Black persons with SLE have the highest mortality rates. People living in poverty have poorer disease outcomes and higher mortality rates than people with low, middle, and high incomes. Low educational attainment is also associated with increased mortality (Peschken, 2020). Lupus nephritis, one of the most serious complications of SLE, has the highest frequency among Black and Hispanic persons. Native American children are three times more likely than children of other groups to develop SLE. People from minority groups and people who are on Medicare have difficulties with accessing primary care and speciality care for SLE and are more likely to require hospitalization than other groups (Brown et al., 2020). Sexual and gender minority status has no known effect on the risk for SLE and DLE.

GLOBAL HEALTH CONSIDERATIONS

The Lupus Foundation of America (2021) estimated that at least 5 million people have a form of lupus. Global data on prevalence vary widely. Prevalence is higher in White people living in Western Europe and in people from the Caribbean living in Europe, and it is lower in Africa and China.

☀ ASSESSMENT

HISTORY. Initial symptoms may involve one organ only or multiple systems. Symptoms vary from mild and infrequent to persistent and life-threatening. Take a careful history with a focus on both systemic and single-organ symptoms. Systemic symptoms include fatigue, malaise, weight loss, anorexia, and fever.

The patient may report musculoskeletal and cutaneous symptoms, including joint and muscle pain, puffiness of hands and feet, joint swelling and tenderness, hand deformities, and skin lesions such as the characteristic "butterfly rash" (fixed reddish and flat rash that extends over both cheeks and the bridge of the nose). Other symptoms may include maculopapular rash (small, colored area with raised red pimples), sensitivity to the sun, photophobia, vascular skin lesions, leg ulcers, oral ulcers, and hair loss.

Other symptoms originate in the genitourinary tract (menstrual abnormalities, amenorrhea, spontaneous abortion) or central nervous system (visual problems, memory loss, mild confusion, headache, seizures, psychoses, loss of balance, depression). Establish a history of symptoms related to the hematological system (venous or arterial clotting, bleeding tendencies), cardiopulmonary system (chest pain, shortness of breath, lung congestion), or gastrointestinal system (nausea, vomiting, difficulty swallowing, diarrhea, and bloody stools).

Ask if there is a family history of SLE. Establish any immune system dysfunction or recent viral infections. Ask if the patient has a history of hormonal abnormality or ultraviolet radiation. Ask if the patient is taking or has taken any of the medications implicated as initiating lupus-like symptoms.

PHYSICAL EXAMINATION. Common symptoms include **fever, joint pain,** and **rash.** Inspect the integumentary system thoroughly, including the mucous membranes, to determine the site of skin rashes and lesions. Check for lesions and necrosis on the fingertips, toes, and elbows; these may be caused by inflammation of terminal arterioles. Examine the hairline for any signs of hair loss. Assess the patient's extremities and joints for signs of arthritis, lymphadenopathy, and peripheral neuropathy. Determine the extent of range of motion and movement of extremities and level of joint discomfort. Auscultate the lungs and heart to determine the presence of a pleural or pericardial friction rub. Palpate the spleen and liver to determine the presence of tenderness, splenomegaly, or hepatomegaly. Examine the patient's urine for hematuria, proteinuria, and casts.

Assess for fever, pallor, and signs of bleeding, including petechiae and bruising. Check the patient's blood pressure because increased blood pressure might indicate kidney involvement. Assess for neurological changes that may include headache, changes in mental status, and seizure activity.

PSYCHOSOCIAL. A patient is facing a chronic and often debilitating disease that can be fatal. The patient may have problems maintaining professional and family roles and may experience loss over a deteriorating health status. The loss of childbearing potential is another loss experience for some patients. Lupus is associated with an increased incidence of spontaneous abortion, fetal death, and prematurity. Assess the patient's and family's ability to cope with a lifelong chronic illness that may affect many organ systems. Determine the level of anxiety, fear, and depression.

PRIMARY NURSING DIAGNOSIS

DIAGNOSIS. Acute pain related to joint or peripheral nerve inflammation or dysfunction as evidenced by self-reports of pain, facial grimacing, and/or protective behavior

OUTCOMES. Comfort status; Knowledge: Pain management; Pain level; Pain control; Symptom severity; Knowledge: Medication; Medication response

INTERVENTIONS. Analgesic administration; Anxiety reduction; Pain management: Acute; Medication management; Medication administration; Teaching: Prescribed medication

☀ PLANNING AND IMPLEMENTATION

Collaborative

Much of the therapy is pharmacologic and guided by the patient's symptoms. General support-ive therapy includes adequate sleep and avoidance of fatigue because mild disease exacerbations may subside after several days of bedrest. A physical therapy program is important to maintain mobility and range of motion without allowing the patient to get overtired. If the kidneys are involved, renal dialysis or transplantation may be required.

Pharmacologic Highlights

Medication or Drug Class	Dosage	Description	Rationale
Hydroxychloro-quine (Plaquenil)	400–600 mg PO daily for 5–10 days, gradually increasing dose until effective; maintenance is usually 200–400 mg/day PO	Antimalarial	Reduces rash, photosensi-tivity, arthralgias, arthritis, alopecia, and malaise
Corticosteroids	Varies with drug	Prednisone, 1–2 mg/kg PO qd; methylpredni-solone 500 mg IV	Control SLE in most severe or life-threatening cases (glomerulonephritis, debili-tation from symptoms)
Disease-modifying anti-rheumatic drugs (DMARDs)	Varies with drug	Nonbiological DMARDs: Cyclophosphamide, methotrexate, azathio-prine, mycophenolate, cyclosporine; biological DMARDs: belimumab	Suppress immune system and reduce consequences of disease
NSAIDs	Varies with drug	Diclofenac, ibuprofen, naproxen	Treat the joint pain and swelling; should be avoided in patients with active nephritis

Other Drugs: Monoclonal antibody (rituximab [Rituxan]). Topical steroids are often used to treat skin rashes. Anticonvulsants may be necessary if seizures occur.

Independent

The pain and discomfort of SLE can be physically and mentally debilitating. Encourage the patient to maintain activity when the symptoms are mild or in remission. Encourage patients to pace all activity and to allow for adequate rest. Hot packs may relieve joint pain and stiffness. If the patient has Raynaud phenomenon (abnormal vasoconstriction of the extremities), use warmth to relieve symptoms and protect the patient's hands from injury.

Support the patient's self-image by encouraging good grooming. Suggest hypoallergenic cosmetics, shaving products, and hair products. Encourage the patient to use a hairstylist or barber who specializes in caring for people with scalp disorders and to protect all body surfaces from direct sunlight. The patient should use sunscreen with a protective factor of at least 20 and wear a hat and long sleeves while in the sun. Note that certain drugs (tetracycline) and foods (figs, parsley, celery) augment the effects of ultraviolet light and therefore should be avoided.

Fatigue and stress can lead to exacerbations of the illness. Explore ways for the patient to get adequate rest. Because the patient's immune system may have a diminished capacity, encourage the patient to avoid exposure to illness.

Explore the meaning of the chronic illness and coping strategies with the patient. Allow adequate time to discuss fears and concerns. A referral to a support group or counselor may also be necessary.

Evidence-Based Practice and Health Policy

Castellano-Rioja, E., Giménez-Espert, M., & Soto-Rubio, A. (2020). Lupus erythematosus quality of life questionnaire (LEQoL): Development and psychometric properties. *International Journal of Environmental Research and Public Health*. Advance online publication. https://doi .org/10.3390/ijerph17228642

- The authors developed and psychometrically tested the Quality of Life of Patients with Lupus Erythematosus Instrument (LEQoL) and studied the quality of life of these patients. They employed a cross-sectional design with a sample of 158 patients recruited from a lupus associ-ation for the psychometric evaluation of the final version of LEQoL.
- The definitive psychometric model was composed of 21 items grouped into five factors. Mean levels of quality of life were observed in patients with systemic LE, with higher values in patients with cutaneous LE. The authors noted that the LEQoL instrument is a useful tool for assessing the quality of life of patients with LE. It allows for the evaluation of current clinical practices, the identification of educational needs, and the assessment of the effec-tiveness of interventions.

DOCUMENTATION GUIDELINES

- Physical changes: Vital signs, particularly blood pressure and temperature; daily weight, intake and output; signs of bleeding or tarry stools, petechiae, bruising, pallor
- Physical changes: Location site and description of any skin lesions or rashes and overall con-dition of the skin
- Physical changes: Presence of any seizure activity, visual disturbances, headaches, personality changes, or memory deficits
- Tolerance to activity, level of pain and fatigue, patient's ability to perform activities of daily living and range of motion of extremities; note the extent of joint involvement and the presence of tingling, numbness, or weakness

DISCHARGE AND HOME HEALTHCARE GUIDELINES

Teach the patient the purpose, dosage, and possible side effects of all medications. Explain to the patient the disease process, the purpose of treatment regimens, and the importance of compli-ance. Teach the patient when to seek medical attention. Teach the patient to wear a Medic Alert bracelet noting the disease and medications so appropriate action can be taken in an emergency. Recommend smoking cessation for patients who use tobacco. Encourage the patient to keep all vaccinations current such as the meningococcal vaccine, pneumococcal vaccine, and routine flu vaccines.

Teach the female patient the importance of planning pregnancies with medical supervision because pregnancy is likely to cause an exacerbation of the disease.

Discuss all precipitating factors that need to be avoided, including fatigue, vaccination, infec-tions, stress, surgery, certain drugs, and exposure to ultraviolet light. Teach the patient how to minimize ultraviolet exposure. Teach the patient to avoid strenuous exercise, instead striving for a balance. Describe pain management strategies. Stress the importance of adequate nutrition. Small, frequent meals may be better tolerated. Any cosmetics should be approved by the physician and should be hypoallergenic. Encourage the patient to contact the Arthritis Foundation, the Lupus Foundation of America, and other appropriate support groups that are available in the area.

Lyme Disease

DRG Category:	868
Mean LOS:	4.6 days
Description:	MEDICAL: Other Infectious and Parasitic Diseases Diagnoses With Complication or Comorbidity

Lyme disease is a tick-borne illness that is an acute recurrent inflammatory disease character-ized by periods of exacerbation and remissions. This disease is named for the town in Connecti-cut where it was first recognized in the 1970s. Although the number of cases varies from year to year, approximately 30,000 cases are reported annually in the United States, making it the leading tick-borne disease in the country. It is also the sixth most common notifiable disease in the United States. Experts estimate that only 30% of patients with early Lyme disease remember a tick bite, making history-taking challenging.

Lyme disease typically begins in summer or early fall and develops in three stages with vary-ing, progressive symptoms over weeks and months if untreated. The most frequent carrier of the disease is the deer tick, a small insect the size of a poppy seed. The deer tick is predominantly found in the New England and mid-Atlantic states, Wisconsin, Minnesota, and northern Cali-fornia, although cases of Lyme disease have been documented in 48 states. Incubation lasts 7 to 10 days, but diagnosis generally must wait for 4 to 6 weeks after the patient is bitten by a tick in order to make laboratory tests reliable. Severe long-term effects occur in fewer than 10% of untreated cases. Complications include pericarditis and myocarditis, cardiac dysrhythmias, encephalitis, peripheral neuropathies, and arthritis.

CAUSES

Lyme disease is caused by a spirochete, *Borrelia burgdorferi*. This organism can be transmitted through the saliva of the tick while it is ingesting blood from a host. Not all ticks carry this spi-rochete, and not all bites from infected ticks lead to Lyme disease. Risk factors include spending time in wooded or grassy areas, living in the Northeast and Midwest, having exposed skin, and not removing ticks promptly and appropriately.

GENETIC CONSIDERATIONS

Heritable immune responses could be protective or increase susceptibility.

SEX AND LIFE SPAN CONSIDERATIONS

The general population of all ages and both sexes are at risk for Lyme disease, especially those who spend time in infested geographic locations. Patterns of exposure seem to parallel the amount of time people spend outside. Children 14 years and under frequently play outside, which likely explains that 25% of Lyme disease cases occur in children of this age range. People can be reinfected throughout their lifetime with new tick bites.

HEALTH DISPARITIES AND SEXUAL/GENDER MINORITY HEALTH

While no differences in susceptibility are known to exist in different races and ethnicities, rashes associated with Lyme disease may be difficult to see in people with a dark skin color. The dis-ease is primarily documented in the White population in the United States, who report about 75% of the cases. Sexual and gender minority status has no known effect on the risk for Lyme disease.

GLOBAL HEALTH CONSIDERATIONS

Lyme disease has been recognized around the globe including in Canada, Europe, and Asia. It may be less prevalent outside of the northern hemisphere but has been reported in the tropics and Australia.

☀ ASSESSMENT

HISTORY. Establish the progression of the disease by noting the progression of stages. The first stage involves skin invasion. A characteristic "bull's-eye" rash (erythema migrans), flu-like symptoms, fatigue, and myalgia may occur within days to weeks of the tick bite. During the second stage, the nerve tissue is invaded, and the patient experiences neurological symptoms and possibly cardiac problems. The most common neurological complications are Bell palsy and aseptic Lyme meningitis, which can progress to encephalitis. Without treatment at this stage, 8% of patients develop cardiac complications such as heart block, pericarditis, congestive heart failure, dizziness, shortness of breath, and palpitations. Final progression of the untreated disease results in arthritis, which sometimes becomes chronic. Establish a history of pain and arthritic symptoms in the tendons, bursae, and joints (most commonly the knees), which may subsequently become infected.

Obtain a thorough history regarding the patient's recall of a tick bite within the past 3 to 30 days and recall of exposure to geographic "hot spots." Determine where the patient lives, works, and vacations. Note that there is a seasonal component to exposure (May to August). Question the patient carefully about presence of malaise, muscle and joint pain, stiff neck, headache, and fatigue, all of which are early symptoms.

PHYSICAL EXAMINATION. Common early symptoms include an **expanding rash at the site, flu-like symptoms**, and **low-grade fever**. Inspect the skin for the characteristic rash (erythema migrans), a reddened expanding ring with a lighter center at the location of the tick bite. The rash may be warm to touch, but it is usually painless and may grow to be inches in diameter. It usually does not appear on the hands and feet but rather in the axillary or gluteal fold, hairline, or beneath the breasts. Children often have the rash on the face, scalp, and hairline. Inspect the face for any signs of paralysis; determine if the patient can open and close the eyes and mouth symmetrically. Determine the patient's temperature. Auscultate the patient's heart rate for irregularity and the presence of tachycardia. Progressive symptoms in untreated patients involve neurological and musculoskeletal symptoms. Perform a complete neurological examination. Assess the range of motion of the neck and other joints, and determine the patient's muscle strength.

PSYCHOSOCIAL. Anxiety of the unknown—both the fear of disease progression and the fear of the potential for reinfection—contributes to the psychological effect of this disease. Patients may be frustrated with experiencing memory loss; determine the family's understanding and ability to support the patient with an altered mental status.

Diagnostic Highlights

Test	Normal Result	Abnormality With Condition	Explanation
Enzyme-linked immunosorbent assay (ELISA)	Nonreactive	Levels of specific IgM antibodies peak during the third to sixth wk after onset and then gradually decline	Measures levels of specific IgM antibodies
IgG Western blot	Negative	Presence of antibodies; positive test with 5–10 bands of antibodies present	Immunoassay that allows visualization of IgG antibodies to a spirochete, *B burgdorferi*, the agent of Lyme disease; more sensitive than ELISA

Diagnostic Highlights (continued)

Other Tests: Note that people living in areas with high exposure to ticks may be treated without blood tests. Culture from skin lesions (impractical and rarely performed). Note: Patients may remain seropositive for long periods, and the ELISA test cannot be used as a proof of cure. A negative Lyme test result does not indicate the absence of disease, nor does a positive result indicate the presence of disease. A positive result is not required to diagnose Lyme disease for someone with clear-cut erythema migrans, and those patients should be treated regardless of test results.

PRIMARY NURSING DIAGNOSIS

DIAGNOSIS. Anxiety related to knowledge deficit of disease progression, treatment, and prevention as evidenced by apprehension, distress, uncertainty, and/or fear

OUTCOMES. Anxiety level; Coping; Symptom control; Symptom severity; Knowledge: Disease process; Knowledge: Medication; Knowledge: Treatment regime

INTERVENTIONS. Anxiety reduction; Calming technique; Coping enhancement; Teaching: Disease process; Teaching: Prescribed medication

PLANNING AND IMPLEMENTATION

Collaborative

Oral antibiotics are usually started as early as possible. Tetracycline is the primary choice, but doxycycline (except for children under the age of 8 years and for pregnant persons), penicillin, or ceftriaxone may be prescribed. Children are usually treated with oral penicillin. Fever is treated with antipyretics and sometimes cooling blankets.

Research is being done on using the protein Osp A from the Lyme spirochete as a potential vaccination for this disease. Surprisingly, Osp A vaccination in mice has kept them free from Lyme disease after infected tick bites, but it also killed the spirochete that was present in the ticks who bit the vaccinated mice. Use of this vaccine might be considered in plant and water supplies to help stop the spread of Lyme disease.

Pharmacologic Highlights

Medication or Drug Class	Dosage	Description	Rationale
Doxycycline	200 mg PO in a single dose for prophylaxis; for treatment, 100 mg PO BID	Antibiotic	Inhibits protein synthesis and bacterial growth; course of antibiotics is generally for 3 wk; drug of choice for adults; may need home IV therapy if chronic Lyme disease occurs
Other antibiotics	Varies with drug	Amoxicillin, tetracycline, erythromycin, azithromycin, clarithromycin, ceftriaxone, cefotaxime, cefuroxime axetil, penicillin G, penicillin VK, chloramphenicol	Combat infection; course of antibiotics is generally for 3 wk; may need home IV therapy if chronic Lyme disease occurs; amoxicillin is drug of choice for children less than 9 yr of age
Analgesics	Varies with drug	Acetaminophen, ibuprofen	Relieve joint discomfort

Independent

The Centers for Disease Control and Prevention (CDC, 2021) recommend removing a tick with a tweezers, grasping the tick at the skin's surface and pulling with a steady pressure. They then suggest cleaning the area with alcohol or soap and water. If the mouth of the tick is not removed from the skin, the CDC recommends leaving it in the skin and allowing the area to heal. Burning a tick off or smothering it with petroleum jelly may cause the tick to regurgitate stomach acids and spirochete into the wound and therefore is not recommended. If the bite is considered high risk by location or other circumstances, prophylactic antibiotics are given.

Nursing care varies, depending on the disease stage. Manage fever with cool sponge baths and limited bedding. Maintain a cool temperature in the environment if possible. Manage fatigue with promotion of rest and comfort. Ice bags are effective for headache. Arthralgia may require immobilization of the painful joint, warm moist applications, and other nonpharmacologic measures to control pain. Assist the patient with range-of-motion exercises and activities to strengthen muscles and joints, being careful not to overexert the patient.

Provide emotional support to patients who are experiencing memory loss and confusion. Determine the patients' chance for injury and plan accordingly by instituting safety measures. Frequently reorient patients to their surroundings. Encourage patients to share any concerns about their mental status. Explain the reason for the mental status changes to patients and significant others, and answer any questions about the long-range complications of the disease. Explain that reinfection is always possible with another tick bite, and discuss preventive measures such as tick prevention lawn care and covering the skin when out of doors.

Evidence-Based Practice and Health Policy

Hirsch, A., Poulsen, M., Nordberg, C., Moon, K., Rebman, A., Aucott, J., Heaney, C., & Schwartz, B. (2020). Risk factors and outcomes of treatment delays in Lyme disease: A population-based retrospective cohort study. *Frontiers in Medicine.* Advance online publication. https://doi.org/10.3389/fmed.2020.560018

- Longer time between symptom onset and treatment of Lyme disease has been associated with poor outcomes. The authors conducted a population-based study to evaluate factors associated with the delayed treatment of Lyme disease and the relationship between delayed treatment and problems that occur after treatment. Participants with Lyme disease ($N = 778$) completed questionnaires ($N = 778$) in a Pennsylvania health system from 2015 to 2017. Time-to-treatment was calculated as time to first medical contact and time under care.
- In the sample, 25% had time to first contact after symptoms appeared of more than 14 days, and 31% had a total time-to-treatment of more than 30 days. Being uninsured and attributing initial symptoms to something other than Lyme disease were positively associated with delayed time to first medical contact. To improve Lyme disease outcomes, prevention efforts should aim to reduce the time before and after seeking care.

DOCUMENTATION GUIDELINES

- Skin assessment: Presence of rash; description and location of rash
- Musculoskeletal assessment: Warmth, tenderness, stiffness, swelling of involved joints, flu-like symptoms
- Cardiac assessment: Rate and regularity of rhythm; presence of chest pain, shortness of breath, palpitations, dizziness
- Neurological assessment: Headache, stiff neck, confusion, sensory loss, memory loss, facial weakness or paralysis, limb weakness
- Response to therapy: Relief of presenting symptoms (fever control, pain relief, resolved neurological and cardiac complications)

DISCHARGE AND HOME HEALTHCARE GUIDELINES

Teach the patient strategies to prevent tick bites by wearing protective clothing, such as long sleeves and long pants (pant legs should also be tucked inside of socks) in at-risk areas, full-cover shoes (not sandals), and light-colored clothing to help make identification of the tiny dark ticks easier. Use chemical repellents such as DEET, but note they may cause respiratory distress if too much is used, especially in children. Stay on cleared paths and avoid wandering through grass and woods. Inspect the body daily with attention to the prime locations for bites: back, axilla, neck, ankle, groin, scalp, and back of the knees. Wash and dry exposed clothing for at least 30 minutes to kill concealed ticks. Inspect pets as well, not only for carrying ticks into the house but also because Lyme disease is a prime cause of animal arthritis.

If a tick is attached to the skin, remove it carefully to avoid causing it to regurgitate saliva and spirochetes into the host. Use tweezers close to the skin to pull the head or jaw out of the skin, if possible. Cleanse the site with antiseptic agent. Do not try to burn off the tick or to smother it with kerosene or petroleum jelly. Emphasize that the patient should finish the entire course of antibiotics, even if the patient is asymptomatic. Inform the physician of recurrent or progressive symptoms for consideration of reinfection.

Lymphoma, Non-Hodgkin

DRG Category:	824
Mean LOS:	7.1 days
Description:	SURGICAL: Lymphoma and Non-Acute Leukemia With Other Procedures With Complication or Comorbidity
DRG Category:	841
Mean LOS:	5.5 days
Description:	MEDICAL: Lymphoma and Non-Acute Leukemia With Complication or Comorbidity

Malignant lymphoma, also called *lymphosarcoma* or *non-Hodgkin lymphoma* (NHL), is a diffuse group of neoplastic diseases characterized by rampant proliferation of lymphocytes, primarily in the lymph nodes. Lymphomas fall into two main categories: Hodgkin and non-Hodgkin lymphomas, based primarily on the presence or absence of the Reed-Sternberg cell; when the cells are absent, the disease is classified as NHL (Table 1).

• **TABLE 1** Comparison of Hodgkin Lymphoma and Non-Hodgkin Lymphoma

CHARACTERISTIC	HODGKIN	LOW-GRADE NON-HODGKIN	ALL OTHER NON-HODGKIN
Site(s) of origin nodal distribution	Nodal axial (centripetal)	Extranodal, about 10% centrifugal	Extranodal, about 35% centrifugal
Nodal spread	Contiguous	Noncontiguous	Noncontiguous
Central nervous system involvement	Rare, < 1%	Rare, < 1%	Uncommon, < 10%
Hepatic involvement	Uncommon	Common, > 50%	Uncommon, < 10%
Bone marrow involvement	Uncommon, < 10%	Common, > 50%	Uncommon
Marrow involvement adversely affects prognosis	Yes	No	Yes
Curable by chemotherapy	Yes	No	Yes

NHL is a common cancer in the United States. The American Cancer Society estimated that 81,560 people will be diagnosed with NHL in 2021, and 20,720 people will die from the cancer. In the past 30 years, the incidence of NHL has increased by more than 80%, making it one of the largest increases of any cancer. This increase is unexpected and is only partially explained by earlier detection because of improved diagnostic techniques or HIV-associated lymphomas.

Malignant lymphoma, or NHL, is a heterogeneous grouping of several disease types that range from the aggressive, rapidly fatal diffuse histiocytic lymphoma to less aggressive nodular types. Still, all have a less promising prognosis than Hodgkin lymphoma. NHL can be divided in two groups based on prognosis: indolent ("lazy") lymphomas and aggressive lymphomas. Indolent lymphomas have a comparatively good prognosis with a survival time of up to 10 years. Most are nodular (or follicular) in nature. People with aggressive lymphoma have a poor overall prognosis, although a number of these patients can be cured with chemotherapy. Complications of NHL include hypercalcemia, increased uric acid levels, and anemia. As tumors grow, they may compress the vital organs and cause organ dysfunction; problems from organ compression include complications such as increased intracranial pressure, spinal cord compression, and gastrointestinal obstruction. Other complications include infections that result from a weakened immune system (meningitis, tuberculosis, pneumonia), infertility, secondary cancers, and depression.

CAUSES

The cause of NHL is unknown, but genetic causes as well as infections, environmental factors, immunodeficiency states, and chronic inflammation have been implicated. Exposures to viruses and immunosuppression are thought to be related to NHL. Organ transplantation, a history of cancer treated with radiation or some chemotherapies, acquired immune deficiencies such as HIV infection, and autoimmune disorders (rheumatoid arthritis, systemic lupus erythematosus, celiac disease) are considered risk factors. Some experts suggest that both Hodgkin lymphoma and NHL result from an immune defect or from the activation of an oncogenic virus. One form of NHL, Burkitt lymphoma, seems to be related to a herpesvirus (Epstein-Barr virus). Exposure to nuclear explosions or reactor accidents, certain pesticides and herbicides, and chemicals (benzene, lead, paint thinner, and formaldehyde) may place patients at risk. Some people with breast implants have developed NHL in their breast.

GENETIC CONSIDERATIONS

A family history of NHL or other cancers increases one's risk of developing the disease, with the highest risk among men who have an affected sibling. Genetic variants in the tumor necrosis factor (*TNF*) gene and interleukin-10 (*IL10*) are associated with NHL risk.

SEX AND LIFE SPAN CONSIDERATIONS

The peak incidence of NHL occurs later than with Hodgkin lymphoma and is five times more common than Hodgkin lymphoma. It is more common in men than in women and is a disease of the middle years. About 25% of cases develop in patients between ages 50 and 59 years. Maximal risk is between ages 60 and 69 years. Small lymphocytic lymphomas occur in older adults, lymphoblastic lymphomas occur most often in males younger than age 20 years, and follicular lymphomas are uncommon in the young. Burkitt lymphoma occurs in children and young adults.

HEALTH DISPARITIES AND SEXUAL/GENDER MINORITY HEALTH

White persons have a higher risk for NHL than Black and Asian persons. Disparities exist with respect to relative survival by race and ethnicity, income, and insurance for many cancer types. The NHL survival rate for White men is higher (74.5%) than for Black men (57%). Being Black or Hispanic, living in high-poverty neighborhoods, and having Medicaid, other government insurance, or no insurance at diagnosis are associated with all-cause mortality

(Murphy et al., 2021), creating a disparity for these groups. Sexual and gender minority status has no known effect on the risk for lymphoma. However, gender and sexual minority persons are a vulnerable group because people with low income, long travel distances to cancer screening sites, or who lack health insurance or paid medical leave are less likely to be treated according to cancer care guidelines (National Institutes of Health, 2021).

GLOBAL HEALTH CONSIDERATIONS

NHL is more common in developed countries than in developing countries, with North America and Europe having the highest levels of disease. Burkitt lymphoma is most common in sub-Saharan Africa, where it is likely responsible for 50% of childhood cancers.

ASSESSMENT

HISTORY. The clinical signs of NHL vary depending on the location of the tumor and the rate of growth. The patient often describes enlarged lymph nodes that are not painful. Because nodes and extranodal sites are more likely to be involved in NHL, the patient may also report vague abdominal distress (bleeding, bowel obstruction, cramping, ascites), symptoms of spinal cord compression, or back pain. Cough, dyspnea, and chest pain occur about 20% of the time and are indicative of lung involvement. Ask about sleep habits to determine if night sweats are a problem. Determine if the patient is experiencing fatigue, fevers, or weight loss. Note any history of infection with HIV, organ transplant, congenital immunodeficiency, autoimmune diseases, or other treatment with immunosuppressive drugs.

PHYSICAL EXAMINATION. Patients often have complaints of **painless enlarged lymph nodes** (commonly in the neck, mediastinum, or chest wall), **fevers, night sweats, weight loss, weakness**, and **malaise**. Carefully inspect all the locations for lymph nodes and the abdomen for signs of hepatosplenomegaly and ascites. Skin lesions that look like nodules or papules with a tendency to ulcerate appear in about 20% of cases. When palpating lymph node chains, examine the submental, infraclavicular, epitrochlear, iliac, femoral, and popliteal nodes. Involved nodes are characteristically painless, firm, and rubbery in consistency; they are in contrast to the rock-hard nodes of carcinoma because they are freely movable and of varying size. Palpate the liver or spleen, which may be enlarged, and the testicles, which may have masses. Assess the patient's weight and nutrition.

PSYCHOSOCIAL. The diagnosis of cancer is devastating at any time of life. Because the disease is most common in the older adult, the patient may be planning retirement. The diagnosis of NHL throws all retirement plans into disarray and may lead to feelings of loss, grief, and anger.

Diagnostic Highlights

Test	Normal Result	Abnormality With Condition	Explanation
Lymph node biopsy; bone marrow biopsy	Normal cells	Positive for lymphoma cells	Determines extent of disease and allows for staging of disease; bone marrow biopsy is generally done only for patients with anemia or fever and night sweats
Computed tomography or magnetic resonance imaging of chest, abdomen, bone, and pelvis	Normal structures	Spread of NHL into organs and body cavities	Used to assist with staging; common sites of extralymphatic involvement include spleen, stomach, small intestine; combined with lymphangiography, can predict nodal involvement in 90% of cases

(highlight box continues on page 774)

Diagnostic Highlights (continued)

Other Tests: Complete blood cell count with peripheral smear and erythrocyte sedimentation rate (shows anemia, fluorescence in situ hybridization [FISH], leukocytosis, elevated platelet count, and erythrocyte sedimentation rate); chest x-ray; positron emission tomography; ultrasonography; tests for liver and renal function, including lactate dehydrogenase, alkaline phosphatase, blood urea nitrogen, and creatinine; gallium scan; HIV, hepatitis B testing; immunophenotype of lymph node, bone marrow, peripheral blood

---

PRIMARY NURSING DIAGNOSIS

DIAGNOSIS. Risk for infection as evidenced by fever, diaphoresis, weakness, and/or malaise

OUTCOMES. Immune status; Knowledge: Infection management; Risk control; Risk detection; Nutritional status; Tissue integrity: Skin and mucous membranes; Self-management: Cancer; Rest

INTERVENTIONS. Infection control; Infection protection; Surveillance; Nutrition management; Medication management; Teaching: Disease process

PLANNING AND IMPLEMENTATION

Collaborative

Treatment is based on classification of the cell and staging of the disease (see **Hodgkin Lymphoma**, Table 2, for staging) as well as symptoms, age, and comorbidities. Some of the indolent types of NHL do well with only supportive therapy. The disease process may be slow enough that treatment is deferred until the disease takes a more aggressive path. Most patients with intermediate-grade and high-grade lymphomas receive combination chemotherapy.

Radiation is effective for many patients with stage I or II NHL. Radiation is delivered to the chest wall, mediastinum, axilla, and neck (the region known as the *mantle field*). Most patients, however, are at stage III or IV at diagnosis. Surgery has limited use in the treatment of NHL. It may be part of the diagnostic and staging process, but diagnostic laparotomy is much less common than in Hodgkin lymphoma. A therapeutic splenectomy may be performed for severe spleen enlargement. Gastric or bowel resection may be done if the patient has a primary gastrointestinal lymphoma or has obstructions from bulky nodes. Stem cell transplantation may be considered for patients who have relapsed, are at high risk for relapse, or have tried conventional therapy without success.

Pharmacologic Highlights

Medication or Drug Class	Dosage	Description	Rationale
Biological therapy	Varies with drug	Interferon and monoclonal antibodies such as rituximab, ibritumomab, alemtuzumab	May slow disease progression; other cytotoxic agents such as chlorambucil, fludarabine, cisplatin
Chemotherapy	Varies with drug	Some common regimens are CHOP (cyclophosphamide doxorubicin, vincristine, prednisone); monoclonal antibody rituximab may be added to CHOP as CHOP-R; BACOP/BACOD (bleomycin, doxorubicin, cyclophosphamide, vincristine, prednisone/dexamethasone); and MACOP-B (methotrexate with leucovorin rescue factor, doxorubicin, cyclophosphamide, vincristine, prednisone, bleomycin, plus trimethoprim-sulfamethoxazole and ketoconazole)	Chemotherapy is used for stage IVA and all stage B patients; usually lasts for 6–8 mo

Pharmacologic Highlights (continued)

Other Drugs: Common side effects are alopecia, nausea, vomiting, fatigue, myelosuppression, and stomatitis. Patients who are receiving chemotherapy are administered antinausea drugs, antiemetics, and pain medicines as needed to help control adverse experiences. New therapies and experimental drugs are being developed and tested, such as paclitaxel, colony-stimulating factor growth factors, topoisomerase-3 inhibitors, chimeric antigen receptor T-cell therapy (CAR-T), interferon alfa, and nucleoside analogues.

Independent

Maintain the patient's comfort, protect the patient from infection, provide teaching and support about the complications of the treatment, and provide emotional support. Fatigue, one of the most common side effects of cancer treatment, can last for several months to several years. During irradiation, the patient may suffer from dry mouth, loss of taste, dysphagia, nausea, and vomiting, which can be managed with frequent mouth care. Explore ways to limit discomfort, such as ice chips. Attempt to provide desired foods to support the patient's nutrition. Keep any foul-smelling odors clear of the patient's environment, particularly during meals. Manage skin irritation and redness by washing the skin gently with mild soap, rinsing with warm water, and patting the skin dry. Encourage the patient to avoid applying lotions, perfumes, deodorants, and powder to the treatment area. Explain that the patient needs to protect the skin from sunlight and extreme cold. Before starting treatments, arrange for the patient to have a wig, scarf, or hat to cover any hair loss, which occurs primarily at the nape of the neck.

If the patient develops bone marrow suppression, institute infection controls. Treat the discomfort that may arise from chemotherapy—joint pain, fever, fluid retention, and a labile emotional state (euphoria or depression)—all of which need specific interventions, depending on their incidence and severity. The complexity of the diagnostic and staging process may make the patient feel lost in a crowd of specialists. It is important for the nurse to provide supportive continuity. Patience and repeated explanations are needed. Provide the patient with information about support groups and refer the patient to a clinical nurse specialist, support groups associated with the American Cancer Society (https://www.cancer.org), or counselors.

Evidence-Based Practice and Health Policy

Vargas-Román, K., Díaz-Rodríguez, C., Cañadas-De la Fuente, G., Gómez-Urquiza, J., Ariza, T., & De la Fuente-Solana, E. (2020). Anxiety prevalence in lymphoma: A systematic review and meta-analysis. *Health Psychology, 39*, 580–588.

- In this review, the authors discuss the prevalence of anxiety among patients with Hodgkin and non-Hodgkin lymphoma and examine the methods used for data collection, intervention frequency, and types of instruments used to recognize anxiety. This systematic review and meta-analysis of the literature was carried out using electronic literature searches.
- The meta-analysis sample was $N = 2,138$, and the overall prevalence of anxiety was 19% in people with lymphoma. The findings demonstrated that patients with Hodgkin and non-Hodgkin lymphoma are vulnerable to suffering anxiety. The psychological effects of anxiety during remission or cancer treatments may affect patient outcomes and require attention.

DOCUMENTATION GUIDELINES

- Emotional and physical response to diagnostic testing; healing of incisions; signs of ineffective coping; response to diagnosis; ability to participate in planning treatment options; response of significant others
- Effects of chemotherapy or radiation therapy; response to treatment of symptoms; presence of complications (weight loss, infection, skin irritation)
- Effectiveness of coping; presence of depression; interest in group support of counseling; referrals made

DISCHARGE AND HOME HEALTHCARE GUIDELINES

Teach the patient the following strategies to limit infections: Avoid crowds; avoid infected visitors, particularly children with colds; wash hands frequently; when an infection occurs, report it to a physician immediately; avoid direct contact with pets to limit the risk of infections from licks, scratches, or bites; do not change cat litter or clean a birdcage.

Maintain a high-calorie and high-protein diet. Take sips of grapefruit juice, orange juice, or ginger ale if nausea persists. Drink at least 2,000 mL of fluid a day unless on fluid restriction.

Perform frequent mouth care with a soft toothbrush, and avoid commercial mouthwashes. Contact support groups, the American or Canadian Cancer Society, or counselors as needed.

Mallory-Weiss Syndrome

DRG Category:	326
Mean LOS:	13.2 days
Description:	SURGICAL: Stomach, Esophageal, and Duodenal Procedures With Major Complication or Comorbidity
DRG Category:	378
Mean LOS:	3.5 days
Description:	MEDICAL: Gastrointestinal Hemorrhage With Complication or Comorbidity

Mallory-Weiss syndrome (MWS) is a tear or laceration, usually singular and longitudinal, in the mucosa at the junction of the distal esophagus and proximal stomach. It is often associated with a hiatal hernia. The primary mechanism creating the tear is a transmural pressure gradient that is greater within the hiatal hernia than in the stomach, leading to tearing of the esophageal-gastric junction. Esophageal lacerations account for between 5% and 15% of upper gastrointestinal (GI) bleeding episodes. Approximately 60% of the tears involve the cardia, the upper opening of the stomach that connects with the esophagus. Another 15% involve the terminal esophagus, and 25% involve the region across the epigastric junction. Most episodes of bleeding stop spontaneously, but some patients require medical intervention. If bleeding is excessive, hypovolemia and shock may result. Esophageal rupture (Boerhaave syndrome) is rare but catastrophic when it does occur. If esophageal perforation occurs, the patient may develop abscesses or sepsis.

CAUSES

The most common cause of MWS is failure of the upper esophageal sphincter to relax during prolonged vomiting, but approximately 25% of people with the condition have no identifiable cause. This poor sphincter control is more likely to occur after excessive intake of alcohol. Any event that increases intra-abdominal pressure can also lead to an esophageal tear, such as persistent forceful coughing, trauma, straining, hiccupping, blunt abdominal trauma, seizures, pushing during childbirth, or a hiatal hernia. Other factors that may predispose a person to MWS are esophagitis, gastritis, and atrophic gastric mucosa. MWS also has been associated with diagnostic procedures such as transesophageal echocardiograph (TEE). Tears may occur in children with predisposing liver conditions such as cirrhosis or portal hypertension.

GENETIC CONSIDERATIONS

MWS is not currently thought to have a genetic association, although it has been seen in identical twins.

SEX AND LIFE SPAN CONSIDERATIONS

MWS, first described in people with alcohol dependence, is now recognized across the life span. The incidence is higher in males than in females. The most typical patient is a male in his 40s or 50s. In women, hyperemesis gravidarum in the first trimester of pregnancy causes persistent nausea and vomiting, which may lead to MWS. Adolescents with MWS should be evaluated for eating disorders or alcohol and drug use.

HEALTH DISPARITIES AND SEXUAL/GENDER MINORITY HEALTH

Ethnicity, race, and sexual/gender minority status have no known effect on the risk for MWS.

GLOBAL HEALTH CONSIDERATIONS

The global incidence of MWS is likely similar to that in the United States, where Mallory-Weiss tears account for up to 15% of people who have upper GI bleeding. Data from developing regions of the world are not available.

ASSESSMENT

HISTORY. The patient may report a history of retching and then vomiting bright red blood. Determine the patient's GI history, including a history of hiatal hernia, gastritis, or esophagitis. Ask the patient about the appearance of the vomitus. Hematemesis has a "coffee-ground" appearance if it is of gastric origin and is often a sign of brisk bleeding, usually from an arterial source or esophageal varices. Ask about passage of blood with bowel movements, either a few hours to several days after vomiting. Although vomiting and retching before the onset of bleeding can be indicative of a Mallory-Weiss tear, some patients with MWS do not present with such a history. Inquire about weakness, fatigue, and dizziness, any and all of which can result with chronic blood loss. Ask about a history of alcohol use, misuse, or abuse. Determine the quantity and frequency of drinking, the number of drinks per day, and when the patient had the last drink. Establish whether the patient has a history of seizures, eating disorders, or a recent severe cough.

PHYSICAL EXAMINATION. The most common symptom is **retching and vomiting** followed by **vomiting bright red blood**. Inspect the patient's nasopharynx to rule out the nose and throat as the source of bleeding. Assess the patient for evidence of trauma to the head, chest, and abdomen as well. Note that manifestations of GI bleeding depend on the source of bleeding, the rate of bleeding, and the underlying or coexisting diseases. Patients with massive bleeding have the clinical signs of shock, such as a heart rate greater than 110 beats per minute, an orthostatic blood pressure drop of 16 mm Hg or more, restlessness, decreased urine output, and delayed capillary refill.

PSYCHOSOCIAL. The sudden admission to an acute care facility for GI bleeding is stressful and upsetting. Assess the patient's anxiety level, along with the patient's understanding of the treatment and intervention plan. Because MWS is associated with alcohol use and abuse, determine if the patient is a problem drinker, and assess the family's and significant others' responses to the patient's drinking.

Diagnostic Highlights

Test	Normal Result	Abnormality With Condition	Explanation
Fiberoptic endoscopy (esophagogastro-duodenoscopy)	Visualization of normal tissue	Mucosal tear at gastroesophageal junction	Small fiberoptic tube is inserted into the esophagus to permit visual inspection and is the best procedure to use both for diagnosis and treatment

(highlight box continues on page 778)

Diagnostic Highlights (continued)

Test	Normal Result	Abnormality With Condition	Explanation
Complete blood count	Red blood cells (RBCs): 3.6–5.8 million/mcL; hemoglobin: 11.7–17.3 g/dL; hematocrit: 36%–52%; white blood cells: 4,500–11,100/mcL; platelets: 150,000–450,000/mcL	Decreased RBCs, Hgb, and Hct because of upper GI bleeding	Serial monitoring to monitor the extent of blood loss; assesses the response to therapy

Other Tests: Arteriography, coagulation studies. Generally, barium or other contrast media such as gastrografin should not be done because they are not sensitive to Mallory-Weiss tears, and they may interfere with other diagnostic tests such as endoscopy.

PRIMARY NURSING DIAGNOSIS

DIAGNOSIS. Ineffective airway clearance related to aspiration of blood as evidenced by coughing, choking, wheezing, and/or respiratory distress

OUTCOMES. Respiratory status: Airway patency; Respiratory status: Gas exchange; Respiratory status: Ventilation; Knowledge: Disease process; Comfort status

INTERVENTIONS. Airway insertion and stabilization; Airway management; Airway suctioning; Oral health promotion; Respiratory monitoring; Ventilation assistance

PLANNING AND IMPLEMENTATION

Collaborative

Bleeding often subsides spontaneously in almost 75% of patients. If bleeding has not stopped, generally treatment is completed during the endoscopy examination. Several choices are available for treating a bleeding tear. Endoscopic band ligation has been shown to be the most effective treatment for severe, active bleeding. Active bleeding may be treated with electrocoagulation or heater probe with or without epinephrine injection to stop bleeding. If epinephrine is administered, the patient needs assessment for cardiovascular complications such as hypertension or tachycardia. Sclerosants such as alcohol may be used. Endoscopic hemoclipping may also be effective for Mallory-Weiss tears, or the patient may need to go to surgery to have the tear oversewn. Generally, the use of balloon tamponade with a Sengstaken-Blakemore or Minnesota tube is no longer considered an effective treatment because it may further widen the tear. For severe cases, embolization of the left gastric artery may be used.

If the patient has excessive blood loss, institute strategies to support the circulation. To stabilize the circulation and replace vascular volume, place a large-bore (14- to 18-gauge) IV catheter and maintain replacement fluids, such as 0.9% sodium chloride, and blood component therapy as prescribed. With continued or massive bleeding, the patient may be supported with blood transfusions and admitted to an intensive care unit for close observation.

Pharmacologic Highlights

Medication or Drug Class	Dosage	Description	Rationale
Epinephrine	1:10,000–1:20,000 dilution injected in small amounts around and into the bleeding point	Catecholamine	To halt bleeding by vasoconstriction
Vasopressin	Titrate to produce the desired clinical outcome	Vasoconstrictor	To halt bleeding by vasoconstriction

Pharmacologic Highlights (continued)

Except for epinephrine, which is sometimes used during endoscopy, no medications are used to manage MWS directly. Patients may be placed on antacids, sucralfate (Carafate), or histamine$_2$ blockers, proton pump inhibitors such as omeprazole (Prilosec), or anti-emetics such as prochlorperazine (Compazine) to reduce nausea and vomiting. In unusual cases of severe hemorrhage, patients may be placed on vasopressin to reduce upper GI bleeding, and fluid resuscitation and vasopressors may be used to support the circulation.

Independent

A major cause of morbidity and mortality in patients with active GI bleeding is aspiration of blood with subsequent respiratory compromise, which is seen in patients with inadequate gag reflexes or those who are unconscious or obtunded. Constant surveillance to ensure a patent airway is essential. Check every 8 hours for the presence of a gag reflex. Maintain the head of the bed in a semi-Fowler position unless contraindicated. If the patient needs to be positioned with the head of the bed flat, place the patient in a side-lying position.

Encourage bedrest and reduced physical activity to limit oxygen consumption. Plan care around frequent rest periods, scheduling procedures so the patient does not overtire. Avoid the presence of noxious stimuli that may be nauseating. Initially, the patient's oral intake will be restricted, but following endoscopy, the patient usually can resume drinking fluids and then, gradually, eating food. Support nutrition by eliminating foods and fluids that cause gastroesophageal discomfort. Encourage the patient to avoid caffeinated beverages, alcohol, carbonated drinks, and extremely hot or cold food or fluids. Help the patient understand the treatments and procedures. Provide information that is consistent with the patient's educational level and that takes into account the patient's state of anxiety.

Evidence-Based Practice and Health Policy

He, L., Li, Z., Zhu, H., Wu, X., Tian, D., & Li, P. (2019). The prediction value of scoring systems in Mallory-Weiss syndrome patients. *Medicine, 98*, e15751.

- The authors wanted to evaluate whether the Glasgow-Blatchford score (GBS), AIMS65 (score that considers albumin, blood clotting, mental status, blood pressure, and age to determine hospital mortality), and shock index are effective in predicting the clinical outcomes of MWS. They enrolled 128 patients from January 2010 to January 2017 diagnosed with MWS by endoscopy. Clinical features including endoscopic treatment and transfusion were analyzed.
- MWS accounted for 6.1% of nonvariceal upper GI bleeding. Patients between ages 40 and 60 years were most commonly affected; 43.8% of MWS was caused by drinking alcohol followed by underlying gastric diseases (33.6%). In female patients alone, underlying gastric diseases were the leading cause (42.9%). GBS system and shock index predicted the need for transfusion.

DOCUMENTATION GUIDELINES

- Physical response: Frequency and amount of hematemesis; laboratory values of interest; presence of blood in the stool; degree of discomfort (location, duration, precipitating factors)
- Response to treatments: Success of interventions to stop bleeding; response to fluids and blood component therapy; function of tamponade tubes; ability to maintain rest and conserve energy
- Ability to tolerate food and fluids; nausea and vomiting

DISCHARGE AND HOME HEALTHCARE GUIDELINES

Teach the patient to avoid foods and fluids that cause discomfort or irritation. Determine the patient's understanding of any prescribed medications, including dosage, route, action or effect, and side effects. Review signs and symptoms of recurrent bleeding and the need to seek immediate medical care. Provide a phone number for the patient to use if complications develop.

Discuss a referral to an alcohol treatment program or for alcohol counseling if appropriate.

Mastitis

DRG Category:	601
Mean LOS:	3.0 days
Description:	MEDICAL: Non-Malignant Breast Disorders Without Complication or Comorbidity or Major Complication or Comorbidity

Mastitis, parenchymatous inflammation of the mammary glands, is seen primarily in lactating women. It can be noninfectious because of a blocked milk duct or infectious because of bacterial proliferation. Approximately 30% of lactating women in the United States develop mastitis, which is more common in primiparas and with infants with short frenulums. Breast abscesses develop in approximately 5% of women with mastitis. Typically, the lactation process is well established before mastitis develops; the highest incidence is seen at 6 weeks' postpartum. It occurs rarely during the antepartum period, particularly with autoimmune diseases of the breast, such as granulomatous lobular mastitis or lupus mastitis. The infection is usually unilateral and is preceded by marked engorgement. If it is left untreated, mastitis may develop into a breast abscess and the infection can progress to sepsis.

Granulomatous mastitis is a rare, chronic inflammatory breast condition with an uncertain cause that is not associated with current lactation. It is associated with immune and connective tissue diseases, fungal infections, or hypersensitivity of the breast. It occurs most often within 5 years of a pregnancy. Although controversial, the condition is usually treated with corticosteroids. Patients with nonlactational mastitis have a higher risk for breast cancer than those without it.

CAUSES

Mastitis is usually caused by the introduction of bacteria from a crack, fissure, or abrasion through the nipple that allows the organism entry into the breast. The source of organisms is almost always the breastfeeding infant's nose and throat; other sources include the hands of the birthing person or birthing personnel and the birthing person's circulating blood. The most common bacterial organism to cause mastitis is *Staphylococcus aureus*; others include beta-hemolytic streptococcus; *Escherichia coli*; *Candida albicans*; and, rarely, streptococcus. Community-acquired *S aureus* and nosocomial methicillin-resistant *S aureus* have also been found to cause mastitis. The actual organism can be cultured from the milk. Common predisposing factors relate to milk stasis. Risks include incomplete or inadequate drainage of a breast duct and alveolus that occurs as a result of missed feedings, prolonged delay in infant feeding, abrupt weaning of the infant, and blocked ducts caused by tight clothing or poor support of pendulous breasts. Other predisposing factors include a history of untreated or undertreated infections and lowered immune function of the birthing person caused by fatigue, stress, or other health problems.

Several risk factors exist for mastitis in nonlactating people. Diabetes mellitus is associated with mastitis in nonlactating people, and cigarette smoking has been linked. Both obesity and nipple piercing are associated with the development of mastitis.

GENETIC CONSIDERATIONS

Heritable immune responses could be protective or increase susceptibility.

SEX AND LIFE SPAN CONSIDERATIONS

Although mastitis can occur in both men and women, it is uncommon in nonlactating women and rare in men.

HEALTH DISPARITIES AND SEXUAL/GENDER MINORITY HEALTH

Ethnicity and race have no known effect on the risk for mastitis. Transgender is a term used to describe persons whose gender identity is different from their sex assigned at birth. Approximately 1% of the U.S. population identify themselves as transgender. Sexual and gender minority persons have higher odds for multiple chronic conditions, cancer, and poor quality of life, and are more apt to have disabilities than cisgender males and females. (Cisgender is a term used to describe persons whose gender identity and gender expression are aligned with their assigned sex listed on their birth certificate.) Gender-affirming hormone therapy is the use of hormone therapy for gender transition or gender affirmation and can be masculinizing or feminizing. Lactation has been induced through hormone therapy in transgender women wishing to breast-feed (Wamboldt et al., 2021). Male-to-female transgender people on gender-affirming hormone therapy are at risk for developing granulomatous mastitis, which is a rare benign inflammatory condition of the breast. It is important during diagnosis to differentiate this condition from breast cancer through breast imaging (Sam et al., 2017).

GLOBAL HEALTH CONSIDERATIONS

Mastitis occurs around the globe, but no prevalence data are available.

ASSESSMENT

HISTORY. Determine the date that the pregnant person delivered. In reviewing breastfeeding history, note if the frequency or regularity of feedings has changed. Investigate (1) the length of time the infant spends feeding; (2) the time between feedings; (3) whether the infant is falling asleep at the breast; (4) whether the infant is sleeping through the night; (5) whether the infant receives supplementary water, juice, or formula; and (6) whether the infant receives bottled breast milk. Elicit a history of systemic and local discomfort. Systemic symptoms include fever, chills, and malaise; localized symptoms include intense pain, tenderness, redness, and heat at the infection site. The birthing person often feels as if they have the flu, with symptoms of muscular aching, fatigue, headache, and continued fever.

Ask if schedule or work changes have occurred that may cause the birthing person to nurse the infant less frequently. In addition, ask if family members have cold or flu symptoms.

PHYSICAL EXAMINATION. Before breast symptoms occur, **chills, fever, and tachycardia** are present. Usually, the **infection is unilateral**. The breast may have a pink or red area that is swollen and often wedge-shaped, resulting from the septal distribution of the connective breast tissue. Most often, the upper outer quadrant is involved, but any area of the breast may be infected. You may also note cracked or sore nipples. Palpation of the area reveals a firm, tender area that is often warm to the touch. During palpation, you may also feel enlarged axillary lymph nodes. When the patient expresses milk, they may express purulent material.

PSYCHOSOCIAL. The transition to parenthood is a time of many changes in the parent's relationships with the infant, the other parent, other children, and grandparents. It is important that the parent realize that mastitis is not a reason to discontinue breastfeeding and that their parenting skills are not inadequate because of it.

Diagnostic Highlights

General Comments: The diagnosis of mastitis is based on the presenting symptoms and lactation history. Mammography is generally not used to diagnose mastitis unless malignancy is suspected.

(highlight box continues on page 782)

Diagnostic Highlights (continued)

Test	Normal Result	Abnormality With Condition	Explanation
Culture of the breast milk	No growth	Shows growth of the organism causing the infection; confirms the diagnosis	Determines the appropriate antibiotic to treat the infection
Bacterial colony count	No growth	> 1,000/mL	Indicates the presence of infection
White blood cells (WBCs)	4,500–11,100/mcL	> 11,100/mcL	Increase in WBCs indicates the magnitude of the infection

PRIMARY NURSING DIAGNOSIS

DIAGNOSIS. Ineffective and/or interrupted breastfeeding related to infection as evidenced by pain and/or changes in feeding patterns

OUTCOMES. Breastfeeding establishment: Infant; Breastfeeding establishment: Maternal; Breastfeeding maintenance; Anxiety level

INTERVENTIONS. Lactation counseling; Nutritional management; Emotional support; Anxiety reduction

PLANNING AND IMPLEMENTATION

Collaborative

Pharmacologic treatment involves the use of antibiotics that are tolerated by the infant and patient. Generally, mastitis is treated with antibiotic therapy for 10 to 14 days. If antibiotic therapy is begun before suppuration begins, the infection usually resolves within 48 hours. Warm compresses, ice packs, and emptying the breast through breastfeeding or pumping should occur every 2 hours. Milk cultures are done prior to starting antimicrobial therapy to identify sensitivities and for successful surveillance on infections. Acetaminophen can be taken for discomfort; NSAIDs can be taken for fever and inflammation. If an abscess develops, it is drained surgically or with needle aspiration.

Pharmacologic Highlights

Medication or Drug Class	Dosage	Description	Rationale
Amoxicillin-clavulanate, dicloxacillin, flucloxacillin, cephalexin	Varies by drug	Broad-spectrum antibiotic	Fight off infection by damaging the cell wall of the infective agent
Vancomycin (used only for resistant, penicillinase-producing staphylococcus), clindamycin, trimethoprim-sulfamethoxazole, doxycycline, ciprofloxacin	Varies by drug	Antibiotic effective against gram-positive bacteria; to manage methicillin-resistant *S aureus*	Interferes with the biosynthesis of the cell

Independent

Prevention is the most important aspect for breastfeeding care. To prevent the development of mastitis, encourage frequent, unrestricted breastfeeding. The infant should be observed while breastfeeding for techniques related to latching on, placement, positions, and suck. At the end of the feeding, evaluate the breast for emptiness. Instruct the patient to rotate feeding position of the infant to promote effective emptying of all lobes and to palpate the breast to evaluate emptiness after each feeding. If clogged ducts are noted, the patient should massage the area before the feeding and assess the area following subsequent feedings to see that it is completely emptied.

If mastitis has developed, encourage the patient to go to bed and stay there. The patient should only provide care for the infant, with a focus on frequent feeding and complete rest for the patient. Encourage the patient to continue breastfeeding frequently because the patient and the baby are colonized with the same organism. If the infected breast is too sore to allow breastfeeding, gentle pumping is recommended; emptying the breasts is an important intervention in preventing an abscess. Recommend that the patient massage the breasts before breastfeeding when the patient feels that the breasts are overly full or were not completely emptied at the previous feeding.

Instruct the patient to apply heat to the affected area or take a warm shower, followed by gentle massage with the palm of the hand, immediately before feeding the infant to promote drainage. Encourage the patient to remove their brassiere/undergarment during feedings so that constriction of the ducts does not occur from pressure. Tell the patient that some infants will not nurse on an inflamed breast. This is due to engorgement and edema, which makes the areola harder to grip; pumping may alleviate this. Note that some infants may not like the taste of the milk from the infected breast because there is increased sodium content. Many patients need encouragement to continue to breastfeed through mastitis.

Infant position during feeding is critical for effective drainage of the breast. Teach the patient to turn the infant fully on the side with the head placed at the patient's breast. The head should face the areola without turning. One or more inches of the areola should be in the infant's mouth, and the infant's chin and nose should rest lightly on the breast. In addition, the infant's lips should be flared during breastfeeding. As the infant nurses, the parent should hear swallowing. Encourage the parent to vary the infant's position (cradle, cross-cradle, football, side-lying) at feedings so that all ducts of the breast are effectively emptied. Feeding should always begin on the affected breast.

Teach the patient that the infant needs to breastfeed a minimum of every 2 to 3 hours around the clock. Frequent feedings may mean that the parent needs to wake the infant during the night. Manage pain through the use of ice packs or warm packs applied to the breast. A supportive, well-fitting brassiere/undergarment may also reduce pain if it does not apply pressure to the infected area. In addition, over-the-counter analgesics may be used. Encourage the patient to drink at least 3,000 mL of fluid per day; light straw-colored urine is an indication of adequate hydration. The patient's diet should meet the nutritional requirements for lactation. Home visits have been shown to decrease breastfeeding complications.

Evidence-Based Practice and Health Policy

Milinco, M., Travan, L., Cattaneo, A., Knowles, A., Sola, M., Causin, E., Cortivo, C., Degrassi, M., Di Tommaso, F., Verardi, G., Dipietro, L., Piazza, M., Scolz, S., Rossetto, M., & Ronfani, L. (2020). Effectiveness of biological nurturing on early breastfeeding problems: A randomized controlled trial. *International Breastfeeding Journal, 15*, 21–25.

- The authors wanted to assess the effectiveness of biological nurturing, compared to usual hospital practices, on the frequency of breast problems and on the prevalence of exclusive breastfeeding at discharge from the maternity ward, after 1 week, 1 month, and 4 months. Women who planned to give birth at the hospital and who expressed the intention to breastfeed were enrolled during pregnancy and randomized to receive breastfeeding support following either the biological nurturing approach ($n = 90$) or the usual care protocol ($n = 98$).
- At discharge from the maternity ward, biological nurturing significantly reduced the risk of breast problems. No statistically significant difference was observed for exclusive breastfeeding at discharge and up to 4 months.

DOCUMENTATION GUIDELINES

• Physical findings: Redness, pain, swelling, appearance of nipples, vital signs
• Ability to nurse: Position, frequency, latching on, sucking
• Emotional status: Anxiety, concern over illness, concern over ability to breastfeed
• Infant's response

DISCHARGE AND HOME HEALTHCARE GUIDELINES

PREVENTION. Teach the patient to prevent mastitis by the following interventions:

• Continue breastfeeding frequently.
• Wash hands before touching breast or beginning breastfeeding.
• Breastfeed every 2 to 3 hours around the clock (wake the baby at night).
• Remove brassiere/undergarment before beginning feeding.
• Always begin breastfeeding on the affected side.
• To promote emptying of the breast at a feeding, apply warmth to the breast immediately before feeding (a disposable diaper may be wet with warm water and wrapped around the breast) and massage the breast before placing the infant at the breast.
• Change the infant's feeding position; use cradle, side-lying, cross-cradle, and football positions to promote emptying of the breast.
• Increase the breastfeeding parent's fluid intake.
• Evaluate the breast after the feeding to see if the infant has completely emptied the breast. If the baby does not completely empty the breast, finish emptying the breast with a breast pump or manual expression.
• Rest and avoid fatigue.

MEDICATIONS. All medications should be taken until the prescription is finished, even if symptoms disappear.

Melanoma Skin Cancer

DRG Category:	580
Mean LOS:	5.2 days
Description:	SURGICAL: Other Skin, Subcutaneous Tissue, and Breast Procedures With Complication or Comorbidity
DRG Category:	595
Mean LOS:	7.5 days
Description:	MEDICAL: Major Skin Disorders With Major Complication or Comorbidity

Melanoma skin cancer is a type of skin cancer that originates from the melanocytes. Melanocytes are melanin-producing cells that are interspersed in the inner layer of the epidermis. Melanin is a dark brown pigment that protects the epidermis and the superficial vasculature of the dermis. It is thought that ultraviolet radiation (UVR) from direct sunlight or tanning beds damages the DNA of melanocytes, impairing the DNA control over how and when cells grow and divide. These skin lesions tend to be hereditary, begin to grow in childhood, and become more numerous in young adulthood.

Skin cancer is the most common cancer in the United States, and melanoma accounts for 1% of all skin cancer cases. Although the lifetime melanoma risk for the overall population is less than 2%, melanoma is responsible for approximately 80% of skin cancer deaths. According to the American Cancer Society, 106,110 new melanomas will be diagnosed and 7,180 people will die of melanoma in 2021. The current lifetime risk for developing an invasive melanoma is 1 in 54. Early diagnosis has led to significant improvement in overall survival. The two most important factors that predict outcomes from treatment are the thickness of the lesion and the status of the regional lymph nodes. In early stages, the 5-year survival rate for melanoma is 99%, and in late stages it is 20% to 30%. Complications include scarring, lymphedema (if lymph nodes were removed during treatment), emotional distress, recurrence, and death.

CAUSES

The majority of melanomas (90%) occur on the skin. Approximately 65% of skin melanomas develop on clear skin, 30% on preexisting moles or nevi (small, circumscribed aggregates of melanocytes), and 5% on age spots. Melanoma cells develop because of gene mutation, followed by inappropriate cell growth and proliferation. Genetic damage occurs for uncertain reasons, but among the theories are exposure to carcinogens in the environment, DNA damage from UV radiation, or heredity. Characteristics associated with an increased risk for melanoma include fair skin that does not tan well and that burns easily, blond or red hair, the tendency to develop freckles, and the presence of a large number of nevi. A strong association exists between exposure to UV light (UV-B radiation) and the development of cutaneous melanoma. Possible mechanisms of damage from UV radiation include suppression of the immune system of the skin, induction of melanocyte cell division, free radical production, and damage of melanocyte DNA. Other risk factors include a positive family history, sunburns early in life, use of tanning beds, and immune suppression because of disease or medications.

GENETIC CONSIDERATIONS

Melanoma has a significant genetic component, with heritability estimated at 58%. A pattern of autosomal dominant transmission is seen in some populations. A person with one first-degree relative affected by melanoma has two to three times the risk of the general population and six times the risk if the relative was affected before age 50 years. The risk increases 13-fold if more than one first-degree relative is affected. Approximately 5% to 10% of melanoma cases are familial. Genes implicated in melanoma susceptibility include *CDKN2A*, *CDK4*, *WNT3*, and *VPS41*.

SEX AND LIFE SPAN CONSIDERATIONS

Men have a 1 in 57 chance of developing melanoma; women have a 1 in 81 chance. The incidence of melanoma increases with age; 50% of cases occur in people who are older than age 50 years and average age of diagnosis is 65 years. Although melanomas are rare in children, the incidence among today's younger people is proportionally higher than among people of the same age decades ago. Melanoma is one of the most common cancers in people who are younger than age 30 years, particularly among young women.

HEALTH DISPARITIES AND SEXUAL/GENDER MINORITY HEALTH

Mortality rates are increasing most rapidly among White men older than age 50 years. White persons have a 1 in 38 lifetime risk for melanoma, Black persons have a lifetime risk of 1 in 1,000, and Hispanic persons have a lifetime risk of 1 in 167. Melanoma most often appears on the trunks of fair-skinned men and the lower legs of fair-skinned women; however, people with more darkly pigmented skin often develop melanoma on their palms and soles, and under the nails. While the prevalence of melanoma is lower in Black and Hispanic persons as compared to White persons, Black persons have a two- to threefold risk for mortality as compared to

White and Hispanic persons. Persons who are Black, Hispanic, over 80 years of age, or who get care at community as compared to university hospitals are less likely to receive the standard of care than other groups (Restrepo et al., 2019 [see Evidence-Based Practice and Health Policy]). Sexual and gender minority status has no known effect on the risk for melanoma, although sexual and gender minority persons may be less likely to have skin cancer screening because of discrimination or the emotional conflict between self-perception and physical anatomy (Gatos, 2018). Gender and sexual minority persons are a vulnerable group because people with low income, long travel distances to cancer screening sites, or who lack health insurance or paid medical leave are less likely to be treated according to cancer care guidelines (National Institutes of Health, 2021).

GLOBAL HEALTH CONSIDERATIONS

The World Health Organization reports that 300,000 melanoma skin cancers occur globally each year, and rates are increasing. It is the 19th most commonly occurring cancer in men and women. One in every three cancers that are diagnosed in the world are skin cancers. The global incidence of melanoma skin cancer is 2.6 per 100,000 females per year and 2.5 per 100,000 males per year. The incidence is 15 times higher in developed than in developing regions, a statistic that may be related to recreational exposure to the sun. The highest rates are in Australia, New Zealand, Norway, and Denmark.

ASSESSMENT

HISTORY. Reports of a change in a nevus or mole or a new skin lesion require careful follow-up. Ask the patient the following questions: When did the lesion first appear or change? What is the specific nature of the change? What symptoms and characteristics of the lesion has the patient noticed? What is the patient's history of exposure to UV light or radiation? What is the history of thermal or chemical trauma? What personal or family history of melanoma or precancerous lesions exists? Determine if melanoma has occurred in any first-degree family relatives.

PHYSICAL EXAMINATION. The most common symptom is a **change in an existing lesion or development of a new lesion**. To identify potentially cancerous lesions, inspect and palpate the scalp, all skin surfaces, and the accessible mucosa in a well-lit room. Examine preexisting lesions, scars, freckles, moles, warts, and nevi closely. Examine all lymph node groups because regional lymph nodes may be involved. The ABCDE rule can be useful in identifying distinguishing characteristics of suspicious lesions (Table 1).

• TABLE 1 ABCDE Rule of Assessment for Melanoma

A = Asymmetry	Change in shape; unbalanced or irregular shape
B = Border irregularity	Indistinct or splayed margins; notching of the borders
C = Color variation	Spread of color from the edge of the lesion into the surrounding skin; multiple shades or colors within a single lesion; dark brown or black, red, white, or blue
D = Diameter	Sudden or continuous increase in size: Diameter > 6 mm (although there has been an increase in 3- to 6-mm melanomas)
E = Evolving	Mole starts to evolve, or change, in size, shape, color, elevation, or a new symptom (bleeding, itching, crusting)

PSYCHOSOCIAL. For many people, the diagnosis of any type of cancer is associated with death. Because cancerous skin lesions are readily visible, the patient with melanoma may experience an altered body image. Ask open-ended questions as you assess the patient's emotional response to the diagnosis of melanoma.

Diagnostic Highlights

Test	Normal Result	Abnormality With Condition	Explanation
Shave biopsy	No cancer cells present	Presence of melanoma cells	Scrapes off the top layers of skin; may not be thick enough to determine the degree of cancer invasion
Punch biopsy	No cancer cells present	Presence of melanoma cells	Removes a deep sample of skin melanoma cells after numbing the site; cuts through all layers of skin
Incisional and excisional biopsy (preferred method)	No cancer cells present	Presence of melanoma cells	Uses a surgical knife to cut through the full thickness of skin and removes a wedge of skin: Incisional biopsy removes only a portion; excisional biopsy removes entire tumor
Fine-needle aspiration biopsy, lymph node biopsy	No cancer cells present	Presence of melanoma cells	Uses a thin needle to remove a very small tissue fragment; may be used to biopsy a lymph node near a melanoma to determine the extent of the disease

Other Tests: Complete blood count, serum chemistries, serum lactate dehydrogenase level, immunohistochemical stains. To diagnose metastases, tests include computed tomography scan, magnetic resonance imaging, positron emission tomography, and x-rays.

PRIMARY NURSING DIAGNOSIS

DIAGNOSIS. Impaired skin integrity related to cutaneous lesions as evidenced by skin changes and/or surgical wounds

OUTCOMES. Tissue integrity: Skin and mucous membranes; Wound healing: Primary intention; Knowledge: Treatment regimen; Nutritional status

INTERVENTIONS. Incision site care; Wound care; Skin surveillance; Skin care: Topical treatment; Medication administration; Infection control; Nutrition management

PLANNING AND IMPLEMENTATION

Collaborative

After diagnostic testing, the cancer is staged. Because the thinner the melanoma, the better the prognosis, the Clark level of a melanoma may be used. This system uses a scale of 1 to 5 to describe which layers of skin are involved. The higher the number, the deeper is the melanoma.

The primary treatment for melanoma is surgical resection. Excision of the cancerous lesion with a 2- to 5-cm margin is recommended when feasible. The width of the surrounding margin should be wider for larger primary lesions. Generally, the margin of the excision should be 10 times as wide as the depth of the tumor. For example, if the penetration of the melanoma is 2.5 mm, the margin should be 2.5 cm around the lesion. When the melanoma is on a finger or toe, surgical treatment is to amputate as much of the finger or toe as is necessary. Elective regional lymph node removal is controversial. While completion lymph node dissection may help control the disease, it does not increase survival. Proponents believe that this procedure decreases the possibility of distal metastases.

The prognosis for metastatic melanoma is poor; it is highly resistant to currently available chemotherapeutic agents. In later stages adjuvant therapy and immunotherapy are used as well as intralesional therapy and chemotherapy. Radiation is not often used to treat the original melanoma but is rather used for symptom management as a palliative measure if the cancer has spread to the brain.

Pharmacologic Highlights

General Comments: Cytokines may cause side effects such as chills, aches, fever, severe fatigue, and swelling. Malignant melanoma is relatively resistant to chemotherapy, but several regimens have shown some activity against the cancer.

Medication or Drug Class	Dosage	Description	Rationale
Chemotherapeutic agents	Varies with drug	Dartmouth regimen: dacarbazine (DTIC), carmustine, cisplatin, and tamoxifen; other: carboplatin, paclitaxel	Decrease replication of malignant cells and kill them
Immunotherapy (adjuvant immunotherapy with cytokines), immunomodulation	Varies with drug	Interferon-alpha; interleukin-2; dabrafenib, trametinib, pembrolizumab	Enhances immune system to recognize and destroy cancer cells; shrinks metastatic melanomas (effective in 10%–20% of patients)

Independent

Patient and family education is the most important nursing responsibility in preventing, recognizing, and treating the disorder. Educational materials and teaching aids are available from various community and national organizations and the local or state branches of the American Cancer Society (https://www.cancer.org) and the National Cancer Institute (https://www.cancer.gov). Nursing care of patients who have had surgery is focused on patient education because most of these patients are treated in an ambulatory or short-term stay setting. Instruct patients to protect the site and inspect the incision and graft sites for bleeding or signs of infection. Immobilize recipient graft sites to promote engraftment. Evaluate limbs that have surgical incisions or local isolated chemotherapy to prevent edema.

Reactions to skin disfigurement that occur with some treatments may vary widely. Determine what the cancer experience means to the patient and how it affects the patient's perception of body image. Help the patient achieve the best possible grooming as treatment progresses. Suggest a support group, or if the patient is coping ineffectively, refer for counseling. If the patient is at a late stage of the disease, discuss with the patient and family if a referral to palliative care is appropriate.

Evidence-Based Practice and Health Policy

Restrepo, D., Huayllani, M., Boczar, D., Sisti, A., Gabriel, E., Lemini, R., Spaulding, A., Bagaria, S., Manrique, O., & Forte, A. (2019). Biopsy type disparities in patients with melanoma: Who receives the standard of care? *Anticancer Research, 39*, 6359–6363.

- The authors aimed to determine whether patient demographics and institutional demographics cause inequality in the type of biopsy performed for people with skin melanoma. They used the National Cancer Database and included all people with cutaneous melanoma and malignant melanoma. They included excisional, punch, shave, or incisional biopsies. Excisional biopsy is the standard of care for lesions that are suspicious for melanoma.
- They found that the likelihood of undergoing an excisional biopsy decreased in patients who were Hispanic, non-White, and older than 80 years of age. And those who were treated at community rather than academic/research cancer treatment centers were less likely to receive excisional biopsies. These groups did not receive standard of care, leading to health disparities.

DOCUMENTATION GUIDELINES

- Description of any suspicious lesions: Specific location, shape, size, color, condition of surrounding skin, sensations reported by the patient

- Description of incision sites: Presence of redness, swelling, drainage, warmth, tenderness
- Pain: Description of the qualities and location of the pain, effectiveness of pain relief measures
- Disease outcomes: Coping, anxiety, stress, patient and family response to diagnosis, need for palliative care

DISCHARGE AND HOME HEALTHCARE GUIDELINES

Teach the patient to protect the incision site from thermal, physical, or chemical trauma. Instruct the patient to inspect the incision site for signs of bleeding or infection. Teach the patient to notify the physician of fever or increased redness, swelling, or tenderness around the incision site. Provide instructions as indicated for specific adjuvant therapy: chemotherapy, radiation, immunotherapy.

Teach the patient strategies for prevention and for modifying the risk factors:

- *Skin self-examination and identification of suspicious lesions:* Moles or nevi that change in size, height, color, texture, sensation, or shape; development of a new mole.
- *Limitation of UV light exposure:* Avoid the sun between the hours of 10 a.m. and 3 p.m. when the UV radiation is the strongest. Wear waterproof sunscreen with a sun protection factor of greater than 15 before going outdoors. Apply sunscreen on cloudy days because roughly 70% to 80% of UV rays can penetrate the clouds. Reapply sunscreen every 2 to 3 hours during long sun exposure. Be aware that the sun's rays are reflected by such surfaces as concrete, snow, sand, and water, thereby increasing exposure to UV rays. Wear protective clothing when outdoors, particularly a wide-brimmed hat to protect the face, scalp, and neck area. Wear wraparound sunglasses with 99% to 100% UV absorption to protect the eyes and the skin area around the eyes. Be aware of medications and cosmetics that increase the sensitivity to UV rays. Minimize UV exposure as much as possible and use sunscreen that contains benzophenones. Avoid tanning booths and sunlamps.

Refer the patient to information about melanoma skin cancer on the American Cancer Society (https://www.cancer.org) and Melanoma Research Foundation (https://www.melanoma.org) Web sites.

Meningitis

DRG Category:	75
Mean LOS:	6.1 days
Description:	MEDICAL: Viral Meningitis With Complication or Comorbidity or Major Complication or Comorbidity
DRG Category:	98
Mean LOS:	7.1 days
Description:	MEDICAL: Non-Bacterial Infection of Nervous System Except Viral Meningitis With Complication or Comorbidity

Meningitis is an acute or subacute inflammation of the meninges (lining of the brain and spinal cord). The bacterial or viral pathogens responsible for meningitis usually come from another site, such as those that lead to an upper respiratory infection, sinusitis, or mumps. The organisms can also enter the meninges through open wounds. Bacterial meningitis is considered a medical emergency because the outcome depends on the interval between the onset of disease and the initiation of antimicrobial therapy. In the United States, approximately 4,000 people contract bacterial meningitis each year, and approximately 500 deaths occur. In contrast, the viral form of meningitis is sometimes called *aseptic* or *serous* meningitis. It is usually self-limiting and, in contrast to the bacterial form, is often described as *benign*.

In the bacterial form, bacteria enter the meningeal space and elicit an inflammatory response. This process includes the release of a purulent exudate that is spread to other areas of the brain by the cerebrospinal fluid (CSF). If it is left untreated, the CSF becomes thick and blocks the normal circulation of the CSF, which may lead to increased intracranial pressure (ICP) and hydrocephalus. Long-term effects of the illness are predominantly caused by a decreased cerebral blood flow because of increased ICP or toxins related to the infectious exudate. If the infection invades the brain tissue itself, the disease is then classified as encephalitis. Other complications include visual impairment, cranial nerve palsies, deafness, chronic headaches, paralysis, and even coma. Treatment complications include hypotension, cardiac dysrhythmias, shock, hyponatremia, syndrome of inappropriate antidiuretic hormone, and stroke.

Of the bacteria that cause meningitis, pneumococcal meningitis has the highest rates of mortality between 20% and 30% in adults and 10% in children. If severe neurological impairment is seen at the time of initial assessment or very early in the clinical course, the mortality rate is 50% to 90%, even when therapy is instituted immediately.

CAUSES

Meningitis is most frequently caused by bacterial or viral agents. In newborns, *Streptococcus pneumoniae* is the most frequent bacterial organism; in other age groups, it is *S pneumoniae* and *Neisseria meningitidis*. *Haemophilus influenzae* is the most common organism in unvaccinated children and adults who contract meningitis. Viral meningitis is caused by many viruses such as West Nile and human immunodeficiency virus. Depending on the cause, isolation precautions may be indicated early in treatment. There has been a decrease in viral meningitis in locations where immunizations have become routine. Risk factors include being immunocompromised (HIV disease, tissue transplantation recipients, autoimmune conditions, and prematurity), alcohol abuse, and cirrhosis.

GENETIC CONSIDERATIONS

Heritable immune responses could be protective or increase susceptibility. Deficiency of complement factor I (*CFI*) causes susceptibility to meningitis.

SEX AND LIFE SPAN CONSIDERATIONS

Meningitis occurs most frequently in young children, older people, and persons in a debilitated state. Infants and the very old are at the most risk for pneumococcal meningitis, whereas children from 2 months to 3 years most frequently have haemophilus meningitis. Male infants have higher rates of infection than female infants. The Centers for Disease Control and Prevention (CDC, 2021) recommend haemophilus vaccine type b conjugate vaccine for infants 2 to 6 months and pneumococcal conjugate vaccine for children under age 2 years. Meningococcal meningitis is most common during childhood after age 3 years and during adolescence. Recommendations are that children receive a meningococcal conjugate vaccine at 11 to 12 years, with a booster dose at age 16 years (CDC, 2021). Now that vaccinations are routine in the United States, bacterial meningitis in children is uncommon. Prognosis is poorest for patients at the extremes of age—the very young and the very old of both sexes.

HEALTH DISPARITIES AND SEXUAL/GENDER MINORITY HEALTH

Black persons are at slightly greater risk than other races and ethnicities for bacterial and viral meningitis, although at this time there is no explanation for those differences in risk. CDC reported in 2018 that 69% of new HIV diagnoses in the United States were in gay and bisexual men. In young people ages 13 to 24 years, young gay and bisexual men account for 83% of all new HIV diagnoses. Persons with HIV are more at risk for meningitis than the general population. These infections may be community-acquired bacterial or viral meningitis, and most commonly are cryptococcal, tuberculous, syphilitic, or lymphomatous meningitis.

GLOBAL HEALTH CONSIDERATIONS

Meningitis is more prevalent in developing than in developed countries because of lower rates of vaccination and less attention to other disease prevention strategies. Experts estimate that the incidence is 10 times higher in developing countries as compared to developed countries because of the lack of preventive services. Causes of viral meningitis around the world include enteroviruses, Japanese B encephalitis virus, mumps or measles virus, and HIV. Many people with these viral infections do not develop symptoms. While it can be found in many countries, meningococcal meningitis is endemic to Africa and India, particularly during hot and dry weather. The area in Northern Africa between Ethiopia to Senegal is considered the "meningitis belt" because of the high prevalence in this area.

ASSESSMENT

HISTORY. The history varies according to which form of meningitis the patient has: acute or subacute. For the subacute form, the patient or family may describe vague, mild symptoms such as irritability, sleepiness, confusion, and loss of appetite. With an acute infection, there may be reports of a headache that became progressively worse, with accompanying neck stiffness, vomiting, disorientation, or delirium. The patient may also note an increased sensitivity to light (photophobia), chills, fever, and even seizure activity.

Ask the patient or family if the patient has traveled recently, because some infections are related to location (Mississippi and Ohio River areas, southwestern United States, Mexico, and Central America, or in the Northeast United States for tick-borne disease). Ask if they have experienced mosquito bites, which may lead to West Nile virus. Frequently, the patient or family describes a recent upper respiratory or other type of infection. A patient with pneumococcal meningitis may have had a recent ear, sinus, or lung infection or endocarditis. It is sometimes associated with other conditions, such as sickle cell disease, basilar skull fracture, splenectomy, or alcoholism. *H influenzae* meningitis is also associated with lung and ear infections.

PHYSICAL EXAMINATION. Classically, the signs of meningitis are **progressive headache, high fever, vomiting, nuchal rigidity** (stiff neck that creates pain when flexed toward chest), and **change in level of consciousness** or disorientation. Other signs include photophobia (sensitivity of eyes to light), a positive Kernig sign (inability to extend legs fully when lying supine) and Brudzinski sign (flexion of the hips when neck is flexed from a supine position), and seizures. Some patients develop signs of increased ICP, such as mental status deterioration with restlessness, confusion, delirium, stupor, and even coma. Patients often experience visual changes; during ophthalmoscopic examination, you may note papilledema and unreactive pupils. Examine babies for bulging fontanels; nuchal rigidity may not be present if the fontanels are open.

An ongoing assessment throughout the patient's hospitalization is important to detect changes in the condition. Serial monitoring for symptoms such as head and neck pain, changes in pupillary response, vomiting, fever, and alterations in fluid and electrolytes is essential. Neurological assessments are completed at timely intervals (every 1 to 2 hours or as indicated by the symptoms), and changes are reported to the physician when appropriate.

PSYCHOSOCIAL. Provide ongoing evaluations to determine the anxiety level and need for information and support. Anxiety is generally present any time there is an illness associated with the brain. Note that some patients or parents feel guilty because of some delay in accessing the healthcare system. Family members may be particularly upset if they witness a seizure.

Diagnostic Highlights

Test	Normal Result	Abnormality With Condition	Explanation
Lumbar puncture for CSF analysis	Red blood cells: 0–10/ mcL; white blood cells: 0–10/mcL; routine culture: no growth; fungal culture: no growth; mycobacteria culture: no growth; color: clear; protein: 15–50 mg/ dL; glucose: 40–80 mg/dL; blood pressure: 5–13 mm Hg; Gram stain: no patho-logical organism seen	Positive cultures with invading microorganism; sensitivities identify antibi-otics that will kill bacteria; cells: 200/mcL; protein: elevated > 50 mg/dL (viral) and > 500 mg/dL (bacterial); glucose: < 45 mg/dL; color: may be cloudy or hazy; blood pressure: elevated; Gram stain: bacteria stain either gram-positive (blue) or gram-negative (red)	Identifies invading micro-organisms; increased protein occurs as the result of the presence of viruses or bacteria; glucose is decreased as microorganisms use glucose for metabolism; lumbar puncture is not done in the presence of known increased ICP

Other Tests: Cultures and sensitivities (blood, nasal swab, urine), C-reactive protein, complete blood count, serum electrolytes and glucose, blood urea nitrogen, creatinine, liver function tests, counter-immunoelectrophoresis (to determine presence of viruses or protozoa in CSF), chest x-ray; computed tomography and magnetic resonance imaging generally do not help with diagnosis but may be done in certain situations such as in people who are immunocompromised or who have seizure disorders.

PRIMARY NURSING DIAGNOSIS

DIAGNOSIS. Risk for infection as evidenced by fever, nuchal rigidity, vomiting, photophobia, and/or headache

OUTCOMES. Infection severity; Immune status; Knowledge: Infection management; Fluid balance; Risk control; Risk detection; Knowledge: Medication

INTERVENTIONS. Infection control; Infection protection; Fluid/electrolyte management; Medication management; Medication administration; Temperature regulation

PLANNING AND IMPLEMENTATION
Collaborative

Assessment and maintenance of airway, breathing, and circulation (ABCs) are essential. Treat-ment with intubation, mechanical ventilation, and hyperventilation may occur if the patient's airway and breathing are threatened, and fluid resuscitation may be needed if the patient is in shock or hypotensive. The most critical treatment is the rapid initiation of antibiotic ther-apy. Generally, people with viral meningitis will recover without antiviral medications, but if encephalitis occurs in conjunction with meningitis, antivirals may be used. Serial neurological assessments and vital signs not only monitor critical changes in the patient but also monitor the patient's response to therapy. Supportive measures such as bedrest and temperature control with antipyretics or hypothermia limit oxygen consumption. Gradual treatment of hyperthermia is required to prevent shivering.

Other strategies to manage increased ICP include osmotic diuretics, such as mannitol, or intraventricular CSF drainage and ICP pressure monitoring. Fluids are often restricted if signs of cerebral edema or excessive secretion of antidiuretic hormone are present. If the patient expe-riences seizures, the physician prescribes anticonvulsant medications. Surgical interventions or CSF drainage may be required to prevent permanent neurological deficits as a result of com-plications such as hydrocephalus or abscesses. The patient is likely to have a severe headache from increased ICP. Because large doses of narcotic analgesia mask important neurological changes, most physicians prescribe a mild analgesic to decrease discomfort. In children, pain relief decreases crying and fretting, which, if left untreated, have the potential to aggravate increased ICP.

Rehabilitation begins with the acute phase of the illness but becomes increasingly important as the infection subsides. If residual neurological dysfunction is present as a result of irritation, pressure, or brain and nerve damage, an individualized rehabilitation program with a multidisciplinary team is required. Vision and auditory testing should be done at discharge and at intervals during long-term recovery because early interventions for these deficits are needed to prevent developmental delays.

Pharmacologic Highlights

Medication or Drug Class	Dosage	Description	Rationale
Antibiotics	High-dose parenteral therapy IV for 2 wk; dosage and drug vary by organism, age, and severity	Choice of antibiotic depends on Gram stain and culture and sensitivities; for suspected bacterial meningitis, a third-generation cephalosporin (ceftriaxone, cefotaxime) is often used while culture results are pending along with vancomycin; in people over age 50 years the therapy may be a combination of vancomycin plus ampicillin plus ceftriaxone or cefotaxime	Cause bacterial lysis and prevent continuation of infection; initial dosages are based on weight or body surface area and then are adjusted according to peak and trough results to maintain therapeutic levels
Antivirals (currently under investigation)	Varies with medication (acyclovir, ganciclovir, foscarnet)	Antiviral agent	Halts viral replication

Other Drugs: Other drugs include analgesics, adjunct corticosteroid therapy (has been reported to decrease the inflammatory process and decrease incidence of hearing loss but is controversial), and anticonvulsants. Vaccinations exist for meningococcal, pneumococcal, and haemophilus meningitis, and the prophylaxis for persons exposed to meningococcal meningitis is rifampin.

Independent

Make sure the patient has adequate ABCs. In the acute phase, the primary goals are to preserve neurological function and to provide comfort. The head of the bed should be elevated 30 degrees to relieve ICP. Keep the patient's neck in good alignment with the rest of the body and avoid hip flexion. Control environmental stimuli such as light and noise and institute seizure precautions. Soothing conversation and touch and encouraging the family's participation are important; they are particularly calming with children who need the familiar touch and voices of parents. Children are also reassured by the presence of a security object.

Institute safety precautions to prevent injury, which may result from either seizure activity or confusion associated with increasing ICP. Take into account an increase in ICP if restraints are used and the patient fights them. Implement measures to limit the effects of immobility, such as skin care, range-of-motion exercises, and a turning and positioning schedule. Note the effect of position changes on ICP, and space activities as necessary.

Explain the disease process and treatments. Alterations can occur in thought processes when ICP begins to increase and the level of consciousness begins to decrease. Reorient the patient to time, place, and person as needed. Keep familiar objects or pictures around. Allow visitation of significant others. Establish alternative means of communication if the patient is unable to maintain verbal contact (e.g., the patient who needs intubation). As the patient moves into the rehabilitative phase, developmentally appropriate stimuli are needed to support normal growth and development. Determine the child's progress on developmental tasks. Make appropriate referrals if the child is not progressing or if the child or family evidence signs of inability to cope.

Evidence-Based Practice and Health Policy

Ellis, D., Zaoutis, T., Thibault, D., Crispo, J., Abraham, D., & Willis, A. (2020). Readmissions after hospital care for meningitis in the United States. *American Journal of Infection Control, 48*, 798–804.

• The authors' objectives were to describe the characteristics of adults hospitalized with meningitis; describe meningitis hospitalization outcomes, including 30- and 90-day readmissions; and determine whether clinical, patient, or hospitalization characteristics were associated with readmission and readmission outcomes. The authors performed a retrospective study of the 2014 National Readmissions Database and extracted data on hospitalized adults ($N = 18,883$) with a principal diagnosis of meningitis.
• Meningitis hospitalizations commonly involved adults 25 to 54 years of age who were insured by private carriers. The readmission rates were 7.0% at 30 days and 11.4% at 90 days. Readmission was associated with greater comorbidity burden, public insurance, and medical error. Readmissions were most often for meningitis, septicemia, or medical complications.

DOCUMENTATION GUIDELINES

• Physiological response: Neurological examination; vital signs; presence of fever; adequacy of ABCs
• Fluid and electrolyte balance: Intake and output, body weight, skin turgor, abnormal serum electrolytes
• Complications: Seizure activity, decreased mental status, fever, increased ICP

DISCHARGE AND HOME HEALTHCARE GUIDELINES

Explain all medications and include the mechanism of action, dosage, route, and side effects. Explain any drug interactions or food interactions. Instruct the patient to notify the primary healthcare provider for signs and symptoms of complications, such as fever, seizures, developmental delays, or behavior changes. Provide referrals and teaching specific to the identified neurological deficits. Encourage the parents to maintain appropriate activities to facilitate the growth and development of the child.

Migraine Headache

DRG Category: 101
Mean LOS: 3.4 days
Description: MEDICAL: Seizures Without Major Complication or Comorbidity

Migraine headache is a recurrent headache syndrome that is episodic, has a neurovascular cause, and may have sensory or visual symptoms known as an aura. Approximately 30 million people have migraine headaches in the United States. It is the most common complaint in healthcare and the fifth leading cause of emergency department visits in the United States. Current thinking is that migraine is a result of neurovascular changes. Experts explaining the neurovascular theory suggest that a complicated series of neural and vascular events lead to migraine, which starts with nervous system changes that then alter cerebral perfusion. Neural excitation causes an aura phase, which then activates a headache phase. In the headache phase, pain-generating substances such as substance P and nitric oxide are released, causing an inflammation response, vasodilation, and, ultimately, pain.

There are two types of migraine headaches: classic migraine and common migraine. Classic migraine has a prodromal (preheadache) phase that lasts approximately 15 minutes and is accompanied by disturbances of neurological functioning such as visual disturbances, speech disturbances, and paresthesias. Neurological symptoms cease with the beginning of the headache, which is often accompanied by nausea and vomiting. Common migraine does not have a preheadache phase but is characterized by an immediate onset of a throbbing headache. Complications include medication overuse to control headaches, depression and mood disorders, chronic migraine, status migrainosus (attacks last longer than 3 days), and stroke.

CAUSES

Both genetic and environmental factors are linked to the development of migraine. With advances in neuroimaging, migraine has been considered a neurovascular process that leads to changes in cerebral perfusion. Hormonal changes in women, stress, sleep disturbance, and head trauma have been linked to migraine. Many studies have also investigated triggers for migraine. These factors include food additives (aspartame, monosodium glutamate), certain food triggers (cheese, salty foods, processed foods), alcohol (particularly wine), smoking, sensory stimuli (bright lights, sun glare, strong smells), changes in barometric pressure, and medications such as nitroglycerine and oral contraceptives. However, while large epidemiological studies have not identified these triggers as causative agents, experts commonly recommend that patients avoid them.

GENETIC CONSIDERATIONS

The inheritance of migraine headaches has been written about since the late 1920s. Twin studies have reported a recurrence risk of migraine with aura at 50% in identical twins and 21% in nonidentical twins. Several loci have been linked or associated with typical migraine. Three genes (*CACNA1A*, *ATP1A2*, and *SCN1A*) have been implicated in the rare disease familial hemiplegic migraine (FHM). FHM is usually transmitted in an autosomal dominant pattern, primarily from the birthing parent, and results in weakness affecting half of the body which can last for a variable amount of time (hours to weeks).

SEX AND LIFE SPAN CONSIDERATIONS

Migraine headaches generally begin in childhood or near puberty and affect females more than males (approximately 75% of people who have migraine are women). Migraine is more severe in women, leads to greater disability than in men, and causes a longer recovery period. Migraine headaches often increase in frequency during pregnancy in the first trimester for those who have experienced them before pregnancy. Oral contraceptives and hormone replacement therapy also increase the frequency of headaches. In children, the incidence of migraine with aura peaks in boys at 5 years of age and in girls at 12 years of age. In adults, the incidence is highest between the ages of 30 and 40 years. Migraine decreases in frequency and severity as people age, and it is uncommon for migraine headaches to occur during old age.

HEALTH DISPARITIES AND SEXUAL/GENDER MINORITY HEALTH

Migraine headaches have a higher prevalence among White persons as compared to Black and Asian persons. Experts note that Black persons are more likely to have inaccurate diagnoses, have more follow-up appointments terminated, and are less likely to have migraine attack medications prescribed according to standards of care than other groups, leading to health disparities in care. In the United States, households with lower educational levels and lower economic resources have higher migraine prevalence. Adults in sexual minority groups have higher odds of experiencing migraine than heterosexual people. Bisexual women (36.8%) and lesbian women (24.7%) have the highest prevalence of migraine followed by heterosexual women (19.7%), gay men (14.8%), and heterosexual men (9.8%). Sexual minority persons may experience discrimination, stigma, and barriers to healthcare access that could trigger or exacerbate migraine and lead to health disparities in the identification and management of migraine (Heslin, 2020; Nagata et al., 2021 [see Evidence-Based Practice and Health Policy]).

GLOBAL HEALTH CONSIDERATIONS

The World Health Organization (WHO) reports that the prevalence of migraine is highest in North America followed by South and Central America. WHO estimates the worldwide prevalence of current migraine to be 10% and lists migraine as 19th among all causes of years lived with disability.

☀ ASSESSMENT

HISTORY. Elicit a description from the patient of all symptoms. Classic migraine is associated with a transient visual, motor, sensory, cognitive, or psychic disturbance or aura that lasts up to 15 minutes and precedes the headache. A second phase occurs with numbness or tingling of the lips, changes in mental status (confusion, drowsiness), aphasia, and dizziness. Common migraine has an immediate onset of throbbing pain. Early warning is often a mood change, and pain is often accompanied by nausea and vomiting. Elicit the timing and pattern of episodes. Two to four attacks a month, often beginning in the mornings and usually lasting a day or two, are a common pattern. Usually migraine does not occur at night.

Generally, migraine headaches are unilateral with pulsating or throbbing pain and are associated with nausea, vomiting, and phonophotophobia (intolerance to light and noise). Duration is from 4 to 72 hours, although the pain often builds over minutes to 1 to 2 hours. Approximately 60% of patients have premonitory or warning symptoms that occur hours to even days before migraine. Determine if the patient has warning symptoms such as food cravings, thirst, fluid retention, lethargy, and heightened sensitivity to light, sound, and smell. If the patient is a female, determine the timing of the menstrual cycle, any birth control pills or hormone replacement therapy, and if the patient is pregnant. Following the migraine, the patient may describe a "washed-out" feeling, weakness, food cravings or food aversions, and euphoria. Ask patients to describe any triggers for migraine that they experience.

PHYSICAL EXAMINATION. The most common symptom is a **throbbing, pulsatile headache**. Perform a neurological assessment to determine focal neurological dysfunction (e.g., drowsiness, vertigo, aphasia, unilateral weakness, confusion) and visual disturbances (e.g., spots, lines, or shimmering light). Test the cranial nerves, particularly cranial nerves V, IX, and X. The patient has no signs and symptoms when the headache is not present, but other disorders need to be ruled out before the initial diagnosis of migraine headache is made. The patient may have tachycardia or bradycardia and hypertension or hypotension.

PSYCHOSOCIAL. Psychosocial assessment should include assessment of the degree of stress people experience and the strategies they use to cope with stress. People with migraine are at risk for depression and mood disorders. Determine the patient's lifestyle patterns, such as exercise patterns, family relationships, rest and work patterns, and substance abuse patterns. Migraine can lead to extensive disability and economic loss. Long-term job counseling may be necessary.

Diagnostic Highlights

No test is diagnostic for migraine headaches; rather, the diagnosis is made by history. The International Headache Society established the following criteria for diagnosis: at least five headache attacks lasting 4 to 72 hours, with at least two of the following characteristics: unilateral location, pulsating quality, moderate or severe pain intensity, and aggravation by or causing avoidance of routine physical activity. The patient also must have one of the following: nausea and/or vomiting; photophobia and phonophobia. The symptoms also must not be related to another disorder. The following tests may be necessary for differential diagnosis: computed tomography scan, skull x-ray, cranial nerve testing, arteriogram, lumbar puncture, cerebrospinal fluid testing, electroencephalogram, and magnetic resonance imaging.

PRIMARY NURSING DIAGNOSIS

DIAGNOSIS. Acute pain related to neurovascular changes, vasoconstriction, and/or vasodilation as evidenced by self-reports of pain, facial grimacing, and/or protective behavior

OUTCOMES. Comfort status; Knowledge: Pain management; Pain level; Pain control; Symptom severity; Knowledge: Medication; Medication response

INTERVENTIONS. Pain management: Acute; Analgesic administration; Medication administration; Medication management; Teaching: Prescribed medication

PLANNING AND IMPLEMENTATION

Collaborative

Migraine treatment is divided into acute and preventive strategies. Acute treatment is focused on reversing the progression of a migraine headache and is usually pharmacologic. Preventive treatment aims to reduce the frequency and severity of migraine. Adequate sleep and stress reduction are important components of prevention. Dietary modification may decrease symptoms; this includes reducing the intake of caffeinated beverages, monosodium glutamate, cheese, sausage, sauerkraut, citrus fruit, chocolate, and red wine. Biofeedback, cognitive behavioral therapy, and relaxation therapy have been shown to be effective along with pharmacologic treatments. Transcranial magnetic stimulator, a device that delivers a pulse of magnetic energy that stimulates the occipital cortex, has been effective for some patients and is approved by the U.S. Food and Drug Administration.

Pharmacologic Highlights

Medication or Drug Class	Dosage	Description	Rationale
Nonnarcotic analgesics	Varies with drug	Either aspirin, acetaminophen, or NSAIDs may abort a migraine headache if taken early; ketorolac tromethamine, ketoprofen, naproxen sodium, flurbiprofen, isometheptene, butalbital with aspirin, and acetaminophen reduce headache pain	Abort or relieve a migraine headache
Serotonin 5-ht-receptor agonists (sumatriptan, naratriptan, zolmitriptan, rizatriptan, almotriptan, frovatriptan, eletriptan)	Varies with drug	Serotonic receptor stimulant; antimigraine that acts by binding with vascular receptors producing a vasoconstrictive effect on cranial blood vessels	Acts on receptors on intracranial blood vessels and sensory nerve endings to relieve migraine headache
Prochlorperazine (Compazine)	5–10 mg IV	Antiemetic, antipsychotic that terminates migraine and helps alleviate nausea	Relieves a migraine headache
Ergotamine	2–3 mg PO; may add additional doses to reach 6 mg in a 24-hr period or 10 mg/wk	Antimigraine that may have an agonist/antagonist action with alpha-adrenergic, serotonergic, and dopaminergic receptors; directly stimulates vascular smooth muscle, constricting arteries and veins	To prevent or abort migraine headache

(highlight box continues on page 798)

Pharmacologic Highlights (continued)

Medication or Drug Class	Dosage	Description	Rationale
Dihydroergotamine (DHE)	1–2 mg IM or SC; during the peak of a headache 5–10 mg or prochlorperazine may be given IV followed by 0.75 mg of DHE IV over 3 min	Venoconstrictor with minimal peripheral arterial constriction; use with caution with patients with cardiac disease	Relieves the pain of migraine headache
Beta blockers, tricyclic antidepressants, calcium channel blockers	Varies with drug	Used to prevent headaches, particularly those that do not respond to acute therapy	To prevent migraine headaches

Independent

Teach the patient to avoid triggers that may lead to headaches. Explain to patients that at the beginning of an attack, they may be able to limit pain by resting in a darkened room. If patients sleep uninterrupted with their eyes covered, symptoms may be alleviated.

A combination of complementary therapies may be successful in managing symptoms. Explain the medication dosage, route, and side effects and the differences among acute therapy (stopping progression), preventive therapy (prophylactic therapy), and rescue therapy (pain relief when acute therapy has not worked). Introduce to the patient the possibility of behavior therapy such as biofeedback, exercise therapy, and relaxation techniques. Explore with the patient some techniques for stress reduction and adequate rest. Discuss family- or work-related stress to determine a regimen that may reduce stress and provide for adequate rest and relaxation. Lifestyle management may be essential to control headaches. Ask a dietician to evaluate the patient's food intake and to work with the patient to develop a diet that will minimize exposure to triggers.

Evidence-Based Practice and Health Policy

Nagata, J., Ganson, K., Tabler, J., Blashill, A., & Murray, S. (2021). Disparities across sexual orientation in migraine among U.S. adults. *JAMA Neurology, 78*, 117–118.

- The authors aimed to determine the association between sexual orientation and migraine in a nationally representative sample of adults ages 31 to 42 years old ($N = 9,894$). Migraine was measured by self-reported responses to the question: "Have you ever had five or more headaches that were at least 4 hours long; one-sided, pulsating, intense, or worsened by activity; and associated with nausea, vomiting, or sensitivity to light or sound?"
- The prevalence of migraine was higher among individuals who reported being mostly heterosexual (30.3%) and lesbian, gay, or bisexual (30.7%) as compared to individuals who reported being exclusively heterosexual (19.4%). The authors concluded that adults in sexual minority groups had higher odds of experiencing migraine than heterosexual people. The authors note that members of sexual minority groups experience prejudice, stigma, and discrimination, which could trigger or worsen migraine.

DOCUMENTATION GUIDELINES

- Discomfort: Timing, character, location, duration, precipitating factors
- Nutrition: Food and fluid intake; understanding of dietary restriction
- Medication management: Understanding of drug therapy; prophylactic, abortive, and rescue protocols; response to medications
- Response to alternative treatments: Success of treatment, interest in developing other, nontraditional management strategies

DISCHARGE AND HOME HEALTHCARE GUIDELINES

Teach the patient how to maintain lifestyle changes with regard to rest, nutrition, and medication management. Make sure the patient and family understand all aspects of the treatment regimen. Review dietary limitations and recommendations, and make sure the patient understands the dosage and side effects of all medications. Provide a referral to a headache clinic that teaches alternative therapies.

Mitral Insufficiency (Regurgitation)

DRG Category:	216
Mean LOS:	15.9 days
Description:	SURGICAL: Cardiac Valve and Other Major Cardiothoracic Procedures With Cardiac Catheterization With Major Complication or Comorbidity
DRG Category:	218
Mean LOS:	6.7 days
Description:	SURGICAL: Cardiac Valve and Other Major Cardiothoracic Procedures With Cardiac Catheterization Without Complication or Comorbidity or Major Complication or Comorbidity
DRG Category:	219
Mean LOS:	10.9 days
Description:	SURGICAL: Cardiac Valve and Other Major Cardiothoracic Procedures Without Cardiac Catheterization With Major Complication or Comorbidity
DRG Category:	221
Mean LOS:	4.7 days
Description:	SURGICAL: Cardiac Valve and Other Major Cardiothoracic Procedures Without Cardiac Catheterization Without Complication or Comorbidity or Major Complication or Comorbidity
DRG Category:	307
Mean LOS:	3.1 days
Description:	MEDICAL: Cardiac Congenital and Valvular Disorders Without Major Complication or Comorbidity

Mitral insufficiency, or mitral regurgitation, is the inadequate closure of the mitral valve, which interferes with expulsion of cardiac output from the left ventricle. It occurs in approximately 20% of middle-aged and older adults, but many are not symptomatic because they have a mild form of the disease. The mitral valve is located between the left atrium and the left ventricle. When the heart contracts, normally blood is moved forward from the left ventricle out through the aortic valve, into the aorta, and ultimately into the systemic circulation. In mitral insufficiency, instead of blood moving to the aorta, a portion of the blood flows backward through the regurgitant mitral valve into the left atrium. Cardiac output, therefore, is separated into forward systemic flow into the aorta and backward regurgitant flow into the left atrium. The amount of forward versus backward flow depends on the severity of the mitral insufficiency and the afterload (impedance to flow against which the left ventricle pumps).

In chronic mitral insufficiency, forward blood flow decreases and blood accumulates in the heart, allowing the left atrium and left ventricle to increase in size. The heart, therefore, tolerates the regurgitant blood flow without engorgement of the pulmonary circulation or significant reduction of cardiac output. In acute mitral insufficiency, the left atrium and ventricle are not able to tolerate the dramatic increase in blood volume, so cardiac output decreases and blood backs up quickly into the pulmonary circulation. Pulmonary congestion and acute illness follow. Complications include heart failure, atrial fibrillation, pulmonary hypertension, and stroke.

CAUSES

Common causes of chronic mitral insufficiency are rheumatic heart disease, coronary artery disease, endocarditis, congenital anomaly, and idiopathic calcification of the mitral annulus, which inhibits valve closure. Calcification associated with aging has been found on autopsies; however, with most patients, there was a minimal functional consequence. Connective tissue diseases (Marfan syndrome, Ehlers-Danlos syndrome) are also associated with mitral insufficiency. Mitral valve prolapse (MVP), a common form of mitral insufficiency, occurs with degeneration of mitral leaflets, which causes a "floppy valve." Acute mitral insufficiency can occur with myocardial infarctions that have been caused by ischemia or necrosis of the papillary muscle or by chordae tendineae that support the mitral leaflets. Other risk factors include a history of mitral stenosis, coronary heart disease, and migraine medications (ergotamine tartrate/ caffeine, cabergoline).

GENETIC CONSIDERATIONS

Mitral insufficiency may be due to congenital valve disorders. MVP is usually considered a sporadic disorder. It can be inherited as an autosomal dominant trait with sex- and age-dependent penetrance. In addition, MVP can be seen as a feature of heritable connective tissue diseases such as Marfan syndrome, Ehler-Danlos syndrome, and osteogenesis imperfecta.

SEX AND LIFE SPAN CONSIDERATIONS

Mitral insufficiency is more common in women than men. The most common causes in women are rheumatic fever and MVP (Barlow disease). MVP is more common in females than males, peaks in the 30s, and is associated with a lower than normal body mass index. Men are more likely to have fibroelastic deficiency and posterior leaflet prolapse than MVP. Women experience health disparities with respect to mitral insufficiency management. Surgical outcomes are worse for women than men and mortality rates are higher, although outcomes are similar for women and men with transcatheter procedures (see Planning and Implementation). MVP is present in approximately 4% of the U.S. population and can be identified through diagnostic tests in about 20% of middle-aged and older adults. Chronic mitral insufficiency increases with age and is therefore more common in the aging population.

HEALTH DISPARITIES AND SEXUAL/GENDER MINORITY HEALTH

Racial disparities exist with the number of procedures performed for structural heart disease. More interventions per population were performed on White persons as compared to Black and Hispanic persons. Black and Hispanic patients also had higher risk profiles than White patients, although there is no difference in complication and mortality rates. In general, Black and Hispanic patients have disparities with respect to access, provision of care, and availability of cardiovascular interventions as compared to White patients (Alkhouli et al., 2019). Sexual and gender minority status has no known effect on the risk for mitral insufficiency.

GLOBAL HEALTH CONSIDERATIONS

Rheumatic fever and related mitral valve disease are more common in developing than in developed countries and are the leading cause of mitral regurgitation globally.

ASSESSMENT

HISTORY. Question the patient about a history of rheumatic fever because 50% of all cases of chronic mitral insufficiency are attributed to rheumatic heart disease. Because MVP, a common form of mitral insufficiency, has a familial association, determine if others in the family have the condition. Coronary heart disease contributes to both chronic and acute disorders; therefore, ask if the patient has chest pain or palpitations or has experienced fatigue or shortness of breath. Symptoms of MVP include orthopnea, palpitations, irregular heartbeat, fatigue, exertional dyspnea, edema, and weight loss.

PHYSICAL EXAMINATION. Determine if the patient has the classic symptoms of **fatigue** and **shortness of breath**. Inspection and palpation of the precordium are usually unremarkable except in extreme cases of mitral insufficiency. Patients may remain asymptomatic for years. Auscultation of the chest usually reveals a **soft first heart sound** and a **systolic murmur**, which is loudest at the apex. In severe mitral insufficiency, you may hear an S_3 gallop. Auscultation of breathing may reveal fine crackles (rales) if pulmonary congestion is present. When the abdomen is palpated, you may note an enlarged liver if the patient has severe right-sided heart failure. The patient may also have jugular vein distention and a prominent alpha wave.

PSYCHOSOCIAL. In an effort to avoid exertional dyspnea and fatigue, patients usually adjust their lifestyles by restricting their activity and resting frequently. They may not notice the increasing fatigue until it gets debilitating. Assess the patient's level of exercise and how the patient copes with activity intolerance.

Diagnostic Highlights

Test	Normal Result	Abnormality With Condition	Explanation
Transesophageal echocardiogram	Normal mitral valve	Incompetent mitral valve	Mitral valve is incompetent, and during the systolic phase, blood flows backward into the left atrium; left-sided heart chambers may be enlarged, with an increased left ventricular end-diastolic volume
Cardiac catheterization	Normal mitral valve	Systolic regurgitant flow from the left ventricle into left atrium; left-sided hypertrophy and/or dilation of heart; may have a decreased left ventricular ejection fraction	Same as above
Doppler echo-cardiography	Normal mitral valve	Incompetent mitral valve	Same as above

Other Tests: Electrocardiogram may show atrial fibrillation, chest radiography, prothrombin time, activated partial thromboplastin time, brain natriuretic peptide level

PRIMARY NURSING DIAGNOSIS

DIAGNOSIS. Decreased activity tolerance related to diminished cardiac output as evidenced by fatigue, shortness of breath, and/or tachycardia

OUTCOMES. Activity tolerance; Energy conservation; Coping; Knowledge: Disease process; Symptom severity; Symptom control; Knowledge: Medication; Knowledge: Treatment regimen

INTERVENTIONS. Energy management; Exercise promotion; Exercise therapy: Ambulation; Medication management; Teaching: Prescribed exercise; Teaching: Prescribed medications

❊ PLANNING AND IMPLEMENTATION

Collaborative

Most patients with mitral insufficiency can compensate or be stabilized with medical treatment for their entire lives. Surgical repair or valve replacement is considered in patients with progressive severe disease. Physicians place most patients with advanced mitral insufficiency on activity restrictions to decrease cardiac workload. Research suggests that if the patient is on bedrest, the use of a bedside commode creates less workload for the heart than using a bedpan. Fluid restrictions and diuretics may be ordered to reduce pulmonary congestion and afterload-reducing agents and beta blockers may be used. Supplemental oxygen enhances gas exchange and oxygenation to decrease dyspnea and chest pain.

Mitral valve repair (valvuloplasty) is preferred over replacement whenever possible. The choice of valve type is based on the patient's age and the potential for clotting problems. Operative mortality is higher for people age 75 years or older; the risks and benefits of surgery are considered on the basis of age and other disease conditions. A biological valve (e.g., a porcine valve from a pig) usually shows structural deterioration after 6 to 10 years and needs to be replaced. A synthetic valve is more durable but is also more prone to thrombi formation. If the incompetent valve is replaced surgically with a synthetic valve, patients are prescribed long-term anticoagulant therapy, such as warfarin (Coumadin). While the techniques have not been perfected to date, percutaneous mitral valve replacement is under study for mitral valve repair and annuloplasty. These techniques are in early stage preclinical and clinical investigation. (See **Coronary Heart Disease (Arteriosclerosis)** for a further discussion of the collaborative and independent management of patients after open heart surgery.)

Pharmacologic Highlights

Medication or Drug Class	Dosage	Description	Rationale
Diuretics	Varies with drug	Thiazides; loop diuretics	Manage fluid overload and congestive symptoms
Angiotensin-converting enzyme inhibitors	Varies with drug	Captopril, enalapril, lisinopril	Decrease preload and afterload; decrease regurgitant blood flow; reduce ventricular size
Warfarin	Initially 10–15 mg, then 2–10 mg/day maintenance	Anticoagulant	Prevents thrombi from forming on the synthetic valve
Heparin or low-molecular-weight heparin	Initially 80 units/kg IV bolus, followed by an infusion of 18 units/kg; serial monitoring of activated partial thromboplastin time to guide future doses	Anticoagulant	Prevents thrombi initially until warfarin therapy is well regulated

Other Drugs: Inotropic agents (dobutamine [Dobutrex], digoxin) are used to enhance the heart's pumping ability. If they are present, dysrhythmias are treated with

Pharmacologic Highlights (continued)

antidysrhythmics, such as propranolol (Inderal) or quinidine. Nitrates may be used to decrease blood pressure and increase coronary artery blood flow. Antibiotics are used prophylactically against bacterial endocarditis and prior to interventional therapies and dental procedures (manipulation of gingival tissue, procedures on the apex of a tooth, or perforation of oral mucosa); common antibiotics are ampicillin, amoxicillin, clindamycin, gentamicin.

Independent

Maintain airway, breathing, and circulation. If the patient is stable, focus on reducing the cardiac workload and psychological stress to reduce the metabolic demands of the myocardium. Provide assistance with activities of daily living and encourage the patient to abide by activity restrictions to allow for adequate rest. Establish a quiet environment with uninterrupted rest periods, if possible. To ease the patient's breathing, elevate the head of the bed. Encourage the patient to avoid sudden changes in position to minimize increased cardiac demand and dizziness. Instruct the patient to sit on the edge of the bed before standing.

Reduce psychological stress by approaching the patient and family in a calm, relaxed manner. Decrease fear of the unknown by providing explanations and encouraging questions. Help the patient maintain or reestablish a sense of control by participating in decisions about aspects of care. If the patient decides to have valve surgery, offer to let the patient speak with someone who already has had the surgery and provide preoperative teaching.

Evidence-Based Practice and Health Policy

Parcha, V., Patel, N., Kalra, R., Suri, S., Arora, G., & Arora, P. (2020). Mortality due to mitral regurgitation among adults in the United States: 1999–2018. *Mayo Clinic Proceedings*, *95*, 2633–2643.

- The authors aimed to evaluate nationwide trends in mortality due to mitral regurgitation in American adults during the years from 1999 to 2018. They used a retrospective cross-sectional analyses of nationwide mortality data from death certificates.
- The authors found that 45,982 deaths due to mitral regurgitation occurred during the study period. Higher mortality rates were found in older White females from the western United States. They also found that mortality rates fell annually by 4% until 2012, and then mortality rates increased by 1.5% annually after 2012. They made no clear explanation for these trends in mortality but suggested further investigation is necessary.

DOCUMENTATION GUIDELINES

- Physical findings: Cardiopulmonary assessment, presence of murmurs and rales, vital signs
- Response to interventions and medications: Diuretics, nitrates, vasodilators, inotropic agents, and antidysrhythmic medications
- Reaction to activity restrictions, fluid restrictions, and cardiac diagnosis
- Presence of complications: Chest pain, bleeding, dyspnea, wound infection

DISCHARGE AND HOME HEALTHCARE GUIDELINES

Be sure the patient understands all medications, including the dosage, route, action, and adverse effects, and the need for routine laboratory monitoring for anticoagulants. Explain the need to avoid activities that may predispose the patient to excessive bleeding; hold pressure on bleeding sites to assist in clotting. Remind the patient to notify healthcare workers of anticoagulant use before procedures. Identify foods high in vitamin K, such as turnips, spinach, liver, and cauliflower, which should be limited so the effect of warfarin is not reversed. Instruct the patient to report the recurrence or escalation of signs and symptoms of mitral insufficiency. The appearance of these symptoms could indicate that the medical therapy needs readjusting or that the replaced valve is malfunctioning. Patients with synthetic valves may hear an audible click from the valve closure. The click sounds like the ticking of a watch.

Patients who have had valvular disorders or valve surgery are susceptible to bacterial endo-carditis, which causes scarring or destruction of the heart valves. Bacterial endocarditis may result from dental work, surgeries, and invasive procedures, so people who have repaired or replaced heart valves should be given antibiotics before and after these treatments.

Mitral Stenosis

DRG Category:	216	
Mean LOS:	15.9 days	
Description:	SURGICAL: Cardiac Valve and Other Major Cardiothoracic Procedures With Cardiac Catheterization With Major Complication or Comorbidity	
DRG Category:	218	
Mean LOS:	6.7 days	
Description:	SURGICAL: Cardiac Valve and Other Major Cardiothoracic Procedures With Cardiac Catheterization Without Complication or Comorbidity or Major Complication or Comorbidity	
DRG Category:	219	
Mean LOS:	10.9 days	
Description:	SURGICAL: Cardiac Valve and Other Major Cardiothoracic Procedures Without Cardiac Catheterization With Major Complication or Comorbidity	
DRG Category:	221	
Mean LOS:	4.7 days	
Description:	SURGICAL: Cardiac Valve and Other Major Cardiothoracic Procedures Without Cardiac Catheterization Without Complication or Comorbidity or Major Complication or Comorbidity	
DRG Category:	307	
Mean LOS:	3.1 days	
Description:	MEDICAL: Cardiac Congenital and Valvular Disorders Without Major Complication or Comorbidity	

Mitral stenosis, a pathological narrowing of the orifice of the mitral valve, occurs when the mitral valve is unable to open fully. The opening of the mitral valve, normally 4 to 6 cm^2 in area, is decreased to half normal size or even smaller because of a series of changes in valve structure. The mitral valve leaflets fuse together and become stiff and thickened by fibrosis and calcification. The chordae tendineae fuse together and shorten, and the valvular cusps lose their flexibility.

The mitral valve is located between the left atrium and the left ventricle. When mitral stenosis occurs, blood can flow from the left atrium to the left ventricle only if it is moved forward by an abnormally elevated left atrial pressure. The elevated left atrial pressure leads to increased pulmonary venous and capillary pressures, decreased pulmonary compliance, and exertional dyspnea. Left atrial dilatation, an increase in pulmonary artery pressure, and right ventricular hypertrophy follow as the heart compensates for the stenotic valve.

Complications of mitral stenosis can be serious. With no surgical intervention, 20 years after the onset of symptoms, the condition can result in an 85% mortality rate. Heart failure with pulmonary edema develops with sudden changes in flow across the mitral valve, such as the increased flow that occurs in exercise. Atrial dysrhythmias, particularly paroxysmal atrial tachycardia, atrial flutter, and atrial fibrillation, occur with more longstanding disease. Pulmonary hypertension can cause fibrosis of the alveoli and pulmonary capillaries. Recurrent pulmonary emboli, pulmonary infections, infective endocarditis, and systemic embolization are all potential complications.

CAUSES

The predominant cause of mitral stenosis is rheumatic fever. Approximately 40% of individuals with rheumatic heart disease have pure or predominant mitral stenosis. A congenital absence of one of the papillary muscles, resulting in a parachute deformity of the mitral valve, is rare. This deformity is observed almost exclusively in infants and young children. Other uncommon causes of mitral stenosis include malignant carcinoid syndrome, systemic lupus erythematosus, rheumatoid arthritis, thrombus formation, and the mucopolysaccharidoses of Hunter syndrome. In addition to rheumatic fever, the other risk factor for mitral stenosis is untreated streptococcal infections.

GENETIC CONSIDERATIONS

Cardiac congenital valve anomalies can produce mitral stenosis, and there have been reports of families with heritable disease affecting the mitral valve.

SEX AND LIFE SPAN CONSIDERATIONS

Approximately two-thirds of the patients with mitral stenosis are female. Two-thirds of all women with rheumatic mitral stenosis are younger than age 45 years.

HEALTH DISPARITIES AND SEXUAL/GENDER MINORITY HEALTH

Racial disparities exist with the number of procedures performed for structural heart disease. More interventions per population were performed on White persons as compared to Black and Hispanic persons. Black and Hispanic patients also had higher risk profiles than White patients, although there is no difference in complication and mortality rates. In general, Black and Hispanic patients have disparities with respect to access, provision of care, and availability of cardiovascular interventions as compared to White patients (Alkhouli et al., 2019). Sexual and gender minority status has no known effect on the risk for mitral stenosis.

GLOBAL HEALTH CONSIDERATIONS

Rheumatic fever and related mitral valve disease are more common in developing than in developed countries because of the rates of rheumatic fever.

ASSESSMENT

HISTORY. Because patients generally have a history of either rheumatic fever or a genetic predisposition to valvular heart disease, ask about specific dates and treatments related to the initial episode of rheumatic fever. Note the use of prophylactic antibiotics against the recurrence of rheumatic fever. Patients may have mitral stenosis for up to 10 to 15 years and remain asymptomatic. Once the valve orifice decreases to less than 2.5 cm, any physiological state that causes an increase in cardiac output (exercise, fever, anxiety, pain, pregnancy) or a decrease in diastolic filling time (tachycardias, atrial fibrillation) may cause the patient to have symptoms such as exercise intolerance, fatigue, or malaise. Approximately 15% of patients with mitral stenosis have a history of thromboembolic phenomena.

PHYSICAL EXAMINATION. The most common signs and symptoms are **excessive fatigue, malaise, decreased tolerance to exercise, dyspnea on exertion, orthopnea, paroxysmal nocturnal dyspnea,** and **dry cough.** As the valve orifice becomes increasingly narrowed, symptoms of right-sided heart failure may occur. Inspect the patient for neck vein distention and pitting peripheral edema. Pulmonary edema may also occur and lead to orthopnea, tachypnea, diaphoresis, pallor, cyanosis, and pink frothy sputum. Palpate the patient's abdomen for hepatomegaly and auscultate the patient's lungs for crackles.

You may note a normal apical pulse or an irregular rate associated with atrial fibrillation when the heart is auscultated. There are four principal findings: (1) a loud apical first heart sound (closure of the stenotic mitral valve); (2) an opening snap (the snapping of the stenotic mitral valve); (3) a rumbling, apical diastolic low-frequency murmur (blood flowing with difficulty and under increased pressure through the stenotic mitral valve); and (4) an increased pulmonic second sound associated with pulmonary hypertension.

PSYCHOSOCIAL. Often, patients have been living with the diagnosis for more than 10 years. The possibility of open heart surgery presents a crisis for patients who fear for their lives. In addition, their symptoms may interfere with activities of daily living. Assess the patient's degree of anxiety and ability to cope with the disease.

Diagnostic Highlights

Test	Normal Result	Abnormality With Condition	Explanation
Transesophageal echocardiogram	Normal mitral valve	Stenotic mitral valve, left atrial enlargement	Opening of mitral valve is narrow, which elevates left atrial pressure and leads to left atrial hypertrophy and right ventricular hypertrophy
Cardiac catheterization	Normal mitral valve	Stenotic mitral valve; elevation of left atrial pressure, elevation of pulmonary capillary pressures and venous pressures, left atrial enlargement	Same as above
Doppler echocardiography	Normal mitral valve	Stenotic mitral valve; left atrial enlargement	Same as above

Other Tests: Electrocardiogram may show atrial fibrillation, chest radiography, prothrombin time, activated partial thromboplastin time

PRIMARY NURSING DIAGNOSIS

DIAGNOSIS. Decreased activity tolerance related to pulmonary congestion and decreased blood supply to meet the demands of the body as evidenced by fatigue, shortness of breath, and/or tachycardia

OUTCOMES. Activity tolerance; Energy conservation; Coping; Knowledge: Disease process; Symptom severity; Symptom control; Knowledge: Medication; Knowledge: Treatment regimen

INTERVENTIONS. Energy management; Exercise promotion; Exercise therapy: Ambulation; Medication management; Teaching: Prescribed exercise; Teaching: medications

PLANNING AND IMPLEMENTATION

Collaborative

Once symptomatic, a patient usually progresses from mild to total disability in 5 to 10 years. This downhill course can be accelerated by conversion from a normal cardiac rhythm to atrial fibrillation or by pregnancy, bacterial endocarditis, or embolization.

Patients with mitral valve area less than 1.5 cm^2 may be considered for percutaneous balloon valvuloplasty if the pulmonary pressure is appropriate and they have reparable valves. The procedure is also used in young patients without calcification, symptomatic pregnant persons, and older individuals who are poor candidates for open heart surgery. While the techniques have not been perfected to date, percutaneous mitral valve replacement is under study for mitral valve repair and annuloplasty. These techniques are in early stage preclinical and clinical investigation. Definitive therapy for mitral stenosis is surgical replacement of the stenotic valve, particularly when the valve has marked stenosis with an orifice less than 1 cm^2. Postoperative anticoagulation is not required. Therefore, even patients with mild symptoms are candidates for surgery. Patients who have more severe, disabling symptoms are more likely to require valve replacement. Either a bioprosthetic or a mechanical valve is used by the surgeon, depending on the patient's condition and the surgeon's preference. (See **Coronary Heart Disease (Arteriosclerosis)** for collaborative and independent interventions for the patient who is undergoing open heart surgery.)

Pharmacologic Highlights

Medication or Drug Class	Dosage	Description	Rationale
Diuretics	Varies with drug	Thiazides; loop diuretics	Manage fluid overload and congestive symptoms
Calcium channel blockers	Varies with drug	Diltiazem	Depresses impulse formation and conduction
Coronary vasodilators	Varies with drug	Nitroglycerine, nitroprusside, captopril, enalapril, hydralazine	Decrease preload and afterload; decrease regurgitant blood flow; reduce ventricular size
Warfarin	Initially 10–15 mg, then 2–10 mg/day maintenance	Anticoagulant	Prevents thrombi from forming on the synthetic valve
Heparin or low-molecular-weight heparin	Initially 80 units/kg IV bolus, followed by an infusion of 18 units/kg; serial monitoring of activated partial thromboplastin to guide future doses	Anticoagulant	Prevents thrombi initially until warfarin therapy is well regulated

Other Drugs: Inotropic agents (dobutamine [Dobutrex], digoxin) are used to enhance the heart's pumping ability. Nitroglycerine may be used to decrease reload and increase coronary artery perfusion. If they are present, dysrhythmias are treated with antidysrhythmics, such as propranolol (Inderal), amriodarone, or quinidine. Antibiotics are used prophylactically against bacterial endocarditis and prior to interventional therapies and dental procedures (manipulation of gingival tissue, procedures on the apex of a tooth, or perforation of oral mucosa); common antibiotics are ampicillin, amoxicillin, clindamycin, and gentamicin.

Independent

Focus on early detection and management of symptoms and the prevention of complications. Interventions depend on the stage of the disease process. If the patient is newly diagnosed, patient teaching becomes important because of the patient's knowledge deficit. If the patient has severe symptoms that interfere with the ability to perform daily functions, strategies to maintain rest and conserve energy become important. If the patient is a surgical candidate, preoperative and postoperative management are the priority.

During periods of activity intolerance, encourage the patient to maintain bedrest and to allow full assistance with hygiene activities. Provide a bedside commode rather than a bedpan to decrease energy expenditure during voiding. Encourage the patient to keep the head of the bed elevated to at least 30 degrees. Support both arms with pillows to ease breathing and to augment chest excursion. Explore with the patient preferred diversionary activities, such as reading, watching television, needlework, listening to the radio, or quiet visitation with friends and family. Monitor the number of visitors to ensure that the patient is not overfatigued.

Encourage the patient and family to discuss their fears about the progress of the symptoms or the possibility of surgery. Answer questions honestly, provide accurate information, and allow the patient and significant others time to digest information before adding additional content. If the patient needs surgical intervention, evaluate the patient's home situation to determine if additional home assistance will be needed after discharge.

Evidence-Based Practice and Health Policy

Mayr, B., Vitanova, K., Burri, M., Lang, N., Goppel, G., Voss, B., Lange, R., & Cleuziou, J. (2020). Mitral valve repair in children below age 10 years: Trouble or success. *Annals of Thoracic Surgery, 110*, 2082–2087.

- The authors sought to determine the outcome of mitral valve repair as compared to mitral valve replacement in children under 10 years of age. They reviewed 40 cases of mitral valve repair for children with congenital mitral valve disease and 10 cases of children with acquired mitral valve disease. Median age at the time of surgery was 1.2 years for congenital disease and 1.9 years for acquired disease.
- In children with congenital mitral valve disease, operative mortality was 5%, and late mortality was 10%. No deaths occurred in children with acquired disease. In patients with congenital mitral valve disease, at 6 years of age, 12 children had required mitral valve replacement. The authors concluded that mitral valve repair is an effective treatment, but it often just delays the time to mitral valve replacement.

DOCUMENTATION GUIDELINES

- Physical findings of the cardiopulmonary and renal systems: Heart and breath sounds, vital signs, capillary refill, pulmonary artery pressure readings if applicable, intake and output, daily weights
- Presence of complications associated with mitral stenosis: Atrial fibrillation, pulmonary edema, heart failure
- Response to medications used to treat the symptoms and complications that are associated with mitral stenosis
- Tolerance to activity
- Response to surgical intervention: Wound healing, fluid balance, pulmonary artery pressures and cardiac output, urine output, chest tube drainage

DISCHARGE AND HOME HEALTHCARE GUIDELINES

Assess the patient's home environment to determine if additional assistance will be needed after discharge. Be sure the patient understands all medications, including the dosage, route, action, and adverse effects. Instruct the patient to report orthopnea, tachypnea, diaphoresis, frothy sputum, irregular pulse, and chest discomfort.

Mononucleosis, Infectious

DRG Category: 866
Mean LOS: 3.4 days
Description: MEDICAL: Viral Illness Without Major Complication or Comorbidity

The term *mononucleosis* refers to the presence of an abnormally high number of mononuclear leukocytes (white blood cells [WBCs]) in the body. Infectious mononucleosis (IM) results from a viral syndrome caused by the Epstein-Barr virus (EBV). The virus is introduced into the host by close contact with another individual who is shedding EBV in the oropharynx. The virus replicates in epithelial cells of the pharynx and salivary glands. A localized inflammatory response produces the pharyngeal exudate. The virus is then carried via the lymphatics to the lymph nodes. Local and generalized lymphadenopathy (swelling of the lymph nodes) develops.

IM is defined by its clinical presentation: fever, pharyngitis, and adenopathy. The EBV infects the B lymphocyte cells of the immune system; circulating B cells spread the infection throughout the liver, spleen, and peripheral lymph nodes. A rapid T-lymphocyte cell response determines whether the infection is controlled or leads (unusually) to uncontrolled B-cell response and, ultimately, to B-cell malignancies (lymphomas). Major complications are rare but may include splenic or liver rupture, aseptic meningitis or encephalitis, pericarditis, or hemolytic anemia. EBV has been linked to Burkitt lymphoma in Africa and to nasopharyngeal carcinoma, particularly in Asians. Mononucleosis can also lead to Guillain-Barré syndrome. Some experts have found an association between IM and the development of multiple sclerosis.

CAUSES

Infection with EBV, a herpes virus, is common throughout the world in humans and leads to IM. EBV is probably spread via the oropharyngeal or respiratory route. EBV is also transmitted by blood transfusion. Risk factors include being 15 to 24 years of age, having intimate contact with someone who has an active EBV infection, and sharing utensils with someone with an active EBV infection. An impaired immune system may increase the risk of serious illness with IM.

GENETIC CONSIDERATIONS

There is an X-linked disorder (X-linked lymphoproliferative disease) that confers high susceptibility to EBV infection, which is caused by mutations in the SH2 domain protein-1A (*SH2D1A*) gene. An autosomal recessive susceptibility to EBV infection has also been reported.

SEX AND LIFE SPAN CONSIDERATIONS

IM rarely occurs in children under age 5 years. EBV infection occurs early in life, however, among individuals of lower socioeconomic groups and in developing countries, which protects them from IM. IM is most often diagnosed in adolescents who come from higher socioeconomic groups and in college students. The peak incidence of IM is ages 16 to 18 years in boys and 14 to 16 years in girls. Approximately 12% to 30% of the total cases of IM occur among university students and military cadets. By adulthood, most individuals have had at least one infection with EBV. Older adults with EBV IM often have few signs and symptoms. There are no known gender considerations, but more than 90% of associated splenic ruptures are found in males.

HEALTH DISPARITIES AND SEXUAL/GENDER MINORITY HEALTH

In the United States, EBV seroprevalence for children and adolescents is approximately 70%, with Black and Hispanic groups having the highest rates. Children in low-income families have the highest rates (81%), and children in high-income families have the lowest rates (54%). In short, when children are exposed to EBV early in childhood, they are protected from having IM during adolescence. In data from the U.S. Armed Forces, the highest rates of mononucleosis occur in non-Hispanic White service members (Stahlman et al., 2019 [see Evidence-Based Practice and Health Policy]). Sexual and gender minority status has no known effect on the risk for IM.

GLOBAL HEALTH CONSIDERATIONS

Globally, a large proportion of the population are exposed to EBV during childhood and adolescence. Precise data on global prevalence of mononucleosis are unknown. In developing regions of the world, approximately 90% of children have had an EBV infection (but not IM) before age 5 years.

ASSESSMENT

HISTORY. Elicit a history of contacts with a person who has had IM. Consider that although children have a short incubation period of about 10 days, symptoms in adults may not appear until 1 to 2 months after exposure to the EBV. The patient with suspected IM typically reports a history of fever and fatigue for 1 week, followed by a sore throat (often described as the most painful the patient has ever experienced). Other symptoms include anorexia, painful swallowing, and swelling of the lymph nodes (adenopathy).

PHYSICAL EXAMINATION. Common symptoms include **fever, sore throat**, and **swollen lymph nodes**. Note the redness of the pharynx and observe for exudate. Observe for petechiae that may appear at the junction of the hard and soft palates (occurs in 25% of patients). Note any facial edema, particularly eyelid and periorbital edema. Facial edema is rarely encountered in other illnesses of young adults and is suggestive of IM. Significant tonsillar enlargement is common and may be exudative or nonexudative. Some patients have a maculopapular rash (discolored patches of skin mixed with elevated red pimples). Palpate for enlarged lymph nodes in the cervical and epitrochlear (around the elbow) areas. Significant adenopathy is almost always present, and its absence should make one doubt the diagnosis of IM. During an abdominal examination, palpate for an enlarged spleen (occurring in 50% of patients) and liver. Use care during the examination and perform a gentle examination.

PSYCHOSOCIAL. The patient with IM has a viral illness that may last up to 4 weeks. Because most cases occur in high school and college students, IM may prevent the student from performing academically at pre-illness levels. If the student falls behind in their studies, the student or parents may feel anxious or stressed. Assess the patient's ability to cope with the interference with school tasks. Determine if the patient has discussed the illness with their teachers or professors and if arrangements have been made to make up work or withdraw from school if needed. If the young adult is employed or in the military rather than in school, determine if the patient has told the employer or superior of their healthcare needs.

Diagnostic Highlights

Test	Normal Result	Abnormality With Condition	Explanation
Monospot	Negative	Presence of heterophil antibodies	Identifies 90% of adult cases with EBV; most common and specific test to confirm diagnosis; detects antibodies 2 to 9 wk after infection

Diagnostic Highlights (continued)

Test	Normal Result	Abnormality With Condition	Explanation
Complete blood count with differential	Red blood cells: 3.6–5.8 million/mcL; hemoglobin: 11.7– 17.3 g/dL; hematocrit: 36%–52%; white blood cells: 4,500–11,100/ mcL; platelets: 150,000–450,000/mcL; segmented neutrophils: 54%–62%; band neutrophils: 3%–5%; eosinophils: 1%–3%; basophils: < 1%; monocytes: 3%–7%; lymphocytes: 25%–33%	Lymphocytosis with characteristic atypical lymphocytes in peripheral blood	Determines extent of viral infection and immune dysfunction
EBV antibodies for EBV antigens	Negative	Viral capsid antigens (VCAs) present at onset 2–6 wk; Epstein-Barr virus (EBV) nuclear antigen appears 6–12 wk after onset; early antigen (EA) appears during acute phase and becomes undetectable at 3–6 mo	Identifies presence of EBV

PRIMARY NURSING DIAGNOSIS

DIAGNOSIS. Risk for infection as evidenced by fever, pharnygitis, adenopathy, anorexia, and myalgia

OUTCOMES. Infection severity; Immune status; Risk control: Infectious process; Symptom severity; Symptom control; Knowledge: Infection management; Knowledge: Disease process

INTERVENTIONS. Infection protection; Temperature regulation; Teaching: Disease process

PLANNING AND IMPLEMENTATION

Collaborative

Most patients require nothing more than supportive therapy, such as acetaminophen for fever and bedrest for fatigue. Pain relief is essential if the patient is to maintain fluid intake to prevent fluid volume deficit and dehydration.

To prevent upper airway obstruction from severe tonsillar enlargement, treatment with corticosteroids (prednisone 40 mg/day for 5–7 days) is sometimes indicated. If the patient is at risk for airway obstruction (a rare complication), endotracheal intubation may be necessary. Generally, patients with streptococcal pharyngotonsillitis are not treated with antibiotics because it represents colonization rather than infection. Ruptured spleen is an unusual but serious complication that causes sudden abdominal pain and is managed surgically by removal of the spleen.

Pharmacologic Highlights

No specific pharmacologic therapy treats mononucleosis; antiviral medications do not limit the EBV infection. Patients usually require analgesia with acetaminophen or even oral narcotics. Some patients may also be placed on corticosteroids or antibiotics for complications such as inflammation, allergy, or infection, although positive throat cultures for group A streptococci are not treated because they are considered colonization rather than infection.

Independent

Most patients do not require hospitalization for IM. Focus on supportive care and teaching. Encourage the patient to use anesthetic lozenges or warm saline gargles for pharyngitis. A soft diet such as milkshakes, sherbets, soups, and puddings provides additional liquid and nutritional supplements. Rest is critically important. Teach patients to avoid strenuous activities and contact sports until liver and spleen enlargement subsides. Make sure patients know to avoid intimate contact with others, including sharing utensils.

Evidence-Based Practice and Health Policy

Stahlman, S., Williams, V., & Ying, S. (2019). Infectious mononucleosis, active component, U.S. Armed Forces, 2002–2018. *Medical Surveillance Monthly Report, 26,* 28–33.

- The authors described the incidence rates, trends, and demographics of IM among active component service members over 16 years. During the period of surveillance, there were 23,780 cases of IM, with the highest rate among the youngest age groups.
- The highest incidence rate was in non-Hispanic White service members compared to other racial and ethnic groups. The rate of recruits was 3.4 times that of other enlisted personnel and 5.6 that of officers. The authors noted that while IM is not a serious illness, it can impact availability for military duty during the acute phase.

DOCUMENTATION GUIDELINES

- Physical findings of pharyngitis, lymphadenopathy, splenomegaly, fever, fatigue
- Reaction to activity and immobility, response to pain medications, understanding of limitations to reduce transmission
- Plan to deal with prolonged confinement and possible suspension of physical, social, and educational activities

DISCHARGE AND HOME HEALTHCARE GUIDELINES

Teach the patient to prevent splenic rupture by avoiding minor trauma, heavy lifting, overexertion, and contact sports for 1 to 2 months. Teach strategies to avoid constipation and straining because these problems cause increased pressure on the spleen. Suggest over-the-counter medications for comfort. Encourage the patient to rest during the acute illness and convalescence period. Note that prolonged fatigue is not uncommon. Encourage students to notify professors about the illness and to arrange for less demanding assignments during the recovery period. Recommend that the patient plan for a recovery period of several weeks before resuming regular activities, academics, or employment.

Instruct the patient to promptly report to the physician any abdominal and upper quadrant pain radiating to the shoulder. In addition, if the patient reports shortness of breath or inability to swallow, the patient should call 911 for emergency help because tracheostomy or intubation may become necessary.

Multiple Myeloma

DRG Category: 841
Mean LOS: 5.5 days
Description: MEDICAL: Lymphoma and Non-Acute Leukemia With Complication or Comorbidity

Multiple myeloma, also known as plasma cell myeloma, malignant plasmacytoma, and myelo-matosis, is a type of cancer formed by malignant plasma cells (a mature, active B lymphocyte normally found in the bone marrow). It is the most common primary neoplasm of the skeletal system and accounts for 10% of all hematological cancers. The American Cancer Society estimates that in 2021, 34,920 new cases will be diagnosed and 12,410 people will die from multiple myeloma.

When a B lymphocyte is stimulated by a T cell, it develops into a mature, antibody-producing factory called a *plasma cell*. Multiple myeloma results from a transformed plasma cell that multiplies and produces antibody unceasingly without stimulation. When plasma cells grow out of control, they generate tumors that infiltrate the bone marrow and other sites. Although multiple myeloma could be considered a lymphoma, it is generally classified differently and discussed separately because it presents a different profile of onset, symptoms, treatment, and prognosis.

The disease infiltrates bone and produces osteolytic lesions throughout the skeleton, destroying bones. In later stages, multiple myeloma infiltrates the body organs and destroys them as well. About 3 to 20 years of plasma cell growth may pass before symptoms become apparent. When patients do report symptoms, the disease is well advanced. Survival rates depend on the stage of initial diagnosis (Table 1). Stage I patients have a median survival rate of 66 months. Stage II patients have a median survival rate of 42 months; stage III patients have a median survival time of 29 months.

• TABLE 1 Revised Staging System for Multiple Myeloma (International Myeloma Working Group, American Society of Clinical Oncology, 2015)

STAGE	EXTENT OF DISEASE
I	Beta-2 microglobulin ≤ 3.5 g/dL and albumin ≥ 3.5 g.dL
	Standard risk for chromosomal abnormalities (cytogenics; CA)
	Normal lactate dehydrogenase (LDH) levels
II	Stage II comprises patients who do not meet criteria for stage I or stage III
III	Beta-2 microglobulin ≥ 5.5 g/dL, and either:
	High risk for CA and/or high LDH

Multiple myeloma causes a number of complications, including infections such as pneumonia. Other complications are pyelonephritis, renal calculi and renal failure, hematological imbalance and gastrointestinal or nasal bleeding, hypercalcemia, hyperuricemia, dehydration, pathological fractures, infection, and sepsis.

CAUSES

The cause is unknown, but several associated factors likely have a role in its etiology. Exposure to radiation; genetic factors; occupational exposure to petroleum products, herbicides, and insecticides; other plasma cell diseases; and chronic antigen stimulation may predispose an individual to the development of the disease. Some patients with multiple myeloma have a history of chronic infections. Other risk factors include frequent viral infections, an increase in body mass index, and exposure to hair dyes over a 20-year period.

GENETIC CONSIDERATIONS

In rare cases, multiple myeloma can affect more than one family member, suggesting a genetic contribution. Studies to identify specific risk genes have not been conclusive, but the human interferon regulatory factor-4 (*IRF4*) gene can function as an oncogene during carcinogenesis and is often aberrantly activated in multiple myeloma.

SEX AND LIFE SPAN CONSIDERATIONS

Multiple myeloma is primarily a disease of late middle age to the older years. The disease may have been developing slowly for many years before diagnosis, however. The average age at diagnosis is 68 years for men and 70 years for women, and it is rare prior to age 40 years; more men than women are affected. Longer survival rates are associated with being female, having a high income and high educational level, living in a rural area, having insurance, and being treated at a cancer center.

HEALTH DISPARITIES AND SEXUAL/GENDER MINORITY HEALTH

For unknown reasons, rates of multiple myeloma for Black persons are twice those for White and Hispanic persons. In a large epidemiology study, the investigators found that Hispanic persons have the youngest age of diagnosis and the worst survival rates as compared to people of other groups. Asian persons have the best overall survival rates. Higher incidence of multiple myeloma occurs in small cities and rural areas as compared to urban areas. Experts suggest this difference may occur because of increased density of agricultural facilities and exposure to pesticides in rural areas. Sexual and gender minority status has no known effect on the risk for multiple myeloma. However, gender and sexual minority persons are a vulnerable group because people with low income, long travel distances to cancer screening sites, or who lack health insurance or paid medical leave are less likely to be treated according to cancer care guidelines (National Institutes of Health, 2021).

GLOBAL HEALTH CONSIDERATIONS

The global incidence of multiple myeloma is 1 to 5 per 100,000 individuals per year. The incidence is eight times higher in developed than in developing regions. Lowest incidence occurs in Asian, Southwest Asian, and South Pacific countries. Highest incidence occurs in Australia, New Zealand, the United States, and Europe.

ASSESSMENT

HISTORY. Establish a history of bone-related pain, particularly the long bones and in the back. Determine if the patient has experienced constant back pain that intensifies with exercise, other aching bone pain, or arthritic-type joint pain. Ask if the patient has experienced any numbness, prickling, or tingling of the extremities (peripheral paresthesia); confusion; fatigue; or weakness. Some patients report bleeding, which is likely due to a low platelet count. Determine if the patient has experienced weight loss, nausea, vomiting, polyuria, or polydipsia. Determine if the patient has had any recent bone fractures. Ask if the patient has been exposed to radiation on the job or has undergone radiation therapy. Establish a history of body height reduction; vertebral collapse may cause a reduction in height of up to 5 inches or more. Find out if the patient has relatives who have been diagnosed with multiple myeloma.

PHYSICAL EXAMINATION. Common symptoms include **bone pain and tenderness**, **pathological fractures**, **anemia**, **fatigue and weakness**, and **infections**. Examine for signs of pathological compression fractures of the vertebral column or long bones. Inspect for joint swelling. Note any joint, long bone, or flat bone tenderness. Note cranial nerve palsies, which may be caused by tumor occlusion of vascular flow. Radiculopathies develop from nerve root compression where there is bone infiltration. Carpal tunnel syndrome is common. In advanced cases, noticeable thoracic deformities may be observable. Thrombocytopenia may lead to purpura around the eyes and on other skin sites. Examine the body for soft tissue masses, which may occur on the ear, anywhere on the skin, within organs, on the tongue, and in the rectum. With patients already on chemotherapy for multiple myeloma, note any signs of infection, such as fever and malaise.

PSYCHOSOCIAL. The psychosocial needs of the patient with multiple myeloma may be complex. The patient faces coping with a chronic, painful, and potentially fatal disease that is treated with potentially painful and uncomfortable regimens. Be sensitive to the enormous psychological strain placed on the patient. Consider the effects of the disease on the patient's job status, personal relationships, financial resources, and body image. Assess the patient's support network.

Diagnostic Highlights

Test	Normal Result	Abnormality With Condition	Explanation
Serum protein electrophoresis; urine protein electrophoresis; assessment for monoclonal protein (densitometer tracing and nephelometric quantitation; confirmation by immunofixation)	Presence of normal immunoglobulins: IgM, IgG, IgE, IgD, IgA	Presence of abnormally low levels of immunoglobulins; presence of abnormal immunoglobulins: monoclonal immunoglobulin (also known as M protein, M spike, paraprotein); presence of abnormal protein, β_2-microglobin	Identifies abnormal proteins (M proteins) produced by cancerous plasma cells as compared with product of normal plasma cells
Bone marrow aspiration; bone marrow biopsy	Presence of normal bone marrow cells	Over 10%–30% of cells in bone marrow sample are plasma cells; biopsy indicates plasma cell tumor	In aspiration, a thin needle is used to draw a small amount of liquid bone marrow; in biopsy, a small cylinder of bone and marrow (about 1/2 in. long) is removed. Site of both samples is usually at back of the hipbone
Serum beta-2 microglobulin (B2M)	0.6–2.4 mg/L	Stage 1: ≤ 3.5 g/dL; stage 3: ≥ 5.5 g/dL	Component of the major histocompatibility complex class I molecule that can aggregate into amyloid fibers that are present in the body; used in staging to determine the level of disease present
Bone x-rays and computed tomography scan	Normal bone size and structure	Bone destruction and bone lesions	Identifies areas of bone destruction and effects of bone-absorbing hormones

Other Tests: Complete blood cell count, serum and ionized calcium, magnetic resonance imaging, serum electrolytes, blood urea nitrogen, serum creatinine, creatinine clearance, serum-free light chain assay protein, albumin, lactate dehydrogenase, metaphase cytogenetics, and fluorescent in situ hybridization (FISH)

PRIMARY NURSING DIAGNOSIS

DIAGNOSIS. Acute and chronic pain related to bone fragility and injury, vertebral collapse, joint swelling, and/or effects of radiation therapy or chemotherapy as evidenced by self-reports of pain, facial grimacing, and/or protective behavior

OUTCOMES. Comfort status; Knowledge: Pain management; Pain level; Pain control; Symptom severity; Knowledge: Medication; Medication response

INTERVENTIONS. Pain management: Acute; Analgesic administration; Medication management; Medication administration; Teaching: Prescribed medication

PLANNING AND IMPLEMENTATION

Collaborative

Treatment depends on staging, treatment decisions are complex, and new drug therapies continue to be available. Clinicians are most interested in the amount of tumor mass, hemoglobin level, calcium level, serum protein levels, and number of lytic bone lesions. Treatment depends on disease staging and generally consists of chemotherapy, radiation, prednisone, and as much ambulation as the patient can tolerate. Autologous bone marrow or peripheral blood stem cell transplantation may be used to allow for more intense treatment with drugs such as melphalan; autologous bone marrow transplant allows the physician to administer what would otherwise be a lethal dose of radiation and chemotherapy.

Severe bone pain may be a problem, and pain management may be difficult; NSAIDs are the best agents for bone pain but are contraindicated with renal dysfunction, which often accompanies multiple myeloma. Low-dose radiation therapy is useful for palliation of bone pain. Radiation therapy may be used for small, local bone lesions or to relieve the pressure caused by compression of nerve roots. Surgical treatments in multiple myeloma are limited to any orthopedic fixation procedures that may need to be done in response to pathological bone fractures. Laminectomy addresses vertebral compression.

Multiple myeloma often leads to bone demineralization and significant amounts of calcium lost into the blood and urine. The patient with multiple myeloma is thus at risk for developing renal calculi, nephrocalcinosis, and renal failure from hypercalcemia. To decrease serum calcium levels that lead to hypercalcemia, the patient is given adequate fluids, diuretics, corticosteroids, or bisphosphonates to decrease demineralization. Plasmapheresis may be used for patients with extremely high immunoglobulin levels that are causing damage to kidneys or patients who have symptoms of hyperviscosity syndrome. Hyperviscosity syndrome results when the plasma proteins (immunoglobulin) contribute more to plasma viscosity than do blood cells.

Pharmacologic Highlights

Medication or Drug Class	Dosage	Description	Rationale
Chemotherapy after transplantation	Varies with drug	Lenalidomide, ixazomib, bortezomib	Suppresses plasma cell growth and controls pain
Biphosphonates	Varies with drug	Pamidronate, zoledronic acid, clodronate	Should be considered for all patients to reduce bone loss
Opioids and NSAIDs	Varies with drug	Morphine sulfate, Demerol, ibuprofen, aspirin	Manage severe bone pain

Other Drugs: Corticosteroids (high-dose dexamethasone), thalidomide, monoclonal antibodies, interferon alfa, erythropoietin, other chemotherapeutic agents (cyclophosphamide, melphalan, daratumumab)

Independent

Encourage the patient to drink 3,000 to 4,000 mL of fluids daily. Provide comfort measures for pain, such as repositioning and relaxation techniques. Always accompany patients as they ambulate and make sure they have a walker or other supportive aid to prevent falls. Provide corsets or braces as appropriate to assist in weight-bearing and to increase bone strength. Provide encouragement and allow the patient to set the pace. If the patient is bedridden, change the patient's position every 2 hours and provide passive range-of-motion exercise. Encourage deep-breathing exercises and promote active exercise when tolerable.

Make sure the patient understands the disease process, diagnostic tests, treatment options, and prognosis as previously explained by the physician. Teach the patient what to expect from the treatment and diagnostic tests, including painful procedures such as bone marrow aspiration and biopsy. Explain to the patient what to expect in the event of surgery, emphasizing the need for deep-breathing and changing position every 2 hours after surgery. Emphasize the need to avoid infection by wearing sufficiently warm clothing and by avoiding crowds and people with infections because chemotherapy causes a sensitivity to cold and diminishes the body's natural resistance to infection. Take precautions to prevent infection. Use sterile technique for all procedures and limit the patient's exposure to visitors, staff, and other patients with infections. Because patients on chemotherapy may develop cold sensitivity, make sure the patient is warm enough.

The patient may experience less anxiety if allowed as much control as possible over the daily schedule. Explaining procedures and keeping the patient informed about the treatment plan and condition may also decrease anxiety. If the patient enters the final phases of multiple myeloma, provide emotional support. Refer the patient and family to the hospice staff or the hospital chaplain. Encourage the patient and family to verbalize their feelings about impending death. Allow for the time needed to adjust, while helping the patient and family begin the grieving process. Assist in the identification of tasks to be completed before death, such as making a will, seeing specific relatives and friends, and attending an approaching wedding, birthday, or anniversary celebration.

Urge the patient to verbalize specific funeral requests to family members. If appropriate, refer the patient and family to the American Cancer Society or another local support group.

Evidence-Based Practice and Health Policy

Cho, Y., & Yoo, Y. (2020). Factors influencing supportive care needs of multiple myeloma patients treated with chemotherapy. *Supportive Care in Cancer, 28,* 1783–1791.

- The authors developed a descriptive survey to identify factors influencing supportive care needs of patients with multiple myeloma treated with chemotherapy. They enrolled patients with multiple myeloma ($N = 141$) who were treated as inpatients or outpatients at one hospital in Korea.
- The mean score of supportive care needs of patients with multiple myeloma was 1.51 out of 4 points. Of supportive care needs, information on future disease outcomes scored the highest, with a mean score of 2.12, followed by easy and candid explanation by healthcare staff (2.11), and information on foods that are healthy for cancer patients (2.02). Anxiety and depression were identified as factors influencing supportive care needs of patients with multiple myeloma.

DOCUMENTATION GUIDELINES

- Response to chemotherapy or radiation treatments
- Physical findings: Fractures; joint swelling; body height; intake and output; level of pain; response to pain medications; breathing patterns; gastrointestinal bleeding
- Presence of complications: Pneumonia, renal calculi, renal failure, hyperuricemia, ineffective patient or family coping
- Laboratory results: Presence or absence of hypercalcemia; complete blood count; presence of Bence-Jones protein; bone marrow aspirations; globulin levels

DISCHARGE AND HOME HEALTHCARE GUIDELINES

If the patient receives outpatient chemotherapy or radiation, teach the patient the purpose, duration, and potential complications of those treatments. Be sure the patient understands any prescribed pain medication, including dosage, route, action, and side effects. Urge the patient to maintain a realistic but positive attitude; the return to an independent lifestyle is possible with the efforts of a rehabilitation team and the patient's cooperation. Provide referrals to palliative care if appropriate.

Multiple Organ Dysfunction Syndrome

DRG Category:	205
Mean LOS:	5.5 days
Description:	MEDICAL: Other Respiratory System Diagnoses With Major Complication or Comorbidity (If the patient develops this syndrome during the hospital stay, the reason for admission will determine the DRG assigned.)

Multiple organ dysfunction syndrome (MODS, formerly known as multiple system organ failure) occurs when altered organ function in an acutely ill patient is present to the extent that homeostasis can no longer be maintained without intervention. MODS was formerly known as multiple system organ failure. The usual sequence of MODS depends somewhat on its cause but often begins with pulmonary failure 2 to 3 days after surgery, followed, in order, by hepatic failure, stress-induced gastrointestinal (GI) bleeding, and renal failure. Other patients begin the organ system cascade with intra-abdominal sepsis, extensive blood loss, pancreatitis, or vascular emergencies. Acute lung injury follows shortly, and the progression might develop over hours rather than 2 to 3 days.

MODS was first associated with traumatic injuries in the late 1960s and has subsequently been associated with infection and decreased perfusion to any part of the body. Primary MODS, the result of a direct injury or insult to the organ itself, is initiated by a specific precipitating event, such as a pulmonary contusion. The injury or insult causes an inflammatory response within that organ system, and dysfunction develops.

Secondary MODS develops as the result of a systemic response to infection or inflammation. Systemic inflammatory response syndrome (SIRS) is an overwhelming response of the normal inflammatory system, producing systemic effects instead of the localized response normally seen. For SIRS to be present, the patient has two or more of the following:

• Temperature > 100.4°F (38.0°C) or < 97°F (36.0°C)
• Heart rate > 90 beats/min
• Respiratory rate > 20 breaths/min or arterial carbon dioxide tension < 32 mm Hg
• White blood cell (WBC) count > 12,000/mcL or < 4,000/mcL or including more than 10% bands

As SIRS progresses to sepsis, septic shock, and MODS, the mortality rate increases from approximately 20% to 75%. The inflammatory response is produced by the activation of a series of mediators and results in alterations in blood (selective vasodilation and vasoconstriction), an increase in vascular permeability, WBC activation, and activation of the coagulation cascade. Mortality rates are high with MODS, and the more organ systems that fail, the higher is the mortality. For example, mortality with two-organ failure is 45% to 55%, higher than 80% with three-organ failure, and approaches 100% if the failure of three or more organs persists longer than several days. Complications include shock, cardiac dysrhythmias, cardiac arrest, and death.

CAUSES

The inflammatory response can be triggered by any event, but it is most often associated with a bacterial infection and sepsis. Experts describe sepsis as a process of malignant intravascular inflammation that leads to a poorly regulated immune response and the release of inflammatory compounds. The events most often associated with the development of SIRS and MODS are shock, trauma, burns, aspiration, venomous snakebites, cardiac arrest, thromboemboli, myocardial infarction, operative procedures, vascular injury, infection, pancreatitis, and disseminated intravascular coagulation. Risk factors include cigarette smoking, stroke, pulmonary infection, immune suppression, chronic illnesses, severe trauma, cancer, alcohol and drug abuse and dependence, and malnutrition.

GENETIC CONSIDERATIONS

Heritable defects in the production of cytokines such as interleukin-6 have been suggested in the etiology of MODS. Animal studies have identified an inherited form of complement deficiency, but clear genetic contributions to MODS have not been elucidated.

SEX AND LIFE SPAN CONSIDERATIONS

Young adults, males twice as often as females, are at particular risk for MODS because they are the primary trauma population. Increased risk in the trauma patient is related to more prolonged hypotension, extensive amounts of tissue damage, and higher infection and sepsis rates. Patients over age 65 years who experience MODS have higher rates of mortality. The normal aging process causes dysfunction of organ systems and, in some patients, immunosuppression. With a significant injury or insult, therefore, it is much easier for organ systems in the older adult to fail. Teenagers, young adults, and adults of all ages who abuse alcohol and who are malnourished are also at risk because of the role of alcohol in immunosuppression.

HEALTH DISPARITIES AND SEXUAL/GENDER MINORITY HEALTH

Ethnicity, race, and sexual/gender minority status have no known effect on the risk for MODS.

GLOBAL HEALTH CONSIDERATIONS

The global prevalence of MODS is unknown, but it frequently results from road traffic injuries and other catastrophic events that can lead to sepsis. The World Health Organization (WHO) estimated in 2021 that more than 1.35 million people die each year from traffic injuries, which is the leading cause of death around the globe for children and young people ages 5 to 29 years of age. Ninety-three percent of those killed in traffic injuries live in low- and middle-income countries. Additionally, the WHO estimated that up to 50 million people experience nonfatal traffic injuries that may lead to infection, MODS, and long-term disability.

ASSESSMENT

HISTORY. The patient with MODS has a history of infection, tissue injury, or a perfusion deficit to an organ or body part. Often, this injury or insult is not life-threatening but exposes the person to bacterial contamination. Question the patient (or, if the patient is too ill, the family) to identify the events in the initial insult and any history of preexisting organ dysfunction, such as chronic lung disease, congestive heart failure, and diabetes mellitus. Ask if the patient has had recent surgery. Elicit a complete medication history and the patient's compliance with medications and ask if the patient has experienced recent weight loss. Determine the patient's dietary patterns to assess the patient's nutritional status. Take a history of the patient's use of cigarettes, alcohol, and other drugs of abuse.

PHYSICAL EXAMINATION. The physical examination of the patient with MODS varies depending on the organ systems involved and the severity of their dysfunction (Table 1). Symptoms vary widely but may include **fever, chills, fatigue, muscle weakness, shortness of breath,** and **mental status changes.** The patient will likely appear acutely ill. Expect the patient to develop signs of pulmonary failure first and then hepatic failure and GI bleeding. Renal failure follows. Note that failures of the central nervous system and the cardiovascular system are late signs of MODS.

• TABLE 1 Organ System Involvement in MODS

ORGAN SYSTEM	SYMPTOMS OF DYSFUNCTION
Central nervous system	Decreased level of consciousness, confusion, lethargy
Cardiovascular system	Hyperdynamic: tachycardic, normotensive, skin warm and flushed, full bounding pulses
	Hypodynamic: tachycardic; hypotensive; skin cool and mottled; weak, thready pulses
Pulmonary system	Crackles or rales, tachypnea
	Cyanosis of the nailbeds and mucous membranes, dyspnea
GI system	Diminished or absent bowel sounds, abdominal distention, intolerance of tube feedings, upper or lower gastrointestinal bleeding, diarrhea
Hepatic system	Jaundice, petechiae, increased bruising
Renal system	Polyuria, oliguria, or anuria
Coagulation system	Oozing or bleeding from IV sites or invasive line sites; bruising and petechiae; bleeding into body parts or cavities; cool, pale to mottled extremities; necrotic digits
General appearance	Weight loss and muscle wasting; temperature > 100.4°F (38.0°C) or < 97°F (36.0°C)

PSYCHOSOCIAL. The patient with MODS may be fully conscious, partially conscious, or unconscious. If patients are oriented, they are likely to be very anxious and fatigued and also confused, lethargic, or comatose. Assess the patient's ability to cope with a prolonged life-threatening illness and the changes in roles that a severe illness brings. The patient and family will likely experience fear because of a real threat to the patient's life.

Diagnostic Highlights

General Comments: Diagnostic data are collected to establish the dysfunction of each of the body's systems (Table 2).

Test	Normal Result	Abnormality With Condition	Explanation
Complete blood count	Red blood cells (RBCs): 3.6–5.8 million/mcL; hemoglobin (Hgb): 11.7–17.3 g/dL; hematocrit (Hct): 36%–52%; WBCs: 4,500–11,100/mcL; platelets: 150,000–450,000/mcL; Differential: neutrophils: 2.7–6.5/mcL (40%–75%); lymphocytes: 2.5–3.7/mcL (12%–44%); monocytes: 0.2–0.4/mcL (4%–9%); eosinophils: 0.05–0.5/mcL (0%–5.5%); basophils: 0–0.1/mcL (0%–1%)	Varies with condition: > 12,000 mm³ or < 4,000 mm³ or > 10% band cells (immature cells); RBCs, Hgb, Hct, blood cells, decreased	Underlying disorder may cause alterations in blood cell counts; SIRS leads to production of inflammatory mediators and alterations in WBC counts; hematological failure may lead to suppression of cell production

Diagnostic Highlights (continued)

Test	Normal Result	Abnormality With Condition	Explanation
Partial thromboplastin time (activated; APTT)	Varies by laboratory; generally 25–35 sec	Prolonged; may be prolonged > 80 sec	May be prolonged if liver failure and hematological failure occurs
Prothrombin time (PT)	Varies by laboratory; generally 10–13 sec	Prolonged > 15 sec	May be prolonged if liver failure occurs

Other Tests: Electrocardiogram, multiple cultures and sensitivities (blood, wound, urine, sputum, catheters), arterial blood gases, pulmonary artery pressure monitoring, cardiac output and index, chest x-ray, ultrasonography, computed tomography, serum lactate levels, ultrasonography, computed tomography, derived oxygen variables (oxygen delivery, oxygen consumption), electrolytes, glucose

• **TABLE 2** Definitions of Organ Failure

ORGAN	DEFINITION OF FAILURE	DIAGNOSTIC FINDINGS
Lungs	Need for ventilator-assisted breathing to treat hypoxemia for 5 days in the postoperative period or until death; acute respiratory distress syndrome requiring positive end expiratory pressure with mechanical ventilation	Decreased Pao_2 and Sao_2 Decreased $Paco_2$ Increased shunt fraction Decreased vital capacity and functional residual capacity Decreased static compliance
Kidneys	Serum creatinine concentration > 2 mg/dL; for patients with preexisting renal disease, doubling of admission serum creatinine level; oliguria	Increased serum creatinine Urine specific gravity < 1.012 Urine sodium > 40 mEq/L
Liver	Serum bilirubin concentration > 2 mg/dL with elevation of either serum aspartate aminotransferase (AST) concentration or lactic dehydrogenase (LDH) concentration above twice normal	Increased bilirubin, AST, LDH
Gastrointestinal (GI) tract	Requirement of two units of blood replacement within 24 hr for presumed stress bleeding or endoscopic confirmation of upper GI bleeding from acute GI ulcers	Dropping Hgb and Hct Visualization of ulcers during surgery or endoscopy

PRIMARY NURSING DIAGNOSIS

DIAGNOSIS. Risk for infection as evidenced by hypothermia/hyperthermia, hypodynamic/hyperdynamic circulation, respiratory distress, and/or mental status changes

OUTCOMES. Infection severity; Immune status; Knowledge: Infection management; Risk control; Risk detection; Fluid balance; Symptom severity; Symptom control

INTERVENTIONS. Infection control; Infection protection; Fluid/electrolyte management; Medication management; Medication administration; Temperature regulation

░ PLANNING AND IMPLEMENTATION

Collaborative

Management of the patient with MODS begins with the recognition of those patients who are at an increased risk for the syndrome. Care must be taken to prevent infection and maintain adequate tissue oxygenation to all body parts. Despite improvement in medical therapies, the mortality rate of MODS remains high.

Treatment of the patient with MODS can be divided into three main areas: anti-infectives, maintenance of tissue perfusion and oxygenation, and maintenance of organ function. Anti-infective therapy is guided by culture and sensitivity reports. Any potential source of infection should be investigated and eliminated. Antifungal and antiviral agents are used primarily with immunocompromised patients, who are especially susceptible to fungal and viral infections. Oral chlorhexidine gluconate may be used for oropharyngeal decontamination to prevent ventilator-associated pneumonia.

Maintaining and monitoring tissue perfusion and oxygenation are crucial to the survival of the patient with MODS. Measurement of oxygen delivery and consumption is necessary to guide fluid replacement therapy and inotropic support of cardiac function. To maximize all components of oxygen delivery (particularly cardiac index, Hgb, and oxygen saturation), the physician maintains the Hct within the normal range or even at a supranormal level with blood transfusions. Mechanical ventilation with positive end expiratory pressure and modes such as pressure-control ventilation and inverse I:E (inspiration-to-expiration) ratio ventilation are used to maintain adequate oxygenation and oxygen delivery. The success of maintaining oxygen delivery is evaluated by following the trend of oxygen consumption. Metabolic demands dramatically increase in MODS. When oxygen delivery cannot meet the body's metabolic demands, these demands may be decreased with sedation, pharmacologic paralysis, and temperature control. The physician will likely follow lactate levels to determine whether the metabolic demands are being met. Generally, blood glucose is kept between 140 mg/dL and 180 mg/dL, which is supported by current outcomes research.

Pharmacologic Highlights

Medication or Drug Class	Dosage	Description	Rationale
Vasopressor therapy	Varies with drug	Dopamine, epinephrine, norepinephrine, phenylephrine, vasopressin	Maintains circulation and tissue perfusion after volume resuscitation has been accomplished
Anti-infective therapy; antifungal agents; antiviral agents	Varies with drug	Therapy focuses on dysfunctional system and culture results; cefotaxime, ceftriaxone, cefuroxime, ticarcillin-clavulanate, piperacillin-tazobactam, imipenem-cilastatin, clindamycin, metronidazole	Prevents and controls infection
H_2 receptor antagonist	Varies with drug	Cimetidine (Tagamet), famotidine (Pepcid), nizatidine (Axid)	Blocks gastric secretion and maintains the pH of gastric contents above 4

Other Drugs: Recombinant human-activated protein C was withdrawn from the market in 2011 for use in sepsis and MODS; corticosteroids (controversial)

Independent

Any potential source of infection should be eliminated if possible. Change the dressing on all invasive line sites and surgical wounds according to protocol to keep the area free of infection and to monitor for early signs of infection. Maintain aseptic technique with all dressing changes and manipulation of IV lines. Institute measures to prevent aspiration when patients are placed on enteral feedings. Keep the head of the bed elevated and check for residual volume and tube placement every 4 hours.

To limit the patient's oxygen expenditure, provide frequent rest periods and create a quiet environment whenever possible. Schedule procedures and nursing care interventions so that the patient has periods of uninterrupted rest. Manage situations of increased metabolic demand—such as fever, agitation, alcohol withdrawal, and pain—promptly so that the patient conserves energy and limits oxygen consumption.

Monitor the patient's environment for sensory overload. Provide purposeful, planned stimuli and keep extraneous, constant noises to a minimum. Provide for planned, uninterrupted rest periods to avoid sleep deprivation. Monitor bony prominences and areas of high risk for skin breakdown. Note that MODS is one of the most critical illnesses that a patient can develop. Although the patient might be well sedated and unresponsive, the family or significant others are generally very anxious, upset, and frightened that the patient might not survive.

These fears are realistic, particularly if multiple organs are involved. Provide the significant others with accurate information about the patient's course and prospects for recovery. Encourage the legal representative to participate in decisions about extraordinary measures to keep the patient alive if the patient cannot speak. Determine if the patient has a living will or has discussed a desire to be kept alive by technology during a potentially terminal illness. If the decision is to terminate life support, work with the significant others to provide a dignified death for the patient in an environment that allows the family to participate and grieve appropriately. Provide referrals to the chaplain, clinical nurse specialist, or grief counselor as needed.

Evidence-Based Practice and Health Policy

Keith, P., Wells, A., Hodges, J., Fast, S., Adams, A., & Scott, L. (2020). The therapeutic efficacy of adjunct therapeutic plasma exchange for septic shock with multiple organ failure: A single-center experience. *Critical Care*. Advance online publication. https://doi.org/10.1186/s13054-020-03241-6

• Sepsis remains a common condition with high mortality when multiple organ failure develops. Therapeutic plasma exchange (TPE), also known as plasmapheresis, removes and replaces blood plasma. In the setting of multiple organ failure, TPA is promising but inconclusive because of the disruption that occurs at the endovascular level. The authors performed a retrospective review of medical records to evaluate the outcomes of adult patients with catecholamine-resistant septic shock and multiple organ failure.

• Patients who received TPE ($n = 40$) were identified and compared to patients who received standard care alone ($n = 40$). The authors found that hemodynamics, organ dysfunction, and fluid balance all improved with TPE, while lengths of stay were increased in survivors who received TPE. They concluded that patients receiving TPE had improved 28-day survival compared to patients receiving standard care alone, even though length of stay was longer.

DOCUMENTATION GUIDELINES

• Physical assessment findings:
  Neurological: Mental status response to stimuli; if pharmacologically paralyzed, then peripheral nerve stimulation testing
  Pulmonary: Respiratory rate, auscultation findings, amount of ventilatory support, oxygen saturation by pulse oximetry
  Hemodynamics: Cardiac output/index, right and left ventricular measures of preload and afterload; oxygen delivery; oxygen consumption, temperature
  Renal function: Fluid intake and urine output
  Hepatic function: Color of skin and sclera, presence of petechiae, bruising, oozing, or frank bleeding
• Response to acute, life-threatening illness: Anxiety level, coping

DISCHARGE AND HOME HEALTHCARE GUIDELINES

Although no specific adaptive structural changes need to be made, assess the patient's individual needs near the time of discharge. Because organ dysfunction or failure is individualized, home-care preparation should be based on meeting the individual's needs. Be sure the patient understands all medications prescribed, including dosage, route, action, and side effects. Make sure the patient understands all follow-up appointments and consultations.

Describe the importance of avoiding fatigue and of taking frequent rests. Teach the patient to eat small, frequent meals to maintain adequate nutrition. Teach the patient any needed postoperative care: incision care, signs and symptoms of infection, pain management, activity restrictions. Also teach the patient when to report signs and symptoms of infection to the primary healthcare provider.

Multiple Sclerosis

DRG Category:	58
Mean LOS:	7.2 days
Description:	MEDICAL: Multiple Sclerosis and Cerebellar Ataxia With Major Complication or Comorbidity

Multiple sclerosis (MS) is a chronic, progressive, degenerative, immune-mediated inflammatory disease that affects the myelin sheath of the white matter of the brain and spinal cord. Each year in the United States, 25,000 people are newly diagnosed with MS, and approximately 400,000 people are living with the disease. It is the most common debilitating disease of young adults. The disease affects quality rather than duration of life. In MS, nerve impulses are conducted between the brain and the spinal cord along neurons protected by the myelin sheath, which is a highly conductive fatty material. When plaques form on the myelin sheath, causing inflammation and eventual demyelination, nerve transmission becomes erratic. Areas commonly involved are the optic nerves, cerebrum, and cervical spinal cord. MS is the most common demyelinating disorder in the United States and Europe.

There are four forms of MS that have varying trajectories. **Clinically isolated syndrome** (CIS) occurs with a first episode of symptoms that lasts for at least 24 hours. The episode is characteristic of MS but does not meet the criteria for diagnosis. People who have brain findings on magnetic resonance imaging may progress to MS. **Relapsing-remitting MS** (RRMS) is the most common disease course with clearly defined attacks of increasing neurological symptoms followed by complete recovery or remission. Following a relapse, new symptoms may disappear, or they may remain and disability may increase. Each person has a unique trajectory. Approximately 85% of people with MS have this course of disease when initially diagnosed. **Secondary progressive MS** (SPMS) initially follows a relapsing-remitting course but then transitions to a progressive course with worsening neurological function and increasing disability. **Primary progressive MS** (PPMS) follows a course of worsening neurological function and accumulating disability from the onset of symptoms. Approximately 15% of people with MS are diagnosed with PPMS. Complications include muscle spasms, leg paralysis and spasticity, urinary tract infections, bladder dysfunction, sexual dysfunction, depression, optic neuritis, myelitis, and seizure disorder.

CAUSES

The cause of MS is unknown. Some evidence suggests that an infective agent causes a predisposition to MS, although that agent has not been identified. Some evidence supports immunological, environmental, or genetic factors as possible causes of the disease. The risk of developing MS is 15 times higher when the disease is present in the patient's immediate family. Conditions such as pregnancy, infection, and trauma seem to precipitate the onset of MS or cause relapses. Risk factors include family history, Epstein-Barr viral infections, low vitamin D levels, cerebrospinal venous insufficiency, and autoimmune diseases (hypothyroidism, type 1 diabetes mellitus, and inflammatory bowel disease).

GENETIC CONSIDERATIONS

Genetics is commonly listed as a risk factor for MS. Clusters of cases in families are not common, but they do occur. Concordance is only slightly higher in identical than in nonidentical twins, but MS is nearly 20 times as common among all relatives of probands than in the general population. Heritability is estimated at 64%. Autosomal recessive transmission with incomplete penetrance has been suggested. It is more likely that one inherits susceptibility to an environmental trigger. Susceptibility is likely associated with certain HLA alleles, with specific evidence for the *HLA-A*, *HLA-DRB1*, *HLA-DR15*, *HLA-DQB1*, and *HLA-DRA* genes.

SEX AND LIFE SPAN CONSIDERATIONS

MS is more prevalent in colder climates and in urban areas. More than 400,000 Americans have MS. MS affects more women than men in a 2.5:1 ratio. Roughly 70% of patients experience the onset of MS when they are between ages 20 and 40 years, while 20% of patients experience the onset of the disease when they are between ages 40 and 60 years. The average age at diagnosis is 29 years for women and 31 years for men.

HEALTH DISPARITIES AND SEXUAL/GENDER MINORITY HEALTH

MS is most common in White persons and almost unknown among Native American and Asian American persons. Analysis of a national database of people with MS found that compared to White persons, Black persons with MS tended to be younger, had a higher level of disability, were less likely to have private insurance, and had higher levels of unemployment or disabled status (Wang et al., 2020). Sexual and gender minority status has no known effect on the risk for MS.

GLOBAL HEALTH CONSIDERATIONS

The National Multiple Sclerosis Society estimates that at least 2.3 million people worldwide have the condition. People of northern European descent have the highest prevalence of MS, and a wide variation in prevalence occurs by global region. Higher prevalence occurs in northern latitudes, and lower prevalence occurs in the tropics and lower altitudes. Low rates occur in people with Asian and African ancestry, and high rates occur in some Mediterranean countries.

ASSESSMENT

HISTORY. Vague and unrelated symptoms often dominate the early period of MS before a definitive diagnosis is made. Brain lesions lead to central nervous system signs. Ask the patient about changes in vision and coordination. Determine whether the patient has experienced slurred speech, impotence, ataxia, facial weakness, or double vision (diplopia). Approximately 70% experience involuntary, rhythmic movements of the eyes (nystagmus).

Spinal cord lesions lead to motor and sensory impairment of the trunk and limbs. Ask if problems have occurred with bowel and bladder or sexual function. Determine if the patient has experienced a feeling of heaviness or weakness, numbness, or tingling in the extremities. Determine the patient's ability to perform activities of daily living with attention to the fine movement of fingers, as when dressing or picking up small objects. Ask if the patient has experienced burning sensation or pain, decreased temperature sensation, intention tremor (a tremor during a voluntary activity), foot-dragging, staggering, dizziness, or loss of balance. Ask if the patient has experienced decreased motor function after taking a hot bath or shower (Uhthoff sign), which is caused by the effects of heat on neuromuscular conduction. Roughly 50% of patients with MS lose the ability to sense position, vibration, shape, and texture.

Symptomatic episodes may occur weeks, months, or years apart and may affect different locations in the body. Some patients may have cognitive changes and others sensory or motor changes. Determine when the patient first noticed any of these difficulties and whether the symptoms later disappeared. Ask about fatigue and its progression throughout the day and what stressors precipitate symptoms. Determine whether there is a family history of the disease. Elicit a history of mild depression and short attention span.

PHYSICAL EXAMINATION. Common symptoms include **tingling and muscle cramping, tremor, ataxia, speech disorders, visual changes,** and **bowel and bladder dysfunction.** Determine the patient's muscle strength and symmetry, arm and leg movement, and gait. To assess arm strength, have the patient use both hands to push against you. Observe for unilateral or bilateral weakness. Ask the patient to open and close the fist and to move each arm without raising it from the bed. If no purposeful movement occurs, apply light tactile pressure to each arm, gradually increasing the pressure in an attempt to elicit a purposeful response. Assess leg movement in the same way. Ask the patient to move each leg and, if the patient cannot, press the Achilles tendon firmly between your thumb and index finger, observing for either a purposeful or a nonpurposeful response. Assess gait by asking the patient to walk away from you; observe for ataxia, shuffling, or stumbling. Stay close to the patient to prevent falls. If the patient is able to perform these tasks well, test balance by having the patient walk heel-to-toe in a straight line. Observe any leaning to one side.

Assess the patient's mental status, speech patterns, attention span, concentration, and memory. Evaluate the patient for eye symptoms such as double vision, loss of vision, loss of color vision, or nystagmus.

PSYCHOSOCIAL. Some patients experience depression, euphoria, or memory loss as symptoms of MS, creating psychological challenges in addition to the difficulties of managing a chronic condition. When a chronic illness with potential for serious debilitation and possible early death is first discovered, a patient goes through a period of grieving. This grief process may take years. Determine the patient's place on the continuum of shock, denial, or anger, and accept the patient's current stage of coping. Role changes because of disability cause stress and place burdens on the patient and family.

Diagnostic Highlights

Test	Normal Result	Abnormality With Condition	Explanation
Magnetic resonance imaging	Normal brain and spinal cord structures	Identifies demyelinating lesions in the brain and spinal cord	Evaluates disease extent and progression; shows brain abnormalities in 90%–95% of patients with MS

Other Tests: No single test reliably diagnoses MS, which is diagnosed based on clinical findings and supporting evidence. Supporting tests include lumbar puncture, electroencephalography, complete blood count, serum chemistries, glucose, evoked potential studies, and computed tomography scan; magnetic resonance imaging with gadolinium may show active lesions in the brain or spine.

PRIMARY NURSING DIAGNOSIS

DIAGNOSIS. Impaired physical mobility related to erratic nerve transmission as evidenced by tingling, muscle cramping, fatigue and/or weakness

OUTCOMES. Self-management: Multiple sclerosis; Ambulation; Joint movement; Mobility; Self-care: Activities of daily living; Balance; Neurological status

INTERVENTIONS. Exercise therapy: Ambulation; Exercise therapy: Balance; Exercise therapy: Joint mobility; Teaching: Prescribed exercise; Energy management; Environmental management; Exercise promotion; Activity therapy

☀ PLANNING AND IMPLEMENTATION

Collaborative

Most medical treatment is designed to slow disease progression and address the symptoms of the disease, such as urinary retention, spasticity, and motor and speech deficits. It focuses on immunomodulation to manage the underlying immune disorder and therapies to manage symptoms. Physicians prescribe steroid therapy to reduce tissue edema during an acute exacerbation. Plasmaphoresis, or plasma exchange, can also be used on a short-term basis for severe exacerbations. Autologous hematopoietic stem cell transplantation may slow the course of MS and repair nervous system damage. A growing number of immunomodulatory therapies are available, and many experimental treatments are in development to manage MS.

Patients may consult with a physical therapist if they need to learn how to use assistive devices or to learn exercises to maintain muscle tone and joint mobility. Muscle stretching for spastic muscles and selective strengthening exercises for weakness are usually prescribed. A social service agency may be required to help the patient and family deal with the often expensive and long-term financial effect of the disease. Vocational redirection may also be required. For a patient who is experiencing depression, consider a referral to a psychiatric clinical nurse specialist. Family counseling is often very helpful.

Pharmacologic Highlights

Medication or Drug Class	Dosage	Description	Rationale
Corticosteroids	Varies with drug	Prednisone (Orasone); methylprednisolone (Solu-Medrol); dexamethasone (Decadron)	Help decrease symptoms and induce remissions through anti-inflammatory effects, particularly during acute relapses; there is no evidence that it changes disease progression
Immunomodulatory agents	Varies with drug	Interferon, glatiramer acetate, alemtuzumab, natalizumab, fingolimod, siponimod, teriflunomide	Help decrease symptoms and induce remissions; treatment includes combination therapy using two or more of these agents
Immunosuppressants	Varies with drug	Cyclophosphamide, mitoxantrone	Suppress immune reactions, delay progression, and extend the time between relapses

Antidepressants and anticonvulsants for pain; baclofen for spasticity; dalfampridine to improve walking

Independent

Sensory perceptual deficits in the visual fields cause dizziness, headaches, and the potential for injury. Patching each eye, alternating with the other several times a day, improves balance and visualization. Peripheral vision may be affected; teach the patient to scan the environment and to remove potential sources of injury. Ask the patient particularly to look out for hot surfaces and hot water to which the patient may not be sensitive.

Be sure the patient understands the need to avoid becoming fatigued or overheated. Instruct the patient to alternate periods of activity with periods of rest, discussing the need for frequent rest periods as a permanent lifestyle change. Explain that baths and showers may prove relaxing but may also exacerbate MS symptoms. Conduct range-of-motion exercises at least twice daily. If necessary, teach the patient how to use a walker or a cane. Care for a neurogenic bladder includes instructing the patient to consume 1,500 mL of fluid daily and void every 3 hours. If urine is retained, teach intermittent self-catheterization with a clean technique to the patient who is capable. Some patients, however, are incontinent.

Teach the patient how to use special pads to avoid skin breakdown. Teach the patient to develop a regular bowel pattern, with bowel elimination about 30 minutes after the morning meal. Insert a glycerine suppository if necessary to stimulate reflex bowel activity. Provide assistance should the patient be unable to perform this self-care.

Teach the patient about the disease process and be sure the patient knows how to contact the local MS Society (https://www.nationalmssociety.org). In addition to information and education, the society holds focus group seminars that study relational issues associated with the disease. The society also provides some ongoing therapy and socialization and support for home maintenance. Helping the patient learn to cope with this chronic illness is a major nursing challenge. Listen to the patient's fears; respect the patient's abilities and provide positive encouragement. The disabled patient not only loses body function but often the patient's role as an active parent and spouse. With the more rapidly progressive forms of MS, the patient may have impairment of cognitive functioning; touch and voice tone can convey concern and care when the meaning of words gets lost.

Evidence-Based Practice and Health Policy

Krysko, K., Graves, J., Dobson, R., Altintas, A., Amato, M., Bernard, J., Bonavita, S., Bove, R., Cavalla, P., Clerico, M., Corona, T., Doshi, A., Fragoso, Y., Jacobs, D., Jokubaitis, V., Landi, D., Llamosa, G., Longbrake, E., Maillart, E., . . . Hellwig, K. (2020). Sex effects across the lifespan in women with multiple sclerosis. *Therapeutic Advances in Neurological Disorders, 13*, 1–30.

- The authors aimed to review the sex effects across the life span in women with MS. The authors note that the female-to-male ratio has increased in recent years, suggesting the possibility that environmental factors affect females more than males. Because onset is often during women's reproductive years, issues such as family planning, including contraceptive and disease-modifying therapy, need to be included in patient care.
- They note that pregnancy decreases the risk of MS relapse, and disease-modifying treatments may be safely stopped during pregnancy. Relapse may instead occur during the postpartum period. Pregnancy is not harmful for long-term prognosis, but as menopause approaches, the disability from MS may progress because of complex hormone interactions. Few studies have addressed menopause in women with MS, and further research in this area is essential.

DOCUMENTATION GUIDELINES

- Physical findings: Muscle strength, gait, muscle symmetry, visual response
- Response to medications, treatments, and special therapies
- Ability to perform self-care, bowel and bladder care
- Presence of complications, infections, contractures

DISCHARGE AND HOME HEALTHCARE GUIDELINES

Be sure the patient understands any pain medication prescribed, including dosage, route, action, and side effects. Be sure the patient understands the need for adequate bladder and bowel elimination. Instruct the patient to notify the primary caregiver of any exacerbation or sudden worsening of the condition. If the patient has difficulty speaking or communicating, be sure the patient has access to a telephone support network or some other means of calling for assistance when at home alone for any length of time. Be sure the patient understands that stress, fatigue, and being overheated stimulate exacerbations. Teach the patient how to avoid situations that produce these reactions. Be sure the patient knows how to contact community agencies such as the MS Society for use of such in-home equipment as beds and wheelchairs and home maintenance support. Determine whether a home-care agency is needed to provide home supervision and ongoing physical therapy support.

Muscular Dystrophy

DRG Category:	92
Mean LOS:	3.9 days
Description:	MEDICAL: Other Disorders of Nervous System With Complication or Comorbidity

Muscular dystrophy (MD) is not a disease; rather, it is a term applied to a number of genetic, noninflammatory disorders characterized by gradual progressive weakness and muscle fiber degeneration without neural involvement. The most significant finding in MD is skeletal muscle deterioration that moves in a proximal to distal direction. Cardiac and other smooth muscles may be involved as well, leading to serious complications and premature death. To date, there is no cure for any of the MDs, but there have been significant research advances related to gene identification for Duchenne MD (a pseudohypertrophic, progressive form that begins in childhood and is transmitted as a sex-linked recessive trait). The genetic abnormality causes an absence of dystrophia, a protein of muscle cells. This deficit prevents adequate cell functioning, which leads to necrosis of muscle fibers. As the muscle undergoes necrosis, fat and connective tissue replace the muscle fibers. Complications include disabilities, contractures, skeletal deformities such as scoliosis, osteoporosis, inability to walk, dysphagia, cardiopulmonary failure, and thoracic muscle weakness. Most experts note that children with Duchenne MD have some degree of intellectual impairment. They are prone to pulmonary complications such as pneumonia and cardiac dysrhythmias and hypertrophy.

CAUSES

MD is a progressive degeneration of skeletal muscles due to an abnormality in the genetic code for muscle proteins. One-third of the people develop the disease because of spontaneous new mutations. Duchenne MD has an incidence of about 3 per 100,000 individuals and is inherited as a recessive single-gene defect on the X chromosome, which means it is transmitted from the mother to her male offspring. Another form of dystrophy, Becker MD, is similarly X-linked but has its onset later in childhood or adolescence and has a slower course. Other heredity disorders include Landouzy-Dejerine dystrophy (fascioscapulohumeral) and Erb MD (limb-girdle dystrophy). The primary risk factor is heredity.

GENETIC CONSIDERATIONS

There are numerous types of MD. The most common, accounting for more than 50% of cases, is Duchenne MD. Both Duchenne MD and a milder form called Becker MD are caused by mutations in the *DMD* gene, which provides instructions for making a protein called dystrophin. Dystrophin is located chiefly in muscle cells and serves a vital role in maintaining muscle fiber integrity. Both Duchenne and Becker MD are inherited in an X-linked recessive pattern. Another form of dystrophy, called myotonic dystrophy, is caused by cytosine-thymine-guanine (CTG) repeats within the genes *DMPK* and *CNBP*. It is inherited in an autosomal dominant pattern. Prenatal testing of at-risk pregnancies is possible if the family mutation has been identified.

SEX AND LIFE SPAN CONSIDERATIONS

In some forms of MD, weakness can appear from infancy to adulthood. The rate of progression varies from rapid to slow, and in many cases, the individual may have a normal life span. Muscular dystrophy can affect children or adults, females and males, depending on the type (Table 1).

• **TABLE 1 Four Types of Muscular Dystrophy**

TYPE	SEX	AGE AT ONSET	CHARACTERISTICS AND PROGRESSION
Duchenne MD (most common type)	Males	Toddler or preschool	Initial loss of pelvic girdle and shoulder muscle control; Gower sign (weakness in hip muscles); rapid progression with death in late adolescence or 20s from cardiac or respiratory complications
Becker MD (second most common type)	Males	Early teens	Similar to Duchenne MD but occurs later in life and is milder; no cardiac involvement; slow, near-normal life span
Autosomal dominant fascioscapulohumeral dystrophy	Males and females	Children through young adults	Weakness and atrophy of shoulder, face, and eye muscles; walking, chewing, and swallowing problems with slow progression, normal life span
Myotonic dystrophy (Steinert disease)	Males and females	Young adults	Muscles remain contracted (myotonia, or prolonged spasm of muscles after use), atrophy occurs; life span into the 30s or 40s; most common form in adults

HEALTH DISPARITIES AND SEXUAL/GENDER MINORITY HEALTH

MD is more common in White persons than Black, Hispanic, and Native American persons. Experts note that nearly one-third of families with children with MD have inadequate insurance coverage, which means that key healthcare needs may not be met (Shing et al., 2018). Sexual and gender minority status has no known effect on the risk for MD.

GLOBAL HEALTH CONSIDERATIONS

The prevalence of MD globally correlates in general with that in the United States. Autosomal dominant fascioscapulohumeral dystrophy tends to occur in Sweden more than other countries. Myotonic dystrophy is more common among French Canadians and in Germany and Finland.

⬜ ASSESSMENT

HISTORY. A complete family and developmental history provides important diagnostic data for the patient with MD. Because it is a genetic disease, determine if anyone in the family has been previously diagnosed with a musculoskeletal or neuromuscular disease. Elicit a history of childhood benchmarks, particularly when the patient began to walk. Elicit the progression of intellect and problem-solving skills. Ask adult patients if they have extremity weakness or difficulty with ambulation. Patients may experience difficulty raising the arms over the head or closing the eyes completely. Other early signs include difficulty in puckering the lips, abnormal facial movements, and the inability of facial muscles to change during laughing and crying.

PHYSICAL EXAMINATION. Children with Duchenne MD have a history of delayed motor milestones, such as sitting, walking, and standing. Adults may report **progressive muscle**

weakness of the legs, face, and shoulder. Most dystrophies involve the hip and shoulder girdle musculature, which leads to functional difficulties. Assess the patient's ability to raise the arms above the head, get up from a chair, or walk. Inspect the patient for scoliosis and contractures. For boys ages 2 to 5 years with Duchenne MD, observe for pelvic and shoulder girdle muscles with distal involvement. Note a waddling, stumbling gait or difficulty climbing stairs. A characteristic sign is the Gower maneuver: patients use their hands to walk up the legs until standing erect. The patients' postures may also be distorted, with a lumbar lordosis and protuberant abdomen. They may toe-walk to compensate for quadriceps weakness. Scoliosis occurs after the child is wheelchair dependent because of weak trunk muscles. Tachycardia occurs as the heart muscle weakens and enlarges. Generally, any cardiac muscle involvement is asymptomatic until late in the course of the disease. Pneumonia and dysphagia develop easily as the child's cough reflex becomes weak and ineffective.

PSYCHOSOCIAL. Because MD is a progressive disease that limits the normal life span, patients and their families will require ongoing emotional support. The genetic nature of the disease frequently creates guilt that often leads to depression. Boys with Duchenne MD often have an IQ below 90. Frustration, depression, and other signs of emotional immaturity may be present because of the intellectual limitation. Family functioning is challenged because of the progressive losses and prognosis.

Diagnostic Highlights

Test	Normal Result	Abnormality With Condition	Explanation
Creatine kinase (CK)	Male: 50–204 units/L; female: 36–160 units/L	Early in process, CK levels may be 50–300 times normal levels, but the levels tend to decrease as the muscle mass decreases	Elevated due to muscle wasting; may also obtain transaminase, lactate dehydrogenase, and aldolase levels
Muscle biopsy	Normal muscle fibers	Muscle cell degeneration with microscopic areas of necrosis and presence of dystrophin	Increased activity of proteolytic enzymes in muscle tissue
Ultrasonography	Normal muscle and bone structure	Increased echogenicity in affected muscles, reduction in underlying bone	Muscle and bone wasting
Electromyogram	No electrical activity at rest; orderly recruitment of voluntary motor unit potentials with gradually increasing voluntary motor muscle effort	Progressive muscle weakness	Destruction and deterioration of muscle function

PRIMARY NURSING DIAGNOSIS

DIAGNOSIS. Impaired physical mobility related to muscle destruction as evidenced by alterations in gait and/or progressive muscle weakness

OUTCOMES. Self-management: Chronic disease; Ambulation; Joint movement; Activity tolerance; Mobility; Self-care: Activities of daily living; Balance

INTERVENTIONS. Exercise therapy: Ambulation; Exercise therapy: Balance; Exercise therapy: Joint mobility; Teaching: Prescribed exercise; Energy management; Exercise promotion; Activity therapy

✳ PLANNING AND IMPLEMENTATION

Collaborative

Currently, there is no cure for MD, and therapeutic management is focused on managing the symptoms and maintaining the highest level of functional independence possible. Patients with MD are managed by a multidisciplinary team because of their complex needs. The goals of treatment are to facilitate ambulation and aggressively manage respiratory and cardiac difficulties. With early diagnosis, interventions such as appropriate diet and exercise and social and psychological counseling can begin to prolong the patient's independence and quality of life.

Physical therapy is directed toward keeping functional muscle strength and preventing contractures by passive stretching. Swimming is frequently recommended as an excellent exercise for keeping limber and for allowing participation in athletic events. Gait training and transfer training are important as the patient loses muscle power. Crutches and the use of a powered wheelchair maintain independent mobility for as long as possible. The occupational therapist may fit the patient with braces or splints to prevent or treat contractures. Long-leg braces are needed to provide stability for weakened muscles that can no longer provide support for ambulation.

Once the patient is in a wheelchair, obesity frequently becomes a problem. A low-calorie, high-protein diet is recommended to avoid this complication because the additional weight places a strain on already compromised muscles. Constipation may also be a problem that can be managed with added dietary fiber, extra fluids, and stool softeners.

The physician may consider surgery to assist the patient in maintaining a higher quality of life. A spinal fusion may correct abnormal spinal curvatures that occur as the trunk muscles weaken to improve comfort, balanced sitting, and body image. Muscle- and tendon-lengthening procedures may be needed to improve decreased function if contractures form. Preoperative and postoperative preparations are essential to prevent complications. Before a surgical procedure is attempted, an electrocardiogram is needed to determine if the cardiac muscle has been affected by the muscle disease. Malignant hyperthermia (a potentially lethal increase in body temperature in response to certain muscle relaxants or anesthetic agents) is a complication that occurs in children with Duchenne MD. Early ambulation is necessary to prevent additional weakness, and aggressive respiratory care prevents pneumonia.

Many new therapies are in the experimental or clinical trial phase of testing. The Muscular Dystrophy Association (MDA; https://www.mda.org) provides updates on MD research. Possible strategies currently being refined include gene therapy, exon skipping, and gene repair. Deflazacort (Emflaza), which is an anti-inflammatory and immunosuppressant, is designed for people age 5 years or older with Duchenne MD. Biological agents are also under study.

Pharmacologic Highlights

No drugs have been found to slow the progression of the disease. Some providers may prescribe corticosteroid therapy, including deflazacort, to help maintain strength.

Independent

Because of the nature of MD, nursing interventions are primarily preventive and supportive. Prevention of complications requires anticipation of problems and systematic monitoring for progression of the disease process. Proper management can increase the length and quality of life. Differences in care can be divided by decreasing mobility into three phases: ambulatory, wheelchair, and bedrest phases.

In the ambulatory phase, when the family first learns of the diagnosis, information about the disease, prognosis, and treatment plans may be overwhelming. Be available to answer questions, provide clarification, and provide emotional support and encouragement related to the family's needs for control in care decisions. The family needs opportunities to express feelings about the genetic transmission, progressive nature, and effect of the disease on the family. The status of younger male children in the family may not be certain; uncertainty creates additional anxiety.

Evaluate safety issues in the home. The child's bedroom should be moved to the first floor if possible, and rugs need to be removed to facilitate mobility. Rubber-soled shoes help prevent slipping. As the disease progresses, home-care equipment may be necessary for assistance with mobility and activities of daily living. Nursing interventions are directed toward preventing contractures and encouraging independence and normal development. The patient needs to be monitored for a tendency toward contracture development and range-of-motion exercises instituted as a preventive measure. Stretching exercises and splinting of the arms and legs at night help to slow the progression of contractures. Assist the child and family in developing a plan for both active and passive range-of-motion exercises to do daily; help make reminder sheets so exercises are consistently done.

As the patient becomes dependent in the wheelchair phase, comfort measures become even more critical. Teach the family to make frequent skin assessments to determine evidence of skin breakdown from prolonged sitting. Support stockings, passive exercises, and elevating the lower extremities may decrease pedal edema for patients in wheelchairs. Provide interventions directed toward attaining the child's maximum growth and development level. In the bedrest phase, eventually the patient will be unable to move without assistance. Frequent position changes and meticulous skin care are essential. Proper body alignment in the bed or chair can be maintained by the use of blanket rolls, sandbags, or pillows. Sheepskin or an alternating pressure mattress may provide comfort. Adequate fluid intake is needed to prevent urinary or bowel complications. Use incentive spirometry and diaphragmatic breathing exercises to maintain gas exchange when respiratory muscles are weak. Percussion and postural drainage are used to facilitate effective airway clearance.

Referral needs to be made to the MDA and other community agencies. These organizations can provide information about the disease, management, and emotional and social support during the long period of illness. They can also provide financial assistance for treatment needs.

Evidence-Based Practice and Health Policy

Tesei, A., Nobile, M., Colombo, P., Civati, F., Gandossini, S., Mani, E., Molteni, M., Bresolin, N., & D'Angelo, G. (2020). Mental health and coping strategies in families of children and young adults with muscular dystrophies. *Journal of Neurology, 267*, 2054–2069.

- The authors wanted to investigate coping profiles of patients with MD and their parents. They aimed to verify whether psychological adaptation of patients can be predicted by coping strategies, taking into account physical impairment, cognitive level, and socioeconomic status. The authors assessed emotional and behavioral factors in patients with MD ($N = 112$).
- They found a high prevalence of intellectual disability and autism spectrum disorders in people with Duchenne MD. Parents tended to rely more on positive reinterpretation and less on disengagement coping. Avoidance coping, whether used by parents or patients, predicted increased emotional and behavioral problems. The authors concluded that interventions should address problems of anxiety and depression that people with MDs experience.

DOCUMENTATION GUIDELINES

- Chronological progression of muscular weakness and decreasing function; cardiac and respiratory involvement
- Responses to treatment plan (exercises, diet, adaptive devices, breathing exercises, growth and development)
- Patient's and family's reactions to disease process, interventions, and role changes

DISCHARGE AND HOME HEALTHCARE GUIDELINES

The child with MD has multiple admissions and discharges. Because MD is a chronic progressive disease, teaching needs to vary according to the interventions and phase of illness. The MD team and the MDA are the best sources of providing information to the patient and family in a timely manner. Encourage the child and parents to maintain peer relationships and foster intellectual development by keeping the child in school as long as possible. Teach the patient and family ways to avoid respiratory problems. Encourage the parents to report respiratory infections as soon as they occur.

Musculoskeletal Trauma

DRG Category:	480
Mean LOS:	7.3 days
Description:	SURGICAL: Hip and Femur Procedures Except Major Joint With Complication or Comorbidity
DRG Category:	507
Mean LOS:	6.0 days
Description:	SURGICAL: Major Shoulder or Elbow Joint Procedures With Complication or Comorbidity or Major Complication or Comorbidity
DRG Category:	562
Mean LOS:	5.0 days
Description:	MEDICAL: Fracture, Sprain, Strain, and Dislocation Except Femur, Hip, Pelvis, and Thigh With Major Complication or Comorbidity

Trauma causes more than 170,000 deaths each year in the United States and leads to both economic and productivity losses for its victims. It is the third leading cause of death in the United States. Experts estimate that 5.6 million fractures occur in the United States annually. The bony skeleton provides the supporting framework for the human body. Its 206 bones are subject to many stressors, which may result in fractures. Fractures vary in complexity and potential harm to the body. Simple fractures occur with no break from the bone to the outside of the body, whereas compound fractures have an external wound, thus creating contamination of the fracture. Complete fractures occur when bone continuity is completely interrupted, whereas partial fractures (incomplete) interrupt only a portion of bone continuity. Fractures can be classified by fragment position or fracture line (Table 1).

• **TABLE 1** Types of Fractures

CLASSIFICATION	TYPE	DEFINITION
Fragment position	Angulated	Bone fragments are at an angle to each other
	Avulsed	Bone fragments are pulled from normal position by muscle spasms, muscle contractions, or ligament resistance
	Comminuted	Bone breaks into many small pieces
	Displaced	Bone fragments separate and are deformed
	Impacted	A bone fragment is forced into another bone or bone fragment

• **TABLE 1** Types of Fractures (continued)

CLASSIFICATION	TYPE	DEFINITION
	Nondisplaced	After the fracture, two sections of the bone maintain normal alignment
	Overriding	Bone fragments overlap, thereby shortening the total length of the bone
	Segmental	Bone fractures occur in two areas next to each other with an isolated section in the center
Fracture line	Linear	Fracture line is parallel to the axis of the bone
	Longitudinal	Fracture line extends longitudinally but not parallel to the axis of the bone
	Oblique	Fracture line crosses the bone at a 45-degree angle to the axis of the bone
	Spiral	Fracture line coils around the bone
	Transverse	Fracture line forms a 90-degree angle to the axis of the bone

Fractures heal in two different ways. Direct healing occurs when anatomic reduction with compression has occurred, which means that anatomic reduction allows for the fractured bone to heal without deformity, and the fragments of bones are realigned to their normal anatomic position. Indirect healing occurs when anatomic reduction is not achieved or compression is not possible. Following the fracture and initial inflammation, granulation tissue forms a soft callus (bony tissue that forms around the ends of a broken bone). The soft callus becomes hard, creating woven bone, with remodeling and bone growth to bridge the gap between bone fragments.

Many complications can occur as a result of musculoskeletal trauma. Arterial damage and bleeding can lead to hypovolemic shock. Nonunion of bones, avascular necrosis, bone necrosis, and peripheral nerve damage can lead to lasting deformities and disabilities. Rhabdomyolysis (destruction of skeletal muscle) can lead to renal failure, and bone injury can lead to fat emboli. Infection is the most common complication of trauma and can lead to sepsis and septic shock.

CAUSES

Traumatic injuries can be intentional (assaults, gunshot wounds, stab wounds) or unintentional (falls, motor vehicle crashes [MVCs] and traffic injuries such as pedestrian, cyclist, and motorcycle injuries). Multiple traumas that result from an MVC often involve several systems of the body and musculoskeletal injury. Falls and traffic injuries account for a high percentage of the fractures seen today. Children at play take falls as a matter of course and only occasionally suffer fractures. Their most common fractures are of the radius, hand, elbow, and clavicle. Adults who fall most often fracture a hip or wrist. Osteoporosis increases the likelihood of fractures from a fall; it even sometimes causes a fracture from a slight shift in the body's position, which then results in a fall, rather than the reverse. Fracture risks include osteoporosis, family history, use of corticosteroids, cigarette smoking, type I diabetes mellitus, alcohol abuse, and rheumatoid arthritis.

GENETIC CONSIDERATIONS

No clear genetic contributions to susceptibility have been defined.

SEX AND LIFE SPAN CONSIDERATIONS

Multiple musculoskeletal traumas can occur at any time in life—no one is exempt. However, young adults are most at risk. Traffic injuries are the leading cause of death for those ages 4 to 34 years. Serious industrial accidents are more common in young men. Men have different patterns of injury than women, and a higher injury severity. Analyses of trauma outcomes indicate that following traumatic injury, males have higher rates of multiple organ failure, pneumonia, and sepsis than females, creating health disparities for men (Marcolini et al., 2019).

Trauma is the third leading cause of death in people ages 45 to 65 years and the seventh leading cause of death in people older than age 65 years. Multiple injuries from falls are especially a problem in older women. Osteoporosis, which occurs in many women past menopause and in men somewhat later in life, accounts for the vulnerability to fractures of those past midlife. Fractures in older people are often of the wrist, hip, and vertebrae. Healing occurs much more rapidly in the young, and older people are more at risk for complications of immobility from both the fracture and its treatment. The high death rate of older adults within a year after a broken hip is largely from complications of immobility.

HEALTH DISPARITIES AND SEXUAL/GENDER MINORITY HEALTH

MVCs and other traffic injuries are one of the leading causes of musculoskeletal trauma. In recent years, Black persons have been killed in traffic crashes at a rate of almost 25% higher than White persons (National Highway Traffic Safety Administration [NHTSA], 2021). Native American persons have the highest rate of MVC injury in the United States, more than twice the rate of Black persons (NHTSA, 2021). Experts have noted that Black and Native American communities tend to be crisscrossed by more dangerous roads than other locations, placing people from those communities at risk for injury. Healthy People 2020 reports that non-Hispanic Black persons have the highest injury death rate in the United States (79.9 injury deaths per 100,000 people), followed by non-Hispanic White people (79.2), Native American people (78.2), Hispanic people (45.5), and Asian/Pacific Islander people (25.6).

Recent work has shown evidence that rural populations have injury mortality rates that are more than twice as high as urban rates. Many factors contribute to these health disparities, including the risk of traffic injury in narrow rural roads, the lack of graded curves and lighted traffic signals on rural highways, and the distance from major trauma centers. Many of the most dangerous occupations, such as mining and agriculture, are found in rural areas and can result in injury, disability, and death. Sexual and gender minority persons have high risk for dating and interpersonal violence, violence related to bullying, and intentional and unintentional injury (Healthy People 2020).

GLOBAL HEALTH CONSIDERATIONS

Musculoskeletal injury often results from both traffic injuries and falls, both of which are the leading causes of unintentional injury globally. For children and young adults ages 5 to 29 years, traffic injuries are the leading cause of death globally. Almost 95% of the world's fatalities occur on the roads in low- and middle-income countries. More than half of all road traffic deaths are among pedestrians, cyclists, and motorcyclists (World Health Organization, 2021). In younger people ages 10 to 49 years, traffic injuries are the leading cause of disease burden, with burden levels higher than infectious diseases, cancer, and heart disease.

ASSESSMENT

HISTORY. Determine the details of the immediate injury. Question the patient if possible, relatives if present, and any witnesses, including bystanders, the police, and the life squad. Note that the obvious injuries may not be the most serious ones. For example, a leg injury may be evident, whereas the pelvic fracture caused by force to the knee or leg during a car crash may be more serious. Obtain information from family or friends about the usual health status. Determine the past medical history, with particular attention to life span considerations such as pregnancy, chronic diseases such as diabetes and hypertension, osteoporosis, and patterns of substance abuse.

PHYSICAL EXAMINATION. Common symptoms are **pain, angulation** (bone fractures are at an angle to each other), **shortening or deformation of limbs, open wounds, bleeding from wounds or into tissues** (ecchymosis), **swelling,** and **muscle spasms.** In the immediate trauma resuscitation, assessment and treatment are merged. Always of first priority is the assessment and management of airway, breathing, and circulation (ABCs). Neurological status becomes part of that initial assessment, because the patient is often in a compromised state of consciousness. Monitor the vital signs every 15 minutes or more often until the patient is stabilized. The patient may demonstrate a wide range of blood pressures and heart rates depending on age, degree of blood loss, baseline vital signs, and degree of alcohol intoxication.

During the physical examination, handle the patient carefully and be aware that any fractures can be made more serious by the manipulation caused by examination. If the cervical spine is injured, movement can lead to lifelong disability. Cervical stabilization is critical until the cervical spine can be evaluated radiographically or with scanning. Broken ribs may not initially pose a serious problem for the patient, but with rough handling, they may become displaced and cause damage to the pleura and lungs. Manipulation of broken bones also causes increased pain and blood loss. Inspect the patient thoroughly for evidence of fractures, including angulation or shortening of limbs, open wounds, and changes in color from the rest of the body. Note any swelling or muscle spasms of the limbs, which may indicate injuries not apparent initially. Palpate any areas suspected of injury, noting the contour of surrounding bones. Check the range of motion of all joints, listening for crepitus and noting any signs of pain from the patient during the examination, but do not move an obviously injured extremity to test for range of motion. Complete a neurovascular examination, checking pulses, capillary refill, and response to sharp and dull pain stimuli.

PSYCHOSOCIAL. The patient with serious musculoskeletal injury is usually seen in the emergency department and may be in hypovolemic shock as well as anxious and in pain. As the patient becomes conscious, the effect of the trauma may be overwhelming; alternatively, the patient may have no memory of the trauma and be distraught to be in the hospital. The older patient who has fallen and suffered a broken hip often becomes confused from the trauma. As the situation becomes clearer, the fears of hospitalization and becoming dependent on others pose a real problem. The patient may deny having a fracture or may not realize that fracture and a broken bone are synonymous. Assess the patient's substance use patterns. If the injury was alcohol or drug related or if the patient has a pattern of misuse, abuse, or dependence, make a referral for further assessment.

The sudden nature of multiple trauma presents serious psychological stressors to the patient, family, and significant others. Often, the victim is young and healthy; parents become extremely anxious, angry, guilty, and even despairing when their child is injured and they cannot protect their child from danger. Peers often rally to support a classmate; their numbers may overwhelm the visiting area and the hospital's resources. A careful assessment of the family's and peer's response to trauma is important if interventions are to be constructive.

Diagnostic Highlights

Test	Normal Result	Abnormality With Condition	Explanation
Urine myoglobin	Negative	Positive; > 20 ng/mL	Myoglobin is a heme-containing, oxygen-binding protein that is present in striated and nonstriated skeletal and cardiac muscle; it is released into the interstitium fluid after injury to a muscle

(highlight box continues on page 838)

Diagnostic Highlights (continued)

Test	Normal Result	Abnormality With Condition	Explanation
X-rays, computed tomography scan, magnetic resonance imaging depending on location of injury	Intact bones, soft tissues, and joints	Visualization of number and location of fractures	Identifies extent and degree of injury; these tests will likely be needed before and after reduction

Other Tests: Blood alcohol level, urine toxic screen, complete blood count, coagulation studies, serum electrolytes, creatinine, blood urea nitrogen, type- and cross-matching for blood

PRIMARY NURSING DIAGNOSIS

DIAGNOSIS. Acute related to inflammation and swelling of the tendon as evidenced by self-reports of pain, facial grimacing, and/or protective behavior

OUTCOMES. Comfort status; Pain control; Pain level; Symptom severity; Knowledge: Pain management

INTERVENTIONS. Comfort; Pain management: Acute; Analgesic administration; Analgesic administration; Anxiety reduction; Teaching: Prescribed medication

PLANNING AND IMPLEMENTATION

Collaborative

In the emergency situation, planning and implementation are related to the priorities of ABCs and neurological status. Unless the musculoskeletal injury is threatening the patient's circulation because of bleeding, management of musculoskeletal injuries usually occurs after the patient is stabilized. When a musculoskeletal injury interrupts a bone or joint, the trauma causes severe muscle spasms that lead to pain, angulation (abnormal formation of angles by the bones), and overriding of the ends of the bones. These complications need to be managed immediately to prevent increased soft tissue injury, decreased venous and lymphatic return, and edema. If the patient has any exposed soft tissue or bone, cover the area with a wet, sterile saline dressing. Prevent reentry of a contaminated bone into the wound if possible.

Early immobilization of the extremity at the trauma scene—which is actually the first step in trauma rehabilitation—preserves the function and prevents further injury. Immobilization limits muscle spasm, decreases angulation and injury from the overriding bone ends, and prevents closed fractures from becoming open fractures. Traction may also be applied to align bone ends in a close-to-normal position. This procedure restores circulatory, nerve, and lymphatic function and limits tissue injury and swelling. Generally, immobilization devices that are applied before the patient is admitted to the hospital are left in place until x-rays are performed.

When the fracture is confirmed by diagnostic testing, the bone is reduced by restoring displaced bone segments to their normal position. When the physician restores the bone to normal alignment, venous and lymphatic return improves, as does soft tissue swelling. The orthopedist may perform a closed reduction in which the bones are manually manipulated to restore alignment. When closed reduction is not possible, a surgical (open) reduction is performed. The method of reduction depends on the grade, type, and location of the fracture.

External fixation devices are now being used frequently for many fractures that would until recently have been treated with traction. External fixation, such as the Hoffmann device, is a metal system of rods designed to maintain alignment of fracture fragments. The patient requires less immobilization and therefore usually suffers fewer of the hazards of immobility. Use the device to position limbs, unless it is being used to stabilize a pelvic fracture. External fixation devices may also cause complications, however. Some patients react to them with local irritation, and a few develop infections. Monitor the area every 8 hours while the patient is hospitalized and clean it according to hospital protocol. The most common method is with half-strength hydrogen peroxide. Use of povidone-iodine (Betadine) or Neosporin ointment around the pins after cleansing may also be indicated to prevent infection. Long-range postoperative care includes staple or suture removal, immobilization with a splint or cast if warranted, weight-bearing at the appropriate time, and physical therapy.

Pharmacologic Highlights

Medication or Drug Class	Dosage	Description	Rationale
Narcotic analgesia	Varies with drug	Codeine, morphine sulfate, meperidine hydrochloride	Relieves pain
Other Drugs: Antibiotics, antispasmodics			

Independent

Follow the priorities of pain management, emotional support to cope with a sudden threat to health status, and prevention of complications. Pain may be caused by ineffective use of some treatment methods for fractures. Casts, traction, and fixation devices, once applied, should not cause pain. Improperly padded casts or ones that have been damaged may cause irritation and pressure to the casted area. Skin traction that causes friction also leads to impaired skin integrity. If the patient has soft tissue wounds that require treatment, a window in the cast may be needed. Maintain the functional integrity of the cast with attention to both immobilization of the fracture and prevention of further damage to the tissues.

Pain that seems extreme when a patient is casted or in skeletal traction may signal the advent of a compartment syndrome, a condition in which an edematous extremity is constricted by the cast. The patient complains of a burning sensation or other paresthesia. Edema may be present; pulses ordinarily remain intact. Even in the presence of substantial edema, the use of ice is contraindicated because of the danger of increased neurovascular compromise. The surgeon may bivalve the cast, remove the traction, or perform a fasciotomy.

The patient and family need a great deal of support to cope with a serious injury. Allow time each day to listen to concerns, discuss the patient's progress, and explain upcoming procedures. If the patient is a young trauma patient, you may need to work out a schedule with the patient's friends so that they can see the patient but also allow the patient adequate rest. Young adults enjoy diversional activities such as watching television and videos and listening to music. Older patients may experience depression and loss if the injury has long-term implications about their self-care. Consult with social workers and advanced practice nurses if the patient's anxiety or fear is abnormal. If the patient is a heavy drinker or was intoxicated at the time of injury, encourage the patient to evaluate drinking patterns and the link between drinking and injury. If needed, refer the patient appropriately for a full evaluation for substance abuse.

Immobilization involving the whole person, rather than one extremity, requires aggressive prevention of the hazards of immobility. Motivate and educate the patient in order to help the patient anticipate and prevent complications. Delayed healing of either wound or bone may occur as a complication of the patient's status at the time of the fracture or as a result of immobility. Encourage a balanced diet with foods that promote healing, such as those that contain protein and vitamin C. Stimulation of the affected area by isometric and isotonic exercises also helps promote healing. Instruct the patient in those techniques, which may not initially seem possible. They provide a partial substitute for the stimulation to bone remodeling that is otherwise provided by weight-bearing. Remember the design adage that is also useful in orthopedics: Form follows function.

Evidence-Based Practice and Health Policy

Hoogervorst, P., Shearer, D., & Miclau, T. (2020). The burden of high-energy musculoskeletal trauma in high-income countries. *World Journal of Surgery, 44*, 1033–1038.

• The authors aimed to review the current epidemiological data on the surgical and economic burden of high-energy musculoskeletal trauma in high-income countries. In 2016, mortality from road traffic injuries between the ages of 15 to 49 years was reported to be 9.5% in high-income countries. Road traffic crashes are the most common mechanism of injury and can serve as a useful indicator of surgical and economic burden.

• In 2009, the global losses were estimated to be $518 billion, costing governments between 1% and 3% of their gross domestic product. In the last decade, costs for those with a musculoskeletal injury in the United States rose 75%. While its impact is large, research on musculoskeletal conditions, including high-energy trauma, is underfunded compared to other specialty areas. An increased awareness among policy makers and healthcare professionals of the importance of care for the high-energy musculoskeletal trauma patient is important.

DOCUMENTATION GUIDELINES

• Physiological response: Adequacy of ABCs, vital signs, serial monitoring of neurological status, urine output, body weight, signs of withdrawal from alcohol or drugs
• History of injury, description, forces applied to the body during the trauma
• Response to treatment/medications: Pain, mobility, range of motion, muscle spasm, response to surgery, tolerance to nutrition
• Presence and response to traction and immobilization devices
• Complications: Infection, bleeding, anxiety, lack of mobility

DISCHARGE AND HOME HEALTHCARE GUIDELINES

Ascertain that the patient is alert and able to care for themselves within the limitations that are imposed by treatment of the fracture (e.g., cast or external fixation device) or has adequate home care available. Make sure the patient and family understand any care that is needed for casts or fixation devices and that they are clear about any limitations on weight-bearing. Arrange with social service for the purchase or rental of any supplies, such as crutches, wheelchairs, or home health devices. Teach the patient the hazards of immobility, the symptoms of complications, and when to seek assistance from a healthcare provider. Teach the patient about the route, dosage, mechanism of action, and side effects of all medications. Make sure the patient understands the basic components of a healthy diet. Explore with the patient the effects of drinking and drug use on long-term health and well-being. Remind the patient that rates of reinjury are very high in those who continue to drink alcohol excessively. Determine that the patient has adequate transportation home and for follow-up appointments.

Myasthenia Gravis

DRG Category:	57
Mean LOS:	5.6 days
Description:	MEDICAL: Degenerative Nervous System Disorders Without Major Complication or Comorbidity

Myasthenia gravis (MG) is an autoimmune disease that produces fatigue and voluntary muscle weakness, both of which become worse with exercise and improve with rest. The underlying pathophysiology of MG occurs because of the formation of antibodies against nicotinic acetylcholine postsynaptic receptors at the neuromuscular junction. At this junction, nervous conduction occurs because of the release of neurotransmitters. When the receptors are blocked or reduced, muscle strength is reduced with repeated use, and then muscle recovery occurs with rest. The muscles that are frequently involved include those for eye and eyelid movement, chewing and swallowing, breathing, and movement of the distal muscles of the extremities. This weakness progressively worsens during the day or at times of stress, so the greatest fatigue is likely to occur at the end of the day. MG frequently accompanies disorders of the immune system or the thyroid gland.

Rapid acute exacerbations result in a 5% mortality rate and are classified as either myasthenic or cholinergic crises. Both crises lead to extreme respiratory distress, difficulty in swallowing and speaking, great anxiety, and generalized weakness, thus making differentiation challenging but crucial for selection of appropriate intensive therapy. Myasthenic crisis is caused by undermedication, whereas a cholinergic crisis results from excessive anticholinesterase medication and is thus likely to occur within 45 to 60 minutes of the last drug dosage. The major complications of MG are respiratory distress or insufficiency, aspiration pneumonia, and poor nutrition linked to eating difficulties.

CAUSES

MG, thought to be an autoimmune disorder, is caused by a loss of acetylcholine receptor (AChR) in the postsynaptic neurons at the neuromuscular junction. About 80% of all patients with MG have elevated titers for AChR antibodies, which can prevent the acetylcholine (ACh) molecule from binding to these receptor sites or can cause damage to them. MG is often associated with thymic tumors. Triggers or situations that exacerbate symptoms include warm weather, surgical procedures or recurrent illnesses, immunizations, emotional stress, pregnancy, and certain medications. The primary risk factor is heredity. Exposure to pesticides can induce symptoms that resemble MG.

GENETIC CONSIDERATIONS

There appears to be genetic susceptibility to autoimmune disorders in general, and MG has occasionally demonstrated some family clustering, most often affecting siblings. The human leukocyte antigen (HLA) region defined by the A1, B8, and DR3 haplotypes are associated with early onset MG with thymus hyperplasia. Late-onset MG is associated with the A3, B7, DR2, DR4, and DRB1 haplotypes.

There is also a congenital form of myasthenic syndrome, which is a nonimmune disorder and is transmitted in an autosomal recessive pattern. This congenital form is associated with many genes including *CHRNE*, *RAPSN*, *CHAT*, *COLQ*, and *DOK7*.

SEX AND LIFE SPAN CONSIDERATIONS

The incidence of MG is estimated to be two cases in 1 million individuals in the United States. In people in the age range of 20 to 30 years, women are more often affected than men; in the later years (over age 40 years), men are more likely to be affected than women. Infants and children are also at risk for MG. Neonatal MG occurs in 10% to 20% of infants with birthing parents who are myasthenic. Symptoms occur within a few days after birth and usually last about 1 to 2 weeks. This short-term form of MG in infants is associated with the circulating maternal antibodies. MG may be congenital; in this case, it occurs in two forms. One form consists primarily of ocular weakness with some extremity weakness. The second form primarily involves bulbar weakness (weakness of the lips, tongue, mouth, larynx, and pharynx) with some ocular impairment; it characteristically is not associated with elevated ACh antibody titers. Juvenile MG begins with symptoms in the preteen years.

HEALTH DISPARITIES AND SEXUAL/GENDER MINORITY HEALTH

Black women have a slightly higher incidence of MG as compared to White women. Black and White men have approximately the same incidence. Sexual and gender minority status has no known effect on the risk for MG.

GLOBAL HEALTH CONSIDERATIONS

Prevalence of MG in the United States and other developed countries is approximately the same, but the prevalence may be slightly higher in Asian children. Few data are available regarding the prevalence in developing countries.

ASSESSMENT

HISTORY. The patient may experience a wide range of signs and symptoms. Elicit a careful history of the patient's symptoms and pay particular attention to changes that involve the eyes, which are often the earliest signs of MG. These changes include ptosis (eyelid drooping), diplopia (double vision), reduced eye closure, and blurred vision. Ask if the patient has to tilt the head back to see properly. Patients describe painless, specific muscle weakness, and in addition to the eye muscles, bulbar (muscles innervated by lower cranial nerves, VII to XII) and proximal limb muscles are involved. Question the patient about weight loss because of problems with chewing and swallowing. Determine the patient's ability to perform sustained or repetitive movements of the extremities, such as brushing the hair or carrying groceries. Determine if the symptoms are milder in the morning, worsen as the day progresses, and subside after short rest periods. Ask the patient if the head bobs when the patient is tired or if the jaw hangs open.

PHYSICAL EXAMINATION. You may note a masklike or "snarling" appearance because of the **involvement of the facial muscles.** Patients may experience **ptosis (drooping eyelids).** Note if the patient has **weak neck muscles that cause difficulty in maintaining head position that increases as the day progresses.** Assess the patient's posture and body alignment because the patient may slouch or walk with a slow gait. The patient's voice may fade during conversation. Determine the symmetry of muscle strength and movement. Perform an eye examination to determine visual acuity and eye movement, which are often abnormal. When you auscultate the patient's lungs, you may hear decreased breath sounds resulting from hypoventilation.

The patient who has confirmed MG may develop acute exacerbations, which can occur in two forms: myasthenic or cholinergic crisis. Myasthenic crisis is caused by undermedication and is also characterized by hypoxia (associated with tachycardia and possible elevated blood pressure), absence of the cough and gag reflexes, ptosis, diplopia and mydriasis (large pupils), and a positive response to the medication edrophonium (Tensilon). In comparison, a cholinergic crisis results from excessive anticholinesterase medication and is likely to occur within 45 to 60 minutes after the last drug dose. Side effects of overmedication include diarrhea and abdominal cramping, bradycardia and possible hypotension, a flushed diaphoretic appearance, miosis (small pupils), and increased secretions (saliva, tears, and bronchial secretions). Response to Tensilon is negative, and twitching and "thick tongue" dysphagia may occur.

PSYCHOSOCIAL. The course of MG is unpredictable because of its exacerbations and remissions. Patients live in fear of not being able to breathe adequately. Depression may occur in patients who experience exacerbations and functional limitations in their lifestyles and role responsibilities. Assess the family's support system and ability to deal with chronic disease and any emergency situation that may occur.

Diagnostic Highlights

Test	Normal Result	Abnormality With Condition	Explanation
Anti-acetylcholine receptor (AChR) antibody	Negative	Positive	Reliable for diagnosing autoimmune MG; positive result for anti-AChR antibody (Ab) in 74% of patients; positive in 90% of patients with generalized myasthenia; positive in 50%–70% of those with ocular myasthenia
Electromyography, motor and sensory nerve conduction studies, compound muscle action potentials, repetitive nerve stimulation, single fiber electromyography	Normal response to repeated nerve stimulation	Decremental response to repetitive nerve stimulation	Skeletal muscle action potential is tested to determine the response to repeated stimulations

Edrophonium (Tensilon) Test: After administration, there is a marked, temporary improvement of strength; administration of 10 mg of edrophonium IV over 30 seconds determines if blocking cholinesterase improves symptoms temporarily. Additional tests include antistriated muscle antibody, anti-MuSK (muscle-specific kinase) antibody, anti-lipoprotein-related protein 4 antibody, antistriational antibody, anti-agrin antibody, radiography, computed tomography.

PRIMARY NURSING DIAGNOSIS

DIAGNOSIS. Ineffective airway clearance related to difficulty in swallowing and aspiration as evidenced by choking, wheezing, and/or respiratory distress

OUTCOMES. Respiratory status: Airway patency; Respiratory Status: Gas exchange; Respiratory status: Ventilation; Symptom severity; Comfort status; Symptom control

INTERVENTIONS. Airway management; Airway suctioning; Oxygen therapy; Airway insertion and stabilization; Cough enhancement; Mechanical ventilation: Invasive/noninvasive; Positioning; Respiratory monitoring

PLANNING AND IMPLEMENTATION

Collaborative

There is no cure for MG; while management is predominantly pharmacologic, MG is treatable. Plasmapheresis is reserved for patients who are refractory to conventional therapy, during myasthenic or cholinergic crisis, for prethymectomy stabilization and possible reduction in postthymectomy ventilator therapy, or if unacceptable drug side effects develop. Plasmapheresis separates and removes circulating AChR antibodies from the patient's blood. A thymectomy is indicated for patients with a thymoma and for other selected patients with generalized MG. Thymectomy increases the chance of remission, increases long-term survival, decreases the chance of relapse after stopping immunosuppressant therapy, and allows better control of the disease. Thymectomy is most effective if it is performed early in the disease course. Improvement is recognized in 60% to 70% of patients who undergo thymectomy and coincides with complete remission in 20% to 40% of cases (although this remission may require several years to occur). In addition to the drugs in the following table, immunoglobulins and monoclonal antibodies may be used.

Pharmacologic Highlights

Medication or Drug Class	Dosage	Description	Rationale
Anticholinesterase drugs	Varies with drug	Pyridostigmine bromide (Mestinon), neostigmine; neostigmine methylsulfate can be given as a continuous infusion if the patient cannot take oral medication, edrophonium (Enlon)	Block the action of the enzyme anticholinesterase, thereby producing symptomatic improvement; atropine must be readily available to treat cholinergic side effects, and medications must be administered on time, or the patient may be too weak or unable to swallow the drug
Prednisone	60–80 mg PO qd followed by tapering to alternate-day regime of lowest effective dose	Prednisone	Suppresses the autoimmune activity of MG; methylprednisolone may be used
Immunomodulators	Varies with drug	Azathioprine (Imuran), cyclophosphamide (Cytoxin), cyclosporine, methotrexate	Suppress autoimmune activity when patients do not respond to prednisone; can produce extreme immunosuppression and toxic side effects

Independent

The primary nursing concerns focus on the adequacy of the patient's airway and breathing. Keep suction equipment and intubation supplies at the patient's bedside.

For meals, place the patient in a completely upright position. Instruct the patient to swallow only when the chin is tipped downward and never to speak with food in the mouth. To prevent pulmonary complications, encourage the patient to perform deep breathing and coughing to enhance ventilation. If the patient requires surgery, instruct the patient on chest splinting during deep-breathing and coughing exercises. Keep the patient's pain under control before all breathing exercises.

Ensure adequate nutritional intake and observe for signs and symptoms of dehydration or malnutrition. Work with the patient and family to plan for foods that are easy to chew and swallow but are still appealing to the patient. Plan mealtime to make the most of the patient's energy peaks. Assist the patient in developing a method for reliable communication. Fear of sudden respiratory distress and the inability to call for help or to reach a call light is very real. If the patient requires hospitalization, locate the patient near the nurses' station, keep a call light nearby at all times, and provide a secondary "call" system (such as a different-toned bell) for use during times of distress. Emphasize clear, honest communication about the realistic expectations of therapy because the time between initiation of the intervention and when the patient experiences improvement can be quite prolonged.

Because treatment and improvement revolve around receiving the optimal dosages of medication, teach patients to recognize their disease status and the indications for self-determined dosage alterations to achieve an optimally effective drug benefit. Also teach the patients how to recognize the early signs of an overdose in order to prevent cholinergic crisis and when to self-medicate with atropine for relief of side effects. Involve the patient in decision making and recognize the patient's ability to manage the disease. Because these patients are frequently responsible for determining drug alterations at home, denying their judgment in determining drug dosages can cause them to feel very vulnerable and insecure. Delays in receiving their medications can cause distrust and may result in significant physical difficulty in swallowing the delayed medication. Incorporate the patient's input on plans for scheduling physical activities around rest periods.

Assist the patient in working through any feelings of depression that can occur because of MG's profound effect on lifestyle, roles, and responsibilities. Depression can also result from the disbelief by others of the MG diagnosis because the patient may appear to have suspiciously fluctuating symptoms. Provide encouragement to these patients to live full, productive lives. Educate the family and significant others on the fluctuation of MG, and place them in contact with support groups and the Myasthenia Gravis Foundation of America.

Evidence-Based Practice and Health Policy

Alanazy, M., Binabbad, R., Alromaih, N., Almansour, R., Alanazi, S., Alhamdi, M., Alazwary, J., & Mualqil, T. (2020). Severity and depression can impact quality of life in patients with myasthenia gravis. *Muscle & Nerve, 61,* 69–73.

- The revised 15-item Myasthenia Gravis (MG) Quality of Life Questionnaire (MGQoL15R) is a validated scale of quality of life in patients with MG. The authors aimed to study the factors causing the variability within the Arabic version of the instrument. The authors administered a standard questionnaire ($N = 118$) and analyzed sociodemographic variables, clinical factors, Patient Health Questionnaire-9 (PHQ9-A), and Generalized Anxiety Disorder-7 (GAD7-A) and compared them to the variability in the MGQoL15R-A.
- The MGQoL15R-A was highly correlated with PHQ9-A and moderately correlated with GAD7-A. The findings suggest that quality of life may be affected by uncontrolled MG status, current relapse, and higher number of MG therapies. MG severity and depressive symptoms can affect the MGQoL15R-A score.

DOCUMENTATION GUIDELINES

- Respiratory status: Rate, quality, depth, ease, breath sounds, arterial hemoglobin saturation with oxygen
- Ability to chew, swallow, and speak (swallowing can be subjectively rated by the patient in anticipating ability to swallow food [0 = unable to swallow liquids to 5 = able to swallow regular diet]), food intake, daily weights
- Muscle weakness and strength, speed and degree of fatigue, ability to perform activities of daily living, response to rest, and plans for modification of activity
- Ptosis (can be rated by the nurse [0 = unable to open lid to 5 = uppermost edge of iris visible])

DISCHARGE AND HOME HEALTHCARE GUIDELINES

Instruct the patient and family on the importance of rest and avoiding fatigue. Be alert to factors that can cause exacerbations, such as infection (an annual flu shot is suggested), surgery, pregnancy, exposure to extreme temperatures, and tonic and alcoholic drinks. Instruct the patient and family about drug actions and side effects, the indications for dosage alteration, and the selective use of atropine for any overdose. Stress the importance of taking the medication in a timely manner. It is advisable to time the dose 1 hour before meals for best chewing and swallowing. Explain the potential drug interactions (especially aminoglycosides and neuromuscular blocking agents, which include many pesticides). Encourage the patient to inform the dentist, ophthalmologist, and pharmacist of the myasthenic condition.

Instruct patients about the symptoms that require emergency treatment and encourage them to locate a neurologist familiar with MG management for any follow-up needs. Suggest that they collect a packet of literature to take to the emergency department in case the available physician is unfamiliar with this disease. (*Myasthenia Gravis: A Manual for the Health Care Provider* is available on request from the MG Foundation of America.)

Instruct patients to wear MG identification jewelry. Suggest having an "emergency code" to alert family if they are too weak to speak (such as ringing the phone twice and hanging up). Instruct the family about cardiopulmonary resuscitation techniques, how to perform the

Heimlich maneuver, how to contact the rescue squad, and how to explain the route to the hospital. Make a referral to a vocational rehabilitation center if guidance for modifying the home or work environment, such as a raised seat and handrail for the toilet, would be beneficial.

Myocardial Infarction

DRG Category:	233
Mean LOS:	12.8 days
Description:	SURGICAL: Coronary Bypass With Cardiac Catheterization With Major Complication or Comorbidity
DRG Category:	234
Mean LOS:	8.6 days
Description:	SURGICAL: Coronary Bypass With Cardiac Catheterization Without Major Complication or Comorbidity
DRG Category:	235
Mean LOS:	9.8 days
Description:	SURGICAL: Coronary Bypass Without Cardiac Catheterization With Major Complication or Comorbidity
DRG Category:	236
Mean LOS:	6.4 days
Description:	SURGICAL: Coronary Bypass Without Cardiac Catheterization Without Major Complication or Comorbidity
DRG Category:	280
Mean LOS:	5.4 days
Description:	MEDICAL: Acute Myocardial Infarction, Discharged Alive With Major Complication or Comorbidity
DRG Category:	315
Mean LOS:	3.8 days
Description:	MEDICAL: Other Circulatory System Diagnoses With Complication or Comorbidity

Myocardial infarction (MI) is myocardial cell death due to prolonged ischemia. Estimates are that approximately 500,000 to 700,000 deaths occur from coronary artery disease in the United States each year, and approximately 1.5 million cases of MI occur each year. It is one of the leading causes of death and is associated with a high mortality rate. One-third of patients die before they arrive at the hospital, and 40% are dead upon arrival. Approximately 5% to 10%

of people following an MI die during their first 12 months after diagnosis, and almost 50% are rehospitalized during the first year post MI. Acute MI is divided into two categories, non–ST-segment elevation MI (NSTEMI) and ST-segment elevation MI (STEMI). NSTEMI resembles unstable angina and has the absence of biomarker elevation. STEMI has the presence of symptoms of myocardial ischemia and injury along with persistent ST-segment elevation and positive biomarkers (see Diagnostic Highlights).

When myocardial tissue is deprived of oxygenated blood supply for a period of time, an area of myocardial necrosis develops; this necrosis is surrounded by injured and ischemic tissue. The area of infarction corresponds with the distribution of the circulation from the obstructed vessel. Pain usually develops from irritation of nerve endings in the ischemic and injured areas. The typical chest pain for adult males is a substernal, crushing pain that radiates down the left arm and up into the jaw. Women and older patients with MIs often experience an indigestion-type discomfort and shortness of breath instead of the "typical" substernal pressure.

Infarctions may be classified according to myocardial thickness and the location of affected tissue. Although the majority of MIs occur in the left ventricle, more right ventricular involvement is being recognized. Left ventricular infarctions are classified as inferior (diaphragmatic), anterior, and posterior. Right ventricular infarctions are usually not differentiated by a specific location. Transmural (full-thickness), or Q-wave, infarctions involve 50% or more of the total thickness of the ventricular wall and are characterized by abnormal Q waves and ST-T wave changes. Partial-thickness infarctions (also called *subendocardial, nontransmural,* and *non–Q-wave* infarcts) are characterized by ST-T wave changes but no abnormal Q waves. Partial-thickness infarctions do not extend through the full thickness of the ventricular wall.

Complications of MI include cardiac dysrhythmias, extension of the area of infarction, heart failure, and pericarditis. Rupture of the atrial or ventricular septum, valvular rupture, or rupture of the ventricles can occur as well. Other complications include ventricular aneurysms, mitral valve regurgitation, and cerebral and pulmonary emboli.

CAUSES

The cause of acute MI is decreased coronary blood flow to the heart muscle. The available oxygen supply cannot meet the oxygen demand, leading to cardiac ischemia. The most common event leading to MI occurs as an atherosclerotic plaque ruptures, leading to thrombosis and decreased blood flow in the coronary arteries. Other causes include spasms of the coronary arteries; cocaine-induced ischemia; and blockage of the coronary arteries by embolism of thrombi, fatty plaques, air, or calcium. MI can also be caused by multiple trauma, vasculitis, aortic dissection, hyperthyroidism, and anemia. Multiple risk factors have been identified for coronary artery disease and MI. Some factors—such as age, family history, and sex—cannot be modified.

Modifiable risk factors include cigarette smoking, which causes arterial vasoconstriction and increases plaque formation. A diet high in saturated fats, cholesterol, sugar, salt, and total calories increases the risk for MIs, as does poor oral hygiene. Elevated serum cholesterol and low-density lipoprotein levels increase the chance for atherosclerosis. Hypertension and obesity increase the workload of the heart, and diabetes mellitus decreases the circulation to the heart muscle. Hostility and stress may also increase sympathetic nervous system activity and pose risk. A sedentary lifestyle diminishes collateral circulation and decreases the strength of the cardiac muscle. Medications can also cause risks. Oral contraceptives may enhance thrombus formation, cocaine use can cause coronary artery spasm, and anabolic steroid use can accelerate atherosclerosis.

GENETIC CONSIDERATIONS

Many MI risk factors such as diabetes mellitus, cholesterol levels, and hypertension have genetic contributions. However, family history is an independent risk factor indicating that susceptibility genes in addition to those involved in producing identified risk factors are probably involved. Heritability is estimated at 50% to 60%, and possibly 45 candidate loci have been identified as possibly influencing risk. Notable polymorphisms that increase risk include those in the connexin 37 gene, the plasminogen-activator inhibitor type 1 gene, and the stromelysin-1 gene. Susceptibility to premature MI has been mapped to the genes *LRP8* and *ALOX5AP*.

SEX AND LIFE SPAN CONSIDERATIONS

Cardiovascular disease is the single largest cause of death among American men and women. The risk of ischemic heart disease increases with age and when predispositions to atherosclerosis (smoking, hypertension, diabetes mellitus, hyperlipoproteinemia) are present. Nearly 10% of MIs occur in people under age 40 years, and 45% occur in people under age 65 years. MIs also occur in young adults, such as individuals who use cocaine, those who are insulin-dependent diabetics, and those who have hypercholesterolemia and a positive family history for early coronary disease.

Both men and women are at risk for MI. Up until age 70 years, more men than women have MIs, and the death rate is three times higher for men than women. Women have higher morbidity rates after MI than men. This increase in morbidity may occur because they are older and have more preexisting diseases than men. Women with chest pain also delay seeking treatment longer than men. Premenopausal women have the benefit of protective estrogens and a lower hematocrit, although heart disease is on the rise in this population, possibly because of an increased rate of smoking in women. Once women become postmenopausal, their risk for MI increases. Gender disparities have been found for women with respect to the management of MI. Women are less likely than men to be treated with evidence-based protocols and less likely to receive coronary angiography, immediate invasive management such as coronary angioplasty, and secondary prevention therapies.

HEALTH DISPARITIES AND SEXUAL/GENDER MINORITY HEALTH

The Centers for Disease Control and Prevention report that 11.5% of White persons, 9.5% of Black persons, 7.4% of Hispanic persons, and 6.0% of Asian persons have coronary heart disease. When considering acute MI, the incidence in Black males exceeds that of White males, and the incidence in Black females exceeds that of White females. Significant health disparities exist in the cardiac care of underrepresented groups as compared to White persons. Black and Hispanic people are known to receive care less often guided by standard cardiac care guidelines than White persons and have higher rates of adverse outcomes. Unless patients have health insurance, White patients are more likely to receive coronary angiograms and other coronary interventions than Black and Hispanic patients, who are also less likely to be referred to cardiologists and cardiac surgeons than White persons (Batchelor et al., 2019).

Transgender is a term used to describe persons whose gender identity is different from their sex assigned at birth. Approximately 1% of the U.S. population identify themselves as transgender. Sexual and gender minority persons have higher odds for multiple chronic conditions, cancer, and poor quality of life and are more apt to have disabilities than cisgender males and females. (Cisgender is a term used to describe persons whose gender identity and gender expression are aligned with their assigned sex listed on their birth certificate.) Gender-affirming hormone therapy is the use of hormone therapy for gender transition or gender affirmation and can be masculinizing or feminizing. It may also affect cardiovascular health in transgender females. In a large sample, researchers have found that transgender men and women are more likely to be overweight than cisgender women. Compared to cisgender women, transgender women reported higher rates of diabetes, ischemic stroke, angina/coronary disease, and myocardial infarction. Gender-nonconforming men and women reported higher odds of MI than cisgender women. Transgender women also had higher rates of any cardiovascular disease than cisgender men (Cacerese, Jackman, et al., 2020; Connelly et al., 2019).

GLOBAL HEALTH CONSIDERATIONS

Cardiovascular diseases (CDs) of all types cause approximately 20 million deaths globally and are the overall global leading cause of death. Experts estimate that 3 million people die of acute MI around the world each year. CDs are the primary cause of death in developed countries and cause an increasing number of deaths in developing countries. More than 75% of cardiovascular deaths in the world occur in low- and middle-income countries. In underresourced regions, experts expect that as deaths from infectious disease decrease and lifestyle becomes similar to high-resourced regions, a growing number of people will die from CDs.

⚛ ASSESSMENT

HISTORY. Symptomatology is very important in diagnosing MIs. Ask about chest, jaw, arm, and epigastric pain. Remember that not all people have the typical chest pain; evaluate the whole clinical picture because some people may experience no pain at all. Typical chest pain associated with an acute MI is intense, steady, and lasts up to an hour. Patients describe the pain as resting beneath the sternum, and on the left side, radiating up to the neck and down the left arm. Ask about shortness of breath, racing heart rate, diaphoresis, clammy skin, dizziness, nausea, and vomiting. Ask about the time the pain occurred. MI occurs most often in the early morning hours when there are increases in blood pressure, coronary artery vascular tone, blood viscosity, and cortisol levels. Note that sudden death and full cardiac arrest may be the first indication of MI.

Elicit a thorough description of the symptoms by using the P, Q, R, S, T approach. *P* stands for palliative or precipitating measures (what was occurring when the symptoms began and what made the symptoms better or worse). *Q* is the quality of the discomfort (sharp, stabbing, or pressure). *R* represents radiating. *S* is the severity of the discomfort on a scale, such as from 1 to 10. *T* stands for time since symptoms and discomfort began. The time is very important because increased time to treatment may mean increased muscle damage; time to treatment dictates management. The timing of asking these questions is also important. If the patient is in acute distress, ask the minimum number of questions necessary to treat the pain effectively and ask the additional questions later. Elicit a medical history, including tobacco and alcohol consumption, exercise patterns, and a history of previous heart disease, hypertension, and diabetes mellitus.

PHYSICAL EXAMINATION. The patient with an MI usually appears acutely ill with **chest discomfort, diaphoresis, clammy skin, nausea and vomiting,** and **shortness of breath,** but the patient may have mild symptoms, such as **epigastric discomfort.** Pain is generally intense and continuous for 30 to 60 minutes and may radiate up the neck and to the shoulder and jaw (referred pain). The patient may describe it as aching, burning, stabbing, or squeezing, but some have only mild discomfort. When you inspect the patient, note the respiratory status, including rate, depth, rhythm, and effort. Observe the patient's skin for color and diaphoresis, and observe the patient's mental status for confusion, dizziness, and anxiety.

When you auscultate the patient's heart, you may hear heart sounds that are irregular if dysrhythmias are present—an S_3 if irregular ventricular filling occurs and an S_4 if irregular atrial filling occurs. A murmur may be heard if the valves are not closing tightly because of ischemia or injury of the papillary muscle. The heart rate may be bradycardic, tachycardic, or normal, and the blood pressure may be hypotensive, hypertensive, or normal depending on the body's response to the MI.

PSYCHOSOCIAL. Inquire about stressors in the patient's life and how the patient deals with them. A diagnosis of heart disease and MI is a life-changing event that carries emotionally laden concerns for most patients. Also assess the patient's ability to cope with a sudden illness and the change in roles that an MI involves. Determine the family's response to a sudden, life-threatening illness.

Diagnostic Highlights

Test	Normal Result	Abnormality With Condition	Explanation
Cardiac troponin I (cTnI); cardiac troponin T (cTnT)	Troponin I: < 0.05 ng/mL; Troponin T: < 0.01 ng/mL	Elevated	Now considered the criterion standard for diagnosis. Cardiac troponin levels have the highest sensitivity and specificity (better than CK-MB levels) in detecting MI; used to differentiate between angina and MI; earliest increases from the onset of chest pain occur in 2–6 hr; peak increase occurs in 15–24 hr; serum levels return to baseline at 5–14 days
Electrocardiogram (ECG)	Normal PQRST pattern	ST-segment elevation, T-wave inversion, and an abnormal Q wave (wider than 0.04 sec or more than 1/3 height of QRS complex); NSTEMI versus ST-elevation myocardial infarction STEMI	Electrical conduction system adversely affected by myocardial ischemia and necrosis; Q wave occurs because necrotic cells do not conduct electrical stimuli; see Planning and Implementation for discussion of NSTEMI and STEMI
B-Type natriuretic peptide	< 100 pg/mL	Elevated	Secreted by the heart in response to excessive stretching of the cardiomyocytes. Helps predict risk for heart failure in patients with MI
Creatine kinase isoenzyme (CK-MB)	0%–4% to total CK	Elevated	Elevations occur resulting from tissue damage

MI has a specific definition based on cardiac troponin values; cardiac troponins are cardiac regulatory proteins that control the interactions between actin and myosin in the cardiac muscle fiber. Myocardial injury occurs when there is evidence of elevated cardiac troponin values with at least one value above the 99th percentile upper reference limit. MI occurs with acute myocardial injury with clinical evidence of acute myocardial ischemia and with detection of rise and fall of cTn values at least one value above the 99th percentile upper reference limit and one of the following: symptoms of myocardial ischemia; new ST-segment changes or a left bundle branch block; presence of pathological Q waves; imaging study showing new regional well motion abnormality; identification of a coronary thrombus at autopsy or angiography (American Heart Association, 2018). Other Tests: Cholesterol (total, low-density lipoprotein, high-density lipoprotein), triglycerides, lactate dehydrogenase, C-reactive protein, complete blood count, serum electrolytes, blood urea nitrogen, creatinine, myoglobin, cardiac catheterization, thallium scan, multidetector computed tomography, coronary angiography, radionuclide ventriculography, two-dimensional echocardiography

PRIMARY NURSING DIAGNOSIS

DIAGNOSIS. Risk for decreased cardiac tissue perfusion as evidenced by chest or referred pain, shortness of breath, and/or dyspnea

OUTCOMES. Cardiac pump effectiveness; Circulation status; Pain control; Pain level; Tissue perfusion: Cardiac

INTERVENTIONS. Cardiac care: Acute; Oxygen therapy; Pain management: Acute; Medication administration

☀️ PLANNING AND IMPLEMENTATION

Collaborative

The primary treatment goals are to restore the balance of oxygen supply and demand to the heart muscle, relieve the pain associated with MI, and prevent complications of MI. On the way to the hospital, the patient should receive aspirin for its antiplatelet effect and have an IV started. Nitroglycerine may be administered for active chest pain. The physician usually prescribes oxygen therapy, often at 2 to 4 L/min to provide increased oxygen to the myocardial tissue. In the initial treatment, it is important to differentiate STEMI and NSTEMI (see Diagnostic Highlights for explanation) because treatment differs. Patients with STEMI need rapid recognition and rapid reperfusion of the myocardium in order to improve outcomes. The goal is to have patients with a STEMI in the cardiac catheterization laboratory within 20 minutes of emergency department admission so that they can receive percutaneous coronary intervention (PCI) or pharmacologic reperfusion as soon as possible. Thrombolytic agents have been shown to improve survival rates in patients with acute MI. If it has been less than 4 to 6 hours since pain began and if the clinical picture suggests an MI, thrombolytic agents may be given to dissolve the coronary thrombus. If percutaneous coronary interventions are not available (see below), then thrombolytics are administered within 12 hours of onset of symptoms for patients with specific ECG changes such as ST-segment elevation, new left bundle-branch block, or ST depression consistent with posterior infarction. Second-generation fibrinolytic drugs such as tenecteplase, alteplase, or reteplase have clot selectivity and are often used.

A cardiac catheterization with PCI may be performed when the patient's condition is stable to identify the areas of blockage in the coronary arteries and to assist in determining treatment. A percutaneous transluminal coronary angioplasty may be performed if the blockages are limited and are accessible with a balloon catheter. The cardiologist inflates the balloon catheter at the area of blockage and compresses the plaque or pushes the arterial wall out to enlarge the arterial lumen. The cardiologist may also place a stent at the area of dilation to maintain patency, although this procedure is under review because of recent outcome studies questioning its usefulness. An arthrectomy, which involves shaving off the plaque in the coronary artery and removing the debris to obtain arterial patency, is another nonsurgical option.

People with NSTEMI are evaluated to determine the risk of hemodynamic and conduction (electrical) stability. They either receive early angiography with possible PCI or surgery or are managed conservatively with medical therapy. Continuous cardiac monitoring, along with intermittent 12-lead ECGs, helps the healthcare team monitor the resolution of ischemic and injured areas. Hemodynamic monitoring may be initiated, and a flow-directed pulmonary artery catheter may be used to measure filling pressures in the ventricles, to determine pulmonary artery pressures, and to calculate the cardiac output. Notify the physician for significant signs of decreased cardiac output, such as hypotension, diminished urine output, crackles in the lungs, cool and clammy skin, and fatigue.

The surgical option for patients with coronary blockages caused by plaque is coronary artery bypass grafting (CABG). To restore blood flow to the heart muscle distal to the blockages, the surgeon uses the left internal mammary artery or the saphenous vein to bypass the areas of blockage within the coronary arteries. Generally, emergency CABG occurs immediately after MI for patients with a failed angioplasty or with complications such as ventricular septal defect or papillary muscle rupture.

Diet restrictions begin in the hospital and should be continued at home. A collaborative effort among the patient, dietician, physician, and nurse plans for a diet low in cholesterol, fat, calories, and sodium (salt). Drinks in the coronary care unit are usually decaffeinated and not too hot or cold in temperature, although some experts question the need to restrict extremes of temperature. Foods with fiber may decrease the incidence of constipation.

Pharmacologic Highlights

Medication or Drug Class	Dosage	Description	Rationale
Antiplatelet therapy	Varies with drug	Aspirin, clopidogrel, ticagrelor, vorapaxar, glycoprotein IIb/IIIa antagonist such as abciximab, eptifibatide, tirofiban	Prevents formation of thrombus; inhibits platelet function by blocking cyclooxygenase
Recombinant tissue plasminogen activator (alteplase, rt-PA)	Protocols vary by drug	Thrombolytic agent; tenecteplase (TNK-tPA) is a genetically engineered variant of rt-PA with lower incidence of mild/moderate bleeding	Less likely to cause hypotension and allergic reaction than other drugs; more expensive than other agents and associated with a higher risk of intracranial hemorrhage but more efficacious
Antithrombic agents	Varies with drug	Bivalirudin, heparin, enoxaparin, dalteparin	Prevents additional thrombus formation in the coronary arteries and inhibits platelet function

Other Drugs: Vasodilators such as nitrates, beta-adrenergic blockers, calcium antagonists, or angiotensin-converting enzyme inhibitors are given to increase coronary perfusion and decrease afterload if the patient's blood pressure is adequate. Usually, the patient requires pain medication, with parenteral morphine being the drug of choice. Antidysrhythmics, sedatives, and stool softeners may be given. Antithrombotic agents include bivalirudin, heparin, enoxaparin, and dalteparin.

Independent

The focus is to control pain and related symptoms, to reduce myocardial oxygen consumption during myocardial healing, and to provide patient/family education. During the acute phase of the illness, constant monitoring of the patients' airway, breathing, and circulation is essential. Changes in cardiovascular status and occurrence of complications such as dysrhythmias or bleeding may appear rapidly and require immediate action. Remember that chest pain may indicate continued tissue damage; therefore, manage chest pain immediately. In addition to the pharmacologic methods mentioned here, a variety of measures can be used to reduce the cardiac workload during periods of chest pain. To decrease oxygen demand, encourage the patient to maintain bedrest for the first 24 hours; encourage rest throughout the entire hospitalization. Create a quiet, restful environment and encourage family involvement in the patient's care. Discourage any straining such as Valsalva maneuver.

Because anxiety and fear are common among both patient and families, encourage everyone to discuss their concerns and express their feelings. Use a calm, reassuring voice; give simple explanations about care and procedures; and stay with the patient during periods of high anxiety if possible. Discuss with the patient and family the diagnosis, activity and diet restrictions, and medical treatment. Numerous lifestyle changes may be needed. A cardiac rehabilitation program is helpful in limiting risk factors and in providing additional guidance, social support, and encouragement. The goals of a cardiac rehabilitation program are to reduce the risk of another MI through reeducation and implementation of a secondary prevention program and to improve the quality of life for the MI victim. The program provides progressive monitored exercise, additional teaching, and psychosocial support. An exercise stress test is used before beginning exercise to evaluate the patient's response to physical activity and to determine an appropriate program. There are usually three phases to cardiac rehabilitation: in hospital, outpatient, and follow-up.

Evidence-Based Practice and Health Policy

McCarthy, C., Murphy, S., Rehman, S., Jones-O'Connor, M., Olshan, D., Cohen, J., Cui, J., Singh, A., Vaduganathan, M., Januzzi, J., & Wasfy, J. (2020). Home-time after discharge among patients with type 2 myocardial infarction. *Journal of the American Heart Association*. Advance online publication. https://doi.org/10.1161/JAHA.119.015978

- Home-time, defined as the time spent alive outside of a healthcare institution, has emerged as a patient-centered health outcome. The authors wanted to learn the discharge locations and distribution of home-time after a type 2 MI, defined as an MI with an identifiable imbalance between myocardial oxygen supply and demand unrelated to a coronary thrombus. The authors reviewed the medical records of 359 patients admitted during an 8-month period.
- Of those discharged alive ($N = 321$), 62.9% were discharged to home, and the remainder went to a facility or hospice. Among those with available follow-up data ($N = 289$), the median home-time was 30 days at 30 days, 171 days at 180 days, and 347 days at 365 days. At 1 year, 29 patients with type 2 MI had spent no time at home, and only 57 patients spent the entire year alive and at home. At 1 year, postdischarge mortality was 23.2%, readmission was 69.2%, and major adverse cardiovascular events (recurrent MI, stroke) was 34.9%. The authors concluded that home-time was low after hospitalization for a type 2 MI.

DOCUMENTATION GUIDELINES

- Response to vasodilators and pain medications, signs of bleeding or complication from medications
- Physical findings of cardiac functions: Vital signs, heart sounds, breath sounds, urine output, peripheral pulses, level of consciousness
- Psychosocial response to treatment and diagnosis
- Presence of complications: Bleeding tendencies, respiratory distress, unrelieved chest pain, constipation

DISCHARGE AND HOME HEALTHCARE GUIDELINES

Be sure the patient understands all the medications, including the dosage, route, action, and adverse effects. Instruct the patient to keep the nitroglycerin bottle sealed and away from heat. The medication may lose its potency after the bottle has been opened for 6 months. If the patient does not feel a sensation when the tablet is put under the tongue or does not get a headache, the pills may have lost their potency.

Explain the need to treat recurrent chest pain or MI discomfort with sublingual nitroglycerin every 5 minutes for three doses. If the pain persists for 20 minutes, teach the patient to seek medical attention. If the patient has severe pain or becomes short of breath with chest pain, teach the patient to take nitroglycerin and seek medical attention right away. Explore mechanisms to implement diet control, an exercise program, and smoking cessation if appropriate.

Myocarditis

DRG Category:	2
Mean LOS:	20.6 days
Description:	SURGICAL: Heart Transplant or Implant of Heart Assist System Without Major Complication or Comorbidity
DRG Category:	315
Mean LOS:	3.6 days
Description:	MEDICAL: Other Circulatory System Diagnoses With Complication or Comorbidity

Myocarditis is an inflammatory condition of the cardiac muscle, with infiltration of the myocardium with lymphocytes, eosinophils, neutrophils, or giant cells that leads to necrosis or degeneration of myocytes (heart muscle cells). It usually occurs in otherwise healthy people and can lead to a range of symptoms from mild to life threatening. The actual incidence of myocarditis is unknown; many people are asymptomatic or have symptoms that may not be attributed to myocarditis. For this reason, a significant number of otherwise unexplained sudden deaths in young people and following childbirth may actually be due to the condition. Some experts suggest that from 1% to 2% of sudden and unexpected deaths can be attributed to myocarditis.

Myocarditis can be acute or chronic. Although it commonly is self-limiting, mild, and asymptomatic, it sometimes induces myofibril degeneration, which leads to right- and left-sided heart failure. When myocarditis recurs, it can produce chronic valvulitis (usually when it results from rheumatic fever), dysrhythmias, thromboembolism, cardiomyopathy, or heart failure, which are the primary complications of the condition.

CAUSES

Myocarditis generally occurs as a result of an infectious agent. In the United States, the most common cause of myocarditis is viral infection (e.g., coxsackie [group B], adenovirus, hepatitis C, cytomegalovirus, Epstein-Barr virus). Estimates are that up to 5% of patients with acute viral infections may have myocarditis. Other causes include a variety of bacterial, protozoal, parasitic, helminthic (e.g., trichinosis), and rickettsial infections that can produce inflammation of the heart. It also can be caused by an autoimmune response in conditions such as celiac disease, Crohn disease, rheumatoid arthritis, and systemic lupus erythematosus. Toxic reactions to radiation or other physical agents, such as lead, may lead to the condition, as may a variety of drugs, such as phenothiazines, lithium, and chronic use of cocaine. Damage occurs because of the toxic effects of the causative agent, a secondary immune response triggered by the causative agent, or an abnormal trigger of cell death (apoptosis).

GENETIC CONSIDERATIONS

Heritable immune responses could be protective or increase susceptibility to myocarditis. Animal studies indicate that inactivation of the *CLU* gene exacerbates the progression of and the damage inflicted by autoimmune myocarditis. Some recent studies have demonstrated some genetic susceptibility loci (*IL1A*, *ITPKC*, *CASP3*, *FCGR2A*, *BLK*, and *CD40*) to developing Kawasaki disease, which often leads to myocarditis.

SEX AND LIFE SPAN CONSIDERATIONS

Myocarditis can occur at any age and in both sexes, but males are slightly more affected than females. In the United States, myocarditis most typically occurs in the fifth decade of life.

HEALTH DISPARITIES AND SEXUAL/GENDER MINORITY HEALTH

A type of myocarditis, peripartum cardiomyopathy, usually develops in the last month of pregnancy or within 5 months after delivery. It is more common in Black women than other women. Experts have found that Black and Hispanic children hospitalized with myocarditis are more likely to die than White children (Olsen et al., 2021). Sexual and gender minority status has no known effect on the risk for myocarditis.

GLOBAL HEALTH CONSIDERATIONS

Myocarditis is diagnosed in all regions of the world. In several South American countries, a common cause of myocarditis is Chagas disease, which is caused by insect bites infected with the parasite *Trypanosoma cruzi*. Infants and immunosuppressed adults are at risk for Chagas disease, particularly in Bolivia, Brazil, El Salvador, Honduras, Paraguay, Ecuador, Argentina, and Chile. Estimates are as high as 18 million people who are infected in those countries, with an estimated 20,000 deaths a year. Children bear the highest burden of mortality from Chagas disease, and death is most commonly caused by myocarditis.

ASSESSMENT

HISTORY. Establish a history of chest pain, fatigue, shortness of breath, muscle pain, and fever. Ask the patient to describe any chest pain or soreness, including the onset, location, intensity, and duration of the pain. Question the patient about recent onset (usually within 1 to 2 weeks) of flu-like symptoms such as fever, joint pain, lethargy, or upper respiratory infection. Some patients may experience a sudden episode of heart failure, syncope, or ventricular dysrhythmias. Determine if the patient has experienced excessive tachycardia, both at rest and with effort. Elicit a history of medication use, particularly the use of phenothiazines, lithium, or cocaine. Ask if the patient has been exposed to radiation or lead or has undergone radiation therapy for lung or breast cancer. Determine if the patient has been previously diagnosed with autoimmune conditions or rheumatic fever, infectious mononucleosis, polio, mumps, trichinosis, sarcoidosis, or typhoid. Develop a history of recent upper respiratory tract infections, including viral pharyngitis and tonsillitis. Ask if the patient has recently traveled to South America.

PHYSICAL EXAMINATION. The most common symptoms are **malaise, fatigue, chest pain, dyspnea, palpitations, myalgias**, and **fever**. Although myocarditis is generally uncomplicated and self-limiting, it may induce myofibril degeneration that results in right and left heart failure. When heart failure progresses, a number of changes can occur. Inspect the patient for signs of cardiomegaly, neck vein distention, dyspnea, resting or exertional tachycardia that is disproportionate to the degree of fever, and supraventricular and ventricular dysrhythmias. Palpation may reveal a left ventricular heave. Auscultate for pericardial friction rub and, with heart failure, crackles in the lungs and an S_3 heart sound. Auscultate breath sounds and heart sounds one to two times every 8 hours. Assess for signs and symptoms of decreased cardiac output (decreased urine output, delayed capillary refill, dizziness, syncope).

PSYCHOSOCIAL. Patients are likely to be experiencing severe anxiety, even fear, because the condition involves their heart. Determine the patients' knowledge of heart disease and the meaning that the diagnosis represents in their life. Assess the patient's emotional, financial, and social resources to manage the disease.

Diagnostic Highlights

Test	Normal Result	Abnormality With Condition	Explanation
Cardiac troponin I (cTnI) and cardiac troponin T (cTnT)	Troponin I: < 0.05 ng/mL; troponin T: < 0.01 ng/mL	Troponin I: > 0.15 ng/mL; troponin T: > 0.01 ng/mL	Sign of inflammation and myocyte necrosis
Endomyocardial biopsy	Normal myocytes	Presence of abnormal numbers of lymphocytes; degeneration of muscle fibers	Viral infection causes damage to myocytes; endomyocardial biopsy should not be undertaken routinely unless exclusion of other causes is critical
Electrocardiogram	Normal PQRST pattern	Nonspecific ST-segment and T-wave abnormalities, sinus tachycardia, bundle branch block, AV conduction delays; evidence of pericarditis: PR-segment depression, ST-segment elevation	Inflammatory response affects the initiation and conduction of the electrical impulses of the heart
Creatine kinase isoenzyme (CK-MB)	< 4% of total CK	Elevated	Elevations occur resulting from tissue damage

Other Tests: Electrocardiogram, chest x-ray, echocardiography, magnetic resonance imaging, viral antigen, IgM antibody titers, erythrocyte sedimentation rate, complete blood count, cytokine levels, complement levels, antiheart antibody levels, troponin levels

PRIMARY NURSING DIAGNOSIS

DIAGNOSIS. Decreased cardiac output related to a reduced mechanical function of the heart muscle or valvular dysfunction as evidenced by chest pain, fatigue, shortness of breath, muscle pain, and/or fever

OUTCOMES. Cardiac pump effectiveness; Circulation status; Tissue perfusion: Pulmonary; Tissue perfusion: Abdominal organs; Tissue perfusion: Peripheral; Vital signs; Electrolyte and acid balance; Energy conservation; Fluid balance

INTERVENTIONS. Cardiac care; Fluid/electrolyte management; Medication administration; Medication management: Oxygen therapy; Vital signs monitoring

☀ PLANNING AND IMPLEMENTATION

Collaborative

The primary goal of treatment of myocarditis is to eliminate the underlying cause: antiviral medication for viral causes, IV immunoglobulin when appropriate. Patients admitted to the hospital are placed in a coronary care unit where their cardiac status can be observed via cardiac monitor. Oxygenation and rest are prescribed in order to prevent dysrhythmias and further damage to the myocardium. Apply intermittent compression boots, as prescribed, to prevent the complications of thrombophlebitis.

Fluid management is important. Congestive heart failure responds to routine management, including digitalization, angiotensin-converting enzyme inhibition, beta-adrenergic blockade, and diuretics. Patients with myocarditis appear to be particularly sensitive to digitalis. Observe for signs of digitalis toxicity such as anorexia, nausea, vomiting, blurred vision, and cardiac dysrhythmias. Patients with a low cardiac output state, which is commonly associated with severe congestive heart failure, require serial monitoring of cardiac filling pressures; a flow-directed pulmonary artery catheter has the capability of measuring cardiac output. Patients may need endotracheal intubation and mechanical ventilation. With severe heart failure, dobutamine appears valuable because of its inotropic effects with limited vasoconstrictor and arrhythmogenic properties. Intractable congestive cardiac failure or shock, or both, in a patient with acute myocarditis may indicate the need for temporary partial or total cardiopulmonary bypass and eventual cardiac transplantation.

Pharmacologic Highlights

Medication or Drug Class	Dosage	Description	Rationale
Antibiotics or antivirals	Varies with drug and causative agent	Varies with drug and causative agent	Kill pathogens

Other Drugs: To manage the primary complications of myocarditis (thromboembolism, dysrhythmia, cardiomyopathy, and heart failure), the following types of drugs might be used: angiotensin-converting enzyme inhibitors, nitroglycerin, nitroprusside, milrinone, calcium channel blockers, loop diuretics, cardiac glycosides, and beta-adrenergic blockers. The use of immunosuppression therapy is indicated for viral immune-mediated myocardial damage; however, precise drug protocols with corticosteroids, azathioprine, or cyclosporine are controversial and are generally limited to use with life-threatening complications such as intractable heart failure. IV immunoglobulins such as Gamimune, Gammagard, Gammar-P, and Sandoglobulin may be used. These preparations neutralize circulating myelin antibodies and downregulate proinflammatory cytokines.

Independent

Focus on maximizing oxygen delivery and minimizing oxygen consumption. Encourage the patient to maintain bedrest with the head of the bed elevated. Stress the importance of bedrest by assisting with bathing, as necessary, and providing a bedside commode to reduce stress on the heart. For patients with enough mobility, encourage active range-of-motion activities to prevent blood stasis. For patients who are acutely ill, extremely weak, or in cardiac failure, perform passive range-of-motion exercises. Provide regular skin care for the patient on bedrest to maintain skin integrity.

In addition to any prescribed analgesics, assist the patient with pain management by teaching relaxation techniques, guided imagery, and distractions. Encourage the patient to sit upright, leaning slightly forward, rather than lying supine. Use pillows to increase the patient's comfort.

Before discharge, be sure to teach the patient about the pathophysiology of myocarditis. Explain the prescribed medications, any potential complications, and lifestyle limitations. Reassure the patient that activity limitations are temporary and that myocarditis is generally a self-limiting condition.

Evidence-Based Practice and Health Policy

Olsen, J., Tjoeng, Y., Friedland-Little, J., & Chan, T. (2021). Racial disparities in hospital mortality among pediatric cardiomyopathy and myocarditis patients. *Pediatric Cardiology, 42,* 59–71.

- The authors proposed to study the impact of racial and ethnic characteristics for children with cardiomyopathy and myocarditis. They employed a review of medical records for children under 18 years of age ($N = 34,617$). Variables in addition to race and ethnicity included age, sex, insurance type, treatment, and noncardiac organ dysfunction.
- They found that Black and Hispanic children had a higher rate of cardiac arrest and mortality during hospitalization than White children. They suggested that these findings may be a result of differences in in-hospital care as well as response to therapy.

DOCUMENTATION GUIDELINES

- Physical findings: Signs of infection, cardiac monitoring results, breath sounds, heart sounds, intake and output, vital signs
- Laboratory results: Hemodynamic results, changes in chest x-ray
- Response to pain: Location, description, duration, response to interventions
- Response to treatment: Change in pain, temperature reduction, increased activity tolerance, understanding of medications
- Presence of complications: Myofibril degeneration, right- and left-sided heart failure

DISCHARGE AND HOME HEALTHCARE GUIDELINES

Be sure the patient and family understand any medication prescribed, including dosage, route, action, and side effects. If the patient is on immunosuppression therapy, review the medications and strategies to limit infection. Review with the patient all follow-up appointments that are scheduled. Review the need to check with the physician before resuming physical activities. Caution the patient to avoid active physical exercise during and after viral or bacterial infection. Review the nature of the disease process and signs and symptoms to report to the physician.

Nephrotic Syndrome

DRG Category:	699
Mean LOS:	4.2 days
Description:	MEDICAL: Other Kidney and Urinary Tract Diagnoses With Complication or Comorbidity

Nephrotic syndrome (NS), a clinical syndrome rather than a disease, is characterized by renal glomerular injury and massive loss of protein in the urine. There is an accompanying loss of serum albumin, an increased level of serum lipids, and massive peripheral edema.

Pathophysiological changes are caused by a defect in the glomerular basement membrane, which results in increased membrane permeability to protein, particularly albumin. Loss of albumin through the glomerular membrane reduces serum albumin and decreases colloidal oncotic pressure in the capillary vascular beds. Subsequently, fluid leaks into the interstitial spaces, collects in body cavities, and creates massive generalized edema and ascites. Interstitial fluid shifts cause a decrease in the fluid volume within the vascular bed. The vascular fluid volume deficits stimulate the renin-angiotensin system and the release of aldosterone. These compensatory mechanisms cause renal tubular reabsorption of sodium and water, which further contributes to edema formation. Some patients become markedly immunosuppressed because of the loss of the immunoglobulin G (IgG) in the urine. Enhanced urinary excretion of transferrin may lead to anemia, and loss of antithrombin III may lead to enhanced coagulation.

Complications occur because of the increased tendency for blood coagulation owing to increased blood viscosity. These changes may result in thromboembolic vascular occlusion in the kidneys, lungs, and lower extremities in particular. Other complications include accelerated atherosclerosis, acute renal failure, malnutrition, and a lowered resistance to infection.

CAUSES

Numerous factors contribute to the development of NS. Causes are classified as idiopathic as in primary disease, secondary from other diseases, and congenital (see Genetic Considerations).

Minimal change NS, the most frequent form in children and a primary cause, is associated with autoimmune changes. Other causes of idiopathic NS are several forms of glomerulonephritis and focal sclerosis of the glomeruli. The most common secondary cause is diabetic nephropathy, which occurs primarily in adults with diabetes mellitus. Secondary NS also occurs during or following a known disease process, such as cancer, HIV infection, or lupus erythematosus. It also follows risk factors such as drug toxicity (biphosphonates such as alendronate [Fosamax] or risondronate [Actonel], lithium, interferon, NSAIDs), insect stings, and venomous animal bites. Children with congenital NS require a kidney transplant for survival.

GENETIC CONSIDERATIONS

Congenital nephrotic syndrome (CNS) is a heterogenous group of disorders that presents in utero or in the first 3 months of life with edema and proteinuria. Mutations in *NPHS1* (encoding nephrin) or *NPHS2* (encoding podocin) are the most common causes of CNS. Other less common forms are caused by mutations in *WT1* or *LAMB2*. Minimal change disease is considered a complex disorder that combines the effects of multiple genes and environment.

SEX AND LIFE SPAN CONSIDERATIONS

In the pediatric population, 80% of the cases of NS are minimal change NS. Congenital NS also occurs in the pediatric population, although it is usually fatal within the first 2 years of life unless the child receives a renal transplant. In younger children (under age 8 years), more males than females develop the disease. Secondary NS occurs in all age groups but is the major causative factor in adults. Overall, more males than females develop NS, just as more males develop diabetes mellitus and chronic renal conditions. Women are more likely to develop NS from systemic lupus erythematosus as compared to chronic renal failure.

HEALTH DISPARITIES AND SEXUAL/GENDER MINORITY HEALTH

Individuals from India and Turkey are known to have an increased potential to develop the disease. Because diabetes mellitus is a major cause of NS, Native American, Hispanic, and Black persons have higher incidence of NS compared with White people, placing them more at risk for NS. Sexual and gender minority persons are also at risk for diabetes mellitus. Transgender is a term used to describe persons whose gender identity is different from their sex assigned at birth. Approximately 1% of the U.S. population identify themselves as transgender. Sexual and gender minority persons have higher odds for multiple chronic conditions, cancer, and poor quality of life, and are more apt to have disabilities than cisgender males and females. (Cisgender is a term used to describe persons whose gender identity and gender expression are aligned with their assigned sex listed on their birth certificate.) In a large sample, researchers have found that transgender men and women are more likely to be overweight than cisgender women. Compared to cisgender women, transgender women reported higher rates of diabetes, ischemic stroke, angina/coronary disease, and myocardial infarction. Transgender men and women are more prone to diabetes mellitus as they age than other groups (Cacerese, Jackman, et al., 2020; Connelly et al., 2019; Gooren & T'Sjoen, 2018) and, therefore, are at risk for NS. HIV nephropathy is a complication of HIV infection that is more common in Black persons than White persons. Because male to male sexual contact is the source for HIV transmission in 66.0% of the cases (Centers for Disease Control and Prevention, 2021), men who have sex with men are at risk for NS related to HIV infection.

GLOBAL HEALTH CONSIDERATIONS

Generally, NS seems to have the same derivation in Western countries as in developing countries. Causes may vary internationally, such as those due to schistosomal infection in Northern Africa and the Middle East.

☀ ASSESSMENT

HISTORY. Patients may report no illness before the onset of symptoms; others have a history of systemic multisystem disease, such as lupus erythematosus, diabetes mellitus, amyloidosis, or multiple myeloma, or have a history of an insect sting or venomous animal bite. Parents may report swelling of the child's face as the first symptom. Adults often report swelling of the feet and legs as the first symptom. Symptoms usually appear insidiously and may include lethargy, depression, and weight gain. The patient may describe gastrointestinal (GI) symptoms of nausea, anorexia, and diarrhea, or they may describe foamy urine. Initially, patients report periorbital edema in the morning and abdominal or extremity edema in the evening. A history of thrombophlebitis or pulmonary embolus may be the initial presenting feature.

PHYSICAL EXAMINATION. In the early stages, inspect the patient's appearance for **swelling of the face** and, particularly, **swelling around the eyes** (periorbital edema), ascites, and peripheral edema. In later stages, inspect the patient for massive generalized edema of the scrotum, labia, and abdomen. Pitting edema is usually present in dependent areas. The patient's skin appears extremely pale and fragile. You may note areas of skin erosion and breakdown. Often, urine output is decreased and may appear characteristically dark, frothy, or opalescent. Some patients have hematuria as well. Patients with severe ascites may be in acute respiratory distress, with an increase in respiratory rate and effort. When you auscultate the patient's lungs, you may hear adventitious breath sounds, such as crackles, or the breath sounds may be distant because of a pleural effusion. When you auscultate the patient's blood pressure, you may find orthostatic changes.

During the acute phases of the illness, assess the patient's fluid status by ongoing monitoring of the patient's weight, fluid intake and output, and degree of pitting edema. Measure the patient's abdominal girth daily and record changes. Monitor for signs of complications, particularly thromboembolic complications such as renal vein thrombosis (sudden flank pain, a tender costovertebral angle, macroscopic hematuria, and decreased urine output) and extremity arterial occlusion (decreased distal pulses, blanched and cold extremities, delayed capillary refill).

PSYCHOSOCIAL. Patients and family members may express fear or display signs of anxiety related to changes in the patient's appearance. The uncertain prognosis and the possibility of lifestyle changes add to their stress. Because of the insidious onset of symptoms, parents and significant others often verbalize guilt over not seeking medical attention sooner.

Diagnostic Highlights

Test	Normal Result	Abnormality With Condition	Explanation
Urinalysis	Minimal red blood cells; moderate clear protein casts; negative for protein	Increased proteinuria	Protein is lost in urine caused by loss of albumin through the glomerular membrane
24-hr urine collection	Minimal red blood cells; moderate clear protein casts; negative for protein	> 3.5 g per day of proteinuria	Protein is lost in urine caused by loss of albumin through the glomerular membrane
Serum albumin	3.4–5.2 g/dL	Decreased	Albumin is lost in urine

Other Tests: Creatinine, blood urea nitrogen, renal biopsy, cholesterol, triglycerides, serum potassium (hypokalemia is common), renal ultrasound

PRIMARY NURSING DIAGNOSIS

DIAGNOSIS. Excess fluid volume related to excessive serum protein loss and resultant volume shifts out of vascular bed as evidenced by facial edema, peripheral edema, and/or ascites

OUTCOMES. Fluid balance; Hydration; Circulation status; Cardiac pump effectiveness; Vital signs; Knowledge: Disease process

INTERVENTIONS. Fluid monitoring; Fluid/electrolyte management; IV therapy; Circulatory care

░ PLANNING AND IMPLEMENTATION

Collaborative

Treatment depends on the cause of NS. For children with idiopathic NS, corticosteroids are the primary treatment along with other immunosuppressive agents. In adults, treatment is also primarily pharmacologic (see Pharmacologic Highlights). Edema is controlled by restricting salt to 2 g/day and administering diuretics. Dietary alterations also include a diet of adequate protein (1 g/kg of body weight/day) with restrictions of cholesterol and saturated fat. Additional dietary protein has not been found to be of value. If the patient has accompanying renal insufficiency, restriction of dietary protein may complicate the dietary plan. Most patients need nutritional consultation with a dietitian to identify an appropriate diet within the restrictions. Involve the patient, parents, or significant others in the meal selection to ensure that the diet is appealing to the patient.

In spite of the excessive edema, patients need to be monitored for dehydration and hypokalemia, particularly when they are on diuretic therapy. Discuss the optimal fluid intake for the patient with the physician so that the patient is well hydrated and yet does not have continued fluid retention. Patients need to maintain an adequate fluid intake and a diet high in potassium (unless they have renal insufficiency).

Pharmacologic Highlights

Medication or Drug Class	Dosage	Description	Rationale
Prednisone (Orasone)	1 mg/kg per day PO until < 3 g protein per day in urine	Glucocorticoid	Decreases permeability of glomerulus to protein; initiated as soon as possible after the diagnosis of NS is confirmed; rituximab (antibody against B cells) is used in children
Cyclophosphamide (Cytoxan)	2 mg/kg per day PO for 8 wk	Antineoplastic; immunomodulators	For patients who respond poorly to glucocorticoids; cyclosporine may also be used
Angiotensin-converting enzyme (ACE) inhibitors and angiotensin II receptor blockers	Varies by drug	ACE inhibitor	Prevents conversion of angiotensin I to angiotensin II; reduces blood pressure by reducing vasoconstriction

Other Drugs: The physician may prescribe diuretics (furosemide, spironolactone) if respiratory compromise from edema occurs or if edema causes tissue breakdown. Some patients may also receive parenteral albumin to raise the oncotic pressure within the vascular bed. Acute thrombolytic episodes may require fibrinolytic agents such as streptokinase or surgical thrombectomy.

Independent

Focus on maintaining the patient's fluid balance, promoting skin care, preventing nosocomial infection, and providing supportive measures. To maintain the patient's skin integrity, turn the patient every 2 hours. Observe the skin closely for areas of breakdown until the edema resolves. Use an eggcrate mattress or specialty bed to limit irritation to skin pressure points and encourage the patient or parents to avoid tight-fitting clothing and diapers.

Note that both the medications and the disease process may lead to immunosuppression. Implement scrupulous infection control measures, such as hand washing, sterile technique with invasive procedures, and clean technique for all noninvasive procedures to reduce the chance of infection. Do not assign patients to rooms with other patients who have infectious processes. Encourage visitation, but ask visitors with infections to wait until they are infection free before visiting. To limit the risk of blood clotting, encourage the patient to be as mobile as possible considering the underlying condition. If the patient is bedridden, use active and passive range-of-motion exercises at least every 4 hours and have the patient wear compression boots when immobile in bed.

Note that some patients have a disturbed body image because of the side effects of steroid therapy (moon face, increased facial and body hair, abdominal distention, and mood swings). Encourage the patient to express these feelings and note that they are temporary until the condition resolves and the steroids are discontinued. If the patient desires, limit visitation to immediate family only until the patient resolves the anxiety over the body image disturbance.

Evidence-Based Practice and Health Policy

Yin, D., Guo, Q., Geng, X., Song, Y., Song, J., Wang, S., Li, X., & Duan, J. (2020). The effect of inpatient pharmaceutical care on nephrotic syndrome patients after discharge: A randomized controlled trial. *International Journal of Clinical Pharmacy, 42*, 617–624.

- The authors planned to evaluate the impact of inpatient pharmaceutical care on medication adherence and clinical outcomes in patients with nephrotic syndrome. They conducted a randomized controlled trial ($N = 61$) with patients with nephrotic syndrome. The intervention consisted of medication reconciliation, pharmacist visits every day, discharge counseling, and education by two certificated pharmacists, while the control group received usual care. Assessments were performed at baseline, 1 month, 3 months, and 6 months after discharge.
- The decline in medication adherence of patients in the intervention group after hospital discharge was decreased at 6 months. However, the groups did not differ in clinical outcomes, medication discrepancies, adverse drug events, and readmission rate. Although pharmaceutical inpatient care improved adherence in patients with nephrotic syndrome after discharge, the effect of the intervention on clinical outcomes, medication differences, adverse drug events, or readmission was not significant.

DOCUMENTATION GUIDELINES

- Fluid volume parameters: Intake and output, urine character, urine specific gravity, urine protein, edema (location and degree of pitting), abdominal girth
- Condition of skin/mucous membranes: Turgor, membrane color and moisture, location of any skin breakdown (location, size, appearance, presence of drainage and character)
- Presence of GI complaints: Nausea, anorexia, diarrhea (if present, amount, frequency, color)
- Respiratory status: Rate and rhythm, lung expansion, presence of retractions or nasal flaring, adventitious breath sounds, type of expectorated secretions
- Comfort level: Type of discomfort, location, and intensity; if pain is present, describe the location, intensity (using a pain scale), and character

DISCHARGE AND HOME HEALTHCARE GUIDELINES

Teach the patient and family about the disease process, prognosis, and treatment plan. Explain that they need to monitor the urine daily for protein and keep a diary with the results of the tests. Have the patient or family demonstrate the testing techniques before discharge to demonstrate their ability to perform these monitoring tasks. Instruct the patient and family to avoid exposure to communicable diseases and to engage in scrupulous infection control measures such as frequent hand washing. Encourage patients with hypercoagulability to maintain hydration and mobility and to follow the medication regimen.

Teach the patient and family the purpose, dosage, route, desired effects, and side effects for all prescribed medications. Inform patients on anticoagulant therapy of the need for laboratory monitoring of activated partial thromboplastin time or prothrombin time. Caution patients who are receiving steroid therapy to take the dosages exactly as prescribed; explain that skipping doses could be harmful or life-threatening. In cases of long-term steroid therapy, explain the signs of complications, such as GI bleeding, stunted growth (children), bone fractures, and immunosuppression. Encourage patients to resume normal activities as soon as possible.

Neurogenic Bladder

DRG Category:	669
Mean LOS:	5.0 days
Description:	SURGICAL: Transurethral Procedures With Complication or Comorbidity
DRG Category:	700
Mean LOS:	3.0 days
Description:	MEDICAL: Other Kidney and Urinary Tract Diagnoses Without Complication or Comorbidity or Major Complication or Comorbidity

The function of the urinary bladder is to store and expel urine in an organized and controlled manner. Neurogenic bladder is defined as an interruption of normal bladder innervation because of lesions on or insults to the nervous system. Neurogenic bladder can be classified with respect to the anatomic location of the lesion that causes the condition, including supraspinal lesions, spinal lesions, and peripheral nerve lesions. Supraspinal lesions occur in the central nervous system above the pons. These conditions include stroke, brain tumor, Parkinson disease, and Shy-Drager syndrome (a rare, progressive degenerative neurological disease of the autonomic nervous system). Spinal cord lesions occur following spinal cord trauma and with multiple sclerosis. Peripheral nerve lesions occur because of chronic conditions such as diabetes mellitus or infections such as neurosyphilis and herpes zoster. Herniated disc disease and pelvic surgery can also lead to peripheral nerve lesions.

The response to these lesions varies. Almost 25% of people with stroke develop urinary retention initially, but after time the bladder may become hyperreflexic with urinary frequency, urgency, and/or incontinence. Brain tumors most commonly cause detrusor (bladder muscle) hyperreflexia, as do Parkinson disease and multiple sclerosis. Following spinal cord injury, spinal shock initially leads to flaccid paralysis below the level of injury and urinary retention, but weeks later detrusor hyperreflexia occurs. In patients with diabetes mellitus, neurogenic bladder dysfunction occurs 10 or more years after diagnosis as nerves undergo demyelination and impaired nerve conduction. Patients lose the sensation of a full bladder and then lose motor function to empty the bladder.

Many complications can result in patients with neurogenic bladder, such as bladder infection and skin breakdown related to incontinence. In addition, urolithiasis (stones in the urinary tract) is a common complication. Patients with spinal lesions above T7 are also at risk for autonomic dysreflexia, a life-threatening complication. Autonomic dysreflexia results from the body's abnormal response to stimuli such as a full bladder or a distended colon. It results in severely elevated blood pressure, flushing, diaphoresis, decreased pulse, and a pounding headache.

Chronic renal failure (CRF) can also result from chronic overfilling of the bladder, causing backup pressures throughout the renal system.

CAUSES

Neurogenic bladder results from a variety of conditions that limit normal bladder function. Supraspinal, spinal, and peripheral lesions all cause neurogenic bladder. The conditions can lead to abnormal filling and/or emptying of the bladder that is caused by diseases such as stroke, brain tumors, diabetes mellitus, and multiple sclerosis or injuries such as spinal cord trauma and pelvic surgery.

GENETIC CONSIDERATIONS

No clear genetic contributions to susceptibility have been defined.

SEX AND LIFE SPAN CONSIDERATIONS

The incidence and manifestations of neurogenic bladder dysfunction do not change with age, except that older people of both sexes are more at risk for strokes, which is a major cause of neurogenic bladder. Older persons also may have had neurological diseases longer, resulting in more sequelae such as neurogenic bladder dysfunction. The treatment plan is unmodified for older patients, except that self-catheterization may need to be modified or not used at all depending on the ability of the individual.

HEALTH DISPARITIES AND SEXUAL/GENDER MINORITY HEALTH

Ethnicity, race, and sexual/gender minority status have no known effect on the risk for neurogenic bladder.

GLOBAL HEALTH CONSIDERATIONS

While no international data are available, neurogenic bladder likely exists as a condition in all regions of the world.

ASSESSMENT

HISTORY. Take a full history of urinary voiding, including night/day patterns, amount of urine voided, and number of urinary emptyings per day. Most patients will describe a history of **urinary incontinence** and **changes in the initiation or interruption of urinary voiding**. Elicit an accurate description of the sensations during bladder filling and emptying. In patients with a hyperreflexic bladder, expect the patient to describe urinary frequency and urgency along with urge incontinence. In patients with flaccid neurogenic bladder, expect overflow urinary incontinence. Also ask patients if they have a history of frequent urinary tract infections, a complication that often accompanies neurogenic bladder.

PHYSICAL EXAMINATION. Evaluate the extent of the patient's central nervous system (CNS) involvement by performing a complete neurological assessment, including strength and motion of extremities and levels of sensation on the trunk and extremities. With a hyperreflexic bladder, the patient may have increased anal sphincter tone so that when you touch the abdomen, thigh, or genitalia, the patient may void spontaneously. Often, the patient will have residual urine in the bladder even after voiding. In patients with a flaccid neurogenic bladder, palpate and percuss the bladder to evaluate for a distended bladder; usually, the patient will not sense bladder fullness in spite of large bladder distention because of sensory deficits. In patients with urinary incontinence, evaluate the groin and perineal area for skin irritation and breakdown. Initiate a voiding diary in which the patient records all bladder activity to determine the voiding pattern.

PSYCHOSOCIAL. The patient will likely view neurogenic bladder dysfunction as one more manifestation of an already uncontrollable situation. Anxiety about voiding will be added to the anxiety about the underlying cause of the dysfunction. Urinary incontinence leads to embarrassment over the lack of control and concern over the odor of urine that often can permeate clothing and linens. Patients who perceive that the only alternative is urinary catheterization have concerns about being normally active with a catheter and may also fear sexual dysfunction.

Diagnostic Highlights

Test	Normal Result	Abnormality With Condition	Explanation
Uroflowmetry	> 200 mL, 10–20 mL/sec, depending on age	Decreased	Measures completeness and speed of bladder emptying, which are both reduced
Cystometry	Absence of residual urine; sensation of fullness at 300–500 mL; urge to void at 150–450 mL	Varies with type of dysfunction; may have residual urine and lack of sensation or urge to void	Evaluates detrusor muscle function and tonicity, determines etiology of bladder dysfunction, and differentiates among classifications of bladder dysfunction

Other Tests: Urethral pressure profile, urinalysis, urine cytology, excretory urogram, voiding cystourethrogram, cystourethroscopy, electromyography of pelvic muscles, postvoid residual bladder volume, uroflow rate, cystogram, ultrasound of bladder, serial sampling of urine for bacterial analysis, blood urea nitrogen, creatinine

PRIMARY NURSING DIAGNOSIS

DIAGNOSIS. Impaired urinary elimination related to trauma or CNS dysfunction as evidenced by difficulty voiding, urinary incontinence and/or urinary retention

OUTCOMES. Urinary continence; Urinary elimination; Infection severity; Fluid balance; Knowledge: Disease process; Knowledge: Treatment regimen; Symptom severity

INTERVENTIONS. Urinary retention care; Fluid management; Fluid monitoring; Urinary catheterization; Urinary elimination management; Urinary incontinence care

PLANNING AND IMPLEMENTATION
Collaborative
The goals for the medical management of patients include maintaining the integrity of the urinary tract, controlling or preventing infection, and preventing urinary incontinence. Many of the nonsurgical approaches to managing neurogenic bladder depend on independent nursing interventions such as the Credé method, Valsalva maneuver, or intermittent catheterization (see subsection Independent). Behavioral modification may be successful in managing urge incontinence.

Overflow incontinence is treated by emptying the bladder with a catheter. Urinary diversion can be accomplished with indwelling urethral catheters, suprapubic catheters, or intermittent catheterization. If all attempts at bladder retraining or catheterization have failed, a surgeon may perform a reconstructive procedure, such as correction of bladder neck contractures, creation of access for pelvic catheterization, or other urinary diversion procedures. Increased outlet resistance can be accomplished with periurethral bulking therapy, sling procedures, or artificial urinary sphincter implantation. Procedures that improve bladder compliance or capacity include sacral neuromodulation, botulinum toxin injection, and bladder augmentation.

Pharmacologic Highlights

Medication or Drug Class	Dosage	Description	Rationale
Anticholinergic and anti-spasmodic drugs	Varies with drug	Atropine; propantheline (Pro-Banthine); darifenacin (Enablex); Solifenacin succinate (VESIcare); dicyclomine hydrochloride (Bentyl), oxybutynin chloride; tolterodine L-tartrate, trospium	Increases bladder capacity and decreases or eliminates urge incontinence; relaxes smooth muscle of the bladder

Other Drugs: Estrogen derivatives; estrogen increases tone of urethral muscle and enhances urethral support; antispasmodic drugs; tricyclic antidepressant drugs increase norepinephrine and serotonin levels and also have a direct muscle relaxant effect on the urinary bladder.

Independent

The patient may notice bladder dysfunction initially during the acute phase of the underlying disorder, such as during recovery from a spinal cord injury. During this time, an indwelling urinary catheter is frequently in place. Ensure that the tubing is patent to prevent urine backflow and that it is taped laterally to the thigh (in men) to prevent pressure to the penoscrotal angle. Clean the catheter insertion site with soap and water at least two times a day. Before transferring the patient to a wheelchair or bedside chair, empty the urine bag and clamp the tubing to prevent reflux of urine. Encourage a high fluid intake (2–3 L/day) unless contraindicated by the patient's condition.

Bladder retraining should stimulate normal bladder function. For the patient with a spastic bladder, the objective of retraining is to increase the control over bladder function. Encourage the patient to attempt to void at specific times. Various methods of stimulating urination include applying manual pressure to the bladder (Credé maneuver), stimulating the skin of the abdomen or thighs to initiate bladder contraction, or stretching the anal sphincter with a gloved, lubricated finger. If the patient is successful, measure the voided urine and determine the residual volume by performing a temporary urinary catheterization. The goal is to increase the times between voidings and to have a concurrent decrease in residual urine amounts. Teach the patient to assess the need to void and to respond to the body's response to a full bladder, as the usual urge to void may be absent. When the residual urine amounts are routinely less than 50 mL, catheterization is usually discontinued. Note that absorbent products designed to protect the skin and clothing from urine are temporary measures until a more permanent solution occurs. Definitive interventions to decrease or eliminate urinary incontinence are available to many patients. Long-term use of absorbent products is appropriate in the care of patients when intractable incontinence persists.

If bladder retraining is not feasible (more frequently experienced when the dysfunction is related to a flaccid bladder), intermittent straight catheterization is necessary. Begin the catheterizations at specific times and measure the urine obtained. Institutions and agencies have varied policies on the maximum amount of urine that may be removed through catheterization at any one time. Self-catheterization may be taught to the patient when the patient is physically and cognitively able to learn the procedure. If this procedure is not possible, a family member may be taught the procedure for home care. Sterile technique is important in the hospital to prevent infection, although home catheterization may be accomplished with the clean technique.

If the patient demonstrates signs and symptoms of autonomic dysreflexia, place the patient in semi-Fowler position, check for any kinking or other obstruction in the urinary catheter and tubing, and initiate steps to relieve bladder pressure. These interventions may include using the bladder retraining methods to stimulate evacuation or catheterizing the patient. The anus should be checked to ascertain if constipation is causing the problem, but perform fecal assessment or evacuation cautiously to prevent further stimulation that might result in increased autonomic dysreflexia. Monitor the vital signs every 5 minutes and seek medical assistance if immediate interventions do not relieve the symptoms.

The patient's psychosocial state is essential for health maintenance. Teaching may not be effective if there are other problems that the patient believes have a higher priority. The need for a family member to perform catheterization may be highly embarrassing for both the patient and the family. Because anxiety may cause the patient to have great difficulty in performing catheterization, a relaxed, private environment is necessary. Some institutions have patient support groups for people who have neurogenic bladders; if a support group is available, suggest to the patient and significant other that they might attend. If the patient has more than the normal amount of anxiety or has ineffective coping, refer the patient for counseling.

Evidence-Based Practice and Health Policy

Wade, D., Cooper, J., Peckham, N., & Belci, M. (2020). Immunotherapy to reduce frequency of urinary tract infections in people with neurogenic bladder dysfunction: A pilot randomised, placebo-controlled trial. *Clinical Rehabilitation, 34*, 1458–1464.

- The authors implemented a feasibility study of a randomized, placebo-controlled trial design to investigate the effect of a specific immunotherapy bacterial lysate OM-89 (Uro-Vaxom) in reducing the frequency of urinary tract infections in people with neurogenic bladder dysfunction. They implemented a randomized, placebo-controlled trial focused on patients with a spinal cord injury, multiple sclerosis, transverse myelitis, or cauda equina syndrome who experienced three or more urinary tract infections treated with antibiotics in the past year. All participants took one capsule of oral OM-89 immunotherapy (6 mg) or a matching placebo. Primary outcome was occurrence of a symptomatic urinary tract infection.
- Over 6 months, 18/25 active group patients had 55 infections, and 18/23 control group patients had 47 infections. Most research and clinical procedures were practical and acceptable to participants. While the trial was not initiated to test for differences, the intervention group had more infections than the placebo group.

DOCUMENTATION GUIDELINES

- Physical findings related to intake, output, residual urine measures, presence of edema or dehydration, incontinence, autonomic dysreflexia, infection
- Response to medications, bladder retraining, and interventions to support bladder function
- Response to treatment, including patient perceptions of comfort, control of bodily functions, and ability to perform bladder evacuation procedures

DISCHARGE AND HOME HEALTHCARE GUIDELINES

The patient and significant others need to understand that although they have achieved a bladder program in the hospital, their daily rhythm may be quite different at home. They need to be encouraged to adapt the pattern of bladder evacuation to the family schedule. Teach the patient the medication dosage, action, side effects, and route of all prescribed medications.

Discuss potential complications, particularly urinary tract infection, and encourage the patient to report signs of infection to the physician immediately. Teach the patient and significant others preventive strategies, such as keeping equipment clean, good hand-washing techniques, and adequate fluid intake to limit the risk of infection. Refer the patient to an appropriate source for catheterization supplies if appropriate or refer the patient to social service for help in obtaining supplies. Discuss the potential for sexual activity with the patient; if possible, have a nurse of the same gender talk with the patient to answer questions and provide support.

Osteoarthritis

DRG Category:	461
Mean LOS:	7.6 days
Description:	SURGICAL: Bilateral or Multiple Major Joint Procedures of Lower Extremity With Major Complication or Comorbidity
DRG Category:	483
Mean LOS:	1.8 days
Description:	SURGICAL: Major Joint or Limb Reattachment Procedures of Upper Extremities
DRG Category:	553
Mean LOS:	4.9 days
Description:	MEDICAL: Bone Disease and Arthropathies With Major Complication or Comorbidity

Osteoarthritis (OA), formerly called degenerative joint disease, is a progressive disorder of movable joints that is associated with aging and accumulated trauma. More than 32 million people in the United States have OA, making it the most common type of joint disease. Weight-bearing joints (knees, hips, cervical and lumbar spine, and feet) are the most affected. Recent evidence suggests that abnormal mechanics and release of inflammatory mediators contribute to joint defects, which are characterized by ulceration of articular (or hyaline) cartilage that leaves the underlying bone exposed. Irritation of the perichondrium (the membrane of fibrous connective tissue around the surface of cartilage) and periosteum (the fibrous membrane that forms the covering of bones except at their articular surfaces) causes a proliferation of cells at the joint margins. Extensive hypertrophic changes produce bony outgrowths or spur formations that expand into the joint, causing considerable pain and limited joint movement when they rub against each other.

Idiopathic OA (primary OA) can occur unilaterally in one or more joints and is usually associated with wear and tear of the hand, wrist, hip, and knee joints. More than half of all persons over age 65 years have evidence of idiopathic OA. Progressive joint deterioration occurs because of age-related changes to collagen and proteoglycans. As a result, joint cartilage has decreased tensile strength and reduced nutrient supply. OA is related to trauma in one or two joints, particularly the knees. The course of the disease is slow and progressive, without exacerbations and remissions. Patients may experience limitations that range from minor finger discomfort to severe disability of the hip or knee joints. Complications include reduced range of motion, pathological fractures, deformities, immobility, and bone necrosis.

CAUSES

Specific causes of OA are not known. While OA was considered a noninflammatory condition, increasingly experts are finding that inflammatory mediators are released into the joint and surrounding cartilage, bone, and synovial fluid. Predisposing factors have been identified. Aging, overweight and obesity, low body weight, trauma, and familial tendencies are known risk factors. Other risk factors include muscle weakness, infection, inflammatory arthritis, Paget disease, joint injuries, bleeding into the joint, joint abnormalities, and excessive joint use, as in certain occupations such as high-impact sports, construction work, and dance. Modifiable risk factors include body weight, cigarette smoking, low physical activity, estrogen deficiency, alcohol abuse, and recurrent falls.

GENETIC CONSIDERATIONS

OA is a complex disorder combining the effects of multiple genes and environment, but the genetic component may be significant. Identical twins have been found to have five times the risk of developing severe OA in the knee or hip than the nonidentical twins with which they were contrasted. Over 90 susceptibility loci for OA have been reported, demonstrating the need for further studies to determine the mechanism of increased risk.

SEX AND LIFE SPAN CONSIDERATIONS

Symptoms of OA generally begin after age 40 years and are more common in women than in men after age 55 years. Approximately 90% of people over age 65 years have evidence on radiography of OA. Women have OA of the distal interphalangeal joints of the hand and the knee joints more frequently than do men, but OA of the hip is more common in men than in women.

HEALTH DISPARITIES AND SEXUAL/GENDER MINORITY HEALTH

Idiopathic OA affects all groups but is more prevalent among Native American persons. Veterans with OA, particularly those who are female, of low income, and Black, have higher rates of reported incidences of discrimination, more severe pain symptoms, and more depression than other groups (McClendon et al., 2021). Researchers have found that Black persons have more radiographic knee changes than other groups. However, Black patients in the United States have lower rates of arthroplasty, which along with knee replacement, is the only curative treatment for OA. This difference in therapy places Black patients at a disadvantage for remaining mobile (Williams et al., 2020). Sexual minority women report a higher number of risk factors for OA as compared to heterosexual women, with primary risks including current smoking and obesity (Caceres et al., 2019).

GLOBAL HEALTH CONSIDERATIONS

Globally, OA is the most common joint disease. In Europe, more people report longstanding problems with their bones and joints than they do with hypertension, headaches, depression, or asthma. Prevalence is highest in Spain, Sweden, and the Netherlands. Few data are available outside of the United States and Western Europe, but OA of the knee is common as people age in China.

ASSESSMENT

HISTORY. Symptom progression is relatively slow, even over decades. Determine if over time the patient has become less active with increasing joint pain. Establish a history of deep, aching joint pain or "grating" joint pain during motion. Determine if the pain intensifies after activity and diminishes after rest and which joints are causing discomfort. Ask if the patient is taking medication for pain and, if so, how much and how often. Ask if the patient feels stiff upon awakening. Determine the relationship of the patient's stiffness to activity or inactivity. Ask if the joints ache during weather changes. Establish a history of altered gait contractures and limited movement. Ask if the patient has a history of loss of height. Determine whether the patient has had a severe injury in the past or has worked at an occupation that may have put stress on the weight-bearing joints, such as construction work or ballet dancing. Ascertain whether a family history of OA exists.

PHYSICAL EXAMINATION. The most common symptoms are **joint pain** and **reduced mobility**. Observe the patient's standing posture and gait. Note any obvious curvature of the spine, shuffling gait, or dowager hump, which are indicators of limited joint movement and existing OA. Note if the patient uses a cane or walker. Determine the patient's ability to flex, hyperextend, and rotate the thoracic and lumbar spine. For a patient with lower back pain, place the patient in a supine position, raise the leg, and have the patient dorsiflex the foot. Intensified pain may indicate a herniated disk; if this occurs, defer the examination and report these findings to the physician. Otherwise, have the patient stand, stabilize the pelvis, and rotate the upper torso 30 degrees to the right and to the left. Support the patient if necessary and ask the patient to bend over from the waist as far as is comfortable. Then ask the patient to bend backward from the waist. Ask the patient to stand up straight and bend to each side. Note the degree of movement the patient is capable of in each maneuver.

Determine the patient's ability to bend the hips. Do not perform this assessment if the patient has had a hip prosthesis. Ask the patient to stand and extend each leg backward with the knee held straight. Have the patient lie on the back and bring each knee up to the chest. Assess internal and external rotation by having the patient turn the bent knee inward and then outward. Have the patient straighten the leg and then adduct and abduct it. Again, note the degree of movement. Listen for crepitus and observe for pain while the joint is moving.

If OA is advanced, flexion and lateral deformities of the distal interphalangeal joints occur. Inspect any nodes for redness, swelling, and tenderness. Observe the patient's hands for deformities, nodules, erythema, swelling, and asymmetry of movement. Grasp the hands and feel for sponginess and warmth. Observe for muscle wasting of the fingers. Ask the patient to extend, dorsiflex, and flex the fingers. Assess for radial and ulnar deviation. Finally, have the patient adduct and abduct the fingers. Ask the patient about the degree of pain during each of these movements.

PSYCHOSOCIAL. If patients have had the disease for some time, explore how it has affected their lives and how well they are adapting to any lifestyle changes. Trauma from occupational or accidental injuries leaves many individuals unable to work. Many older patients look forward to retirement and leisure and become depressed about the prospect of pain and limited movement.

Diagnostic Highlights

Test	Normal Result	Abnormality With Condition	Condition
X-rays	Normal structure of bones and joints	Joint deformity with deterioration of articular cartilage and formation of reactive new bone at articular surface	Joint disease leads to tissue destruction, scarring, and laying of new bone
Dual-energy x-ray-absorptiometry (DXA)	T score > 1 standard deviation (SD)	T score –1 to –2.5 SD: osteopenia; T score < –2.5 SD: osteoporosis	Measures bone mineral density and risk of fracture to determine progression of disease

Other Tests: Serum calcium, serum albumin, ionized calcium, parathyroid hormone levels, bone-specific alkaline phosphatase, erythrocyte sedimentation rate, computed tomography scan, magnetic resonance imaging, bone scan

PRIMARY NURSING DIAGNOSIS

DIAGNOSIS. Chronic pain related to joint irritation and destruction as evidenced by self-reports of pain, facial grimacing, and/or protective behavior

OUTCOMES. Comfort status; Pain control; Pain level; Symptom control; Symptom severity; Knowledge: Disease process; Knowledge: Medication; Knowledge: Pain management

INTERVENTIONS. Pain management: Chronic; Analgesic administration; Cutaneous stimulation; Heat or cold application; Exercise promotion

PLANNING AND IMPLEMENTATION

Collaborative

MEDICAL. Initial medical treatment consists of prescribing pharmacologic therapy. An appropriate ongoing exercise program, which includes teaching proper body mechanics, is prescribed by the physical therapist. Therapy may include the use of moist heat in the form of soaks and whirlpools. Hot soaks and paraffin dips may be used to relieve hand pain, and a cervical collar and hand splints may be used for painful joints. A transcutaneous electric nerve stimulator (TENS) may be particularly helpful for vertebral pain relief. The physical therapist teaches the patient to use a walker and cane if indicated. Occasionally, the patient needs to learn to manage activities of daily living in the home with the help of assistive technical aids. If considerable help is required in learning these skills, the occupational therapist becomes part of the team effort.

If the patient is overweight or obese, discuss the feasibility of weight loss and provide a referral. Reducing weight places less wear and tear on joints and may reduce symptoms. Recommend a nutritional consultation.

SURGICAL. Surgical treatment may be undertaken to restore joint function when conservative treatment is ineffective. Patients who are in relatively good physical and mental condition may be candidates for joint reconstructive surgery (arthroplasty). Other surgical procedures include débridement, to remove loose debris within a joint, and osteotomy, which involves cutting the bone to realign the joint and shift the pressure points to a less denuded area of the joint. An osteotomy requires internal fixation with wires, screws, or plates as well as limited joint movement with restricted weight-bearing for a prescribed period of time. Fusion of certain joints (arthrodesis) may be done for the vertebrae and certain smaller joints when other types of procedures have not been successful in eliminating pain. Fusion eliminates movement in the joint and therefore is undertaken as a last resort. Patients who undergo knee replacement surgery are sometimes placed on a continuous passive motion machine, which is set to put the patient's leg through an increasing range of motion and thus prevent scar tissue. Rehabilitation is essential to regain and restore joint function.

Pharmacologic Highlights

Medication or Drug Class	Dosage	Description	Rationale
NSAIDs	Varies by drug	Ibuprofen, piroxicam, fenoprofen, phenylbutazone, indomethicin, naproxen	Relieve pain and decrease inflammation
Calcium metabolism modifiers	Varies by drug	Alendronate, risedronate, calcitonin, ibandronate, zoedronic acid	Inhibits osteoclastic resorption, prevents dissolution of bone
Prednisone	10–150 mg PO qd	Corticosteroids	Decreases joint inflammation; used only for severe cases

Other Drugs: Amlodipine/celecoxib may be given in combination when treatment for both hypertension and joint pain are needed. It provides the combination of a calcium channel blocker to dilate arteries and NSAIDs to reduce inflammation. Raloxifene, a selective estrogen receptor modulator, may be used to block resorption of bone. Salicylates may be given for pain. Glucosamine and chondroitin have shown some success in reducing the pain; intra-articular injection of high-molecular-weight visco supplements, particularly hyaluronic acid, has been successful in decreasing knee pain with OA. Capsaicin (Dolorac, Capsin, Zostrix) has been used with some success for topically treating pain. Some patients may require opioids to maintain quality of life.

Independent

Teach the patient assistive techniques to manage joint pain, such as meditation, biofeedback, and distraction. When the pain is reduced and mobility improves, encourage the patient to assume more responsibility for self-care. Recommend a firm mattress or bed board for lumbar and sacral spine pain. Apply moist heat pads to relieve hip pain, and assist with gentle range-of-motion exercises. A total or partial hip replacement requires limited joint movement and restricted weight-bearing depending on the type of prosthesis and surgical approach. Preventing dislocation of the hip prosthesis is extremely important. Keep the patient from lying on the affected side. Place three pillows between the patient's legs while the patient is sleeping and when you turn the patient. Avoid hip flexion. Keep the cradle boot in place except for a brief period during a bath. Once the patient is allowed up, instruct the patient not to cross the legs while sitting and to avoid wearing shoes and stockings or bending over. After the recovery time is over, teach the patient to wear well-fitting supportive shoes and to replace worn-out heels.

Teach patients who have undergone knee replacement surgery to use a walker or crutches with limited weight-bearing. Advise the patient to use special equipment in the home, such as grab bars, shower seats, and elevated toilet seats. Assist the patient in arranging for a home health nurse to visit and evaluate the patient's functioning in the home. Assist the patient in arranging ongoing physical therapy in the home. Assist the patient with activities of daily living and teach strategies for managing self-care in the home. Teach the patient to carry out therapeutic regimens, including energy conservation. Suggest the use of a firm mattress and straight-back chairs with armrests. Show the patient how to avoid flexion contractures of the large muscle groups while sleeping and sitting. Teach the patient to avoid putting pillows under the legs while sitting and to avoid sitting in low chairs, which can cause hip flexion.

Evidence-Based Practice and Health Policy
Singh, J., & Cleveland, J. (2021). Hospitalized infections in people with osteoarthritis: A national U.S. study. *Journal of Rheumatology*, *48*, 933–939.

- The authors aimed to study the incidence, time-trends, and outcomes of serious infections in people with OA. Using a national database, they examined the epidemiology of five serious infections (opportunistic infections, skin and soft tissue infections, urinary tract infection, pneumonia, and sepsis/bacteremia) in people with OA. They analyzed factors associated with healthcare utilization (hospital charges, length of hospital stay, discharge to nonhome setting), and in-hospital mortality.
- Of approximately 50 million serious infection hospitalizations, roughly 6.5% of the cases had OA. Patients with OA were 16 years or older, more likely to be female, White, have Medicare, and be less likely to receive care at an urban teaching hospital. Serious infection rates increased from 1998–2000 to 2015–2016 in all five types of infection. In multivariable-adjusted analyses, older age, sepsis, Northeast region, urban hospital, and medium or large hospital bed size were significantly associated with higher healthcare utilization outcomes and in-hospital mortality, and Medicaid insurance, non-White race, and female sex with higher healthcare utilization. The authors concluded that serious infection rates have increased in people with OA.

DOCUMENTATION GUIDELINES

- Physical findings: Deformed joints, swollen nodes, location and duration of pain, gait, range of motion
- Response to medication, treatments, and recommendations for weight loss
- Ability to perform self-care, degree of mobility

DISCHARGE AND HOME HEALTHCARE GUIDELINES

PATIENT TEACHING. Ensure that the patient understands the need to rest every hour, space work out over several days, and get at least 8 hours of sleep at night. Ensure that the patient knows whom to call in the event of sudden severe pain (as in a subluxation) or general worsening of the existing condition. Determine whether a home-care agency needs to evaluate the home for safety equipment, such as rails and grab bars, and whether ongoing supervision is required. Explain the recommended level of activity and strategies to maintain mobility.

MEDICATIONS. Instruct patients on calcium metabolism modifiers, NSAIDs, and salicylates because they may need periodic laboratory monitoring of liver and kidney functioning. Patients need to consider drug interactions. Instruct the patient not to take over-the-counter drugs or change the dosage of NSAID medications without consulting the primary caregiver. Advise the patient to take medications with food or after meals to avoid gastrointestinal discomfort.

The Arthritis Foundation, which publishes information about arthritis, is engaged in a national education program about living with the condition. Help the patient get in touch with this organization by writing to Arthritis Foundation, 1355 Peachtree Street N.E., Suite 600, Atlanta, GA 30309, or visiting online at https://www.arthritis.org.

Osteomyelitis

DRG Category:	515
Mean LOS:	8.3 days
Description:	SURGICAL: Other Musculoskeletal System and Connective Tissue Operating Room Procedures With Complication or Comorbidity
DRG Category:	539
Mean LOS:	7.8 days
Description:	MEDICAL: Osteomyelitis With Major Complication or Comorbidity

Osteomyelitis is an infection of bone, bone marrow, and the soft tissue that surrounds the bone. It is generally caused by pyogenic (pus-producing) bacteria but may be the result of a viral or fungal infection. Osteomyelitis may be an acute or chronic condition. Acute osteomyelitis refers to an infection that is less than 1 month in duration from the time of the initial infection. Chronic osteomyelitis refers to a bone infection that persists for longer than 4 weeks or represents a persistent problem with periods of remission and exacerbations; the prevalence of chronic osteomyelitis is two cases per 10,000 people.

Osteomyelitis most commonly occurs in the long bones and, in particular, the tibia, femur, and fibula. The metaphysis (growing portion of a bone) of the distal portion of the femur and the proximal portion of the tibia are the most frequent sites because of the sluggish blood supply that occurs in those areas. After gaining entrance to the bone, the bacteria grow and form an abscess, which spreads along the shaft of the bone under the periosteum. Pressure elevates the periosteum, destroying its blood vessels and causing bone necrosis. The dead bone tissue (sequestra) cannot easily be liquefied and removed. The body's healing response is to lay new bone (involucrum) over the sequestra. However, the sequestra is a perfect environment for bacteria, and chronic osteomyelitis occurs if the bacteria are not eliminated. Complications from osteomyelitis include deep vein thrombosis, chronic infection, skeletal and joint deformities, altered growth and development, immobility, septic arthritis, septic pulmonary embolus, sepsis, and septic shock.

CAUSES

The causes of osteomyelitis are organized by primary and secondary causes. Primary osteomyelitis is hematogenous, or disseminated through the bloodstream. These are indirect infections caused by organisms that are transported through the circulation from an infection in a distant site, such as otitis media, tonsillitis, or a furuncle (boil). Hematogenous osteomyelitis may occur in an adult who has undergone surgery or examination of the genitourinary tract or whose resistance has been lowered by debilitating illness. With older patients, the infection may become localized in the vertebrae. Approximately 20% of adult osteomyelitis cases are hematogenous. Secondary osteomyelitis occurs because of trauma, surgery, or sepsis of any etiology. Any break in the skin, which normally acts as a protective barrier, can lead to direct infection. These breaks may be caused by abrasions, open fractures, or surgical instrumentation, such as the insertion of pins for skeletal traction. The most common organisms responsible for osteomyelitis are *Staphylococcus aureus*, followed by pseudomonas, Enterobacteriaceae, and hemolytic streptococcus species.

Previous trauma to a bone may predispose the area to osteomyelitis. Any delay in treatment of a fracture may also contribute to the development of osteomyelitis. Other risk factors include skin infections, diabetes mellitus, peripheral vascular disease, immune deficiency, joint replacement surgery, IV drug abuse, sickle cell anemia, and cancer.

GENETIC CONSIDERATIONS

Heritable immune responses could be protective or increase susceptibility to osteomyelitis. There is, however, a syndrome called chronic recurrent multifocal osteomyelitis (CRMO) that appears not to be infectious. CRMO with pustulosis is a recessive disorder associated with mutations in the *IL1RN* gene. Although the exact mechanism of CRMO is unknown, it appears to be related to defects in the TLR4/MAPK/inflammasome signaling cascade.

SEX AND LIFE SPAN CONSIDERATIONS

The acute form of osteomyelitis is most frequently found in children, while the chronic form is most commonly observed in adults. For unknown reasons, more males than females develop osteomyelitis. Hematogenous osteomyelitis generally occurs in boys from the ages of 1 to 12 years. Osteomyelitis in a joint is more common in children than in adults. If the epiphyseal plate is heavily infected in the child, one extremity may develop longer than the other. Adults may experience an infection as a result of malignancy, burns, pressure sores, urinary tract infections, or infections as a result of atherosclerosis and diabetes mellitus.

HEALTH DISPARITIES AND SEXUAL/GENDER MINORITY HEALTH

Ethnicity, race, and sexual/gender minority status have no known effect on the risk for osteomyelitis.

GLOBAL HEALTH CONSIDERATIONS

The overall prevalence of osteomyelitis is higher in developing regions of the world as compared to the United States and Western Europe. While the reasons for this difference are unknown, they may be associated with unavailability of appropriate treatment and increasing levels of traumatic injury in developing countries.

ASSESSMENT

HISTORY. Question the patient about any previous bone trauma, open injuries, or surgical procedures. Elicit information about the patient's general well-being, level of fatigue, and previous illnesses, specifically any infections. In the acute phase, the patient may report the characteristic signs of an infection: high temperature, chills, fever, increased pulse, nausea, diaphoresis, general weakness, and malaise. In the chronic phase, the patient may report an exacerbation characterized by low-grade fever, fatigue, pain, local redness and swelling, and purulent drainage from a sinus tract. Weight-bearing may be disturbed.

PHYSICAL EXAMINATION. Common symptoms of long bone osteomyelitis are **restricted movement of the limb, abrupt onset of fever, fatigue,** and **redness, swelling, and tenderness of the limb.** Some forms of osteomyelitis have a more insidious onset with more subtle symptoms. Examination of the area reveals local infectious symptoms, such as redness or swelling and increased warmth. A foul-smelling draining wound may be present, with an intense pain or tenderness over the affected bone; you may note muscle spasms as well. The examination may reveal problems with range of motion or limb deformity. The patient often protects the extremity by intentionally limiting movement in the joint closest to the affected area. Observe the patient's gait to identify a limp or abnormal gait.

PSYCHOSOCIAL. If the patient has an acute condition, assess the level of anxiety related to treatment plans or potential of the illness to become chronic. In the chronic condition, the patient may be depressed and discouraged. A mistrust of the healthcare team may develop if interventions do not result in permanent resolution of the infection. Chronic pain and decreased mobility can lead to long-term disability, resulting in financial burdens, changes in body image or self-image, and alteration in family or social roles.

Diagnostic Highlights

Test	Normal Result	Abnormality With Condition	Explanation
Bone scan, bone computed tomography, bone radiography	Normal bony structures	Bone changes caused by inflammation and infection	Identifies areas of infection; identifies changes in blood flow resulting from inflammation
Bone biopsy	Cultures and sensitivities are negative	Positive for infecting organism	Identifies organisms; identifies bacterial sensitivities to antibiotics
Blood cultures and sensitivities	Negative	Positive for infecting organism	Identify organisms; identify bacterial sensitivities to antibiotics; blood cultures are positive in only 50% of cases of osteomyelitis

Other Tests: Tests include complete blood count, erythrocyte sedimentation rate, C-reactive protein (an acute-phase protein), renal, bone, and hepatic blood profiles, ultrasound, and x-rays. In early stages, magnetic resonance imaging is particularly helpful.

PRIMARY NURSING DIAGNOSIS

DIAGNOSIS. Acute pain related to swelling and inflammation as evidenced by self-reports of pain, facial grimacing, and/or protective behavior

OUTCOMES. Comfort status; Pain control; Pain level; Symptom control; Symptom severity; Knowledge: Medication; Knowledge: Pain management

INTERVENTIONS. Pain management: Acute; Analgesic administration; Cutaneous stimulation; Heat/cold application; Exercise therapy: Joint mobility; Medication administration

PLANNING AND IMPLEMENTATION
Collaborative
The most critical factor in eliminating osteomyelitis is prevention. To prevent direct infections, early care of injuries that break the skin and aseptic care of surgical wounds are essential. Acute osteomyelitis is considered a surgical and medical emergency. Immediate

treatment includes antibiotic therapy, surgical drainage, and other surgical procedures as needed. Early débridement of open fractures to remove necrotic tissue limits bacterial growth. Administration of prophylactic antibiotics in patients with open fractures and after surgery to reduce fractures decreases the incidence of posttraumatic and chronic osteomyelitis. It is important for antibiotics to reach the bone before bone necrosis occurs. If treatment is delayed and necrotic bone develops, there is a decrease in effectiveness of the antibiotic to combat infection. With early treatment, the chances of effectively controlling acute osteomyelitis are quite good.

Usually patients self-limit their activity because of pain, but the joints above and below the affected part are often immobilized. A splint or a bivalved cast decreases pain and muscle spasm and supports wound healing. No weight-bearing is permitted on the affected part. Physical therapy consultation is important during the acute, chronic, and recovery phases. A diet high in calories, protein, calcium, and vitamin C is started as soon as possible to promote bone healing. If there is pus formation under the periosteum, the physician performs a needle aspiration and possibly insertion of a drainage tube to evacuate the subperiosteum area. If the response to antibiotics is slow and an abscess develops, an incision and drainage (I and D) may be done. The surgeon may place catheters in the wound for irrigation or for direct antibiotic instillation. Treatment for chronic osteomyelitis may include surgical débridement of devitalized and infected tissue so that permanent healing can take place. This operation, called a sequestrectomy, consists of the removal of the sequestrum and the overlying involucrum (sheath or covering).

Pharmacologic Highlights

Medication or Drug Class	Dosage	Description	Rationale
Antibiotics: nafcillin, ceftriaxone, cefazolin, ciprofloxacin, ceftazidime, cephalexin, clindamycin, vancomycin, linezolid, rifampin, trimethoprim-sulfamethoxazole	Varies with drug: S aureus: Nafcillin, cefazolin or cloxacillin. Methicillin-resistant S aureus: Vancomycin, ciprofloxacin. Group A or B streptococci: Clindamycin. Broad spectrum: ceftriaxone, ceftazidime. Enterococci or Escherichia coli: Ampicillin and gentamicin	Depends on cultures and sensitivities; parenteral antibiotic therapy may be continued for 4–8 wk, followed by oral antibiotics for 2–3 wk	Kill bacteria and decrease spread of infection; after open fractures and surgery, used to reduce fractures

Independent

Osteomyelitis often includes a prolonged hospital stay and in-depth preparation for long-term care in the home. Several strategies exist to manage the discomfort of fever and pain nonpharmacologically. Heat applications may decrease discomfort. Frequent positioning and distractions help with pain control. Use imagery and relaxation techniques to help control discomfort. Encourage oral fluids to prevent dehydration because of the elevated temperature and infectious process.

To prevent contamination to other areas of the body, use various types of sterile dressings to contain the exudate from draining wounds. The most common are dry, sterile dressings; dressings saturated in saline or antibiotic solution; and wet-to-dry dressings. Use aseptic technique when you change dressings and dispose of contaminated dressings appropriately. Universal precautions are extremely important to prevent cross-contamination of the wound or spread of the infection to other patients.

Handle the involved extremity carefully to avoid increasing pain and the risk of a pathological fracture. To provide support, immobilization, and comfort, the extremity may be splinted. Proper application of the splint is extremely important because an improperly applied device can result in pressure ulcers or nerve damage. Regular skin assessments and conscientious skin care are important to prevent pressure sores from bedrest. Good body alignment, appropriate positioning of the affected extremity, and frequent position changes for the rest of the body prevent complications and promote comfort. Flexion deformity or contractures may occur if the patient is permitted to maintain a position of comfort instead of a position of function. Footdrop can develop quickly in the lower extremity if the foot is not correctly supported. Promote range-of-motion, isotonic, and isometric exercises for the rest of the body to maintain joint flexibility and muscle strength.

Evidence-Based Practice and Health Policy

Matharu, J., Taylor, H., Sproat, C., Kwok, J., Brown, J., & Patel, V. (2020). Diffuse sclerosing osteomyelitis: A case series and literature review. *Oral and Maxillofacial Surgery, 129*, 437–446.

- The authors retrospectively evaluated bisphosphonate treatment outcomes in patients with diffuse sclerosing osteomyelitis (DSO) of the mandible and compared outcomes with cases using alternative treatment modalities and those reported in the current literature. They identified 11 cases and collected data on all treatment modalities with a focus on patients who underwent management with oral bisphosphonates.
- Eight of 11 patients who continued to have symptoms after failure of previous interventions were prescribed alendronic acid (70 mg once weekly) for an average of 16 months. All patients reported improvement or resolution of symptoms within 72 hours. Oral bisphosphonates appear to provide prolonged symptom relief in patients with DSO compared with previously attempted treatment strategies. The exact regimen and length of use is still being debated.

DOCUMENTATION GUIDELINES

- Appearance of extremity and wound
- Physical signs of infection: Vital signs, appearance of area, presence of weakness or malaise
- Response to medications: Pain, antipyretic, stool softeners
- Response to interventions such as surgery or débridement

DISCHARGE AND HOME HEALTHCARE GUIDELINES

Patient education varies with the etiology of osteomyelitis; an individualized teaching plan needs to be developed for each patient. Regardless of the etiology, prolonged bedrest and parenteral antibiotic therapy are usually a part of the treatment plan. Discuss the cause and treatment of osteomyelitis with the patient, along with the importance of following the treatment plan. The major issues that need to be addressed are medication administration, activity, and signs and symptoms that may require notification of the physician. Discuss the need to contact the physician if increased pain, temperature, drainage, redness, or swelling develops. Also make certain the patient understands the signs of allergic drug reactions.

Emphasize the importance of long-term antibiotics that the patient requires, including the need to continue the medication even after the symptoms disappear. If IV or central line antibiotics are prescribed at home, arrange for assistance from home healthcare nurses. Also include the family in all patient teaching. Note that significant others are often responsible for delivering the care. Have the patient or significant other not only explain all procedures but also demonstrate all techniques.

Osteoporosis

DRG Category:	553
Mean LOS:	4.9 days
Description:	MEDICAL: Bone Disease and Arthropathies With Major Complication or Comorbidity

O steoporosis is an age-related, chronic, progressive metabolic disease defined as low bone mass with structural deterioration leading to bone fragility. It is the most common metabolic bone disease in the United States, as 10 million Americans have the condition and another 43 million have low bone mass, or osteopenia. While osteoporosis can lead to devastating, life-changing consequences, long-term bone health is not always emphasized because there are no symptoms until a fracture occurs. With the aging of the U.S. population, osteoporosis is expected to increase, and hip fractures are expected to rise to 750,000 per year by 2050. Common sites for fractures are the wrist, hip, and vertebral column.

Bone demineralization results in decreased density and subsequent fractures as bone resorption occurs faster than bone formation. The general reduction in skeletal bone mass occurs as bones lose calcium and phosphate, become brittle and porous, and develop an increased susceptibility to fractures. Osteoporosis can be classified as primary or secondary. Primary osteoporosis is more common and is not associated with an underlying medical condition. Conditions such as juvenile, idiopathic postmenopausal, and age-associated osteoporosis are forms of primary osteoporosis. Secondary osteoporosis results from congenital causes or is associated with hypogonadal conditions such as anorexia nervosa and Turner syndrome, endocrine disorders, deficiency states, inflammatory diseases, neoplastic disorders, and medications such as anticonvulsants, antipsychotic drugs, furosemide, glucocorticoids, and endocrine therapies. Complications of osteoporosis include pathological, stress, and traumatic bone fractures; osteonecrosis (bone death); chondrolysis (loss of cartilage in joints); hemarthrosis (bleeding into joints); joint infection; and deterioration of tendons and ligaments.

CAUSES

The exact cause of osteoporosis is unknown, but multiple mechanisms are involved. A mild but prolonged negative calcium balance, resulting from an inadequate dietary intake of calcium, may be an important contributing factor. Declining gonadal adrenal function, faulty protein metabolism because of estrogen deficiency, and a sedentary lifestyle may also contribute. Risk factors that increase the likelihood of osteoporosis also include smoking, advanced age, heavy caffeine consumption, vitamin D deficiency, excess alcohol consumption, long-term heparin or corticosteroid use, being underweight, and the use of laxatives or antacids. In addition, patients who are postmenopausal are more susceptible to osteoporosis. Patients who have Cushing disease, Parkinson disease, rheumatoid arthritis, scoliosis, or anorexia or those who have had bilateral oophorectomy are also at greater risk. Paradoxically, both a sedentary lifestyle and excessive exercise are thought to be risk factors for osteoporosis.

GENETIC CONSIDERATIONS

It is clear that osteoporosis runs in families, with heritability estimates from 50% to 85%. Polymorphisms in the *VDR*, *COL1A1*, *CALCR*, and *PDLIM4* genes are linked to osteoporosis, along with numerous others. Currently, over 90 candidate genes have been associated with bone mineral density and osteoporosis.

SEX AND LIFE SPAN CONSIDERATIONS

Osteoporosis is the 12th leading cause of death in the United States (generally due to complications from a bone fracture), and it accounts for more than $19 billion in health-related costs each year. More than 1.5 million fractures per year occur in persons over age 45 years. The incidence in women is five times greater than in men, and approximately 50% of all women over age 65 years have symptomatic osteoporosis.

Postmenopausal osteoporosis occurs in women between ages 60 and 70 years, with wrist and vertebral fractures a common injury. In people over age 70 years, women are affected twice as often as men. One in three women over age 50 years will have a bone fracture related to osteoporosis. The mortality rate for older patients with hip fractures is more than 50%, and the resulting disability for those who live can be devastating.

HEALTH DISPARITIES AND SEXUAL/GENDER MINORITY HEALTH

White, Hispanic, and Asian persons have the highest prevalence of osteoporosis, and White women have the highest rate of hip fractures compared to other groups. Transgender is a term used to describe persons whose gender identity is different from their sex assigned at birth. Approximately 1% of the U.S. population identify themselves as transgender. Gender-affirming hormone therapy is the use of hormone therapy for gender transition or gender affirmation and can be masculinizing or feminizing (Cacerese, Jackman, et al., 2020; Connelly et al., 2019). It can also affect bone health because both sex steroids, estrogen and testosterone, are important for bone formation in puberty and bone turnover in adulthood. Current thinking is that gender-affirming therapy for adults seems to maintain or improve bone health. In children and adolescents, hormone therapy used to delay puberty (gonadotropin-releasing hormone agonists) may lead to bone loss if given without sex hormone replacement (Stevenson & Tangpricha, 2019).

GLOBAL HEALTH CONSIDERATIONS

Osteoporosis is the most common metabolic bone disease in the world. Experts estimate that osteoporosis affects over 200 million people around the globe, and up to 75 million people in developed regions have osteoporosis. In 40 years, experts expect that the global prevalence of hip fractures will more than double, and many suggest that 50% of these fractures will occur in Asia.

ASSESSMENT

HISTORY. Take a careful history of all traumatic injuries, with a particular focus on previous bone fractures. Ask if there is a family history of osteoporosis. Collect data about risk factors: age, sex, race, body frame, age of menopause onset, diet, patterns of alcohol intake, caffeine use, smoking, medications, concurrent medical conditions, and exercise habits. Ask if the patient has any hearing or vision limitations. Inquire about complaints of back pain while lifting or bending, particularly when assessing older women. Determine if there has been a loss in height. Often, patients report a height reduction of 2 to 3 inches over 20 years. If the patient has vertebral collapse, the patient may describe backache or pain that radiates around the lower trunk and is aggravated by movement.

PHYSICAL EXAMINATION. Diagnosis of osteoporosis is typically made after the patient sustains a vertebral, wrist, or hip fracture. Often, the patient is asymptomatic before admission with a bone fracture. A typical first sign of osteoporosis is vertebral collapse on bending over; sudden lower back pain that radiates around the trunk is a common symptom. Inspection of the vertebral column reveals curvature of the dorsal spine, the classic "dowager's hump." Palpation of the vertebrae that is accompanied by back pain and voluntary restriction of spinal movement is indicative of a compression vertebral fracture, which is the most common type of osteoporotic fracture. The most common area for fracture occurrence is between T8 and L3.

Evaluate the patient's gait and balance and note any pain with ambulation. Evaluate the patient's range of motion and note any limitations and pain. Gently palpate the radius to determine if Colles fracture has occurred. Palpate the hip and femur to assess for pain and fracture. Point of maximum tenderness may occur over the fracture site.

PSYCHOSOCIAL. Assess the patient's concept of body image and self-esteem if there is severe curvature of the spine. Inquire about the patient's ability to find clothing to fit, any decrease in social activity, or alterations in sexuality. Evaluate the patient's home environment; inquire about fall risks in the environment—for example, stairs, waxed floors, and scatter rugs.

Diagnostic Highlights

Test	Normal Result	Abnormality With Condition	Explanation
Dual-energy x-ray absorptiometry (DXA)	No bone loss	Bone loss > 3%; T-scores are the number of standard deviations (SD) from the mean bone density values in healthy young adults: T-score of –1 to –2.5 SD indicates osteopenia; T-score of less than –2.5 SD indicates osteoporosis; T-score of less than –2.5 SD with fragility fracture(s) indicates severe osteoporosis. Z-scores are the number of standard deviations from the normal mean value for age- and sex-matched controls	Measures bone mineral density (BMD) at several sites; for each SD reduction in BMD, the relative fracture risk increases 1.5–3 times
Bone x-rays	No bone loss	Bone loss; cannot determine bone loss until 25%–40% has occurred	Determine structure of bone

Other Tests: Complete blood count, chemistry screening, thyroid-stimulating hormone level, urinalysis, serum protein electrophoresis, serum and urine calcium levels, vitamin D level, serum phosphorus levels, alkaline phosphatase, computed tomography scan; bone-specific alkaline phosphatase, osteocalcin, carboxyterminal propeptide of type I collagen, aminoterminal propeptide of type I collagen

PRIMARY NURSING DIAGNOSIS

DIAGNOSIS. Acute pain related to fracture or joint destruction as evidenced by self-reports of pain, facial grimacing, and/or protective behavior

OUTCOMES. Comfort status; Pain control; Pain level; Symptom control; Symptom severity; Knowledge: Medication; Knowledge: Pain management

INTERVENTIONS. Pain management: Acute; Analgesic administration; Exercise therapy: Joint mobility; Exercise therapy: Ambulation; Exercise therapy: Balance; Medication administration

PLANNING AND IMPLEMENTATION

Collaborative

Nonsurgical management is directed to measures that retard bone resorption, form new bone tissue, and reduce the chance of fracture. These goals are often met through pharmacologic therapy. For the patient who has had a fracture, pain medication is prescribed to relieve pain, and a diet high in protein, vitamin C, and iron is recommended to promote bone healing. Orthotic devices are ordered to stabilize the spine and reduce pain. All patients with osteoporosis should have adequate calcium (dairy products, sardines, nuts, sunflower seeds, tofu, green leafy vegetables) and vitamin D (eggs, liver, butter, fatty fish) intake.

Consult with the physical therapist to develop an exercise plan that includes weight-bearing and strengthening exercises. Consult with the occupational therapist if self-care assistive devices are needed. Low-impact exercises, such as walking and biking, are recommended three to five times a week for 45 to 60 minutes. Balance training to reduce the risk of falls has shown to be helpful. Generally, bowling and horseback riding are discouraged. If your assessment indicates that the patients' home environment places them at risk for falls, consult with social services or a home health nurse.

Pharmacologic Highlights

Medication or Drug Class	Dosage	Description	Rationale
Calcium and vitamin supplements	1,200 mg/day PO	Mineral supplement	Prevents bone loss and supplements calcium; calcium should be taken in conjunction with vitamin D; adults should receive 800 international units (IU) of vitamin D daily
Alendronate (Fosamax)	5 mg/day PO prevention and 10 mg/day PO treatment	Bone resorption inhibitor; similar preparations with different doses are risedronate (Actonel), etidronate (Didronel), and ibandronate (Boniva)	Prevents bone loss and inhibits bone resorption

Other Drugs: Androgens and calcitonin may be ordered to decrease bone resorption. Parathyroid hormone analogues, selective estrogen receptor modulator, monoclonal antibodies. Analgesics may also be needed to manage the pain. Estrogen may be given to decrease bone resorption and halt bone loss (not used to treat postmenopausal women).

Independent

Stress the need for routine exercise of the upper and lower body and a diet high in calcium (not to exceed 1,200 mg/day) and vitamin D for all middle-aged and older women and men. If the female patient is placed on estrogen, encourage the patient to complete monthly breast self-examinations and immediately report any lumps to the physician. Teach the patient to report abnormal vaginal bleeding immediately. Emphasize the need for regular gynecological examinations. Careful monitoring of patient medications with side effects of weakness and dizziness is also warranted.

To prevent falls and other activities that could cause a fracture, a hazard-free environment is required. If the patient is hospitalized, assist the patient during ambulation in a well-lighted room and provide nonskid shoes. Maintain the patient's activity at the highest level possible. Encourage the patient to perform as many of the activities of daily living as the pain allows. Check the patient's skin daily for redness, warmth, and new sites of pain, which are all indicators of new fractures. Explain to the patient's family how easily an osteoporotic patient's bones can fracture. Check orthotic devices for proper fit, patient tolerance, and skin irritation. If surgery is needed to repair fractures, encourage verbalization of feelings about surgery, change in body image, or inability to cope with the disease progression. The patient may need reassurance to help cope with limited mobility. If possible, arrange for the patient to interact with others who have osteoporosis. Be sure to include the family or significant other in the interactions.

Evidence-Based Practice and Health Policy

Cornelissen, D., deKunder, S., Si, L., Reginster, J., Evers, S., Boonen, A., & Hiligsmann, M. (2020). Interventions to improve adherence to anti-osteoporosis medications: An updated systematic review. *Osteoporosis International, 31,* 1645–1669.

- The authors aimed to perform a systematic literature review on interventions to improve adherence to anti-osteoporosis medications. The authors conducted a review using electronic databases to search for original studies that assessed interventions to improve adherence. Variables include initiation, implementation, discontinuation, and persistence to anti-osteoporosis medications among patients with osteoporosis.
- Fifteen studies fulfilled the inclusion criteria, of which 12 were randomized controlled trials. Interventions were classified as patient education ($n = 9$), drug regimen ($n = 3$), monitoring and

supervision ($n = 2$), and interdisciplinary collaboration ($n = 1$). In most subtypes of interventions, mixed results on adherence and persistence were found. Multicomponent interventions based on patient education and counseling were the most effective interventions when aiming to increase adherence and/or persistence to osteoporosis medications. The authors concluded that patient education, monitoring and supervision, change in drug regimen, and interdisciplinary collaboration have mixed results on medication adherence and persistence, with more positive effects for multicomponent interventions with active patient involvement.

DOCUMENTATION GUIDELINES

• Physical findings of musculoskeletal assessment: Pain, mobility, numbness, curvature of the spine
• Response to pain medications, nutrition recommendations
• Reaction to exercise plan and orthotic devices

DISCHARGE AND HOME HEALTHCARE GUIDELINES

Reinforce the medication, exercise, and diet plan. Provide a hazard-free environment to prevent falls. Apply orthotic devices correctly. If appropriate, recommend that the patient remove scatter rugs, provide good lighting, and install handrails in the bathroom to reduce the risk for falls. Be sure the patient understands all medications, including the dosage, route, action, and side effects. If the patient is placed on estrogen therapy, she needs routine gynecological checkups to detect early signs of cervical cancer. Consider placement in a rehabilitation facility if a patient cannot return home. The need for physical or occupational therapy, social work, and homemaking personnel can be assessed at discharge. Facilitate the procurement of needed orthotic devices or ambulation aids before the patient goes home. The Bone Health and Osteoporosis Foundation (https://www.bonehealthandosteoporosis.org) provides information to clients regarding the disease and its treatment.

Otitis Media

DRG Category:	145
Mean LOS:	2.4 days
Description:	SURGICAL: Other Ear, Nose, Mouth, and Throat Operating Room Procedures Without Complication or Comorbidity or Major Complication or Comorbidity
DRG Category:	153
Mean LOS:	2.9 days
Description:	MEDICAL: Otitis Media and Upper Respiratory Infection Without Major Complication or Comorbidity

O titis media (OM), the most common reason for antibiotic prescription in the United States, is an infection of the middle ear that can occur in several forms. Acute otitis media (AOM) has a rapid onset with fever, otorrhea (ear discharge), otalgia (ear pain), and other signs of acute infection. OM with effusion (OME) is a middle ear effusion that lacks the signs and symptoms of an infection, whereas chronic, suppurative (pus-forming) OM is related to chronic inflammation of the middle ear that lasts 6 weeks or more. OM is common, and at least half of children have their first episode before their first birthday.

The eustachian tube protects the middle ear from secretions and allows for drainage of secretions into the nasopharynx. It also permits equalization of air pressure with atmospheric pressure in the middle ear. A mechanical obstruction of the eustachian tube can result in infection and middle ear effusion (MEE). A functional obstruction can occur with persistent collapse of the eustachian tubes, particularly in infants and young children, because the amount and stiffness of their cartilage is less than that of older children and adults. Eustachian tube obstruction leads to negative middle ear pressure and a sterile MEE. Drainage of the effusion is inhibited by impaired mucociliary action and sustained negative pressure. Contamination of the middle ear may occur from nasopharyngeal secretions and lead to infection. Because infants and young children have a shorter eustachian tube than older children, they are more susceptible to reflux of nasopharyngeal secretions into the middle ear and development of infection. Complications include persistent AOM, tympanic membrane perforation, mastoiditis, hearing loss for several months, speech delay, and cerebral thrombophlebitis. When people have chronic suppurative OM during childhood, they may experience adult tinnitus and hearing loss in adulthood.

CAUSES

Bacteria pulled into the eustachian tube leads to the accumulation of purulent fluid in the middle ear. Common bacteria include *Streptococcus pneumoniae*, *Haemophilus influenzae*, and *Moraxella catarrhalis*. The most common type of infection (40%–50% of all cases) is *S pneumoniae*, and it is the least likely to resolve without antibiotic treatment. Risk factors include upper respiratory infections, allergies, Down syndrome, bottle propping during feedings, daycare attendance, and parental smoking.

GENETIC CONSIDERATIONS

Substantial evidence supports a familial contribution to OM susceptibility. Twin studies suggest a genetic contribution between 60% and 70%. Heritability is also suggested by ethnic group variations. The frequency of infection is unusually high in American Indians and Australian aborigines and comparatively low in Africans. Some families may also be predisposed because of inherited anatomic variations in ear construction.

SEX AND LIFE SPAN CONSIDERATIONS

AOM is most common in infants and children. Approximately 70% of children younger than age 3 years develop AOM, and 20% of children have recurrent problems with otitis media. The peak number of infections occurs between 6 to 36 months and 4 to 6 years of age. Children who develop AOM during their first 12 months of life have higher risk of recurrent acute or chronic disease. Boys have more infections than girls, and there is also an increased incidence in children with cleft palates and other craniofacial anomalies.

HEALTH DISPARITIES AND SEXUAL/GENDER MINORITY HEALTH

OM is more common in Native American children than other children. Other factors, such as children attending day care, children with poor nutrition, and children living in crowded conditions seem to be related to the number of infections that children experience. Sexual and gender minority status has no known effect on the risk for OM.

GLOBAL HEALTH CONSIDERATIONS

While there are some differences in prevalence globally by region, they are primarily influenced by socioeconomic factors and climate. OM is common around the world during childhood and contributes to global childhood mortality because of intracranial complications when children are assessed late in the disease course. Developing countries bear a disproportionate burden of OM.

☀ ASSESSMENT

HISTORY. Determine the presence of risk factors by observing the child and asking the parents questions. If the child is not able to speak, ask the parents if the child has had evidence of ear pain (otalgia). In infants and young children, ear pain is often manifested by irritability, inability to sleep, and ear pulling. Parents may report that the child has more symptoms when lying down, probably due to increased eustachian tube dysfunction during a recumbent position. Discharge may drain from the inner ear if the tympanic membrane is perforated or if the child has a pre-existing tympanostomy tube. Ask if the child has demonstrated headache, lethargy, dizziness, tinnitus, and unsteady gait. Other symptoms include diarrhea, vomiting, fever, cough, sudden hearing loss, stuffy nose, rhinorrhea, and sneezing.

PHYSICAL EXAMINATION. Common symptoms include **irritability, feeding difficulty in infants, persistent fever**, and **ear tugging**. In older children and adults, **hearing loss** and **ear fullness** often occur. During an examination with an otoscope, the clinician can see a reddened, bulging tympanic membrane with poor mobility and obscured or absent landmarks. The tympanic membrane is often hypervascular and red, yellow, or purple in color rather than the normal color, which is a translucent, pale gray. Note that redness alone should not be used to diagnose AOM, particularly in a crying child. The tympanic membrane may demonstrate thin-walled, sagging bullae (bubble-like cavity) filled with yellow fluid if the child has chronic suppurative OM. Differential diagnosis includes mastoiditis, dental abscesses, sinusitis, parotitis, peritonsillar abscess, trauma, impacted teeth, and immune deficiency.

It is important for practitioners to distinguish between AOM and OME, which is more common than AOM. Antibiotics may be prescribed unnecessarily for OME, which is fluid in the middle ear without signs or symptoms of infection and is usually caused when the eustachian tube is blocked. When infection follows, the child develops signs and symptoms of AOM.

PSYCHOSOCIAL. Evaluate the parent-child interaction to determine how well the parent follows up on the child's cues. Determine the extent of the parent's knowledge about risk factors. Determine the child's feeding patterns to see if they are related to AOM risk.

Diagnostic Highlights

Test	Normal Result	Abnormality With Condition	Explanation
Tympanocentesis	Negative for fluid and infection	Positive for bacteria and fluid	Not recommended for routine screening; performed on children < 2 mo old; in older infants and children, the procedure is rarely done unless (1) the child is in a toxic state or is immunocompromised, (2) resistant infection is present, (3) there is acute pain from suppurative OM, or (4) there is no response to antibiotic therapy
Pneumatic otoscopy	Mobility of tympanic membrane	Immobility of tympanic membrane when slight pressure is applied	Used as the primary diagnostic test for OME if the child has otalgia, hearing loss, or both. A tympanometry is recommended for unclear diagnosis of OME

Other Tests: Complete blood count, tympanometry (test to examine condition of middle ear, mobility of tympanic membrane, and conduction bones by creating variations of air pressure in the ear canal)

PRIMARY NURSING DIAGNOSIS

DIAGNOSIS. Risk for infection as evidenced by fever, irritability, feeding difficulty, crying, hearing loss, and/or ear tugging

OUTCOMES. Infection severity; Immune status; Knowledge: Infection management; Symptom severity; Symptom control; Knowledge: Medication

INTERVENTIONS. Infection protection; Medication administration; Medication management; Temperature regulation; Teaching: Prescribed medication; Teaching: Disease process

▧ PLANNING AND IMPLEMENTATION

Collaborative

Once AOM is diagnosed, the primary treatment is pharmacologic. However, a current debate exists as to whether antibiotics are appropriate because of growing rates of antibiotic-resistant bacteria. Many physicians support the idea that because 60% to 90% of the infections resolve without antibiotics, treatment for all AOM may not be necessary. The American Academy of Pediatrics recommends the following protocols (Table 1):

• TABLE 1

CHILDREN'S AGES	TREATMENT
Children 6–23 mo	Antibiotics for children with a diagnosis of bilateral AOM; antibiotics for children older than 6 mo with severe signs or symptoms of pain lasting 48 hr or longer and temperature of 102.2°F (39°C) or higher
Children 6–23 mo	Antibiotics or close observation for children with nonsevere unilateral AOM
Chidren 24 mo or older	For children with unilateral or bilateral AOM, antibiotics are recommended or the provider may use close observation with follow-up. Parents should be informed to notify the provider for worsening or no improvement of symptoms after 48–72 hr of symptom onset.

Recommendations for children with OME not at risk for infection should include the watchful waiting approach for 3 months from time of onset or diagnosis. Decongestants and antihistamines are not considered helpful unless the child has allergies. Intranasal or systemic steroids are not recommended treatments for OME.

In patients with severe pain, therapeutic drainage (myringotomy) may be necessary to provide immediate relief. An incision is made that is large enough to allow for adequate drainage of the middle ear. Children who undergo this procedure need to be evaluated after approximately 14 days to determine that the infection and otoscopic signs are resolving.

Pharmacologic Highlights

Medication or Drug Class	Dosage	Description	Rationale
Amoxicillin	40 mg/kg per 24 hr tid for 10 days	Antibacterial	Treats AOM because it is usually effective against the most commonly encountered bacteria
Antibacterials	Varies with drug	Many appropriate drugs, including cefuroxime, clavulanate potassium (Augmentin), ceftriaxone, erythromycin, clarithromycin, azithromycin, sulfonamide, cefaclor	Eradicate the bacterial infection

(highlight box continues on page 886)

Pharmacologic Highlights (continued)

Other Treatments: Antimicrobial ototopical drops are indicated if the tympanic membrane is ruptured. Analgesic eardrops may help with the pain if there has been no perforation of the membrane. Acetaminophen is usually used to reduce fever. Ibuprofen may be used for moderate pain. Other drugs include antihistamine-decongestants, intranasal steroids, and mycolytics.

Independent

Explain to the parents that the symptoms should begin to resolve in 24 to 48 hours as the antibiotics take effect. If the acute signs increase in the first 24 hours despite antibiotics, the parents need to bring the child back for a return examination to rule out severe infections such as meningitis or suppurative complications. Make sure the parents understand that the child needs to receive the entire course of therapy to prevent recurrent infections. Teach the parents that supportive therapy with relief of pain and fever will increase the child's comfort. Application of heat may provide pain relief.

Instruct the parents about bottle propping, feeding infants while they are recumbent, and passive smoke exposure, all of which are risk factors for developing AOM. Breastfeeding until at least 6 months or longer has a protective effect against AOM. Encourage patients to attend follow-up appointments and to avoid requesting antibiotics unless it is absolutely necessary. If repeated infections occur and the child attends day care, parents may want to consider another situation. Pneumococcal conjugate vaccine and annual influenza vaccine administration should be based on current recommendations. Hearing tests may be recommended for additional follow-up if OME persists for longer than 3 months or if the child is at risk.

Evidence-Based Practice and Health Policy

Scott, A., Clark, J., Julien, B., Islam, F., Roos, K., Grimwood, K., Little, P., & Del Mar, C. (2019). Probiotics for preventing acute otitis media in children. *Cochrane Database of Systematic Reviews.* https://doi.org/10.1002/14651858.CD012941.pub2

- The authors aimed to assess the effects of probiotics to prevent the occurrence and reduce the severity of otitis media in children. They performed searches of electronic databases to locate randomized controlled trials of children up to age 18 years comparing probiotics with placebo, usual care, or no probiotics.
- Children taking probiotics and who were not prone to acute middle ear infections had lower infection rates, but the authors suggested that there may not be any additional benefit to probiotics in those children prone to acute middle ear infections. Probiotics decreased the proportion of children taking antibiotics for any type of infection. The authors noted that the type, duration, frequency, and administration timing of the probiotics still needs to be determined.

DOCUMENTATION GUIDELINES

- Discomfort: Character, location, duration, severity, nonverbal indicators, strategies that reduce discomfort
- Behavior: Manifestations, signs of irritability, gait, amount of crying
- Patterns of rest and activity: Sleep patterns, presence of lethargy or restlessness
- Medication management: Parents' understanding of drug therapy, response to medications
- Response to teaching: Response to parenting suggestions, understanding of follow-up appointments

DISCHARGE AND HOME HEALTHCARE GUIDELINES

Make sure the parents understand all aspects of the treatment regimen, with particular attention to taking the full course of medication therapy. Make sure the parents understand the necessity of any follow-up visits.

Ovarian Cancer

DRG Category:	737
Mean LOS:	5.0 days
Description:	SURGICAL: Uterine and Adnexa Procedures for Ovarian or Adnexal Malignancy With Complication or Comorbidity
DRG Category:	755
Mean LOS:	4.1 days
Description:	MEDICAL: Malignancy, Female Reproductive System With Complication or Comorbidity

Ovarian cancer is the primary cause of death from reproductive system malignancies in women. It ranks as fifth in cancer deaths among women (American Cancer Society [ACS], 2021). In 2021, the ACS estimates that in the United States, 21,140 new cases of ovarian cancer will be diagnosed, and 13,770 women will die. The 5-year survival rate for localized ovarian cancer is 93% and for distant ovarian cancer is 31%. Only 20% of the cases are diagnosed before metastasis has occurred (ACS, 2021). In the last 10 years, the death rate from ovarian cancer has been decreasing 2% each year.

Three types of ovarian cancers exist owing to three main types of tissue in the ovary: primary epithelial tumors, germ cell tumors, and gonadal stromal (sex cord) tumors. Primary epithelial tumors comprise approximately 90% of all ovarian cancers and include serous and mucinous cystadenocarcinomas, endometrioid tumors, and mesonephric tumors. They arise in the ovarian epithelium (known as *müllerian epithelium*). Germ cell tumors, which arise from an ovum, include endodermal sinus malignant tumors, embryonal carcinoma, immature teratomas, and dysgerminoma. Sex cord tumors, which arise from the ovarian stroma (the foundational support tissues of an organ), include granulosa cell tumors, thecomas, and arrhenoblastomas.

Because of the location of the ovaries in the abdominal cavity, ovarian cancers grow and spread silently until they affect the surrounding organs or cause abdominal distention. At the appearance of these symptoms, metastases to the fallopian tubes, uterus, ligaments, and other intraperitoneal organs occur. Tumors can spread through the lymph system and blood into the chest cavity. As the disease progresses, the patient experiences multiple system complications. Peripheral edema, ascites, and intestinal obstruction can complicate the course of the disease. Patients develop severe nutritional deficiencies, electrolyte disturbances, and cachexia. If the lungs are involved, the patient develops malignant recurrent pleural effusions.

CAUSES

Although several theories exist, the exact cause of ovarian cancer is unknown; many factors, however, seem to play a role in its development. Experts have recently suggested that the majority of tumors originate in the fimbria, the threadlike structures at the end of the fallopian tube that reach toward the ovary. During ovulation, the fibers get incorporated into the ovary, where they grow into a tumor. A family history of ovarian cancer places the patient at risk, as does a diet high in saturated fats. It appears that ovarian cancer occurs in patients who have more menstrual cycles (i.e., early menarche, late menopause, nulliparity, infertility, and celibacy). Exposure to asbestos and talc may place the patient at risk. Late menarche, early menopause, pregnancy, and oral contraception may offer a protective benefit by effecting ovulation suppression. Other factors that have been associated with ovarian cancer risk include use of talcum powder on the vulva, high lactose consumption, smoking, the experience of posttraumatic stress syndrome, endometriosis, and an increased height and weight.

GENETIC CONSIDERATIONS

Only 10% of ovarian cancer cases are believed to be genetic in etiology. Susceptibility to ovarian cancer coexists with breast cancer susceptibility when *BRCA1* or *BRCA2* mutations are present and may be associated with Lynch syndrome. Breast/ovarian cancer can be transmitted through families as an autosomal dominant trait from either the mother's or the father's side of the family. The likelihood that ovarian cancer is inherited increases if two or more relatives are affected with ovarian cancer or if several relatives are affected with breast and/or ovarian cancer. Genetic risk is also increased if breast and ovarian cancer occur in the same person, if there is Ashkenazi Jewish heritage, or if there are family members who carry the *BRCA1*, *BRCA2*, or *HNPCC* gene mutations. New studies have demonstrated a link between *HOX* transcription factor genes and ovarian cancer risk.

SEX AND LIFE SPAN CONSIDERATIONS

The incidence of ovarian cancer is highest in postmenopausal women, with 50% of the cases occurring in women who are older than age 63 years. In rare instances, the disease can occur in childhood and during pregnancy. In the general population, ovarian cancer occurs in 1 in 70 women; the risk is increased to 5% if one first-degree relative has the disease.

HEALTH DISPARITIES AND SEXUAL/GENDER MINORITY HEALTH

White women have higher rates of ovarian cancer than other groups, and Asian women have increased rates of ovarian cancer when they immigrate to North America or Europe from Asia. However, Black women are disproportionately affected with ovarian cancer when compared to White women, and the 5-year survival rate for Black women is 45% as compared to 38% for White women. The National Institutes of Health (https://www.cancer.gov) in the United States provide statistics and information about cancer disparities. People with low income, low health literacy, long travel distances to cancer screening sites, or who lack health insurance or paid medical leave are less likely to be treated according to cancer care guidelines. Rural women also have a poorer survival rate and are more likely to be diagnosed at a late stage of the disease (Petersen et al., 2021; Weeks et al., 2020). People who live in communities that lack clean water and clean air may be exposed to cancer-causing substances. These factors all contribute to inequities in ovarian cancer diagnosis, treatment, and outcome.

Sexual and gender minority persons have higher odds for multiple chronic conditions, cancer, and poor quality of life, and are more apt to have disabilities than cisgender males and females. (Cisgender is a term used to describe persons whose gender identity and gender expression are aligned with their assigned sex listed on their birth certificate.) Lesbian women are more likely to be overweight/obese or to smoke as compared to their heterosexual counterparts, placing them at risk for ovarian cancer (Office on Women's Health, 2019). Transgender is a term used to describe persons whose gender identity is different from their sex assigned at birth. Approximately 1% of the U.S. population identify themselves as transgender. Cancer disparities are perpetuated because sexual and gender minority people receive poor quality of care due to stigma, lack of healthcare providers' awareness, and insensitivity to the unique needs of this community. Transgender men may delay or avoid having symptoms of ovarian cancer evaluated because of discrimination based on gender identity or the emotional conflict between self-perception and physical anatomy (Cacerese, Jackman, et al., 2020; Connelly et al., 2019; Gatos, 2018).

GLOBAL HEALTH CONSIDERATIONS

The global incidence of ovarian cancer is approximately 7 per 100,000 females per year. Women who live in developed countries have a higher risk than those in developing countries, where women have high parities. Epithelial ovarian cancer occurs primarily in White women living in developed countries. The incidence is five times higher in developed than in developing countries. Scandinavian women have high rates as compared to women in other regions of Europe, and women from India and Asian countries have low risk.

ASSESSMENT

HISTORY. The patient's history may be very nonspecific, which is a reason the diagnosis often comes late. Elicit a detailed personal and family history of all cancer-related illnesses, paying particular attention to the history of female relatives. The patient's descriptions of the signs and symptoms vary with the tumor's size and location; symptoms usually do not occur until after tumor metastasis. The symptoms patients most commonly report are back and abdominal pain, fatigue, indigestion, bloating, constipation, and urinary urgency. Most patients with ovarian cancer have at least two of these symptoms. Other symptoms include urinary frequency, abdominal distention, pelvic pressure, vaginal bleeding, leg pain, and weight loss. Pelvic discomfort and acute pelvic pain may occur, and if infection, tumor rupture, or torsion has resulted, the pain may resemble that of acute appendicitis.

PHYSICAL EXAMINATION. Early signs are vague such as **bloating, abdominal distention, pelvic pain, changes in bowel patterns,** and **vaginal bleeding.** The patient often appears **thin and chronically ill.** The patient's **abdomen may be grossly distended (ascites),** but **extremities are thin and even wasted.** When you palpate the abdominal organs, you may be able to feel masses. During the vaginal examination, you may be able to palpate an ovary in postmenopausal patients that feels like the size of an ovary in premenopausal patients. An ovarian tumor may feel hard like a rock or pebble, may feel rubbery, or may have a cyst-like quality. Palpation of an irregular, nodular ("handful of knuckles"), insensitive bilateral mass in the pelvis strongly suggests the presence of an ovarian tumor. Note that swelling of a leg may be due to a venous thrombosis, and the patient may have a pleural effusion with shortness of breath, tachypnea, and cough.

PSYCHOSOCIAL. If the patient is young and needs to undergo surgery and will lose childbearing ability, determine the meaning of children to the patient and the patient's partner. Consider the patient's developmental level, financial resources, job responsibilities, home-care responsibilities, and degree of independence of any current children in the home. If the patient is a child, determine whether the parents have told the child that the child has cancer. If the prognosis of the patient's cancer is poor, determine the patient's degree of understanding of the gravity of the prognosis. Determine the effect of the patient's religion and spirituality on the course of the disease. If the patient is older, the diagnosis may make the patient and family think about their end-of-life wishes.

Diagnostic Highlights

General Comments: None of the tumor markers is specific enough to be considered for routine screening, but they are helpful in differential diagnosis of pelvic masses and to follow up treated cases.

Test	Normal Result	Abnormality With Condition	Explanation
Cancer antigen 125 (CA-125)	0–35 units/mL	Elevated in 80% of the patients	Glycoprotein antigen detected by using mouse monoclonal antibody; serial measured; elevation indicates tumor progression; decrease indicates effective antitumor treatment; limited value for screening

(highlight box continues on page 890)

Diagnostic Highlights (continued)

Test	Normal Result	Abnormality With Condition	Explanation
Transvaginal ultrasound and computed tomography scan	No masses noted	Mass visible	Uses sound waves to detect and evaluate ovarian masses
Human chorionic gonadotropin; serum α-fetoprotein	Normally are not present in nonpregnant persons	Elevated in embryonal cell carcinoma and dysgerminoma	Serially measured; elevation indicates tumor progression; decrease indicates effective antitumor treatment
Exploratory laparotomy	Negative study	Tumor is visualized	Accurate diagnosing and staging

Other Tests: Magnetic resonance imaging and sonography are useful for monitoring the course of the disease. Mammography. Upper and lower endoscopy and bowel series and IV pyelography are done to determine the extent of the disease and whether the cancer is primary or metastatic. Liver function studies, blood chemistries, and chest x-rays are also done.

PRIMARY NURSING DIAGNOSIS

DIAGNOSIS. Acute pain related to tumor invasion, tissue destruction, and organ compression as evidenced by self-reports of pain, facial grimacing, and/or protective behavior

OUTCOMES. Pain control; Comfort status; Pain level; Symptom control; Symptom severity; Knowledge: Pain management; Knowledge: Disease process; Knowledge: Medication

INTERVENTIONS. Analgesic administration; Pain management: Acute; Teaching: Prescribed medication; Medication administration

PLANNING AND IMPLEMENTATION

Collaborative

SURGICAL. Laparoscopic surgery may be used for diagnostic purposes in low-risk patients and to remove masses if the tumor is small, has a distinct border, there is no ascites present, the serum CA-125 level is normal, and there is no family history of ovarian cancer. Aggressive surgical treatment is usually used and may be followed with chemotherapy. If there is a desire to preserve the fertility of young patients, however, a conservative approach may be used if they have a unilateral encapsulated tumor. In this approach, the surgeon may resect the ovary, biopsy structures such as the omentum and uninvolved ovary, and perform peritoneal washings for cytological examination of pelvic fluid. These patients need careful follow-up with periodic diagnostic tests to determine if the tumor is metastasizing.

More typically, the surgeon performs a total abdominal hysterectomy and bilateral salpingo-oophorectomy with tumor resection. In addition, the surgeon performs an omentectomy, appendectomy, lymph node palpation with possible lymphadenectomy, and other biopsies and washings as necessary. Sometimes, the surgeon is unable to remove the tumor completely if it is wrapped around or has invaded vital organs. Monitor the patient carefully after surgery for complications such as wound infection, hemorrhage, fluid and electrolyte imbalance, and poor gas exchange. If a young patient has had both ovaries removed, the patient needs hormonal replacement beginning at puberty so that the patient develops secondary sex characteristics.

Most patients are not treated with surgery alone. In late stages, chemotherapy after surgery prolongs survival time but is primarily palliative rather than curative, although it does provide remissions in some patients. Although radiation therapy is uncommon because it depresses the bone marrow, sometimes patients receive it as an option to other treatments.

PAIN MANAGEMENT. No matter which treatment is chosen to manage the patient's cancer, pain management is an issue. Monitor the patient's pain (location, duration, frequency, precipitating factors) and administer analgesics as needed. Determine the patient's response to analgesia by asking the patient to rate pain on a scale of 0 to 10, with 0 indicating no pain and 10 indicating the worst pain the patient has experienced. Collaborate with the physician to develop a pain-management strategy that effectively keeps the patient free of pain and yet awake and alert without respiratory complications. Consider patient-controlled analgesia (PCA) as a possibility if IV medications are needed. If the patient's disease is terminal, manage the pain so that the patient has a comfortable and dignified death.

Pharmacologic Highlights

Medication or Drug Class	Dosage	Description	Rationale
Carboplatin plus paclitaxel (preferred) or cisplatin plus paclitaxel or paclitaxel and carboplatin	Varies with drug	Standard postoperative initial chemotherapy	Used after surgery to destroy cancer cells that may have spread into the abdominal cavity
Antineoplastic agents	Varies with drug	Etoposide, topotecan, gemcitabine, docetaxel, vinorelbine, ifosfamide, fluorouracil, melphalan, altretamine, bevacizumab	Inhibits cell growth and proliferation
Acetaminophen; NSAIDs; opioids; combination of opioid and NSAID	Depends on the drug and patient condition and tolerance	Analgesics	Analgesics used are determined by the severity of pain

Independent

Prevention and early detection are difficult in ovarian cancer because of the disease's lack of obvious signs and symptoms. Encourage all adolescent girls and women to have regular pelvic examinations as part of an annual checkup. When the patient is diagnosed with ovarian cancer, the patient has to manage a host of physical and emotional problems. Help the patient manage any accompanying physical discomfort with nonpharmacologic strategies and pain medications. Teach the patient relaxation techniques or guided imagery. Explain the role of diversions as a mechanism to control pain. If the patient requires hospitalization for surgery or chemotherapy, teach the patient about the route, dosage, action, and complications of analgesics so that the patient can manage pain at home knowledgeably. If the patient is discharged with a PCA system, arrange for the patient to rent the equipment and obtain the prescriptions needed to continue using it. If the patient's family does not have the financial resources to manage the needed equipment, discuss the patient's needs with a social worker or contact the American or Canadian Cancer Society for assistance.

Depression, grief, and anger are common in patients who have been diagnosed with ovarian cancer. To determine the patient's ability to cope, encourage the patient to discuss feelings, and monitor the patient for the physical signs of inability to cope, such as altered sleep patterns. Encourage the patient to express feelings without fear of being judged. Note that surgery and chemotherapy may profoundly affect the patient's and partner's sexuality. Answer any questions honestly, provide information on alternatives to traditional sexual intercourse if appropriate, and encourage the couple to seek counseling if needed. If the patient's support systems and coping mechanisms are insufficient to meet the patient's needs, help the patient find other support systems and coping mechanisms. Provide a list of support groups.

Evidence-Based Practice and Health Policy

Babic, A., Sasamoto, N., Rosner, B., Tworoger, S., Jordan, S., Risch, H., Harris, H., Rossing, M., Doherty, J., Fortner, R., Chang-Claude, J., Goodman, M., Thompson, P., Moysich, K., Ness, R., Kjaer, S., Jensen, A., Schildkraut, J., Titus, L., . . . Terry, K. (2020). Association between breastfeeding and ovarian cancer risk. *JAMA Oncology*. Advance online publication. https://doi.org/10.1001/jamaoncol.2020.0421

- The authors aimed to determine the association between breastfeeding (ever/never, duration, timing) and ovarian cancer risk overall. They compared women with ovarian cancer from a large database with control women to answer the research question. Data were collected on breastfeeding history, duration of breastfeeding, at first and last breastfeeding, and years since last breastfeeding.
- A total of 9,973 women with ovarian cancer and 13,843 controls were included. Breastfeeding was associated with a 24% lower risk of invasive ovarian cancer. Ever having breastfed was associated with reduction in risk of invasive ovarian cancer. For a single breastfeeding episode, mean breastfeeding duration of 1 to 3 months was associated with 18% lower risk, and breastfeeding for 12 or more months was associated with a 34% lower risk. The findings suggest that breastfeeding is a potentially modifiable factor that may lower the risk of ovarian cancer independent of pregnancy alone.

DOCUMENTATION GUIDELINES

- Physiological response: Vital signs, intake and output if appropriate, weight loss or gain, sleep patterns, incisional healing
- Comfort: Location, onset, duration, and intensity of pain; effectiveness of analgesics and pain-reducing techniques
- Response to therapy: Drugs, surgery, radiation, signs of postoperative complications

DISCHARGE AND HOME HEALTHCARE GUIDELINES

PREVENTION. Teach the patient the need to have regular gynecological examinations and to report any symptoms to the healthcare provider.

MEDICATIONS. Ensure that the patient understands the dosage, route, action, and side effects of any medication the patient is to take at home. Note that some of the medications require the patient to have routine laboratory tests following discharge to monitor the response.

COPING. Discuss with the patient helpful coping mechanisms. Encourage the patient to be open with the patient's partner, family, and friends about concerns. Help the patient cope with hair loss. Teach the patient cosmetic techniques to deal with hair and body changes. Explore alternative methods to medication to manage nausea and vomiting. Discuss with the family and patient whether they desire to begin end-of-life planning and hospice care.

POSTOPERATIVE. Discuss any incisional care. Encourage the patient to notify the surgeon of any unexpected wound discharge, bleeding, poor healing, or odor. Teach the patient to avoid heavy lifting, sexual intercourse, and driving until the surgeon recommends resumption.

RADIATION. Teach the patient to maintain a diet high in protein and carbohydrates and low in residue to decrease bulk. If diarrhea remains a problem, instruct the patient to notify the physician or clinic because antidiarrheal agents can be prescribed. Encourage the patient to limit exposure to others with colds because radiation tends to decrease the ability to fight infections. To decrease skin irritation, encourage the patient to wear loose-fitting clothing and avoid using heating pads, rubbing alcohol, and irritating skin preparations.

Paget Disease

DRG Category: 553
Mean LOS: 4.9 days
Description: MEDICAL: Bone Disease and
Arthropathies With Major
Complication or Comorbidity

Paget disease, or osteitis deformans, is a slowly progressing condition of bone structure characterized by increased and disorganized bone turnover. It affects approximately 4% of the U.S. population older than age 40 years. The bones affected vary, but those most commonly involved are the femur, tibia, lower spine, pelvis, and skull. It can involve only one bone (monostotic) or multiple bones (polyostotic). Initially, there is an increase in the number of osteoclasts, which leads to excessive bone resorption and a compensatory increase in osteoblastic activity to repair bone matrix. As a result, the bone is enlarged and distorted, with areas of poor mineralization that resemble a mosaic pattern. Ultimately, the bone is larger, more vascular, mechanically weaker, and therefore less able to withstand stresses and strains.

Paget disease causes bones to fracture easily, often after only a minor trauma; these fractures heal slowly and often incompletely. If the spine is involved, the vertebrae may collapse, causing paraplegia. If the skull is involved, bony impingements on the cranial nerves can lead to blindness, hearing loss, tinnitus, or vertigo. Other complications of Paget disease include osteoarthritis, hypocalcemia, renal calculi, bone sarcoma, amputation, hypertension, and gout. The disease is life threatening when it is combined with congestive heart failure because of the need for increased cardiac output to supply increased blood flow to the bones.

CAUSES

The cause of Paget disease is not known, but experts suggest that both genetics and the environment pay a role in its development. One theory suggests that it is the result of a slow viral infection, possibly measles, with a long dormant period. Autoimmune, connective tissue, and vascular disorders are possible causes. A familial tendency has also been noted. Regional differences suggest that it may have an environmental cause. Older age and heredity are the primary risk factors.

GENETIC CONSIDERATIONS

Paget disease appears to have a hereditary component. Family studies have demonstrated that there are multiple predisposition genes, including *TNFRSF11A*, *TNFRSF11B*, *ZNF687*, and *SQSTM1*, with additional loci at 5q31, 6p21.3, and 18q23. However, families with affected members have been small, making genetic studies difficult.

SEX AND LIFE SPAN CONSIDERATIONS

Paget disease occurs most frequently in people over age 40 years and is slightly more common in men than in women. The highest prevalence is in people over 65 years of age. Prevalence is difficult to determine because many people with the condition have no symptoms. Experts estimate that as many as 10% of people over age 80 years have the disease. For unknown reasons, Paget disease occurs more often in the northern United States than in southern regions, perhaps because of a higher proportion of people with Western European ancestry who live there (see Global Health Considerations).

HEALTH DISPARITIES AND SEXUAL/GENDER MINORITY HEALTH

Ethnicity, race, and sexual/gender minority status have no known effect on the risk for Paget disease.

GLOBAL HEALTH CONSIDERATIONS

Paget disease is more common in North America, Western Europe (England, France, Spain, Italy, Greece, and Germany but not Scandinavia), Australia, and Argentina near Buenos Aires than in other regions of the globe, perhaps because those areas were settled by people from Western Europe. Paget disease is more common in Black people living in the United States than in Africa, but whether that difference occurs because of genetic or environmental reasons is unknown. Paget disease is rare in Asian countries.

ASSESSMENT

HISTORY. Because many people are asymptomatic, Paget disease is frequently discovered as a result of x-rays taken during a routine physical examination. Ask if the patient has experienced deep, dull, constant bone pain. Establish a history of bone fractures. The femur is the most common site for fracture in Paget disease. Ask if the patient's hat size has changed or if the patient has experienced headaches or tinnitus. Elicit any history of decreased hearing or vision or of vertigo. Find out if the patient has noticed any changes in gait while walking or has experienced any difficulty breathing (possibly caused by kyphosis of the spine).

PHYSICAL EXAMINATION. **Although most people with Paget disease are asymptomatic, some present with bone pain.** Assess the patient's skeleton for deformities. Inspect the skull for enlargement, particularly in the frontal and occipital areas. Check for cranial nerve compression by testing for decreased hearing and vision, difficulty swallowing, and problems with balance. Examine legs and arms for bowing and subsequent deformities. Ask the patient to walk across the room and back to observe a characteristic waddling gait.

Observe for signs of kyphosis. Note if the patient is bent forward with the chin resting on the chest or has a barrel chest. Kyphosis can compromise chest excursion and cause dyspnea. Palpate the affected areas for increased warmth. Paget disease causes an increase in vascularity of the affected bones, causing the skin temperature to rise. Elderly patients or those with large, highly vascular lesions may develop congestive heart failure because of the heart's attempt to pump more blood through bones with increased vascularity. Assess the patient's apical pulse, respirations, and blood pressure. Note the presence of peripheral edema and neck vein distention from right-sided heart failure and pulmonary congestion.

PSYCHOSOCIAL. Because the diagnosis of Paget disease is unexpected, the patient and family may experience increased anxiety levels. There may be fear related to possible falls with fractures and the possibility of self-care deficits. Social isolation may also occur as a result of increasing bone pain and deformities.

Diagnostic Highlights

Test	Normal Result	Abnormality With Condition	Explanation
X-rays	Normal structure of the skeletal system	Disordered and architecturally unsound	Disease causes increased osteoclastic bone resorption
Computed tomography; bone scan	Normal structure of the skeletal system	Enlarged bones with trabecular (small interconnecting rods of bone making up mass of spongy bone) coarsening and increased cortical thickness	Disease causes increased osteoclastic bone resorption; often used to diagnose complications
Serum alkaline phosphatase (AP); bone-specific alkaline phosphatase (BSAP)	AP: 25–142 units/L; BSAP: ≤ 22 mcg/L	Elevated	Increased osteoblastic activity and bone formation causes elevations; BSAP is more specific to Paget disease than total serum AP

Other Tests: Magnetic resonance imaging, bone biopsy, serum calcium, complete blood cell count, urinary N-telopeptide, α-C telopeptide

PRIMARY NURSING DIAGNOSIS

DIAGNOSIS. Acute pain related to fractures and nerve compression as evidenced by self-reports of pain, facial grimacing, and/or protective behavior

OUTCOMES. Comfort status; Pain control; Pain level; Symptom control; Symptom severity; Knowledge: Pain management; Knowledge: Medication

INTERVENTIONS. Pain management: Acute; Analgesic administration; Teaching: Prescribed medication; Heat application; Exercise promotion

▒ PLANNING AND IMPLEMENTATION
Collaborative

MEDICAL. Generally, patients with Paget disease who are asymptomatic require no specific treatment but need careful ongoing monitoring. Pharmacologic therapy is used when there is metabolically active bone disease, in preparation for bone surgery or joint replacement, and/or if the patient has hypercalcemia. Calcitonin and bisphosphonates are used to treat Paget disease. Patients should also receive calcium (1000–1500 mg/day) and vitamin D supplements (400 units/day). Mild pain is usually controlled successfully with NSAIDs. Nonpharmacologic treatment modalities are also prescribed for patients with Paget disease. Heat therapy and massage can help decrease pain. A physical therapy consultation can provide a protocol of simple strengthening and weight-bearing exercises. Braces and other ambulation aids may help support deformities and improve function.

SURGICAL. Surgery may be needed to reduce or prevent pathological fractures, to correct secondary deformities, and to relieve neurological impairment. Unfortunately, joint replacement is difficult because methyl methacrylate (a gluelike bonding material) does not set properly on bone that is affected by Paget disease.

Pharmacologic Highlights

Medication or Drug Class	Dosage	Description	Rationale
Bisphosphonates: alendronate (Fosamax), etidronate, pamidronate, tiludronate, risedronate, zoledronic acid	40 mg/day for 6 mo; may also use etidronate, risedronate, pamidronate, tiludronate	Bisphosphonates; calcium regulator	Slows rate of bone turnover in pagetic lesions; lowers serum alkaline phosphatase; reduces elevated cardiac output by decreasing vascularity of bone, thereby averting high-output cardiac failure
Calcitonin	100 International Unit SC or IM qd	Calcium regulator	Decreases the number and availability of osteoclasts, thereby retarding bone resorption; relieves bone pain; helps the remodeling of pagetoid bone into lamellar bone

Independent

Focus on reducing pain and immobility, preventing injury, and educating the patient about the disease and treatment regimen. Correlate the patient's pain with the patient's activities and modify schedules as needed. Instruct the patient in the use of relaxation techniques, such as guided imagery and music therapy. Evaluate the patient's level of functioning and encourage the patient to remain as active as possible. Perform range-of-motion exercises to joints, unless contraindicated, progressing from passive to active exercise as tolerated. Encourage the patient to perform self-care activities independently.

For patients on extended bedrest, reposition the patient frequently and use a flotation mattress. Prevent pressure ulcers by providing meticulous skin care.

Institute measures to prevent injury. Instruct the patient to move slowly and avoid sudden movements. Keep the environment free of clutter. Encourage the use of ambulation aids, such as walkers or canes, as needed. Carefully plan exercise protocols and activity regimens to minimize fatigue.

Evidence-Based Practice and Health Policy

Reid, I. (2020). Management of Paget's disease of bone. *Osteoporosis International, 31,* 827–837.

• The author defines Paget's disease as a progressive focal bone condition that can lead to pain, low quality of life, bone deformity, and other complications. The progression of the disease can be slowed or halted with bisphosphonates, which slow the rate of bone turnover, lower serum alkaline phosphatase, and decrease the vascularity of bone. These medications improve quality of life and pain control.

• The author notes that bisphosphonates normalize bone cell activity and prevent disease progression at a low cost. Patients who are symptomatic or at risk for complications have the opportunity to improve their quality of life and halt disease progression when on this medication.

DOCUMENTATION GUIDELINES

• Physical findings: Kyphosis, mobility, gait, presence of skeletal deformities
• Description of physical pain, comfort measures used, and response to interventions
• Sensory disturbances: Vision loss, hearing loss
• Level of tolerance of activity
• Laboratory results: Serum calcium and alkaline phosphatase levels
• Reaction to changes in body image

DISCHARGE AND HOME HEALTHCARE GUIDELINES

Encourage the patient to follow a recommended moderate exercise program. Suggest the use of a firm mattress or bed board to minimize spinal deformities. Emphasize the importance of attending physical therapy sessions and routine follow-up visits with the physician. Stress the importance of assessing the home environment for safety. Teach the patient to maintain adequate lighting, remove scatter rugs, and keep the home uncluttered. Instruct the patient to avoid abrupt movements and to report any increases in bone pain. Teach the patient to use assistive devices for ambulation.

Be sure the patient understands the dosage, route, action, and side effects of all prescribed medications. Instruct the patient in proper self-injection techniques for calcitonin. Educate the patient about side effects, such as nausea, vomiting, itchy hands, fever, inflammation of the injection site, and facial flushing, as well as the signs and symptoms of hypercalcemia. Teach the patient to take bisphosphonate medication with water on an empty stomach at least 30 minutes before eating or drinking other than the water taken with the medication. Ask the patient to stand or sit upright for up to an hour afterward to prevent gastric irritation and reflux. Tell the patient to call the physician if the patient experiences stomach cramps, diarrhea, or new bone pain. Tell the patient to report any easy bruising, bleeding, nausea, or anorexia. Provide information about Bone Health and Osteoporosis Foundation (https://www.bonehealthandosteoporosis.org).

Pancreatic Cancer

DRG Category:	436
Mean LOS:	4.5 days
Description:	MEDICAL: Malignancy of Hepatobiliary System or Pancreas With Complication or Comorbidity

Pancreatic cancer is currently the third most common cause of cancer-related deaths in the United States (Centers for Disease Control and Prevention, 2021). Pancreatic cancer includes carcinomas of the head of the pancreas, the ampulla of Vater, the common bile duct, and the duodenum. The American Cancer Society reported that in 2021, 60,430 people will be diagnosed with pancreatic cancer, and 48,220 people will die from the disease. Depending on stage, the 5-year survival rate ranges from 3% to 39%. Most patients (52%) are diagnosed when the disease is fairly advanced because the symptoms are nonspecific and subtle. Pancreatic cancer is a fatal disease.

Tumors can develop in both the exocrine and the endocrine tissue of the pancreas, although 95% arise from the exocrine parenchyma (functional tissue) and are referred to as adenocarcinomas. The remaining 5% of pancreatic tumors develop from endocrine cells of the pancreas; they are named according to the hormone they produce (i.e., insulinomas, glucagonomas). Adenocarcinoma of the ductal origin is the most common exocrine cell type (75%–92%), and it occurs most frequently in the head of the pancreas. Pancreatic adenocarcinoma grows rapidly, spreading to the stomach, duodenum, gallbladder, liver, and intestine by direct extension and invasion of lymphatic and vascular systems. Further metastatic spread to the lung, peritoneum, and spleen can occur. Metastatic tumors from cancers in the lung, breast, thyroid, or kidney or skin melanoma have been found in the pancreas. In addition to metastatic cancer, other complications include weight loss, bowel obstruction, liver failure, and death.

CAUSES

Diabetes mellitus, obesity, and chronic pancreatitis, as well as genetic mutations that are both inherited and acquired after birth, have been suggested as possible causes. Risk factors that have known association with pancreatic cancer are cigarette smoking (incidence is more than twice as high for smokers as for nonsmokers) and diets high in fat, meat, dehydrated foods, fried foods, refined sugars, soybeans, and nitrosamines. Estimates are that 30% of cases of pancreatic cancer are related to smoking. Persons who have occupational exposure to gasoline derivatives, naphthylamine, and benzidine are considered to be at higher risk. High coffee consumption and alcohol intake have been implicated; however, many believe a direct effect of these substances on the development of pancreatic cancer is questionable.

GENETIC CONSIDERATIONS

Pancreatic cancer is generally not heritable (with estimated heritability of ~9%), but there are several familial cancer syndromes and hereditary pancreatitis. There have also been families with isolated heritable pancreatic cancer that is transmitted in an autosomal dominant fashion, showing early onset and a penetrance greater than 80%. Heritable (germline) mutations in *BRCA2* are the most common seen in familial pancreatic cancer. Mutations in *PALB2* and *CDKN2A* have also been associated with a predisposition to developing pancreatic cancer. Other genetic syndromes that can cause pancreatic cancer include familial pancreatitis (*PRSS1*), Lynch syndrome (*MLH1* or *MLH2*), and Peutz-Jeghers syndrome (*STK11*).

SEX AND LIFE SPAN CONSIDERATIONS

Pancreatic carcinoma can occur in persons of all ages but is rare before age 45 years. Its peak incidence is between the ages of 60 and 70 years. The incidence in men and women is now equal and is attributed to the increase in smoking among women.

HEALTH DISPARITIES AND SEXUAL/GENDER MINORITY HEALTH

Pancreatic cancer occurs more frequently among Black than White persons, with the highest incidence in the United States among people who immigrated from Eastern Europe. Significant research supports that Black patients receive less treatment and have more instances of delayed treatment than other groups, creating health disparities and decreased survival rates for Black patients. Patients with private insurance and higher education receive earlier treatment than those with public insurance or no insurance and lower education attainment. Experts have also found that Black and Hispanic patients and their families are less likely than White patients to ask for and receive hospice care when they are dying from pancreatic cancer (Paredes et al., 2021; Zhu et al., 2020). These differences create unequal care.

Sexual and gender minority persons have higher odds for multiple chronic conditions, cancer, and poor quality of life, and are more apt to have disabilities than cisgender males and females. (Cisgender is a term used to describe persons whose gender identity and gender expression are aligned with their assigned sex listed on their birth certificate.) Lesbian women are more likely to be overweight/obese or to smoke as compared to their heterosexual counterparts, placing them at risk for pancreatic cancer (Office on Women's Health, 2019). Transgender is a term used to describe persons whose gender identity is different from their sex assigned at birth. Approximately 1% of the U.S. population identify themselves as transgender. Transgender people are less likely to be treated for pancreatic cancer than their cisgender counterparts (Jackson et al., 2021). Cancer disparities are perpetuated because sexual and gender minority persons receive poor quality of care due to stigma, lack of healthcare providers' awareness, and insensitivity to the unique needs of this community (Cacerese, Jackman, et al., 2020; Connelly et al., 2019; Gatos, 2018).

GLOBAL HEALTH CONSIDERATIONS

Pancreatic cancer is the 11th most common cancer globally but ranked 7th as a cancer cause of death. The global incidence of pancreatic cancer is approximately 1 to 15 cases per 100,000 individuals per year. The overall incidence of pancreatic cancer is five to six times higher in developed than in developing countries. India in particular has a low incidence, and countries in Eastern Europe have a high incidence.

ASSESSMENT

HISTORY. Cancer of the pancreas has been called a "silent" disease; one reason for the poor survival rate is that cancer is often not detected during its early stages because of its insidious onset. The signs and symptoms are vague and frequently disregarded or they are attributed to some minor ailment. The patient may report anorexia, malaise, nausea, fatigue, and midepigastric pain. Unplanned weight loss and epigastric pain that may radiate to the back are common complaints. Abdominal or back pain is a common sign of advanced pancreatic cancer. Cancer of the body of the pancreas impinges on the celiac ganglion, causing pain. Patients often report a dull, intermittent pain that has become more intense. Ask the patient to describe the type and intensity of the pain and also aggravating and relieving factors. Eating and activity often precipitate pain, whereas lying supine or sitting up and bending forward may offer relief. Question the patient as to the presence of any nausea and vomiting (especially that worsens after eating), anorexia, flatulence, diarrhea, constipation, or unusual fatigue. Check to see if the patient has been diagnosed with diabetes mellitus within the past year; if the patient has no risk factors for diabetes, pancreatic cancer is a possibility.

PHYSICAL EXAMINATION. The diagnosis of pancreatic cancer based on symptoms is difficult because **early symptoms are vague and nonspecific.** Symptoms may include **weight loss, anorexia, fatigue,** and **epigastric pain.** Inspect the patient for the presence and extent of jaundice, which is the presenting symptom in 80% to 90% of patients with cancer of the pancreatic head. The jaundice may have preceded or followed the onset of pain, but it usually progresses along a distinctive pattern: beginning on the mucous membranes, then on the palms of the hands, and finally becoming generalized. If the cancer blocks the release of pancreatic juices into the intestines, the patient may have difficulty digesting fatty foods; this will result in pale, bulky, greasy stools that tend to float in the toilet. Assess for the presence of pruritus and dark urine, which is caused by a buildup of bilirubin in the skin and blood, respectively.

Early tumors usually cannot be palpated, but auscultate, palpate, and percuss the abdomen. If the tumor involves the body and tail of the pancreas, an abdominal bruit may be heard in the left upper quadrant (indicating involvement of the splenic artery), and a large, hard mass may be palpated in the subumbilical or left hypochondrial region. Note the presence of liver or spleen enlargement. Dullness on percussion may indicate the presence of ascites or gallbladder enlargement.

PSYCHOSOCIAL. Unfortunately, pancreatic cancer is a lethal diagnosis, and the mean survival time of all patients is 4 to 6 months because diagnosis most often occurs at an advanced stage of disease. Assess for the presence of denial, irritability, depression, and personality changes. The sudden onset of characteristic symptoms can precipitate these emotional responses. Families and patients often display profound grief and disbelief upon receiving the diagnosis of pancreatic cancer and a poor prognosis. Assess the specific feelings and fears of the patient and family as well as the support systems available and previous coping strategies.

Diagnostic Highlights

Test	Normal Result	Abnormality With Condition	Explanation
Computed tomography (CT) scan	Normal structure of the pancreas and surrounding organs and structures	Identifies size and location of tumors	Provides detailed images with multiple cross sections of the pancreas
Magnetic resonance imaging	Normal structure of the pancreas and surrounding organs, structures, and vessels	Identifies size and location of tumors; determines if vessels are compressed by tumor	Uses radio waves and strong magnets; computer translates pattern of radio waves into detailed images
Abdominal sonogram (ultrasound)	Normal structure of the pancreas	Although CT is more accurate in locating tumors, may be used to rule out pancreatic pseudocysts	Creates oscilloscopic picture from echoes of high-frequency sound waves passing over pancreatic area
Tumor marker antigen; CA 19-9	< 37 units/mL	Elevated; a value of > 100 units/mL is specific for malignancy and > 1,000 units/mL may indicate metastasis	Elevated levels occur in 80% of patients with late-stage pancreatic cancer; also used after treatment to determine effectiveness or reoccurrence

Other Tests: Upper gastrointestinal (GI) series, positron emission tomography, biopsy of pancreatic tissue, angiography, endoscopic retrograde cholangiopancreatography

PRIMARY NURSING DIAGNOSIS

DIAGNOSIS. Acute pain related to the effects of tumor invasion and surgical incision as evidenced by self-reports of pain, facial grimacing, and/or protective behavior

OUTCOMES. Comfort status; Pain control; Pain level; Symptom control; Symptom severity; Knowledge: Pain management; Knowledge: Medication

INTERVENTIONS. Pain management: Acute; Analgesic administration; Teaching: Prescribed medication; Medication administration; Patient-controlled analgesia assistance

▒ PLANNING AND IMPLEMENTATION

Collaborative

Surgery is the primary mode of treatment, but radiotherapy and chemotherapy have a role. A distal pancreatectomy, used more often with islet cell tumors than with exocrine cancer, removes only the tail of the pancreas or the tail and part of the body. The spleen is also removed. A total pancreatectomy or a pancreatoduodenectomy (Whipple procedure) is used when cure is the objective. In a total pancreatectomy, the entire pancreas and spleen are removed. The Whipple procedure involves removal of the head of the pancreas, distal stomach, gallbladder, pancreas, spleen, duodenum, proximal jejunum, and regional lymph nodes. The procedure induces exocrine insufficiency and insulin-dependent diabetes. A pancreatojejunostomy, hepaticojejunostomy, and gastrojejunostomy are performed with the Whipple procedure to reconstruct the GI system. A vagotomy is usually done in both procedures to decrease the risk of peptic ulcer. A stent may be used for bile duct obstruction.

Careful postoperative management is essential for providing comfort and reducing surgical mortality. Observe vital signs, prothrombin times, drainage from drains, and wounds for signs of infection, hemorrhage, or fistula formation. Report immediately any evidence of increasing abdominal distention; shock; hematemesis, bloody stools; or bloody, gastric, or bile-colored drainage from incision sites. Vitamin K injections and blood components may be needed.

Monitor GI drainage from the nasogastric (NG) or gastrostomy tubes carefully. These tubes are strategically placed during surgery to decompress the stomach and prevent stress on the anastomosis sites. Maintain the tube's patency by preventing kinks or dislodgment; maintain suction at the prescribed level (usually low continuous suction for an NG tube). Secure gastrostomy tubes in a dependent position. Monitor the color, consistency, and amount of drainage from each tube. The presence of serosanguineous drainage is expected, but clear, bile-tinged drainage or frank blood could indicate disruption of an anastomosis site and should be reported immediately. Do not irrigate the NG or gastrostomy tube without specific orders. When irrigation is ordered, gently instill 10 to 20 mL of normal saline solution to remove an obstruction.

Because postoperative nutritional requirements for adequate tissue healing are approximately 3,000 calories per day, parenteral hyperalimentation is often ordered. Monitor the blood and urine glucose levels every 6 hours and administer insulin as needed. Once oral food and fluids are allowed, the patient is placed on a bland, low-fat, high-carbohydrate, high-protein diet. Administer pancreatic enzyme supplements (pancrelipase [Viokase, Cotazym] and lipase for metabolism of long-chain triglycerides) with each meal and snack. Observe and report any evidence of diarrhea or frothy, floating, foul-smelling stools (an indication of steatorrhea) because an adjustment in the enzyme replacement therapy may be needed.

A combination of adjuvant chemotherapy and radiation therapy with surgery may increase survival time 6 to 11 months. In patients with metastatic disease, combination therapy with gemcitabine and erlotinib have improved survival rates. Most patients receive chemotherapy and radiation therapy on an outpatient basis. Palliative surgical procedures can be used to relieve the obstructive jaundice, duodenal obstruction, and severe back pain that are characteristic of advanced disease.

Pharmacologic Highlights

Medication or Drug Class	Dosage	Description	Rationale
Chemotherapy	Varies with drug	Gemcitabine; erlotinib, fluoro-uracil (5-FU); cisplatin; irinote-can, paclitaxel; capecitabine; oxaliplatin; streptozocin	Kills cancer cells
Pancreatic enzyme supplements	Varies with drug	Pancrelipase; lipase	Aid in digestion of proteins, carbohydrates, and fats

Other Drugs: Narcotic analgesics delivered via a patient-controlled analgesic device or an epidural catheter are usually ordered postoperatively. Monitor the patient's response to these devices and encourage their usage to maintain pain at a tolerable level. Administer prophylactic antibiotics as ordered.

Independent

Provide emotional support and information as treatment goals and options are explored. Patients who are newly diagnosed with pancreatic cancer are often in shock, especially when the disease is diagnosed in the advanced stages. Encourage the patient and family to verbalize their feelings surrounding the diagnosis and impending death. Allow for the time needed to adjust to the diagnosis, while helping the patient and family begin the grieving process. Assist in the identification of tasks to be completed before death, such as making a will; seeing specific relatives and friends; or attending an approaching wedding, birthday, or anniversary celebration. Urge the patient to verbalize specific funeral requests to family members.

Help family members identify the extent of physical home care that is realistically required by the patient. Arrange for visits by a home health agency. Suggest that the family seek supportive counseling (hospice, grief counselor) and, if necessary, make the initial contact for them. Local units of the American Cancer Society offer assistance with home care supplies and support groups for patients and families.

Following any surgical procedure, direct care toward preventing the associated complications. Use the sterile technique when changing dressings and emptying wound drainage tubes. Place the patient in a semi-Fowler position to reduce stress on the incision and to optimize lung expansion. Help the patient turn over in bed and perform coughing, deep-breathing, and leg exercises every 2 hours to prevent skin breakdown and pulmonary and vascular stasis. Teach the patient to splint the abdominal incision with a pillow to minimize pain when turning or performing coughing and deep-breathing exercises. As soon as it is allowed, help the patient get out of bed and ambulate in hallways three to four times each day. Be alert for the sudden onset of chest pain or dyspnea (or both), which could indicate the presence of a pulmonary embolism.

As the disease progresses and pain increases, large doses of narcotic analgesics may be needed. Instruct the patient on the effective use of the pain scale and to request pain medication before the pain escalates to an intolerable level. Consider switching as-needed pain medication to an around-the-clock dosing schedule to keep pain under control. Encourage the patient and family to verbalize any concerns about the use of narcotics and stress that drug addiction is not a consideration.

Evidence-Based Practice and Health Policy

Segel, J., Hollenbeak, C., & Gusani, N. (2020). Rural-urban disparities in pancreatic cancer stage of diagnosis: Understanding the interaction with medically underserved areas. *Journal of Rural Health, 36*, 476–483.

- The authors wished to estimate the differences in pancreatic cancer diagnosis stage by the rural nature of their residence and the impact of living in a medically underserved area. The authors used a statewide database (Pennsylvania) to analyze adults ($N = 14,888$) diagnosed with pancreatic cancer. They categorized each patient's residence by rural-urban continuum: metro, nonmetro adjacent with population 20,000 or greater; nonmetro adjacent with population less than 20,000; nonmetro nonadjacent; and completely rural. They examined the percentage of patients diagnosed with early and late stages of disease.
- No patients with pancreatic cancer living in completely rural areas were diagnosed at the earliest stage of cancer. Patients living in completely rural areas have significantly lower rates of early and middle range stages of pancreatic cancer at diagnosis as compared to more urban patients. If pancreatic cancer is diagnosed at a later stage, survival rates are lower. Therefore, rural patients are at an important disadvantage compared to their urban counterparts with respect to early cancer diagnosis and treatment.

DOCUMENTATION GUIDELINES

- Response to the diagnosis of pancreatic cancer, the diagnostic tests, and recommended treatment regimen; communication of patient and family plans for end-of-life care
- Description of all dressings, wounds, and drainage collection devices: Location of drain, color and amount of drainage, appearance of incision, color and amount of GI drainage
- Physical findings related to the pulmonary assessment, abdominal assessment, presence of edema, and condition of extremities
- Response to pain medications, oral intake, and activity regimen
- Presence of complications: Hemorrhage, infection, pulmonary congestion, activity intolerance, unrelieved discomfort, absence of return of bowel sounds and function, decrease in urinary output
- Bowel pattern: Presence of constipation, diarrhea, steatorrhea

DISCHARGE AND HOME HEALTHCARE GUIDELINES

Reinforce the need for small, frequent meals. Warn against overeating at any one meal, which places too great a demand on the pancreas, and encourage the patient to limit caffeine and alcohol. Instruct the patient to inspect the stools daily and report to the physician any signs of steatorrhea. Teach the patient and family the care related to surgically induced diabetes: symptoms and appropriate treatment for hypoglycemia and hyperglycemia, procedure for performing blood glucose monitoring, and administration of all medications including insulin injections. Teach the patient or significant other to change the dressing over the abdominal incision and empty the drains daily (if present).

Make sure the patient and family are comfortable with all planning for end-of-life care and strategies to keep the patient at rest and pain free. Work with social service and hospice to ensure a safe and coordinated transition to home or facility.

Teach the patient care of skin in the external radiation field. Instruct the patient to do the following:

- Wash the skin gently daily with mild soap, rinse with warm water, and pat the skin dry
- Not wash off the dark ink markings outlining the radiation field
- Avoid applying any lotions, perfumes, deodorants, or powder in the treatment area
- Wear nonrestrictive, soft, cotton clothing directly over the treatment area
- Protect the skin from sunlight and extreme cold

Pancreatitis

DRG Category:	439
Mean LOS:	3.8 days
Description:	MEDICAL: Disorders of Pancreas Except Malignancy With Complication or Comorbidity
DRG Category:	405
Mean LOS:	12.6 days
Description:	SURGICAL: Pancreas, Liver, and Shunt Procedures With Major Complication or Comorbidity

Pancreatitis, acute or chronic, is an inflammation and potential necrosis of the pancreas. The pancreas is responsible for secretion of enzymes the body needs for digestion (exocrine function) as well as for the production of insulin and glucagon (endocrine function). Tissue damage from pancreatitis occurs because of activation of proteolytic and lipolytic pancreatic enzymes that are normally activated in the duodenum. Proteolytic enzymes, such as trypsin, elastase, and phospholipase, break down protein; lipolytic enzymes break down fats. The enzymes cause autodigestion (destruction of the acinar cells and islet cell tissue) of the pancreas, with leakage of the enzymes and fluid into surrounding tissues. At the same time, molecular fragments act as triggers for inflammatory cells, which worsen the problem by releasing oxygen radicals and cytokines into the area, enhancing the immune response and inflammation. Hemorrhage, edema, and possibly infection from the gastrointestinal (GI) tract lead to multiple organ involvement. With successful treatment, the pancreas can return to normal after an attack of acute pancreatitis, or it may progress to a state of chronic inflammation and disease.

The mortality rate of people with acute pancreatitis is as high as 15%, but in patients with severe disease, it can reach 30%, particularly when people develop multiple organ dysfunction syndrome. In chronic pancreatitis, there is permanent destruction of the pancreatic gland with irreversible morphological changes. Precipitation of proteins causes pancreatic duct obstruction. Edema and distention cause damage and loss of the acinar cells, which normally produce digestive enzymes. The normal cells are replaced with fibrosis and necrosis. As the autodigestion process of the pancreas progresses, the cells form walls around the fluid that contains enzymes and the necrotic debris. These pseudocysts can rupture into the peritoneum and surrounding tissues, resulting in complications of infection, abscesses, and fistulae. The islet cells within the pancreas may also be damaged and destroyed, leading to diabetes mellitus. Other complications include massive pancreatic hemorrhage and shock, acute respiratory distress syndrome, atelectasis, pleural effusion, pneumonia, paralytic ileus, and rarely, cancer.

CAUSES

Three factors cause premature enzyme activation: mechanical causes, metabolic causes, and miscellaneous causes. Mechanical causes—such as pancreatic duct damage and obstruction—may result from gallstones migrating into the duct, bile reflux from the duodenum into the duct, tumors, radiation therapy, abdominal trauma, ulcer disease, or inflammation. Endoscopic retrograde cholangiopancreatography (ERCP) is known to cause pancreatitis. Some experts state that many cases of pancreatitis that are attributed to unknown causes may actually be due to microlithiasis, very small gallstones. Metabolic causes result from changes in the secretory processes of the acinar cells in conditions such as alcoholism (35% of the cases of pancreatitis overall), diabetic ketoacidosis, hyperlipidemia, hypercalcemia, and drugs (acetaminophen, estrogen). Miscellaneous causes include infectious diseases (mumps, hepatitis B, coxsackie viral infections) and ischemic injury as a result of lupus erythematosus, cardiopulmonary bypass surgery, post-transplantation complications, or shock. Risk factors include alcohol misuse, abuse, and dependence; tobacco smoking (Aune et al., 2019); biliary tract disease; trauma; drugs (a few examples are azatioprine, sulfonamides, tetracycline, estrogens, fursemide, and corticosteroids); acute biliary infections; viral infections; and heredity.

GENETIC CONSIDERATIONS

Mutations in the trypsinogen gene *PRSS1*, *PRSS2*, *CTRC*, *SPINK1*, or the cystic fibrosis gene (*CFTR*) have been associated with heritable forms of pancreatitis in an autosomal dominant manner. Because genetic testing for the *PRSS1* gene produces many false negatives, persons considered vulnerable are often instructed to make lifestyle adaptations, such as avoiding alcohol and smoking and being vigilant about follow-up and screening, which will protect the pancreas. Mutations in other genes regulating pancreatic enzyme secretion have been seen in patients with chronic pancreatitis.

SEX AND LIFE SPAN CONSIDERATIONS

The main cause of pancreatitis is alcohol abuse and dependence in adult males and cholelithiasis and biliary tract disturbances in adult females. Alcohol-related pancreatitis has an average onset of 39 years of age, whereas biliary tract–related pancreatitis has an average onset of 69 years of age. The overall incidence is approximately the same in males and females. The principal cause in children is cystic fibrosis. Because pancreatic secretions decrease with age, older persons have decreased ability to tolerate dietary fat and have an increased risk of gallstones that may lead to pancreatitis. As people age, hospitalization rates increase for females compared to males.

HEALTH DISPARITIES AND SEXUAL/GENDER MINORITY HEALTH

The risk for pancreatitis among middle-aged Black persons is 10 times higher than for White or Native American persons, and the racial/ethnic differences are more pronounced in men than in women. Black persons are less likely to receive the standard of care with respect to invasive diagnostic testing, creating health disparities for that group (Chouairi et al., 2021 [see Evidence-Based Practice and Health Policy]). Sexual and gender minority people have higher rates of alcohol consumption and tobacco use than the general population (Centers for Disease Control and Prevention, 2021), which may place them at risk for pancreatitis.

GLOBAL HEALTH CONSIDERATIONS

Pancreatitis is an international disease. The range of the worldwide incidence of acute pancreatitis varies across countries, with the highest rates in the developed regions of North America, Australia, and Western Europe. In the United States, pancreatitis is most likely to be associated with alcohol abuse, but in Asia and Western Europe, it is more likely associated with gallstones.

ASSESSMENT

HISTORY. Determine the onset and severity of symptoms. Patients often seek medical attention for severe upper abdominal pain they describe as knifelike, twisting, and deep in the mid-epigastrium or umbilical region. The pain may radiate to the dorsal area of the back or around the costal margins. Pain begins 12 to 48 hours after excessive alcohol intake or, with gallstone-related pancreatitis, can occur after a large fatty meal. Nausea and vomiting are present in up to 90% of the cases.

Obtain a detailed history of alcohol use and ingestion patterns. Assess for a family history of pancreatitis or a history of external abdominal trauma, surgery, cancer, recent bacterial infections, and biliary or GI disease. Ask if the patient recently underwent any diagnostic testing. Obtain a complete medication profile of prescribed and over-the-counter drugs.

PHYSICAL EXAMINATION. The patient appears acutely ill with **severe upper abdominal pain** as well as **restlessness, apprehensiveness**, and **agitated behavior**. Some become confused and, if shock or hypoxemia is impending, unresponsive. Respirations are often rapid and shallow. The patient may assume a fetal position with legs drawn upward to relieve abdominal pain. You may note mottled or jaundiced skin. You may see a bluish discoloration in the flanks (Grey Turner sign) and around the umbilicus (Cullen sign), which indicates blood accumulation in these areas. Skin may be cold and diaphoretic, but the patient is likely febrile. During periods of pain, the patient may be hypertensive, but as hypovolemic shock progresses to late stages, blood pressure may fall. Patients usually have rapid heart rates; rapid, thready pulses; and decreased breath sounds in the lower lobes because of shallow respirations, pain, and increased abdominal size. You may also note coarse tremors of the extremities as a sign of low calcium. Other findings include tea-colored or foamy urine (indicating the presence of bile) and gray, foul-smelling, foamy stools that indicate the presence of undigested fat.

Auscultate the abdomen before palpation and percussion to check for decreased bowel sounds, which is a common finding in patients with pancreatitis. On palpation, note extreme abdominal tenderness, distention, guarding, and rigidity. Ascites and rebound tenderness are present in severe disease. When you percuss the abdomen, you may find abdominal tympany.

PSYCHOSOCIAL. Assess the patient's anxieties and coping abilities related to the demands of an acute care environment and a sudden illness. The patient with chronic pancreatitis may express feelings of hopelessness and apathy that may result from chronic pain and general debilitation. Assess the family's coping with role changes and responsibilities. Alcohol abuse counseling may be necessary. The patient's condition may change rapidly as the disease progresses. Communicate with the family about the seriousness of the disease and the patient's instability.

Diagnostic Highlights

Test	Normal Result	Abnormality With Condition	Explanation
Serum amylase	100–300 units/L	> 300 units/L	Enzyme produced by pancreas that aids digestion of complex carbohydrates; increases 12–24 hr after acute inflammation; amylase three times the referenced range indicates acute pancreatitis
Serum calcium	8.2–10.2 mg/dL	< 8.2 mg/dL	Necrosis of fat from release of pancreatic enzymes leads to binding of free calcium
Computed tomography and magnetic resonance imaging	Normal pancreas	Pancreatic enlargement, inflammation, fluid collection	Inflammation, necrosis, swelling, fluid collection changes the configuration of the pancreas; most reliable imaging method for severe pancreatitis
Abdominal ultrasonography; endoscopic ultrasonography; ERCP	Normal pancreas	Presence of gallstones that have migrated into pancreatic duct	Determines cause of pancreatitis; if acute cholangitis occurs, patient should have an ERCP within 24 hr if choledocholithiasis is suspected
Serum lipase	0–60 units/L	> 60 units/L	Enzyme produced by pancreas that aids digestion of fat; specific marker for inflammation of pancreas; begins to elevate within 2 hr of the inflammation
Serum glucose	60–100 mg/dL	> 100 mg/dL	Interference with insulin release and B-cell injury leads to hyperglycemia in some patients

(highlight box continues on page 906)

Diagnostic Highlights (continued)

Other Tests: Complete blood count (generally leukocytosis occurs), serum electrolytes, blood urea nitrogen, creatinine, ionized calcium, C-reactive protein, liver function tests, lactate dehydrogenase, serum bilirubin, alkaline phosphatase, trypsinogen activation peptide, serum trypsinogen–2, trypsin 2-α-1 antitrypsin complex, abdominal ultrasound

---

PRIMARY NURSING DIAGNOSIS

DIAGNOSIS. Acute pain related to inflammation, edema and peritoneal irritation as evidenced by self-reports of pain, facial grimacing, and/or protective behavior

OUTCOMES. Comfort status; Pain control; Pain level; Symptom severity; Symptom control; Knowledge: Pain management; Knowledge: Medication

INTERVENTIONS. Analgesic administration; Pain management: Acute; Medication administration; Teaching: Prescribed medication

PLANNING AND IMPLEMENTATION

Collaborative

The immediate goal of therapy is to control and decrease the inflammation of the pancreas. The fluid lost into the retroperitoneal space can be as much as 4 to 12 L with severe disease. The patient is kept NPO (nothing by mouth) with IV volume replacement (lactated Ringer injection or normal human serum albumin) to restore blood volume and prevent hypovolemic shock. There is controversy about which fluids to choose. Normal human serum albumin is often used if low albumin levels lead to a loss of osmotic pressure in the vascular system. Urinary output is monitored hourly to measure volume status: Less than 1 mL/kg per hour is a sign of hypoperfusion. The physician may insert a pulmonary artery catheter for hemodynamic monitoring to assess the adequacy of the volume replacement and cardiac output. Patients who develop sepsis and shock may not respond to fluid volume replacement and remain hypovolemic. This complication requires vasoactive parenteral medications.

Hypocalcemia is a common electrolyte imbalance that accompanies pancreatic necrosis and requires calcium replacement. It may cause tetany, seizures, respiratory complications, and myocardial changes. Magnesium deficits often accompany hypocalcemia and need replacement as well. Loss of potassium through vomiting, fluid loss in the third spaces, acidosis, and renal insufficiency can lead to ventricular dysrhythmia. The blood glucose is monitored as a part of the renal profile every 6 hours to determine the need for exogenous insulin replacement. Respiratory support involves administering oxygen by a variety of routes, which may include mechanical ventilation. Because of inadequate breathing patterns and the risk of laryngospasm, the patient may require endotracheal intubation; also, positive end expiratory pressure, pressure control ventilation, and inverse inspiratory-to-expiratory ratio ventilation (increasing inspiratory time) may be used.

The goal of therapy is to reduce the secretion of pancreatic enzymes, which stops the inflammatory process. The inflammation leads to nerve irritation and pain. Obtain a baseline pain assessment and reassess every 4 hours using a pain rating scale; provide narcotic analgesia as needed. Bedrest is important to decrease the basal metabolic rate, which, in turn, decreases pancreatic secretions. Insertion of a nasogastric tube for intermittent suction also contributes to this goal by preventing the release of secretion in the duodenum. NPO status is strictly maintained, with no ice chips or sips of water during the acute phase. Nutritional support to restore the damaged pancreatic cells is provided by initiating total parenteral nutrition within 3 days of the onset of the acute phase.

Surgical interventions may be indicated for managing the complications associated with pancreatic necrosis. The procedures include pancreatic drainage, pancreatic resection or débridement, and removal of obstructions (biliary stones). The current therapy for removal of stones is early endoscopic retrograde cholangiopancreatography and endoscopic sphincterotomy. Peritoneal lavage is used for patients who do not respond to intensive treatment after 3 days; it has significantly decreased the incidence of complications and the mortality rate.

Pharmacologic Highlights

Medication or Drug Class	Dosage	Description	Rationale
Antibiotics	Varies with patient	Ceftriaxone (Rocephin), ampicillin, imipenem, and cilastatin	Antibiotics are not routinely administered unless infection is present. For microorganisms causing biliary pancreatitis and acute necrotizing pancreatitis; therapy is based on idea that enteric anaerobic and aerobic gram-bacilli microorganisms are often the cause of pancreatic infections
Opiates	Varies with drug	Meperidine (Demerol); fentanyl (Sublimaze); tramadol (Ultram)	Relieve pain; narcotic analgesics that do not cause spasms of the sphincter of Oddi may falsely elevate amylase level, so amylase levels need to be drawn before the pain therapy begins; meperidine is thought to produce less muscle spasm than other opiates

Other Drugs: Antacids to neutralize gastric secretions; histamine antagonists to decrease gastric acid production; dopamine to improve myocardial contractility, increase cardiac output, and decrease inflammation by reducing permeability in pancreatic ducts. Chronic therapy may include a low-fat diet and oral pancreatic enzyme supplements. Insulin may be needed to control hyperglycemia.

Independent

Patients with acute pancreatitis deteriorate quickly and need continuous cardiopulmonary monitoring. Monitor fluid balance carefully, and balance pain medication with the need for the patient to maintain an adequate blood pressure. During the acute phase of pancreatitis, focus on continued monitoring. Monitor the patient's pain to determine intensity, location, characteristics, and factors that aggravate or relieve the pain. Frequent doses of analgesics are required. Other measures to provide comfort include positioning the patient in a knee-chest posture, stress reduction, and relaxation exercises. Provide a restful environment, but also initiate diversional activities. Monitor the patient's respiratory status continually. Place the patient in high Fowler position to improve lung expansion and use other mechanisms to enhance gas exchange unless the patient develops shock and severe hypotension. If the patient is not intubated, keep emergency intubation equipment close by in case tetany and laryngospasm occur. The risk of tetany is enhanced if the patient hyperventilates. Maintain a calm environment, a constant presence, and medications to assist the patient with quiet breathing.

After the removal of the nasogastric tube, the diet progresses slowly from liquids to a diet high in calories and low in fat. During the immediate recovery period, arrange for small, frequent meals. Explain the need to avoid food and drinks with caffeine, spicy foods, and heavy meals that stimulate pancreatic secretion. Develop a realistic weight gain goal. Assist with dietary teaching by planning a week's menu, incorporating the patient's specific dietary needs and restrictions. If the patient has abused or misused alcohol, make appropriate referrals to assist the patient to reduce drinking.

Evidence-Based Practice and Health Policy

Chouairi, F., McCarty, T., Hathorn, K., Sharma, P., Aslanian, H., Jamidar, P., Thompson, C., & Muniraj, T. (2021). Evaluation of socioeconomic and healthcare disparities on same admission cholecystectomy after endoscopic retrograde cholangiopancreatography among patients with acute gallstone pancreatitis. *Surgical Endoscopy*. Advance online publication. https://doi .org/10.1007/s00464-020-08272-2

• Despite scientific evidence recommending same admission cholecystectomy (CCY) after ERCP for patients with acute gallstone pancreatitis, clinical practice varies. The authors aimed to investigate the role of clinical and sociodemographic factors in the management of acute gallstone pancreatitis. The authors used a national database to review patients with acute gallstone pancreatitis who underwent ERCP and classified them by treatment strategy: ERCP + same admission CCY ($N = 118,318$) versus ERCP alone ($N = 86,694$).
• A majority of patients in the ERCP alone group were at urban-teaching hospitals. Length of stay was longer with higher associated costs for patients with same admission CCY. Mortality was decreased significantly for patients who underwent ERCP + CCY. Female gender, Black race, Medicare payer status, urban-teaching hospital location, and household income decreased the odds of undergoing same admission CCY + ERCP. These groups therefore are less likely to receive accepted standard care.

DOCUMENTATION GUIDELINES

• Patient's description of pain and response to medications and alternative comfort measures
• Physical findings: Respiratory rate and rhythm, stability of blood pressure and signs of shock, adequacy of oxygenation, use of accessory muscles, character of breath sounds, mentation, pertinent laboratory findings, presence of fever
• Intake and output, fluid balance, weight changes, vital signs, results of renal profile laboratory studies
• Presence of nausea and vomiting, nasogastric tube, weight loss to 20% under ideal
• Presence of complications: Hemorrhage, sepsis, shock, respiratory distress syndrome, tetany, hyperglycemia

DISCHARGE AND HOME HEALTHCARE GUIDELINES

Prevention involves correcting the initiating events. If the disease is related to alcohol use, reinforce the importance of abstaining, and provide appropriate referrals. If the patient smokes tobacco, refer them to a smoking cessation program. Teach the patient to recognize early symptoms that may indicate recurrence and when to contact the physician. Emphasize the importance of follow-up care. Teach the rationale, action, dosage, and side effects of all prescribed medications. Instruct the patient to take prescribed pancreatic enzyme replacements with or immediately after meals and to swallow them whole and not with hot liquids that would disrupt the protective coating. If the patient is being discharged with the requirement for continued insulin injections, the patient and family should demonstrate the injection technique and the procedure for blood glucose self-monitoring. Provide a log and show them how to keep a record of glucose levels and insulin dosages. The patient with a loss of pancreatic endocrine function requires extensive ongoing diabetic teaching after discharge; refer for additional counseling if necessary. Encourage the patient to seek nutritional follow-up with clinic or physician visits, especially for hyperglycemic management.

Parkinson Disease

DRG Category: 57
Mean LOS: 5.6 days
Description: MEDICAL: Degenerative Nervous System Disorders Without Major Complication or Comorbidity

Parkinson disease (PD), also known as *paralysis agitans*, is a neurological disorder that affects 1% of older adults beyond the seventh decade of life. It is a common clinical condition characterized by gradual slowing of voluntary movement (bradykinesia); muscular rigidity; stooped posture; distinctive gait with short, accelerating steps; diminished facial expression; and resting tremor. The disabilities that occur in PD can be slowed but not halted with treatment. The disease occurs with progressive parkinsonism in the absence of a toxic or known etiology.

PD is caused by a degeneration of the substantia nigra in the basal ganglia of the midbrain, which leads to depletion of the neurotransmitter dopamine (DA). DA is normally produced and stored in this location and promotes smooth, purposeful movements and modulation of motor function. Depletion of DA leads to impairment of the extrapyramidal tracts and consequent loss of movement coordination. Almost 80% of DA neurons are lost before the patient begins to have the motor signs of PD. Complications of PD include injuries from falls, skin breakdown from immobility, pneumonia, and urinary tract infections. Death is usually caused by aspiration pneumonia or other infection.

CAUSES

The cause of PD is unknown, but most experts suggest that the cause is a combination of heredity and environmental exposure. The majority of cases of classic PD are primary, or idiopathic, Parkinson disease (IPD), which is suspected to be due to heredity. Secondary, or iatrogenic, PD is drug or chemical related. Dopamine-depleting drugs such as reserpine, phenothiazine, metoclopramide, tetrabenazine, and the butyrophenones (droperidol and haloperidol) can lead to secondary PD. Pesticide exposure may increase the risk of PD by 80%. Risk factors include living in a rural environment, using well water, and exposure to pesticides and toxins. Interestingly, both smoking and caffeine have protective effects for PD.

GENETIC CONSIDERATIONS

PD, like other neurodegenerative diseases, has both sporadic (no clear etiology) and familial forms. Familial cases of PD are caused by mutations in the *SNCA* gene, encoding alpha-synuclein, and the *LRRK2* gene, encoding leucine-rich repeat kinase 2. These mutations follow an autosomal dominant pattern. There is also a juvenile form of PD that follows an autosomal recessive pattern and is caused by mutations in the gene Parkin (*PRKN*). In sporadic PD, where there is no clear inheritance pattern, genetic contributions appear much less prominent (heritability is only 5%–30%). Mutations that appear to increase susceptibility include the genes *HTRA2, LRRK2, NR4A2, NDUFV2, ADH3, FGF20, GBA*, and *MAPT*.

SEX AND LIFE SPAN CONSIDERATIONS

PD occurs in 1% of the population over age 60 years. Juvenile parkinsonism, however, is associated with people younger than age 40 years who have Wilson disease, progressive lenticular degeneration, or Huntington disease. The lenticular nucleus is the part of the brain that contains the putamen and globus pallidus. PD affects men slightly more often than it does women. Approximately 15% of people with IPD develop dementia as they age.

HEALTH DISPARITIES AND SEXUAL/GENDER MINORITY HEALTH

Hispanic and White people have a higher incidence of PD than other groups. Sexual and gender minority status has no known effect on the risk for PD.

GLOBAL HEALTH CONSIDERATIONS

The global incidence of PD is 10 to 20 cases per 100,000 individuals per year. Environmental factors in different global regions most likely explain the variation in incidence by location.

ASSESSMENT

HISTORY. Obtain a family, medication, and occupational history. Elicit a description of PD progression; determine where in the progressive stages of PD the patient's symptoms occur: (1) mild unilateral dysfunction; (2) mild bilateral dysfunction, as evidenced by expressionless face and gait changes; (3) increasing dysfunction, with difficulties in walking, initiating movements, and maintaining equilibrium; (4) severe disability, including difficulties in walking and maintaining balance and steady propulsion, rigidity, and slowed movement; and (5) invalidism, which requires total care. Note the timing of progression of all symptoms.

Determine if the patient has experienced any of the three cardinal signs of PD: involuntary tremors, akinesia (loss or impairment of voluntary movement), and progressive muscle rigidity. The first sign of PD is a coarse, rest tremor of the fingers and thumb (pill-rolling movement) of one hand. It occurs during rest and intensifies with stress, fatigue, cold, or excitation. This tremor disappears during sleep or purposeful movement. The tremor can occur in the tongue, lip, jaw, chin, and closed eyelids. Eventually, the tremor can spread to the foot on the same side and then to the limbs on the other side of the body. Note if the arm does not swing during walking and if the foot on the same side drags. Ask if the patient has a reduction in the sense of smell.

PHYSICAL EXAMINATION. The diagnosis of PD is made on the basis of two out of the four important symptoms: **resting tremor**, **bradykinesia** (slowing down or loss of voluntary muscle movement), **cogwheel rigidity** (rigidity of a muscle that gives way in a series of little jerks when passive stretching occurs), and **postural instability**; one of the two symptoms must be resting tremor or bradykinesia. Dystonia, which is inversion, or turning in or down of a foot accompanied by cramping or aching, may occur. Generally, the onset of symptoms is asymmetric and may begin with a resting tremor in one arm.

Assess the patient for signs of bradykinesia. Perform a passive range-of-motion examination, assessing for rigidity. Rigidity of the antagonistic muscles, which causes resistance to both extension and flexion, is a cardinal sign of PD. Flexion contractures develop in the neck, trunk, elbows, knees, and hips. Note alterations in the respiratory status because rigidity of the intercostal muscles may decrease breath sounds or cause labored respirations. Observe the patient's posture, noting if the patient is stooped, and assess gait dysfunction. Note involuntary movements, slowed movements, decreased movements, loss of muscle movement, repetitive muscle spasms, an inability to sit down, and difficulty swallowing.

Observe the patient's face, noting an expressionless, masklike appearance, drooling, and decreased tearing ability; note eyeballs fixed in an upward direction or eyelids completely closed, which are rare complications of PD. Assess for defective speech, a high-pitched monotone voice or soft voice, trouble with speech initiation, stuttering, and parroting the speech of others. Autonomic disorders that are manifested in PD include hypothalamic dysfunction, so assess for decreased or Parkinson perspiration, heat intolerance, seborrhea, and excess oil production. Observe the patient for orthostatic hypotension, which manifests in fainting or dizziness. Note constipation or bladder dysfunction (urgency, frequency, retention).

PSYCHOSOCIAL. PD does not usually affect intellectual ability, but 20% of patients with PD develop dementia similar to that of Alzheimer disease. The patient with PD commonly develops depression later in the disease process, and this is characterized by withdrawal, sadness, loss of appetite, and sleep disturbance. Patients may also demonstrate problems with social isolation, ineffective coping, potential for injury, and sleep pattern disturbance.

Diagnostic Highlights

The diagnosis of PD is usually made through clinical findings rather than diagnostic tests because there is no specific biological marker that exists for PD. The key to diagnosis is the patient's response to levodopa (see Pharmacologic Highlights).

Test	Normal Result	Abnormality With Condition	Explanation
Positron emission tomography and single photon emission computed tomography	Normal dopamine uptake in basal ganglia	Decreased dopamine uptake in the basal ganglia	Degeneration of substantia nigra in the basal ganglia of midbrain leads to depletion of dopamine. Note that these scans are useful but not routinely required because the diagnosis is made by symptoms

Other Tests: Magnetic resonance imaging and computed tomography scan are usually normal in people with PD.

PRIMARY NURSING DIAGNOSIS

DIAGNOSIS. Impaired physical mobility related to rigidity and tremors as evidenced by altered gait, decreased fine motor skills, decreased range of motion, and/or movement-induced tremor

OUTCOMES. Self-care: Activities of daily living; Self care: Bathing; Self care: Hygiene; Self care: Dressing; Comfort status; Energy conservation; Mobility; Exercise participation

INTERVENTIONS. Exercise therapy: Ambulation; Exercise therapy: Balance; Exercise therapy: Joint mobility; Exercise therapy: Muscle control; Environmental management; Self-care assistance; Exercise promotion

PLANNING AND IMPLEMENTATION
Collaborative
The goals of treatment are to provide control of symptoms and minimize adverse effects of treatment. At this time there is no proven treatment that modifies or cures the disease. To control tremor and rigidity, pharmacologic management is the treatment of choice. Generally, people have good control of their symptoms for about 5 years. After that time, their disability progresses with long-term motor complications; difficulty with their balance; and, for some, dementia. Long-term levodopa therapy can result in drug tolerance or drug toxicity. Symptoms of drug toxicity are confusion, hallucinations, and decreased drug effectiveness. Treatment for drug tolerance and toxicity is either a change in drug dosage or a drug holiday. Autologous transplantation of small portions of the adrenal gland into the brain's caudate nucleus of PD patients is offered on an experimental basis in some medical centers as a palliative treatment. In addition, if medications are ineffective, stereotaxic neurosurgery (deep brain stimulation) may be done to treat intractable tremor. A new procedure that allows for infusing a carbidopa/levodopa enteral suspension into the jejunum by a portable pump may provide more continuous release of medication.

Physical and occupational therapy consultation is helpful to plan a program to reduce flexion contractures and to maximize functions for the activities of daily living. To prevent impaired physical mobility, perform passive and active range-of-motion exercises and muscle-stretching exercises. In addition, include exercises for muscles of the face and tongue to facilitate speech and swallowing. Use of a cane or walker promotes ambulation and prevents falls.

Pharmacologic Highlights

Medication or Drug Class	Dosage	Description	Rationale
Antiparkinson	Varies with drug	Levodopa (L-dopa); carbidopa levodopa (Sinemet); other dopamine agonists: apomophine, pramipexole, ropinirole, amantadine, rotigotine	Controls tremor and rigidity; converted to dopamine in the basal ganglia; dopamine replacement therapy
Amantadine hydrochloride (Symmetrel)	100 mg bid PO	Antiviral	Controls tremor and rigidity by increasing the release of dopamine to the basal ganglia
Monoamine oxidase B (MOA-B) inhibitors	Varies with drug	Rasagiline, salfinamide, selegiline	MAO-B inhibitors inhibit the activity of MAO-B oxidases that inactivate dopamine; supports sympathetic activity and as an adjunct to levodopa
Synthetic anticholinergics	Varies with drug	Trihexyphenidyl (Artane); benztropine mesylate (Cogentin)	Block acetylcholine-stimulated nerves that lead to tremors

Other Drugs: Antihistamines are sometimes prescribed with the anticholinergics to inhibit dopamine uptake; bromocriptine mesylate, a dopamine antagonist, is ordered to stimulate dopaminergic receptors. Selegiline may have a neuroprotective effect if started at the time of diagnosis. Safinamide serves as an "add-on" treatment for patients on levadopa/carbidopa.

Independent

Promote independence in the patient. Encourage maximum participation in self-care activities. Allow sufficient time to perform activities and schedule outings in late morning or in the afternoon to avoid rushing the patient. Reinforce occupational and physical therapy recommendations. Use adaptive devices as needed. If painful muscle cramps threaten to limit the patient's mobility, consider warm baths or muscle massage.

To facilitate communication, encourage the patient with PD to speak slowly and to pause for a breath at appropriate intervals in each sentence. Teach deep-breathing exercises to promote chest expansion and adequate air exchange. Be alert to nonverbal clues and supplement interactions with a communication board, mechanical voice synthesizer, computer, or electric typewriter.

To maintain nutritional status, monitor the patient's ability to chew and swallow. Monitor weight, intake, and output. Position the patient in the upright position for eating to facilitate swallowing. Offer small, frequent meals; soft foods; and thick, cold fluids. Supplemental puddings or nutritional shakes may be given throughout the day to maintain weight.

Help the patient maintain a positive self-image by emphasizing the patient's abilities and by reinforcing success. Encourage the patient to verbalize feelings and to write in a journal. Help the patient maintain a clean, attractive appearance. Caregivers may need a great deal of emotional support. Explore strategies for long-term care with the patient and significant others.

Evidence-Based Practice and Health Policy

Tan, S., Williams, A., Tan, E., Clark, R., & Morris, M. (2020). Parkinson's disease caregiver strain in Singapore. *Frontiers in Neurology*, *11*, 1–10.

• Because caregiver strain is recognized globally with Parkinson disease (PD), the authors wanted to investigate strain for families caring for people living with PD. Ninety-four

caregivers of people living with idiopathic PD were recruited for the study. They were mostly cohabiting spouses, partners, or offspring. Around half employed foreign domestic helpers.
• Mean caregiving duration was 5.9 years with an average of 8 hours per day spent in caregiving roles. Most care providers were comparatively healthy. Caregivers reported significant levels of strain that increased with greater level of disability. Most caregivers in this Singapore sample reported high levels of strain, despite comparatively good physical function.

DOCUMENTATION GUIDELINES

• Ability to ambulate, perform the activities of daily living, progress in an exercise program
• Use of verbal and nonverbal communication
• Statements about body image and self-esteem
• Discomfort during activity

DISCHARGE AND HOME HEALTHCARE GUIDELINES

Be sure the patient or caregiver understands all medications, including the dosage, route, action, and adverse reactions. Avoid the use of alcohol, reserpine, pyridoxine, and phenothiazine while taking levodopa. In general, recommend massage and relaxation techniques and reinforce exercises recommended by the physical therapist. Several techniques facilitate mobility and enhance safety in PD patients. Instruct the patient to try the following strategies: (1) To assist in maintaining balance, concentrate on taking larger steps with feet apart, keeping back straight and swinging the arms; (2) to overcome akinesia, tape the "frozen" leg to initiate movement; (3) to reduce tremors, hold objects (coins, keys, or purse) in the hand; (4) to obtain partial control of tremors when seated, grasp chair arms; (5) to reduce rigidity before exercise, take a warm bath; (6) to initiate movement, rock back and forth; (7) to prevent spine flexion, periodically lie prone and avoid using a neck pillow; and (8) teach the patient to eliminate loose carpeting, install grab bars, and elevate the toilet seat. Use of chair lifts can also be beneficial.

Explore coping strategies with the patient and family. Support groups for the PD patient and family are available in most cities. Contact the American Parkinson Disease Association (APDA) at https://www.apdaparkinson.org. Encourage the patient to be independent in the activities of daily living. Use devices and assistance as necessary. Provide ample time to complete self-care.

Pelvic Fractures

DRG Category:	535
Mean LOS:	4.7 days
Description:	MEDICAL: Fractures of Hip and Pelvis With Major Complication or Comorbidity

The pelvis, or pelvic ring, consists of two innominate bones connected anteriorly at the symphysis pubis and posteriorly at the sacrum. These structures form a ring of bones with ligaments that are designed to accommodate weight distributed from the trunk to the pelvis across both the sacrum and the joints at the S1 vertebra. The bony structures protect vascular structures, nerves, and organs. A pelvic fracture is a break in the integrity of either the innominate bones or the sacrum. Pelvic fractures account for approximately 3% of all fractures, with an associated mortality rate that ranges from 3% for low-risk fractures to 25% for high-risk fractures.

The iliac vascular structures, lumbosacral plexus, lower genitourinary tract, reproductive organs, portions of the small bowel, distal colon and rectum, iliofemoral vessels, and lumbosacral plexus bilaterally all may be affected by a pelvic fracture. The pelvic area is highly vascular, and bleeding can occur from exposed fractures, soft tissue injury, and local venous and arterial bleeding. The most immediate, serious complications associated with pelvic fractures are hemorrhage and exsanguination, which together cause up to 60% of the deaths from pelvic injuries because they can lead to the loss of 2 or 3 L of blood. Pelvic fractures associated with sacral and sacroiliac disruption may cause sciatic and sacral nerve injuries. Other complications include gait disturbances, erectile dysfunction, genitourinary tract trauma, hip dislocation, and thromboembolic phenomena including fat emboli. A variety of classification systems have been developed to describe pelvic fractures. See Table 1 for one such classification.

• TABLE 1 Functional Classification of Pelvic Fractures (other classification systems also exist)

CLASSIFICATION	DESCRIPTION/STABILITY
Lateral compression	Rotationally unstable but vertically stable
	Posterior elements are stable
	May cause soft tissue and genitourinary tract injury
Anterior-posterior compression	"Open book injury" with symphysis pubis disruption
	Posterior element stability is variable
	May be associated with genitourinary tract injury
Vertical shear	Virtually always instability in the posterior elements
	Commonly associated with soft tissue, skin, vascular, genitourinary, gastrointestinal, and neurological injury
Acetabular disruption (Combined Mechanism)	Includes simple fractures, dislocations, and implosion of the head of the femur into the pelvis
	Generally unstable
	May be associated with genitourinary and neurovascular injuries

CAUSES

Two out of three occurrences of pelvic fractures are associated with traffic crashes, which are high-energy events. Fractures associated with traffic crashes generally have the greatest morbidity and mortality as compared to other causes because of the significant forces involved. Combat blast injuries are also high injury events that can lead to pelvic fracture. They may also occur from low-energy events such as falls, sports injuries, or direct blows to bony prominences. Industrial accidents, crush injuries, and assaults also cause pelvic fractures. In older persons, the most common cause is a fall from a standing position. Risk factors for a pelvic fracture include old age, osteoporosis, visual dysfunction, corticosteroid use, vitamin deficiency, physical inactivity, alcohol abuse, and tobacco use.

GENETIC CONSIDERATIONS

Genetic disorders, such as osteogenesis imperfecta (OI), that decrease bone strength can increase the likelihood of pelvic fractures. Mutations in collagen genes *COL1A1* and *COL1A2* cause OI.

SEX AND LIFE SPAN CONSIDERATIONS

Pelvic fractures may occur at any age, from infants to older adults. Traffic crashes are the most common cause of pelvic fractures in young children as well as in young adults 15 to 28 years of age. During young adulthood, more males than females have pelvic fractures. Complex pelvic fractures (pelvic fractures with soft tissue injury) are more common in men and women younger than age 35 years and are less frequent in patients older than age 65 years. The overall incidence of pelvic fractures is similar for men and women, with an increase in incidence in women older than age 85 years, perhaps because of their increased incidence of osteoporosis.

HEALTH DISPARITIES AND SEXUAL/GENDER MINORITY HEALTH

In recent years, Black persons have been killed in traffic crashes at a rate almost 25% higher than White persons (National Highway Traffic Safety Administration [NHTSA], 2021). Native American persons have the highest rate of traffic crash injury in the United States, more than twice the rate of Black persons (NHTSA, 2021). Experts have noted that Black and Native American communities tend to be crisscrossed by more dangerous roads than other locations, placing people from those communities at risk for injury. Recent work has shown evidence that rural populations have injury mortality rates that are more than twice as high as urban rates. Many factors contribute to these health disparities, including the risk of traffic injury in narrow rural roads, the lack of graded curves and lighted traffic signals on rural highways, and the distance from major trauma centers. Many of the most dangerous occupations, such as mining and agriculture, are found in rural areas and can result in injury, disability, and death. Sexual and gender minority persons have high risk for dating and interpersonal violence, violence related to bullying, and intentional and unintentional injury (Healthy People 2020).

GLOBAL HEALTH CONSIDERATIONS

Specifically with respect to abdominal and pelvic trauma, traffic crashes are the leading cause of injury, and they occur most commonly in males ages 14 to 30 years. According to the World Health Organization, falls from heights of less than 5 meters are the leading cause of injury globally, but estimates are that only 6% of those are related to abdominal or pelvic trauma.

ASSESSMENT

HISTORY. Establish a history of the mechanism of injury, along with a detailed report from prehospital professionals. In cases of traffic crashes and pedestrian injuries, include the type of vehicle and speed at the time of the crash. Determine whether the patient was a driver or passenger and whether the patient was using a safety restraint. If the patient was a pedestrian, ask for a description of the site of the injury and the anatomic location of the impact. If the patient experienced a fall, determine the point of impact, distance of the fall, and type of landing surface. Ask if the patient experienced suprapubic tenderness, the inability to void, or pain over the iliac spikes. Determine if the patient has any underlying medical disorders, such as polycystic kidney disease, frequent urinary tract infections, osteoporosis, or rheumatoid arthritis. Take a medication history, ask if the patient is taking corticosteroids, and determine if the patient has a current tetanus immunization.

PHYSICAL EXAMINATION. The initial evaluation or primary survey of the trauma patient is centered on assessing the airway, breathing, circulation, disability (neurological status), and exposure (completely undressing the patient). Make sure that the cervical spine is immobilized. Inspection may reveal **abrasions; pain and tenderness; ecchymosis; or contusions or lacerations over bony prominences, the groin, genitalia, and suprapubic area. Ecchymosis or hematoma formation over the pubis or blood at the urinary meatus** is significant for associated lower genitourinary tract trauma. Palpation of the iliac crests and anterior pubis may suggest underlying injury; however, "rocking of the pelvis" is discouraged because it may cause an increase in vascular injury and bleeding. Internal rotation of the lower extremity or "frog leg positioning" is suggestive of pelvic ring abnormalities. Instability on hip adduction and pain on hip motion may indicate an acetabular fracture with or without an associated hip fracture. Detection of neurovascular injury that accompanies pelvic fracture is important, particularly lower sacral nerve root injuries that may lead to bowel and bladder dysfunction.

Perform complete rectal and pelvic examinations to assess for bleeding; rectal tone; and, in women, the presence of vaginal wall disruptions. Check the position of the prostate gland in men and palpate for a "high-riding" prostate, which may indicate genitourinary tract injury. Assess the lower extremities for paresis, hypoesthesia, alterations in distal pulses, and abnormalities in the plantar flexion and ankle jerk reflexes. Inspect the perineum, groin, and buttocks for lacerations that may have been caused by open pelvic fractures. Note that from one-third to one-half of all trauma patients have an elevated blood alcohol level, which complicates assessments and may mask abdominal pain.

Monitor hourly fluid volume status, including hemodynamic, urinary, and central nervous system parameters. Notify the physician if delayed capillary refill, tachycardia, urinary output less than 0.5 mL/kg per hour, or alterations in mental status (restlessness, agitation, and confusion) occur. Body weights are helpful in indicating fluid volume status over time.

PSYCHOSOCIAL. The patient who has a pelvic fracture faces stressors that range from the unexpected nature of the traumatic event and acute pain to potential life-threatening complications. The traditional means of verbal communication are often limited or absent, thus leading to the patient's fear, loss of control, and isolation. Significant lifestyle and functional changes may occur in patients with pelvic fractures and their associated injuries. Assess patients' and families' coping strategies, level of anxiety, and overall understanding of their injuries. Assess patients' ability to adapt to their current circumstances.

Diagnostic Highlights

Test	Normal Result	Abnormality With Condition	Explanation
Pelvic x-rays	Intact bony structure	Evidence of fractures and dislocations	Demonstrates radiographic evidence of pelvic injury; uncovers 90% of pelvic fractures with initial screening
Ultrasound; focused assessment with sonography for trauma (FAST)	Intact bony structure of pelvis with no hemorrhage	Intrapelvic bleeding and fluid accumulation; intraperitoneal bleeding is also possible	Noninvasive test that shows location of bleeding to explain shock
Retrograde urethrography; cystography	Intact urethra and bladder	Injured or transected urethra or bladder	Shows location and extent of genitourinary injury
Computed tomography scan	Intact bony structure	Evidence of fractures, dislocations, and sacral injuries	Assesses pelvis and sacroiliac joint and sacral injuries; best study to evaluate pelvic anatomy and amount of bleeding within and around the pelvic cavity; confirms hip dislocation associated with acetabular fracture

Other Tests: Pregnancy test, hematocrit, hemoglobin, platelet count, prothrombin time

PRIMARY NURSING DIAGNOSIS

DIAGNOSIS. Risk for bleeding as evidenced by active or occult hemorrhage, hypotension, and/or tachycardia

OUTCOMES. Blood loss severity; Fluid balance; Circulation status; Cardiac pump effectiveness; Hydration; Vital signs; Fluid balance

INTERVENTIONS. Bleeding reduction; Fluid resuscitation; Blood product administration; IV therapy; Shock prevention; Shock management

░ PLANNING AND IMPLEMENTATION

Collaborative

Maintenance of airway, breathing, and circulation are the highest priority. Many patients are in hypovolemic shock (see **Hypovolemic/Hemorrhagic Shock**) and require fluid resuscitation. FAST facilitates a timely diagnosis for patients with blunt abdominal trauma and pelvic fractures and often occurs simultaneously with emergency care. FAST decreases the time to diagnosis, demonstrates the location and severity of hemoperitoneum (intra-abdominal hemorrhage), and can be repeated to assess further bleeding. During care, avoid excessive movement of the pelvis whether the fracture is stable or unstable. Patients with stable pelvic fractures can be managed with bedrest alone, and early ambulation is guided by their level of pain or associated injuries. Patients with unstable pelvic fractures can also be managed with bedrest, spica casts, or sling traction, but there is an increasing risk of complications associated with prolonged bedrest. Movement, weight-bearing restrictions, and head of bed elevation are prescribed by the orthopedic surgeon. The physician often prescribes sequential compression devices to prevent venous stasis. Prevention of venous thrombosis is a critical part of care.

External immobilization helps decrease pain, reduce the amount of blood transfusions, and facilitate early ambulation. Immobilization can be achieved through the use of several devices that can be applied externally or percutaneously to the pelvis through the skin into the bony structure. This type of fixation can be performed at the scene of the injury in an attempt to decrease bleeding and to immediately immobilize bony deformities. A pneumatic antishock garment (PASG) immobilizes unstable bony injuries and provides a tamponade effect, but it is a controversial intervention because its use has been associated with an increase in prehospital time and hemodynamic abnormalities. External stabilization can also be accomplished through the use of an external skeletal fixation device.

There is a growing trend to use early surgical treatment to decrease blood transfusion requirements, decrease systemic complications, prevent deformities, and improve survival. Surgical open reduction and internal fixation of pelvic ring disruptions are accomplished with the use of a variety of plates and screws that are secured internally. The goal of internal fixation is to restore the pelvis to its original anatomic configuration. When to perform the open reduction and internal fixation is controversial. Monitor for erythema, drainage, and edema at all wound sites, incision sites, and external fixator appliance insertion sites every 4 hours. Perform pin care as prescribed every 4 to 6 hours.

Pharmacologic Highlights

General Comments: Surgeons may choose to follow cultures of wounds, urine, blood, and sputum rather than use prophylactic antibiotics. A tetanus booster may be administered to patients, depending on their history.

Medication or Drug Class	Dosage	Description	Rationale
Narcotic analgesics	Varies with drug but generally given IV in the early phases	Morphine sulfate, fentanyl, meperidine	Provide relief of pain

Other Drugs: Antibiotics such as gentamicin, ampicillin, vancomycin, metronidazole; other analgesics such as hydrocodone bitartrate and acetaminophen, oxycodone and acetaminophen; anticoagulants or antiplatelet drugs as appropriate

Independent

Maintain the patient in a supine position if it is not contraindicated because of other injuries. Ensure adequate airway and breathing in this position. Because Trendelenburg position may have negative hemodynamic consequences, may increase the risk of aspiration, and may interfere with pulmonary excursion, it is not recommended. If the PASG has been applied to stabilize the bony fractures and tamponade bleeding, protect the extremities with towels.

Wound care varies, depending on the severity of wounds, the presence of an open fracture, and the type of fixation device applied. Initial débridement may be done in the operating room at the time of the exploratory laparotomy. Wounds and any exposed soft tissue and bone are covered with wet sterile saline dressings. Avoid povidone-iodine (Betadine)–soaked dressings to limit iodine absorption and skin irritation. Use universal precautions to avoid exposing patients to infection.

Extensive periods of bedrest increase the risk of complications. Remove devices every shift to assess the underlying skin and provide skin care. Sequential compression devices may be applied to the upper extremities if the lower extremities are fractured or in skeletal traction. Provide active or passive range-of-motion exercises to uninjured extremities every shift, as appropriate. Maintain traction by keeping it free-hanging; do not remove weights when moving or repositioning the patient. Some patients may benefit from the use of specialty beds, such as a rotating bed that may improve pulmonary status while maintaining bony stability. Do not use external fixation devices to move or turn patients. Maintain skin integrity by using specialty mattresses with pressure-releasing components. Protect the patient from injury by covering all wire ends with plastic tips, corks, or gauze. When positioning the patient with an external fixation device, protect the skin with padding. Keep the patient's skin clean and dry. Gently massage the patient's bony prominences every 4 hours.

Evidence-Based Practice and Health Policy

Chaijareenont, C., Krutsri, C., Sumpritpradit, P., Singhatas, P., Thampongsa, T., Lertsithichai, P., Choikrua, P., & Poprom, N. (2020). FAST accuracy in major pelvic fractures for decision-making of abdominal exploration: Systematic review and meta-analysis. *Annals of Medicine and Surgery, 60*, 175–181.

• The authors wanted to determine the accuracy of FAST in diagnosing significant intra-abdominal hemorrhage following pelvic fracture to determine if therapeutic abdominal exploration was necessary. They reviewed electronic databases and found 677 cases, and they added 28 cases from their own institution.
• Leading mechanisms of injury were motor vehicle collision, fall from height, and motorcycle collision. Overall mortality rate was 11.65%. The pooled sensitivity, specificity, and accuracy of FAST to identify significant intra-abdominal hemorrhage was 79%, 90%, and 93%, respectively. The authors concluded that FAST in major pelvic fracture accurately detected significant intra-abdominal hemorrhage. It also allowed practitioners to determine whether to perform abdominal exploration with the expectation of finding significant intra-abdominal hemorrhage that required surgical control.

DOCUMENTATION GUIDELINES

• Physical findings: Vital signs, urine output, body weight, capillary refill, mental status, quality of peripheral pulses, urethral bleeding, bowel sounds, wound healing, bruising
• Response to bedrest and immobility, position of external fixation device, degree of range of motion, progress toward rehabilitation
• Presence of complications: Infection; pressure sores; inadvertent injury from external fixation devices, hemorrhages
• Pain: Location, duration, precipitating factors, responses to interventions

DISCHARGE AND HOME HEALTHCARE GUIDELINES

To prevent complications of prolonged immobility, encourage the patient to participate in physical and occupational therapy as prescribed. If compression stockings are prescribed, teach the patient or family the correct application. Verify that the patient has demonstrated safe use of assistive devices such as wheelchairs, crutches, walkers, and transfers. Teach the patient the purpose, dosage, schedule, precautions, potential side effects, interactions, and adverse reactions of all prescribed medications. Review with the patient all follow-up appointments that are arranged. If home care is necessary, verify that appropriate arrangements have been completed.

Pelvic Inflammatory Disease

DRG Category:	744
Mean LOS:	5.8 days
Description:	SURGICAL: Dilation & Curettage, Conization, Laparoscopy and Tubal Interruption With Complication or Comorbidity or Major Complication or Comorbidity
DRG Category:	758
Mean LOS:	4.4 days
Description:	MEDICAL: Infections, Female Reproductive System With Complication or Comorbidity

Pelvic inflammatory disease (PID) is a polymicrobial infectious disease of the pelvic cavity and the female reproductive organs. The Centers for Disease Control and Prevention estimate that one million women experience PID each year in the United States. PID may be localized and confined to one area or it can be widespread and involve the whole pelvic region including the uterus (endometritis), fallopian tubes (salpingitis), ovaries (oophoritis), pelvic peritoneum, and pelvic vascular system. The infection can be acute and recurrent or chronic. The first stage of the disease is either vaginal or cervical infection with an organism. The second phase, which is when the disease becomes symptomatic, is the movement of the organism into the upper genitourinary tract, with resulting infection and inflammation of organs and tissues. Intercourse may speed the movement due to orgasm, and hormonal changes during ovulation and menstruation may aid the movement upward.

PID can be a life-threatening and life-altering condition. Complications of PID include pelvic (or generalized) peritonitis and abscess formations, with possible obstruction of the fallopian tubes. Obstructed fallopian tubes can cause infertility or an ectopic pregnancy. Other complications of PID are bacteremia with septic shock, thrombophlebitis with the possibility of an embolus, chronic abdominal pain, and pelvic adhesions.

CAUSES

The causes of PID vary by geographic location and population. Many types of microorganisms, such as a virus, bacteria, fungus, or parasite, can cause PID. Common organisms involved in PID include *Chlamydia trachomatis*, *Neisseria gonorrheae*, staphylococci, streptococci, coliform bacteria, mycoplasmas, and *Clostridium perfringens*. The means of transmission is usually by sexual intercourse, but PID can also be transmitted by childbirth or by an abortion. Organisms enter the endocervical canal and proceed into the upper uterus, tubes, and ovaries. During menses, the endocervical canal is slightly dilated, facilitating the movement of bacteria to the upper reproductive organs. Bacteria multiply rapidly in the favorable environment of the sloughing endometrium. Douching increases the risk for PID because it destroys the protective normal flora of the vagina, and it could flush bacteria up into the uterus. Risk of reoccurrence of PID is possible with the use of latex condoms if they are not used correctly. *Actinomyces* bacteria may lead to PID cases when linked with the use of an intrauterine device (IUD). Risks for PID include young age at first intercourse, multiple sex partners, history of sexually transmitted infections (STIs), previous PID infections, frequent sexual intercourse, use of an intrauterine device, history of HIV disease, and having unprotected sexual intercourse.

GENETIC CONSIDERATIONS

Heritable immune responses could be protective or increase susceptibility.

SEX AND LIFE SPAN CONSIDERATIONS

PID is the most common cause for hospitalization of reproductive-age women. It predominantly affects women who are sexually active, particularly those who have multiple partners or who change partners frequently. In the future, men may be screened for chlamydia to decrease PID in females.

HEALTH DISPARITIES AND SEXUAL/GENDER MINORITY HEALTH

For women who have had PID previously, there are no ethnic and racial differences in PID prevalence. In women who have never had PID diagnosed, Black women have a lifetime prevalence that is 2.2 times that of White women. Women with lower median income and no insurance, both of which may decrease access to and use of healthcare, have the highest percentage of emergency department visits due to PID. In a large study of female Veterans, Black, Hispanic, and Native American/Pacific Islander women were more likely to have experienced PID, more likely to report infertility, and less likely to report receiving infertility treatments than White women (Goossen et al., 2019). Sexual and gender minority status has no known effect on the risk for PID.

GLOBAL HEALTH CONSIDERATIONS

PID is a serious problem internationally. The causative organism is highly dependent on geographical region. While no international data are available on PID prevalence, the World Health Organization estimates that 448 million cases of curable STIs occur each year in people 14 to 49 years of age. Experts suggest that in rural areas of developing countries, rates of PID are higher than in urban areas because of increased parity, multiple sexual contacts, and associated pelvic organ prolapse.

ASSESSMENT

HISTORY. A thorough history of past infections, a sexual history, and a history of contraceptive use are essential to evaluate a patient with PID. The patient may describe a vaginal discharge, but the characteristics of the discharge (e.g., color, presence of an odor, consistency, amount) depend on the causative organism. For example, a gonorrhea or staphylococcus infection causes a heavy, purulent discharge. With a streptococcus infection, however, the discharge is thinner with a mucoid consistency. The patient may also experience pain or tenderness, described as aching, cramping, and stabbing, particularly in the lower abdomen, pelvic region, or both. Low back pain may also be present. Other symptoms include dyspareunia (painful sexual intercourse); fever greater than 101°F (38.3°C); general malaise; anorexia; headache; nausea, possibly with vomiting; urinary problems such as dysuria, frequency, urgency, and burning; menstrual irregularity; and constipation or diarrhea.

PHYSICAL EXAMINATION. Observe closely for **vaginal discharge** and the characteristics of this discharge. Common symptoms include **pain or tenderness, described as aching, cramping, and stabbing, particularly in the lower abdomen or pelvic region.** Inspect the vulva for signs of maceration. Note if the patient has experienced pruritus that has led to irritated, red skin from scratching. When the cervix is manipulated, the patient may complain of pain in this area. Uterine tenderness and adnexal tenderness (tenderness in those structures next to the uterus such as the ovaries and fallopian tubes) is usually present. Auscultate the bowel; at first, the bowel sounds are normal, but as the disease progresses, if it is not treated, the bowel sounds are diminished or even absent if a paralytic ileus is present. Rebound tenderness may be noted. If vomiting is reported, inspect the skin for signs of fluid deficit, such as dryness or poor skin turgor.

PSYCHOSOCIAL. Because PID may be a life-threatening and life-altering disease, assess the patient's emotional ability to cope with the disease process. Explore the patient's and partner's concerns about fertility. Because sexual partners need to be treated to prevent reinfection, the patient may have concerns about discussing the illness with the patient's partner or partners. Studies show that many teens with PID are reinfected within 48 months. Notify the patient that some STIs need to be reported to the state public health department and that their partners will be notified.

Diagnostic Highlights

General Comments: A variety of tests, along with clinical symptoms and sexual history, support the diagnosis of PID. All females of childbearing age should have a pregnancy test.

Test	Normal Result	Abnormality With Condition	Explanation
White blood cell (WBC) count	4,500–11,100/mm³	> 10,500/mm³	Infection and inflammation elicit an increase in WBCs
Erythrocyte sedimentation rate	Up to 25 mm/hr	> 25 mm/hr	Inflammation increases the protein content of plasma, thus increasing the weight of red blood cells and causing them to descend faster
C-reactive protein	Negative to trace	Elevated	Indicates inflammation
Laparoscopy (the gold standard)	Normal-appearing reproductive organs	Pelvic structures are red and inflamed; possible adhesions and scarring	Direct visualization of the pelvic cavity
Transvaginal ultrasound or magnetic resonance imaging	Normal-appearing reproductive organs	Thickened, fluid-filled fallopian tubes, pelvic fluid, tubo-ovarian abscess	Indicates infectious disease of reproductive organs
Falloposcopy	Normal-appearing fallopian tubes	Tubes are red and inflamed; possible adhesions and scarring	Visual inspection of the tubes to detect damage

Other Tests: Transvaginal sonography or magnetic resonance imaging; endometrial biopsy with histopathological evidence of infection, culture and sensitivity

PRIMARY NURSING DIAGNOSIS

DIAGNOSIS. Acute pain related to infectious process as evidenced by self-reports of pain, facial grimacing, and/or protective behavior

OUTCOMES. Pain control; Pain level; Comfort status; Symptom control; Symptom severity; Knowledge: Pain management; Knowledge: Disease process; Knowledge: Medication

INTERVENTIONS. Medication administration; Pain management: Acute; Heat/cold application; Analgesic administration; Teaching: Prescribed medication; Teaching: Disease process

PLANNING AND IMPLEMENTATION

Collaborative

Without treatment, this disease process can be lethal. The goal is to rid the patient of infection and preserve fertility if possible. Because no single antibiotic is active against all possible pathogens, the Centers for Disease Control and Prevention (CDC) recommend combination regimens. These regimens vary if the patient is hospitalized or treated on an outpatient basis. Usually, the treatment is with broad-spectrum antibiotics. Both the affected patient and sexual partner(s) should be treated with antibiotics. Patients with PID are usually treated as outpatients, but if they become acutely ill, they may require hospitalization. Patients should be followed up in an outpatient setting within 72 hours to check on the effectiveness of treatment. The hospitalized patient with PID usually is placed on bedrest in a semi-Fowler position to promote vaginal drainage. Priority should be given to timely administration of IV antibiotics to maintain therapeutic blood levels. IV fluids may be initiated to prevent or correct dehydration and acidosis. If an ileus or abdominal distention is present, a nasogastric tube is usually inserted to decompress the gastrointestinal tract. Urinary catheterization is contraindicated to avoid the spread of the disease process; tampons are also contraindicated.

Laparoscopy allows for direct visualization of the pelvis and collecting of cultures. PID can sometimes be managed with laparoscopic surgery. If antibiotic therapy is not successful and the patient has an abscess, hydrosalpinx (distention of the fallopian tube by fluid), or some type of obstruction, a hysterectomy with bilateral salpingo-oophorectomy (removal of ovaries and fallopian tubes) may be done. A laparotomy may be done to incise adhesions and to drain an abscess. Signs of peritonitis, such as abdominal rigidity, distention, and guarding, need to be reported immediately so that medical or surgical intervention can be initiated. If the patient is poorly nourished, a dietary consultation is indicated.

Analgesics are prescribed to manage the pain that accompanies PID. Comfort measures can include the use of heat applied to the abdomen or, if they are approved by the physician, warm douches to improve circulation to the area. (See other interventions for pain in the following section.)

Several oral/oral-parenteral antibiotic regimens are also newly recommended by the CDC. For example, an oral and intramuscular regimen is ceftriaxone 250 mg IM, single dose, plus doxycycline 100 mg bid PO for 14 days with or without metronidazole 500 mg PO bid for 14 days; a parenteral regimen is cefotetan 2 g IV q12 hours plus doxycycline 100 mg PO or IV every 12 hours.

Pharmacologic Highlights

Medication or Drug Class	Dosage	Description	Rationale
Cefoxitin or cefotetan and doxycycline	Varies with drug, but course is 14 days	Cephalosporin, second-generation cephalosporin, second-generation tetracycline antibiotic	Inpatient treatment recommended by the CDC
Clindamycin and gentamycin	Varies with drug	Antibiotic, aminoglycoside	Inpatient treatment recommended by the CDC

Independent

Monitor vital signs and the patient's symptoms to evaluate the course of the infection and its response to treatment. Always follow universal precautions; ensure that any item used by the patient is carefully disinfected. Provide perineal care every 2 to 4 hours with warm, soapy water to keep the area clean. Teach the patient that these procedures need to be done as well. Allow the patient time to express concerns. If appropriate, include the patient's partner in a question-and-answer session about the couple's potential to have children. Note that the inability to bear children is a severe loss for most couples, and they may need a referral for counseling.

Interventions that can help relieve pain include having the patient lie on the side with the knees flexed toward the abdomen. Massaging the lower back also increases comfort. Use diversions such as music, television, and reading to take the patient's mind off the discomfort.

Teach the patient interventions to prevent the recurrence of PID: using condoms, having all current sexual partners examined, washing hands before changing pads or tampons, and wiping the perineum from front to back. Encourage the patient to obtain immediate medical attention if fever, increased vaginal discharge, or pain occurs. Discuss with the patient when sexual intercourse or douching may be resumed (usually at least 7 days after hospital discharge).

Evidence-Based Practice and Health Policy

Falconer, H., Yin, L., Salehi, S., & Altman, D. (2021). Association between pelvic inflammatory disease and subsequent salpingectomy on the risk for ovarian cancer. *European Journal of Cancer, 145*, 38–42.

- The authors aimed to determine the relationships among ovarian cancer, salpingectomy, and PID. In a population-based cohort study using a nationwide registry, data were obtained for women diagnosed with PID with or without a subsequent salpingectomy compared to an undiagnosed population.
- Of the women with a diagnosis of PID who underwent a salpingectomy, there was a significant decrease in ovarian cancer compared to women who had a diagnosis of PID and did not have a salpingectomy. Chronic inflammation of the fallopian tubes has been implicated in malignancies of the reproductive organs, particularly ovarian cancer. The authors note that cells in the fallopian tubes from PID can be a source of precancerous transformation and could contribute to the rise in ovarian cancer.

DOCUMENTATION GUIDELINES

- Physical findings: Vital signs, abdominal assessment, condition of integument
- Occurrence of pain: Location, intensity, duration, triggers, response to pain interventions
- Presence of vaginal discharge: Characteristics, amount of discharge

DISCHARGE AND HOME HEALTHCARE GUIDELINES

PREVENTION. To prevent a recurrence of PID, teach the patient the following:

- Take showers instead of baths
- Wear clean, cotton, nonconstrictive underwear
- Avoid using tampons if they were the problem
- Do not douche
- Change sanitary pads or tampons at a minimum of every 4 hours
- If using a diaphragm, remove it after 6 hours
- If any unusual vaginal discharge or odor occurs, contact a healthcare provider immediately
- Maintain a proper diet, with exercise and weight control
- Maintain proper relaxation and sleep
- Have a gynecological examination at least annually
- Use a condom if there is any chance of infection in the sexual partner
- Use a condom if the sexual partner is not well known or has had another partner recently
- Obtain prompt treatment for any STI and complete the medication prescribed by the healthcare provider

MEDICATIONS. Ensure that the patient knows the correct dosage and time that the medication is to be taken and that the patient understands the importance of adhering to this regimen.

COMPLICATIONS. Teach all patients who have had PID the signs and symptoms of an ectopic pregnancy, which are pain, abnormal vaginal bleeding, faintness, dizziness, and shoulder pain. Explain alternative means of contraception to the patient if the patient previously used an IUD. Ensure that the patient is familiar with the manifestation of PID so the patient can report a recurrence of the disease.

Pelvic Organ Prolapse

DRG Category:	748
Mean LOS:	2.0 days
Description:	SURGICAL: Female Reproductive System Reconstructive Procedures
DRG Category:	760
Mean LOS:	3.4 days
Description:	MEDICAL: Menstrual and Other Female Reproductive System Disorders With Complication or Comorbidity or Major Complication or Comorbidity

Pelvic organ prolapse (POP) is the abnormal descent from their original position, or herniation, of organs in the pelvic cavity. The prolapse may occur through the vaginal opening. Current terminology is to divide the pelvis into anterior, posterior, and middle (apical) compartments to discuss prolapse. Older terminology may refer to the structures themselves: uterus (uterine prolapse) or vaginal apex (apical vaginal prolapse), anterior vagina (cystocele), or posterior vagina (rectocele). A cystocele is a structural problem of the genitourinary tract that occurs in women. The urinary bladder presses against a weakened anterior vaginal wall, causing the bladder to protrude into the vagina. The weakened vaginal wall is unable to support the weight of urine in the bladder, and this results in incomplete emptying of the bladder and cystitis. A rectocele is a defect in the rectovaginal septum, causing a protrusion of the rectum through the posterior vaginal wall. The rectum presses against a weakened posterior vaginal wall, causing the rectal wall to bulge into the vagina. The pressure against the weakened wall is intensified each time the woman strains to have a bowel movement; feces push up against the vaginal wall and intensify the protrusion. Frequently, a rectocele is associated with an enterocele, a herniation of the intestine through the cul-de-sac. Complications include urinary tract infection (UTI), constipation, and dyspareunia.

CAUSES

Pelvic floor defects occur as a result of labor and childbirth when structures are torn or stretched during delivery. It also can be caused by pregnancy itself. Other causes are impaired nerve transmission to the muscles of the pelvic floor from conditions such as diabetes, genital atrophy from low estrogen levels, pelvic tumors, and sacral nerve disorders. Conditions associated with increases in intra-abdominal pressure increase risk: obesity, constipation, or chronic pulmonary disease may lead to POP as well. Women who smoke and have a chronic cough are also at risk. In comparison studies, pregnant persons who deliver vaginally are more likely to have POP than those who have cesarean delivery without labor.

GENETIC CONSIDERATIONS

No clear genetic contributions to susceptibility have been defined.

SEX AND LIFE SPAN CONSIDERATIONS

The disorders tend to occur in middle-aged and older women who have had children by vaginal birth, and incidence increases with age and parity. In postmenopausal women, POP is associated with a higher burden of climacteric symptoms.

HEALTH DISPARITIES AND SEXUAL/GENDER MINORITY HEALTH

Nursing home residents compared to community-dwelling women have worse short- and long-term outcomes related to POP, perhaps explained by multiple vulnerabilities. After surgery for POP, Black women experience a higher complication rate and higher readmission rate than White women. Several factors may contribute to this disparity including surgeon training and experience, institutional factors, and clinician bias (Brown et al., 2022). Sexual and gender minority status has no known effect on the risk for POP.

GLOBAL HEALTH CONSIDERATIONS

In all regions of the globe, up to 50% of parous women have some degree of POP, with even higher prevalence of POP in multiparous, postmenopausal, and older women.

ASSESSMENT

HISTORY. Ask about symptoms such as vaginal fullness or pressure, pain or discomfort during sexual intercourse, or lower back or abdominal pain. Patients may describe frequent and urgent urination, history of UTIs, and urinary incontinence. Ask about the pattern and extent of incontinence: Does incontinence occur during times of stress, such as laughing and sneezing? Is it a constant, slow seepage? Is the amount such that the patient needs to use a peripad or incontinence underwear?

Patients with rectocele may describe a history of constipation, hemorrhoids, low back pain, and problems with evacuation of the bowel. Symptoms may be worse when standing and lifting and are relieved somewhat when lying down. Obstetric history often reveals a forceps delivery, a large fetus, and prolonged pushing during delivery. Some report that they are able to facilitate a bowel movement by applying digital pressure along the posterior vaginal wall when defecating to prevent the rectocele from protruding.

PHYSICAL EXAMINATION. The most common symptoms of POP are **vaginal fullness or pressure, pain or discomfort during sexual intercourse**, and **lower back or abdominal pain**. Patients with a cystocele have **frequent and urgent urination, frequent UTIs, difficulty emptying the bladder**, and **stress incontinence**. Patients with a rectocele have a history of **constipation, hemorrhoids, pressure sensations**, and **difficulty controlling and evacuating the bowel**. Upon inspection, the bulging of the bladder and/or rectum may be visualized when the patient is asked to bear down. This bulge may also be palpated. In addition, inspect the patient for hemorrhoids and assess sphincter tone. Levator ani muscles are tested by inserting two fingers in the vagina and asking the patient to tighten or close the introitus.

The International Continence Society has proposed a classification using the following POP Quantification (POP-Q) system.

STAGE	DESCRIPTION
0	No prolapse
I	Descent of the most distal prolapse to more than 1 cm above the level of the hymen
II	Descent between 1 cm above and 1 cm below the hymen
III	Descent beyond stage II but not complete
IV	Total or complete vaginal eversion

PSYCHOSOCIAL. Assess feelings regarding stress incontinence and the patient's knowledge of the problem. Explore the effects on the patient's social life, ability to travel, ability to meet occupational demands, and sexual function. Patients may describe anxiety about their sexual functioning as they age.

Diagnostic Highlights

General Comments: No specific laboratory tests are indicated unless the patient has the symptoms of a UTI. The healthcare provider may evaluate blood urea nitrogen, creatinine, glucose, and calcium and may order magnetic resonance imaging, urodynamic testing, or cystoscopy.

Test	Normal Result	Abnormality With Condition	Explanation
Bimanual examination	No bulging or protrusions felt along anterior or posterior vaginal walls	Bulging of anterior vaginal wall felt with cystocele; bulging of posterior vaginal wall felt with rectocele	Cystoceles and rectoceles result in prominent protrusions into the vaginal canal
Transvaginal ultrasound	No bulging or protrusions into the vaginal wall	Detailed locations and extent of tissue changes can be visualized	Allows for visualization of identified changes of the endopelvic fascia

PRIMARY NURSING DIAGNOSIS

DIAGNOSIS. Impaired urinary elimination related to weakened vaginal wall and/or bladder protrusion into the vagina as evidenced by frequent urination, urgent urination, urinary stasis, stress incontinence, and/or bladder pressure

OUTCOMES. Urinary continence; Urinary elimination; Knowledge: Treatment regimen; Symptom control; Symptom severity

INTERVENTIONS. Urinary incontinence care; Urinary elimination management; Teaching: Procedure/treatment; Teaching: Disease process

PLANNING AND IMPLEMENTATION
Collaborative

Conservative management is recommended for POP. Mild symptoms of a POP may be relieved by Kegel exercises to strengthen the pelvic musculature. If the patient is postmenopausal, estrogen therapy may be initiated to prevent further atrophy of the vaginal wall. Sometimes, the bladder can be supported by use of a pessary, a device shaped like a diaphragm, cube, or donut inserted into the vagina that exerts pressure on the bladder neck area to support the bladder. Pessaries can cause vaginal irritation and ulceration and are better tolerated when the vaginal epithelium is well estrogenized. When the symptoms of cystoceles and rectoceles are severe, surgical intervention is indicated. For a cystocele, an anterior colporrhaphy (or anterior repair), which sutures the pubocervical fascia to support the bladder and urethra, is done. A posterior colporrhaphy (or posterior repair), which sutures the fascia and perineal muscles to support the perineum and rectum, is performed to correct a rectocele. A newer surgical technique for rectoceles involves the use of a dermal allograft to augment the defect repair. Newer methods also include the use of a synthetic mesh to strengthen the vaginal wall. While the procedure is associated with success rates of over 75%, rates of complication are relatively high, and long-term outcomes are being evaluated.

Preoperative care specifically for posterior repairs includes giving laxatives and enemas to reduce bowel contents. If the new allograft technique is used, postmenopausal patients need to be told to apply estrogen cream for 3 to 4 weeks preoperatively to improve intraoperative handling and postoperative healing.

Postoperatively monitor the patient's vaginal discharge, which should be minimal, as well as the patient's pain level and response to analgesics. Sitz baths may be used for comfort. In an anterior repair, an indwelling urethral catheter is inserted and left in place for approximately 4 days. Encourage fluid intake to ensure adequate urine formation. After a posterior repair, stool softeners and low-residue diets are often given to prevent strain on the incision when defecating.

Pharmacologic Highlights

Medication or Drug Class	Dosage	Description	Rationale
Stool softeners; laxatives	Varies with drug	Drug depends on patient and physician preference	Assist with bowel movement in patients with rectocele
Antibiotics	Varies with drug	Broad-spectrum antibiotic	Prophylaxis for infection related to surgery
Nonsalicylates; opioid analgesics	Varies with drug	Analgesics	Maintain comfort related to mild preoperative pain and more severe postoperative discomfort

Independent

Preventive measures include teaching the patient to do Kegel exercises 100 times a day for life to maintain the tone of the pubococcygeal muscle. Menopausal patients should be encouraged to evaluate the appropriateness of estrogen replacement therapy, which can help strengthen the muscles around the vagina and bladder. If the patient has symptoms that are managed conservatively, teach the patient the use of a pessary—how to clean and store it, how to prevent infections—and to report any complications that may be associated with pessary use, including discomfort, leukorrhea, or vaginal irritation. Answer questions about treatment options and explain the procedures and possible complications.

Listen to the patient's and partner's concerns and assist them in decision making about care. For additional support, have the patient speak to others who have undergone similar treatments.

Evidence-Based Practice and Health Policy

Mattsson, N., Karjalainern, P., Tolppanen, A., Heikkinen, A., Sintonen, H., Harkki, P., Nieminen, K., & Jalkanen, J. (2020). Pelvic organ prolapse surgery and quality of life: A nationwide cohort study. *American Journal of Obstetrics & Gynecology, 222,* E1–10.

- The authors aimed to evaluate the effect of female POP surgery on health-related quality of life and patient satisfaction. They employed a prospective nationwide cohort design of 3,515 women undergoing surgery for POP. The outcomes were measured by health-related quality of life instruments at 6 months and 2 years postoperatively.
- Results suggested a clinically important improvement at 6 months but not at 2 years. However, an improvement in sexual activity, discomfort and symptoms, and urinary excretion was observed during both follow-up assessments. The strongest predictive factors for a favorable outcome were advanced apical prolapse and vaginal bulge. Given that surgical treatment of POP effectively improves quality of life, these results could be used in patient counseling on whether to undergo surgical treatment of POP. Smoking was associated with an unfavorable outcome, so patients should be encouraged to stop smoking to avoid an unfavorable outcome.

DOCUMENTATION GUIDELINES

- Level of comfort and response to pain medication
- Physical response: Fluid intake and output, urinary continence, ability to have a bowel movement, amount and type of vaginal discharge
- Presence of complications: Bleeding, inability to urinate after urethral catheter is removed, infection

DISCHARGE AND HOME HEALTHCARE GUIDELINES

MEDICATIONS. Instruct the patient on all medications, including the dosage, route, action, and adverse effects.

COMPLICATIONS OF SURGERY. Instruct the patient to notify the physician if signs of infection or increased vaginal bleeding are noted. If the patient is discharged with a catheter, be sure the patient understands that the catheter must remain patent and to notify the physician if the catheter fails to drain urine. If the catheter is removed and must be reinserted because the patient cannot urinate, an experienced nurse should replace the catheter to prevent damage to the insertion site.

PATIENT TEACHING. Instruct the patient to avoid enemas, heavy lifting, prolonged standing, and sexual intercourse for approximately 6 weeks. Note that it is normal to have some loss of vaginal sensation for several months. Emphasize the importance of keeping follow-up visits.

Peptic Ulcer Disease

DRG Category:	326
Mean LOS:	13.2 days
Description:	SURGICAL: Stomach, Esophageal, and Duodenal Procedures With Major Complication or Comorbidity
DRG Category:	383
Mean LOS:	4.9 days
Description:	MEDICAL: Uncomplicated Peptic Ulcer With Major Complication or Comorbidity

Peptic ulcer disease refers to ulcerative disorders in the lower esophagus, upper duodenum, and lower portion of the stomach. Approximately 4 to 5 million people in the United States have peptic ulcers. The types of peptic ulcers are gastric and duodenal, both of which are chronic diseases. The ulcer represents the development of a circumscribed defect in the gastric or duodenal mucosa that is exposed to acid and pepsin secretion. The ulcer may extend through the tissue layers of the muscle and serosa into the abdominal cavity. Stress ulcers, which are caused by a physiological response to major trauma, are clinically distinct from chronic peptic ulcers.

Gastric ulcers are less common than duodenal ulcers and usually occur in the lesser curvature of the stomach within 1 inch of the pylorus. The ulcer formation is caused by an inability of the mucosa to protect itself from damage by acid pepsin in the lumen (which is caused by a breakdown of the defensive factors). Duodenal ulcers occur in the proximal part of the duodenum (95%), are often less than 1 cm in diameter, and are round or oval. A higher number of parietal cells in the stomach causes hypersecretion, or rapid emptying of the stomach; this may lead to a larger amount of acid being delivered to the first part of the duodenum and may result in the formation of an ulcer. Hemorrhage, peritonitis, and septic shock can occur if the peptic ulcer erodes through the intestinal wall. Other complications include abdominal or intestinal infarction or erosion of the ulcer into the liver, pancreas, or biliary tract.

CAUSES

The *Helicobacter pylori* bacterium and the use of NSAIDs are the principal causative agents of peptic ulcers. *H pylori* grows in the gastrointestinal (GI) tract, attacks the stomach lining, and creates chronic gastritis. The gastric epithelium becomes inflamed and infiltrated with immune cells, and immune chemicals create more tissue damage. NSAIDs disrupt the mucosal lining of the GI tract, making it more vulnerable to injury. Associated diseases include hyperparathyroidism, chronic lung disease, and alcoholic cirrhosis. Risk factors include a genetic predisposition to ulcer formation, poor cell restitution, excessive acid secretion, stress, excessive alcohol intake, smoking, depression, and chronic use of drugs such as steroidal, potassium, or iodine compounds.

GENETIC CONSIDERATIONS

A polymorphism in the interferon-gamma receptor-1 gene (*IFNGR1*) is associated with an increased likelihood of *H pylori* infection. Another susceptibility factor is a variation in the Lewis (b) blood group antigen, an epithelial receptor for *H pylori*. Autosomal dominant transmission of elevated serum pepsinogen I (PGI) levels has been seen in families with a history of duodenal ulcer. Peptic ulcer is also seen as a component of other genetic conditions, including Zollinger-Ellison syndrome.

SEX AND LIFE SPAN CONSIDERATIONS

The incidence of duodenal ulcers is highest in people ages 40 to 50 years and is equally common in men and women. Gastric ulcers, which occur most often in people ages 60 to 70 years, are more common in men. Mortality with gastric ulcer perforation is three times greater than that with duodenal ulcer perforation, partly because of the increased age of the patients. Duodenal ulcers occur in approximately 10% of the population at some time in their lives. More than half of the people who have duodenal ulcers heal spontaneously but have a high incidence of recurrence within 2 years.

HEALTH DISPARITIES AND SEXUAL/GENDER MINORITY HEALTH

Hospitalization rates for peptic ulcer disease are highest in Black and Asian persons. Experts have noted that persons who are uninsured have higher rates of perforation and higher mortality rates than persons who are insured. Sexual and gender minority status has no known effect on the risk for peptic ulcer disease. However, sexual and gender minority persons have higher rates of alcohol and tobacco consumption than the general population (Centers for Disease Control and Prevention, 2021), which may place them at risk for peptic ulcer disease.

GLOBAL HEALTH CONSIDERATIONS

In developed countries, the incidence of peptic ulcer disease is decreasing with the recognition of the role of *H pylori* bacteria in its development. Additionally, developed countries have reduced the use of NSAID agents. The incidence of peptic ulcer disease in developing countries is increasing depending on the association with *H pylori* and NSAID patterns of use.

▓ ASSESSMENT

HISTORY. Epigastric pain is a common symptom. Assess the patient's pain by obtaining a history of the onset, duration, and characteristics in relation to food intake and medications. Patients may describe pain as sharp, burning, or gnawing, or it may be achy and perceived as abdominal pressure. Pain with duodenal ulcer occurs from 90 minutes to 3 hours after eating, is relieved with food or antacids, and may awaken a person at night. It is located to the right of the midline epigastrium with duodenal ulcers and to the left of the midline with gastric ulcers. Gastric ulcer pain is precipitated by food and is not relieved by antacid use to the same extent as duodenal ulcer pain is. Some patients have constant pain or no clear pattern of discomfort. As a result of the pain, weight loss and anorexia may occur with gastric ulcers. Weight gain may result with duodenal ulcers because food relieves the pain.

Question the patient about a family history of ulcer disease; smoking and alcohol habits; presence of other symptoms, such as nausea and vomiting; heartburn; and changes in stool color, level of energy, appetite, and body weight. Review the patient's medication profile, both prescribed and over the counter (OTC). Ask about the amounts of caffeinated beverages taken daily. Determine the foods that aggravate the symptoms. Assess the patient's level of stress and coping skills.

PHYSICAL EXAMINATION. Epigastric pain is the major symptom. Some patients have pain that is so severe, even slight movement greatly worsens the pain. On inspection, you may note pale mucous membranes and skin because of anemia from acute or chronic blood loss. Some patients have hematemesis and others black or tarry stools that test positive for blood. Currant-colored or bright red stools occur only with massive bleeding. During auscultation, you may note that bowel sounds are hyperactive initially but diminish because of a paralytic ileus with ulcer perforation and peritonitis. Palpation in the midline may reveal epigastric tenderness. If perforation occurs, bacteria and stomach content contaminates the abdominal cavity, and septic shock may occur with fever, hypotension, and tachycardia.

PSYCHOSOCIAL. Researchers have not been able to establish a characteristic duodenal ulcer personality. Chronic stress and anxiety, however, are believed to increase gastric secretions and may be factors in exacerbating ulcer recurrence. Assess the patient's response to the disease and note any unusual stressors that have an effect on the patient's or significant other's life.

Diagnostic Highlights

Test	Normal Result	Abnormality With Condition	Explanation
Esophagogastro-duodenoscopy	Normal GI mucosa	Presence of mucosal ulcerations in the stomach or duodenum; ulcers tend to be solitary and are 1–2.5 cm in size	Flexible endoscopy to allow visualization of mucosa

Note: Experts suggest that in patients older than age 45 to 50 years who have dysphagia, recurrent vomiting, weight loss, or bleeding should have an endoscopy as soon as possible because of risk of hemorrhage. Other Tests: Serum gastrin levels, hemoglobin, hematocrit, complete blood count; serum electrolytes, blood urea nitrogen, and creatinine; coagulation profile; tests for *H pylori*: (1) antibody detection (immunoglobulin G) to *H pylori* is measured in serum, plasma, urine, or whole blood; (2) urea breath tests detect active *H pylori* infection by identifying enzymatic activity of bacterial urease; and (3) fecal antigen testing detects presence of *H pylori* antigens in stools.

PRIMARY NURSING DIAGNOSIS

DIAGNOSIS. Acute pain related to inflammation and irritation as evidenced by self-reports of pain, facial grimacing, and/or protective behavior

OUTCOMES. Comfort status; Pain control; Pain level; Symptom severity; Symptom control; Knowledge: Pain management; Knowledge: Medication

INTERVENTIONS. Analgesic administration; Pain management: Acute; Medication administration; Patient-controlled analgesia assistance; Teaching: Prescribed medication

PLANNING AND IMPLEMENTATION
Collaborative

The treatment of choice for patients with peptic ulcers is generally pharmacologic. Drugs can be used to buffer or inhibit acid secretion that leads to ulceration and causes symptoms. Nutritional therapy is also prescribed. The current treatment is to eliminate foods that cause discomfort and symptoms. There is no evidence that bland or soft diets reduce gastric acid, promote healing, or relieve symptoms. Instruct the patient to avoid alcohol, coffee, and other caffeine-containing beverages. Refer patients with significant weight loss to a dietitian.

Fewer than 5% of patients require surgery. However, in the event of the primary complications of hemorrhage, perforation, or obstruction, surgery may be necessary. Hemorrhage occurs in 15% of patients with duodenal ulcers and occurs more frequently in patients with NSAID-associated ulcers who have no prior symptoms. Perforation into the peritoneal cavity, which occurs in 6% of patients, happens when the ulcer erodes through the entire thickness of the gastric or duodenal wall. Obstruction occurs in 2% to 4% of patients with duodenal or pyloric ulcers. Treatment begins conservatively with gastric suction and fluid and electrolyte therapy. Pyloroplasty may follow.

Pharmacologic Highlights

General Comments: Most duodenal ulcers heal in 4 to 6 weeks, and treatment seldom extends past 8 weeks. Maintenance drug therapy is indicated for at least 1 year for patients with frequent recurrences. Gastric ulcers should heal in 8 to 12 weeks, and more rapidly when acid is completely suppressed with use of a proton pump inhibitor such as omeprazole (Prilosec). If gastric ulcers do not heal with treatment, malignancy is suspected.

Medication or Drug Class	Dosage	Description	Rationale
H$_2$ antagonist	Varies with drug	Cimetidine, famotidine, nizatidine	Reduces acid secretion to optimize ulcer healing
Proton pump inhibitors	Varies with drug	Omeprazole, esomeprazole, lansoprazole, rabeprazole, pantoprazole	Optimizes ulcer healing by binding to the proton pump of parietal cell and inhibiting secretion of hydrogen ions into gastric lumen
Triple therapies: Antibiotics (for patients with H pylori bacteria) and proton pump inhibitor	Omeprazole (Prilosec), 20 mg PO bid for 14 days with clarithromycin (Biaxin) 500 mg PO bid for 14 days and amoxicillin (Amoxil) 1 g PO bid for 14 days and metronidazone or omeprazole, tetracycline, and metronidazole	Other protein pump inhibitors may be used: Lansoprazole (Prevacid); rabeprazole (Aciphex); esomeprazole (Nexium)	Antibiotics eradicate H pylori and protein pump inhibitor reduces acid secretion; triple therapy may also consist of antibiotics and bismuth-based therapy such as Pepto-Bismol

Other Drugs: Antacids (aluminum and magnesium hydroxide), prostaglandins

Independent

Provide information about the cause and contributing factors as they pertain to the individual patient. Explain the relationship of gastric acidity, mucosal damage, and the significance of the symptoms of ulcer formation (pain, bleeding, nausea and vomiting, black stools). Discuss possible complications of peptic ulcer disease as it progresses: hemorrhage, perforation, and obstruction because of repeated ulcerations and scarring. Emphasize the need to adhere to the medication schedule, even when symptoms subside, to ensure complete healing and to prevent recurrence. Encourage the patient to avoid aspirin and other NSAIDs for aches and pains and suggest alternatives, such as acetaminophen (Tylenol). Provide a list of OTC drugs that contain aspirin.

Explore ways to reduce stress and emphasize the importance of emotional and physical rest to reduce gastric secretion. Teach relaxation exercises to use during rest periods that fit into daily routines. Explain why elimination of smoking facilitates healing and reduces recurrence. Provide a list of community agencies that have smoking-cessation programs. Discuss patterns of alcohol use, and if alcohol is a contributing factor, discuss options for alcohol counseling. Discuss the patient's concerns openly. Identify attitudes and situations that could interfere with the needed lifestyle changes. Involve the family or significant others in these discussions and plans to gain their support.

Evidence-Based Practice and Health Policy

Wijarnpreecha, K., Panjawatanan, P., Leelasinjaroen, P., & Ungprasert, P. (2020). Statins and risk of peptic ulcer disease: A systematic review and meta-analysis. *Arab Journal of Gastroenterology, 21*, 135–138.

- The author wanted to summarize all available data from recent epidemiological studies that have suggested that there is a protective effect of statins against the development of peptic ulcer disease. Previous work in this area has been inconsistent. Online databases were used to identify studies that evaluated the risk of peptic ulcer disease among statins users versus nonusers.
- They found the risk of peptic ulcer disease was numerically lower among statins users compared with nonusers. However, the result did not achieve statistical significance in part because of a small sample size. Further work is needed to understand the relationship between statins and peptic ulcer disease.

DOCUMENTATION GUIDELINES

- Physical findings of epigastric or abdominal pain, nausea, vomiting, tarry stools, bleeding, infection, presence of complications (hemorrhage, perforation, obstruction)
- Response to medication therapy, nutritional therapy, emotional/physical rest; response to alcohol and smoking counseling
- Response to surgical interventions

DISCHARGE AND HOME HEALTHCARE GUIDELINES

Advise the patient that recurrence is greater than 50% with noncompliance. Reinforce the need to avoid the following: aspirin products and NSAIDs, alcohol intake, caffeine products, and smoking. Provide information about smoking cessation to patients, and refer patients with alcohol abuse to an outpatient treatment program. Review signs and symptoms that should be reported—those that may indicate recurrence or complications, including pain, nausea, vomiting, black tarry stools, fatigue, and frank bleeding. Stress the importance of eating three meals at approximately the same time each day. Put patient in contact with the Helicobacter Foundation (https://helico.com).

Postoperatively, tell the patient what to expect if infection occurs so the patient can tell the healthcare provider when the first signs occurred. The symptoms include pain, redness, swelling, and drainage at the incisional site. After a Billroth II surgical procedure, the patient may develop symptoms of dumping syndrome. Explain the reason and timing of the symptoms that may occur, noting that the episodes will subside in 6 to 12 months. Teach the patient how to control the problems with the following suggestions: (1) Take fluids only between meals and none with meals; (2) eat smaller amounts more frequently in a semirecumbent position; (3) eat a low-carbohydrate diet, concentrating on high-protein and moderate-fat foods; (4) avoid refined sugars (sweets); (5) lie down after meals for 30 minutes; (6) take anticholinergic drugs 30 minutes before meals as prescribed; and (7) reinforce the need to stop smoking to promote healing and prevent recurrence.

Pericarditis

DRG Category:	315
Mean LOS:	3.6 days
Description:	MEDICAL: Other Circulatory System Diagnoses With Complication or Comorbidity

Pericarditis is an inflammation of the pericardium, which is the membranous sac that encloses the heart and great vessels. The inflammatory response causes an accumulation of leukocytes, platelets, fibrin, and fluid between the parietal and the visceral layers of the pericardial sac, producing a variety of symptoms depending on the amount of fluid accumulation, how quickly it accumulates, and whether the inflammation resolves after the acute phase or becomes chronic. Normally, it contains approximately 20 to 50 mL of fluid and can stretch to accommodate approximately 100 mL of fluid that accumulates rapidly. If additional fluid accumulates, it places pressure on the chambers of the heart, reducing atrial and ventricular filling and markedly decreasing cardiac output. Decreased peripheral perfusion occurs, and if it continues, the patient can develop hypotension and shock.

Chronic constrictive pericarditis usually begins as an acute inflammatory pericarditis and progresses over time to a chronic, constrictive form because of pericardial thickening and stiffening. The thickened, scarred pericardium becomes nondistensible and decreases diastolic filling of the cardiac chambers, and cardiac output falls. Chronic pericardial effusion is a gradual accumulation of fluid in the pericardial sac. The pericardium is slowly stretched and can accommodate more than 1 L of fluid at a time. Complications of pericarditis include cardiac tamponade, heart failure, shock, and death.

CAUSES

Between 25% and 90% of people with pericarditis have illnesses that are considered idiopathic (occurring without a known cause). Pericarditis may also be classified etiologically into three broad categories: infectious pericarditis, noninfectious pericarditis, and pericarditis presumably related to hypersensitivity or autoimmunity. Infectious pericarditis may be caused by tuberculosis (TB) and a viral infection such as the coxsackie B virus. Pyrogenic, tuberculous, mycotic, syphilitic, and parasitic infections may also cause pericarditis. Noninfectious pericarditis may be caused by a number of factors, including acute myocardial infarction, trauma, aortic aneurysm (with leakage into the pericardial sac), sarcoidosis, and myxedema. Uremic pericarditis occurs in up to 10% of people with end-state renal failure. Both primary tumors, either benign or malignant, and metastatic tumors in the pericardium may cause pericarditis. Other causes include cholesterol and chylopericardium.

Pericarditis is also thought to be related to hypersensitivity or autoimmunity. Rheumatic fever and collagen vascular disease, such as systemic lupus erythematosus, rheumatoid arthritis, and scleroderma, may cause pericarditis. Other cardiac-related and miscellaneous causes include postcardiac injury (Dressler syndrome, postpericardiotomy syndrome) and drugs such as procainamide, isoniazid, reserpine, and hydralazine.

GENETIC CONSIDERATIONS

Although currently genetic contributions to pericarditis are unknown, recurrent pericarditis can be seen as a feature of a heritable problem such as familial Mediterranean fever, an autosomal recessive disease that primarily affects Jews, Turks, Armenians, and Arabs. There is also an autosomal recessive syndrome called CACP (camptodactyly arthropathy coxa vara pericarditis) that is caused by mutations in the gene *PRG4*.

SEX AND LIFE SPAN CONSIDERATIONS

Pericardial disease can occur at any age. Idiopathic (viral) inflammatory pericarditis occurs most frequently in adults and is more common in men than in women. Tuberculous (bacterial) pericarditis occurs most often in children and in immunosuppressed patients.

HEALTH DISPARITIES AND SEXUAL/GENDER MINORITY HEALTH

Ethnicity and race have no known effect on the risk for pericarditis. The Centers for Disease Control and Prevention (CDC) reported in 2018 that 69% of new HIV diagnoses in the United States were in gay and bisexual men. In young people ages 13 to 24 years, young gay and bisexual men account for 83% of all new HIV diagnoses. HIV places people at risk for tuberculosis and tuberculosis-related pericarditis.

GLOBAL HEALTH CONSIDERATIONS

Pericarditis is a global health problem. In developed countries, malignancy is the most common cause of pericardial effusions secondary to pericarditis. In developing countries, TB is an important cause of pericarditis.

░ ASSESSMENT

HISTORY. Establish a history of recent surgeries, injuries, infections, and other illnesses. Acute inflammatory pericarditis is most frequently idiopathic; however, the patient may have a history of a viral, bacterial, fungal, or parasitic infection. Take a detailed history of the patient's symptoms, especially pain. Ask the patient to describe the pain: Is it dull or sharp, and is it persistent? Is the location of the pain retrosternal or left precordial and radiating to the neck, left arm, and trapezius ridge? Ask if the pain is worsened by trunk movement, position, and deep inspiration. Palpitations are often the presenting symptom as well. Ask about fever, cough, dyspnea, dysphagia, hiccups, nausea, and abdominal pressure (because of the compression of surrounding tissues by the enlarged pericardial sac).

The patient with a chronic pericardial disease may reveal a history of myocardial infarction (Dressler syndrome, an inflammatory response after a myocardial infarction), TB, chronic renal failure, radiation therapy, malignancies, connective tissue disease, and HIV disease. Note a history of increasing dyspnea, fatigue, loss of appetite, nausea, and cough. Chest pain is not usually associated with chronic pericarditis.

PHYSICAL EXAMINATION. The most common symptoms are **precordial or retrosternal chest pain, tachycardia, tachypnea, cough**, and **fever**. If there is an effusion, the blood pressure may be low and a pulsus paradoxus (an abnormal drop in systolic pressure with inspiration) may be present. Inspect the patient's neck for vein distention because of elevated jugular venous pressures caused by chronic pericarditis. Auscultate for heart sounds to establish a pericardial friction rub, which is a scratching or grating sound that occurs at different points during systole and diastole in about 50% of people with pericarditis. Although the presence of a pericardial friction rub is a significant finding, the absence of a rub is not, because pericardial friction rub is transient.

PSYCHOSOCIAL. Because of severe chest pain, patients with acute pericarditis are likely in distress. The patient may be fearful of having a myocardial infarction. Assess the patient's ability to cope with a sudden illness and severe pain.

Diagnostic Highlights

Test	Normal Result	Abnormality With Condition	Explanation
Transthoracic echocardiography	Normal	Abnormal amount of fluid in pericardial sac	Inflammatory response causes accumulation of leukocytes, platelets, fibrin, and fluid between the parietal and the visceral layers of the pericardial sac

Diagnostic Highlights (continued)

Test	Normal Result	Abnormality With Condition	Explanation
Electrocardiogram	Normal PQRST pattern	PR segment depression; ST-T wave elevation and eventually T-wave inversion when ST segment returns to baseline	Results of pericardial thickening and diminished diastolic filling
Computed tomography scan or magnetic resonance imaging	Normal cardiac structures	Pericardial thickening	Radiography and three-dimensional evidence of inflamed pericardium

Other Tests: White blood cell count (elevated), serum electrolytes, blood urea nitrogen, creatinine, erythrocyte sedimentation rate, C-reactive protein, cardiac enzymes (creatine kinase, troponin), TB testing, HIV testing, thyroid function tests, liver function tests, chest x-ray, intracardiac pressure measurements, cardiac catheterization, echocardiography

PRIMARY NURSING DIAGNOSIS

DIAGNOSIS. Acute pain related to swelling and inflammation of the heart or surrounding tissue as evidenced by self-reports of pain, facial grimacing, and/or protective behavior

OUTCOMES. Comfort status; Pain control; Pain level; Symptom control; Symptom severity; Rest; Knowledge: Pain management; Knowledge: Disease process; Knowledge: Medication

INTERVENTIONS. Analgesic administration; Pain management: Acute; Oxygen therapy; Medication administration; Teaching: Prescribed medication

PLANNING AND IMPLEMENTATION
Collaborative

Pericarditis is treated by correcting the underlying cause and therefore relieving the signs and symptoms. Acute pericarditis is treated with analgesic and anti-inflammatory agents. Acute pericardial effusions are treated according to the hemodynamic effect on the myocardium. An acute effusion that causes a decreased cardiac output is an indication for pericardiocentesis. An echocardiographically guided percutaneous pericardiocentesis is considered the procedure of choice because the intended needle direction is guided by echocardiography to confirm the direction for needle advancement and removal of fluid from the pericardial sac. Pericarditis caused by renal failure may be treated by intensifying dialysis. Cardiac compression is relieved, and cardiac output returns. Other alternatives are a pericardiotomy, which is a surgical incision in the pericardial sac, or pericardial window (fenestration), which is the removal of one or more small portions of the pericardial sac. These surgical procedures are used when pericardiocentesis is unsuccessful or must be repeated because of continued accumulation of fluid.

Chronic pericarditis, with or without an effusion, may require a pericardectomy, which involves a thoracotomy incision and carries a much higher mortality (5%–14%) than the other procedures. Note that to halt the hemorrhage, a rapidly accumulating tamponade from hemorrhage into the pericardiac space should be managed surgically rather than by pericardiocentesis.

Pharmacologic Highlights

Medication or Drug Class	Dosage	Description	Rationale
NSAIDs	Varies with drugs	Aspirin, indomethacin, ibuprofen, ketorolac	Reduce pain and inflammation

(highlight box continues on page 936)

Pharmacologic Highlights (continued)

Other Drugs: Other choices include anti-inflammatories such as colchicine, alone or in combination with an NSAID, or aspirin for treatment of pericarditis associated with myocardial infarction. Corticosteroids can create gastrointestinal disturbances, which may increase the likelihood of the patient's failure to adhere to the prescribed medical therapy. Bacterial pericarditis is treated with antibiotics.

Independent

Place the patient in a high Fowler position. Use pillows to increase the patient's comfort and encourage the patient to sit upright and lean slightly forward rather than lie supine. If the upright position does not alleviate the pain, have the patient try a side-lying position for 10 minutes. If the patient needs to perform coughing and deep-breathing exercises, provide instruction on splinting the chest with pillows to decrease the pain.

Remain with the patient during periods of increased pain and discomfort. Encourage the patient and family to verbalize their fears and concerns and to ask questions about the treatment and course of the disorder. Inform the patient and family about pericarditis and its causes. Explain all procedures. Assist the patient and family in distinguishing acute pericarditis from myocardial infarction. Teach them about continuing medications as prescribed even after the pain is gone but to taper use of steroids.

Evidence-Based Practice and Health Policy

Huang, J., Zhu, P., Zhong, F., Yu, G., Ye, B., & Fang, L. (2020). Clinical significance of pulse index contour continuous cardiac output monitoring in patients with constrictive pericarditis undergoing pericardiectomy. *Interactive Cardiovascular and Thoracic Surgery, 31*, 364–368.

- The usefulness of pulse index contour continuous cardiac output (PiCCO) monitoring in patients with constrictive pericarditis undergoing pericardiectomy is unclear. The authors aimed to explore whether PiCCO monitoring could improve clinical outcomes such as postoperative and survival outcomes in 74 patients with an intervention and control group. The baseline characteristics were comparable between the two groups, 33 in the experimental and 41 in the control group.
- The PiCCO group showed more intraoperative fluid infusion and higher postoperative central venous pressure as well as lower levels of postoperative brain natriuretic peptide, and a lower incidence of postoperative complications. The PiCCO group showed significantly shorter duration of chest drainage, length of stay in the intensive care unit, and postoperative hospital stay. The authors noted that PiCCO monitoring in the recovery of patients with constrictive pericarditis provides new options for monitoring that may positively affect outcomes.

DOCUMENTATION GUIDELINES

- Physical findings: Vital signs, signs of pulsus paradoxus or pericardial friction rub, breath sounds, quality of heart tones
- Response to treatments like pericardiocentesis, status of puncture site, status in symptoms after the procedure (usually symptoms subside after fluid drainage)
- Assessment of pain: Precipitating factors, quality, radiation, associated signs and symptoms, relief
- Response to medication: Body temperature, pain control

DISCHARGE AND HOME HEALTHCARE GUIDELINES

Be sure the patient understands any pain medication prescribed, including dosage, route, action, and side effects. The patient and family or significant other need to understand the importance of decreased activity until the chest pain is completely gone. If the patient has undergone a surgical procedure, follow the activity restrictions for a thoracotomy.

Peritonitis

DRG Category:	394
Mean LOS:	3.8 days
Description:	MEDICAL: Other Digestive System Diagnoses With Complication or Comorbidity
DRG Category:	357
Mean LOS:	5.9 days
Description:	SURGICAL: Other Digestive System Operating Room Procedures With Complication or Comorbidity

Peritonitis is the inflammation of the peritoneal cavity. The peritoneum is a double-layered, semipermeable sac that lines the abdominal cavity and covers all the organs in the abdominal cavity. Between its visceral and its parietal layers is the peritoneal cavity. Although the peritoneum walls off areas of contamination to prevent the spread of infection, if the contamination is massive or continuous, this defense mechanism may fail, resulting in peritonitis. Peritoneal infections are classified as primary, secondary, or tertiary. Primary infections usually occur in people who are immunocompromised, and they occur by spread of bacteria from the blood. Secondary infections are related to a pathological process such as a perforated abdomen or abdominal injury. Tertiary peritonitis is a persistent infection after appropriate initial treatment. Peritonitis can also occur by chemical irritants such as bile, blood, or other substances that enter the peritoneal cavity without an accompanying bacterial infection. The inflammatory response that occurs with chemical peritonitis is similar to secondary peritonitis.

Normally, the peritoneum is sterile. When there is spillage of the contents of the gastrointestinal (GI) tract into the peritoneum, which occurs from secondary peritonitis, bacteria enter the sterile peritoneum, proliferate, and create an immune response. A cascade of events leads to production of cytokines and hormones that cause cellular damage, shock, and even organ failure. One of the most serious complications caused by peritonitis is intestinal obstruction, which results in death in 10% of patients. Other complications include abscess formation, bacteremia, respiratory failure, sepsis, and septic shock.

CAUSES

The most common cause is infection with *Escherichia coli*, but streptococci, staphylococci, and pneumococci may also cause the inflammation. The main sources of inflammation are the GI tract, external environment, and bloodstream. Entry of a foreign body—such as a bullet, knife, or indwelling abdominal catheter—and contaminated peritoneal dialysate may precipitate peritonitis. Acute pancreatitis may also cause peritonitis. Risk factors for peritonitis include immune suppression, appendicitis, stomach ulcers, pancreatitis, alcohol abuse, liver cirrhosis, renal failure, inflammatory bowel disease, trauma, peritoneal dialysis, and surgical procedures.

GENETIC CONSIDERATIONS

Heritable immune responses could be protective or could increase susceptibility. Peritonitis is associated with familial Mediterranean fever, which is caused by mutations in the *MEFV* gene.

SEX AND LIFE SPAN CONSIDERATIONS

Peritonitis can occur at any age. Older patients with peritonitis are at greater risk for developing life-threatening complications as compared to children and young adults. Older patients with cirrhosis who have secondary peritonitis have a poor long-term prognosis. In contrast, the young adult male population is particularly at risk because of the prevalence of peritonitis related to multiple trauma.

HEALTH DISPARITIES AND SEXUAL/GENDER MINORITY HEALTH

Ethnicity, race, and sexual/gender minority status have no known effect on the risk for peritonitis.

GLOBAL HEALTH CONSIDERATIONS

While peritonitis exists in all regions of the world, no prevalence data are available.

ASSESSMENT

HISTORY. Obtain a thorough history and try to determine the possible sources of peritoneal infection. Ascertain any history of GI disorders, penetrating or blunt trauma to the abdomen, or recent abdominal surgery. Ask if the patient has any inability to pass flatulence or stools. Ask if the patient has experienced any weakness, nausea, vomiting, or diarrhea or a recent history of dehydration and high temperatures.

The parietal peritoneum is well supplied with somatic nerves, whereas the visceral peritoneum is relatively insensitive. With peritonitis, stimulation of the parietal peritoneum causes sharp, localized pain, whereas stimulation of the visceral peritoneum results in a more generalized abdominal pain. The pain is a steady ache that occurs directly over the area of inflammation. The intensity depends on the type and amount of foreign substances that are irritating the peritoneum and the somatic nerves supplying the parietal peritoneum. Peritoneal pain is almost always increased by pressure or tension of the peritoneum, such as coughing, sneezing, and palpation. Ask whether abdominal pain is generalized or localized. Inflamed diaphragmatic peritonitis can cause shoulder pain as well.

PHYSICAL EXAMINATION. Common symptoms include **abdominal pain and distention, fever, chills, changes in mental status,** and **diarrhea.** Note that as many as 20% of patients have few or no symptoms. Some patients may develop ascites, acute renal failure, and paralytic ileus. Visually inspect the abdomen for size and shape. Peritonitis leads to abdominal distention. When assessing the GI system, auscultate before palpation. Bowel sounds are decreased or absent. Palpation reveals abdominal rigidity and elicits rebound tenderness with guarding. The patient may keep movement to a minimum to reduce the pain. Well-localized pain may cause rigidity of the abdominal muscles. The patient is generally in a knee-flexed position with shallow respirations in an attempt to minimize pain.

Check the patient for signs of dehydration, such as a dry and swollen tongue, dry mucous membranes, and thirst. High fever may result in rapid heart rate. The patient may experience hiccups in cases of diaphragmatic peritonitis. Observe the patient for pallor, excessive sweating, or cold skin, which are signs of electrolyte and fluid loss.

PSYCHOSOCIAL. Patients with peritonitis have often been coping with a serious illness or traumatic injury to the abdomen and may already be weary of discomfort and pain. Besides dealing with intensified pain and new complications, the patient with peritonitis is also at risk for life-threatening complications such as shock, renal problems, and respiratory problems. Assess the patient's and family's anxiety and feelings of powerlessness about the illness and potential complications.

Diagnostic Highlights

Test	Normal Result	Abnormality With Condition	Explanation
White blood cell (WBC) count	Adult males and females: 4,500–11,100/mm^3	Elevated	Detects the presence of an infectious process

Diagnostic Highlights (continued)

Test	Normal Result	Abnormality With Condition	Explanation
Abdominal and chest x-rays	Normal structures	Dilation, edema, inflammation, fluid or free air in abdominal cavity	Inflammation leads to accumulation of fluid, perforation, or even rupture
Diagnostic peritoneal lavage	Clear return	WBCs: > 500 mm³; red blood cells: > 50,000/mL; presence of bacteria on Gram stain; bile-stained fluid	Identifies presence of infection, bleeding, or in the case of bile, ruptured gallbladder or intestines

Other Tests: Tests include serum electrolytes, blood urea nitrogen, creatinine, hemoglobin, hematocrit, blood cultures and sensitivities. Experimental diagnostic test: Rapid diagnosis of spontaneous bacterial peritonitis through bedside reagent strips analyzed by a portable spectrophotometric instrument. Generally, the diagnosis can be made clinically, and abdominal ultrasound and computed tomography (CT) are not used because they delay surgical treatment. CT scan may be used to locate a peritoneal abscess or other pathology.

PRIMARY NURSING DIAGNOSIS

DIAGNOSIS. Acute pain related to inflammation of the peritoneal cavity as evidenced by self-reports of pain, facial grimacing, and/or protective behavior

OUTCOMES. Comfort status; Pain control; Pain level; Symptom severity; Symptom control; Rest; Knowledge: Pain management; Knowledge: Medication

INTERVENTIONS. Analgesic administration; Pain management: Acute; Medication administration; Patient-controlled analgesia assistance

▓ PLANNING AND IMPLEMENTATION

Collaborative

Interventions are supportive and include fluid and electrolyte replacement. To rest the GI tract, a nasogastric (NG) or intestinal tube is inserted to reduce pressure within the bowel. Food and fluids are prohibited. Parenteral nutrition is often indicated for nutritional support. Monitor fluid volume by checking the patient's skin turgor, urine output, weight, vital signs, mucous membrane condition, and intake and output, including NG tube drainage.

If the peritonitis has been caused by a perforation of the peritoneum, surgery is necessary as soon as the patient's condition is stabilized. Surgery will eliminate the source of the infection by removing the foreign contents from the peritoneal cavity and inserting drains. Paracentesis (abdominocentesis) to remove excess fluids may be necessary as well. Some patients may undergo percutaneous and endoscopic stent placement for drainage or laparoscopic surgery. After surgery, it is important to assess the patient frequently for peristaltic activity. Auscultate for bowel sounds and check for flatus, bowel movements, and a soft abdomen. When peristalsis resumes and the patient's temperature and pulse rate become normal, treatment generally calls for a decrease in parenteral fluids and an increase in oral fluids. If the patient has an NG tube in place, clamp it for short intervals. If the patient does not experience nausea or vomiting, begin oral fluids as ordered and tolerated.

Pharmacologic Highlights

Medication or Drug Class	Dosage	Description	Rationale
Antibiotics	Varies with drug	Third-generation cephalosporin cefotaxime; other antibiotics might be used such as cefoxitin, cefuroxime, ceftriaxone, or ampicillin with an aminoglycoside; amoxicillin, piperacillin, tazobactam, ticarcillin, clindamycin	Halt the growth of bacteria and cause bacterial lysis
Analgesics	Varies with drug	Meperidine (Demerol), morphine, fentanyl	Relieve pain; until a firm diagnosis is made, analgesia may be withheld to prevent its masking significant changes in the patient's condition

Independent

Nursing care focuses on providing a stable, comfortable environment for the patient, who is experiencing both physical and psychological stress. To provide relief from pain, maintain bedrest and place the patient in the semi-Fowler position, which helps the patient breathe more deeply. Offer regular oral hygiene and lubrications to counteract mouth and nose dryness caused by fever, dehydration, and NG intubation. Provide psychological support by encouraging questions and verbalization of the patient's anxieties and concerns. Teach the patient about peritonitis and what caused it in the patient's case, explaining the necessary treatment.

For patients who are undergoing surgery, provide teaching before surgery. Answer questions about the surgical procedure and the potential complications. Review postoperative care procedures. Teach the patient deep-breathing and coughing exercises. Explain the duration of the patient's hospital stay after surgery, which varies depending on the underlying cause. Postoperatively, because even slight movements intensify the patient's pain, move the patient carefully. Keep the bed's side rails up and implement other safety measures, particularly if fever and pain disorient the patient. Teach the patient how to care for the incision; describe signs of infection. If convalescent services are required after discharge, refer the patient to the hospital's social service department or to a home healthcare agency.

Evidence-Based Practice and Health Policy

Collard, M., Lefevre, J., Batteux, F., & Parc, Y. (2020). COVID-19 health crisis: Less colorectal resections and yet no more peritonitis or bowel obstructions as a collateral effect? *Colorectal Disease, 22*, 1229–1230.

- The authors note that during the early days of the COVID health crisis, hospitals declared that nonessential surgical procedures should be postponed. They aimed to determine changes in surgical volume when emergencies led to postponing surgical procedures. They analyzed GI surgical data from 14 public hospitals in France during the months of April and May 2020 and compared them to data from the same months in the previous year.
- In 2019, 4,678 surgical procedures were carried out, as compared to 1,847 procedures in 2020, an overall reduction of 61%. Major emergency procedures (peritonitis; intra-abdominal abscess; bowel obstruction, ischemia, or perforation) decreased from 56% to 46%. The authors suggest this decrease in emergency GI surgeries occurred because of a decrease in road traffic crashes and the use of nonsurgical treatment such as antibiotic therapy to manage uncomplicated cases of appendicitis.

DOCUMENTATION GUIDELINES

- Physical response: Vital signs; signs of pain, guarding, abdominal rigidity; bowel sounds
- Response to medications, including antibiotics and analgesics, blood values (WBC count, electrolytes)
- Presence of complications: Respiratory distress, shock, inadequate renal output, unrelieved discomfort
- Appearance of dressing or wound: Bleeding, drainage, appearance of incision
- Level of activity: Activity tolerance, ability to ambulate

DISCHARGE AND HOME HEALTHCARE GUIDELINES

Be sure the patient understands all medications, including the dosage, route, action, and adverse effects. If the patient is to be discharged while still on antibiotics, emphasize the need to complete the medication regimen. Teach the patient the signs of resistance (new onset of fever and abdominal pain) and superinfection (oral *Candida* infection, yeast infection in the moist areas of the skin).

Teach the patient to report any nausea; vomiting; abdominal pain; abdominal distention, bloating, or swelling; or bleeding, odor, redness, drainage, or warmth from a surgical incision. Advise the patient to seek emergency treatment for respiratory problems such as dyspnea. Teach the patient to avoid heavy lifting for 6 weeks. Review dietary and activity limitations.

Pernicious Anemia

DRG Category:	812
Mean LOS:	3.4 days
Description:	MEDICAL: Red Blood Cell Disorders Without Major Complication or Comorbidity

Anemia is a condition of reduced hemoglobin levels. Pernicious anemia is the most prevalent form of vitamin B_{12} deficiency in the United States and is most common in the Great Lakes region and New England, possibly due to the number of people with Northern European ancestry who live there. Pernicious anemia (also known as *Addison anemia*) is a megaloblastic anemia (large cells with an arrest in maturation) caused by a deficiency of or inability to use vitamin B_{12}, also known as *cobalamin*. Historically, it was named "pernicious" (tending to cause death or serious injury) because it was fatal before treatment became available.

Normally, vitamin B_{12} combines with the intrinsic factor, a substance secreted by the gastric mucosa, and then follows a path to the distal ileum, where it is absorbed and transported to body tissues. In pernicious anemia, intrinsic factor deficiency impairs vitamin B_{12} absorption. The deficiency of vitamin B_{12} inhibits the growth of red blood cells (RBCs) and leads to the production of insufficient and deformed RBCs with poor oxygen-carrying capacity. Because these deformed RBCs are known as *megaloblasts* (primitive, large, macrocytic cells), pernicious anemia is characterized as one of the megaloblastic anemias. Pernicious anemia is also caused by a deficiency of gastric hydrochloric acid (hypochlorhydria).

Complications caused by pernicious anemia include macrocytic anemia and gastrointestinal (GI) disorders. Pernicious anemia impairs myelin formation and thus alters the structure and disrupts the function of the peripheral nerves, spinal cord, and brain. Patients have a high incidence of benign gastric polyps, peptic ulcers, and gastric carcinoma. Low hemoglobin levels and consequent hypoxemia of long duration can result in congestive heart failure and angina pectoris in older persons. If left untreated, pernicious anemia can cause psychotic behavior or even death.

CAUSES

Two causes lead to deficiency of vitamin B_{12}: inadequate intake or poor absorption. Inadequate intake may result from dietary deficiencies. Failure to absorb occurs from a deficiency in intrinsic factor. Pernicious anemia is significantly more common in patients with autoimmune-related disorders, such as thyroiditis, myxedema, and Graves disease, which, in theory at least, decrease the hydrochloric acid production essential for intrinsic factor formation. Gastric resection can also result in the absence of intrinsic factor. Other causes include bacterial overgrowth in the intestine (bacteria compete with cobalamin) and problems with blood transport of cobalamin. Risks for pernicious anemia include family history, type I diabetes mellitus, Crohn disease, GI surgery, vegetarian or vegan diets, and lack of vitamin supplementation.

GENETIC CONSIDERATIONS

Congenital pernicious anemia is a rare condition. Some evidence points to its being an autosomal recessive disorder characterized by a polymorphism in the coding region of the gene for the gastric intrinsic factor (GIF).

SEX AND LIFE SPAN CONSIDERATIONS

Pernicious anemia occurs in only 0.1% of the population. This disorder most commonly affects people older than age 50 years, and the incidence rises as the age increases. Juvenile pernicious anemia, however, has been found in children younger than 10 years; generally, it is caused by a congenital stomach disorder that secretes abnormal intrinsic factor. Because their life span is longer, women are more prone to develop pernicious anemia.

HEALTH DISPARITIES AND SEXUAL/GENDER MINORITY HEALTH

Pernicious anemia occurs most often in people with Celtic (English, Irish, Scottish) or Scandinavian backgrounds. It is less common in other groups, but it occurs in all races and ethnicities. Experts suggest that the prevalence in Black, Indigenous, and other people of color is likely underestimated due to the complexity of the diagnosis and low index of suspicion of healthcare providers. While the mean onset is 60 years of age, Black persons, and Black women in particular, have an earlier onset. Sexual and gender minority status has no known effect on the risk for pernicious anemia.

GLOBAL HEALTH CONSIDERATIONS

In the past, experts thought that pernicious anemia occurred primarily in people of Northern European ancestry, but recent research demonstrates that it is common in all global regions and across all populations.

ASSESSMENT

HISTORY. Because large stores of vitamin B_{12} are present in the body, signs and symptoms of pernicious anemia may not appear for some time, and the report of symptoms may be vague. Elicit a complete history of medical conditions, especially autoimmune-related disorders, such as thyroiditis, myxedema, and Graves disease. Ask if the patient has undergone a gastric resection or if any family members have had pernicious anemia. Take a diet history and ask about vitamin supplements. Weight loss of 10 to 15 pounds occurs in approximately half of patients with pernicious anemia. Ask if the patient has experienced repeated infections. Elicit a history of severe fatigue, weakness, anorexia, nausea, vomiting, flatulence, diarrhea, or constipation. Ask if the patient has experienced a sore tongue or heart palpitations or recent difficulties in breathing after exertion.

Central nervous system findings are a hallmark of this anemia. Establish a history of sensory organ disturbance; ask if the patient has experienced blurred or altered vision, altered taste, or altered hearing. Ask if the patient has experienced numbness, tingling, lack of coordination, or lack of position sense. Ask male patients about recent experiences with impotence. Elicit any history of lightheadedness, memory lapses, faulty judgment, irritability, or paranoia.

PHYSICAL EXAMINATION. The patient may appear listless. Common symptoms are **weakness, sore tongue,** and **tingling of the extremities (paresthesias).** Note any premature graying or whitening of the hair. The patient may have waxy, pale to light lemon-yellow skin and jaundiced sclera. Inspect the patient's mouth and check for pale lips and gums and a beefy, red, smooth tongue as a result of papillary atrophy. Note any incidence of leg edema. Weight loss may be apparent.

Percussion or palpation of the abdomen may reveal an enlarged spleen and liver. Congestive heart failure and coronary insufficiency may occur and may necessitate more intensive care. You may note tachycardia and a rapid pulse rate. Auscultation of the heart may reveal a systolic murmur. Neurological symptoms such as paresthesias, weakness, clumsiness, and an unsteady gait may occur and place the patient at risk for falls and injury. Spinal degeneration may occur, and positive Romberg and Babinski signs may be a clinical finding.

PSYCHOSOCIAL. Pernicious anemia produces a variety of distressing signs and symptoms, such as changes in the function of the sensory organs, dietary habits, excretory function, and sexual performance. Appearance changes may disturb the patient as well. Neurological complications may cause paranoia, disorientation, or delirium.

Diagnostic Highlights

Test	Normal Result	Abnormality With Condition	Explanation
RBC count	3.6–5.8 million/mcL	Macrocytic anemia; decreased RBC: < 3.6 million/mcL	Development of abnormally large RBCs because of vitamin deficiency
Vitamin B_{12} level (cobalamin level)	200–900 pg/mL	Decreased less than 150 pg/mL diagnostic for deficiency	Deficit in absorption or intake; cobalamin is the family of chemicals that includes vitamin B_{12}
Peripheral blood smear	Normal cell volume and cell hemoglobin	Increased cell volume and cell hemoglobin	Inadequate absorption and metabolism of vitamin B_{12} leads to diminished DNA synthesis and abnormal development of RBCs
Serum antibodies to intrinsic factor	Negative	Positive	Type I and type II antibodies occur in 50% of patients with pernicious anemia

Other Tests: Complete blood count, indirect bilirubin, serum lactic dehydrogenase, serum folic acid, bone marrow biopsy, peripheral blood smear, evaluation of gastric secretions. The Shilling test is no longer performed at most medical centers because of lack of availability of the substances needed for the test, and other mechanisms are available for diagnosis.

PRIMARY NURSING DIAGNOSIS

DIAGNOSIS. Imbalanced nutrition: less than body requirements related to vitamin deficiency as evidenced by a sore tongue, fatigue, anorexia, diarrhea, weight loss, and/or numbness and tingling of the extremities

OUTCOMES. Nutritional status: Biochemical measures; Nutritional status: Food and fluid intake; Nutritional status: Nutrient intake; Endurance; Knowledge: Disease process

INTERVENTIONS. Nutrition management; Nutrition therapy; Nutritional counseling; Nutritional monitoring; Fluid/electrolyte management; Medication management; Medication administration

☀ PLANNING AND IMPLEMENTATION

Collaborative

Primary intervention focuses on locating and correcting the contributing causes. Medical therapy centers on vitamin B_{12} replacement. Oral vitamin B_{12} is indicated for rare dietary deficiencies when intrinsic factor is intact. More often, vitamin B_{12} is given parenterally, but because of the risk of allergic reactions, it should be started slowly. A generally well-balanced diet with emphasis on vitamin B_{12}–rich foods, such as animal protein, eggs, and dairy products, is important. Soy milk may be offered as a source of vitamin B_{12} for strict vegetarians. A low-sodium diet may be imposed. Blood transfusions are rarely necessary.

If the patient has significant cardiac symptoms, begin bedrest to combat fatigue. To reduce the cardiac workload, elevate the head of the bed and administer oxygen as ordered. Oral care may include antifungal preparations and special mouth rinses with hydrogen peroxide and salt water and topical anesthetics, such as magnesium hydroxide and viscous lidocaine, for mouth pain. Ensure that meals do not irritate the patient's mouth by being too hot or cold or too difficult to chew.

Pharmacologic Highlights

Medication or Drug Class	Dosage	Description	Rationale
Vitamin B_{12} (cyanocobalamin)	100 mcg IM or SC daily for 1 wk, followed by 100 mcg IM/SC twice weekly for 5–6 wk, then 100 mcg IM/SC every mo for life; alternatively, 25–250 PO mcg/day	Vitamin	Replaces vitamin for a vitamin deficiency

Other Drugs: Multivitamins, antidysrhythmics, cardiotonics, diuretics, or vasodilators may be prescribed. Stool softeners are sometimes ordered to reduce straining during bowel movements. Antibiotics may be prescribed to combat accompanying infections. For critically ill patients with cardiopulmonary distress, blood transfusions and digitalis may be ordered. Higher doses are administered until RBC regeneration occurs, after which monthly injections are given for life. Iron replacement may be given initially to combat lowered hemoglobin levels.

Independent

Plan undisturbed rest periods to help the patient conserve energy. Provide a safe environment to prevent injury caused by neurological effects. Provide assistance for walking and activities of daily living if necessary. Provide a safe environment because fine motor skills are diminished and paresthesias and balance difficulties occur. Allow time each day to sit with the patient to talk about the response to the illness and to answer questions.

If the patient's mouth and tongue discomfort make speech difficult, provide an alternative means of communication, such as a pad and pencil. Encourage fluid intake. Monitor dietary patterns carefully to determine if the patient is eating easily and tolerating meals.

Patient teaching and discharge planning are priorities. Teach the patient about the disease process of pernicious anemia and its chronic nature. Explore acceptable alternatives to activities of daily living that make living with pernicious anemia easier. Teach the patient to pace all activities and take rest periods. Encourage the patient to avoid extremes in temperature. Recommend that if the patient has developed problems with fine motor control, the patient may have an easier time dressing if clothing is designed without small buttons or hooks. Teach the patient and family to recognize and report immediately any signs of infection or complications (difficulty breathing, chest pain, dizziness, tingling in the extremities). Social service and home care referrals may be needed for follow-up.

Evidence-Based Practice and Health Policy

Seage, C., Glover, E., & Mercer, J. (2020). Receiving a diagnosis of pernicious anemia: Exploring experiences of relationships with health professionals. *Journal of Patient Experience, 7,* 1386–1390.

* The authors planned to explore patients' lived experiences of diagnosis and treatment of pernicious anemia. Participants were recruited by advertising on Pernicious Anaemia Society's Web site and social media page. They conducted semistructured interviews with patients with pernicious anemia ($N = 11$), covering participants' diagnostic and treatment journeys, the responses of others to their diagnosis, and the role health professionals played in their medical care. Interviews were analyzed for recurrent themes using interpretative phenomenological analysis.
* The authors identified three superordinate themes: "The struggle to achieve a diagnosis," "The significance of a diagnosis," and "Battling for sufficient treatment." Participants were dissatisfied with their care due to diagnostic delay, insufficient treatment, and poor relationships with health professionals. Many experienced stigma, which led to a reduced quality of life and withdrawal from the medical profession.

DOCUMENTATION GUIDELINES

* Physical findings: Red, swollen tongue; pale yellow lips and gums; skin tone
* Laboratory results: Decreased RBCs, white blood cells, platelets, vitamin B_{12}
* Presence of complications: Neurological deficits, congestive heart failure
* Disturbed sensorium: Delirium, irritation, disorientation, paranoia
* Response to vitamin B_{12} therapy

DISCHARGE AND HOME HEALTHCARE GUIDELINES

Teach the patient the relationship between vitamin B_{12} injections and the resolution of signs and symptoms of pernicious anemia. Instruct the patient how to self-administer a B_{12} injection and establish a calendar for regular monthly injections. Discuss the need for a well-balanced diet.

Teach the route, dosage, side effects, and indications for use of medications. Instruct the patient to report any recurrent episodes of signs and symptoms of pernicious anemia. Patients with pernicious anemia are at risk for developing gastric carcinoma, so encourage twice-a-year complete physical examinations.

If the patient has experienced permanent neurological disabilities, refer the patient to a physical therapist for an intensive program of rehabilitation.

Pheochromocytoma

DRG Category: 644
Mean LOS: 4.3 days
Description: MEDICAL: Endocrine Disorders With Complication or Comorbidity

Pheochromocytoma is a rare tumor, most often located in the adrenal gland, that arises from catecholamine-producing chromaffin cells. Although pheochromocytoma occurs in only 0.05% to 0.2% of all hypertensive patients, hypertension may be fatal if the pheochromocytoma goes unrecognized. These tumors secrete large quantities of epinephrine and norepinephrine, resulting in persistent or paroxysmal hypertension. Pheochromocytomas are vascular tumors that contain hemorrhagic or cystic areas and are most often well encapsulated, with 90% of the tumors being benign. The tumors are generally less than 6 cm in diameter and usually weigh less than 100 g.

Some 80% of these tumors arise from the adrenal medulla and are unilateral. These tumors follow the rule of 10s: 10% occur in children, 10% are bilateral or multiple, 10% are familial, 10% are malignant, 10% recur after surgical removal, and 10% are extra-adrenal. The 10% located in extra-adrenal sites are known as *paragangliomas*. Complications include cerebrovascular accident, retinopathy, heart disease, cardiac dysrhythmias, metastatic cancer, and renal failure. Patients with pheochromocytoma are also at higher risk for complications during operative procedures, pregnancy, and diagnostic testing.

CAUSES

Most patients develop a pheochromocytoma from unknown causes, but approximately 10 genes have been located as sites of mutations that are associated with the disease. Approximately 30% of pheochromocytomas may be associated with an inherited autosomal dominant trait, which can result in two familial multiple endocrine neoplasia (MEN) syndromes. Type IIa MEN combines pheochromocytoma with hyperparathyroidism and medullary carcinoma of the thyroid. Type IIb MEN combines pheochromocytoma and medullary carcinoma of the thyroid with multiple neuromas, Marfan syndrome, hypertrophic corneal nerves, and ganglioneuromas. In addition to heredity, risks for pheochromocytoma include conditions that cause hypoxemia, hypertension, and congenital heart disease.

GENETIC CONSIDERATIONS

Current estimates predict that up to 40% of all pheochromocytomas are related to an inherited germline mutation. Pheochromocytoma occurs as a feature of several heritable syndromes including neurofibromatosis I (NF1), von Hippel-Lindau syndrome (VHL), tuberous sclerosis, hereditary paraganglioma syndromes, and MEN (MEN IIa-medullary thyroid cancers, pheochromocytoma, parathyroid tumors, and neuromas). MEN II is a cancer syndrome that has an autosomal dominant transmission pattern. Pheochromocytoma may be seen in about half the individuals in families with MEN-IIa, and in some of these families, pheochromocytoma can cause up to 30% of deaths. Individuals with MEN II have mutations in the *RET* proto-oncogene. Familial pheochromocytoma is associated with mutations in the succinate dehydrogenase complex (*SDHB* and *SDHD*). Isolated pheochromocytoma can also be caused by mutations in *RET*, *KIF1B*, *MAX*, and *TMEM127*, while susceptibility has also been linked to mutations in *GDNF*.

SEX AND LIFE SPAN CONSIDERATIONS

Pheochromocytoma occurs equally in men and women and most commonly occurs between the early 20s and after 55 years of age. Approximately 10% occur in children, where the tumors are more likely to occur bilaterally and in an extra-adrenal location. Pheochromocytoma can occur during pregnancy, most often during the third trimester, and can cause the death of the birthing parent and the fetus.

HEALTH DISPARITIES AND SEXUAL/GENDER MINORITY HEALTH

Ethnicity, race, and sexual/gender minority status have no known effect on the risk for pheochromocytoma.

GLOBAL HEALTH CONSIDERATIONS

Pheochromocytoma occurs in people with all ancestries around the world. No specific prevalence data are available.

☀ ASSESSMENT

HISTORY. Although some patients with pheochromocytoma are asymptomatic, about 50% have a history of experiencing "spells" characterized by the 5 Ps: sudden increase in blood pressure, palpitations, pallor, profuse perspiration, and pain (chest pain, headache, and abdominal pain). The spells may last 1 minute to several hours and may occur from several times a day to once every several months. The attacks may also be precipitated by heavy lifting, exercise, or distention of the urinary bladder. Medications, such as opiates, histamine, and corticotropin, can also lead to attacks; therefore, take a complete medication history. Ask if the patient has experienced weight loss or constipation because of excessive catecholamine secretion.

A patient's history may include failure to respond to a multiple antihypertensive drug regimen, unusual fluctuations of blood pressure, cardiac dysrhythmias that are resistant to treatment, signs of cardiomyopathy, and a family history of pheochromocytoma or MEN. Hypertension (diastolic pressure higher than 115 mm Hg), which is the single most characteristic clinical sign, is sustained in 50% of the patients and is paroxysmal in the other 50%.

PHYSICAL EXAMINATION. Common symptoms are **nausea, weakness, headache, diaphoresis, pallor, palpitations,** and **tremor** in conjunction with hypertension. Patients may experience **chest pain, headache,** and **abdominal pain.** Perform an ophthalmic examination to assess for retinal changes. Note if the patient has a tremor or if the skin feels unusually warm and appears flushed. Auscultate the patient's blood pressure to determine any orthostatic changes (two-thirds of patients with pheochromocytoma experience significant decreases in blood pressure when they stand up). Inspect the patient's urine for hematuria, which is associated with pheochromocytoma of the urinary bladder.

Throughout the time the patient is under your care, monitor serial blood pressures to determine if high or low levels occur. Monitor the heart rate and rhythm, assessing for sinus tachycardia and other cardiac dysrhythmias. Avoid palpation over the bladder or deep palpation of the kidneys and the adrenal gland, which can lead to a severe hypertensive attack.

PSYCHOSOCIAL. If the tumor is resectable, determine the patient's degree of anxiety about the illness, surgery, and recovery. If the tumor is malignant, assess the patient's ability to cope with lifestyle changes, possibly including early retirement. Assess the patient for extreme anxiety, emotional lability, personality changes, and psychosis.

Diagnostic Highlights

Test	Normal Result	Abnormality With Condition	Explanation
Computed tomography scan (recommended for adults) or magnetic resonance imaging (recommended for children)	Normal adrenal structure	Location and size of tumor and metastases	Identifies tumor
Free urine catecholamines, vanillylmandelic acid (VMA) and metanephrines (24 hr)	Epinephrine: 0–15 mcg; norepinephrine: 0–100 mcg; VMA: < 7 mcg/mg; metanephrines: < 1 mg/day	Elevated	Elevated amount of catecholamines are excreted in the urine
Plasma catecholamine levels and fractionated free plasma metanephrine (metabolite of epinephrine)	Epinephrine: 0–110 pg/mL; norepinephrine: 70–750 pg/mL; fractionated free plasma metanephrine: 12–60 pg/mL	Increased	Tumor releases epinephrine and norepinephrine

Other Tests: Serum calcitonin, serum ionized calcium, serum electrolytes and glucose, complete blood count, sonography, genetic testing

PRIMARY NURSING DIAGNOSIS

DIAGNOSIS. Risk for ineffective cerebral tissue perfusion as evidenced by headache, nausea, weakness, and/or palpitations

OUTCOMES. Circulation status; Cognition; Neurological status: Consciousness; Neurological status: Peripheral; Tissue perfusion: Cerebral

INTERVENTIONS. Cerebral perfusion promotion; Neurological monitoring; Resuscitation; Vital signs monitoring; Hemodynamic regulation; Teaching: Disease process

☀ PLANNING AND IMPLEMENTATION

Collaborative

More than 90% of pheochromocytomas can be cured by surgical removal, which usually results in cure of the hypertension. Many tumors can be removed by minimally invasive (laparoscopic) adrenalectomy unless the tumor is very large and invasive. Patients who do not have operative tumors are treated pharmacologically. Preoperative treatment goals are to lower blood pressure, increase intravascular volume, and prevent paroxysmal hypertension. Before surgery, the patient's blood pressure needs to be controlled pharmacologically. To prevent intraoperative and postoperative hypotension, the patient may require IV plasma volume expanders or blood transfusions. In addition, a high-salt diet is recommended to help expand blood volume.

Postoperatively, the patient is usually admitted to an intensive care unit for continuous cardiac and respiratory monitoring. Because of the rapid decrease in circulating catecholamines, hypovolemic shock and hypotension are critical concerns; however, most patients have persistent hypertension in the immediate postoperative period. Often, the patient requires continuous pulmonary and systemic arterial monitoring to determine the hemodynamic response to tumor removal. Hypoglycemia can occur after the tumor is removed because of excessive insulin secretion; close monitoring of blood glucose and sustained infusion of glucose-containing fluids are necessary for several days after surgery. If a bilateral adrenalectomy is performed, iatrogenic adrenocortical insufficiency results, necessitating adrenocortical hormone replacement for life. In this instance, glucocorticoids are administered during and after surgery.

Monitor the blood pressure continuously after surgery and expect it to be labile. The patient may need IV antihypertensives but may also be sensitive to IV analgesics, which may cause hypotension. Observe the patient for complications such as paralytic ileus (absent bowel sounds, abdominal distention), hemorrhage (delayed capillary blanching, piloerection [gooseflesh], diminished urinary output, increased heart rate), infection (wound drainage, poor wound healing, fever), and low glucose (dizziness, irritability, tachycardia, palpitations).

Pharmacologic Highlights

Medication or Drug Class	Dosage	Description	Rationale
Alpha-adrenergic blocking agent	Varies with drug	Phenoxybenzamine hydrochloride (Dibenzyline), doxazosin mesylate (Cardura), phentolamine mesylate (Regitine), prazosin, terazosin	Produces and maintains a chemical sympathectomy; lowers blood pressure; used preoperatively to control blood pressure and prevent intraoperative hypertensive crisis, followed by administration of beta blockers (see next row)
Beta-adrenergic blockers	Varies with drug	Labetalol, propranolol, metaprolol, esmolol, or atenolol	Manage hypertension for patients with a heart rate > 110, history of dysrhythmias, or epinephrine-secreting tumor; instituted several days after the alpha-adrenergic blockade; use of labetalol preoperatively is controversial

> **Pharmacologic Highlights** (continued)
>
> Other Drugs: Calcium channel blockers, angiotensin receptor blockers. Vasodilators: nitroprusside; patients for whom surgery is not an option can be managed with metyrosine, which controls hypertensive episodes by decreasing catecholamine synthesis. If malignancy occurs, the patient can be treated with radiation therapy followed by chemotherapy, consisting of cyclophosphamide (Cytoxan), vincristine, and decarbazine.

Independent

Before the surgical procedure, document the number and type of attacks the patient experiences. Ask the patient to immediately report signs such as headache, palpitations, and nervousness. Remain with the patient during the acute attack and monitor serial vital signs. Maintain a quiet environment to limit the development of stressful episodes, which could precipitate a spell. If the patient experiences signs and symptoms, document the duration, type of symptoms, and precipitating factors. Promote rest, and encourage the patient to avoid stressors; explore relaxation techniques such as breathing exercises, music therapy, and guided imagery.

If the patient is facing surgery, encourage the patient to verbalize feelings and concerns about the surgery. Explain the procedure, what the patient can expect preoperatively and postoperatively, and how long the patient should anticipate being in an intensive care unit. Answer any questions the patient and family might have about the differences among the types of surgery. Explore how the patient may feel postoperatively, and remind the patient that pain medication is available to manage postoperative discomfort.

Expect the postoperative patient to have a labile blood pressure for the first 48 hours, and hypoglycemia may occur as well. Maintain a quiet environment because increased noise and stress may precipitate a hypertensive episode. Postoperative diaphoresis and intolerance to heat often occur; if possible, lower the room temperature to fit the patient's comfort level and assist the patient with dry linens at least every 8 hours. Before the patient's discharge, make sure the patient and significant others understand all medications and postoperative home care.

Evidence-Based Practice and Health Policy

Ma, W., Mao, Y., Zhuo, R., Dai, J., Fang, C., Wang, C., Zhao, J., He, W., Zhu, Y., Xu, D., & Sun, F. (2020). Surgical outcomes of a randomized controlled trial compared robotic versus laparoscopic adrenalectomy for pheochromocytoma. *European Journal of Surgical Oncology*, *46*, 1843–1847.

* The authors wanted to compare perioperative outcomes of robotic-assisted laparoscopic adrenalectomy (RA) versus traditional laparoscopic adrenalectomy (LA) for pheochromocytoma. For 3 years, all patients with pheochromocytoma ($N = 140$) suitable for laparoscopic adrenalectomy were assigned randomly to RA or LA. The primary outcome was the operative time. Secondary outcomes were estimated blood loss and postoperative recovery.
* The RA group had a shorter median operative time, but it had higher total hospitalization cost. Demographics and other perioperative outcomes were similar in both groups. The RA group showed a significantly lower blood loss and operative time than the LA group. Patients benefit from less blood loss and operative time when a robotic surgery system was used, but RA had a significant higher cost.

DOCUMENTATION GUIDELINES

* Physical findings related to pheochromocytoma: Blood pressure and heart rate; presence of flushing or pallor; nausea and vomiting; palpitations; pain (headache, chest pain, abdominal pain); profuse perspiration, orthostatic hypotension, and significant changes in blood pressure; hypoglycemic reactions; fever; extreme anxiety; changes in mental capacity
* Response to alpha-adrenergic and beta-adrenergic drug therapy, fluid replacement, and pain medications

• Response to the removal of the tumor: Severe hypotension, signs and symptoms of adrenal insufficiency, hypoglycemia, absence of symptoms
• Presence of complications: Hemorrhage, hypovolemia, shock, profound hypotension, adrenal insufficiency, infection

DISCHARGE AND HOME HEALTHCARE GUIDELINES

Teach the patient the importance of compliance with reevaluation studies of catecholamine and metanephrine levels. Teach the patient that pheochromocytoma can recur and that pheochromocytoma left undetected can cause encephalopathy, high-grade fever, multisystem failure, and death. Teach patients to monitor their blood pressure at home, to report subnormal measurements or diastolic pressures over 115 mm Hg, and to notify the physician immediately for other symptoms of an attack. Be sure the patient understands all medications, including the dosage, route, action, and adverse effects.

Pituitary Tumor

DRG Category:	614
Mean LOS:	4.8 days
Description:	SURGICAL: Adrenal and Pituitary Procedures With Complication or Comorbidity or Major Complication or Comorbidity
DRG Category:	644
Mean LOS:	4.3 days
Description:	MEDICAL: Endocrine Disorders With Complication or Comorbidity

Pituitary tumors, which are generally anterior lobe adenomas, make up from 10% to 15% of all intracranial neoplasms. The American Cancer Society (ACA, 2021) reports that about 10,000 new pituitary tumors are diagnosed each year in the United States, but very few are fatal or cancers, and most are adenomas. Microadenomas are smaller than 1 cm, and macroadenomas are larger than 1 cm. While microadenomas may cause complications because of overproduced pituitary hormones, they generally do not damage surrounding tissue. Because of their size, macroadenomas can be locally invasive, often damaging normal pituitary tissue and nearby nerves and parts of the brain. Most pituitary tumors are nonmalignant, but because of their invasiveness, they are considered neoplastic conditions. The ACA notes that as many as one in four people have a pituitary adenoma, but most are small and never cause symptoms, so they go unrecognized.

Some 75% of pituitary adenomas are functional (hormone-producing) tumors. The hormone produced by an adenoma strongly influences its signs and symptoms and thus the choice of diagnostic tests and treatment. Adenomas are classified as prolactinomas, or prolactin-producing adenomas (30% of pituitary tumors); somatotropin-secreting adenomas (15% to 20%); corticotropin, or adrenocorticotropic hormone (ACTH)–secreting adenomas (10% to 15%); gonadotropin-secreting adenomas (very small percentage); thyrotropin-secreting adenomas (very small percentage); null cell adenomas (15% to 20%); and plurihormonal (mixed-cell) adenomas. The outlook for survival also varies, depending on what kind of adenoma exists. Other types of tumors include craniopharyngiomas (benign tumors that develop next to the pituitary that do not make pituitary hormones but can disrupt hormone production by compressing the pituitary gland); teratomas, germinomas, and choriocarcinomas (uncommon tumors that occur most often in children or young adults); and Rathke cleft cysts and gangliocytomas (uncommon tumors that are usually found in adults).

Pituitary tumors lead to hormone excess, hormone deficiencies, or any combination of imbalances. In addition, as the tumor grows, it replaces normal pituitary gland tissue. Complications from pituitary tumors include loss of hormonal function in all systems of the body and compression of central nervous system (CNS) structures such as the hypothalamus, including vision loss. Complications of surgery include hemorrhage, infection, cerebrospinal fluid (CSF) leak, and diabetes insipidus.

CAUSES

Although the cause of pituitary tumors is unknown, the genetic mutations may predispose people to a tumor. Genes likely determine whether the tumor is benign or cancerous. The ACA (2021) notes that pituitary tumors have not been linked with any outside risk factors.

GENETIC CONSIDERATIONS

Most pituitary tumors are sporadic; however, the heritable disorder multiple endocrine neoplasia type I (MEN I) is associated with parathyroid, pancreatic, and pituitary tumors. MEN I is transmitted in an autosomal dominant pattern through germline mutations in the *MEN1* gene. Pituitary tumors occur in 15% to 42% of patients with MEN I patients, 25% to 90% of which are prolactinomas. Low expression of various tumor suppressor genes has been implicated in pituitary tumor growth. Mutations in the aryl hydrocarbon receptor-interacting protein (*AIP*) or *GNAS1* can also cause pituitary adenomas.

SEX AND LIFE SPAN CONSIDERATIONS

Approximately 70% of pituitary tumors occur in people between ages 30 and 50 years. Only 3% to 7% occur in people younger than age 20 years, and twice as many females as males have the condition. Women of childbearing age have a higher prevalence of pituitary adenomas than do men.

HEALTH DISPARITIES AND SEXUAL/GENDER MINORITY HEALTH

Black persons seem to have slightly higher rates of pituitary tumors than other groups. People who are uninsured or on Medicaid insurance have been found to have larger tumors, longer postoperative lengths of stay, and higher rates of complication than people with private insurance. This health disparity may occur because they were at a later stage of disease when the tumor was identified. Sexual and gender minority status has no known effect on the risk for pituitary tumor.

GLOBAL HEALTH CONSIDERATIONS

Although no specific data are available, experts note that the global incidence of pituitary tumors is probably similar to that of the United States.

⬛ ASSESSMENT

HISTORY. Ask the patient to describe any endocrine or neurological symptoms. Usually, patients give a history of slowly developing, progressive symptoms. Ask about headaches or visual changes because more than half of patients have visual symptoms due to compression of the optic nerve. Depending on the tumor type, they may report weight loss or weight gain. Family members may report CNS changes, such as anxiety, personality changes, seizure activity, and even dementia. Depending on tumor type, patients may describe weakness, fatigue, sensitivity to cold, and constipation.

PHYSICAL EXAMINATION. They frequently complain of **headaches, visual disturbances** (blurred vision or double vision progressing to blindness), **decreased sexual interest, menstrual irregularities**, and **impotence.** You may note that the skin has a waxy appearance; fewer than normal wrinkles for the patient's age; and a decreased amount of body, pubic, and axillary hair. Assess the patient's skin for hyperpigmentation, oiliness, acne, and diaphoresis. Assessment of visual function is important because pituitary tumors may press on the optic chiasm. Assess the patient's visual fields, visual acuity, extraocular movements, and pupillary reactions. A classic finding is bitemporal hemianopsia (blindness in the temporal field of vision). Perform an assessment of the cranial nerves. The tumor may involve cranial nerves III (oculomotor, which regulates pupil reaction), IV (trochlear, which along with the abducens regulates conjugate and lateral eye movements), and VI (abducens). Examine the patient's musculoskeletal structure, determining whether foot and hand size are appropriate for body size; whether facial features are altered, such as thick ears and nose; and whether the skeletal muscles are atrophied.

PSYCHOSOCIAL. The patient may have personality changes such as irritability and even occasional hostility. Assess the patient's interpersonal relationships, the response of significant others, and the patient's and significant others' abilities to cope with a potentially serious illness. Patients may be concerned about body image, fertility, and sexual performance.

Diagnostic Highlights

Test	Normal Result	Abnormality With Condition	Explanation
Growth hormone	≤ 10 ng/mL	Elevated	Functional (hormone-producing) tumor elevates levels of various hormones
Gonadotropins: Follicle-stimulating hormone	Adult male: 1.4–15.5 International Unit/L; adult female: 1.4–9.9 International Unit/L (follicular or luteal), 6.2–17.2 International Unit/L (midcycle peak); postmenopausal female: 19–100 International Unit/L	Elevated	Functional tumor elevates levels of various hormones
Luteinizing hormone	Adult male: 2–18 International Unit/L; adult female: 5–12 International Unit/L (follicular or luteal), 30–250 International Unit/L (midcycle peak)	Elevated	Functional tumor elevates levels of various hormones
Prolactin	4–30 ng/mL	Elevated	Functional tumor elevates levels of various hormones
Thyrotropin (thyroid-stimulating hormone)	0.4–4.2 microunit/mL	Elevated	Functional tumor elevates levels of various hormones
ACTH	< 70 pg/mL	Elevated	Functional tumor elevates levels of various hormones
Magnetic resonance imaging	No visual evidence of tumors; normal brain structure	Provides visual evidence of tumors	Standard imaging test to identify pituitary tumors; can identify macroadenomas and microadenomas > 3 mm; can locate small abnormalities in pituitary gland unrelated to symptoms; 5%–25% of patients have unrelated minor abnormalities of pituitary gland

Other Tests: Biopsy of pituitary tissue, glucose, electrolytes, ophthalmological examination

PRIMARY NURSING DIAGNOSIS

DIAGNOSIS. Acute pain related to pressure from a space-occupying lesion as evidenced by self-reports of headache or blurred vision, facial grimacing, and/or protective behavior

OUTCOMES. Comfort status; Pain control; Pain level; Symptom control; Symptom severity; Knowledge: Pain management; Knowledge: Disease process; Knowledge: Medication

INTERVENTIONS. Pain management: Acute; Analgesic administration; Medication administration; Medication management; Teaching: Procedure/treatment; Teaching: Medication

PLANNING AND IMPLEMENTATION

Collaborative

The treatment of a pituitary tumor is guided by whether it is a carcinoma or an adenoma. Treatment of adenomas is guided by whether the adenoma is functional, whether it is a microadenoma or a macroadenoma, and which hormone is being secreted. The main treatment for many pituitary tumors is surgery, while medications can relieve symptoms and sometimes shrink the tumor. With larger and more invasive tumors, the likelihood of cure by surgery decreases. The usual operation for pituitary tumors is a transsphenoidal hypophysectomy (removal of the pituitary gland through a surgical incision in the sphenoid bone). The surgery has a low neurological complication rate and leaves no visible scar. Cure rates for microadenomas are greater than 80% but are lower if the tumor is large or if it has invaded nearby nerves or brain tissue.

In a newer procedure, surgeons use endoscopic surgery, operating through a fiberoptic device inserted through an incision in the lining of the nose. This procedure takes less time and causes fewer complications than transsphenoidal hypophysectomy. For larger or more complicated tumors, a craniotomy is required to remove the tumor, but the surgery exposes patients to a higher incidence of permanent neurological complications than with transsphenoidal hypophysectomy. The overall surgical cure rate for patients with growth hormone–secreting adenomas is about 60%. The cure rate is slightly higher for corticotropin-secreting adenomas because these tend to be smaller tumors. Only complicated prolactinomas are treated surgically.

Complications of pituitary surgery can be serious but, fortunately, are extremely rare. If large arteries, nearby nerves, or nearby brain tissue is damaged, a stroke or blindness is possible. Meningitis can result from damage to the membranes that surround the brain. Much more likely is a temporary onset of diabetes insipidus, which usually resolves itself within 1 to 2 weeks after surgery. Damage to the pituitary leading to hypopituitarism may be unavoidable when treating some macroadenomas, but such damage can be treated by medication.

Postprocedural or postsurgical monitoring of the patient is crucial. Make sure the patient has an adequate airway and is breathing at all times. If you suspect airway compromise (changes in mental status, restlessness, confusion, shortness of breath, stridor, apnea), notify the physician immediately. Check with the surgeon to determine the preferred protocol for endotracheal suctioning. Perform serial neurological assessments to identify changes in mental status, pupil reaction, and strength and motion of the extremities. After surgery, maintain the subarachnoid drainage systems, and note the amount, color, and consistency of all drainage. Position the patient by elevating the head of the bed to 30 to 45 degrees to decrease edema and to promote CSF flow to the lumbar cistern. If the patient is not responsive, position the patient in a side-lying position to facilitate drainage from the mouth.

Explain that the patient needs to avoid leaning forward, blowing the nose, and sneezing. Do not remove the nasal packing until the surgeon requests it. Withhold oral fluid intake in the immediate postoperative period because it may stimulate the vomiting center and contribute to increased intracranial pressure. Provide analgesics to manage pain relief, and if the patient does not experience relief, notify the surgeon so that the medication type or dosage can be altered. If CSF drains from the nose, notify the surgeon immediately, and monitor the patient for signs of a CNS infection (changes in level of consciousness, irritability, fever, foul drainage) or pulmonary infection (fever, pulmonary congestion, yellow or white pulmonary secretions). Monitor the patient for diabetes insipidus owing to a lack of antidiuretic hormone; maintain intake and output records, and notify the physician if a fluid deficit occurs.

Pharmacologic Highlights

Medication or Drug Class	Dosage	Description	Rationale
Prolactin-inhibitor, dopamine agonists	Varies with drug	Bromocriptine (Alphagan, Parlodel); cabergoline (Dostinex)	Shrinks prolactin-secreting tumors in 1–6 mo; ineffective for treating acromegaly; side effects such as nausea and orthostatic hypotension may preclude use of bromocriptine in some patients

Other Drugs: Octreotide, lanreotide is used to inhibit growth hormone (somatotropin) secretion; cyproheptadine is used to inhibit corticotropin.

Independent

To limit the risk of injury before surgery, discuss with the patient the best mechanisms to provide a safe environment if vision is impaired. Provide an uncluttered room with a clear pathway to the bathroom. Encourage the patient to wear well-fitting shoes or slippers when ambulating. Keep the call light within reach of the patient at all times.

Postoperatively, elevate the patient's head to facilitate breathing and fluid drainage. Do not encourage the patient to cough, as this interferes with the healing of the operative site. Monitor the patient's fluid balance carefully to identify if diabetes insipidus occurs during the first 14 days after surgery. Provide frequent mouth care and keep the skin dry. To promote maximum joint mobility, perform or assist with range-of-motion exercises. Encourage the patient to ambulate within 1 to 2 days of the surgery. To ensure healing of the incision site, explain the need to avoid activities that increase intracranial pressure, such as tooth brushing, coughing, sneezing, nose blowing, and bending. Provide a well-organized and stress-free environment. Explain the treatment options and answer questions. Provide periods of uninterrupted rest each day, and schedule diagnostic procedures to allow the patient to recover.

Encourage the patient to use nonpharmacologic methods to control any discomfort. Both patients requiring surgery and patients being managed medically have many emotional needs. Provide privacy so that the patient is able to ask questions about sexual function. Expect that patients may experience loss, grief, or anger if they are dealing with sexual dysfunction such as impotence or infertility. The patient may require support and assistance to develop coping strategies.

Evidence-Based Practice and Health Policy

Pertichetti, M., Serioli, S., Belotti, F., Mattavelli, D., Schreiber, A., Cappelli, C., Padovani, A., Gasparotti, R., Nicolai, P., Fontanella, M., & Doglietto, F. (2020). Pituitary adenomas and neuropsychological status: A systematic literature review. *Neurosurgical Review, 43*, 1065–1078.

* Neurocognitive and psychological dysfunctions associated with pituitary adenomas are probably underreported. The aim of this review was to provide an update on the neuropsychological status, psychopathology, and perceived quality of life (QoL) in patients with pituitary adenomas. The authors performed a systematic review with electronic databases to identify reports on neurocognitive, psychiatric, and psychological disorders in pituitary adenomas.
* They found that the prevalence of neurocognitive dysfunctions was 15% to 83% in Cushing disease, and 2% to 33% in acromegaly. Memory was altered in 22% of nonfunctioning pituitary adenomas. Worsened QoL was reported in 40% of patients with Cushing disease. Psychiatric disorders in Cushing disease reached 77% and in acromegaly 63%, involving depression, psychosis, and anxiety. These data suggest the importance of a multidisciplinary evaluation for an optimal management of neuropsychological outcomes in pituitary adenomas.

DOCUMENTATION GUIDELINES

- Physical findings of hormone excesses or deficiencies: Decreased body hair, hirsutism, altered secondary sexual characteristics, acromegaly, galactorrhea; vital signs; neurological assessment; visual examination
- Response to therapy: Surgery, radiation, medications, counseling
- Postoperative management: CSF drainage, nasal packing, wound drainage, fluid balance, signs of complications (diabetes insipidus, infection, increased intracranial pressure, hemorrhage, CSF leak, airway compromise)

DISCHARGE AND HOME HEALTHCARE GUIDELINES

Be sure the patient understands all medications, including dosage, route, action, and adverse effects. Explain the symptoms of a CSF leak to the patient. Instruct the patient to notify the physician of fluid drainage from the nares or down the back of the throat, increased temperature, unrelieved headaches, photophobia, nausea and vomiting, or a stiff neck. Explain the risk for massive fluid loss through urination (diabetes insipidus) and the need to replace this fluid volume. Instruct the patient on a diet that replaces fluid and electrolytes. Instruct the patient to notify the physician of any excess urination.

Placenta Previa

DRG Category:	786
Mean LOS:	6.3 days
Description:	SURGICAL: Cesarean Section Without Sterilization With Major Complication or Comorbidity
DRG Category:	787
Mean LOS:	4.0 days
Description:	SURGICAL: Cesarean Section Without Sterilization With Complication or Comorbidity
DRG Category:	805
Mean LOS:	4.0 days
Description:	MEDICAL: Vaginal Delivery Without Sterilization or Dilation & Curettage With Major Complication or Comorbidity
DRG Category:	806
Mean LOS:	2.7 days
Description:	MEDICAL: Vaginal Delivery Without Sterilization or Dilation & Curettage With Complication or Comorbidity

Placenta previa occurs in 1.9 per 1,000 primiparous singleton pregnancies and 3.9 per 1,000 multiparous singleton pregnancies. Normally, the placenta implants in the body (upper portion) of the uterus. Implantation allows for delivery of the infant before the delivery of the placenta. With placenta previa, the placenta is implanted in the lower uterine segment over or near the internal os of the cervix. As the uterus contracts and the cervix begins to efface and dilate, the villi of the placenta begin to tear away from the uterine wall, and bright red, painless, vaginal bleeding occurs. The bleeding is facilitated by the poor ability of the myometrial fibers of the lower uterine segment to contract and constrict the torn vessels. Bleeding can occur antepartum or during labor and delivery. Hemorrhage from the placental site may continue into the postpartum period because the lower uterine segment contracts poorly, contrasted with the fundus and body of the uterus. Placenta previa is classified in four ways depending on the degree of placental encroachment on the cervical os (Box 1).

The degree of the previa depends largely on the cervical dilation. For example, a marginal previa at 2 cm may become a partial previa at 8 cm because the dilating cervix uncovers the placenta. Sometimes, a placenta may correct itself, especially if it is low lying; as the uterus enlarges, the placenta moves cephalad. Depending on the amount of blood loss and gestational age of the fetus, placenta previa may be life-threatening to both the birthing parent and the fetus. Complications for the birthing parent include infection, thromboembolic phenomenon, shock, and death. Complications for the fetus include slow fetal growth due to insufficient blood supply, anemia, and fetal distress due to hypoxemia.

• BOX 1 Classification of Placenta Previa

LOW LYING

The placenta implants in the lower uterine segment but does not reach the cervical os; often this type of placenta previa moves upward as the pregnancy progresses, eliminating bleeding complications later.

MARGINAL

The edge of the placenta is at the edge of the internal os; the birthing parent may be able to deliver vaginally.

PARTIAL

The placenta partially covers the cervical os; as the pregnancy progresses and the cervix begins to efface and dilate, bleeding occurs.

TOTAL

The placenta covers the entire cervical os; this usually requires an emergency cesarean section.

CAUSES

The cause of placenta previa is unknown. Risks include birthing parents of advanced age (over age 35 years); those who have a history of uterine surgeries (cesarean sections, dilation and curettage, abortions) and infections with endometritis, and those who have had a previous placenta previa. It is also more common in birthing parents with previous pregnancies and those who currently have a multiple gestation with a large placenta. Smoking and cocaine use are also contributing factors.

GENETIC CONSIDERATIONS

No clear genetic contributions to susceptibility have been defined.

SEX AND LIFE SPAN CONSIDERATIONS

Placenta previa is more common in birthing parents of advanced age and in patients with multiparity. It is more strongly associated with advanced age of birthing parent than placental abruption and occurs in approximately 1 of 1,500 deliveries of patients who are age 19 years and 1 in 100 deliveries of those over age 35 years. The incidence of placenta previa has increased over the past 30 years; this increase is attributed to the shift in older birthing parents having infants. Overall incidence is 1 in 200 deliveries; risk for recurrence may be as high as 10% to 15%. The birthing parent mortality rate from previas is 0.3%.

HEALTH DISPARITIES AND SEXUAL/GENDER MINORITY HEALTH

Nurses have a significantly higher risk of anemia, placenta previa, and pregnancy-associated hypertensive diseases and preeclampsia during the antenatal period than nonmedical working birthing parents. Ethnicity, race, and sexual/gender minority status have no known effect on the risk for placenta previa.

GLOBAL HEALTH CONSIDERATIONS

While no global data are available, placenta previa occurs around the world.

ASSESSMENT

HISTORY. Although many patients who develop placenta previa have an unremarkable obstetric or gynecologic history, some have had previous uterine surgeries or infections. The prenatal course of the current pregnancy is often uneventful until the patient experiences a bout of bright red, painless bleeding. Question the patient as to the onset and amount of bleeding first noticed. The initial bleeding in placenta previa is often scant because few uterine sinuses are exposed.

PHYSICAL EXAMINATION. The classic sign of placenta previa is **painless, bright red bleeding**; assess the amount and character of blood loss. Most often this bleeding occurs between 28 and 34 weeks when the lower uterine segment thins and the low implantation site is disrupted, but it may occur as early as 16 to 24 weeks. If heavy bleeding occurs at this point, there is over a 50% chance of pregnancy loss. With a marginal or low-lying placenta previa, the bleeding may not start until the patient is in labor. Assess the uterus for contractions; unless the patient is in labor, the uterus is relaxed and nontender. A vaginal examination should not be performed because even the gentlest examination can cause immediate hemorrhage.

Check the vital signs; note any symptoms of hypovolemic shock (restlessness; agitation; increased pulse; delayed capillary blanching; increased respirations; pallor; cool, clammy skin; hypotension; and oliguria). Monitor the baseline fetal heart rate and the presence or absence of accelerations, decelerations, and variability in the electronic fetal monitoring (EFM).

Ask if the patient feels the fetus move. Assess the fetal position and presentation by using Leopold maneuvers. Monitor the patient's contraction status, and palpate the fundus to determine the intensity of contractions. View the fetal monitor strip to assess the frequency and duration of the contractions; more often, the uterus is soft and nontender, unless the patient is in labor. Throughout the patient's hospitalization, continue to monitor for signs of hypovolemic shock and the amount and character of bleeding. Maintain continuous EFM until bleeding ceases; then, if hospital policy permits, monitor the fetus for 30 minutes every 4 hours.

PSYCHOSOCIAL. The heavy, bright red bleeding that often accompanies placenta previa is anxiety producing for the patients and significant others. The patients are concerned not only for themselves but also for the well-being of the infant. Determine the patients' support system because many of these patients have been on complete bedrest for an extended period of time. Assess the effect of prolonged bedrest on the patients' job, childcare, interpersonal, financial, and social responsibilities.

Diagnostic Highlights

General Comments: Vaginal examinations are contraindicated for a pregnant patient who is bleeding until a previa is ruled out by ultrasound visualization.

Test	Normal Result	Abnormality With Condition	Explanation
Transvaginal ultrasound (preferred); transabdominal ultrasound is also done	Placental implantation visualized in fundus of uterus	Placental implantation visualized in lower uterine segment	Visualization of placenta determines location and can rule out other causes of bleeding (e.g., abruption, cervical lesion, excessive show); transvaginal ultrasound can diagnose a placenta previa with 100% accuracy

(highlight box continues on page 958)

Diagnostic Highlights (continued)

Test	Normal Result	Abnormality With Condition	Explanation
Red blood cell count	3.6–5.8 mL/mm³	Decreases several hours after significant blood loss has occurred	Active bleeding causes decrease
Hemoglobin	11.7–17.3 g/dL	Decreases several hours after significant blood loss has occurred	Active bleeding causes decrease
Hematocrit	36%–52%	Decreases several hours after significant blood loss has occurred	Active bleeding causes decrease

Other Tests: Blood type and crossmatch; coagulation studies if bleeding is excessive

PRIMARY NURSING DIAGNOSIS

DIAGNOSIS. Risk for bleeding as evidenced by frank or occult hemorrhage, hypotension, and/or tachycardia

OUTCOMES. Blood loss severity; Fluid balance; Hydration; Circulation status; Symptom severity; Symptom control; Vital signs

INTERVENTIONS. Bleeding reduction; Blood product administration; Fluid resuscitation; Fluid monitoring; IV therapy; Shock management: Volume; Vital signs monitoring

PLANNING AND IMPLEMENTATION
Collaborative

Management of a patient with placenta previa depends on the admission status of the birthing parent and the fetus, the amount of blood loss, the likelihood that the bleeding will subside on its own, and the gestational age of the fetus. If both the birthing parent and the fetus are stable and the fetus is immature (less than 37 weeks), delivery may be put off and an IV infusion started with lactated Ringer solution. In addition, the patient is maintained on bedrest with continuous EFM. Closely monitor the fetal heart rate. If any signs of fetal distress are noted (flat variability, late decelerations, bradycardia, tachycardia), turn the patient to the left side, increase the rate of IV infusion, administer oxygen via face mask at 10 L/min, and notify the physician. Once the bleeding has ceased for 24 to 48 hours, the patient may be discharged to home on bedrest before delivery. This conservative treatment gives the preterm fetus time to mature. If the patient is in labor and a marginal placenta previa that is at least 10 mm from the cervical os is present, the practitioner allows the patient to labor and deliver vaginally, with careful surveillance of patient and fetal status throughout the labor. Postpartum, the patient will require oxytocics to prevent hemorrhaging, owing to the poor ability of the lower uterine segment to contract.

If fetal distress is present or if the patient has lost a significant amount of blood, an immediate cesarean section and, possibly, blood transfusions are indicated. If the patient delivers (vaginally or by cesarean), monitor the patient for postpartum hemorrhage because contraction of the lower uterine segment is sometimes not effective in compressing the uterine vessels that are exposed at the placental site. Although medication is not given to treat a previa, pharmacologic treatment may be indicated to stop preterm labor (if it is occurring and if bleeding is under control), enhance fetal lung maturity if delivery is expected prematurely, or prevent

Rh disease, if the patient delivers. Patients with placenta previa have an increased chance of complications and hysterectomy.

Pharmacologic Highlights

Medication or Drug Class	Dosage	Description	Rationale
Magnesium sulfate	4–5 g IV loading dose, 1–2 g/hr of IV maintenance	Central nervous system depressant	Effective tocolytic, has fewer side effects than beta-adrenergic drugs; administered only if bleeding is under control and preterm labor is evident
Betamethasone (Celestone)	12 mg IM q 24 hr × two doses	Glucocorticoid	Hastens fetal lung maturity; given if delivery is anticipated between 24 and 34 wk
RhD immunoglobulin (RhoGAM)	1,500 IM within 72 hr (prepared by the blood bank)	Immune serum	Prevents Rh isoimmunizations in future pregnancies; given if birthing parent is Rh-negative and infant is Rh-positive

Independent

If the patient is actively bleeding and patient and fetus are stable, maintain the patient on bedrest in the lateral position (preferably left lateral) to maximize venous return and placental perfusion. Because the patient may be on bedrest for an extended period of time, comfort can be increased with back rubs and positioning with pillows. Provide diversional activities and emotional support. The nurse should make every attempt to explain the condition, treatment, and potential outcomes to the patient. Often, if a preterm delivery is unavoidable, a special care nursery nurse comes in and discusses what the birthing parent can expect to happen to the infant on admission to the neonatal intensive care unit.

Evidence-Based Practice and Health Policy

Chen, M., Liu, X., You, Y., Wang, X., Li, T., Lua, H., Qu, H., & Xu, L. (2020). Internal iliac artery balloon occlusion for placenta previa and suspected placenta accreta: A randomized controlled trial. *Obstetrics & Gynecology*, *135*, 1112–1119.

- The authors aimed to study the effect of intraoperative balloon occlusion of the internal iliac arteries in women with placenta previa and antenatally diagnosed with placenta accreta. Placenta accreta occurs when all or part of the placenta attaches abnormally to the uterine wall and is associated with placenta previa. They used a single center, randomized control design with 100 women, 50 assigned to a usual care group and 50 with intraoperative balloon catheter placement and occlusion of bilateral internal iliac arteries. The primary outcome was the number of packed red blood cell units transfused.
- The numbers of packed red blood cells that were transfused were not significantly different in the two groups. Hospitalization costs and the number of postoperative fevers were significantly higher in the balloon group. The authors concluded that the balloon procedures did not improve outcomes for women with placenta previa and suspected placenta accreta.

DOCUMENTATION GUIDELINES

- Amount and character of blood loss; vital signs; presence or absence of signs of hypovolemic shock; fetal heart rate baseline, variability, and presence or absence of accelerations or decelerations; intake and output
- Frequency, intensity, and duration of contractions
- Emotional well-being; patient's response to high-risk situation

DISCHARGE AND HOME HEALTHCARE GUIDELINES

If the patient is discharged undelivered, provide the following instructions:

• Notify the physician of any vaginal bleeding, spontaneous rupture of membranes, decreased fetal movement, or regular labor contractions.
• Monitor fetal kick counts each day. Healthy babies should take less than 2 hours for 10 kicks.
• Maintain continuous bedrest with bathroom privileges.
• Avoid the supine position; use the lateral or semi-Fowler position.
• Abstain from sexual intercourse.
• Be sure to have the ability to contact help at the hospital at all times and the ability to be transported to the hospital.

Pneumocystis Jirovecii Pneumonia

DRG Category:	177
Mean LOS:	6.9 days
Description:	MEDICAL: Respiratory Infections and Inflammations With Major Complication or Comorbidity
DRG Category:	975
Mean LOS:	5.5 days
Description:	MEDICAL: HIV With Major Related Condition With Complication or Comorbidity

P*neumocystis jirovecii* pneumonia (PJP), also known as *Pneumocystis carinii* pneumonia, is an acute or subacute pulmonary infection that can be fatal. The causative organism, originally named *Pneumocystis carinii*, has been renamed *P jirovecii* after the scientist (Otto Jirovec), who isolated the organism from humans. While it is classified as a fungal infection, it does not respond to antifungal therapy. It occurs in 5% to 10% of transplant patients; in addition, it is the most common opportunistic infection in people infected with HIV and is the leading cause of death in this population. PJP is viewed as an opportunistic infection because normal cell-mediated immunity protects most humans from infection. With prophylactic medications, an estimated 1% to 20% of people with HIV infection develop PJP at some point in their lifetimes. Epidemiological surveys have found that by age 3 to 4 years, most humans have been exposed to the pathogen.

Early in the infection, the organisms line up along the alveolar wall near the type I pneumocytes. The alveoli become infiltrated with a fluid that contains proteins, organisms in varying states of development, cellular debris, and surfactant. As the alveoli become clogged with fluid and wastes, gas exchange is impaired. As the disease progresses, alveoli hypertrophy, type I pneumocytes die, and the patient has markedly diminished gas exchange. PJP affects both lungs and can lead to complications such as pulmonary insufficiency, respiratory failure, pneumothorax, and death. People infected with HIV have a 10% to 20% mortality rate, whereas other immunocompromised individuals have a 40% mortality rate.

CAUSES

Although the causative agent, *P jirovecii*, is often classified as a protozoa, its structure and function are closer to a unicellular fungus. Organisms in this family are often found in the lungs of healthy people, and airborne exposure in healthy children occurs globally. PJP occurs when a person become immunocompromised and the fungus multiplies aggressively in the alveoli. Incubation is approximately 4 to 8 weeks. Risk factors include any condition that causes immunodeficiency, such as cancer (e.g., lymphoma, leukemia, multiple myeloma), hereditary immune deficiencies, premature birth, HIV infection, medications that cause immunosuppression (corticosteroids, neoplastic agents), connective tissue disorders, and organ transplantation. PJP used to be common in lung transplant patients, but it is now very rare because of prophylactic treatment.

GENETIC CONSIDERATIONS

Heritable immune responses could be protective or could increase susceptibility.

SEX AND LIFE SPAN CONSIDERATIONS

The Centers for Disease Control and Prevention (CDC, 2020) report that approximately 10,000 people are hospitalized with PJP each year in the United States. Premature infants are at risk for PJP, as are children with immunodeficiency diseases. People who take corticosteroids for conditions such as chronic lung diseases, cancer, inflammatory/autoimmune diseases, solid organ transplants, and stem cell transplants are at risk across the life span. Because people with HIV disease are immunosuppressed, they are also at risk. Individuals can contract HIV at any time during their life span, including infancy. The patterns of HIV-related deaths have changed during the past 20 years. In the late 1990s, HIV was the second leading cause of death in the United States in men ages 25 to 44 years and the third leading cause of death in women of the same age range. The most recent mortality statistics from the CDC (2020) indicate that in 2018, 15,820 deaths in the United States and U.S.-dependent areas were directly attributed to HIV disease, a much lower death rate.

HEALTH DISPARITIES AND SEXUAL/GENDER MINORITY HEALTH

About 40% to 50% of persons who acquire PJP have HIV disease. Before the use of highly active antiretroviral therapy, up to 80% of persons with HIV contracted PJP, and although it remains the most common opportunistic infection they acquire, a far smaller number of persons now become infected. Black and Hispanic persons bear a disproportionate burden of HIV disease compared with other populations. In addition, 65% of women with newly diagnosed HIV disease are Black, and many live in the southern parts of the United States. The CDC reported in 2018 that 69% of new HIV diagnoses in the United States were in gay and bisexual men. In young people ages 13 to 24 years, young gay and bisexual men account for 83% of all new HIV diagnoses, and therefore, they are the group that is most at risk for PJP.

GLOBAL HEALTH CONSIDERATIONS

PJP occurs around the globe. In developed countries with wide availability of antiretroviral therapy, the prevalence of PJP has decreased markedly in the last several decades, but in some developing countries, rates are increasing. In Africa, approximately 80% of infants with HIV infection and pneumonia have pneumocystic organisms present in their lungs. In sub-Saharan Africa, tuberculosis and PJP often are comorbidities. Some experts note that in developing countries, rates of PJP are likely higher than reported because of lack of diagnostic tools to determine when the disease is present.

⚕ ASSESSMENT

HISTORY. Patients with PJP often appear acutely ill and weak. They often report weight loss and fatigue on exertion and become short of breath even when speaking. Determine if the patient has a history of leukemia, lymphoma, connective tissue disorders, organ transplantation, or HIV infection, all of which compromise the immune system and increase the risk of PJP. Because symptoms of PJP develop over a period of weeks (4–8 weeks, generally), initial symptoms may be vague and may be confused with other conditions.

Determine if the patient has experienced nonproductive cough or increasing shortness of breath, which are frequent initial symptoms of PJP. Ask about a recent history of anorexia, nausea, vomiting, weight loss, or a low-grade intermittent fever. Note that before PJP prophylaxis in HIV-positive patients, this disease was the first indication of HIV infection in 60% of HIV-positive patients.

PHYSICAL EXAMINATION. Common symptoms include **fever, dyspnea on exertion, nonproductive cough, stridor, nasal flaring,** and **chest tightness.** Patients usually have tachypnea and tachycardia. If the patient has a cough, note the type. Examine the patient's skin, noting its color, turgor, temperature, and whether it is dry and flaky. Check for pallor, flushing, cyanosis, and signs of hypoxemia such as mental status changes and agitation. Note the type, amount, and color of sputum, which is commonly blood tinged. Observe the patient's level of consciousness and irritability. Note any muscle wasting or guarding of painful areas. Auscultate the lungs for abnormal breath sounds, crackles, or diminished or absent breath sounds, either unilaterally or bilaterally. Late in PJP, when you percuss the chest, you may hear dullness from lung consolidation, and the patient may have nasal flaring and intercostal retractions.

PSYCHOSOCIAL. PJP is a serious and life-threatening infection; in addition, it may be the defining condition for diagnosis of HIV disease, according to the CDC. The patient may experience anxiety, depression, or difficulty in coping with the change in health status. Identify the patient's support system and evaluate its effectiveness. The diagnosis of HIV disease or the other conditions associated with PJP presents many complex familial and societal issues.

Diagnostic Highlights

Test	Normal Result	Abnormality With Condition	Explanation
Lactic dehydrogenase	50–150 units/L	> 220 units/L	Reflects onset of infection; 90% of patients with HIV and PJP have elevations
Bronchoscopy and bronchoalveolar lavage	Normal pulmonary structures and negative cultures	Washings positive for *P carinii* on immunofluorescent stain	Used to view the pulmonary structures and obtain bronchoalveolar washings (more sensitive than standard sputum specimens)
Serum immunofluorescent antibodies	< 1:16; no organisms observed	Presence of organisms	Used to identify antibodies that circulate in blood, formed in response to antigens in protozoan bacterial cell wall
Chest x-ray	Clear lung fields	Diffuse bilateral infiltrates; may be normal in early stages of PJP	Findings reflect areas of infection and consolidation

Other Tests: High-resolution computed tomography, arterial blood gases, gallium scan, pulmonary function tests, HIV testing, complete blood count

PRIMARY NURSING DIAGNOSIS

DIAGNOSIS. Risk for infection as evidenced by fever, dyspnea on exertion, nonproductive cough, and/or stridor

OUTCOMES. Infection severity; Immune status; Symptom severity; Knowledge: Infection management; Respiratory status: Gas exchange; Respiratory status: Ventilation; Risk control: Infectious process

INTERVENTIONS. Infection control; Infection protection; Respiratory monitoring; Oxygen therapy; Medication management; Medication administration

▓ PLANNING AND IMPLEMENTATION

Collaborative

Patients require pharmacologic treatment to eradicate the organism. PJP infections may be treated with incentive spirometry, percussion and postural drainage, and humidified oxygen. Some patients may require intubation and mechanical ventilation to maintain gas exchange. If the patient is not intubated and is able to take oral nutrition, a high-calorie, protein-rich diet is recommended. If the patient cannot tolerate large amounts of food, smaller, more frequent meals can be offered. IV fluids and total parenteral nutrition may be needed to maintain fluid balance if the patient cannot tolerate oral enteral feedings.

Pharmacologic Highlights

Medication or Drug Class	Dosage	Description	Rationale
Trimethoprim sulfamethoxazole (Bactrim, Septra, TMP/SMX)	5 mg/kg PO/IV every 6–8 hr for 21 days for HIV, 14 days for all other diagnoses	Antibacterial	Inhibits bacterial synthesis of essential elements
Antibiotics, anti-infectives	Varies with drug	Primaquine phosphate; trimetrexate and leucovorin; pentamidine isethionate (Nebupent) aerosol treatment or IV; clindamycin	Bactericidal
Prednisone	40 mg PO bid for 5 days and then taper	Corticosteroid	Decreases pulmonary inflammation; only for patients with severe disease

Other Drugs: Antipyretics, antitussives, and analgesics are prescribed as needed. Oral narcotics may be given to reduce the respiratory rate and control anxiety, thereby improving comfort and gas exchange. Some people are successfully treated with the antifungal agent caspofungin.

Independent

Patients with PJP infection are often weak and debilitated. They may become short of breath even when speaking, and their dyspnea is severe. Discuss your concerns with the physician if the patient remains uncomfortable. Alterations in the medication regimen may be necessary.

Discuss with the patient the chance or recurrence and when to report signs and symptoms of a recurrence of PJP. Position patients so that they are comfortable and breathe with as little effort as possible. Usually, if you elevate the bed and support the patient's arms on pillows, the respiration eases. A major nursing responsibility is to coordinate periods of activity and rest. Schedule diagnostic tests and patient care activities with ample rest periods between them. As the patient gains strength, encourage coughing and deep-breathing exercises and teach the patient how to perform incentive spirometry. Evaluate the patient's gait, and if it is steady, encourage periods of ambulation interspersed with periods of rest.

Reduce the patient's anxiety by providing a restful environment, including diversionary activities. Teach the patient guided imaging or relaxation techniques for nonpharmacologic relief of discomfort. Provide time each day to allow the patient to ask questions and explore fears. Include the family and significant others in all teaching activities as appropriate.

Evidence-Based Practice and Health Policy

Tasaka, S. (2020). Recent advances in the diagnosis and management of *Pneumocystis* pneumonia. *Tuberculosis and Respiratory Diseases, 83*, 132–140.

• In people with human immunodeficiency virus (HIV) disease, PJP is opportunistic infection with established management strategies. However, PJP is an emerging threat to immunocompromised patients without HIV infection, such as those receiving immunosuppressive therapeutics for malignancy, organ transplantation, or connective tissue diseases. Clinical manifestations of PJP are different between patients with and without HIV infections. In patients without HIV infection, PJP rapidly progresses, is difficult to diagnose correctly, and causes severe respiratory failure with a poor prognosis. Differences in clinical and radiological features are due to severe inflammatory responses that are caused by a relatively small number of organisms in patients without HIV infection. Although corticosteroids and anti-*Pneumocystis* agents have been shown to be beneficial in some patients, the optimal dose and duration remain to be determined. Because a variety of novel immunosuppressive therapeutics are now available, further innovations in the diagnosis and treatment of PJP are needed for people with PJP and either HIV disease or other conditions.

DOCUMENTATION GUIDELINES

• Physical changes: Breath sounds, breathing patterns, sputum production
• Nutritional status: Appetite, body weight, food tolerance
• Complications, changes in oxygen exchange or airway clearance, respiratory status
• Response to medications, understanding of medication
• Tolerance to activity, level of fatigue, ability to sleep at night, comfort

DISCHARGE AND HOME HEALTHCARE GUIDELINES

Advise the patient to quit smoking, rest, avoid excess alcohol intake, maintain adequate nutrition, and avoid exposure to crowds and others with upper respiratory infections. Teach the patient appropriate preventive measures, such as covering the mouth and nose while coughing when in contact with susceptible individuals. Be sure the patient understands all medications, including the dosage, route, action, and adverse effects. Teach the patient to recognize symptoms, such as dyspnea, chest pain, fatigue, weight loss, fever and chills, and productive cough, that should be reported to healthcare personnel. If the patient is newly diagnosed with HIV disease, make sure the patient is aware of safe sex precautions, strategies to maintain health, and the appropriate medication regime.

Pneumonia

DRG Category:	177
Mean LOS:	6.9 days
Description:	MEDICAL: Respiratory Infections and Inflammations With Major Complication or Comorbidity
DRG Category:	193
Mean LOS:	5.2 days
Description:	MEDICAL: Simple Pneumonia and Pleurisy With Major Complication or Comorbidity
DRG Category:	207
Mean LOS:	13.9 days
Description:	MEDICAL: Respiratory System Diagnosis With Ventilator Support > 96 Hours
DRG Category:	208
Mean LOS:	6.7 days
Description:	MEDICAL: Respiratory System Diagnosis With Ventilator Support ≤ 96 Hours
DRG Category:	3
Mean LOS:	30.3 days
Description:	SURGICAL: ECMO or Tracheostomy With Mechanical Ventilation > 96 Hours or Principal Diagnosis Except Face, Mouth, and Neck With Major Operating Room Procedures

An increasing global awareness now exists because of the threat of epidemics of pneumonia, the severity of which can range from a mild illness to a life-threatening condition. Viral diseases such as severe acute respiratory syndrome (SARS), the novel coronavirus 2019 disease (COVID-19), avian influenza (A/H5N1), and H1N1 (swine flu) are examples of viral pneumonias associated with high mortality and morbidity. Bacterial pneumonia is also a significant problem. In the United States, acute lower respiratory infections cause more disease and death than any other bacterial infection. Bacterial pneumonia can occur in several settings: community-acquired pneumonia (CAP), nursing home–acquired pneumonia (NHAP), healthcare-associated pneumonia (HCAP), hospital-acquired pneumonia (HAP), and ventilator-associated pneumonia (VAP). *Nosocomial pneumonia* is an older term that incorporates HAP and VAP.

Pneumonia is an inflammatory condition of the interstitial lung tissue in which fluid and blood cells escape into the alveoli. Even when no epidemic such as COVID-19 exists, more than 3 million people in the United States are diagnosed each year with pneumonia. The disease process begins with an infection in the alveolar spaces. As the organism multiplies, the alveolar spaces fill with fluid, white blood cells, and cellular debris from phagocytosis of the infectious agent. The infection spreads from the alveolus and can involve the distal airways (bronchopneumonia), part of a lobe (lobular pneumonia), or an entire lung (lobar pneumonia). The inflammatory process causes the lung tissue to stiffen, resulting in a decrease in lung compliance and an increase in the work of breathing. The fluid-filled alveoli cause a physiological shunt, meaning that venous blood passes unventilated portions of lung tissue and returns to the left atrium unoxygenated. As the arterial oxygen tension falls, the patient begins to exhibit the signs and symptoms of hypoxemia. In addition to hypoxemia, pneumonia can lead to complications such as respiratory failure, lung abscess, and septic shock. Infection may spread via the bloodstream and cause endocarditis, pericarditis, meningitis, or bacteremia.

CAUSES

Primary pneumonia is caused by the patient's inhaling or aspirating a pathogen, such as bacteria or a virus. Bacterial pneumonia, often caused by staphylococcus, streptococcus, or *Klebsiella*, usually occurs when the lungs' defense mechanisms are impaired by such factors as suppressed cough reflex, decreased cilia action, decreased activity of phagocytic cells, and the accumulation of secretions. Viral pathogens account for up to a fourth of CAPs in adults and are most commonly caused by the influenza virus. Viral pneumonia occurs when a virus attacks bronchiolar epithelial cells and causes interstitial inflammation and desquamation, which eventually spread to the alveoli. In addition to the influenza viruses mentioned earlier, other common viruses include respiratory syncytial virus (RSV); influenza A; parainfluenza 1, 2, and 3; and adenovirus (see **Emerging Infectious Diseases [COVID-19]** for an explanation of COVID-19).

Secondary pneumonia ensues from lung damage that was caused by the spread of bacteria from an infection elsewhere in the body or by a noxious chemical. Aspiration pneumonia is caused by the patient inhaling foreign matter, such as food or vomitus, into the bronchi. Factors associated with aspiration pneumonia include old age, impaired gag reflex, surgical procedures, debilitating disease, and decreased level of consciousness.

The most common causes of CAP are *Streptococcus pneumoniae* (pneumococcus), *Mycoplasma pneumoniae*, *Haemophilus influenzae*, *Chlamydia pneumoniae*, and respiratory viruses. CAP in the intensive care unit is most commonly caused by *S pneumoniae*, *Staphylococcus aureus*, *Legionella* species, and gram-negative bacilli such as *Escherichia coli* and *Klebsiella pneumoniae*. Risk factors for the development of pneumonia include cigarette smoking, chronic obstructive pulmonary disease, asthma, immunosuppression, protein pump inhibitors, alcohol abuse, major surgery, drug dependence or abuse, altered mental status, seizure disorder, and recent pulmonary infections with the flu or cold.

GENETIC CONSIDERATIONS

Heritable immune responses could be protective or could increase susceptibility.

SEX AND LIFE SPAN CONSIDERATIONS

Children and young adults up to age 30 years are at risk for several forms of viral pneumonia, including mycoplasma pneumonia, adenovirus pneumonia, rubeola pneumonia, and RSV pneumonia. Neonates with multisystem disease are also at risk for viral pneumonia caused by cytomegalovirus. Pregnant patients with viral pneumonia have a higher risk for severe disease than other patients. Adults are at risk for varicella viral pneumonia. As people age past 65 years, rates of viral pneumonia again increase. More than 60% of hospitalizations and 85% of deaths from viral pneumonia occur in older adults. People over age 40 years are at greater risk to contract all forms of bacterial pneumonia, with older men more susceptible to streptococcal bacterial pneumonia and *Klebsiella* bacterial pneumonia. Staphylococcal pneumonia tends to strike those who are debilitated or who have a history of influenza or IV drug abuse.

HEALTH DISPARITIES AND SEXUAL/GENDER MINORITY HEALTH

Black men are more likely to die from bacterial pneumonia than White men, although little is known about the reasons for this disparity. Black and White women have similar mortality rates with respect to bacterial pneumonia. Sexual and gender minority status has no known effect on the risk for pneumonia except for *Pneumocystis jirovecii* pneumonia (see ***Pneumocystis jirovecii*** **Pneumonia**).

GLOBAL HEALTH CONSIDERATIONS

The World Health Organization (WHO, 2019) states that pneumonia is the single largest infectious cause of death in children in the world. It occurs around the world but is most prevalent in South Asia and sub-Saharan Africa. Serious pneumonia in children and overall deaths from pneumonia for all ages occur more often in developing than in developed countries. WHO reported that in 2017, approximately 800,000 children died from pneumonia and accounted for 15% of all deaths in children under 5 years of age. Environmental factors that contribute to pneumonia in children are indoor cooking with biomass fuels such as wood or dung, living in crowded homes, and parental smoking (WHO, 2019).

✳️ ASSESSMENT

HISTORY. Ask if the patient has experienced recent air travel, exposure to contaminated air-conditioning or water systems, exposure to crowds or overcrowded institutions (jails, homeless shelters), or exposure to animals such as cattle, rabbits, rodents, sheep, turkeys, or chickens. The patient may have a history of a recent upper respiratory infection, influenza, or a viral syndrome. The patient may report a productive cough, fever, chest pain, or difficulty breathing. Elicit a history of a chronic pulmonary disease, such as asthma, bronchitis, or tuberculosis; prolonged immobility; sickle cell anemia; neurological disorders that cause paralysis of the diaphragm; surgery of the thorax or abdomen; smoking; alcoholism; IV drug therapy or abuse; and malnutrition. Establish any history of exposure to noxious gases, aspiration, or immuno-suppressive therapy. Determine if the patient recently underwent general anesthesia. Ask the patient to describe the type of cough and the nature of the sputum production. Determine the location of any pain, especially chest pain. Ask about sore throat or chills, vomiting, diarrhea, and anorexia. Ask if the patient has comorbid conditions such as diabetes mellitus, stroke, or autoimmune diseases.

PHYSICAL EXAMINATION. The major symptoms of pneumonia are **cough, fever, sputum production, chest pain**, and **shortness of breath**. Observe the patient's general appearance and respiratory pattern to determine level of fatigue, presence of cyanosis, and presence of dyspnea, tachypnea, or tachycardia. Examine the patient's extremities, torso, and face for rash. Assess vital signs for rapid, weak, thready pulse; fever; and blood pressure changes such as hypotension and orthostasis (postural hypotension). Palpate the chest to determine any areas of consolidation or tactile fremitus. Percuss the chest to detect dullness over the area of consolidation. When you auscultate the patient's breathing, listen for rales, crackles, rhonchi, and wheezes; "E" to "A" changes; and whispered pectoriloquy.

PSYCHOSOCIAL. The patient with pneumonia may be anxious, fatigued, and in pain from the constant coughing. Assess the patient's ability to cope with a sudden, debilitating illness. The patient and family will likely be very anxious because of difficulty breathing and distressed over purulent sputum. Pneumonia can be life threatening if not treated promptly, and the family and patient will likely recognize this serious situation.

Diagnostic Highlights

Test	Normal Result	Abnormality With Condition	Explanation
Rapid detection test: Reverse-transcriptase-polymerase chain reaction	Negative for influenza, RSV, rhinoviruses, parainfluenza, and other viruses	Positive for virus	Obtained through nasal swabs; sensitivity for influenza in adults ranges between 50% and 60%, and specificity is greater than 90%
Sputum cultures and sensitivities	Negative cultures and sensitivities (other than normal bacterial flora)	Presence of infecting organisms	Cultures identify organism; sensitivity testing identifies how resistant or sensitive the bacteria are to antibiotics
Chest x-ray	Clear lung fields	Areas of increased density; can be a lung segment, lobe, one lung, or both lungs	Findings reflect areas of infection and consolidation

Other Tests: Arterial and venous blood gases, complete blood count, coagulation profile, blood cultures, serum lactate level, serum free cortisol value, serum electrolytes, blood urea nitrogen, creatinine, glucose, bronchoscopy. Chest computed tomography and chest ultrasound may be completed.

PRIMARY NURSING DIAGNOSIS

DIAGNOSIS. Ineffective airway clearance related to increased production of secretions and increased viscosity as evidenced by cough, wheezing, dyspnea, and/or shortness of breath

OUTCOMES. Respiratory status: Airway patency; Respiratory status: Gas exchange; Respiratory status: Ventilation; Symptom severity; Medication response; Knowledge: Treatment regimen

INTERVENTIONS. Airway management; Oxygen therapy; Airway suctioning; Airway insertion and stabilization; Cough enhancement; Mechanical ventilation: Invasive; Mechanical ventilation: Noninvasive; Respiratory monitoring; Medication management

PLANNING AND IMPLEMENTATION
Collaborative

Patients have a range of symptoms, which may be mild to severe. Bacterial pneumonia is treated with antibiotics as the mainstay of therapy, but some patients need oxygen and noninvasive or invasive ventilatory support for hypoxemia and fluid resuscitation for volume depletion. Physicians may request regular measurements of peak and trough levels of antibiotics, especially for patients who are receiving aminoglycosides, which can produce severe side effects such as renal failure and hearing loss. High fever may be treated with antipyretics or IV hydration to replace fluid loss. The patient's condition may change rapidly; continuous monitoring of cardiovascular parameters and oxygenation is critical. Percussion and postural drainage may be prescribed to assist the patient in expectorating secretions. Appropriate nutrition and early mobilization speed recovery and reduce complications.

Pharmacologic Highlights

Medication or Drug Class	Dosage	Description	Rationale
Antibiotics	Varies with drug	Depends on bacteria. Initial antibiotic: Macrolides including erythromycin, azithromycin, roxithromycin, and clarithromycin. Other antibiotics: Penicillin G for streptococcal pneumonia; nafcillin or oxacillin for staphylococcal pneumonia; aminoglycoside or a cephalosporin for *Klebsiella* pneumonia; penicillin G or clindamycin for aspiration pneumonia. Cephalosporins: Cefepime, cefotaxime, cefuroxime. Alternatives: Amoxicillin and clavulanate (Augmentin); doxycycline; trimethoprim and sulfamethoxazole (Bactrim DS, Septra); levofloxacin (Levaquin); cefazolin, aztreonam, cefepime, ciprofloxacin	Macrolides provide coverage for likely organisms in community-acquired bacterial pneumonia
Antivirals	Varies with drug	Acyclovir may be used for varicella and herpes simplex pneumonia; ganciclovir and immunoglobulin are used in immunocompromised patients with cytomegalovirus pneumonia	Few specific antiviral agents are available to manage pneumonia

Independent

Make sure the patient coughs and uses deep-breathing exercises at least every 2 hours. Encourage drinking 3 L of fluid daily, unless contraindicated, to help expectorate secretions. If the patient cannot cough up secretions, you may have to perform nasotracheal or orotracheal suction to maintain an open airway. Turn and position patients on bedrest to help keep the airway open and free of secretions and to reduce the risk of pulmonary aspiration. Elevate the head of the bed to at least 45 degrees to help the patient maintain an open airway and find positions that ease breathing. Place the patient in an upright position with both arms well supported on pillows or position the patient to lean forward and rest the arms on the overbed table.

Involve the patient in as much decision making as possible and, when possible, include the family in teaching situations. Explain all procedures, particularly intubation and suctioning. Teach the importance of adequate rest and the deep-breathing and coughing exercises that are designed to clear lung secretions.

Teach proper ways to dispose of secretions and proper hand-washing techniques to minimize the risk of spreading infection. Advise annual influenza vaccinations or avoidance of using antibiotics indiscriminately because such use creates a risk for upper airway colonization by antibiotic-resistant bacteria.

Evidence-Based Practice and Health Policy

Yamagata, A., Ito, A., Nakanishi, Y., & Ishida, T. (2020). Prognostic factors in nursing and healthcare-associated pneumonia. *Journal of Infection and Chemotherapy, 26,* 563–569.

• Nursing and healthcare-associated pneumonia (NHCAP) is a category of healthcare-associated pneumonia used in Japan. The authors implemented a prospective study to determine the prognostic factors related to 30-day mortality in patients with NHCAP by analyzing prospective data. They analyzed patients hospitalized for NHCAP ($N = 817$) and collected data on age, sex, comorbidities, vital signs, and laboratory findings, with primary outcome as the 30-day mortality.

- The mean age was 78.0, 71% were men, and 30-day mortality was 13.1%. Male sex, malignancy, temperature, heart rate, respiratory rate, serum albumin, and blood urea nitrogen were predictive factors for mortality. The risk of drug-resistant pathogens was not necessarily related to poor prognosis.

DOCUMENTATION GUIDELINES

- Physical findings of chest assessment: Respiratory rate and depth, auscultation findings, chest tightness or pain, vital signs
- Assessment of degree of hypoxemia: Lips and mucous membrane color, oxygen saturation by pulse oximetry
- Response to deep-breathing and coughing exercises, color and amount of sputum
- Response to medications: Body temperature, clearing of secretions

DISCHARGE AND HOME HEALTHCARE GUIDELINES

Be sure the patient understands all medications, including dosage, route, action, and adverse effects. The patient and family or significant others need to understand the importance of avoiding fatigue by limiting activity and taking frequent rests. Advise small, frequent meals to maintain adequate nutrition. Fluid intake should be maintained at approximately 3,000 mL/day so that the secretions remain thin. Teach the patient to maintain pulmonary hygiene measures of coughing, deep breathing, and incentive spirometry at home. Provide information about how to stop smoking.

Pneumothorax

DRG Category:	199
Mean LOS:	6.7 days
Description:	MEDICAL: Pneumothorax With Major Complication or Comorbidity

Pneumothorax occurs when there is an accumulation of air in the pleural space. Normally, the pleural space is a "potential space," a space that occurs between two adjacent structures that are normally pressed together. The area between the visceral and parietal pleura has a negative atmospheric pressure, creating a vacuum as well as containing a small amount of protective fluid to lubricate the tissues. In pneumothorax, air accumulates in the pleural space, and the pressure rises, leading to atelectasis (collapsed lung) and ineffective gas exchange. There are three major types of pneumothorax: spontaneous, traumatic, and tension. Spontaneous pneumothorax is not life threatening and occurs when a portion of the lung collapses without a known cause. Most experts suspect that it is due to the formation of small sacs of air that rupture, causing air to leak into the pleural space. Traumatic pneumothorax can be further classified as either open (when atmospheric air enters the pleural space) or closed (when air enters the pleural space from the lung). Traumatic pneumothoraces are most often associated with an injury resulting in a wound or puncture, disrupting the pleural space by changing the vacuum into a positive-pressure space. When the wound seals off, the air is trapped in the pleural space. In open traumatic pneumothorax, a chest wall defect creates an opening that connects the outside atmospheric air to the pleural space. A gunshot or stab wound that leaves a hole in the chest wall is one cause of an open pneumothorax.

The degree of distress and compromise that the patient experiences depends on the degree of collapse on the affected side. When the air in the pleural space cannot escape, tension pneumothorax occurs. If air accumulation is not stopped, the entire mediastinum shifts toward the unaffected side, causing bilateral lung collapse, which is a life-threatening condition. Tension pneumothorax is a life-threatening complication that can lead to shock, low blood pressure, and cardiopulmonary arrest. Other complications include respiratory failure, hypoxemia, and pneumonia.

CAUSES

The cause of a closed or primary spontaneous pneumothorax is the rupture of a bleb (sac or vesicle) on the surface of the visceral pleura, allowing air from the lungs to enter the pleural space. Secondary spontaneous pneumothorax can result from chronic obstructive pulmonary disease (COPD), which is related to hyperinflation or air trapping, or from the effects of cancer, which can result in the weakening of lung tissue or erosion into the pleural space by the tumor. Associated conditions include HIV disease, asthma, cancer, cystic fibrosis, and inhaled drug use. Blunt chest trauma and penetrating chest trauma are the primary causes of traumatic and tension pneumothorax. Other possible causes include therapeutic procedures such as thoracotomy, thoracentesis, and insertion of a central line. Risk factors for spontaneous pneumothorax include smoking; a tall, thin stature; Marfan syndrome; pregnancy; and family history.

GENETIC CONSIDERATIONS

Spontaneous pneumothorax (SP) is known to be associated with certain heritable disorders of connective tissue, particularly Marfan syndrome and Ehlers-Danlos syndrome, but it may occur as an isolated familial disorder without other signs of connective tissue disease. Familial SP appears to follow an autosomal dominant transmission pattern with incomplete penetrance and variable expression, with some cases of SP associated with mutations in folliculin (*FLCN*). *FLCN* mutations are also associated with Birt-Hogg-Dubé syndrome which is characterized by lung cysts, spontaneous pneumothorax, fibrofolliculomas, and renal cell cancer.

SEX AND LIFE SPAN CONSIDERATIONS

Pneumothorax can occur at any age. It occurs in 2% of neonates and has a rate of approximately 20% in infants with neonatal respiratory distress syndrome. Older people with COPD and younger people with paraseptal emphysema are susceptible to spontaneous pneumothorax. Spontaneous primary pneumothorax occurs most often in tall, thin men between ages 20 and 30 years. Traumatic injuries are more common in adolescent and young adult males than in other populations.

HEALTH DISPARITIES AND SEXUAL/GENDER MINORITY HEALTH

Ethnicity and race have no known effect on the risk for pneumothorax. Smoking increases the risk of a first spontaneous pneumothorax by more than 20-fold in men and by nearly 10-fold in women as compared to nonsmokers. The Centers for Disease Control and Prevention (2021) report that 13.8% of heterosexual adults smoke cigarettes, whereas 19.2% of lesbian, gay, and bisexual adults smoke, as do 35.5% of trans adults. Smoking places sexual and gender minority people at risk for pneumothorax.

GLOBAL HEALTH CONSIDERATIONS

Globally, more men than women experience pneumothorax because men are more likely than women to experience traumatic injuries. Traditional Chinese medicine with acupuncture may lead to pneumothorax, which is the most serious complication reported in the literature, with an incidence of 1 in 5,000 individuals after acupuncture in the area of the lungs.

ASSESSMENT

HISTORY. Ask about chest pain; determine its onset, intensity, and location. Question if the patient has had shortness of breath, difficulty breathing, cough, or fatigue. Elicit a history of COPD or emphysema or if the patient has had a thoracotomy, thoracentesis, or insertion of a central line. Determine if the patient has had a previous pneumothorax because recurrence is common. Ask if the patient smokes cigarettes.

For patients who have experienced chest trauma, establish a history of the mechanism of injury by including a detailed report from the prehospital professionals, witnesses, or significant others. Specify the type of trauma (blunt or penetrating). If the patient has been shot, ask the paramedics for ballistic information, including the caliber of the weapon and the range at which the person was shot. If the patient was stabbed, ask about the size of the knife and the angle of the attack. If the patient was in a motor vehicle crash, determine the type of vehicle (truck, motorcycle, car); the speed of the vehicle; the victim's location in the car (driver versus passenger); and the use, if any, of safety restraints. Determine if the patient has had a recent tetanus immunization.

PHYSICAL EXAMINATION. The patient may present in a number of ways, from being asymptomatic to having profound cardiopulmonary instability. The most common symptoms are **sharp or stabbing chest pain that may increase with inspiration, shortness of breath, anxiety,** and **cough.** The severity of the symptoms depends on the extent of any underlying disease and the amount of air in the pleural space. Examine the patient's chest for a visible wound that may have been caused by a penetrating object. Patients with an open pneumothorax also exhibit a sucking sound on inspiration. Inspect the patient with pneumothorax for cyanosis, nasal flaring, asymmetrical chest expansion, dyspnea, tachypnea, and intercostal retractions. Observe whether the patient has a flail chest, a condition in which the patient has paradoxical chest movement with the chest wall moving outward during expiration and inward during inspiration. On palpation, note any tracheal deviation toward the unaffected side, subcutaneous emphysema (also known as *crepitus*; a dry, crackling sound caused by air trapped in the subcutaneous tissues), or decreased to absent tactile fremitus over the affected area. Percussion may elicit a hyperresonant or tympanic sound. Auscultation reveals decreased or absent breath sounds over the affected area and no adventitious sounds other than a possible pleural rub.

Examine the thorax area, including the anterior chest, posterior chest, and axillae, for contusions, abrasions, hematomas, and penetrating wounds. Note that even small penetrating wounds can be life-threatening if vital structures are perforated. Observe the patient carefully for pallor. Take the patient's blood pressure and pulse rate, noting the early signs of shock or massive bleeding, such as a falling pulse pressure, a rising pulse rate, and delayed capillary refill. Continue to monitor the vital signs frequently during periods of instability to determine changes in the condition or the development of complications.

The signs of tension pneumothorax are more intense than those of spontaneous pneumothorax; they include chest pain, shortness of breath, anxiety, and confusion. Patients show signs of hypotension and hypoxemia, with absent breath sounds on the affected side, and the trachea deviates away from the affected side. There may be hyperresonance on auscultation, tachycardia, and jugular vein distention.

PSYCHOSOCIAL. Patients with a pneumothorax may be confused, anxious, or restless. They may be concerned about their pain and dyspnea and could be in a panic state. Determine the patient's past ability to manage stressors and discuss with the significant others the most adaptive mechanisms to use. Note that approximately one-half of all traumatic injuries are associated with alcohol and other drugs of abuse.

Diagnostic Highlights

Test	Normal Result	Abnormality With Condition	Explanation
Chest x-ray, computed tomography scan	Clear lung fields	Lung collapse with air between chest wall and visceral pleura	Lungs are not filled with air but rather are collapsed; confirms diagnosis
Ultrasound; focused assessment with sonography for trauma (FAST)	Intact bony structure with intact lungs	Absence of lung sliding during breathing	Normal movement of the visceral pleura against parietal pleura does not occur

Diagnostic Highlights (continued)

Other Tests: Complete blood count, plasma alcohol level, arterial blood gases, pulse oximetry, esophagography, rib x-rays, ultrasonography

PRIMARY NURSING DIAGNOSIS

DIAGNOSIS. Impaired gas exchange related to decreased oxygen diffusion capacity as evidenced by restlessness, agitation, anxiety, cough, air hunger, dyspnea, and/or tachycardia

OUTCOMES. Respiratory status: Gas exchange; Respiratory status: Ventilation; Comfort level; Anxiety control; Symptom severity; Symptoms control; Vital signs

INTERVENTIONS. Airway insertion and stabilization; Airway management; Respiratory monitoring; Oxygen therapy; Mechanical ventilation; Anxiety reduction

PLANNING AND IMPLEMENTATION

Collaborative

The priority is to maintain airway, breathing, and circulation. The most important interventions focus on reinflating the lung by evacuating the pleural air. Patients with a primary spontaneous pneumothorax that is small with minimal symptoms may have spontaneous sealing and lung reexpansion. Some patients receive outpatient care as long as they have reliable follow-up and clear instructions about when to return to the emergency department if they worsen. The patient may be observed for 4 to 6 hours in the emergency department or for a longer period as an inpatient without chest drainage. For patients with jeopardized gas exchange, chest tube insertion or other strategies may be necessary to achieve lung reexpansion.

An ambulatory device that incorporates a one-way valve is available for stable patients in some situations (Hallifax et al., 2020 [see Evidence-Based Practice and Health Policy]), or simple aspiration with a small-bore catheter may be used. A chest tube system with a closed chest drainage system may be used if the patient is unstable or needs continuous fluid and/or air evacuation. Regulate suction according to the chest tube system directions; generally, suction does not exceed 20 to 25 cm H_2O negative pressure. Monitor a chest tube unit for any kinks or bubbling, which could indicate an air leak, but do not clamp a chest tube without a physician's order because clamping may lead to tension pneumothorax. Stabilize the chest tube so that it does not drag or pull against the patient or against the drainage system. Maintain aseptic technique, changing the chest tube insertion site dressing and monitoring the site for signs and symptoms of infection such as redness, swelling, warmth, and drainage.

Oxygen therapy and mechanical ventilation are prescribed as needed. Some patients may be managed with video-assisted thoracic surgery (VATS), which allows for closure of leaks and is less invasive than other more traditional surgical procedures. Surgical interventions include removing the penetrating object, exploratory thoracotomy if necessary, thoracentesis, and thoracotomy for patients with two or more episodes of spontaneous pneumothorax or patients with pneumothorax that does not resolve within 1 week.

Pharmacologic Highlights

No routine pharmacologic measures will treat pneumothorax, but the patient may need antibiotics, local anesthesia agents for procedures, and analgesics, depending on the extent and nature of the injury. Analgesia is administered for pain once the patient's pulmonary status has stabilized.

Independent

Place the patient in a semi-Fowler position to improve lung expansion. Change the patient's position every 2 hours to prevent infection and allow for lung drainage. For a patient with a traumatic closed pneumothorax, turn the patient onto the unaffected side to improve the ventilation-to-perfusion ratio. Encourage coughing and deep breathing to remove secretions.

For patients with traumatic open pneumothorax, prepare a sterile occlusive dressing and cover the wound. Monitor carefully for a tension pneumothorax (absent breath sounds, tracheal deviation) because the occlusive dressing prevents air from escaping the lungs. Teach alternative pain relief techniques. Explain all procedures in advance to decrease the patient's anxiety.

Evidence-Based Practice and Health Policy

Hallifax, R., McKeown, E., Sivakumar, P., Fairbairn, I., Peter, C., Leitch, A., Knight, M., Stanton, A., Ijaz, A., Marciniak, S., Cameron, J., Bhatta, A., Blyth, K., Reddy, R., Harris, M., Maddekar, N., Walker, S., West, A., Laskawiec-Szkonter, M., . . . Rahman, N. (2020). Ambulatory management of primary spontaneous pneumothorax: An open-label, randomised controlled trial. *The Lancet, 396*, 39–49.

• The authors note that the optimal management of primary spontaneous pneumothorax is not defined. They tested an ambulatory device that incorporates a one-way valve as compared to the standard chest tube system with outcomes including the duration of hospitalization and safety of ambulatory management. Their study design was an open-label, randomised controlled trial of adults (aged 16–55 years) with symptomatic primary spontaneous pneumothorax, recruited from 24 hospitals over a period of 3 years. Patients were randomly assigned to treatment with either an ambulatory device or standard guideline-based management (aspiration, standard chest tube insertion, or both).
• After 30 days, the median hospitalization was significantly shorter in the ambulatory treatment group. More patients in the standard care group had adverse events, but all serious adverse events occurred in patients who received ambulatory care, including an enlarging pneumothorax, asymptomatic pulmonary edema, and the device malfunctioning, leaking, or dislodging. The authors concluded that ambulatory management of primary spontaneous pneumothorax significantly reduced the duration of hospitalization, including readmissions in the first 30 days, but at the expense of increased adverse events.

DOCUMENTATION GUIDELINES

• Physical findings: Breath sounds, vital signs, level of consciousness, urinary output, skin temperature, amount and color of chest tube drainage, dyspnea, cyanosis, nasal flaring, altered chest expansion, tracheal deviation, absence of breath sounds
• Response to pain: Location, description, duration, response to interventions
• Response to treatment: Chest tube insertion—type and amount of drainage, presence of air leak, presence or absence of crepitus, amount of suction, presence of clots, response to fluid resuscitation; response to surgical management
• Complications: Infection (fever, wound drainage); inadequate gas exchange (restlessness, dropping Sao_2); tension pneumothorax

DISCHARGE AND HOME HEALTHCARE GUIDELINES

Review all follow-up appointments, which often involve chest x-rays, arterial blood gas analysis, and a physical examination. If the injury was alcohol related, explore the patient's drinking pattern. Refer for counseling, if necessary. Teach the patient when to notify the physician of complications (infection, an unhealed wound, and anxiety) and to report any sudden chest pain or difficulty breathing.

Polycystic Kidney Disease

DRG Category:	659
Mean LOS:	8.1 days
Description:	SURGICAL: Kidney and Ureter Procedures for Non-Neoplasm With Major Complication or Comorbidity
DRG Category:	699
Mean LOS:	4.2 days
Description:	MEDICAL: Other Kidney and Urinary Tract Diagnoses With Complication or Comorbidity

Polycystic kidney disease is a progressive, inherited disease characterized by the development and enlargement of large cysts in the kidney and other organs. Although inherited polycystic diseases are not the only types of cystic diseases of the kidney, all types are a major contributor to chronic renal failure. Infantile autosomal recessive polycystic kidney disease (RPK) and autosomal dominant polycystic kidney disease (ADPKD) are two types of inherited polycystic kidney disease. Infantile (RPK) disease affects both kidneys, leads to renal failure, and causes biliary dilation and fibrosis in the liver. The basic pathology of cyst development is a weakening of the basement membrane, which possibly is caused by an abnormality of the extracellular connective tissue cells. The cyst then fills with fluid from the glomerular filtrate. Adult-onset disease (ADPKD) is a bilateral disorder, although it may have asymmetrical progression with multiple expanding cysts that destroy renal function. Renal deterioration eventually leads to uremia, chronic renal failure, and the need for chronic renal dialysis.

Complications include liver, pancreatic, spleen, and lung cysts; aneurysms of the cerebral artery or abdominal aorta; colonic diverticula; and mitral valve prolapse. Approximately 45% of adult patients die of coronary or hypertensive heart disease, and 15% die from infections. About 10% to 40% of people with ADPKD have berry aneurysms, and 10% die as a result of subarachnoid hemorrhages.

CAUSES

RPK and ADPKD are inherited conditions. In RPK, siblings of either sex have one chance in four of having the disease. ADPKD has a 100% incidence because it is an autosomal dominant trait. An average of half of the affected individuals have children with ADPKD.

GENETIC CONSIDERATIONS

ADPKD is characterized by renal cysts, liver cysts, and intracranial aneurysm. It is primarily caused by mutations in the genes, *PKD1* (accounting for 85% of ADPKD) and *PKD2* (15% of ADPKD cases). ADPKD accounts for approximately 90% of polycystic kidney cases with average onset between ages 30 and 40 years. Autosomal recessive polycystic kidney disease (ARPKD) is much less common, with symptoms beginning in the earliest months of life or prenatally. ARPKD is caused by mutations in the fibrocystin (*PKHD1*) gene.

SEX AND LIFE SPAN CONSIDERATIONS

RPK always becomes apparent during childhood in boys and girls, usually before age 13 years. An infant born with active RPK usually dies within the first 2 months of life as a result of uremia or pulmonary complications. Renal failure and hypertension develop more slowly when the disease occurs later in childhood. Most patients with ADPKD are identified between ages 30 and 50 years, although newborns can be diagnosed with the disease. A neonate with ADPKD is likely to be stillborn or die from renal failure within 9 months. In most men and women with ADPKD, the disease progresses to end-stage renal failure by the time the patient reaches the age of 40 to 50 years. ADPKD is more severe in males than in females.

HEALTH DISPARITIES AND SEXUAL/GENDER MINORITY HEALTH

Black patients with ADPKD wait longer for kidney transplants as compared to patients from other groups and are more likely to be on dialysis. Being Black is also a risk factor for delayed graft function but is not associated with graft failure after transplantation. Racial disparities exist for Black renal transplant patients, and there need to be strategies to improve transplant equity (Williams et al., 2021 [see Evidence-Based Practice and Health Policy]). Sexual and gender minority status has no known effect on the risk for polycystic kidney disease.

GLOBAL HEALTH CONSIDERATIONS

Globally, 4 to 7 million people have ADPKD. Polycystic kidney disease is responsible for up to 10% of cases of end-stage renal disease in developed countries and is the most common cause of inherited end-stage renal disease. Worldwide, slightly more men than women have ADPKD, which rarely occurs in children. Few data are available for developing countries.

⬛ ASSESSMENT

HISTORY. Take a complete medical history from parents of children with RPK; the children are apt to have a lengthy medical history, including multiple system complications and frequent hospitalizations. Ask the parents or children whether the patient has had abdominal, flank, or back pain; hematuria; or urinary tract infections (UTIs). Because children with ADPKD usually experience cardiopulmonary complications, ask the parents about respiratory distress or increased blood pressure during checkups. The child can also have bleeding varices; ask the parents if the child has ever spit up blood.

When you take a history from adults with ADPKD who are approximately 30 to 40 years old, note that they may have one of two forms of presenting symptoms: pain or hypertension. Pain can occur in one or both kidneys and can vary from a vague sense of heaviness or a dull ache to severe, knifelike pain. Some patients describe flank pain from renal colic, bloody urine from the passage of renal calculi, signs of a UTI (burning or pain on urination, urinary frequency and urgency, fever), and gastrointestinal symptoms (nausea, vomiting, diarrhea, constipation) from compression by the enlarged kidneys. Patients with the second type of ADPKD often develop hypertension as the initial clinical sign. Changes in urinary output and concentration may accompany hypertension because of developing renal insufficiency. Some children have a history of UTIs and perinephric abscesses.

PHYSICAL EXAMINATION. The most common symptom is **abdominal pain**. The infant with RPK has pronounced epicanthal folds (vertical skin folds that extend from the root of the nose to the median end of the eyebrow), a pointed nose and small chin, and low-set ears. When you palpate the child's kidneys, you are able to feel huge, tense, bilateral masses on both flanks. These children usually have multiple assessment findings from many malfunctioning organ systems, such as bleeding esophageal varices, pulmonary congestion, hypertension, and oliguria or anuria.

Adult patients with ADPKD may have a healthy appearance but may have urine that is foul-smelling, cloudy, or bloody because of a UTI. If the blood vessels that surround the kidney cysts rupture into the renal pelvis, the patient may have moderate to severe hematuria. The patient probably has had hypertension for years before any renal damage occurs. As the disease progresses, the patient develops a widening abdomen, which is tender when palpated. In advanced stages, palpation reveals grossly enlarged kidneys.

PSYCHOSOCIAL. When a child is diagnosed with RPK, assess the siblings for the disease as well. With both types of polycystic disease, the patient and partner need genetic counseling. Children of parents diagnosed with ADPKD should have an ultrasound or genetic testing because approximately half also have ADPKD. There is a great strain on individuals and their families with both types of polycystic kidney disease because of the poor prognosis of children with RPK and the knowledge that ADPKD worsens throughout life.

Diagnostic Highlights

Test	Normal Result	Abnormality With Condition	Explanation
Genetic testing	No mutations on genes of interest	*PKD1, PKD2,* and *PKD3* genes may have mutations that lead to ADPKD	Genetic alterations lead to ADPKD
Renal ultrasound	Normal renal structure	Markedly enlarged kidney with dilated cysts	Cyst development leads to altered tubular epithelium, cell proliferation, and fluid secretion

Other Tests: Computed tomography, magnetic resonance imaging, magnetic resonance angiography, serum chemistries, uric acid, serum blood urea nitrogen and creatinine, urinalysis, glomerular filtration rate, IV pyelogram

PRIMARY NURSING DIAGNOSIS

DIAGNOSIS. Acute pain related to compression of tissues, trauma to structures from renal colic, inflammation of cysts, calculi, and infection as evidenced by self-reports of pain, facial grimacing, and/or protective behavior

OUTCOMES. Comfort status; Pain control; Pain level; Symptom severity; Symptom control; Knowledge: Pain management; Knowledge: Medication

INTERVENTIONS. Pain management: Acute; Analgesic administration; Medication administration; Medication management; Teaching: Prescribed medication

PLANNING AND IMPLEMENTATION
Collaborative

Because there is no cure for polycystic kidney disease, care focuses on alleviating symptoms and slowing the onset of renal impairment. Infants with RPK need management of airway, breathing, and circulation because of the extent of the multiple system involvement. Patients who survive past infancy need treatment for hypertension, congestive heart failure, renal failure, and hepatic failure.

Rigorous blood pressure control is important for patients with ADPKD and should start early in the disease. Infections need to be prevented when possible and treated vigorously because they are difficult to cure, and the residual scarring can further worsen the disease. As renal impairment progresses, patients require hemodialysis and renal transplantation. Allografts from siblings may be used only after appropriate genetic screenings have ruled out the possibility that the sibling also has the disease. For those with ADPKD, surgery may decrease the pressure caused by enlarging cysts. This procedure sometimes removes functioning nephrons and may contribute to the loss of renal function, but it also controls hypertension and decreases pain. An alternative is percutaneous aspiration of the cysts.

Metabolic problems, including hyperkalemia, hypocalcemia, hyperphosphatemia, hyper-parathyroidism, and metabolic acidosis, also occur during the course of the disease and need to be managed. Usually, the patient needs a diet high in carbohydrate content and with prescribed limits of fluid, sodium, potassium, phosphorus, and protein.

Pharmacologic Highlights

Medication or Drug Class	Dosage	Description	Rationale
Tolvaptan	45–60 mg PO in a.m. and 15–30 mg in p.m.	Selective vasopressin V2–receptor antagonist	Slows kidney function decline

Medications are administered to manage complications: hypertension, infection, renal insufficiency, and end-stage renal disease. Analgesic drugs may be needed for control of the flank pain associated with enlarged kidneys, and hypertension may be controlled with angiotensin-converting enzyme inhibitors and angiotensin II receptor antagonist blockers or by calcium channel blockers. Patients are encouraged to avoid NSAIDs because of their nephrotoxic effects.

Independent

One of the most important nursing roles is to promote the patient's comfort. Encourage tepid baths, relaxation techniques, and other nonpharmacologic methods to improve comfort. Because many patients retain fluid from impaired renal regulatory mechanisms, fluid restriction may be necessary. Work with the patient to determine a personal schedule for fluid intake. If the patient desires, allot some of the fluid intake for ice chips. If possible, administer medications with meals to allow the patient to consolidate fluid intake.

The disease can be emotionally draining for the patient and family. Try to provide quiet time each day to talk with the patient. Answer questions, provide teaching materials, and listen to concerns. If the patient or family is not able to cope effectively, refer for counseling.

Teach the patient to use measures to prevent UTIs. Explain the need to empty the bladder completely when voiding. Encourage female patients to wipe from front to back after having a bowel movement. Explain the mechanism of action of all antibiotics to the patient and stress the need to take them on schedule to maintain blood levels and to take all of them. Teach the patient to notify the primary healthcare provider if any of the following symptoms recur: burning, fre-quency, urgency, cloudy or red urine, foul-smelling urine.

Evidence-Based Practice and Health Policy

Williams, N., Korneffel, K., Koizumi, N., & Ortiz, J. (2021). African American polycystic kid-ney patients receive higher risk kidneys, but do not face increased risk for graft failure or post-transplant mortality. *American Journal of Surgery, 221*, 1092–1103.

- The authors studied people with ADPKD with respect to race to determine if racial disparities exist. They used a national database including 10,842 renal transplant recipients with ADPKD to perform a retrospective analysis.
- Black patients waited longer for transplants (942 days as compared to 747 days) as compared to patients from other groups and were more likely to be on dialysis. Being Black was also a risk factor for delayed graft function but was not associated with graft failure. The authors concluded that racial disparities exist for Black renal transplant patients and there is a need to improve transplant equity.

DOCUMENTATION GUIDELINES

• Physical findings: Pain, fluid intake and output, daily weights, serial vital signs, laboratory findings (renal function tests and electrolytes in particular), appearance of urine
• Response to pain medications and nonpharmacologic methods of pain relief, fluid and dietary restrictions
• Presence of complications: UTI, edema, cardiac disease, intracranial hemorrhage

DISCHARGE AND HOME HEALTHCARE GUIDELINES

Teach the patient how to recognize a UTI and prevent its recurrence: Maintain fluid intake as allowed; complete perineal cleansing; avoid long, hot baths; empty the bladder completely. Teach the patient to notify the physician about the following because of possible deterioration in renal function: nausea, vomiting, and weight loss; changes in the pattern of urinary elimination; pruritus; headaches; a weight gain of more than 5 pounds in 1 week; edema; difficulty in breathing; and decreasing urine output. Stress the need to keep follow-up appointments. Teach the patient how to maintain any prescribed diet restrictions and include the family. Explain all medications, including the dosage, action, side effects, and route.

Polycythemia

DRG Category: 841
Mean LOS: 5.5 days
Description: MEDICAL: Lymphoma and Non-Acute Leukemia With Complication or Comorbidity

Polycythemia as a generic term refers to an increased concentration of red blood cells (RBCs, or erythrocytes). This blood disorder has several causes and can be classified as primary, secondary, or relative polycythemia (Table 1).

• **TABLE 1** Types of Polycythemia

TYPE	DEFINITION	SIGNS AND SYMPTOMS	PHYSICAL EXAMINATION
Primary polycythemia (polycythemia vera)	Chronic proliferative stem cell disorder of the bone marrow that leads to overproduction of RBCs, white blood cells (WBCs), and platelets; results in increased blood viscosity and platelet dysfunction	Early: Feeling of fullness in the head, tinnitus, headache, dizziness, hypertension, blurred vision, night sweats, epigastric pain, joint pain, pain on walking Late: Pruritus (abnormal histamine metabolism), abdominal fullness, pleuritic pain, epistaxis, gingival bleeding, angina, intermittent	Engorged veins in the fundus and retina of the eye on fundoscopic examination, congestion of conjunctiva, congested oral mucous membranes, tenderness of ribs and sternum on palpation, ruddy cyanosis, enlarged liver and spleen

(table continues on page 980)

• TABLE 1 Types of Polycythemia (continued)

TYPE	DEFINITION	SIGNS AND SYMPTOMS	PHYSICAL EXAMINATION
Secondary polycythemia	Excessive production of RBCs because of an underlying condition such as hypoxemia, tumors; often triggered by overproduction of erythropoietin (hormone produced primarily in the kidney and necessary for RBC production)	Shortness of breath from underlying pulmonary disease, symptoms from underlying disease processes	Ruddy cyanosis, ecchymosis, spoon-shaped nails, clubbing of fingers
Relative polycythemia	Caused by reduced plasma volume; actual RBC count is normal or even reduced; increased blood concentration occurs because of increased concentration of cells compared with plasma	Symptoms often vague: headache, dizziness, fatigue, dyspnea, diaphoresis, claudication, ruddy appearance, enlarged liver and spleen, hypoventilation	Ruddy appearance, enlarged liver and spleen, hypoventilation

Most complications of all types of polycythemia occur as a result of increased blood viscosity (hyperviscosity) or sudden blood loss (hemorrhage). Hyperviscosity may lead to thromboembolic events, such as organ thromboses or splenomegaly. Hemorrhage in any system can occur from platelet dysfunction. Hemorrhage and vasculitis may occur together because an excessive number of RBCs exert pressure on capillary walls. Specific complications include gangrene of the fingers and toes, hypertension, peptic ulcer disease, and cerebrovascular accident. Life expectancy for patients with polycythemia is decreased if it is left untreated and is roughly 2 years.

CAUSES

The cause of primary polycythemia is unknown, but a current theory is that the disease is caused by a genetic mutation (*JAK2*) that affects intracellular signaling and stem cell hypersensitivity or mutations related to erythropoietin production. Secondary polycythemia is caused by excessive production of erythropoietin. Decreased oxygen delivery leads to appropriate overproduction of erythropoietin in the following diseases: chronic obstructive pulmonary disease, sleep apnea, cyanotic heart disease, congestive heart failure, drug toxicities inducing hypoventilation, and prolonged exposure to high altitudes. Overproduction of erythropoietin occurs inappropriately in the following conditions: renal carcinoma, renal cysts, hepatoma, uterine fibroids, and endocrine disorders.

Relative polycythemia is caused by dehydration from the following conditions: decreased plasma volume because of diuretic therapy, persistent nausea and vomiting, decreased fluid intake, diabetic ketoacidosis, diabetes insipidus, plasma loss after thermal injury, and excessive drainage from drains or tubes. Risk factors include smoking, sleep apnea, carbon monoxide exposure, high altitudes, and heredity leading to genetic mutations.

GENETIC CONSIDERATIONS

Primary familial and congenital polycythemia (PFCP) is inherited as an autosomal dominant trait and has been associated with mutations in the genes encoding *VHL*, ECYT3, erythropoietin (*EPO*), or the erythropoietin receptor (*EPOR*). Somatic mutations in a single hematopoietic stem cell in the *JAK2* or *TET2* gene can also lead to polycythemia vera.

SEX AND LIFE SPAN CONSIDERATIONS

The incidence of primary polycythemia is the highest in middle-aged and older people, with a median onset age of 60 years. Some sex differences occur in primary polycythemia as males have a 12% increase in hemoglobin as compared to females. Sex differences seem particularly important with respect to symptom burden. Women report more severe and frequent individual symptoms such as abdominal discomfort and microvascular disturbances (headache, dizziness) and have higher symptom severity scores as compared to men (Palandri et al., 2021 [see Evidence-Based Practice and Health Policy]). It is rare in children except in those with cyanotic heart disease. Babies who are small for their gestational age and infants of diabetic mothers may also be at risk.

HEALTH DISPARITIES AND SEXUAL/GENDER MINORITY HEALTH

Ethnicity, race, and sexual/gender minority status have no known effect on the risk for polycythemia.

GLOBAL HEALTH CONSIDERATIONS

No global data are available, but polycythemia exists around the world.

ASSESSMENT

HISTORY. The history, symptoms, and clinical findings vary slightly with the three types of polycythemia and degree of increased blood viscosity. Ask if the patient has experienced any headaches, visual changes, ringing in the ears, shortness of breath, pleuritic pain, or hypoventilation. Some patients experience itching after a bath or shower due to increased histamine levels. The patient may report a recent weight loss because of feeling full (satiety) because of enlargement of the spleen. A thorough family, environmental, and occupational history is necessary. Many patients with polycythemia have a history of cardiac and pulmonary disease, particularly emphysema, and they may describe fatigue, night sweats, and bone pain.

PHYSICAL EXAMINATION. Common symptoms include **headache, diaphoresis, ringing in the ears, visual changes,** and **dizziness**. The patient's skin may have a red or purple tinge. Other patients might have no symptoms at all. Check the patient's pupil response to light. Examine the nose, gums, and skin for signs of bleeding or bruising or for evidence of scratching because of skin irritation and itchiness. Check all peripheral pulses to determine if the patient is experiencing thrombotic complications, and note that hypertension is common. Check the fingers for spoon-shaped nails or clubbing of fingers. The patient may have enlargement of the liver and spleen.

PSYCHOSOCIAL. Assess the effects of a chronic illness on the patient and family; if the patient does not get enough rest or relaxation, suggest lifestyle changes that might decrease stress. Determine the patient's and family's coping styles, since long-term management of the disease is likely. Heavy smokers may acquire certain hemoglobin abnormalities that can lead to secondary polycythemia, and they will benefit from smoking cessation.

Diagnostic Highlights

Test	Normal Result	Abnormality With Condition	Explanation
Bone marrow biopsy	Normal bone marrow cells	Hypercellular bone marrow with residual fat; increased erythroid progenitors, increased maturing granulocytic precursors and megakaryocytes	Thin needle is used to draw up small amount of liquid bone marrow; a small cylinder of bone and marrow (about 1/2 in. long) is removed; site of both samples is usually at the back of the hipbone
Complete blood count	RBCs: 3.6–5.8 million/mcL; hemoglobin (Hgb): 11.7–17.3 g/dL; hematocrit (Hct): 36%–52%; WBCs: 4,500–11,100/mcL; platelets: 150,000–450,000/mcL	Hgb: > 16.5 g/dL; Hct: ≥ 49%; RBC ≥ 6 million/mm^3; WBCs: 12,000–50,000 cells/mm^3; platelet count: > 400,000/mm^3	Increased proliferation and production of bone marrow elements

Other Tests: Vitamin B$_{12}$ level, ultrasound or computed tomography scanning to evaluate the spleen, leukocyte alkaline phosphatase, arterial oxygen saturation, total red cell mass, genetic testing, serum uric acid level

PRIMARY NURSING DIAGNOSIS

DIAGNOSIS. Ineffective protection related to abnormal blood profiles (coagulation) as evidenced by visual changes, dizziness, bleeding from mucous membranes, and/or bruising

OUTCOMES. Circulation status; Tissue integrity: Skin and mucous membranes; Tissue perfusion; Fluid balance; Knowledge: Disease process; Knowledge: Medication

INTERVENTIONS. Bleeding precautions; Fluid management; Surveillance; Medication management; Teaching: Disease process; Teaching: Prescribed medication; Wound care

PLANNING AND IMPLEMENTATION
Collaborative

Table 2 contains the collaborative interventions for primary, secondary, and relative polycythemia. The primary goals are to reduce the risk of thrombosis, prevent bleeding events, reduce the risk of blood cancers, and reduce the symptom burden. Splenectomy may be done for patients with painful splenomegaly or repeated splenic infarction.

• TABLE 2   Interventions for Polycythemia

TYPE	OBJECTIVE	INTERVENTIONS
Primary polycythemia	Reduce blood viscosity	Periodic phlebotomies (removing approximately 350–500 mL of blood) to help the patient maintain hemoglobin below 45%; usually every other day

• TABLE 2 Interventions for Polycythemia (continued)

TYPE	OBJECTIVE	INTERVENTIONS
		Bone marrow suppression for patients over age 50 years with chemotherapy (hydroxyurea) can usually control the disease process (medications can cause leukemia and therefore only used in most seriously ill patients); phosphorus-32 may be used in patients over age 80 years with comorbid conditions
		Ruxolitinib, a *JAK1/JAK2* inhibitor if there was inadequate response to hydroxyurea
		Pheresis techniques are used to remove RBCs, WBCs, and platelets and to return plasma to blood
Secondary polycythemia	Treat disease that acts as a hypoxic trigger or causes increased production of erythropoietin	Change of location for those who live at high altitudes if that is the hypoxic trigger
		May be treated by phlebotomy or pheresis if the patient has not responded to treatment or if increased blood viscosity is considered dangerous
Relative polycythemia	Prevent dehydration and thromboembolic conditions; to correct fluid volume deficits	Rehydration with fluids and replacement of electrolytes to manage dehydration
		Treat underlying cause
		Low-cholesterol, low-fat, low-sodium diet; low-purine diet modifies high uric acid levels and limits the risk of calculus formation

Pharmacologic Highlights

Medication or Drug Class	Dosage	Description	Rationale
Hydroxyurea	10–15 mg/kg/day	Antimetabolites	Induces hematologic remission, inhibits DNA synthetics and cell replication
JAK inhibitors: ruxolitinib, fedratinib	Varies by drug	JAK1/JAK2 kinase inhibitor to limit signaling of cytokines and growth factors	To prevent myelofibrosis, a neoplasm associated with JAK signaling

Other Drugs: Anagrelide hydrochloride may be used for platelet anti-aggregation. Aspirin may be given for the antiplatelet effect. For symptom management, increased serum uric acid levels can be treated with allopurinol or cyproheptadine, and pruritus can be managed with antihistamines or phenothiazines.

Independent

The patient's activity level is a primary concern. Allow for periods of rest because the patient may have both hypoxemia and a low hemoglobin count. At the same time, the patient needs to maintain mobility to prevent thrombosis because of increased blood viscosity. If rest and activity are balanced, the patient has the energy to be active for part of the day to limit complications. If the patient is bedridden, a program of active and passive range-of-motion exercises is essential. If the patient's appetite is dulled, encourage small, frequent feedings followed by a rest period to decrease nausea and vomiting. Fluid intake should be at least 3,000 mL/day to decrease blood viscosity and limit uric acid calculus formation; work with the patient to determine the best method to prevent fluid volume deficit.

Monitor the patient carefully for signs of bleeding tendencies. Common bleeding sites include the nose, gingiva, and skin. Teach the patient to monitor these sites carefully after hospital discharge and to report any increased bleeding immediately. If the patient experiences minor trauma, teach the patient to apply pressure to the puncture site. In addition, encourage the patient to avoid razors and handling sharp objects. If the patient has received antimetabolites, protect the patient from infection. Make sure that the patient's environment is safe to limit the risk of falls or injury. If the patient develops pruritus, discourage scratching of the skin, use skin emollients, and work with the patient to determine a medication schedule that limits discomfort.

Evidence-Based Practice and Health Policy

Palandri, F., Mora, B., Gangat, N., & Catani, L. (2021). Is there a gender effect in polycythemia vera? *Annals of Hematology, 100*, 11–25.

- Polycythemia vera is characterized by excessive red cell production and the release of proinflammatory cytokines. The authors note that sex-based discrepancies have been described in terms of incidence, response to treatment, and prognosis.
- Some sex differences occur as males have a 12% increase in hemoglobin as compared to females. Sex differences seem particularly important with respect to symptom burden. Women report more severe and frequent individual symptoms such as abdominal discomfort and microvascular disturbances (headache, dizziness) and have higher symptom severity scores as compared to men. Factors such as anemia or adverse prognosis were comparable between men and women, and women had a similar quality of life as men. Risk of thrombotic events and the effectiveness of treatment do not seem to vary by sex. Although the data are complicated, most experts note that women have longer survival times than men. The authors note that sex is a potential disease modifier, but the mechanisms by which sex influences the disease remain to be clarified.

DOCUMENTATION GUIDELINES

- Physical findings of skin and mucous membranes: Presence of redness, tenderness, swelling, temperature changes, scratch marks, bleeding ecchymosis
- Response to medications, fluids, diet, and treatments such as phlebotomy or pheresis
- Presence of complications: Bleeding tendencies, respiratory distress, mental status changes, gastric distress, infections

DISCHARGE AND HOME HEALTHCARE GUIDELINES

Teach the patient to avoid the following: crossing the legs, prolonged periods of sitting or standing, and leg positions that put pressure on the popliteal space. Be sure the patient understands all medications, including the dosage, route, action, and adverse effects. Be sure the patient understands all diet and fluid therapy.

Instruct the patient to report leg pain or swelling, skin discoloration, bleeding, decreases in peripheral skin temperature, or signs of possible infection to the physician. For patients with primary polycythemia, genetic counseling may be necessary.

Postpartum Hemorrhage

DRG Category:	786
Mean LOS:	6.3 days
Description:	SURGICAL: Cesarean Section Without Sterilization With Major Complication or Comorbidity
DRG Category:	787
Mean LOS:	4.0 days
Description:	SURGICAL: Cesarean Section Without Sterilization With Complication or Comorbidity
DRG Category:	805
Mean LOS:	4.0 days
Description:	MEDICAL: Vaginal Delivery Without Sterilization or Dilation & Curettage With Major Complication or Comorbidity
DRG Category:	806
Mean LOS:	2.7 days
Description:	MEDICAL: Vaginal Delivery Without Sterilization or Dilation & Curettage With Complication or Comorbidity

A postpartum hemorrhage (PPH) is frequently defined as a blood loss of greater than 500 mL after giving birth vaginally or a blood loss of greater than 1,000 mL after a cesarean section. Because many women lose at least 500 mL of blood during childbirth and do not experience any symptoms, a more accurate way to define PPH is losing 1% or more of the body weight after delivering a baby (1 mL of blood weighs 1 g). For example, a patient weighing 175 pounds (80 kilograms) would need to lose 800 mL of blood to be classified as having a PPH. Greater than a 10% decrease in the prenatal hematocrit is another means used to suggest that PPH has occurred; this value needs to be used cautiously because hematocrit is affected by factors other than blood loss, such as dehydration. It is estimated that 2% to 4% of all deliveries end in PPH, and it is a major contributor to maternal morbidity and mortality.

PPH is classified as either an early hemorrhage (occurring during the first 24 hours after delivery) or a late hemorrhage (occurring more than 24 hours after delivery). With the current trend in obstetric practice of sending postpartum patients home in 48 hours or less after delivery, the significance of PPH, particularly late hemorrhage, is profound. Often, the severity of the hemorrhage depends on the expediency with which it is diagnosed and treated; if the patient hemorrhages at home, the risk increases significantly. Complications include anemia, hemorrhagic/hypovolemic shock, and death.

CAUSES

There are several causes of PPH, particularly uterine atony, trauma, retained placental tissue, and thrombosis. Several predisposing factors related to these causes can be found in Box 1. The number one cause of early PPH is uterine atony, a condition in which the uterus does not adequately contract, allowing increased blood loss from the placental site of implantation. After the placenta is delivered, the uterus needs to contract to seal off the iliac arteries. If the uterus is contracted, the placental site is smaller, causing less bleeding.

• BOX 1 Predisposing (risk) Factors for Postpartum Hemorrhage

Overdistention of the uterus (multiple gestation and delayed-interval delivery in twin and triplet pregnancies, hydramnios)	Obesity
	Forceps or vacuum delivery; prolonged or rapid labor
Use of anesthetic agents, especially halothane	Extended used of oxytocin (Pitocin) during labor
Delivery of large infant	Maternal malnutrition or anemia
Manual removal of the placenta	Uterine infections
Placenta previa	Pregnancy-induced hypertension
Placenta accreta (separation of the placenta is difficult or impossible)	Maternal history of hemorrhage or blood coagulation problems
Mismanaged/prolonged (> 30 min) third stage of labor	Hypopituitarism (rate of PPH increases to 8.7%)
Lacerations	

Lacerations of the perineum, vagina, and cervix can occur during a vaginal birth. Lacerations of the cervix occur with rapid dilation or with pushing before complete dilation. During the second stage of labor, vaginal, perineal, and periurethral tears occur. Failure to repair these lacerations adequately can result in a slow, steady trickle of blood.

The most common cause of late PPH is retained placental tissue. If parts of the placenta remain in the uterus after delivery, small clots (thrombosis) form around the retained parts, sealing off the bleeding. After a while, the clots slough, and heavy bleeding occurs. Subinvolution (delayed involution) can also be a causative factor in a late PPH.

GENETIC CONSIDERATIONS

Several genetic coagulopathies could predispose a woman to postpartum hemorrhage (PPH), including familial hypofibrinogenemia or Scott syndrome. Von Willebrand disease is the most commonly inherited bleeding disorder. It is usually transmitted in an autosomal dominant fashion but can rarely be transmitted autosomal recessively. It results in mild to moderate risk of bleeding, but in some cases, bleeding can be severe and similar to that of hemophilia. Von Willebrand disease affects men and women equally and is caused by mutations in the *VWF* gene.

SEX AND LIFE SPAN CONSIDERATIONS

PPH is linked not to age but to risk factors (see Box 1).

HEALTH DISPARITIES AND SEXUAL/GENDER MINORITY HEALTH

Jehovah's Witnesses are at a 44-fold increased risk of death owing to hemorrhage during and after delivery because of decisions against blood transfusion when it is recommended. Black, Asian, and Hispanic women have a higher rate of PPH than White women. Women with severe maternal complications are more likely to be Black, multiparous, and/or 35 years or older. They are also likely to have public health insurance and receive inadequate prenatal care. The most common causes of severe maternal morbidity are hemorrhage (48%) and preeclampsia/eclampsia (20%). Sexual and gender minority status has no known effect on the risk for PPH (Geller et al., 2021).

GLOBAL HEALTH CONSIDERATIONS

Although rates of PPH have declined in the developed regions of the globe, it is the leading cause of maternal mortality in the world, accounting for 25% of all maternal deaths. Experts at the World Health Organization and other agencies estimate that 100,000 to 140,000 women die from PPD each year, with the majority of them from developing and underresourced regions. Reasons for the high rates of maternal death in developing regions include availability of medication and blood transfusion, lack of experienced caregivers present during birth, lack of operating room services, and increased prevalence of nutritional deficiencies.

✳ ASSESSMENT

HISTORY. Take a complete reproductive history. Because PPH can be repeated in subsequent pregnancies, always ask if a multipara had a previous PPH. Inquire about a family history of coagulation disorders or excessive bleeding with surgical procedures or menses.

PHYSICAL EXAMINATION. The most common symptom is **heavy vaginal bleeding**. Observe the amount and characteristics of blood loss; sometimes there is a pooling of blood and the passage of large clots. Usually, complete saturation of one perineal pad within 15 minutes or saturation of two or more pads in 1 hour suggests hemorrhage. A bimanual examination may be done to determine tone, uterine enlargement, or presence of pelvic hematomas. Palpate the fundus, noting if it is firm or boggy, if it is midline or deviated laterally, and if it is above or below the umbilicus. Normally, after delivery, the fundus is firm, midline, and at the level of the umbilicus. A fundus above the umbilicus and deviated laterally may indicate a full bladder. A boggy uterus is indicative of uterine atony and, if it is not corrected, results in a PPH. If the fundus is firm, midline, and at or below the umbilicus and if there is steady, bright red bleeding, further assessment for trauma is necessary. Inspect the perineum carefully to discern any unrepaired lacerations or bleeding from a repaired episiotomy. If a hematoma is suspected, the patient is placed in lithotomy position and the vagina and perineal area are carefully inspected. Ask if the patient has perineal pain. Although some discomfort is expected after a vaginal delivery, severe pain or pressure is uncommon and often indicates a hematoma. A bulging and discoloration of the skin is noted if a hematoma is present. Assess the patient's vital signs. A temperature above 100.4°F (38°C) may indicate uterine infection, which decreases the myometrium's ability to contract and makes the patient more susceptible to PPH. Note any foul vaginal odor that may accompany the fever with infection. Elevated heart rate, delayed capillary refill, decreased blood pressure, and increased respiratory rate may be noted if PPH is occurring. Assess the patient's color and skin temperature; pallor and cool, clammy skin also indicate hypovolemic shock.

PSYCHOSOCIAL. PPH is a traumatic experience because medical complications are unexpected during what is anticipated as a happy time. Assess the anxiety level of the patient; the patient going into hypovolemic shock is highly anxious and then may lose consciousness. The significant others experience a high level of anxiety as well and need a great deal of support.

Diagnostic Highlights

General Comments: Diagnosis of PPH is usually based on the estimated blood loss, which eventually is reflected in serum laboratory tests. Coagulation studies and typing and crossmatching are done if bleeding remains excessive. Serial monitoring of serum electrolytes, blood urea nitrogen, and creatinine is important.

Test	Normal Result	Abnormality With Condition	Explanation
Complete blood count	Red blood cells (RBCs): 3.6–5.8 million/mcL; hemoglobin (Hgb): 11.7–17.3 g/dL; hematocrit (Hct): 36%–52%; white blood cells: 4,500–11,100/mcL; platelets: 150,000–450,000/mcL	RBC count, Hgb, and Hct decrease several hours after significant blood loss has occurred	Active bleeding causes decrease

PRIMARY NURSING DIAGNOSIS

DIAGNOSIS. Risk for bleeding as evidenced by frank or occult hemorrhage, thirst, oliguria, hypotension, and/or tachycardia

OUTCOMES. Blood loss severity; Fluid balance; Hydration; Circulation status; Shock severity: Hypovolemic; Vital signs

INTERVENTIONS. Bleeding reduction: Postpartum uterus; Blood product administration; Fluid resuscitation; IV therapy; Shock prevention; Shock management: Volume; Vital signs monitoring

☀ PLANNING AND IMPLEMENTATION
Collaborative

The goal of treatment is to correct the cause and replace the fluid loss. Resuscitation occurs first, followed by identification and management of the underlying cause of PPH. Patients should have nothing by mouth until hemostasis is established. Expedient diagnosis and treatment of the cause reduce the likelihood of a blood transfusion. Treatment for uterine atony involves performing frequent fundal massage, sometimes bimanual massage (by the medical clinician only), and pharmacologic therapy. Fluid replacement with normal saline solution, lactated Ringer injection, or volume expanders is essential, and administration of blood may be necessary. Raising the patient's legs will improve venous return. Multiple venous access sites, 100% oxygen, and a Foley catheter are often needed. If uterine atony is not corrected quickly, a life-saving hysterectomy is indicated.

Serial laboratory measures to monitor the patient's hemoglobin and RBC count are essential, along with ensuring that blood products are readily available for transfusion. Monitor the hematocrit and hemoglobin to determine the success of fluid replacement and the patient's intake and output. If an infection is the cause of the atony, the physician prescribes antibiotics. PPH caused by trauma requires surgical repair with aseptic technique. Hematomas may absorb on their own; however, if they are large, an incision, evacuation of clots, and ligation of the bleeding vessel are necessary. Administer analgesics for perineal pain. If retained fragments are suspected at the time of delivery, the uterine cavity should be explored. If manual removal or expression of clots/placental fragments is unsuccessful, cervical dilation and curettage is indicated to remove retained fragments. A type of compression suture, Meydanli, may decrease PPH of cesarean deliveries with abnormal placental attachments or atony. The suture is placed from the lower end of the uterus to the top on both sides to assist in uterine compression.

Pharmacologic Highlights

Medication or Drug Class	Dosage	Description	Rationale
Oxytocin (Pitocin)	Mix 10–40 units in 1,000 mL, give 20–40 milliunit/min	Oxytocic	Controls bleeding by producing uterine contractions
Methylergonovine (Methergine)	0.2 mg IM	Oxytocic	Controls bleeding by producing uterine contractions
Carboprost	259 mcg IM	Prostaglandin	Controls bleeding by producing uterine contractions
Misoprostol	1,000 mcg PR	Prostaglandin	Causes sustained uterine contraction

Independent

Be alert for PPH in any postpartum patient, especially those who have any of the predisposing factors. It is often the nurse who discovers the hemorrhage. For the first 24 hours postpartum, perform frequent fundal checks. Fundal check should be every 15 minutes for the first hour, then every 30 minutes the next hour, then every 2 hours for 4 hours, then every 4 hours and progressing to every 8 hours if there are no problems with involution. If the fundus is boggy, massage until it feels firm; it should feel like a large, hard grapefruit. When massaging the fundus, keep one hand above the symphysis pubis to support the lower uterine segment, while gently but firmly rubbing the fundus, which may lose its tone when the massage is stopped. Explain that cramping or feeling like "labor is starting again" is expected with liberal administration of the oxytocic drugs used to manage the bleeding. Monitor for hypertension if oxytocics and prostaglandins are used. Encourage the patient to void; a full bladder interferes with contractions and normal uterine involution. If patients are unable to void on their own, straight catheterization is necessary.

Monitor vaginal bleeding; the lochia is usually dark red and should not saturate more than one perineal pad every 2 to 3 hours. Blood loss is frequently underestimated. If unsure, weigh the perineal pads and any blood-soaked underpads or sheets. One gram of weight is equal to 1 mL of blood loss volume. Notify the physician if the bleeding is steady and bright red in the presence of a normal firm fundus; this usually indicates a laceration. Ice packs and sitz baths may relieve perineal discomfort. The patient is usually on complete bedrest. Rooming in with the infant may be difficult; provide for safe care for the infant while it is in the birthing parent's room. Assist the patient and significant others as much as possible with newborn care to facilitate quality time between the parent and the newborn. Assist the patient with ambulation the first few times out of bed; syncope is common after a large blood loss. Ensure adequate rest periods.

Evidence-Based Practice and Health Policy

Almutairi, W., Ludington, S., Griffin, M., Burant, C., Al-Zahrani, A., Alshareef, F., & Badr, H. (2021). The role of skin-to-skin contact with breastfeeding on atonic postpartum hemorrhage. *Nursing Reports, 11*, 1–11.

- The authors aimed to conduct a retrospective chart review using codes for atonic postpartum hemorrhage to determine the incidence of PPH, the amount of estimated blood loss, and the duration of the third stage of labor in women with and without PPH. The cases were from medical records of patients who received care in a large university-based tertiary healthcare setting.
- The postpartum hemorrhage rate due to atonic uterus increased by 47.5% from 2009 to 2015, and the third stage of labor was longer for the postpartum hemorrhage patients. Women who had skin-to-skin contact and breastfed their newborns immediately after birth had a shorter third stage of labor, and estimated blood loss was lower than for women who did not have that experience.

DOCUMENTATION GUIDELINES

- Bleeding: Amount, characteristics, precipitating factors
- Fundus: Location (above or below umbilicus, midline or lateral) and firmness
- Vital signs and any signs and symptoms of hypovolemic shock
- Appearance of the perineum, episiotomy, laceration repair (use REEDA [redness, edema, ecchymosis, drainage, approximation] to guide the documentation); fluid intake and output
- Absence or presence of vaginal odor

DISCHARGE AND HOME HEALTHCARE GUIDELINES

TEACHING. Teach the patient how to check the fundus and do a fundal massage; this is especially important for patients at risk who are discharged early from the hospital. Advise the patient to contact the physician for the following: a boggy uterus that does not become firm with massage, excessive bright red or dark red bleeding, many large clots, fever above 100.4°F (38°C), persistent or severe perineal pain or pressure.

MEDICATIONS. If iron supplements are provided, teach the patient to take the drug with orange juice and expect some constipation and dark-colored stools. If oxytocics are ordered, emphasize the importance of taking them around the clock as prescribed. If antibiotics are ordered, teach the patient to finish the prescription, even though the symptoms may have ceased.

Preeclampsia

DRG Category:	786
Mean LOS:	6.3 days
Description:	SURGICAL: Cesarean Section Without Sterilization With Major Complication or Comorbidity
DRG Category:	787
Mean LOS:	4.0 days
Description:	SURGICAL: Cesarean Section Without Sterilization With Complication or Comorbidity
DRG Category:	807
Mean LOS:	2.2 days
Description:	MEDICAL: Vaginal Delivery Without Sterilization or Dilation & Curettage Without Complication or Comorbidity or Major Complication or Comorbidity

Preeclampsia is a pregnancy-specific syndrome of reduced organ perfusion secondary to vasospasm and endothelial activation that affects approximately 7% of all pregnant persons. It is characterized by hypertension (blood pressure [BP] > 140/90), oliguria, and proteinuria (300 mg in 24 hours or 1+ dipstick) after 20 weeks' gestation. Although it is often present, edema is no longer included as a diagnostic criterion for preeclampsia because it is an expected occurrence in pregnancy and has not been shown to be discriminatory.

If untreated (or sometimes even with aggressive treatment), the symptoms get progressively worse. Symptoms relate to decreased perfusion to the major organs: kidneys (proteinuria, oliguria), liver (epigastric pain, elevated enzymes), brain (headache, blurred vision, hyperreflexia, clonus, seizures), and the placenta (fetal distress, intrauterine growth restriction). Two different progressions of preeclampsia are (1) eclampsia (seizure occurs) and (2) HELLP syndrome (hemolysis, elevated liver enzyme levels, low platelet count). Eclampsia and HELLP may or may not occur together. Another complication can be disseminated intravascular coagulation, which is often fatal. Not only is preeclampsia life-threatening for the mother, but it can also cause intrauterine growth retardation, decreased fetal movement, chronic hypoxia, or even death in the fetus caused by decreased placental perfusion. If seizures occur, the patient has a risk of complications such as placental abruption, neurological deficits, aspiration pneumonia, pulmonary edema, cardiopulmonary arrest, acute renal failure, and death. Fetal bradycardia is typical during the seizure, usually with slow recovery to the baseline heart rate upon the seizure ending.

Preeclampsia is one of the hypertensive disorders that can complicate a pregnancy. In addition to preeclampsia, there are four other categories of hypertension disorders in pregnancy: (1) gestational hypertension—BP of 140/90 or higher for the first time during pregnancy, and blood pressure returns to normal in less than 12 weeks after delivery; (2) chronic hypertension—BP of 140/90 or higher before pregnancy or occurring before 20 weeks' gestation; (3) eclampsia—includes the symptoms of preeclampsia with the development of seizures; and (4) HELLP syndrome—symptoms of preeclampsia and/or eclampsia with elevated liver enzymes, elevated uric acid, low platelet count, and upper right quadrant abdominal pain.

CAUSES

The cause of preeclampsia is unknown; it is often called the "disease of theories" because many causes have been proposed, yet none has been well established. Experts suggest that the primary pathophysiology of hypertension disorders in pregnancy is related to the placenta, likely poor implantation leading to decreased placental perfusion. Hypoxia of the placenta leads to a release of antiangiogenic proteins that enter the pregnant person's circulation, damaging endothelial cells and leading to vasospasm. Other theories include immune maladaptation to paternal antigens associated with the fetus that leads to a situation similar to acute graft rejection. Another theory is that decreased levels of prostaglandins and a decreased resistance to angiotensin II lead to a generalized arterial vasospasm that then causes endothelial damage. The brain, liver, kidney, and blood are particularly susceptible to multiple dysfunctions. Several risk factors have been identified that may predispose a pregnant person to developing preeclampsia: age of pregnant person; obesity; nulliparity; familial history; multiple gestation; patient history of diabetes mellitus, chronic hypertension, renal disease, urinary tract infection, trophoblastic disease, periodontal disease, and malnutrition. Calcium deficiency is also linked to hypertensive disorders in pregnancy. Bariatric surgery for obese pregnant persons may decrease their chances of becoming preeclamptic.

GENETIC CONSIDERATIONS

There is a genetic component in the development of both preeclampsia and pregnancy-induced hypertension (PIH). Several genes, including the angiotensin II type 1 receptor and the *SERPINE1/PAI1* gene, have been associated with susceptibility. Mutations in the *STOX1* gene have been found to cause preeclampsia in some Dutch families. Further studies are needed to determine the mechanism of these genetic mutations.

SEX AND LIFE SPAN CONSIDERATIONS

Preeclampsia tends to occur most frequently in pregnant adolescents, in birthing parents over age 35 years, and in primigravidas. Pregnancies at an advanced age have been associated with higher complication rates but without differences in placental pathology. Worse outcomes associated with advanced age and preeclampsia are usually related to chronic conditions rather than issues with the placenta.

HEALTH DISPARITIES AND SEXUAL/GENDER MINORITY HEALTH

Black women have the highest rates of severe maternal mortality as compared to other groups, with maternal mortality rate 2.5 to 3 times higher than White women. Native American women and Alaskan Native women are also disproportionately affected by preeclampsia (Johnson & Louis, 2020). Well-established risk factors for preeclampsia, such as obesity, diabetes, and hypertension, disproportionately affect Black, Native American, and Hispanic women, placing them at risk. Preeclampsia and eclampsia are second only to postpartum hemorrhage as morbidity postpartum for Black women (Geller et al., 2021). Nurses have a significantly higher risk of anemia, placenta previa, and pregnancy-associated hypertensive diseases and preeclampsia during the antenatal period than nonmedical working women. Sexual and gender minority status has no known effect on the risk for preeclampsia.

GLOBAL HEALTH CONSIDERATIONS

The global incidence of preeclampsia ranges from 2% to 15% of all pregnancies, with developing regions in Africa having the highest incidence.

☼ ASSESSMENT

HISTORY. Obtain a thorough medical and obstetric history early in the pregnancy to determine if the patient has any of the risk factors. If the patient had a previous delivery, obtain information on any problems that occurred. Assess the patient's level of consciousness and orientation because the patient's mental status may deteriorate as preeclampsia progresses. Ask if the patient has noticed an increase in edema, especially in the face; nondependent edema is more significant than dependent edema. The significant other may report that the patient's face is "fuller." Ask if the patient's hands and feet swell overnight and if rings feel tight; the patient may even report being unable to take off the rings. Question the patient about any nausea, headaches, visual disturbances (blurred, double, spots), or right upper quadrant pain. Ask the patient and significant others if the patient has had seizures.

PHYSICAL EXAMINATION. Common symptoms include **hypertension, proteinuria, pitting edema, headache,** and **oliguria**. Although most pregnant people experience some edema, it has a more abrupt onset in preeclampsia. Weigh the patient daily in the same clothes and at the same time to help estimate fluid retention; often, the patient gains several pounds in 1 week. BP should be taken on the right arm while the patient is supine and in the left lateral position, which promotes optimal placental perfusion. Compare BP readings to determine increasing trends.

A funduscopic inspection of the retina may reveal vascular constriction and narrowing of the small arteries. Auscultate the patient's lungs bilaterally to assess for pulmonary edema. Assess the deep tendon reflexes and assign a rating from 1 to 4; with PIH, reflexes are brisker than normal. Check for clonus bilaterally by dorsiflexing the foot briskly and checking if the foot comes back and taps your hand. Count the beats of clonus present; presence of clonus is indicative of central nervous system involvement. Perform a sterile vaginal examination to determine if the patient is in labor or to determine the ripeness of the cervix for labor. Also note if the amniotic sac is intact or ruptured and if there is any bloody show, which signals the onset of labor. If the amniotic sac is ruptured, note the color, amount, and presence of odor of the fluid. A yellow-green color and foul odor indicate possible fetal distress or infection. Assess the uterus for the presence of contractions, noting the frequency, duration, and intensity. Place the patient on the fetal monitor immediately to determine the status of the fetus. Provide ongoing assessments of the baseline fetal heart rate and of the presence or absence of variability, accelerations, and decelerations in the heart rate. Often, a nonstress test (NST) is done on admission to assess the fetus's well-being.

PSYCHOSOCIAL. Many expect pregnancy to be a happy and normal process; hospitalization is unexpected. Assess the patient's ability to cope with the disorder and the patient's social supports. In addition to concern about the pregnancy, the patient may have other children or occupational responsibilities that need management while the patient is hospitalized. Assess the resources of the patient and significant others to manage job, childcare, financial, and social responsibilities.

Diagnostic Highlights

General Comments: The minimum diagnostic criteria for preeclampsia are BP > 140/90 mm Hg after 20 weeks' gestation and proteinuria > 300 mg in 24 hours or > 1+ dipstick. Other evidence to support the diagnosis of preeclampsia includes elevated serum creatinine, lactate dehydrogenase (LDH), alanine aminotransferase (ALT), or aspartate transaminase (AST); low platelets; persistent headache or visual disturbance; persistent epigastric pain; and increasing BP and proteinuria. Serial laboratory tests are done to assist with diagnosis and monitoring of the disease. Increasing and decreasing trends indicate improvement or worsening of the disease state and help diagnose multiorgan involvement.

Diagnostic Highlights (continued)

Test	Normal Result	Abnormality With Condition	Explanation
Dip/24-hr urine for protein and creatinine	Dip–negative 80–125 mL/min	2+ or higher > 3 g/L for 24 hr elevated	Increase in protein and creatinine in the urine indicates renal disease
Uric acid	2.5–7 mg/dL	Elevated	Indicates renal disease
Blood urea nitrogen (BUN)	10–31 mg/dL	Elevated	Indicates renal disease
Liver enzymes • AST • ALT • LDH • Bilirubin	• 15–30 International Unit/L • 5–24 International Unit/L • 90–156 International Unit/L • 0.1–1.0 mg/dL	Elevated	Increases indicate liver involvement
Platelets	140,000–400,000/mm³	Decreased	Decrease caused by endothelial damage and activation of thrombin

Other Tests: Tests include complete blood count and coagulation studies. Starting at the 26th week of gestation, fetal testing assesses well-being and includes modified biophysical profiles (BPP), daily fetal kick counts, and with decreased amniotic fluid or lack of fetal reactivity, a full BPP (ultrasonography to measure fetal breathing, fetal movement, fetal tone, and amniotic fluid volume); contraction stress or Doppler velocimetry; for patients in labor, continuous fetal monitoring and possible scalp pH. If the fetus is premature, an amniocentesis may be done to obtain amniotic fluid for fetal lung maturity tests. If cerebral edema or intracranial bleeding is suspected, computed tomography scanning and magnetic resonance imaging are used.

PRIMARY NURSING DIAGNOSIS

DIAGNOSIS. Risk for decreased cerebral tissue perfusion as evidenced by hypertension, visual disturbance, and/or headache

OUTCOMES. Vital signs; Hypertension severity; Urinary elimination; Fluid balance; Neurological status; Tissue perfusion: Cerebral; Fetal status: Intrapartum; Medication response

INTERVENTIONS. Vital signs monitoring; Fluid monitoring; Fluid management; Fluid/electrolyte management; Seizure precautions; Medication administration; Medication management; Electronic fetal monitoring: Intrapartum

PLANNING AND IMPLEMENTATION
Collaborative
Tight BP control in both mild chronic essential and gestational nonproteinuric hypertension in pregnancy leads to better perinatal outcomes and less severe hypertension. Often, preeclampsia occurs before the fetus is term. The goals of treatment are to prevent seizures, intracranial hemorrhage, and serious organ damage in the birthing parent and to deliver a healthy term infant. The only cure for preeclampsia is delivery of the infant; however, if the infant is preterm, care is balanced between preventing parental complications and allowing the fetus more time in utero. If the symptoms in preeclampsia are mild, often the patient is treated at home on bedrest, with careful instructions and education on the danger signs and frequent prenatal visits to monitor progression of the disorder. The patient should be instructed to remain on bedrest and to perform daily kick counts to monitor fetal well-being. Antihypertensives are usually not prescribed

for mild preeclamptics; no differences in gestational age or birthweight have been noted, and growth-restricted infants were twice as frequent in patients who took labetalol than in those treated with bedrest/hospitalization alone. Mild preeclampsia is really a misnomer because it can become severe very rapidly. Frequent tests of fetal well-being are done throughout the pregnancy, including an NST and BPP, to detect the effects of preeclampsia on the fetus.

If symptoms of preeclampsia worsen, hospitalization is mandatory. Maintain the patient on complete bedrest. If the urine output is below 30 mL per hour, suspect renal failure and notify the physician. Readings of 2+ to 4+ protein in the urine and urine-specific gravities of greater than 1.040 are associated with proteinuria and oliguria. Hemodynamic monitoring with a central venous pressure catheter or a pulmonary artery catheter may be initiated to regulate fluid balance. Respiratory monitoring (respiratory rate, breath sounds) along with cardiac monitoring is important for ongoing assessments. Magnesium sulfate is given via IV infusion to prevent seizures. Serum magnesium levels are done to determine if the level has reached the therapeutic level; serum levels also alert the caregiver of a move toward toxicity. If the magnesium sulfate infusion does not prevent seizure, the physician may order phenobarbital or benzodiazepines. Using either low doses of aspirin or dietary calcium supplementation is being explored as means to prevent preeclampsia.

If the patient is alert and is not nauseated, a high-protein, moderate-sodium diet is appropriate. Low-salt diets are not indicated. Glucocorticoids may be given to the patient intramuscularly at least 48 hours before delivery to assist in maturing fetal lungs to decrease the severity of respiratory difficulties in the preterm neonate. A cesarean section is indicated if the fetus is showing signs of distress or if preeclampsia is severe and the patient is not responding to aggressive treatment. All efforts are made to stabilize the patient's condition before surgery.

Pharmacologic Highlights

Medication or Drug Class	Dosage	Description	Rationale
Magnesium sulfate	4–5 g IV piggyback (PB) loading dose; 1–2 g/hr IV maintenance dose for 12 to 24 hr	Anticonvulsant	PIH can progress to eclampsia; drug of choice to prevent seizures
Calcium gluconate	1 g IV push (IVP) slowly over 3 min	Antidote for magnesium sulfate	Respiratory depression occurs with magnesium toxicity
• Methyldopa (Aldomet) • Labetalol (Normodyne) • Nifedipine (Procardia) • Hydralazine (Apresoline)	Varies with drug • PO • PO • PO • PO or IV	Antihypertensive	Given if diastolic is > 110 mm Hg; IV medication is used if oral is ineffective

Independent

Remember that the patient's condition can deteriorate rapidly. Monitor for signs and symptoms of progressive disease and impending eclampsia and HELLP. Assess the blood pressure, pulse, respirations, and urine output hourly. Check deep tendon reflexes and for clonus hourly or as ordered. Report upward trends. Be alert for signs and symptoms of impending eclampsia such as accelerating hypertension, headache, epigastric pain, nausea, visual disturbances, altered sensorium, and increased bleeding tendencies.

Maintain the patient on bedrest in the left lateral position as much as possible. This position assists with venous return, organ perfusion, and optimal placental perfusion. Maintain a quiet, dim environment for rest, close to the nurse's station, and maintain a calm demeanor to prevent increasing anxiety in the patient. Eliminate extraneous noises, lights, visitors, and interruptions that might increase cerebral irritation and precipitate a seizure. Plan assessments and care to ensure optimal rest. Pad the side rails and always keep the bed in the low position with the call light in reach. To be prepared for emergencies, keep a "toxemia kit," which includes an artificial airway, calcium gluconate (antidote for magnesium sulfate), syringes, alcohol pads, and other medications, at the bedside. If the patient is receiving magnesium sulfate, monitor for signs of magnesium toxicity: hyporeflexia, decreased respirations, and oliguria. Expect the patient receiving magnesium sulfate to be lethargic.

If the patient is in labor, closely monitor fetal heart rate patterns and contractions. If the fetal heart rate shows signs of stress, turn the patient to the left side, increase the rate of the IV fluids, administer humidified oxygen per mask at 10 L/min, and notify the physician. Because abruptio placentae is a potential complication of preeclampsia, be alert for any of the following signs of placental detachment: profuse vaginal bleeding, increased abdominal pain, and a rigid abdomen. The fetus also shows signs of distress (late decelerations, bradycardia).

Provide emotional support to the patient and family. The onset and severity of preeclampsia, along with its potential outcomes for the infant, are worrisome. If delivery of a preterm infant is imminent, educate the family on the environment and care given in the neonatal intensive care unit (NICU). Tour the NICU with the parents, and explain what can be expected after the birth. This preparation helps alleviate some of the new parents' fears after the delivery.

After delivery, complications of preeclampsia can still manifest over the next 48 hours. Continue ongoing monitoring; be alert for seizures and indications that the patient is going into HELLP syndrome.

Evidence-Based Practice and Health Policy

Rana, S., Lemoine, E., Granger, J., & Karumanchi, S. A. (2019). Preeclampsia pathophysiology, challenges, and perspectives. *Circulation Research, 124,* 1094–1112.

- Women with a history of preeclampsia are at increased risk for cardiovascular disease and dementia later in life including myocardial infarction without the progressive forewarning of symptoms of acute coronary syndrome. Preeclampsia is also associated with a 4.7-fold risk for end-stage renal disease late in life.
- Research has also shown that children born to women with preeclampsia have an increased risk for cardiovascular disease. Early risk identification and treatment are essential to prevent preeclampsia, and more research is needed for its treatment.

DOCUMENTATION GUIDELINES

- Vital signs: BP (value and patient's position); heart rate; respiratory rate; daily weights; intake and output; daily fetal kick counts
- Edema: Location, presence or absence of pitting, numerical rating (1–4)
- Reflexes rated on a 1 to 4 scale and presence or absence of clonus
- Presence or absence of headache, visual disturbances, altered sensorium, epigastric discomfort, nausea
- Response to treatment: Anticonvulsants, antihypertensives, sedatives, bedrest
- Fetal assessment: Baseline heart rate; presence or absence of accelerations, decelerations, variability, fetal movement; response to movement
- Patient's response to pain during labor and to pain relief measures (analgesics, epidural)

DISCHARGE AND HOME HEALTHCARE GUIDELINES

HOME CARE IF UNDELIVERED. If the patient is discharged undelivered, emphasize that follow-up appointments are important for timely diagnosis of progressive preeclampsia. Educate the patient on the importance of the left lateral position for bedrest. Tell the patient to notify the physician immediately for any of the following symptoms: headache; visual disturbance; right upper quadrant pain; change in level of consciousness or "feeling funny"; decreased urine output; increase in edema, especially facial; or any decrease in fetal movement. Tell the patient to obtain weight daily and notify the physician of a sudden weight gain. Be sure the patient understands the seriousness of the disorder and the potential complications to the patient and infant.

HOME CARE IF DELIVERED. Because preeclampsia does not resolve immediately after delivery, if the patient is discharged after delivery, the patient needs to receive similar teaching.

Premature Rupture of Membranes

DRG Category:	786
Mean LOS:	6.3 days
Description:	SURGICAL: Cesarean Section Without Sterilization With Major Complication or Comorbidity
DRG Category:	787
Mean LOS:	4.0 days
Description:	SURGICAL: Cesarean Section Without Sterilization With Complication or Comorbidity
DRG Category:	807
Mean LOS:	2.2 days
Description:	MEDICAL: Vaginal Delivery Without Sterilization or Dilation & Curettage Without Complication or Comorbidity or Major Complication or Comorbidity

Premature rupture of membranes (PROM) is the spontaneous rupturing of the amniotic membranes ("bag of water") before the onset of true labor. While it can occur at any gestational age, PROM usually refers to rupture of the membranes (ROM) that occurs after 37 weeks' gestation prior to the onset of labor. Preterm premature rupture of membranes (PPROM) occurs between the end of the 20th week and the end of the 36th week. PPROM occurs in 30% to 40% of all preterm births and is a major contributor to perinatal morbidity and mortality owing to the lung immaturity and respiratory distress. PROM can result in two major complications. First, if the presenting part is ballotable (still floating, not engaged) when PROM occurs, there is risk of a prolapsed umbilical cord. Second, the birthing parent and fetus can develop an infection. The amniotic sac serves as a barrier to prevent bacteria from entering the uterus from the vagina; once the sac is broken, bacteria can move freely upward and cause infection in the birthing parent and the fetus. Furthermore, if the labor must be augmented because of PROM and the cervix is not ripe, the patient is at a higher risk for a cesarean delivery.

CAUSES

Although the specific cause of PROM is unknown, there are many predisposing factors. An incompetent cervix leads to PROM in the second trimester. Infections such as cervicitis and amnionitis—and placenta previa, abruptio placentae, and a history of induced abortions—may be involved with PROM. In addition, any condition that places undue stress on the uterus, such as multiple gestation, polyhydramnios, or trauma, can contribute to PROM. Fetal factors involved are genetic abnormalities and fetal malpresentation. A defect in the membrane itself is also a suspected cause. Factors associated with PPROM include tobacco use, preterm labor history, human papillomavirus (HPV) infection, urinary tract infection, low body mass index, and low socioeconomic status.

GENETIC CONSIDERATIONS

PROM may occur with some of the hereditary connective tissue disorders, such as Ehlers-Danlos syndrome, a class of six conditions resulting in skin fragility, skin extensibility, and joint hypermobility, that can be inherited in either an autosomal dominant or an autosomal recessive pattern. Mutations often occur in genes encoding for collagen or proteins that process or interact with collagen.

SEX AND LIFE SPAN CONSIDERATIONS

While estimates vary, PROM occurs in approximately 3% to 10% of all deliveries. It also occurs in 30% to 40% of preterm deliveries in the United States and Western Europe. It is not associated with age of the birthing parent, but women with HPV infections have a higher risk for PPROM and PROM at term compared with noninfected women. However, HPV does not increase the risk of preterm delivery beyond those deliveries caused by PPROM.

HEALTH DISPARITIES AND SEXUAL/GENDER MINORITY HEALTH

Low socioeconomic status is a factor associated with PPROM and is a health disparity for those women with low incomes. Ethnicity, race, and sexual/gender minority status have no known effect on the risk for PROM.

GLOBAL HEALTH CONSIDERATIONS

The World Health Organization states that PROM occurs in 3% of all pregnancies.

ASSESSMENT

HISTORY. Ask the patient the date of the last menstrual period to determine the fetus's gestational age. Ask if the patient has been feeling the baby move. Review the prenatal record if it is available or question the patient about problems with the pregnancy, such as high blood pressure, gestational diabetes, bleeding, premature labor, illnesses, and trauma. Have the patient describe the circumstances leading to PROM. Determine the time the rupture occurred, the color of the fluid and the amount, and if there was an odor to the fluid. **Patients may report a sudden gush of fluid** or a feeling of "always being wet." Inquire about any urinary, vaginal, or pelvic infections. Ask about cigarette, alcohol, and drug use and exposure to teratogens.

PHYSICAL EXAMINATION. The most common sign is ROM and **gushing, leaking, or pooling of amniotic fluid**. The priority assessment is auscultation of the fetal heart rate (FHR). Fetal tachycardia indicates infection. FHR may be decreased or absent during early pregnancy or if the umbilical cord prolapsed through the cervix. If absent heart rate or bradycardia is noted, perform a sterile vaginal examination to check for an umbilical cord. If a cord is felt, place the patient in Trendelenburg position, lift the presenting part off of the umbilical cord, and notify the physician immediately.

Note the frequency, duration, and intensity of any contractions. With PROM, contractions are absent. Perform a sterile vaginal examination if the patient is term (> 37 weeks), and note the dilation and effacement of the cervix and the station and presentation of the fetus. If the patient is preterm, notify the physician before doing a vaginal examination, which is often deferred in preterm patients to decrease the likelihood of introducing infection.

It is important in the initial examination to determine if PROM occurred. A sterile speculum vaginal examination can be done to confirm ROM. Pooling of amniotic fluid in the vagina or leakage from the cervix can be noted by the examiner (see Diagnostic Highlights for amniotic fluid analysis). Often, urinary incontinence, loss of the mucous plug, and increased leukorrhea, which are common occurrences during the third trimester, are mistaken for PROM. Inspect the perineum and vaginal vault for presence of fluid, noting the color, consistency, and any foul odor. Normally, amniotic fluid is clear or sometimes blood-tinged with small white particles of vernix. Meconium-stained fluid, which results from the fetus passing stool in utero, can be stained from a light tan to thick green, resembling split pea soup. Take the patient's vital signs. An elevated temperature and tachycardia are signs that infection is present because of PROM. Auscultate the lungs bilaterally. Palpate the uterus for tenderness, which is often present if infection is present. Check the patient's reflexes and inspect all extremities for edema.

PSYCHOSOCIAL. If the pregnancy is term, most patients are elated with the occurrence of ROM, even though they are not having contractions. If the patient is preterm, PROM is extremely upsetting. Assess the patient's relationship with the significant other and available support.

Diagnostic Highlights

Test	Normal Result	Abnormality With Condition	Explanation
Nitrazine test tape	Yellow to olive green indicates acidic and intact membranes	Blue-green to deep blue indicates alkaline; membranes probably ruptured	Amniotic fluid is alkaline and thus turns the yellow paper blue
Speculum examination and fern test	No fluid is seen in vaginal vault; fern pattern is not noted on slide	Fluid is visualized at cervical os; microscope slide reveals fern pattern	Amniotic fluid possesses ferning capacity evident by microscopic examination of a prepped slide

Other Tests: Complete blood count, cervical cultures for infections, amniocentesis (to check lung maturity if the patient is preterm when PPROM occurs), ultrasound

PRIMARY NURSING DIAGNOSIS

DIAGNOSIS. Risk for infection as evidenced by fever, tachycardia, and/or changes in color or odor of vaginal discharge or amniotic fluid

OUTCOMES. Immune status; Risk control: Infectious process; Risk detection; Symptom severity; Symptom control; Knowledge: Infection control

INTERVENTIONS. High-risk pregnancy care; Infection control; Labor induction; Electronic fetal monitoring: Intrapartum

⁂ PLANNING AND IMPLEMENTATION
Collaborative

Treatment varies, depending on the gestational age of the fetus and the presence of infection. Healthcare providers may immediately induce labor or implement expectant management to allow the patient to begin labor naturally. If infection is present, the fetus is delivered promptly regardless of gestational age. Delivery can be vaginal (induced) or by cesarean section. IV antibiotics are begun immediately. The antibiotics cross the placenta and are thought to provide some protection to the fetus.

If the patient is preterm (< 37 weeks) and has no signs of infection, the patient is maintained on complete bedrest. A weekly nonstress test, contraction stress test, and biophysical profile are done to continually assess fetal well-being. If the gestational age is between 28 and 32 weeks, glucocorticoids are administered to accelerate fetal lung maturity. Use of tocolysis to stop contractions if they begin is controversial when ROM has occurred. Some patients are discharged on bedrest with bathroom privileges if the leakage of fluid ceases, no contractions are noted, and there are no signs and symptoms of infection; however, most physicians prefer to keep the patient hospitalized because of the high risk of infection.

If the patient is term and PROM has occurred, the labor can be augmented with oxytocin. It is always desirable to deliver a term infant within 24 hours of ROM because the likelihood of infection increases significantly at 12 and 16 hours. Some patients and physicians prefer to wait 24 to 48 hours and let labor start on its own without the use of oxytocin. If this is the case, inpatient monitoring for signs and symptoms of infection and fetal well-being is recommended.

Pharmacologic Highlights

Medication or Drug Class	Dosage	Description	Rationale
Ampicillin, or other antibiotics (ampicillin, erythromycin)	1–2 g every 6 hr IV piggyback (PB); dosage varies with drug; given for a maximum of 5 days, followed by oral antibiotics	Antibiotic	Prophylaxis; treatment for infection

Independent

Teach every prenatal patient from the beginning to call the healthcare provider if ROM is suspected. If ROM occurs, monitor for signs and symptoms of infection and the onset of labor. Maintain the patient in the left lateral recumbent position as much as possible to provide optimal uteroplacental perfusion. Vaginal examinations should be held to an absolute minimum, and strict sterile technique should be used to avoid infection.

If the patient is discharged to home and undelivered, make sure the patient understands home healthcare guidelines and directions. The patient should maintain bedrest, check temperature four times per day, abstain from intercourse, not douche or use tampons, and have a white blood cell count drawn every other day. Tell the patient to notify the physician immediately of any fever, uterine tenderness or contractions, leakage of fluid, or foul vaginal odor.

Evidence-Based Practice and Health Policy

Kole-White, M., Neson, L., Lord, M., Has, P., Werner, E., Rouse, D., & Hardy, E. (2021). Pregnancy latency after preterm premature rupture of membranes: Oral versus intravenous antibiotics. *American Journal of Obstetrics & Gynecology.* Advance online publication. https://doi.org/10.1016/j.ajogmf.2021.100333

- The purpose of the study was to determine pregnancy latency after PROM following treatment with antibiotics. Prophylactic IV antibiotics have been shown to increase the time from ROM to delivery (termed latency in obstetrics). They used a retrospective historic control study comparing women with preterm premature rupture of membranes with two groups: oral only antibiotics ($n = 37$) and IV antibiotics for 48 hours followed by 5 days of oral antibiotics ($n = 79$).
- The groups had similar baseline characteristics with regard to gestational age, rate of rectovaginal colonization, and pregnancy latency. There was no significant difference in the relative risk of maternal infection or neonatal infection between the two groups. Oral antibiotic treatment had comparable outcomes to IV and oral antibiotic therapy and could be considered as an acceptable alternative for patients who would prefer to wait for labor onset at home.

DOCUMENTATION GUIDELINES

- Time of ROM, color of fluid, amount of fluid, presence of any odor
- Contractions: Frequency, duration, intensity, pattern, patient's response
- Fetal heart rate assessment: Baseline, accelerations, decelerations, variability
- Patient's comfort level in labor, response to medications, vital signs
- Signs and symptoms of infection: Elevated birthing parent heart rate and temperature; malodorous amniotic vaginal discharge/fluid; fetal tachycardia

DISCHARGE AND HOME HEALTHCARE GUIDELINES

HOME CARE IF DELIVERED. Teach the patient to be aware of signs and symptoms that indicate postpartum complications. Teach the patient not to lift anything heavier than the baby and not to drive until after the postpartum checkup with the physician.

Pressure Injury

DRG Category:	573
Mean LOS:	15.4 days
Description:	SURGICAL: Skin Graft for Skin Ulcer or Cellulitis With Major Complication or Comorbidity
DRG Category:	593
Mean LOS:	5.3 days
Description:	MEDICAL: Skin Ulcers With Complication or Comorbidity

Approximately 1 million pressure injuries (formerly *pressure ulcer*) occur each year in the United States, and the incidence of pressure injury in hospitalized patients ranges from 2% to 30%, with patients in the intensive care unit likely having a higher incidence. Experts estimate that 60,000 people die each year as a direct result of a pressure injury. The National Pressure Ulcer Advisory Panel recommends the term *pressure injury*, defined as localized damage to the skin and underlying soft tissue, usually over a bony prominence or related to a medical or other device.

A pressure injury is an irregularly shaped, depressed area that results from damage or necrosis of the epidermis and/or dermis layers of the skin. Pressure is exerted on the skin and soft tissue by the person's weight against the surface beneath. If the pressure exceeds capillary filling at approximately 32 mm Hg, inadequate circulation occurs with ischemic ulceration and tissue breakdown. Muscle tissue seems particularly susceptible to ischemia. Pressure injuries may occur in any area of the body but occur mostly over bony prominences that can include the occiput, thoracic and lumbar vertebrae, scapula, coccyx, sacrum, greater trochanter, ischial tuberosity, lateral knee, medial and lateral malleolus, metatarsals, and calcaneus. Some 96% of pressure injuries develop in the lower part of the body, with the hip and buttock region accounting for almost 70% of all pressure injuries.

Pressure injuries are the direct cause of death in 7% to 8% of all patients with paraplegia, and of those patients who develop pressure injuries in the hospital, more than half will die within a year. Complications include scarring, cellulitis, bone and joint infection, sepsis, septic shock, and death. Pressure injuries have been staged by the National Pressure Ulcer Advisory Panel (Table 1), but the stages serve as a description only and do not necessarily provide an order for progression.

• TABLE 1 Staging of Pressure Injuries

STAGE OF PRESSURE INJURY	DESCRIPTION
I: Pressure injury: Intact skin	Localized area of nonblanchable erythema; may look different in darkly pigmented skin; blanchable erythema or changes in sensation, temperature, or firmness may occur before visual changes; should not have purple or maroon discoloration
II: Pressure injury: Partial-thickness skin loss with exposed dermis	Wound bed is viable; pink or red; moist; may also be an intact or ruptured serum-filled blister; adipose and deeper tissues are not visible; granulation, slough, and eschar are not present
III: Pressure injury: Full-thickness skin loss	Adipose tissue is visible in the ulcer, and granulation tissue with or without rolled wound edges is often present; slough and/or eschar may be visible; depth of tissue damage varies by anatomical location; undermining and tunneling may occur
IV: Pressure injury: Full-thickness skin and tissue loss	Full-thickness skin and tissue loss with exposed or directly palpable fascia, muscle, tendon, ligament, cartilage, or bone in the ulcer; slough and/or eschar may be visible; rolled edges, undermining, and/or tunneling often occur; depth varies by anatomical location

CAUSES

The most important mechanism that causes pressure injury formation is unrelieved pressure, leading to tissue compression and prolonged ischemia. When external pressure exceeds normal capillary pressure of 32 mm Hg, blood flow in the capillary beds is decreased. When the external pressure surpasses arteriole pressure, blood flow to the area is impaired. Ischemia occurs when the pressure exceeds 50 mm Hg and blood flow is completely blocked. Pressure from the bony prominence is transmitted from the surface of the body to the underlying bone, and all underlying tissues are compressed.

Pressure injury caused by shearing or friction results when one tissue layer slides over another. Shearing results in stretching and angulating of blood vessels, causing injury and thrombosis to the area. Friction occurs when two surfaces move across one another, leading to tissue drag and injury. These injuries commonly occur when the head of the bed is elevated, causing the torso to slide downward, or when people are moved across bed sheets. Risks include immobility, malnutrition and alcohol dependence, tobacco use, dehydration, lack of sensory perception, diabetes, vascular disease, and corticosteroid use.

GENETIC CONSIDERATIONS

No clear genetic contributions to susceptibility have been defined.

SEX AND LIFE SPAN CONSIDERATIONS

Pressure injuries can occur at any age and in males and females but are more prevalent in the older population over age 70 years. Pressure injuries are also common in individuals who are neurologically impaired and immobile; most younger individuals suffering from pressure injury are males, which reflects the greater number of young men suffering traumatic spinal cord injuries.

HEALTH DISPARITIES AND SEXUAL/GENDER MINORITY HEALTH

There are no known racial and ethnic considerations, but patients with dark skin may have more severe pressure injury and a higher rate of complication than patients with light skin due to difficulty visualizing blanching and redness in early stage injury. Sexual and gender minority status has no known effect on the risk for pressure injury.

GLOBAL HEALTH CONSIDERATIONS

Pressure injury occurs around the globe and has a higher incidence in older people and people who are immobilized because of chronic conditions such as stroke or spinal cord injury. In developing countries where malnutrition is common, pressure injury is more common.

ASSESSMENT

HISTORY. Generally, patients have a history of a condition that causes decreased circulation and sensation leading to inadequate tissue perfusion. Establish a history of associated diseases and conditions, such as diabetes mellitus, arterial insufficiency, peripheral vascular disease, and decreased activity and mobility or spinal cord injury. Determine the name and dose of all medications and ask about dietary habits, weight loss, or weight gain. Assess the continence status of the patient. Ask about patterns of alcohol and drug use as well as tobacco use. Patients with casts, braces, and splints are also predisposed to developing pressure injury.

PHYSICAL EXAMINATION. The most common symptom is **an area of breakdown or lesion on the skin** resulting from unrelieved pressure. The clinical manifestations of pressure injury are generally described in four stages that reflect the amount of tissue injury and the degree of underlying structural damage. Assess the wound to determine the precise location, along with size and depth. The color of the wound (whether pink, red, yellow, or black) indicates the stage of healing and the presence of epithelial tissue. A beefy red color signifies the presence of granulation tissue and denotes adequate healing. Black tissue indicates necrotic and devitalized tissue and signifies delayed healing. Observe for areas of sinus tracts and undermining, which indicate deeper involvement under intact wound margins. Determine the amount of drainage and the type, color, odor, consistency, and quantity. Assess the area around the wound for redness, edema, indurations, tenderness, and breakdown of healed tissues to identify signs and symptoms of infection.

PSYCHOSOCIAL. The patient may exhibit signs of anxiety and depression because of the potential setback in an already long list of medical problems. The condition may slow the patient's progress toward independence or necessitate a move from home to a nursing home for an older patient.

Diagnostic Highlights

Test	Normal Result	Abnormality With Condition	Explanation
Skin or wound culture and sensitivity	Negative for microorganisms	Positive for microorganisms	Some pressure injuries become infected, which slows healing

Other Tests: Supporting tests include complete blood count, transferrin level, albumin and total protein levels, skin biopsy, blood culture, bone scan or x-ray if osteomyelitis is suspected.

PRIMARY NURSING DIAGNOSIS

DIAGNOSIS. Impaired skin integrity related to pressure over bony prominences or shearing forces as evidenced by firmness, color changes, blanchable erythema, and/or wound formation

OUTCOMES. Tissue integrity: Skin and mucous membranes; Wound healing: Primary intention; Immobility consequences: Physiological; Knowledge: Treatment regimen; Nutritional status; Tissue perfusion: Peripheral

INTERVENTIONS. Wound care; Skin surveillance; Positioning; Pressure injury care; Pressure injury prevention; Medication administration; Circulatory precautions; Infection control; Nutrition management

PLANNING AND IMPLEMENTATION

Collaborative

In the early stages, pressure injuries are best handled by nursing rather than medical interventions. Surgical intervention may be necessary to excise necrotic tissue in late stages of ulcer development. Skin grafts or musculocutaneous flaps may be indicated in very deep wounds in which healing is difficult or has been unsuccessful in completely covering the area. Drains may be inserted to prevent fluid buildup in the wound. The drains facilitate the removal of blood and bacteria from the wound that can increase the risk of infection. Cleaning solutions include normal saline solution (when there is no infection present); diluted povidone-iodine for bacteria, spores, fungi, and viruses; acetic acid (0.5%) for *Pseudomonas aeruginosa*; and sodium hypochlorite (2.5%) for cleansing and débridement.

Mechanical débridement by an enzymatic agent (collagenase [Santyl]) may be ordered. Other types of wound care dressings include hydrocolloid, hydrogels, calcium alginates, film dressings, and topical agents and solutions. The type of dressing depends on the depth of the wound and the amount of débridement of necrotic tissue or support of granulation tissue required. In general, the following guidelines are helpful in pressure injury management, although management may depend on the particular pressure injury and patient:

Stage I pressure injury requires no type of dressings; approximately 70% to 90% of pressure injuries heal with reduction of pressure.

Stage II pressure injury is treated with moist or occlusive dressings to maintain a moist, healing environment.

Stage III pressure injury requires débridement, usually with an enzymatic agent or wet-to-moist normal saline soak.

Stage IV pressure injury is treated like stage III ulcers or by surgical excision and grafting.

All wounds are assessed before treatment because all wounds are different, and similar treatments may not be successful for dissimilar wounds. Other therapies include supplementing the patient's nutrition, hyperbaric oxygen therapy for wounds that are deep and difficult to treat, and electrotherapy to deliver low-intensity direct current to wounds in attempts to assist the healing process.

Pharmacologic Highlights

Medication or Drug Class	Dosage	Description	Rationale
Hydrocolloids	No dosage; prepackaged wafers	Occlusive, adhesive wafers such as Duo-DERM (ConvaTec)	Provides a moist, occluded, and protective environment for shallow wounds with light exudates; may remain in place for 3–5 days; retains moisture, absorbs exudates, and causes auto-débridement
Hydrogels	No dosage; topical gel	Glycerin-based gel such as IntraSite	Gel promotes healing by rehydrating necrotic tissue, facilitating débridement, and absorbing exudates to maintain moist environment; retains moisture and causes auto-débridement

(highlight box continues on page 1004)

Pharmacologic Highlights (continued)

Medication or Drug Class	Dosage	Description	Rationale
Alginates	No dosage; prepackaged pads	Pads formed from brown seaweed; Kaltostat	Absorbent; used to treat deep wounds with heavy drainage
Adhesive films	No dosage; prepackaged pads	Plastic, self-adhering membrane; Tegaderm	Self-adhering but waterproof wafers that are permeable to oxygen and water vapor; appropriate for partial-thickness wounds; useful as secondary dressings for wounds treated with hydrocolloids or alginates; retains moisture and causes auto-débridement
Foams	No dosage; prepackaged	Sheets and fillers	Obliterates dead space in the ulcer; retains moisture, absorbs exudates, and causes auto-débridement

Experimental Treatments: Cytokine growth factors such as recombinant platelet–derived growth factors and basic fibroblast growth factors and skin equivalents

Independent

The most important nursing intervention is prevention. Identify patients who are at risk by using assessment tools such as the Braden scale or the Norton scale, which determine the sensory and physiological factors that increase the incidence of pressure injuries. The high-risk patient needs turning and proper positioning at least every 2 hours. Pressure-relieving devices, such as silicone-filled pads, or gel and foam mattresses, may be helpful. Dynamic devices include specialty beds (low air loss, air fluidized, and air cushions). Airflow pressure mattresses are also useful preventive strategies.

Keep the patient's skin dry. Patients who are incontinent of feces and urine should be cleaned as soon as possible to prevent skin irritation. When soiling of the skin cannot be controlled, use absorbent underpads and topical agents that act as moisture barriers. Avoid the use of hot water and use a mild cleansing agent to minimize dryness and irritation in high-risk patients. Treat dry skin with moisturizers, but use care in massaging bony prominences as this may impede capillary blood flow and increase the risk of deep tissue injury. Lift high-risk patients up in bed instead of pulling them, which increases the risk of shearing and friction forces on the skin's surfaces. To prevent the patient from sliding down in bed, do not elevate the patient's head more than 20 degrees unless this angle is contraindicated because of other medical problems or treatment modalities. Keep linens dry and wrinkle-free. When skin breakdown occurs, apply appropriate dressings using clean technique or, in cases in which infection is present, sterile technique.

Teach the caregiver preventive strategies and determine if the patient's situation is in jeopardy because of inadequate care. Note that the caregiver may have feelings of guilt because of the failure to prevent complications of immobility; the caregiver may need support rather than teaching, depending on the situation.

Evidence-Based Practice and Health Policy

Tschannen, D., & Anderson, C. (2020). The pressure injury predictive model: A framework for hospital-acquired pressure injuries. *Journal of Clinical Nursing, 29*, 1398–1421.

• The authors note that pressure injuries are a source of significant pain and delayed recovery for patients and cause substantial quality control and cost issues for hospitals. If current thinking about pressure injury risk is reevaluated to improve risk assessments, new nursing interventions may be created to reduce pressure injuries. The authors used Walker and Avant's (2005)

theory synthesis framework to examine the relevance of existing pressure injury models and determine how they align with the current literature.
- A synthesis of an extensive literature search culminated in a new pressure injury risk model. Gaps in previous models include lack of attention to the environment, contributing episode-of-care factors, and the dynamic nature of injury risk for patients. The authors identified the need for a new model and developed the Pressure Injury Predictive Model, a representation of the complex and dynamic nature of pressure injury risk that builds on previous models and addresses new patient, contextual, and episode-of-care process influences.

DOCUMENTATION GUIDELINES
- Physical findings of assessment for potential skin breakdown: Pressure injury stage, redness and dryness
- Physical findings of direct wound assessment: Size, depth, type of tissue present (granulation, necrotic), drainage; signs of infection
- Type and frequency of dressing changes with sequencing of how the wound was cleaned and the dressing applied
- Response to treatments: Surgery, wound débridement, dressing, medication application

DISCHARGE AND HOME HEALTHCARE GUIDELINES
Refer patients at increased risk for skin breakdown to a home healthcare agency to assist with monitoring skin and providing pressure-relieving devices in the home environment. Teach the patient or caregiver about frequent turning and positioning, how to keep the skin clean and dry, signs and symptoms of early breakdown and complications of existing pressure injuries, strategies to manage redness or skin breakdown, and appropriate wound care and dressing techniques. Use a return demonstration before discharge to assess the understanding and ability to perform wound care.

Preterm Labor

DRG Category:	807
Mean LOS:	2.2 days
Description:	MEDICAL: Vaginal Delivery Without Sterilization or Dilation & Curettage Without Complication or Comorbidity or Major Complication or Comorbidity
DRG Category:	818
Mean LOS:	4.0 days
Description:	MEDICAL: Other Antepartum Diagnoses With Operating Room Procedures With Complication or Comorbidity
DRG Category:	832
Mean LOS:	3.7 days
Description:	MEDICAL: Other Antepartum Diagnoses Without Operating Room Procedures With Complication or Comorbidity

Preterm labor (PTL) occurs after the completion of the 20th week and before the beginning of the 37th week of gestation. To be considered PTL, the uterine contractions must occur at a frequency of four in 20 minutes or eight in 60 minutes. Spontaneous rupture of the membranes often occurs in PTL. If the membranes are intact, documented cervical change (80% effacement or > 1 cm dilation) must be noted during a vaginal examination for the situation to be classified as PTL.

PTL has a poorly understood etiology, unclear mechanisms, and an absence of medical consensus related to diagnosis and treatment. This is unfortunate because preterm birth is the second-highest cause of the high infant morbidity and mortality rate in the United States (birth defects is the first). Preterm birth occurs in approximately 12% of pregnancies in the United States, and the risk of having a recurrent preterm birth after one, two, or three occurrences is 15%, 30%, and 45%, respectively. The major fetal risk of preterm delivery is related to immaturity of the lungs and respiratory system. Preterm infants can have many other problems as well, such as neurological complications, thermoregulation problems, and immaturity of major organ systems. Risks of PTL in the birthing parent are related to the pharmacologic treatment involved in stopping the labor.

CAUSES

In many cases, the cause cannot be identified. Preterm premature rupture of membranes occurs in about one-third of the cases, but its causes are also unknown. Intrauterine, genital tract, and/or periodontal infection can precede or follow premature rupture of membranes. Infectious processes that occur prior to and early in pregnancy are thought to be linked to PTL/rupture of membranes owing to the inflammatory response that weakens the fetal membranes. There is also evidence that an idiopathic, undiagnosed PTL leads to microbial invasion owing to a breakdown in the cervical barrier function, and this eventually manifests itself as chorioamnionitis and true clinical PTL.

Stress is known to be an important risk factor. Increased stress causes an increase in the release of corticotropin-releasing hormone (CRH) from the hypothalamus and adrenocorticotropic hormone (ACTH) from the pituitary gland, causing excessive cortisol secretion. Stress also suppresses the immune system and increases the production of cytokines. The combined hormonal and cytokine release related to stress is associated with prostaglandin secretion, relaxation of the uterus, and preterm birth (Mete & Ozbert, 2020). Several risk factors for PTL have been identified (Box 1).

• BOX 1   Risk Factors for PTL

HISTORICAL	OBSTETRIC RELATED
Preterm labor	Cervical incompetence
Preterm delivery	Placenta previa or abruption
Cone biopsy	Uterine distention (hydramnios, twins, large
Induced or habitual abortions	for gestational age [LGA] fetus)
Diethylstilbestrol exposure	Maternal infection (periodontal, genital
Uterine leiomyomas or cervical anomalies	tract, chorioamnionitis)
Renal disease	Abdominal surgery during pregnancy
Hypertension	Smoking, alcohol, drug use during pregnancy
Stress	
Prepregnancy weight < 100 lb	FETAL RELATED
	Multiple gestation
	Fetal anomalies

GENETIC CONSIDERATIONS

No clear genetic contributions to susceptibility have been defined.

SEX AND LIFE SPAN CONSIDERATIONS

Women who are younger than age 17 years or older than age 35 years are more likely to have PTL.

HEALTH DISPARITIES AND SEXUAL/GENDER MINORITY HEALTH

PTL is more prevalent in Black and Hispanic women than White women and is also associated with low socioeconomic status, low educational level, domestic violence, and single parenthood. There are significant health disparities with respect to the administration of antenatal corticosteroids before preterm birth. Black and Hispanic women receive lower rates of corticosteroid administration during 23 to 34 weeks of gestation for fetal lung maturation as compared to White women (Gulersen et al., 2020). Sexual and gender minority status has no known effect on the risk for PTL.

GLOBAL HEALTH CONSIDERATIONS

No data are available.

⬛ ASSESSMENT

HISTORY. Ask the date of the patient's last menstrual period to estimate delivery date. If the patient reports using cigarettes, alcohol, or other substances, determine the amount and frequency. Ask about the onset of contractions; their frequency, duration, and intensity; whether they are painful or painless; or whether the patient feels cramping and lower back pain or pelvic pressure or fullness. Sometimes false labor is felt in the lower abdomen and is irregular. Ask if the patient has bloody show. Determine if the patient has nausea, vomiting, diarrhea, discomfort, a sense of "just feeling bad," or a sensation that the baby is "balling up." Ask about presence and leakage of amniotic fluid and its character. Determine the history of any medical problems because some pharmacologic treatment may be contraindicated in certain instances (cardiac disease, hypertension, renal disease, uncontrolled diabetes, and asthma).

PHYSICAL EXAMINATION. The most common symptoms are **uterine contractions of sufficient frequency and intensity to cause progressive cervical dilation and effacement**. An initial examination is needed to help determine if the patient is in PTL or in false labor. Apply a fetal monitor to determine the frequency and duration of contractions. Palpate the fundus of the uterus; if the patient is having PTL, note uterine firmness. Obtain the fetal heart rate with an electronic fetal monitor, noting baseline, presence or absence of accelerations or decelerations, and variability (see Diagnostic Highlights for fetal fibronectin test). A sterile vaginal examination to determine dilation, station, and effacement can be performed after the fetal fibronectin test. Note any vaginal bleeding, bloody show, or leakage of amniotic fluid. Nitrazine (pH) paper can be used during the examination to detect if the membranes have ruptured (paper turns blue because pH is alkaline). Note that an elevated temperature indicates infection or dehydration.

PSYCHOSOCIAL. The reality of a premature delivery and an unstable newborn in a neonatal intensive care unit (NICU) creates a tremendous amount of stress and emotion for the parents and significant others. Assess the patient's and the significant others' abilities to cope. Patients may experience guilt, suspecting that they did something wrong during the pregnancy to precipitate the labor.

Diagnostic Highlights

General Comments: PTL is generally diagnosed by the presence of contractions accompanied by cervical change. Testing is done to examine the possibility of delivery and cervical ripeness.

(highlight box continues on page 1008)

Diagnostic Highlights (continued)

Test	Normal Result	Abnormality With Condition	Explanation
Fetal fibronectin (fFn) by vaginal swab	Absent in cervico-vaginal secretions between 20 and 37 wk	Positive; fFn is a protein produced by fetal cells found at the interface of the chorion and decidua; binds the fetal sac to uterine lining	Predicts likelihood of preterm birth; if positive, 60% will deliver within 1 wk; if negative, 99.3% will not deliver within 1 wk; fFn test should be done before a digital cervical examination or vaginal probe ultrasound because manipulation of cervix may cause release of fFn, yielding a false-positive test
Cervical length (via transvaginal ultrasound)	> 30 mm at 24 wk; no evidence of a bulging bag of water or leakage of fluid	< 25 mm (10th percentile) or evidence of funneling at 24 wk or leaking of the amniotic fluid at the internal os	Cervical effacement labor

Other Tests: Pregnancy test, abdominal ultrasound to assess the size and well-being of the infant, Doppler fetal heart tones, amniocentesis to obtain amniotic fluid to perform tests to determine fetal lung maturity (lecithin-to-sphingomyelin ratio, phosphatidyl-glycerol, surfactant-to-albumin ratio), complete blood count, vaginal/cervical/urine cultures (infections often precede PTL)

PRIMARY NURSING DIAGNOSIS

DIAGNOSIS. Fear related to uncertainty of outcome and complexity of treatments as evidenced by apprehension, restlessness, avoidance behavior, anxiety, and/or muscular tension

OUTCOMES. Fear level; Anxiety level; Comfort status; Coping; Knowledge: Labor & delivery

INTERVENTIONS. Anxiety reduction; Anticipatory guidance; Labor suppression; High-risk pregnancy care; Resuscitation: Neonate

PLANNING AND IMPLEMENTATION
Collaborative

The goals of treatment are to stop the contractions and to prevent the cervix from dilating, thereby avoiding delivery until at least 34 weeks. Once the cervix reaches 4 cm in dilation, treatment to stop contractions is ended, and the delivery is allowed to occur. Ideally, delivery is in a hospital with the expertise necessary to treat a preterm neonate.

Although they are the first strategies often employed to halt PTL, bedrest, hydration, and sedation are not supported in the literature as effective means of stopping PTL. IV fluids, usually a crystalloid such as lactated Ringer solution and a sedative if the patient is anxious, are used. Magnesium sulfate, indomethacin, and nifedipine are the first-line medications used to stop PTL. If the contractions stop and the labor is not progressing, patients are discharged home on complete bedrest. Home monitoring of uterine contractions with transmission of data to the physician is possible.

If labor continues, IV medications are indicated. Tocolysis (inhibition of uterine contractions) is contraindicated in cases of maternal infection, pregnancy-induced hypertension, hypovolemia, and fetal distress. During the initial period of infusion of tocolytic drugs, auscultate the patient's lungs for rales and rhonchi; observe for dyspnea and chest discomfort; determine the fetal heart rate, maternal pulse, blood pressure, and respiratory rate; and monitor the status of contractions every 10 minutes. Fluid restriction, accurate monitoring of intake and output, and daily weights are indicated to monitor fluid balance.

Administer glucocorticoids concurrently with tocolytics. The incidence of respiratory distress is lower if the birth is delayed for at least 24 hours after the initiation of glucocorticoids. The effect on the lung maturity persists for 1 week after the therapy is completed. If glucocorticoids are administered concurrently, monitor the patient for signs and symptoms of pulmonary edema. If magnesium sulfate is used for tocolysis, closely monitor deep tendon reflexes; hyporeflexia occurs if the patient is becoming toxic and precedes respiratory depression. If tocolysis is successful and contractions are under control, the infusion is discontinued by gradually decreasing the rate and converting to oral administration.

Monitor the fetal heart rate variability and for the absence or presence of accelerations and decelerations. If signs of fetal stress occur, turn the patient on the left side, increase the rate of the IV hydration, administer oxygen at 10 L/minute per mask, and notify the physician. Delivery of the preterm infant can be done vaginally or by cesarean. The decision for the method of delivery is often made jointly by the physician, neonatologist, and parents. If the fetus is very premature, often the neonatologist suggests a cesarean to prevent trauma to the fetal head and an increased risk of intraventricular hemorrhage.

Pharmacologic Highlights

Medication or Drug Class	Dosage	Description	Rationale
Nifedipine	20 mg loading dose, 20 mg every 3–8 hr for 48–72 hr	Calcium channel blocker; tocolytic	Inhibits contraction of smooth muscles by reducing intracellular calcium influx
Indomethacin	100 mg PR, then 50 mg PO every 6 hr for eight doses	Prostaglandin synthetase inhibitor; tocolytic (labor repression)	Reduces prostaglandin synthesis and decreases inflammation
Magnesium sulfate (contraindicated in myasthenia gravis): Note: This is off-label use	4–6 g IV loading dose, 1–4 g/hr of IV maintenance	Central nervous system depressant; tocolytic	Decreases contraction of smooth muscles by reducing intracellular calcium influx; some controversy about its effectiveness
Betamethasone (Celestone)	12 mg IM every 24 hr × 2	Glucocorticoid	Hastens fetal lung maturity; indicated if delivery is anticipated between 24 and 34 wk

Independent

Prevention of PTL is an important function of the nurse. During the initial prenatal visit, educate the patient on the signs and symptoms of PTL and on subsequent visits ask if the patient is experiencing any of these indicators. If a patient reports alcohol, cigarette, or drug use any time during the pregnancy, work with the patient to modify behavior. A referral to a drug-treatment, smoking-cessation, or alcohol counseling program may be indicated. Encourage patients to stay well hydrated, especially during the warm weather, because dehydration can cause contractions. In addition, nurses can become involved in community education of pregnant people about the symptoms, risk factors, and consequences of PTL.

Admission to the hospital for PTL is often a first hospitalization for many young patients. Provide emotional support and educate the patient on simple procedures that may seem routine (drawing laboratory work, frequent assessments done by nurses and physicians, mealtimes and menus). Discuss the implications and expectations of preterm delivery. Be realistic in the discussions, and if possible, arrange for a visit to the neonatal intensive care unit and a talk with the neonatologist. Include the family in conversations with the patient and encourage them to assist with caring for the patient while the patient is on bedrest. Often, the patient is on bedrest for several days in the hospital and at home. While the patient is in the hospital, suggest diversional activities, such as videos, special visitors, and games. Encourage the pregnant person to lie on the side to increase placental perfusion and reduce pressure on the cervix.

Evidence-Based Practice and Health Policy

Mete, S., & Oxberk, H. (2020). Relaxation-focused nursing care in threatened preterm birth: Can it be a complementary treatment? *International Journal of Caring Sciences, 13*, 2110–2122.

* In this study, the authors developed a program for pregnant women at high risk for preterm labor to promote relaxation and reduce stress. The authors presented a conceptual model demonstrating the links between physiology, stress, and uterine contractions. The program was composed of initiating positive communication and creating a safe environment, teaching deep relaxation in a calm environment with identification of stressors, visualization, endorphin massage, breathing exercises, and positive self-talk.
* The authors presented the program over 16 hours for women who were pregnant and had threatened preterm birth. The authors noted that patients report that practicing the relaxation techniques reduced stress, and the durations of the patients' pregnancies were extended.

DOCUMENTATION GUIDELINES

* Contraction status: Frequency, intensity, duration
* Fetal heart rate: Baseline, variability, accelerations, decelerations
* Patient's response to bedrest and hydration
* Patient's response to tocolysis: Vital signs, anxiety, ability to sleep, deep tendon reflexes, lung sounds, intake and output

DISCHARGE AND HOME HEALTHCARE GUIDELINES

HOME CARE IF UNDELIVERED. Discuss the importance of maintaining bedrest in the lateral position. Teach the patient to remain well hydrated, take all medications exactly as prescribed, and report any uncomfortable side effects to the physician. Teach the patient to avoid any activity that could possibly initiate labor (sexual intercourse, nipple stimulation). Explain that the patient should check daily to determine whether the fetus is moving or the uterus is contracting. Review the warning signs of PTL and when the patient should call the physician.

HOME CARE IF DELIVERED. Teach the patient to be aware of signs and symptoms that indicate postpartum complications: a hard, reddened area on the breast; pain in the calf of the leg; increase in bleeding; foul odor to vaginal discharge; fever; burning with urination; or persistent mood change. Teach the patient not to lift anything heavier than the baby and not to drive a car until after the postpartum checkup with the physician. Encourage the patient to maintain a healthy diet and adequate nutrition and to schedule rest time around the baby's sleeping times. Elicit the help of family members if needed.

Prostate Cancer

DRG Category:	713
Mean LOS:	4.0 days
Description:	SURGICAL: Transurethral Prostatectomy With Complication or Comorbidity or Major Complication or Comorbidity
DRG Category:	715
Mean LOS:	6.2 days
Description:	MEDICAL: Other Male Reproductive System Operating Room Procedures for Malignancy With Complication or Comorbidity or Major Complication or Comorbidity

Other than skin cancer, prostate cancer is the most common type of cancer in men and the second leading cause of death after lung cancer among men in the United States. The American Cancer Society (ACS) estimates that in 2021, there will be 248,530 new cases of prostate cancer and approximately 34,130 deaths from the disease. Overall, 1 in 8 men is diagnosed with prostate cancer and 1 in 41 dies from this disease. According to the ACS, the 5-year survival rate with all stages combined is 98%. Prostate cancer may begin with a condition called *prostatic intraepithelial neoplasia* (PIN), which can develop in men in their 20s. In this condition, there are microscopic changes in the size and shape of the prostate gland cells. The more abnormal the cells look, the more likely that cancer is present. It has been noted that 50% of men have PIN by the time they are age 50 years.

Adenocarcinomas compose 90% of the prostate cancers. They most frequently begin in the outer portion of the posterior lobe in the glandular cells of the prostate gland. Local spread occurs to the seminal vesicles, bladder, and peritoneum. The cancer develops when the rates of prostate cell division increase when compared to cell death, leading to uncontrolled tumor growth. Further genetic mutation occurs, and the tumors progress and ultimately metastasize. Prostate cancer metastasizes to other sites via the hematologic and lymphatic systems, following a fairly predictable pattern. The pelvic and perivesicular lymph nodes and bones of the pelvis, sacrum, and lumbar spine are usually the first areas to be affected. Metastasis to other organs usually occurs late in the course of the disease, with the lungs, liver, and kidneys being most frequently involved. Other complications include incontinence and erectile dysfunction.

The ACS in 2016 made the following recommendations for prostate cancer screening: Men should be screened if they so choose after they receive information about the uncertainties, risks, and benefits of prostate cancer screening. This discussion should occur at the following time points: age 50 years for men with average risk, age 45 years for men at high risk (African American men, men with a first-degree relative diagnosed with prostate cancer before the age of 65 years), and age 40 years for men with a first-degree relative who had prostate cancer at an early age. Screening should include the prostate-specific antigen (PSA) and digital rectal examination.

CAUSES

The cause of prostate cancer remains unclear, but age, viruses, family history, diet, and androgens are thought to have contributing roles. A high-fat diet may alter the production of sex hormones and growth factors, increasing the risk of prostate cancer. Environmental exposure to cadmium (an element found in cigarettes and alkaline batteries) is also considered a risk factor. Other possible risks that have sometimes been supported by research include cigarette smoking, exposure to Agent Orange (used during the Vietnam War), obesity, and prostatitis.

GENETIC CONSIDERATIONS

Prostate cancer has one of the most significant heritable components of any cancer (heritability of ~38%–57%). The risk of developing prostate cancer is approximately 40% higher in men with three or more affected relatives. There are now almost 100 loci that are associated with susceptibility to prostate cancer. Several of these include *BRCA1, BRCA2, ATM, CHEK2, RNASEL, MXI1, KAI1, PCAP, HOXB13*, and *MED12*. Ongoing studies are needed to identify the most significant drivers of prostate cancer risk.

SEX AND LIFE SPAN CONSIDERATIONS

The incidence of prostate cancer increases as men age, but it can occur even in the teenage years. The peak incidence of prostate cancer is in men between ages 65 and 75 years; 85% of the cases are diagnosed in men over age 65 years. Prostate cancer is rare in men under age 40 years, but when the disease occurs in younger men, it is generally more aggressive.

HEALTH DISPARITIES AND SEXUAL/GENDER MINORITY HEALTH

One in seven Black men will develop prostate cancer in his lifetime. The highest incidence of prostate cancer among all groups occurs in Black men, who also have it diagnosed at a later stage than other groups. Prostate cancer mortality is twofold higher in Black persons as compared to White persons. Scientists suggest that these differences occur because of racial bias; Black men are less likely than White men to be offered a PSA testing and may not receive adequate treatment for early-stage disease. Persons of Asian and Native American ancestry have the lowest rate. Sexual and gender minority persons have higher odds for multiple chronic conditions, cancer, and poor quality of life and are more apt to have disabilities than cisgender males and females. (Cisgender is a term used to describe persons whose gender identity and gender expression are aligned with their assigned sex listed on their birth certificate.) Transgender is a term used to describe persons whose gender identity is different from their sex assigned at birth. Approximately 1% of the U.S. population identify themselves as transgender. Cancer disparities are perpetuated because sexual and gender minority persons receive poor quality of care due to stigma, lack of healthcare providers' awareness, and insensitivity to the unique needs of this community. Transgender women may delay or avoid having symptoms of prostate cancer evaluated because of discrimination based on gender identity or the emotional conflict between self-perception and physical anatomy (Cacerese, Jackman, et al., 2020; Connelly et al., 2019).

GLOBAL HEALTH CONSIDERATIONS

Worldwide, Black and Caribbean men of African descent have the highest incidences of prostate cancer. Prostate cancer occurs in the countries with the highest socioeconomic levels, with the highest rates in North America, Western Europe, and Australia and the lowest rates in Africa, South and Central America, and Asia.

ASSESSMENT

HISTORY. The majority of prostate cancer is identified not by symptoms but by prostate cancer screening. Most people are asymptomatic at the time of diagnosis. Ask about family history of prostate cancer, an occupational exposure to cadmium, and the usual urinary pattern. A patient may report symptoms such as urinary urgency, frequency, nocturia, dysuria, urinary retention, slow urinary stream, impotence, back pain, or hematuria if the disease has spread beyond the periphery of the prostate gland or if benign prostatic hypertrophy is also present. Presenting symptoms of late-stage disease include weight loss, back pain, anemia, bone pain, overdistended bladder, and shortness of breath, which are indicative of advanced or metastatic disease.

PHYSICAL EXAMINATION. Most men with early-stage prostate cancer are asymptomatic. When symptoms occur, they include **urinary complaints (retention, urgency, frequency, nocturia, dysuria, hematuria)** and **back pain**. The physician palpates the prostate gland via a digital rectal examination (DRE). A normal prostate gland feels soft, smooth, and rubbery. Early-stage prostate cancer may present as a nonraised, firm lesion with a sharp edge, or be asymmetric or boggy. An advanced lesion is often hard and stonelike with irregular borders. A suspicious prostatic mass is further evaluated by extending the examination to the groin to look for the presence of enlarged or tender lymph nodes.

PSYCHOSOCIAL. Men have reported not having a rectal examination because of embarrassment. In addition, treatment for prostate cancer can be accompanied by distressful side effects, such as sexual dysfunction and urinary incontinence. Assess the patient's knowledge and feelings related to these issues and the presence of support systems. Note the coping strategies the patient has used in the past to manage stressors. Include the patient's spouse or significant other in conversations.

Diagnostic Highlights

General Comments: Positive findings during the DRE and an elevated PSA suggest the diagnosis. Other tests may be needed to confirm and determine metastasis.

Test	Normal Result	Abnormality With Condition	Explanation
PSA	< 4 ng/mL	Increased levels, > 10 ng/mL; a small proportion of men will have cancer even with levels as low as 1 ng/mL	The higher the level, the greater the tumor burden; can be used to monitor response to treatment or recurrent cancer
Transrectal ultrasound	Prostate gland is of normal size, contour, and consistency	Enlarged, solid prostate mass is noted	Used to direct the biopsy procedure; not helpful as a screening tool
Biopsy	Benign	Malignant	Confirms the diagnosis

Other Tests: Computed tomography scan of the abdomen and pelvis, magnetic resonance imaging, lymphangiogram, IV pyelogram, chest x-ray, bone scan, laparoscopic pelvic lymphadenectomy, serum reverse transcriptase–polymerase chain reaction, acid phosphatase level

PRIMARY NURSING DIAGNOSIS

DIAGNOSIS. Chronic pain related to metastatic spread of disease as evidenced by gait disturbances, self-reports of pain, facial grimacing, and/or protective behavior

OUTCOMES. Comfort status; Pain control; Pain level; Symptom severity; Symptom control; Knowledge: Pain management; Knowledge: Medication

INTERVENTIONS. Analgesic administration; Pain management: Chronic; Medication administration; Transcutaneous electric nerve stimulation (TENS); Patient-controlled analgesia assistance

✸ PLANNING AND IMPLEMENTATION
Collaborative

Treatment is determined in consultation with the patient. It depends on the overall life expectancy (How old is the patient? Does the patient have other diseases that will shorten the life span?) and the nature of the tumor. It also is determined by the patient's wishes and concerns about the permanent lifestyle changes that can occur as a result of some of the treatments. The steps of treatment include active surveillance, watchful waiting, radical prostatectomy, and radiation therapy.

CONSERVATIVE. The goal of active surveillance is to protect quality of life during the early management of prostate cancer by delaying invasive therapy. The healthcare team closely monitors the disease, sometimes for years, with the potential of avoiding radical treatment. Periodic observation, or "watchful waiting," may be proposed to a patient with early-stage, less-aggressive prostate cancer. With this option, no specific treatment is given, but the progression of the disease is monitored via periodic diagnostic tests. Large-scale clinical trials show that men who opt for conservative treatment have a slightly higher risk for death and significantly higher rate of metastasis than those who have a radical prostatectomy. Note that patients who ingest diets high in omega-3 fatty acids and low in glycemic index as well as weight loss may have slowed tumor growth and improved prognosis.

SURGICAL. New surgical treatments have changed prostate cancer care quite a bit. Nerve-sparing techniques, laparoscopic procedures, robotically assisted procedures, and more traditional procedures such as retropubic prostatectomy and perineal prostatectomy are all potential avenues for treatment. Radical prostatectomy has been the recommended treatment option for patients with middle-stage disease because of high cure rates. This procedure removes the entire prostate gland, including the prostatic capsule, the seminal vesicles, and a portion of the bladder neck. Two common side effects of prostatectomy are urinary incontinence and impotence. The urinary incontinence usually resolves with time and after performing Kegel exercises, although 10% to 15% of patients continue to experience incontinence 6 months after surgery. Impotence occurs in 85% to 90% of patients. All patients who undergo radical prostatectomy lack emission and ejaculation because of the removal of the seminal vesicles and transection of the vas deferens. A newer surgical technique (nerve-sparing prostatectomy) preserves continence in most patients and erectile function in selected cases. Cryosurgery (cryoablation of the prostate) with liquid nitrogen is less invasive and may be associated with fewer long-term consequences (impotence and incontinence). Both techniques are under study for their long-term outcomes. Other options for localized prostate cancer are radiation therapy, active surveillance, and androgen deprivation therapy.

Transurethral resection of the prostate (TURP) may be recommended for patients with more advanced disease, especially if it is accompanied by symptoms of bladder outlet obstruction. This procedure is not a curative surgical technique for prostate cancer but does remove excess prostatic tissue that is obstructing the flow of urine through the urethra. The incidence of impotence following TURP is rare, although retrograde ejaculation (passage of seminal fluid back into the bladder) almost always occurs because of the destruction of the internal bladder sphincter during the procedure. Many patients equate ejaculation with normal sexual functioning, and to some, the loss of the ejaculatory sensation may be confused with the loss of sexual interest or potency. Also, a bilateral orchiectomy may be done to eliminate the source of the androgens since 85% of prostatic cancer is related to androgens.

Patients return from surgery with a large-lumen, three-way Foley catheter. The large lumen of the catheter and the large volume in the balloon (30 mL) help splint the urethral anastomosis and maintain hemostasis. Blood-tinged urine is common for several days after surgery, but dark red urine may indicate hemorrhage. If continuous urinary drainage is used, maintain the flow rate to keep the urine light pink to yellow in color and free from clots, but avoid overdistention of the bladder.

Antispasmodics may be ordered for bladder spasms. Anticholinergic and antispasmodic drugs may also be prescribed to help relieve urinary incontinence after the Foley catheter is removed. Because of the close proximity of the rectum and the operative site, trauma to the rectum should be avoided as a means of preventing hemorrhage. Stool softeners and a low-residue diet are usually ordered to limit straining with a bowel movement. Rectal tubes, enemas, and rectal thermometers should not be used.

RADIATION THERAPY. Multiple forms of radiation therapy are used, including conventional radiation therapy, three-dimensional conformal radiation therapy, intensity-modulated radiation therapy, proton beam radiation, and stereotactically guided radiation. Radiation therapy is also used in areas of bone metastasis. The goal in extensive disease is palliation: reduce the size of the prostate gland and relieve bone pain. Brachytherapy involving the permanent (iodine-125 or gold-198) or temporary (iridium-192) placement of radioactive isotopes can be used alone or in combination with external radiation therapy.

Patients who receive permanently placed radioisotopes are hospitalized for as long as the radiation source is considered a danger to persons around them. The principles of time, distance, and shielding need to be implemented. Care needs to be exerted so that the radioisotope does not become dislodged. Dressings and bed linens need to be checked by the radiation therapy department before these items are removed from the patient's room.

HORMONAL THERAPY. Medication choices for hormone therapy include gonadotropic-releasing hormone (GnRH) agonists, luteinizing hormone-releasing hormone analogues (LHRH), or antagonists and antiandrogens.

Pharmacologic Highlights

Medication or Drug Class	Dosage	Description	Rationale
Acetaminophen/ NSAIDs, opioids, combination opioids/ NSAIDs	Varies by drug	Analgesic	Analgesic is determined by severity of pain; pain may be postoperative or caused by metastasis
Antimicrotubular antineoplastics	Varied by drug	Docetaxel, cabazitaxel	Improves survival in patients with metastatic disease
GnRH agonists	Depends on stage of cancer and treatment combination; given every mo or every 3, 4, 6, or 12 mo	Antineoplastic hormonal agent; leuprolide, triptorelin, goserelin	Provides medical castration ultimately by decreasing testosterone levels; blocks the action/secretion of androgens that stimulate tumor growth (causes temporary tissue flare)
Antineoplastic, hormonal agent; antiandrogen	Varies by drug	Flutamide (Eulexin), nilutamide (Nilandron), bicalutamide (Casodex), abiraterone	Blocks androgens; often given with other similar agents

Other Drugs: Leuprolide and triptorelin are antineoplastic agents used for advanced disease. Finasteride (Proscar), an androgen hormone inhibitor currently being used to treat benign prostatic hyperplasia, may reduce the risk of developing prostate cancer by 25%. Ketoconazole is an adrenal androgen synthesis inhibitor. Zoledronic acid is a bisphosphonate used to treat bone metastases.

Independent

Dispel misconceptions and explain all diagnostic procedures. Patients with early-stage disease need support while they make decisions about the many treatment options. Encourage the patient and partner to verbalize their feelings and fears. Clarify the differences between the various treatment options and reinforce the treatment goals. Support the patient's treatment decisions; the number of options, tied to specific patient lifestyle outcomes, necessitates an individual plan of care for the patient and family or partner. Provide written materials, such as *Facts on Prostate Cancer* published by the ACS or *What You Need to Know About Prostate Cancer* published by the National Cancer Institute (NCI). Suggest that the patient write down questions that arise so they are not forgotten during visits with the physician.

Ask about pain regularly and assess pain systematically. Believe the patient and family in their reports of pain. Inform the patient and family of options for pain relief as proposed by the NCI (pharmacologic, physical, psychosocial, and cognitive-behavioral interventions), and involve the patient and family in determining pain relief measures.

If the patient has surgery, implement postoperative strategies to decrease complications. Patients are usually able to ambulate on the first day after surgery. Help the patient to get out of bed and walk in the halls to the patient's tolerance level, usually three or four times a day. Once nausea has passed, bowel sounds are present, and fluids are allowed, encourage a fluid intake of 2,500 to 3,000 mL/day to maintain good urine output. Adequate fluid intake, and thus output, minimizes the formation of blood clots in the urinary bladder that can obstruct the Foley catheter.

Be alert for behavior indicating denial, grief, hostility, or depression. Inform the physician of any ineffective coping behaviors and the patient's need for more information or a referral for counseling. Postoperative incontinence and impotence may be difficult for patients to discuss. Inform patients of exercises, medications, and products that can assist with incontinence. Suggest alternative sexual behaviors, such as touching and caressing. Patients who are undergoing orchiectomy need extensive emotional support. Establish a therapeutic relationship to promote the expression of feelings. Be sensitive to the patient's fear of loss of masculinity. Reinforce that having the testes removed in adulthood does not affect the ability to have an erection and orgasm.

During hospitalization for insertion of a radioactive implant, in-person interactions with family and healthcare staff will occur during a short period of time to limit their radiation exposure. Shortened personal interactions may be disturbing to patients. Attempt to relieve feelings of abandonment and isolation by communicating with the patient via the hospital intercom system. Once the temporary implant has been removed or the permanent radioactive substance has decayed, remind the patient that they are no longer a danger to others.

Evidence-Based Practice and Health Policy

Carlsson, S., & Vickers, A. (2020). Screening for prostate cancer. *Medical Clinics of North America, 104,* 1051–1062.

- The authors note that PSA screening can reduce the risk of metastatic prostate cancer and death from the disease. However, it is also associated with major harms, including overdiagnosis and overtreatment, with accompanying urinary, sexual, and bowel dysfunction. They suggest seven steps that will reduce the harms of PSA screening while still preserving its benefits.
- (1) Get consent for prostate cancer screening. (2) PSA screening is only for healthy men ages 45 to 70 years. (3) Tailor screening frequency based on PSA level and cease screening of men older than 60 years unless the PSA is higher than the median. (4) For men with elevated PSA, repeat the PSA. (5) Use secondary test, such as marker or imaging, before biopsy or only refer to urologists who do so. (6) Only refer to urologists who recommend active surveillance

to almost all patients with low-grade cancer. (7) Refer to urologists at major academic centers. The authors concluded that primary care physicians need to develop relationships with urologists who advocate conservative approaches to biopsy and treatment.

DOCUMENTATION GUIDELINES

- Description of all dressings, wounds, drainage collection devices, and urinary output; location, color, and amount of drainage; appearance of incision; color and amount of urine; presence of clots in the urine; urinary pattern after catheter removal
- Physical findings related to the pulmonary assessment, abdominal assessment, presence of edema, condition of extremities, bowel patterns, presence of complications (hemorrhage, infection, pulmonary congestion, activity intolerance, unrelieved discomfort, blockage of Foley catheter)
- Urinary pattern following removal of Foley catheter
- Response to potential for alteration in sexual function
- Description of the skin in the radiation field or site of insertion of radiation implant

DISCHARGE AND HOME HEALTHCARE GUIDELINES

TEACHING. Provide the following instructions to patients who have undergone a radical prostatectomy:

- Perform Kegel exercises to enhance sphincter control after the Foley catheter is removed. Establish a voiding pattern of every 2 hours during the day and every 4 hours during the night. With each voiding, contract the pelvic muscles to start and stop urinary flow several times. Contract the pelvic floor muscles and the muscle around the anus as though to stop a bowel movement 10 to 20 times, four times each day.
- Maintain an oral fluid intake of 2,000 to 3,000 mL/day. Avoid alcoholic and caffeinated beverages.
- Eat high-fiber foods and take stool softeners to prevent constipation. Avoid straining with bowel movements and do not use suppositories and enemas.
- Avoid strenuous exercise, heavy lifting, and driving an automobile until the physician allows.
- Avoid sitting with the legs in a dependent position for 3 to 4 weeks and avoid sexual intercourse for 6 weeks.

CARE OF SKIN IN EXTERNAL RADIATION FIELDS. Instruct the patient to do the following:

- Wash the skin gently with mild soap, rinse with warm water, and pat dry daily.
- Leave (not wash off) the dark ink markings that outline the radiation field.
- Avoid applying any lotions, perfumes, deodorants, or powder to the treatment area.
- Wear soft, nonrestrictive cotton clothing directly over the treatment area.
- Protect the skin from sunlight and extreme cold.

CARE AFTER THE INSERTION OF A PERMANENT RADIOISOTOPE. Instruct the patient to observe for lost seeds in bed linens. Teach the patient to use tweezers to place lost seeds in aluminum foil, wrap them tightly, and take them to the radiation oncology department at the hospital. Teach the patient to call the physician if the patient experiences a temperature over 100°F (37.8°C), burning or difficulty with urination, excessive bleeding or clots in urine, or rectal bleeding.

FOLLOW-UP CARE. Teach the patient when to see the physician for follow-up care and to watch for any sign of recurrent disease.

Prostatitis

DRG Category:	713
Mean LOS:	4.0 days
Description:	SURGICAL: Transurethral Prostatectomy With Complication or Comorbidity or Major Complication or Comorbidity
DRG Category:	728
Mean LOS:	3.6 days
Description:	MEDICAL: Inflammation of the Male Reproductive System Without Major Complication or Comorbidity

Prostatitis, an inflammation of the prostate gland, is classified in four categories. Acute bacterial prostatitis is an acute, usually gram-negative, bacterial infection of the prostate gland, generally occurring in conjunction with acute bacterial cystitis. Chronic bacterial prostatitis is a subclinical chronic infection of the prostate by bacteria that can be localized in prostatic secretions and is the most common recurrent urinary tract infection (UTI) in men. Chronic prostatitis/chronic pelvic pain syndrome (CPPS) occurs in the absence of a UTI and in the presence of urological pain and can be inflammatory or noninflammatory. Asymptomatic inflammatory prostatitis occurs when the prostate becomes inflamed but no genitourinary symptoms occur. Generally, this condition is diagnosed during examinations for infertility or an elevated prostate-specific antigen (PSA) level.

Prostatitis leads to approximately 2 million outpatient visits each year. CPPS is the most common category diagnosed and accounts for more than 90% of cases of prostatitis. Approximately 8% of men have prostatitis at some point in their lives. The most common complication of prostatitis is a UTI. If it is left untreated, a UTI can progress to complications such as prostatic edema, urinary retention, pyelonephritis, epididymitis, erectile dysfunction, prostatic abscess, and sepsis.

CAUSES

Both acute and chronic prostatitis can result from the ascent of bacteria in the urethra, the reflux of infected urine, or the spread of bacteria from the rectum via the lymph nodes. Instrumentation (the process of spreading infection during procedures such as cystoscopy or urinary catheterization) is a less common cause. Prostatitis can also occur from sexual intercourse. Gram-negative bacteria such as *Escherichia coli* and *Enterobacter* cause approximately 80% of bacterial prostatitis. In younger patients, *Neisseria gonorrhoeae* and *Chlamydia trachomatis* infections may occur. Risk factors for prostatitis include a recent UTI, use of a urinary catheter, urological procedures, sexually transmitted infections, unprotected anal and vaginal intercourse, and immune suppression.

GENETIC CONSIDERATIONS

Heritable inflammatory and immune responses could be protective or could increase susceptibility.

SEX AND LIFE SPAN CONSIDERATIONS

In older men, acute bacterial prostatitis occurs because of the enlargement of the prostate gland with age. Acute bacterial prostatitis should also be considered as a source of infection in all men with fever of unknown origin. Chronic prostatitis affects up to 35% of all men over age 50 years but is not necessarily associated with infection. Prostatitis occurs in younger men who are immunocompromised.

HEALTH DISPARITIES AND SEXUAL/GENDER MINORITY HEALTH

Bacterial prostatitis or abscesses are more prevalent in people with HIV-related diseases than in other individuals. Black and Hispanic people bear a disproportionate burden of HIV disease compared with other populations and are at risk for prostatitis. Acute bacterial prostatitis occurs more frequently in men age 35 years and younger, in part because of the HIV disease prevalence in younger men. The Centers for Disease Control and Prevention (CDC) reported in 2018 that 69% of new HIV diagnoses in the United States were in gay and bisexual men. In young people ages 13 to 24 years, gay and bisexual men account for 83% of all new HIV diagnoses. Therefore, gay and bisexual men are the group that is most at risk for prostatitis because people with HIV disease are immunosuppressed.

GLOBAL HEALTH CONSIDERATIONS

The incidence of mycobacterial (tuberculosis) prostatitis is increasing in developing regions, particularly in conjunction with HIV-related diseases. In developing regions with widespread sexually transmitted infections and large numbers of sex workers, the incidence of acute bacterial prostatitis is higher than in other regions of the world.

ASSESSMENT

HISTORY. Take a careful history to elicit genitourinary symptoms and a list of all recent urinary procedures such as catheterization or urological procedures. Generally, patients with suspected acute bacterial prostatitis have symptoms similar to those of a UTI: dysuria, frequency, urgency, and nocturia. In addition, patients report perineal pain radiating down to the sacral region of the back, down the penis and suprapubic area, and possibly into the rectal area. Hematuria or a purulent urethral discharge may be present. The patient may also complain of fever, chills, myalgia (muscle aches), arthralgia (painful joints), and malaise. Patients with chronic bacterial prostatitis are usually asymptomatic but complain of chronic cystitis. Take a sexual history to determine usual practices and also birth control strategies or condom use. Ask if the patient has ejaculatory pain or erectile dysfunction. Determine if the patient has a history of conditions that can lead to immunosuppression, such as HIV disease.

PHYSICAL EXAMINATION. Although some patients are asymptomatic, the patient may appear acutely ill with **fever, chills, muscle and joint ache, weakness**, and **malaise**. Patients may complain of perineal pain and urinary symptoms such as **frequency, urgency, dysuria, nocturia, hesitance**, and **retention**. Inspect the urethra for redness, swelling, or discharge. Inspect the urine for cloudiness, purulence, or hematuria. The practitioner palpates the prostate rectally to determine the degree of tenderness and consistency of the gland and to rule out the presence of a perirectal abscess, tumor, or foreign body. In acute bacterial prostatitis, the prostate may feel warm, firm, indurated, swollen, and tender to palpation. In chronic prostatitis, the prostate may be normal or feel boggy or indurated. Prostatic massage should not be performed because of the risk of bacteremia. Patients with chronic bacterial prostatitis have varying symptoms, often symptoms similar to those of acute bacterial prostatitis but milder. They may have dysuria, pelvic pain, ejaculatory pain, and erectile dysfunction.

PSYCHOSOCIAL. Discuss the patient's fear of sexually transmitted disease and impotence related to this illness. Assess the patient's ability to cope with a painful, prolonged illness with a high probability of recurrence or chronicity. If the patient has chronic bacterial prostatitis, assess the patient's and partner's coping strategies and support systems. Conditions that interfere with sexual functioning can be very anxiety-producing.

Diagnostic Highlights

General Comments: Prostatitis is primarily diagnosed by symptoms; however, a urine culture will confirm the diagnosis and identify the causative organism. Although prostatic massage is not recommended to obtain prostatic fluid, if this is done and leukocytes are present with a negative culture, a diagnosis of nonbacterial prostatitis can be made.

Test	Normal Result	Abnormality With Condition	Explanation
Urine culture	Negative findings	Positive for bacteria growth, > 10,000 bacteria/mL of urine	The causative pathogen is identified

Other Tests: Complete blood count, transrectal ultrasound, computed tomography, blood urea nitrogen and creatinine level

PRIMARY NURSING DIAGNOSIS

DIAGNOSIS. Acute pain related to prostate inflammation and infection as evidenced by self-reports of pain and dysuria, facial grimacing, and/or protective behavior

OUTCOMES. Pain control; Pain level; Symptom severity; Symptom control; Knowledge: Pain management; Knowledge: Medication

INTERVENTIONS. Analgesic administration; Medication administration; Pain management: Acute; Teaching: Prescribed medication; Teaching: Disease process

PLANNING AND IMPLEMENTATION
Collaborative

Most physicians prescribe antibiotic therapy based on the results of the bacterial cultures; sometimes parenteral antibiotics are required if the infection is systemic. Bedrest and local measures such as 20-minute sitz baths two or three times a day can assist in reducing pain. Regular sexual intercourse or ejaculation helps drainage of prostatic secretions and lessens infection and pain after the acute inflammation subsides. For acute episodes, and once antibiotics have been started, some physicians recommend regular prostatic massage for several weeks.

If drug therapy for chronic bacterial prostatitis is unsuccessful, on rare occasions the patient may undergo a transurethral resection of the prostate (TURP) to remove all infected tissue. Because this procedure may lead to retrograde ejaculation and sterility, it is usually done on older men. A total prostatectomy also has the risk of causing impotence and incontinence and is performed only when necessary.

Pharmacologic Highlights

Medication or Drug Class	Dosage	Description	Rationale
Combination of ceftriaxone, azithromycin, and doxycycline	Single-dose IM ceftriaxone, and cotreatment with single-dose oral azithromycin or 7 days of oral doxycycline	Antibiotic	Based on CDC treatment guidelines for gonococcal infections
Trimethoprim sulfamethoxazole (Bactrim, Septra)	1 DS tablet bid for 30 days; may also use an aminoglycoside and ampicillin for 1 wk followed by 4–6 wk of oral antibiotics	Antibacterial	Eliminates causative organism; for nonbacterial prostatitis caused by Chlamydia and Ureaplasma species, a trial of doxycycline or erythromycin may be used

Pharmacologic Highlights (continued)

Medication or Drug Class	Dosage	Description	Rationale
Ciprofloxacin hydrochloride (Cipro), levofloxacin, ofloxacin	Dose varies, course is generally 14–28 days	Fluoroquinolone anti-infective	Eliminates causative organism
Nitrofurantoin (Macrodantin)	100 mg daily for 4–16 wk	Urinary antiseptic	Given for chronic prostatitis along with Bactrim

Other Drugs: Alpha-adrenergic antagonists such as terazosin, tamsulosin to release bladder outlet obstruction; stool softeners to manage constipation, which is very painful; analgesics to relieve pain

Independent

The most important nursing interventions for patients with acute or chronic bacterial prostatitis focus on preventing complications. Monitor for urinary retention; for persistence of fever, perineal pain, or difficulty voiding; and for recurring UTI. If the patient is not on fluid restriction, encourage the patient to drink at least 3 L of fluid a day to facilitate elimination. Management of constipation may reduce discomfort.

Suggest strategies to increase comfort. If the patient exhibits a decreased ability to void, encourage the patient to void while in a warm-water bath with the pelvic muscles relaxed. To assist with pain control, use relaxation techniques and diversionary activities.

Patient teaching is essential. Some patients prefer to have someone of the same sex talk about sexual functioning. In periods of acute infection and inflammation, the patient is usually encouraged to abstain from sexual intercourse. If the patient has chronic bacterial prostatitis, encourage the patient to be sexually active to promote drainage of the prostate gland. During periods of known infection, the patient should use a condom. Answer the patient's and partner's questions thoroughly. If possible, encourage the patient to speak with others with prostatitis to learn how they have coped with the illness.

Evidence-Based Practice and Health Policy

Su, Z., Zenilman, J., Sfanos, K., & Herati, A. (2020). Management of chronic bacterial prostatitis. *Current Urology Reports, 21*, 29.

- The authors conducted a review of the literature describing the most current diagnosis and treatment options for chronic bacterial prostatitis. They noted that recurrence after taking oral antibiotics is common, due in part to increasing rates of antimicrobial resistance and the patient's inability to completely clear the bacteria from the prostate.
- They suggest various treatment options for chronic bacterial prostatitis refractory to conventional antibiotics. These treatments include the use of alternative agents such as fosfomycin, direct antimicrobial injections into the prostate, surgical removal of infected prostatic tissue, and chronic oral antibiotic suppression. They also discuss an emerging therapy using bacteriophages to target antibiotic-resistant bacteria.

DOCUMENTATION GUIDELINES

- Physical findings: Pain, bladder distention, hematuria, enlarged and tender prostate
- Response to therapy: Pain medication, sitz baths, fluids, antibiotics, ability to resume sexual functioning
- Urinary output: Characteristics, color, amount
- Presence of complications: Urinary retention, persistence of fever, perineal pain, dysuria
- Response to treatment: TURP or surgery

DISCHARGE AND HOME HEALTHCARE GUIDELINES

PREVENTION. Explain the need to drink fluids to facilitate kidney function and to avoid food and drinks that have diuretic action or are prostatitic. If the physician has prescribed sitz baths, the patient or family needs to know that sitz baths should be taken for 10 to 20 minutes several times daily.

MEDICATIONS. Be sure the patient understands the need to take all prescribed antibiotics. The patient should understand all medications, including the dosage, route, action, and any adverse effects. Remind the patient that the entire course of antibiotics should be completed before stopping the drug.

COMPLICATIONS. Instruct the patient to report fever, hematuria, urinary retention, or difficulty voiding. The patient needs to understand the need for prolonged follow-up to avoid recurrence.

POSTPROCEDURE. If the patient has had surgery or a TURP, teach that urinary dribbling, frequency, and occasional hematuria are not unusual. Explain that the patient will gradually regain urinary control. Remind the patient to avoid heavy lifting, strenuous exercise, or long automobile or plane trips. These situations may place the urinary system under high pressures from bladder distention or abdominal pressure that may lead to bleeding. Usually, the physician requests that the patient abstain from sexual activity for several weeks after the procedures.

Psychoactive Substance Abuse

DRG Category: 895
Mean LOS: 12.4 days
Description: MEDICAL: Alcohol, Drug Abuse or Dependence With Rehabilitation Therapy

Psychoactive substances are drugs or chemicals that have an effect on the central nervous system (CNS). The National Institute on Drug Abuse (NIDA) defines drug misuse as improper or unhealthy use and implies use that can cause harm to the user or their friends or family. It is roughly equivalent to the term "abuse" but is believed to be a less stigmatizing description. Physical dependence is a condition in which the body adapts to regular use (develops tolerance) and is accompanied by withdrawal symptoms when the substance is taken away. Addiction is a broader term describing a chronic disorder characterized by drug seeking and use that is compulsive, despite negative consequences. The *Diagnostic and Statistical Manual of Mental Disorders, Fifth Edition* (*DSM-5*) describes (and replaces) all of the above terms as varying degrees of a substance use disorder. Harmful drug use impairs one's ability to perform daily activities of living and function in work environments. Relationships with family and friends become impaired and dysfunctional.

Most of the misused drugs fall into two main categories: CNS depressants and CNS stimulants. CNS depressants include narcotics, sedatives, barbiturates, tranquilizers, and inhalants. The desired effect by the user is a sense of increased self-esteem, euphoria, relaxation, and relief from pain and anxiety. CNS stimulants include amphetamines, hallucinogens, and cocaine. The desired effect by the user is a sense of well-being, alertness, excitation, overconfidence, and increased initiative.

In 2019, the U.S. National Survey on Drug Use and Health (NSDUH) estimated that 5.5 million people age 12 years or older were past users of cocaine, including about 778,000 users of crack and 2 million users of methamphetamine in the past year. Approximately 1 million people had a methamphetamine use disorder. Overdose deaths have increased for both cocaine and methamphetamines; methamphetamine overdose deaths quadrupled from 2011 to 2017 and in 2020 during the COVID-19 pandemic, overdose deaths from psychostimulants (like methamphetamine) increased by almost 35%.

NIDA (2020) reported significant increases in vaping among teenagers with as high as 40.6% admitting to use within the past year. Vaping of marijuana among teenagers has doubled in the past 2 years. Reports of serious respiratory illness secondary to vaping have raised additional safety concerns. Inhalant use (such as fuels, solvents, adhesives, aerosol propellants, and paint thinners, many of which contain toluene) has been increasing among teenagers over the last several years with significant increases among eighth graders.

Opioid misuse, overdose, and death continue to be a national epidemic in the United States. The CDC (2020) report that on average 128 Americans die per day from opioid overdose. While prescription misuse and heroin use have been primary sources of opioid addiction in the past, illicitly manufactured synthetic opioids such as fentanyl (30 to 50 times more potent than pure heroin) and carfentanil (100 times more potent than fentanyl) are primary drivers of the current epidemic. Mixtures of fentanyl and heroin are particularly lethal. According to the CDC, opioid overdose deaths increased by over 38% in the 12-month period ending in May 2020.

According to the most recent NSDUH, in 2018, 2% of Americans age 12 years and older reported using hallucinogens in the past year (NIDA, 2020). Lysergic acid diethylamide (LSD), like other hallucinogens, does not lead to the development of physical addiction or withdrawal symptoms. However, tolerance for LSD and other hallucinogens develops quickly and to a high degree. In fact, tolerance is complete after 3 to 4 consecutive days of use. Recovery from the tolerance also occurs very rapidly (in 4 to 7 days), so that the individual is able to achieve the desired effect from the drug repeatedly and often. LSD, psilocybin, and ketamine are all being explored for potential benefits in treatment-resistant depression. Currently, only ketamine has approval from the U.S. Food and Drug Administration for this use, and its administration must be in certified medical clinics with a Risk Evaluation and Mitigation Strategy (REMS). Chronic misuse of psychoactive substances may lead to complications, including pulmonary emboli, respiratory infections, trauma, musculoskeletal dysfunctions, psychosis, malnutrition disturbances, gastrointestinal disturbances, hepatitis, thrombophlebitis, bacterial endocarditis, gangrene, coma, and death.

CAUSES

The causes of substance misuse are complex and multifactorial, influenced by the type and availability of the drug, personality type, environmental factors, peer pressure, coping abilities of the individual, genetic factors, and sociocultural influences. Cocaine dependence is thought to be associated with a deficiency in dopamine and norepinephrine neurotransmitters. Use of narcotics and opiates may interfere with the biochemical factors related to the body's own production of opiate-like substances.

Psychological factors include low self-esteem, feelings of inadequacy, loneliness, shame, guilt, depression, hopelessness, and despair. Sociocultural factors include relationships with individuals and groups where drug use is an accepted practice, isolation, unemployment, and poverty. Teenagers and young adults often begin experimenting as a result of peer pressure and the easy availability of drugs. Risk factors for substance misuse include family history of addiction, mental health disorders, peer pressure, lack of family involvement, exposure to use at an early age, exposure to violence and sexual assault, and posttraumatic stress disorder.

GENETIC CONSIDERATIONS

The ways in which genes influence behavior are complex, and definitive studies have proved elusive. Finding genetic causes of susceptibility to substance misuse has been difficult, but twin studies estimate that a susceptibility to substance misuse is highly genetic (heritability of ~60% to 80%). Genes associated with predisposition to dependence and risky behaviors include those encoding the dopamine D4 receptor, phosphodiesterase 1B, the AMPA receptor subunit GluR1, 5HT1B receptor, protein kinase C, and the transcription factor FosB. Variations in monoamine oxidase B (*MAOB*) influence a behavioral response to novelty. Some evidence has shown that a decreased expression of the gene encoding the *5-HTT* transporter may be associated with an increased risk for substance use disorders.

SEX AND LIFE SPAN CONSIDERATIONS

Drug use and misuse are prevalent across the life span from young adolescents to the oldest of the old. Increasing numbers of older adults are abusing drugs as a way of coping with the stressors of aging. Young teens are vulnerable to experimentation as they attempt to conform to group norms and peer pressure. Club drugs such as MDMA (Ecstasy, Adam, clarity, Eve, lover's speed, etc.), flunitrazepam (Rohypnol, forget-me pill, roofies), and gamma-hydroxybutyrate (GHB, G, Georgia home boy, liquid ecstasy) are used primarily by adolescents and young adults at bars, nightclubs, concerts, and parties.

HEALTH DISPARITIES AND SEXUAL/GENDER MINORITY HEALTH

Rates of substance misuse vary by race and ethnicity, depending on the substance, geography, and a variety of sociocultural factors. Socioeconomic vulnerability seems to be less important to substance misuse patterns than mental health issues. Transgender is a term used to describe persons whose gender identity is different from their sex assigned at birth. Approximately 1% of the U.S. population identify themselves as transgender. The CDC report that when compared to heterosexual individuals, gay and bisexual men, and lesbian and transgender individuals are more likely to use drugs and have higher rates of substance misuse. They suggest that drug use may be a reaction to homophobia, discrimination, marginalization, and violence they experience. Experts suggest that the exclusion of transgender persons from the substance use literature makes it difficult to determine their substance use prevalence.

GLOBAL HEALTH CONSIDERATIONS

According to the 2019 World Drug Report, an estimated 35 million people have drug use disorders requiring treatment. The report estimates that 53 million people worldwide are opioid users (up 56% from previous estimates), and two-thirds of the 585,000 people who died from drug use in 2017 had deaths related to opioid overdose. Fentanyl and its analogues are the primary driver of the synthetic opioid crisis in North America, but West and Central and North Africa are experiencing a crisis of another synthetic opioid, tramadol. Cannabis continues to be the most widely used psychoactive substance with an estimated 188 million users.

ASSESSMENT

HISTORY. The physiological signs and symptoms of use or intoxication vary, depending on the substance. Consequently, when a person is admitted in an intoxicated state or in withdrawal, it is important to know what drug or drugs have been used, the route used, and if possible, the amount of drug used. Determine if alcohol is also being used because there is a synergistic effect that increases the effect of both drugs.

Some patients may be misusing psychoactive drugs through ignorance. Others may have begun using them as part of a physician-prescribed treatment regimen and then became addicted. If the individual is unable to give a history because of overdose, friends or family members may provide needed information, and clothing can be checked for drug paraphernalia. Elicit a history of previous detoxification treatments, effectiveness, length of recovery, and what influenced a return to drug usage.

PHYSICAL EXAMINATION. The most common symptoms depend on the illicit drug (see Table 1). If the patient is admitted with intoxication and a drug history cannot be obtained, signs and symptoms can be indicators of the type of drug used (Table 1). Inspect the patient for evidence of how the drug is used, such as needle marks from mainlining, nasal irritation caused by snorting, ulcerations on lips and tongue from chewing, cellulitis from injecting drugs and missing the vein, and infections from sites used for mainlining.

• TABLE 1 Signs and Symptoms of Drug Use and Withdrawal

DRUG	OVERDOSE	WITHDRAWAL
Marijuana (cannabis)	Euphoria, fatigue, decreased coordination, paranoia, panic, psychosis	Cravings, appetite loss
Narcotics	Small pupils, shallow respirations, increasing unresponsiveness, seizure activity	Tearing of the eyes, runny nose, anorexia, nausea, abdominal cramping and pain, irritability, shaking chills, diaphoresis
Depressants/barbiturates	Dilated pupils, shallow breathing, diaphoresis, thready and rapid pulse, increasing unresponsiveness	Shakiness, anxiety, sleeplessness, shaking, seizure activity
Stimulants/amphetamines, cocaine	Fever, anxiety, restlessness, hypertension, agitation, hallucinations, seizure activity	Depression, sleepiness, fatigue, apathy, irritability, weight gain
Hallucinogens	Dilated pupils, hypertension and tachycardia, sweating, vomiting, flushing, tremors and seizures, coma, stroke, organ failure, muscle necrosis, death	Flashbacks, anxiety, problems with concentration, confusion, depersonalization, depression, paranoia, delusions

PSYCHOSOCIAL. Obtain information on how patients perceive the effect drugs have on their life, work, and relationship with family and friends. Identify strengths and limitations. Assess the patient's emotional state before admission, especially noting depression and thoughts about suicide. If the patient is involved in a relationship, determine the degree of stability. Ask whether the partner or significant others use drugs and what their attitude is toward the patient's drug use. If the patient is a parent, find out the children's ages and investigate how the children are affected by the patient's drug use.

Elicit an employment history, including the type and length of employment. Determine how the use of drugs has affected the patient's work. Determine how much time off from work has been caused by the drug use. Establish a history of the financial effects of the drug use; ask how much the patient spends on drugs, and if there are other sources of income besides the primary job that were developed to gain income for drugs. Determine how the use of drugs has affected the patient's financial resources.

Diagnostic Highlights

Test	Normal Result	Abnormality With Condition	Explanation
Serum and urine drug screens	Negative for screened substance	Positive for screened substance	Identify drugs that have been ingested

Other Tests: Gas chromatography–mass spectrometry. For unresponsive patients with suspected drug overdose—serum glucose, complete blood count, blood urea nitrogen, serum electrolytes, arterial blood gases, electrocardiogram, chest x-ray.

PRIMARY NURSING DIAGNOSIS

DIAGNOSIS. Risk for injury as evidenced by seizures, difficulty breathing, delirium, or anxiety (potential overdose) or nervousness, trouble sleeping, or flu-like symptoms (potential withdrawal)

OUTCOMES. Coping; Role performance; Mood equilibrium; Risk control: Drug use

INTERVENTIONS. Counseling; Substance use treatment: Withdrawal; Substance use treatment: Overdose; Therapy group; Support group; Emotional support; Mood management

PLANNING AND IMPLEMENTATION

Collaborative

The immediate goal after depressant ingestion is to keep the individual safe during a drug overdose or withdrawal. The long-term goal is for the patient to remain drug free. In the acute phase, the immediate effects of narcotics can be reversed with naloxone (Narcan). In the case of barbiturate overdose when the patient is conscious, mild intoxication can be treated by letting the individual "sleep it off." More severe cases of overdoses need to be handled in an acute or critical care environment where continuous monitoring can occur. Of paramount importance is to make sure the patient has adequate airway, breathing, and circulation (ABCs) during the time period that depressants may lead to severe respiratory depression.

Generally, if the patient is unconscious and the substance is unknown, the following steps are taken in management: (1) Begin supplemental oxygen; (2) insert an IV line with saline infusion or dextrose in water; (3) administer dextrose, thiamine, and naloxone; (4) protect airway with endotracheal intubation; (5) pass orogastric tube, lavage, and administer activated charcoal; and (6) admit the patient for ongoing observation and management. Activated charcoal is produced from the destructive distillation of organic materials. The substance absorbs toxic substances because of large external pores and a large internal surface area that binds with toxic ions. A cathartic such as magnesium citrate is given to help gastrointestinal excretion of the toxic substance bound with activated charcoal. Activated charcoal is also given for overdoses when the substance is known, such as phenobarbital, carbamazepine, cyclic antidepressants, amphetamines, and cocaine. Lipid emulsion therapy may be used to treat drug toxicities from tricyclic antidepressants and cocaine.

Management of stimulants can be similar to that of depressants, with the administration of activated charcoal. Seizures are a possibility in the case of an overdose with stimulants, but note that amphetamines and cocaine have a short duration time of 2 to 4 hours. Phenytoin (Dilantin) can be ordered to prevent seizure activity, and benzodiazepines are also used to treat agitation or seizures. External cooling may be used to reduce hyperthermia, and IV fluids may be used to replace fluid loss and to prevent myoglobin damage in the kidneys. All patients with substance misuse and overdoses need counseling and therapy to manage their substance use patterns.

Pharmacologic Highlights

Medication or Drug Class	Dosage	Description	Rationale
Naloxone	2 mg IV; use smaller doses for patients who are not apneic to avoid withdrawal; 4 mg nasal spray and may repeat using new nasal spray in alternating nostrils, every 2 to 3 min if the patient does not respond, or responds and then relapses into respiratory depression	Opioid antagonist	Blocks the action of opioids that can lead to respiratory depression and apnea

Pharmacologic Highlights (continued)

Medication or Drug Class	Dosage	Description	Rationale
Dextrose	100 mL IV 50% solution	Sugar	Rules out hypoglycemia as a cause for coma; given to patients who are known not to be hyperglycemic
Benzodiazepines	Varies with drug	Chlordiazepoxide, clorazepate, diazepam, lorazepam, oxazepam	Controls seizures and anxiety
Haloperidol	2–5 mg IV or IM	Antipsychotic	Controls combative or agitated behavior during withdrawal or treatment
Clonidine	0.1–0.3 mg every 4–6 hr	Antihypertensive	Opioid withdrawal; treats hypertension and tachycardia
Pentobarbital	100–200 initially PO and then in decreasing doses over 10 days	Barbiturate	Protects the patient from seizure activity
Phenytoin	300–400 mg daily in divided doses PO or IV	Anticonvulsant	Prevents and limits seizures related to drug withdrawal

Other Drugs: Desipramine hydrochloride (Norpramin), bromocriptine mesylate (Parlodel), amantadine hydrochloride (Symmetrel), and melphalan (phenylalanine mustard) have been prescribed to decrease the craving for cocaine during withdrawal. Naltrexone (ReVia [oral] or Vivitrol [injectable]) and methadone (an opioid partial agonist) are medications used to prevent relapse in opioid use disorders. Phenothiazines in low doses may be ordered to control the flashbacks that can occur after the last dose of a hallucinogen. Because the patient has built up a tolerance for drugs, the amount of medication needed to keep the patient safe may be more than what is considered a safe dosage.

Independent

During the acute phase, keep the patient safe. Use strategies for continuous monitoring of ABCs and implement emergency measures as needed to support life. Monitor for seizure activity and place the patient on the seizure precautions regimen. Examine the environment for safety risks such as falls from the bed or self-discontinuation of tubes. Assess the potential for a suicide attempt and, if necessary, initiate suicide precautions and never leave the patient unattended.

Meet the self-care deficits related to hygiene, nutrition, and elimination. Promote a sense of security: Approach the patient in a calm, nonthreatening, and nonjudgmental way. Building a trusting relationship with the patient provides a foundation for addressing the more long-term goals associated with becoming drug free.

Following the acute phase, initiate the process of rehabilitation and implement a treatment plan to maintain abstinence. The first goal is to work toward getting the individual to break through the denial of drug misuse and take responsibility to begin the recovery process. Motivational interviewing is an evidence-based strategy for promoting patient engagement in the change process. Provide educational materials and arrange a consultation with an addictions counselor to begin the process before discharge from an acute care setting. Often, individuals are admitted from an acute care setting to an inpatient or outpatient treatment facility where nursing staff and other healthcare providers can begin specialized treatment programs. These programs include peer group programs in which confrontation, support, and hope are part of the treatment process. Treatment goals for the individual include development of a healthy self-concept, self-discipline, adaptive coping strategies, strategies to improve interpersonal relationships, and ways of filling leisure time without the use of drugs.

Evidence-Based Practice and Health Policy

Wang, Q., Kaelber, D., Xu, R., & Volkow, N. (2021). COVID-19 risk and outcomes in patients with substance use disorders: Analyses from electronic health records in the United States. *Molecular Psychiatry, 26*, 130–139.

- This retrospective case-control study of 73,099,850 electronic health records, 12,030 of whom had COVID-19, sheds light on the following risks and outcomes for patients with substance use disorders. The findings support that screening for and treating substance use disorders has implications as one of the strategies for controlling the COVID-19 pandemic. Patients with a recent (within the past year) diagnosis of substance use disorders were at significantly increased risk for COVID-19, especially those with opioid use disorder (followed by those with tobacco use disorder).
- Compared to patients without substance use disorder, patients with substance use disorder had significantly higher prevalence of chronic kidney, liver, and lung diseases; cardiovascular diseases; type 2 diabetes; obesity; and cancer. Among patients with recent diagnosis of substance use disorder, Black persons had significantly higher risk of COVID-19 and worse outcomes than White persons. COVID-19 patients with substance use disorder had significantly worse outcomes (death: 9.6%, hospitalization: 41.0%) than general COVID-19 patients (death: 6.6%, hospitalization: 30.1%).

DOCUMENTATION GUIDELINES

- Physical findings: Vital signs; adequacy of ABCs; response to medication protocols for overdose or withdrawal, nutrition, intake and output, elimination patterns
- Mental/neurological findings: Anxiety levels, depression, delusions, hallucinations, presence or absence of seizures
- Understanding of the need for consultation with addictions counselor
- Understanding of the need for continued treatment for self and family

DISCHARGE AND HOME HEALTHCARE GUIDELINES

The patient should be discharged to an inpatient or outpatient treatment program to address the long-term effects of substance misuse or addiction. After discharge from a treatment program, the individual may continue with groups such as Narcotics Anonymous, Cocaine Anonymous, or Alcoholics Anonymous. Family dynamics often play a role in the use of drugs. It is important for the family to be involved in the treatment plan through individual and family therapy and support groups that address issues dealing with family members who misused drugs. NIDA provides a wealth of information on drugs and drug misuse for healthcare professionals, teachers, and families at https://www.drugabuse.gov.

Pulmonary Embolism

DRG Category:	175
Mean LOS:	5.1 days
Description:	MEDICAL: Pulmonary Embolism With Major Complication or Comorbidity or Acute Cor Pulmonale

Pulmonary embolism (PE) is a potentially life-threatening condition in which a free-flowing blood clot (embolism) becomes lodged within the pulmonary vasculature. PEs are frequent occurrences with the incidence of venous thromboembolism as high as 1 per 1,000 people.

While estimates vary, from 600,000 to 800,000 cases of PE are reported yearly, and approximately 60% of patients who die in a hospital are found to have a PE on autopsy. PE is therefore the third most common cause of death in hospitalized patients, and it is viewed as the most commonly missed diagnosis in older adults.

When an embolism becomes lodged within a pulmonary vessel, platelets accumulate around the thrombus and trigger the release of potent vasoactive substances. The pulmonary vasculature constricts, which leads to an increased pulmonary vascular resistance, increased pulmonary arterial pressure, and increased right ventricular workload. Blood flow abnormalities result in a ventilation/perfusion mismatch that is initially dead-space ventilation (ventilation with no perfusion) and hyperventilation. As atelectasis occurs, shunting (perfusion without ventilation of the alveolus) and hypoxemia result. If the right side of the heart (accustomed to pumping out against a relatively low-resistance pulmonary circuit) cannot empty its volume against the increased pulmonary vascular resistance, right-sided heart failure occurs. Ultimately, cardiac function may deteriorate with decreased cardiac output, decreased systemic blood flow, profound hypoxemia, and shock.

CAUSES

A thrombus forms, usually on the valves of the veins of the lower extremities, with the accumulation of platelets and fibrin. A PE usually occurs when a thrombus in the deep veins of the lower extremities loosens or dislodges and begins to move in the bloodstream. The thrombus (now an embolus because it is moving in the bloodstream) floats to the heart, moves through the right side of the heart, and enters the pulmonary circulation through the pulmonary artery. Major risk factors for the development of PE include any condition that produces venous stasis or turbulent blood flow, increased blood coagulability, or venous endothelial (vessel wall) injury. Situations resulting in these pathological changes include immobility, dehydration, injury, or decreased venous return. Conditions associated with these risk factors include varicosities, pregnancy, obesity, tumors, thrombocytopenia, atrial fibrillation, multiple trauma, presence of artificial heart valves or vessels, sepsis, and congestive heart failure. Reflecting the major factors, recent studies of patients with the novel coronavirus 2019 disease (COVID-19) have found that from 18% to 24% of hospitalized patients with COVID-19 have a PE.

GENETIC CONSIDERATIONS

Susceptibility to PE can be caused by various inherited thrombophilias, including factor V Leiden, prothrombin G20210A mutations, protein C deficiency (*PROC*), protein S deficiency (*PROS1*), and antithrombin deficiency (*SERPINC1*).

Workup for these hereditary coagulopathies should be considered when a person has VTE meeting any of the following criteria: onset before age 50 years, idiopathic VTE at any age, recurrent VTE, and venous thrombosis at unusual sites (e.g., cerebral, mesenteric, portal, and hepatic veins). Testing has also been recommended when VTE occurs during pregnancy, in the postpartum period, or in association with oral contraceptive use or hormone replacement therapy.

SEX AND LIFE SPAN CONSIDERATIONS

PE may occur in any age group. PE causes sudden death for 60,000 to 100,000 people each year in the United States. PE in children is associated with cardiac conditions and coagulopathic diseases such as sickle cell anemia and cancer. Young women are at risk for PE during pregnancy or while they take birth control pills with a high estrogen content. Adults, particularly older adults, are at risk for PE because of deep vein thrombosis (DVT), cardiac conditions, and increased blood coagulability. Some experts suggest that death rates are about 30% higher for men than for women.

HEALTH DISPARITIES AND SEXUAL/GENDER MINORITY HEALTH

Mortality rates are higher for Black persons than for other groups and higher for White persons than for Asian and Native American persons. Black men and women have a twofold higher adjusted mortality rate due to PE compared with White men and women (Martin et al., 2020 [see Evidence-Based Practice and Health Policy]). Sexual and gender minority status has no known effect on the risk for PE.

GLOBAL HEALTH CONSIDERATIONS

The incidence of DVT and PE is approximately the same across all regions globally; the average annual incidence of VTE in the United States is 1 per 1,000 individuals. Global differences are likely due to accuracy of diagnosis and consistency of reporting rather than true differences in incidence.

ASSESSMENT

HISTORY. Many patients with PE report a history of DVT, surgery, or some other condition that results in vascular injury or increased blood coagulability. Establish a history of recent travel (4 hours or more of sitting down), malignancy and lung cancer, or trauma to the legs or pelvis. Ask if the patient uses tobacco products. Patients may describe a sudden onset of dyspnea and chest pain for no apparent reason. Some patients report severe symptoms, such as severe pain, wheezing, diaphoresis, and a sense of impending doom. The severity of the symptoms partly depends on the size, number, and location of the emboli.

PHYSICAL EXAMINATION. The patient may demonstrate a variety of symptoms. They may have a complete **cardiopulmonary collapse requiring resuscitation** or have **gradually progressing shortness of breath, diaphoresis, pleuritic chest pain, cough, and hemoptysis**. They may be febrile, or their skin may be cold and clammy. Those in critical condition may develop severe chest pain, syncope, and chest splinting and may cough up bloody sputum. Not all patients become hypoxemic because the increased respiratory rate increases their minute volume and thereby maintains gas exchange. However, some patients have signs of hypoxemia, such as confusion, agitation, central cyanosis, and decreasing level of consciousness. Others may have atypical symptoms such as seizures, abdominal pain, wheezing, cardiac dysrhythmias, and flank pain.

More than 90% of people with PE have tachypnea with a respiratory rate greater than 16/minute, and more than half have rales and an accentuated heart sound upon chest auscultation. Just less than half have tachycardia with a heart rate greater than 100/minute and fever. About a third have diaphoresis. Thus, when you auscultate the patient's chest, you may note decreased breath sounds, wheezing, crackles, or a transient pleural friction rub. You may also note tachycardia, a third heart sound, or a loud pulmonic component of the second heart sound. You may note a warm, tender area in the leg. Ongoing monitoring during an acute episode of PE is essential for patient recovery. Monitor the patient's vital signs, including temperature, pulse, blood pressure, and respiratory rate, every hour or as needed. Observe the patient continuously for signs of right ventricular failure as evidenced by neck vein distention, rales, peripheral edema, enlarged liver, dyspnea, increased weight, and increased heart rate. Monitor the patient for signs of shock, such as severe hypotension, mottling, cyanosis, cold extremities, and weak or absent peripheral pulses.

PSYCHOSOCIAL. Depending on the severity of symptoms, patients and their families usually display some degree of anxiety. Because PE is life threatening, their fears are justified and appropriate. The disease process can make the patient feel anxious with a sense of impending doom as hypoxemia increases; many patients have significant fear and anxiety during an acute PE. Assess the patient's and family's ability to cope and intervene as necessary.

Diagnostic Highlights

Notes: No one study is diagnostic for a PE.

Test	Normal Result	Abnormality With Condition	Explanation
Arterial blood gases	Pao_2: 80–95 mm Hg; $Paco_2$: 35–45 mm Hg; SaO_2: > 95%	Pao_2: < 80 mm Hg in a majority of patients; $Paco_2$ varies but often < 35 mm Hg; SaO_2: < 95%	Arterial oxygenation is not a good predictor of suspected PE because of compensatory mechanisms. However, low arterial oxygenation accompanied by dyspnea is a better predictor. Theoretically, poor gas exchange and shunting lead to hypoxemia, and hypocapnia occurs from increased respiratory rate; arterial blood gases provide important data but do not allow a "rule out" or "rule in" of a diagnosis of PE.
High-resolution multidetector computed tomographic angiography	Patent arteries and veins; negative for emboli/thrombi	Obstruction to blood flow by clot	Can detect flow in small arteries and veins; imaging test of choice if available
Ventilation/perfusion scan; nuclear scintigraphic ventilation-perfusion; pulmonary angiography	Negative for emboli/thrombi; uniform uptake of particles and equal gas distribution	Wash out of radioactivity in embolized areas; ventilation defects in embolized areas	Emboli/thrombi lead to lack of perfusion and shunting

Other Tests: Complete blood count, ischemia modified albumin levels, prothrombin time, partial thromboplastin time, international normalized ratio (INR) of prothrombin time, echocardiogram, pulmonary angiogram, D-dimer, troponin levels, chest x-ray, computed tomography, electrocardiogram, impedance plethysmography and compression ultrasonography for diagnosis of DVT, contrast-enhanced spiral chest computed tomography

PRIMARY NURSING DIAGNOSIS

DIAGNOSIS. Impaired gas exchange related to impaired pulmonary blood flow and alveolar collapse as evidenced by restlessness, agitation, anxiety, dyspnea, tachypnea, diaphoresis, and/or tachycardia

OUTCOMES. Respiratory status: Gas exchange; Respiratory status: Ventilation; Blood coagulation; Cardiopulmonary status; Vital signs; Tissue perfusion

INTERVENTIONS. Airway management; Anxiety reduction; Oxygen therapy; Airway suctioning; Airway insertion and stabilization; Mechanical ventilation; Respiratory monitoring; Teaching: Disease process

PLANNING AND IMPLEMENTATION
Collaborative

Anticoagulation is the primary treatment for PE, although the medications of choice vary depending on the severity of the condition. In patients without symptoms, an oral factor Xa inhibitor (see Pharmacologic Highlights) will not reduce the clot but will keep it from getting larger and reduce the formation of other clots. Generally these patients are not hospitalized. Symptomatic patients are hospitalized and usually receive an IV heparin bolus followed by a continuous heparin infusion monitored by activated partial thromboplastin time (aPTT) levels to adjust dosage.

Massive PE is a medical emergency. The priority is to make sure that the patient's airway, breathing, and circulation (ABCs) are maintained. Oxygen is administered immediately to support gas exchange, and patients may need intubation and mechanical ventilation. IV access for administration of fluids and pharmacologic agents occurs so that anticoagulation can proceed. Thrombolytic therapy is used without delay for patients with hypotension who are not at high risk for bleeding or for people whose clinical status indicates a high risk for hypotension. While controlled trials have not indicated that thrombolytic therapy is superior to heparin, most experts suggest its use in the setting of PE and hypotension. Before administration of thrombolytic agents, a coagulation profile and complete blood count are obtained at baseline. Long-term anticoagulation continues after discharge with warfarin.

Although it is rare, severe cases of PE that are unresponsive to anticoagulant or thrombolytic therapy may require surgery. The least invasive technique is the insertion of a transvenous catheter into the pulmonary vasculature. If the procedure is unsuccessful, however, a thoracotomy may be required to remove the obstructing embolism. Patients prone to PE seeded from deep vein thrombi may have a prosthetic umbrella inserted into the inferior vena cava to trap the emboli.

Pharmacologic Highlights

Medication or Drug Class	Dosage	Description	Rationale
Thrombolytic agents	Varies with drug	Reteplase, alteplase	Break down clots previously formed and hasten resolution of clots but have not been shown to reduce mortality
Anticoagulants	Varies with drug and patient weight; low-molecular-weight heparin (LMWH); fondaparinux, enoxaparin (Lovenox)	Fractionated LMWH subcutaneously; warfarin maintenance therapy initiated after 1–3 days of effective heparinization	Reduce further formation of clots
Direct thrombin inhibitors and factor Xa inhibitors	Varies with drug: Rivaroxaban, apixaban, dabigatran, edoxaban, betrixaban	Direct thrombin inhibitors prevent thrombus development, block conversion of fibrinogen to fibrin; factor Xa inhibitors prevent conversion of prothrombin to thrombin	Keeps clot from getting larger and reduces further formation of clots
Warfarin	2–5 mg QD for 2 days and adjusted according INR level	Interferes with the liver synthesis of vitamin K–dependent coagulation factors	Used for prevention and treatment of thromboembolic events; dose is tailored to maintain an INR between 2.5 and 3.5.

Other Drugs: Morphine sulfate to manage pain and anxiety, diuretics to reduce edema, inotropic agents for heart failure

Independent

The primary concern for the nurse who is caring for a patient with PE includes the maintenance of ABCs by support of the cardiopulmonary system. The most important independent measure before PE is prevention of thrombus formation. To prevent PE in high-risk patients, encourage early chair rest and ambulation as the patient's condition allows. Even patients who are intubated and mechanically ventilated with multiple catheters can be gotten out of bed without physiological risk for periods of chair rest. Provide active and passive range-of-motion exercises at least every 8 hours for all patients on bedrest. Teach the family and significant others of an immobile patient how to perform passive range-of-motion exercises. If the patient is not on fluid restriction, encourage drinking at least 2 L of fluids a day to decrease blood viscosity. Use compression boots for patients who are on bedrest to increase venous return.

During anticoagulant or thrombolytic therapy, protect patients from injury. Report any signs of increased bleeding, such as ecchymosis, epistaxis, hematuria, mucous membrane bleeding, decreasing hemoglobin or hematocrit, and bleeding from puncture sites. Restrict parenteral injections and venipunctures to essential procedures only. If the patient is ambulatory, provide a safe environment.

Provide information about the diagnosis and prognosis of PE and explain all procedures and diagnostic tests. Set aside time each day to talk with the patient and family to allow for expression of their feelings. If the patient is a child, monitor the patterns of growth and development using age-appropriate milestones and developmental tasks. Provide age-appropriate play activities for children.

Evidence-Based Practice and Health Policy

Martin, K., Molsberry, R., Cuttica, M., Desai, K., Schimmel, D., & Khan, S. (2020). Time trends in pulmonary embolism mortality rates in the United States, 1999–2018. *Journal of the American Heart Association, 9*. Advance online publication. https://doi.org/10.1161/JAHA.120.016784

- The authors aimed to describe trends in death rates caused by PE in the United States, describing overall statistics and also by sex and race. They used nationwide death certificate data from the Centers for Disease Control and Prevention. They found that PE mortality has increased over the last 10 years.
- Black men and women had a twofold higher adjusted mortality rate compared with White men and women. Mortality rates increased for younger adults 25 to 64 years of age, and remained stable for people 65 years and older. The authors noted that both health disparities between Black and White people and the rising rate of mortality in younger people needed to be remedied.

DOCUMENTATION GUIDELINES

- Respiratory response: Rate and rhythm, presence of adventitious breath sounds; retractions or nasal flaring (pediatric); oxygen saturation; character and amount of expectoration; type, location, and patency of the artificial airway
- Cardiovascular response: Skin and oral mucosa color; heart rate and rhythm; peripheral pulses; location and degree of edema
- Presence of pain (chest or extremity), location, character, and intensity; swelling or warmth of the patient's extremities
- Complications: Hematuria, epistaxis, hemoptysis, bloody vomitus, bleeding
- Response to treatment: Anticoagulation, oxygen, sedation, surgery

DISCHARGE AND HOME HEALTHCARE GUIDELINES

Teach the patient and family methods of prevention. Because of the association of DVT and PE, instruct patients to avoid factors that cause venous stasis. Explain that patients should avoid prolonged sitting, crossing of their legs, placing pillows beneath the popliteal fossae, and wearing tight-fitting clothing such as girdles. Encourage hospitalized patients to ambulate as soon as possible after surgery and to wear antiembolic hose or pneumatic compression boots while they are bedridden. Encourage patients to drink at least 2 L of fluid a day unless they are on fluid restriction. Suggest that obese patients limit calorie intake to reduce their weight.

Discuss all medications with the patient and family. Patients are usually discharged on warfarin. Remind the patient to keep appointments with the healthcare professional. Note that the patient needs periodic blood specimens to monitor drug levels. Explain that warfarin is continued unless the patient consults with the healthcare professional. Explain that the patient cannot take any over-the-counter drug preparations that contain salicylates without consulting the healthcare provider. Encourage the patient to avoid foods that are rich in vitamin K, such as dark green vegetables, which counteract the effects of warfarin. Encourage the patient to wear a Medic Alert bracelet that shows the patient is on anticoagulant therapy. Describe the complications of anticoagulant therapy. Instruct the patient to avoid activities that might predispose to injury or bleeding. Children may require helmets and other protective equipment. Encourage the patient to use a soft toothbrush and, for shaving, an electric razor. Instruct the patient to report any orange or pink-red urine discoloration, blood in the stool, excessive bruising, heavy menses, excessive gum bleeding, hemoptysis, bloody vomitus, and abdominal or flank pain. Encourage the patient to inspect the back in the mirror each day to check for bruising. Instruct the patient to inform dentists and other healthcare providers about the anticoagulant therapy before any procedure.

Instruct the patient and family about possible complications. If leg pain or swelling, decreased pulses in the lower extremities, shortness of breath, chest pain, or anxiety occurs, the patient or family should report to an emergency department as soon as possible.

Pulmonary Fibrosis

DRG Category:	196
Mean LOS:	6.2 days
Description:	MEDICAL: Interstitial Lung Disease With Major Complication or Comorbidity

Pulmonary fibrosis is a restrictive lung disease in which alveolar inflation is reduced, thus impairing lung function. The alveoli are affected by fibrotic tissue, which may develop after inflammation, infection, or tissue damage. The resulting scarring and distortion of pulmonary tissue lead to serious compromise in gas exchange. Fibrosis leads to decreased lung compliance and increased elastic recoil, which increases the overall work of breathing and inefficient exchange of gases.

Usually, the onset of the disease is gradual, over approximately 6 months, and the disease is more common in people 50 years of age and older. Symptoms are slow to develop, and patients are often referred to a cardiologist because of exertional dyspnea and nonproductive cough rather than to a pulmonologist. The disease has a poor prognosis because, to date, there are no effective therapies. The mean survival time is 2 to 5 years after diagnosis. Complications include venous thromboembolism, heart failure, coronary heart disease, lung cancer, and pneumonia.

CAUSES

Idiopathic pulmonary fibrosis (IPF) is of unknown etiology. Current thinking is that exposure to an inciting agent such as smoke, pollutants, or viral infections may lead to alveolar damage. After injury, instead of normal healing, aberrant activation of alveolar epithelial cells leads to fibroblastic activity with scarring and destruction of functional lung tissue. Pulmonary conditions that can result in pulmonary fibrosis include pneumonia, atelectasis, alveolar cell cancer, pulmonary edema, and lung surgery or trauma. Nonpulmonary causes include neuromuscular disease such as Guillain-Barré syndrome, amyotrophic lateral sclerosis, myasthenia gravis, and muscular dystrophy. Approximately one-third of patients can trace their initial episodes of dyspnea to a viral respiratory illness. Deformities of the bones, such as ankylosing spondylitis and scoliosis, can result in pulmonary fibrosis. Risk factors include use of tobacco products (cigarettes, cigars, and pipes), viral infections, exposure to environmental pollutants, gastroesophageal reflux disease (GERD), radiation therapy for breast cancer, autoimmune diseases (rheumatoid arthritis, lupus, scleroderma), obstructive sleep apnea, and certain medications (chemotherapy, amiodarone, methotrexate).

GENETIC CONSIDERATIONS

Genetic contribution to pulmonary fibrosis is suggested by familial cases of the disease. Variants in the gene encoding pulmonary surfactant protein A1 (*SFTPA1*) have increased susceptibility to idiopathic pulmonary fibrosis in nonsmokers. Mutations in *SFTPA2* can also cause idiopathic pulmonary fibrosis. Mutations in the gene encoding surfactant protein C (*SFTPC*) have been identified in some families with idiopathic pulmonary fibrosis but not in others. Finally, variants in the mucin B gene (*MUC5B*) have been shown to increase susceptibility to pulmonary fibrosis.

SEX AND LIFE SPAN CONSIDERATIONS

Although it is possible for pulmonary fibrosis to occur at any age, approximately 60% of patients are 60 years or older at the time of diagnosis. Older patients or those exposed to risk factors for a prolonged period of time are at the greatest risk. Pulmonary fibrosis has a higher prevalence in men than in women.

HEALTH DISPARITIES AND SEXUAL/GENDER MINORITY HEALTH

Ethnicity, race, and sexual/gender minority status have no known effect on the risk for pulmonary fibrosis.

GLOBAL HEALTH CONSIDERATIONS

Around the world, the prevalence is reported as 10 to 20 cases per 100,000 individuals. The influences of geographical region, environmental exposure by region, and regional culture such as dietary habits and differences in smoking patterns are unknown.

ASSESSMENT

HISTORY. Ask the patient to provide a complete medical history with particular attention to recent viral diseases and any autoimmune disorders or breast cancer. Many patients report exertional dyspnea as their first sign. A nonproductive cough is common. Establish a history of work or lifestyle that may have caused the disease. Ask if the patient has worked as a coal miner or with materials such as asbestos or silica or whether the patient has lived near industrial plants that use such materials. Determine if the patient has had respiratory complications or conditions such as pneumonia, atelectasis, alveolar cell cancer, pulmonary edema, and lung surgery or trauma. Ask if the patient has experienced pain while breathing or shortness of breath. Determine if the patient has a history of obstructive sleep apnea, which may be related to pulmonary fibrosis. Ask if the patient smokes cigarettes, pipes, or cigars. There is some suspicion that genetic factors may determine susceptibility to the disease, so take a family history of pulmonary conditions, including pulmonary fibrosis.

PHYSICAL EXAMINATION. Although the symptoms of pulmonary fibrosis are nonspecific, the patient may have **progressive dyspnea on exertion and a dry cough**. Observe the patient's respiratory status, noting rate, depth, rhythm, and ease of breathing. In the initial phases of the disease, the physical examination may be normal and the lungs may be clear on auscultation. As the disease progresses, individuals with pulmonary fibrosis frequently develop shallow, rapid breathing patterns in an attempt to conserve energy. Auscultate the patient's lungs; listen for diminished or absent breath sounds or coarse crackles, particularly at the lung bases on inspiration. Note chest excursion and symmetry. Check for digital clubbing, which occurs in 25% to 50% of patients with pulmonary fibrosis. Some patients develop weight loss, fatigue, fever, and muscle pain. Because pulmonary fibrosis in its late stages can cause cor pulmonale, check for signs of cardiac failure, such as elevated neck veins, liver distention, and swelling of the lower extremities (pedal edema). When you auscultate the heart, you may hear a loud P2 component of the second heart sound; a fixed, split S2 heart sound; and a systolic murmur from tricuspid regurgitation.

PSYCHOSOCIAL. Patients may experience a lowering of self-esteem with increased dependence on others and changing roles. In addition, shortness of breath and difficulty in breathing usually cause increased anxiety. If the disease has an occupational source, financial concerns may play an important role if the patient is unable to return to work.

Diagnostic Highlights

Test	Normal Result	Abnormality With Condition	Explanation
Chest x-ray	Clear lung fields	Identification of interstitial infiltrates or ground glass pattern	Fibrotic areas have a changed appearance
High-resolution computed tomography	Normal lung structures	Reticular opacities, traction bronchiectasis, honeycombing, and alveolar distortion; ground-glass pattern	Fibrotic areas have a changed appearance
Forced expiratory flow: Maximal flow rate attained during the middle (25%–75%) of forced vital capacity maneuver	Varies by body size	25% of the predicted value	Predicts obstruction of smaller airways
Residual volume (RV): Volume of air remaining in lungs at end of a maximal expiration	1.2 L	Increased up to 400% normal	Increased RV indicates obstruction
Rheumatoid factor, antinuclear antibodies	Negative	Rheumatoid factor > 30 International Unit/mL; antinuclear antibodies > 1:8	Identifies autoimmune response and connective tissue disease

Other Tests: Hemoglobin may be elevated due to chronic hypoxemia; erythrosedimentation rate may be elevated; C-reactive protein, gallium scan, serological tests, histological analysis, high-resolution computed tomography

PRIMARY NURSING DIAGNOSIS

DIAGNOSIS. Ineffective breathing pattern related to scarring and distortion of pulmonary tissue as evidenced by shortness of breath, cough, and/or dyspnea on exertion

OUTCOMES. Respiratory status: Gas exchange; Respiratory status: Ventilation; Symptom severity; Symptom control; Respiratory status; Knowledge: Disease process

INTERVENTIONS. Airway management; Anxiety reduction; Oxygen therapy; Airway suctioning; Airway insertion and stabilization; Cough enhancement; Mechanical ventilation management: Invasive and noninvasive; Respiratory monitoring

PLANNING AND IMPLEMENTATION

Collaborative

No effective treatment exists at this time. Comorbid conditions can contribute to pulmonary fibrosis and should be managed to minimize symptoms that may contribute to ineffective breathing patterns. These conditions include chronic obstructive pulmonary disease, obstructive sleep apnea, gastroesophageal reflux disease, and coronary artery disease. To relieve breathing difficulties and correct hypoxia, most physicians prescribe low-flow oxygen therapy (2–4 L/min). Bronchodilators may improve wheezing and airway obstruction. Because the current thinking is that idiopathic pulmonary fibrosis is an epithelial-fibroblastic disease, antifibrotic therapies have been developed (see Pharmacologic Highlights). Patients who do not respond to conventional therapy and whose life expectancy is less than 18 months may be candidates for lung transplantation. If cor pulmonale develops, the patient may be placed on diuretics and digitalis. Infections need to be identified and treated promptly. Pneumococcal and influenza vaccines are important. Corticosteroids have shown no benefit in randomized controlled trials and are no longer recommended for pulmonary fibrosis.

Pharmacologic Highlights

Medication or Drug Class	Dosage	Description	Rationale
Nintedanib	150 mg PO Q12 hr	Tyrosine kinase inhibitor	Blocks intracellular signals for proliferation, migration, and transformation of fibroblasts
Pirfenidone	Dose is titrated upward beginning with 267 mg PO tid ultimately to 801 mg PO tid	Antifibrotic agent	Anti-inflammatory and antifibrotic effect, reduces fibroblast proliferation and inhibits collagen synthesis

Independent

Focus on relieving respiratory difficulties and caring for the patient's emotional condition. To assist with breathing, assist the patient to attain an upright, supported position to enhance respiratory excursion. Assist the patient into a Fowler or semi-Fowler position. Provide assistance with the activities of daily living as appropriate, and help the patient conserve energy by alternating rest periods with periods of activity. Plan rest time of at least 1 hour after meals before engaging in activities. Teach the patient deep-breathing and coughing exercises. Use humidified air. Provide regular oral hygiene to combat dry mouth.

Because there is no cure for pulmonary fibrosis, dealing with a chronic debilitating disease requires many psychosocial adjustments for the patient and family members. Encourage the patient to verbalize concerns and fears. Encourage the patient to identify actions and care measures that help make the patient comfortable and relaxed. As much as possible, try to include the patient and family in decision making about care measures. Lifestyle changes for the patient may be necessary. A well-balanced diet with adequate fluid intake is important. If the patient smokes cigarettes, cigars, or pipes, smoking cessation is an essential intervention for the patient's survival. A job counseling session may be helpful if the patient needs to change occupations. If the patient is having trouble coping with role changes, counseling may be helpful. If the patient is at the end of life, a referral to hospice care is appropriate.

Evidence-Based Practice and Health Policy

Jeganathan, N., Smith, R., & Sathananthan, M. (2021). Mortality trends of idiopathic pulmonary fibrosis in the United States from 2004 through 2017. *Chest, 159,* 228–238.

• The authors aimed to determine the trends in idiopathic pulmonary fibrosis (IPF)–related mortality rates in the United States from 2004 through 2017. They used the Multiple Cause of Death Database available through the Centers for Disease Control and Prevention Web site, which contains data from all deceased U.S. residents. IPF-related deaths were identified using *International Classification of Diseases* codes and examined annual trends in age-adjusted mortality rates stratified by age, sex, race, and state of residence.

• The age-adjusted mortality decreased in both men and women, with the rate of decline three times greater in women. The overall decrease was driven by a decline in IPF-related mortality in patients younger than 85 years and in all races except White men, in whom the rate remained stable. The most common cause of death was pulmonary fibrosis.

DOCUMENTATION GUIDELINES

• Physical changes: Skin color, respiratory patterns, breath sounds, breathing difficulties, chest symmetry and excursion, pulse oximetry
• Reaction to diagnosis and coping strategies
• Frequency of oxygen use, noting liter flow and type of delivery device, activity tolerance

DISCHARGE AND HOME HEALTHCARE GUIDELINES

Teach energy conservation methods and relaxation, breathing, and coughing techniques. Explain the importance of pacing activities, avoiding strenuous activity, and providing rest periods. Teach the patient positions that can provide relief during acute episodes of dyspnea. To prevent infection, encourage the patient to receive flu and pneumococcal vaccines and to avoid crowds and people with known respiratory infections. Be sure the patient understands all medications, including the dosage, route, action, and adverse effects. If the patient is using oxygen therapy at home, teach the patient and family appropriate safety precautions. Help the patient understand the equipment and liter flow and provide information on how to obtain all the necessary equipment. Work with social services to provide for equipment in the home or referral to hospice care if appropriate.

Pulmonary Hypertension

DRG Category:	315
Mean LOS:	3.6 days
Description:	MEDICAL: Other Circulatory System Diagnoses With Complication or Comorbidity

Pulmonary hypertension is a rare disease that is diagnosed when the systolic pressure in the pulmonary artery exceeds 25 mm Hg without an identifiable cause. It is most commonly seen in preexisting pulmonary or cardiac disease but may occur (although rarely) as a primary condition when it is produced by fibrosis and thickening of the vessel intima. The World Health Organization divided pulmonary hypertension into five classifications: Group 1, Idiopathic pulmonary artery hypertension (IPAH), also known as primary PAH; Group 2, Pulmonary hypertension due to left-sided heart disease; Group 3, Pulmonary hypertension due to lung disease and hypoxemia; Group 4, Chronic thromboembolic pulmonary hypertension; and Group 5, Pulmonary hypertension with unclear origins.

IPAH occurs because of trauma to the endothelium, resulting in a series of events leading to scarring, endothelial dysfunction, and smooth muscle growth. As the pulmonary artery pressure increases, thrombosis may occur along with remodeling of the pulmonary vasculature and replacement of normal vessel structures. When hypertension in the pulmonary system (measured as pulmonary vascular resistance) is greater than the ability of the right side of the heart to pump, the cardiac output falls and may cause shock. Other complications include cardiac dysrhythmias, thromboembolic phenomenon, and palpitations.

CAUSES

The cause of IPAH is unknown, but the disease tends to occur in families. Secondary pulmonary hypertension is caused by conditions that produce hypoxemia, such as chronic obstructive pulmonary disease (COPD), obesity, alveolar hypoventilation, smoke inhalation, and high altitude. Associated diseases include connective-tissue diseases, thyroid disease, liver cirrhosis, stimulant abuse, and HIV disease. Risk factors are family history, high altitude, substance abuse, obstructive sleep apnea, systemic lupus erythematosus, pregnancy, and COPD.

GENETIC CONSIDERATIONS

IPAH typically shows an autosomal dominant mode of inheritance with reduced penetrance and is more common in women than in men. Autosomal recessive transmission has also been documented. When pulmonary hypertension is inherited, it demonstrates the genetic concept of anticipation, where subsequent generations often have severe cases of the disease. IPAH is also seen in conjunction with other genetic problems, such as hereditary hemorrhagic telangiectasia type 2, caused by mutations in the type III receptor *ENG*. Mutations in the *BMPR2* gene are the most common genetic cause of IPAH and are also associated with sporadic forms of the disease. Other gene mutations that have been demonstrated to cause autosomal dominant familial IPAH are the caveolin 1 gene (*CAV1*) and the two-pore potassium channel (*KCNK3*).

SEX AND LIFE SPAN CONSIDERATIONS

Groups 2 and 3 pulmonary hypertension are most commonly seen in the older person with cardiac or pulmonary disease. They may occur at any age, however. IPAH tends to occur more often in women between ages 20 to 40 years; women are also more likely than men to be symptomatic. Estrogens and estrogen metabolites may play a role in the pathophysiology of the condition, increasing the risk for women. Both women and men with IPAH have a shortened life span. Congenital causes may lead to occurrence in the pediatric population.

HEALTH DISPARITIES AND SEXUAL/GENDER MINORITY HEALTH

Black and White persons have similar rates of IPAH. Outcome studies have shown that people with IPAH without private health insurance or on Medicaid have higher mortality rates than those with private health insurance, creating a health disparity for those without coverage (Parikh et al., 2017). HIV is considered a risk factor for the development of IPAH. The CDC reported in 2018 that 69% of new HIV diagnoses in the United States were in gay and bisexual men. In young people ages 13 to 24 years, young gay and bisexual men account for 83% of all new HIV diagnoses. Therefore, they are a group that is at risk for IPAH.

GLOBAL HEALTH CONSIDERATIONS

The global incidence rate is approximately two to six cases per 1 million individuals per year. Pulmonary hypertension exists around the globe at approximately the same incidence as in the United States.

ASSESSMENT

HISTORY. Patients are usually without symptoms until late in the disease. Up to 50% of the pulmonary circulation may be impaired before significant hypertension is produced. Determine the presence of risk factors. Ask if the patient has experienced chest pain, labored and painful breathing (dyspnea), fatigue, or syncope. Some patients have sleep disturbance, possibly from dyspnea. Occasionally, the enlarged pulmonary artery compresses the left recurrent laryngeal nerve, producing hoarseness. Some patients may describe periods of heart palpitations. Ask about other comorbid conditions such as HIV disease and connective tissue disease.

PHYSICAL EXAMINATION. Signs of right ventricular failure are common, such as **dyspnea, weakness,** and **recurrent syncope likely accompanied by jugular venous distention, increased central venous pressure,** and **peripheral edema.** Low cardiac output may produce central cyanosis, fatigue, syncope, or chest pain. Auscultation of the heart may therefore reveal atrial gallop at the lower left sternal border, narrow splitting of S_2 or increased S_2 intensity, or ejection click at the second intercostal space, left sternal border. A murmur from tricuspid regurgitation may be present. When palpating the precordium, you may detect a heave over the right ventricle or an impulse from the pulmonary artery itself. Signs of left ventricular failure, such as systemic hypotension (low blood pressure) and low urinary output, may coexist. Presentation may include hyperventilation, coughing, and eventually rapid breathing (tachypnea) or dyspnea. Initially, breath sounds may be clear or decreased, but you may hear crackles or wheezing.

PSYCHOSOCIAL. The patient is experiencing a potentially life-threatening condition that requires the use of complex medical technology. Assess the anxiety level of the patient and plan interventions to place a minimum demand on the patient's energy. Support of the patient is essential throughout hospitalization, from routine care such as placement and maintenance of the pulmonary artery catheter to attempts at averting a cardiac arrest.

Diagnostic Highlights

Test	Normal Result	Abnormality With Condition	Explanation
Echocardiogram	Normal lung structures and circulation	Right-to-left shunting across a patent foramen ovale (occurs in approximately 33% of patients with pulmonary hypertension)	Estimate ventricular functioning; pulmonary hypertension may occur because of right-to-left shunting
Pulmonary artery pressure and pulmonary vascular resistance (PVR) (measurements made with a pulmonary artery catheter)	Systolic: 15–20 mm Hg; diastolic: 8–15 mm Hg; PVR: 180–285 dynes/sec per cm^{-5} per m^2	Pressures elevated, with systolic pressure < 25 mm Hg; pulmonary artery systolic pressure may approach systemic arterial pressure	Sustained elevation of pulmonary vascular pressures

Other Tests: Antinuclear antibody to exclude autoimmune disorders, thyrotropin, HIV testing, antinuclear antibody, pulmonary function tests, exercise testing, electrocardiogram, ventilation perfusion scan, pulmonary angiogram, chest x-rays, echocardiogram, high-resolution computed tomography, genetic testing

PRIMARY NURSING DIAGNOSIS

DIAGNOSIS. Impaired gas exchange related to changes in the alveolar membrane structure and increased pulmonary vascular resistance as evidenced by dyspnea on exertion, fatigue, weakness, and/or syncope

OUTCOMES. Respiratory status: Gas exchange; Respiratory status: Ventilation; Cardiopulmonary status; Vital signs; Knowledge: Disease process; Anxiety control

INTERVENTIONS. Airway insertion and stabilization; Airway management; Respiratory monitoring; Oxygen therapy; Mechanical ventilation; Anxiety reduction; Teaching: Disease Process

▓ PLANNING AND IMPLEMENTATION

Collaborative

IPAH has limited therapy, and patients tend to have hemodynamic deterioration in spite of therapy. The median survival rate after diagnosis is 2.5 years. Supportive measures include supplemental oxygen for people who are hypoxemic and the use of diuretics in people who are fluid-overloaded. Relief of hypoxemia helps reduce pulmonary vasoconstriction. If the origin of the problem is structural, surgery may be attempted. A single or double lung transplant may be recommended for patients who are unresponsive to medical treatment. Heart-lung transplantation may be a consideration for severe conditions.

Pharmacologic Highlights

Medication or Drug Class	Dosage	Description	Rationale
Diuretics	Varies by drug	Loop diuretics, thiazide diuretics	Reduce both right and left ventricular failure
Sodium warfarin (Coumadin)	5 mg PO initially, guided by coagulation studies	Anticoagulant	Prevents microvascular thrombosis, venous stasis, and limitation of physical activity
Vasodilators	Varies by drug	Nitrates; calcium channel blockers; prostacyclin analogs: Epoprostenol (Flolan), treprostinil (Remodulin), iloprost (Ventavis); endothelin antagonists: bosentan (Tracleer), ambrisentan (Letairis)	Improve muscle tone in pulmonary vascular bed and reduce right ventricular workload
PAH-specific therapies	Varies by drug	Epoprostenol, treprostinil, iloprost, sildenafil, tadalafil, riociguat, macitentan	Promotes selective smooth muscle relaxation

Other Drugs: Bronchodilators to improve hypoxemia and reduce pulmonary vascular resistance (note that use of vasodilators is limited because it may produce systemic hypotension); oral prostacyclin (PG12) treprostinil extended-release tablets to cause vasodilation. Other prostaglandin-related medications are selexipag and bosentan.

Independent

If the patient is critically ill, to minimize the risk of infection, use the sterile technique during setup and maintenance of the pulmonary artery catheter. Dressings should be changed according to policy, usually every 72 hours. Ask the patient to evaluate chest pain using a scale from 1 to 10 and provide comfort measures in addition to any ordered medication. Reduce energy demands by assisting the patient to a position of comfort, such as the semi-Fowler or Fowler position. Document pulmonary artery catheter readings and report significant changes to the medical team. Monitor the patient for the development of cardiac dysrhythmias.

Allow the patient to verbalize fears and assist in the development of a realistic perception as the patient appears ready. Because this is a disease that may affect young women in their 20s and 30s, consider the effects on their lifetime goals. Family considerations, especially if the patient is the parent of young children, require sensitivity and possible referral. Incorporate family members and other support system members as appropriate. Help the patient adjust to the limitations imposed by this disorder. Advise against overexertion during acute illnesses, but after recovery mild aerobic activity and exercise training are recommended. The patient may need diversionary activities during periods of restricted activity. Low sodium and low fluid diet is recommended. Be sure the patient understands dietary limitations and medication regimens.

Evidence-Based Practice and Health Policy

Medrek, S., Sahay, S., Zhao, C., Selej, M., & Frost, A. (2020). Impact of race on survival in pulmonary arterial hypertension: Results from the REVEAL registry. *Journal of Heart and Lung Transplantation*, *39*, 321–330.

- The authors aimed to evaluate the relationships among race, ethnicity, and survival in a large U.S.-based registry of people ($N = 3,046$) with PAH. Baseline hemodynamic and clinical characteristics as well as medication use were described.
- White patients had the lowest survival rates, and Black patients were more likely to have connective tissue disease–associated PAH. Hispanic patients were more likely to have portopulmonary hypertension, and Asian patients were more likely to have congenital heart disease–associated PAH. However, the authors did not find that race and ethnicity were significant predictors of mortality in people with PAH.

DOCUMENTATION GUIDELINES

- Vital signs, including pulmonary artery catheter readings
- Cardiovascular and pulmonary physical assessment data, including breath and heart sounds as noted in previous sections, response to exercise training
- Responses to therapies and disease status, including medication, diet, fluids, oxygen administration, and psychological/family coping

DISCHARGE AND HOME HEALTHCARE GUIDELINES

Risk for recurrent pulmonary embolism can be reduced by teaching the patient to minimize hypercoagulability, to reduce venous stasis, and to control risk factors such as obesity. Teach the patient to drink 2,000 mL of fluid a day unless restricted, to rest between activities, and to avoid overexertion. Teach the patient about the prescribed dosage, route, action, and follow-up laboratory work needed for all medications. If the patient is discharged on potassium-wasting diuretics, encourage a diet that is rich in high-potassium foods, such as apricots, bananas, oranges, and raw vegetables. The patient may also need instruction on a low-sodium diet. If the patient needs home oxygen, instruct the patient and significant others in oxygen use and oxygen safety. Arrange with social services for the delivery of oxygen equipment. If the patient smokes, teach strategies for smoking cessation or provide a referral for smoking-cessation programs. Assess the family situation and the effects of a chronic and debilitating disease that will affect occupational goals, child care, role fulfillment, and long-term health.

Pyelonephritis

DRG Category:	689
Mean LOS:	4.8 days
Description:	MEDICAL: Kidney and Urinary Tract Infections With Major Complication or Comorbidity

Pyelonephritis is an inflammation of the renal pelvis and of the renal tissue; it is caused by an invasion of microorganisms. More than 250,000 cases are diagnosed each year in the United States, and approximately 200,000 hospitalizations result. The cost of pyelonephritis is estimated to exceed $2 billion each year. It can be either acute (also known as *acute infective tubulointerstitial nephritis*) or chronic in nature, as differentiated by the clinical picture and long-term effects. The infection, which primarily affects the renal pelvis, calyces, and medulla, progresses through the urinary tract as organisms ascend the ureters from the bladder because of vesicoureteral reflux (reflux of urine up the ureter during micturition) or contamination.

Acute pyelonephritis occurs within 24 to 48 hours after contamination of the urethra or after instrumentation such as a catheterization. Acute pyelonephritis is potentially life threatening and often causes scarring of the kidney with each infection. Complications include calculus formation, renal abscesses, renal failure, septic shock, and chronic pyelonephritis. Chronic pyelonephritis is a persistent infection that causes progressive inflammation and scarring. It usually occurs after chronic obstruction or because of vesicoureteral reflux. This destruction of renal cells may alter the urine-concentrating capability of the kidney and can lead to acute kidney injury or chronic renal failure or conditions such as sepsis and septic shock.

CAUSES

The causative organisms are usually bacteria but can be fungi or viruses. Patients with diabetes, hypertension, chronic renal calculi, chronic cystitis, and congenital or abnormal urinary tract, and pregnant persons are more likely to acquire pyelonephritis than other groups. *Escherichia coli* is responsible for 90% of the episodes in a normal anatomic urinary tract system. *Proteus*, *Klebsiella*, and occasionally gram-positive cocci account for the rest. People with structural and functional abnormalities of the urinary tract, metabolic abnormalities such as diabetes mellitus, pregnancy, recent antibiotic use, and recent urinary tract instrumentation are at risk for pyelonephritis.

GENETIC CONSIDERATIONS

While no clear genetic determinants are known, a family history of urinary tract infections (UTIs) may increase the risk for pyelonephritis, especially among young women.

SEX AND LIFE SPAN CONSIDERATIONS

Pyelonephritis occurs more often in women than in men because the female urethra is much shorter than the male urethra. The incidence of pyelonephritis is highest in females, particularly adolescent and young adult females between the ages of 15 and 35 years who are sexually active and/or pregnant. Men, however, are more susceptible if they have an obstruction from prostatic hypertrophy, cancer, urinary stones, or urethral stenosis and may have more insidious symptoms than women. Pyelonephritis is also seen in older men with indwelling catheters. Both men and women over age 65 years have a higher risk of mortality than their younger counterparts.

HEALTH DISPARITIES AND SEXUAL/GENDER MINORITY HEALTH

Ethnicity and race have no known effect on the risk for pyelonephritis. Men who have unprotected anal sexual intercourse are at risk for a UTI, which may progress to pyelonephritis.

GLOBAL HEALTH CONSIDERATIONS

While pyelonephritis occurs in all countries around the globe, no international prevalence statistics are available. Some evidence suggests that the incidence is higher in regions with warm temperatures.

ASSESSMENT

HISTORY. Determine if the patient has experienced fever, pain, dysuria, frequency, and urgency (signs of an irritative urinary tract) before seeking care. Ask if the patient is voiding in small amounts or experiencing nocturia. It is important to determine if these symptoms are a change from the patient's usual voiding patterns. Ask for a description of the urine, which may be foul smelling, cloudy, or bloody; gross hematuria is present in approximately 40% of women seeking care. Elicit a description of pain or discomfort, which usually occurs in the flank, groin, or suprapubic areas. Also question the patient about any flu-like symptoms, such as malaise, nausea, vomiting, chills, headache, and fatigue. The pain may radiate down the ureter toward the epigastrium and may be colicky if it is associated with a renal calculus. Discuss the patient's sexual history and practices to determine if they contribute to the infection.

PHYSICAL EXAMINATION. The most common symptoms are **fever, costovertebral angle pain, nausea and vomiting**, and **hematuria**. Not all of these signs may be present. If you suspect acute pyelonephritis, determine if the patient is febrile. Inspect the urine for color, cloudiness, blood, or presence of a foul odor. Percussion or deep palpation over the costovertebral angle (located on the back, it is the angle between the 12th rib and the spine, directly over the kidney) elicits marked tenderness. Lower urinary tract symptoms are absent in approximately 15% of women. Flank pain, tenderness, and fever may also be absent. In chronic pyelonephritis, the early symptoms are minimal. Assess the blood pressure because often these patients present with hypertension. There may be irritating urinary tract symptoms, but they are milder in nature than in acute pyelonephritis.

PSYCHOSOCIAL. To prevent permanent kidney damage, acute and chronic pyelonephritis need to be diagnosed promptly and treated appropriately. Assess the patients' ability to care for themselves, as well as their learning capabilities, support systems, financial resources, and access to healthcare. Identify and alleviate barriers to ensure a prompt, efficient plan of care to help the patient regain a sense of wellness.

Diagnostic Highlights

Test	Normal Result	Abnormality With Condition	Explanation
Urine culture and sensitivity	Negative cultures	Presence of bacteria	Identifies bacterial contaminants; most common is E coli
Urinalysis	Minimal red and white blood cells; moderate clear protein casts; negative for protein	Pyuria, leukocyte castes	Shows the presence of white blood cells and pus

Other Tests: Blood cultures; complete blood count; x-ray of kidney, ureter, bladder; blood urea nitrogen; creatinine; renal ultrasound; IV pyelogram; cystourethrogram; contrast enhanced helical/spiral computed tomography (imaging study of choice if the symptoms are insidious or if the patient has HIV disease, poorly controlled diabetes, or is immunosuppressed). Imaging may also be completed if fever persists or the patient's condition worsens.

PRIMARY NURSING DIAGNOSIS

DIAGNOSIS. Risk for infection (urinary tract) as evidenced by fever, pain, nausea, vomiting, and/or hematuria

OUTCOMES. Immune status; Infection severity; Knowledge: Infection management; Knowledge: Disease process; Symptom severity; Symptom control; Pain level

INTERVENTIONS. Infection control; Infection protection; Medication prescribing; Medication administration; Pain management: Acute

PLANNING AND IMPLEMENTATION

Collaborative

If patients are ambulatory and have uncomplicated pyelonephritis, they may be treated as outpatients. Hospitalization is usually reserved for patients who are severely ill, pregnant, with comorbidities, or frail. The goal of therapy is to rid the urinary tract of the pathogenic organisms and to relieve an obstruction if present. The antibiotics chosen depend on the urine culture and sensitivity. Urinary catheterization is used only when absolutely necessary. Oral or parenteral fluids are needed to manage fever and dehydration. Surgery is performed only if an underlying defect is causing obstruction, reflux, calculi, or an abscess. Hypertension is common in patients with chronic pyelonephritis and needs to be controlled with medication. In addition, supportive care is important. If the cause of pyelonephritis is renal calculi, dietary management, such as limiting calcium, oxalate, or purines, may be necessary.

Pharmacologic Highlights

Medication or Drug Class	Dosage	Description	Rationale
Antibiotics	Varies by drug; generally parenteral antibiotics for 3–5 days until the patient is afebrile for 24–48 hr, followed by oral administration for 2–4 wk	Depends on urine culture and sensitivity; common drugs include ciprofloxacin (Cipro), levofloxacin (Levaquin), ceftriaxone (Rocephin), cefaclor, ceftazidime, gentamicin, ampicillin, vancomycin, trimethoprim, sulfamethoxazole trimethoprim/sulfamethoxazole; (Bactrim), and amoxicillin-clavulanate potassium	Eradicate bacteria and maintain adequate blood levels; provide accurate results in serum peak and trough levels

Other Drugs: Most patients are admitted with nausea and vomiting, and the physician may prescribe IV fluids to balance hydration. Patients are given analgesics, antipyretics, and antiemetics to control pain, fever, and nausea. Urinary analgesics such as phenazopyridine (Pyridium) may be administered.

Independent

Provide comfort measures for the patient with flank pain, headache, and irritating urinary tract symptoms. Back rubs may provide some relief of flank pain. Sitz baths may provide some relief if perineal discomfort is present. It is helpful to use a pain management flowsheet and alternative distractions and comfort measures (massage, music, positioning, verbal support, imagery). Because the patient is usually febrile, employ measures that promote heat reduction (cool packs, limited bedding, cool room temperature). To promote nutrition and adequate fluid balance, ask for the patient's fluid preferences. Encourage the patient to drink at least 2,000 mL/day to help empty the bladder and to prevent calculus formation but not more than 4,000 mL/day, which would dilute the antibiotic concentration and lessen its effectiveness. Initiate measures to ensure complete emptying of the bladder, such as running water or spraying the perineum with warm water. Ensure the patient's privacy during voiding.

Teach women in the high-risk groups strategies to limit reinfection. Encourage the patient to clean the perineum by wiping from the front to the back after bowel movements. Encourage men who have sex with men to have protected anal sexual intercourse. Stress the need for frequent hand washing. Explain the need for routine checkups if the patient experiences frequent UTIs. Encourage patients to notify the physician if they note cloudy urine, burning on urination, and urinary frequency or urgency.

Evidence-Based Practice and Health Policy

Kim, B., Myung, R., Kim, G., Lee, M., Kim, J., & Pai, H. (2020). Diabetes mellitus increases mortality in acute pyelonephritis patients: A population study based on the National Health Insurance Claim Data of South Korea for 2010–2014. *Infection, 48*, 435–443.

- Diabetes mellitus has been suspected to increase mortality in people with acute pyelonephritis (APN). As such, the authors sought to determine whether data from a nation-wide sample in South Korea supported the association. They analyzed demographic and clinical information including comorbidities of patients with APN and compared the in-hospital mortality and recurrence of APN across a diabetes group ($N = 105,085$) and nondiabetes group ($N = 740,571$).
- The mean age of the diabetes group was 65 years and the nondiabetes group was 47 years. Approximately 90% of the cases in both groups were female. The in-hospital mortality rate was higher in the diabetes group. The authors concluded that mortality of patients with APN is higher than those without diabetes, and this effect becomes stronger for young patients.

DOCUMENTATION GUIDELINES

- Physical appearance of urine: Cloudy, bloody, or malodorous
- Presence of flank or perineal pain, duration of pain, frequency of pain, response of pain to interventions
- Presence of dysuria; frequency and urgency of urination
- Presence of complications: Increasing blood urea nitrogen and creatinine, unresolved infection, urinary tract obstruction, uncontrolled pain or fever

DISCHARGE AND HOME HEALTHCARE GUIDELINES

Instruct the patient on ways to reduce the risk of subsequent infections: Increase fluid intake to 2,000 to 3,000 mL/day to wash the bacteria out of the bladder; avoid caffeine and alcohol; drink juices that acidify the urine (cranberry, plum, and prune); void at the first urge and at least every 2 to 3 hours during the day to prevent bladder distention; void immediately and drink two glasses of water as soon as possible after sexual intercourse; and practice good perineal hygiene (wipe labia from front to back).

Explain to the patient that the entire prescription of antibiotics should be taken even if the patient feels better. Emphasize the importance of following the special instructions that accompany the antibiotic. Emphasize the importance of follow-up urine cultures and examinations. Note that recurrent infection may require prolonged antibiotic therapy.

Respiratory Distress Syndrome, Acute

DRG Category:	189
Mean LOS:	4.6 days
Description:	MEDICAL: Pulmonary Edema and Respiratory Failure
DRG Category:	207
Mean LOS:	13.9 days
Description:	MEDICAL: Respiratory System Diagnosis With Ventilator Support > 96 Hours
DRG Category:	208
Mean LOS:	6.7 days
Description:	MEDICAL: Respiratory System Diagnosis With Ventilator Support ≤ 96 Hours
DRG Category:	3
Mean LOS:	30.3 days
Description:	SURGICAL: ECMO or Tracheostomy With Mechanical Ventilation > 96 Hours or Principal Diagnosis Except for Face, Mouth, and Neck With Major Operating Room Procedures

The term adult respiratory distress syndrome was first coined by Ashbaugh and Petty in 1969. Since World War I, terms such as stiff lung, wet lung, shock lung, adult hyaline-membrane disease, and others were used to describe the acute respiratory distress that occurs after catastrophic events such as major surgical procedures, serious injuries, or other inflammatory conditions such as severe pancreatitis. In 1992, the American-European Consensus Conference on ARDS recommended changing the name back to what Ashbaugh and Petty originally named it, *acute respiratory distress syndrome* (ARDS), because this condition affects children, teenagers, and adults.

ARDS, the most severe form of acute lung injury, is defined as noncardiogenic pulmonary edema that occurs despite low to normal pressures in the pulmonary capillaries. Patients with ARDS are characterized as having high-permeability pulmonary edema (HPPE) in contrast to cardiogenic pulmonary edema. They have bilateral pulmonary infiltrates and severe hypoxemia, but these changes are not due to heart failure. In ARDS, the alveolar-capillary membrane is damaged, and both fluid and protein leak into the interstitial space and alveoli. Recent research has focused on likely mediators of capillary endothelial damage, such as the proteins released during the inflammatory process, including tumor necrosis factor (TNF), leukotrienes, and macrophage inhibitory factor. Other contributors include bacterial toxins and oxygen free radicals, among others. Recent research suggests that the use of positive pressure ventilation may promote the development of ARDS by causing ventilator-assisted lung injury. The onset of symptoms generally occurs within 24 to 72 hours of the original injury or illness.

As ARDS progresses, patients exhibit decreased lung volumes, markedly decreased lung compliance, and diffuse alveolar damage. Type II pneumocytes, the cells responsible for surfactant production, are damaged. This deficiency is thought to be partly responsible for the alveolar collapse and the decrease in lung volumes that occur. In addition, fibroblasts proliferate in the alveolar wall, migrate into the intra-alveolar fluid, and ultimately convert the exudate (fluid with high concentration of protein and cellular debris) into fibrous tissue. Refractory hypoxemia occurs as the lungs are perfused but not ventilated (a condition called capillary shunting) owing to the damage to the alveoli and developing fibrosis. As ARDS progresses, respiratory failure and cardiopulmonary arrest can develop. Complications include pneumothorax, infection, ventilator-associated pneumonia, inadequate nutrition, hemorrhage, and deep vein thrombosis.

CAUSES

Although approximately 20% of patients who develop ARDS do not have risk factors identified, many conditions can predispose a patient to ARDS. These conditions represent a sudden catastrophic situation and can be classified into two categories: direct lung injury and indirect lung injury. Direct injury occurs from situations such as gastric aspiration, near drowning, chemical inhalation, and oxygen toxicity. Indirect injury occurs from mediators released during sepsis, multiple trauma, thermal injury, pancreatitis, hypoperfusion or hemorrhagic shock, disseminated intravascular coagulation, drug overdose, and massive blood transfusions. The novel coronavirus 2019 disease (COVID-19) leads to severe acute respiratory syndrome and ARDS due to indirect injury. The most common risk factor for ARDS is sepsis from an abdominal source and most are associated with pneumonia. Approximately 200,000 new cases of ARDS occur each year in the United States, and it is responsible for one in 10 admissions to intensive care units. Mortality rates vary and have been estimated to be between 30% and 40%, but older patients and patients with severe infections have a higher rate. Survivors generally have almost normal lung function a year after the acute illness.

GENETIC CONSIDERATIONS

While there are no single mutations that have been identified to cause ARDS, there are genetic factors that influence both the susceptibility and progression of ARDS. Survivors are more likely than nonsurvivors to have certain alleles of the genes that code for angiotensin-converting enzyme (ACE) and interleukin (*IL6*). Other genes implicated in ARDS are those involved in vascular injury response (*VEGFA, ANGPT2, MYLK*) and innate immune response (*IRAK3, TLR1, NFKB1, NFKBIA, FAS, PI3*).

SEX AND LIFE SPAN CONSIDERATIONS

ARDS can occur at any age, including during childhood, to those who have been subjected to severe physiological stresses such as sepsis, burns, or trauma. As of January 2021, 93% of patients who died from COVID-19 in the United States were 55 years of age or older. People over 70 years of age have a higher incidence and rate of mortality than younger persons.

HEALTH DISPARITIES AND SEXUAL/GENDER MINORITY HEALTH

Some authorities have reported that in female patients, ARDS related to trauma may have a higher incidence than in males. Following traumatic injury, Black patients have a higher risk of developing ARDS than White patients. Uninsured patients have a higher risk of developing ARDS and dying from ARDS than patients with private insurance (Chou et al., 2021). During the first year of the COVID-19 pandemic, Hispanic people had a disproportionately high number of people who died compared to other groups (Centers for Disease Control and Prevention, 2021). Sexual and gender minority status has no known effect on the risk for ARDS.

GLOBAL HEALTH CONSIDERATIONS

People who live in developing countries without well-developed emergency medical systems may not survive the initial insult (trauma, sepsis, burns), and therefore, ARDS may not occur. If critical care is not available to manage ARDS, mortality will be very high. In Europe, investigators have reported an incidence of 18 cases per 100,000 individuals for acute lung injury and 14 cases per 100,000 individuals for ARDS.

⬛ ASSESSMENT

HISTORY. The patient with ARDS appears in acute respiratory distress with a marked **increase in the work of breathing** that may lead to **nasal flaring**, the **use of accessory muscles** to breathe, and profound diaphoresis. The respiratory rate may be more than 30 to 40 breaths per minute. If ARDS has progressed, the patient may have a dusky appearance with cyanosis around the lips and nailbeds, or the patient may be very pale. **Hypoxemia** usually leads to **restlessness, confusion, agitation**, and even combative behavior.

PHYSICAL EXAMINATION. Palpation of the peripheral pulses reveals rapid, sometimes thready, pulses. Body temperature may be elevated, normal, or low. Blood pressure may be normal or elevated initially and then decreased in the later stages. Auscultation of the lungs differs depending on the stage of ARDS. In the early stage, the lungs have decreased breath sounds. In the middle stages of ARDS, the patient may have basilar crackles or even coarse crackles. In the late stage of ARDS, if the disease has been left untreated, the patient may have bronchial breath sounds or little gas exchange with no breath sounds. If airway and breathing are not maintained, the patient becomes fatigued and apneic. When the patient is intubated and mechanically ventilated, the lungs may sound extremely congested, with wheezes and coarse crackles throughout.

Diagnosis involves excluding other causes of acute respiratory failure. A consensus conference has defined ARDS as having the following features: acute (within 1 week of clinical insult or onset of respiratory symptoms) bilateral lung infiltrates on x-ray not fully explained by effusions, consolidations, or lung collapse; noncardiac edema; and severity determined by the ratio of Pao_2 to inspired oxygen concentration (Fio_2) when the patient is on at least 5 cm H_2O of positive end-expiratory pressure (PEEP) or continuous positive airway pressure (CPAP). Three categories of ARDS severity are mild (ratio = 200–300), moderate (ratio = 100–200), and severe (ratio of ≥ 100).

PSYCHOSOCIAL. Patients may exhibit anxiety and fear because of hypoxemia and the real threat of death. Feelings of social isolation and powerlessness can occur as the patient is placed on mechanical ventilation and is unable to verbalize. Pain relief and sedation are essential for patient comfort (see Pharmacologic Highlights). The family and significant others will exhibit anxiety, fear, and significant concern.

Diagnostic Highlights

General Comments: The diagnosis of ARDS can be controversial and is one of exclusion. There are no specific markers that identify alveolar-capillary membrane damage. Early in ARDS, the pH is elevated and the $Paco_2$ is decreased because of hyperventilation. In the later stages, the $Paco_2$ is elevated, and the pH is decreased. Other supporting tests include pulmonary function tests, pulse oximetry, and pulmonary artery catheters with measurement of capillary wedge pressures to guide fluid balance. Computed tomography is more sensitive than routine chest radiography but may not be needed and may present safety issues if the patient is unstable. Supporting tests to evaluate organ systems include complete blood count, electrolytes, renal and hepatic function tests, and cytokine levels. Echocardiogram and electrocardiogram may be included to the work-up to assess cardiac function.

Test	Normal Result	Abnormality With Condition	Explanation
Chest x-ray	Clear lung fields	Diffuse bilateral infiltrates without cardiomegaly or pulmonary vascular redistribution	Findings reflect noncardiogenic pulmonary edema

(highlight box continues on page 1050)

Diagnostic Highlights (continued)

Test	Normal Result	Abnormality With Condition	Explanation
Arterial blood gases (ABGs)	Pao_2 80–95 mm Hg; $Paco_2$ 35–45 mm Hg; SaO_2 > 95%	Pao_2 < 80 mm Hg; $Paco_2$ varies; SaO_2 < 95%	Poor gas exchange leads to hypoxemia and, as respiratory failure progresses, to hypercapnea. When the $Paco_2$ is divided by the Fio_2, the result is 200 or less.

PRIMARY NURSING DIAGNOSIS

DIAGNOSIS. Impaired gas exchange related to increased alveolar-capillary permeability, interstitial edema, and decreased lung compliance as evidenced by abnormal ABGs, dyspnea, abnormal breathing pattern, confusion, hypoxemia, and/or irritability

OUTCOMES. Respiratory status: Gas Exchange; Respiratory status: Ventilation; Respiratory status: Airway patency; Symptom severity; Fluid balance; Comfort status: Physical; Anxiety level

INTERVENTIONS. Airway insertion and stabilization; Airway management; Respiratory monitoring; Oxygen therapy; Mechanical ventilation management; Anxiety reduction; Fluid management

PLANNING AND IMPLEMENTATION
Collaborative

MECHANICAL VENTILATION. The treatment for ARDS is directed toward the underlying cause and maintaining gas exchange to maintain the arterial oxygen saturation 88% to 95%, the PaO_2 of 55 to 80 mm Hg, and the arterial pH 7.30 to 7.50. To this end, almost all patients with ARDS require endotracheal intubation and mechanical ventilation with a variety of positive-pressure modes and low tidal volumes (6 mL/kg of ideal body weight). Common methods for mechanical ventilation include pressure-controlled ventilation with an inverse inspiratory-expiratory ratio. This mode alters the standard inspiratory-expiratory ratio of 1:2 to 1:3 by prolonging the inspiratory rate and changing the ratio to 1:1 or even higher. It also controls the amount of pressure in each breath to stabilize the alveoli and to reestablish the functional residual capacity (FRC) to normal levels. If possible, the physician attempts to limit the fraction of inspired oxygen (Fio_2) to less than 0.50 (50%) to reduce complications from oxygen toxicity. PEEP is often added to the ventilator settings to increase the FRC and to augment gas exchange. Lung-protective, pressure-targeted ventilation, a method whereby controlled hypoventilation is allowed to occur, minimizes the detrimental effects of excessive airway pressures and has also been used in ARDS with positive outcomes.

Another strategy includes improving oxygenation by turning patients from the supine to a prone position, with care to keep all tubes and IV devices intact. Prone positioning should occur in 16-hour sessions, followed by 8 hours in supine position, and should be initiated within 48 hours of the onset of severe ARDS with refractory hypoxemia. Experts continue to debate the best fluid management strategies for patients with ARDS. Aggressive fluid resuscitation may be needed in the early stages, particularly in septic shock patients, but as the condition evolves, a neutral fluid balance may be associated with improved outcomes. Nutrition support, generally with enteral nutrition delivered by a feeding tube, is recommended after 48 hours of the start of mechanical ventilation. A serious consideration is missing a treatable underlying cause of ARDS, so an ongoing search for infection is part of management.

Pharmacologic Highlights

General Comments: Use of genetically engineered surfactant has been studied in ARDS but has not demonstrated the success that has occurred in premature infants with surfactant deficiency. Although high- and low-dose corticosteroids have been used in ARDS, studies have not demonstrated improvement in patient outcomes, and their use remains controversial. Simvastatin, a hydroxymethylglutaryl-coenzyme A reductase inhibitor, may improve oxygenation and respiratory mechanics in some patients. While inhaled nitric oxide may improve oxygenation, its administration has not improved survival rates. Short-acting nonopioid analgesics (ketamine), short-acting opioid analgesics (fentanyl, sufentanil, remifentanil), or sedatives (dexmedetomidine) may be added to the treatment plan below for pain and sedation.

Medication or Drug Class	Dosage	Description	Rationale
Neuromuscular blocking agents: Vecuronium (Norcuron), rocuronium (Zemuron), atracurium (Tracrium), cisatracurium (Nimbex)	Dosage varies with drug	Increases chest wall compliance and minimizes the work of breathing	Used to paralyze the skeletal muscles when patients are difficult to ventilate with poor gas exchange; must be used with analgesics and sedation
Propofol (Diprivan)	0.005 mg/kg/min IV for 5 min, then titrated to desired clinical effect. Can be increased by 5–10 mcg/kg/min over 5- to 10-min intervals IV to desired clinical effect. Maintenance: 0.005–0.05 mg/kg/min IV	General anesthetic	To sedate the patient to decrease work of breathing and decrease stress of the intensive care unit and mechanical ventilation experience

Independent

To augment gas exchange, the patient needs endotracheal suctioning periodically. Prior to suctioning, hyperventilate and hyperoxygenate the patient to prevent the ill effects of suctioning, such as cardiac dysrhythmias or hypotension. Turn the patient as often as possible, even every hour, to increase ventilation and perfusion to all areas of the lung. If the patient has particularly poor gas exchange, consider a rocking bed that constantly changes the patient's position. Placing patients in prone position, which may improve oxygenation, requires significant expertise to keep the patient safe and maintain the ventilator connections. Experts suggest that the patient be placed in the prone position for 16 hours/day and supine for 8 hours/day. As the patient improves, get patients out of bed for brief periods, even if they are intubated and on a ventilator.

If the patient requires neuromuscular blocking agents for skeletal muscle paralysis, provide complete care and make sure the medical management includes sedation. Use artificial tears to moisten the patient's eyes because the patient loses the blink reflex. Provide passive range-of-motion exercises every 8 hours to prevent contractures. Reposition the patient at least every 2 hours for comfort and adequate gas exchange and to prevent skin breakdown. Provide complete hygiene, including mouth care, as needed. Assist the patient to conserve oxygen and limit oxygen consumption by spacing all activities, limiting interruptions to enhance rest, and providing a quiet environment.

The patient and family are likely to be fearful and anxious. Acknowledge their fear without providing false reassurance. Explain the critical care environment and technology, but emphasize the importance of the patient's humanness over and above the technology. Maintain open communication among all involved. Answer all questions and provide methods for the patient and family to communicate, such as a magic slate or point board.

Evidence-Based Practice and Health Policy

Ding, L., Wang, L., Wanhong, M., & He, H. (2020). Efficacy and safety of early prone positioning combined with HFNC or NIV in moderate or severe ARDS: A multi-center prospective cohort study. *Critical Care, 24*, 2738–2745.

- Prone position can improve oxygenation and reduce mortality in ARDS. The authors studied patients with the early use of prone position in two groups of patients: those with noninvasive ventilation or high-flow nasal cannula. The outcome measure was endotracheal intubation rate.
- Two hospitals served as study sites, where the authors enrolled 20 moderately to severely ill patients with ARDS. Eleven patients did not require intubation (major outcome variable).
- Seven of the intubated patients with low oxygenation had noninvasive ventilation. Early application of prone position with high-flow nasal cannula in patients with moderate ARDS may help prevent endotracheal intubation.

DOCUMENTATION GUIDELINES

- Respiratory status of the patient: respiratory rate, breath sounds, and the use of accessory muscles; ABG levels; pulse oximeter and chest x-ray results
- Response to treatment, mechanical ventilation, immobility, prone position, and bedrest
- Response to medications, level of pain, level of consciousness, level of anxiety
- Presence of any complications (depends on the precipitating condition leading to ARDS)

DISCHARGE AND HOME HEALTHCARE GUIDELINES

PREVENTION. Prompt attention for any infections may decrease the incidence of sepsis, which can lead to ARDS.

COMPLICATIONS. If patients survive ARDS, few residual effects are seen. Complications are directed to any other conditions the patient may have. Patients may need physical therapy to restore muscular strength after a debilitating illness.

Retinal Detachment

DRG Category:	117
Mean LOS:	2.7 days
Description:	SURGICAL: Intraocular Procedures Without Complication or Comorbidity or Major Complication or Comorbidity
DRG Category:	124
Mean LOS:	5.2 days
Description:	MEDICAL: Other Disorders of the Eye With Major Complication or Comorbidity

A retinal detachment occurs when the retina is pulled away from or out of its normal position. Approximately 6% of the U.S. population has retinal breaks, but most do not lead to retinal detachment, which has a prevalence of 0.3%. Estimates are that 15% of people with retinal detachments in one eye develop detachment in the other eye, and the risk of bilateral detachment increases to 30% in people who have had bilateral cataract surgery. Retinal detachments are classified as rhegmatogenous, tractional, and exudative. A rhegmatogenous retinal detachment, the most common form, is a retinal tear leading to fluid accumulation and separation of the neurosensory retina from the underlying retinal pigment epithelium. With a tractional detachment, contractile membranes pull the neurosensory retina away from the retinal pigment epithelium. Exudative detachment occurs with a change in the inflow or outflow of fluid from the vitreous cavity that leads to fluid accumulation in the subretinal space.

The retina is the innermost lining of the eye and contains millions of photoreceptors, light-sensitive nerve fibers, and cells that are responsible for converting light energy into nerve impulses. The retina functions as film does in a camera: The light enters through the lens to the retina, and an image is transmitted to the brain via the optic nerve. The retina is attached to the choroid (vascular coat of the eye between the sclera and the retina) at two locations: at the optic nerve and at the ciliary body. The remaining retina relies on the vitreous (jellylike mass that fills the cavity of the eyeball) to apply pressure against the lining to maintain its position. The detachment can occur spontaneously as a result of a change in the retina or vitreous; this detachment is referred to as a primary detachment. Secondary detachment occurs as a result of another problem, such as trauma, diabetes, or pregnancy-induced hypertension. Complications from retinal detachment include visual impairment and blindness.

CAUSES

The most common cause of retinal detachment is the formation of a hole or tear, which can occur as part of the normal aging process or during cataract surgery or trauma. The hole allows the vitreous fluid to leak out between the layers, thus separating the sensory retinal layer from its blood supply in the choroid. Traction from inflammatory membranes may lead to separation of the retina from the retinal pigment epithelium, or exudate may occur behind the retina due to hypertension, venous occlusion, or papilledema. Patients who have had previous cataract surgery, severe injury, or a family history of detachment, glaucoma, and nearsightedness are more likely to experience a retinal detachment. People who engage in contact sports such as boxing and paintball games have increased prevalence of retinal detachment.

GENETIC CONSIDERATIONS

Some forms of retinopathy leading to detachment are heritable, such as familial exudative vitreoretinopathy. Snowflake vitreoretinal degeneration is an autosomal dominantly inherited retinal degeneration that produces yellow-white spots on the retina and retinal detachment. Autosomal dominant and X-linked forms of retinal detachment have been described. Genetic diseases such as osteoporosis-pseudoglioma and Norrie disease are typified by retinal detachment and are caused by mutations in the *LRP5* and *NDP* genes, respectively. A recent genome-wide association study in the United Kingdom implicated 11 candidate loci that were associated with retinal detachment, including *BMP3, COL22A1, COL2A1, DLG5, EFEMP2, FAT3, LOXL1, PLCE1, TRIM29, TYR*, and *ZC3H11B*.

SEX AND LIFE SPAN CONSIDERATIONS

A retinal detachment most often occurs in women and men ages 50 to 70 years. For those less than age 45 years, the prevalence is higher in males than in females. It can also occur infrequently in children who were born prematurely and are experiencing retinopathies as a result of prolonged oxygenation.

HEALTH DISPARITIES AND SEXUAL/GENDER MINORITY HEALTH

The incidence of retinal detachment is relatively frequent in Jewish persons and relatively low in Black persons. Sexual and gender minority status has no known effect on the risk for retinal detachment.

GLOBAL HEALTH CONSIDERATIONS

Retinal detachment occurs around the globe with a prevalence approximately the same as that in North America. The most common associated factors globally are nearsightedness (young adults), cataract removal with lens implant (older adults), and traumatic injury (young people).

ASSESSMENT

HISTORY. Establish a history of eye disease or eye surgery or trauma to the eye. Patients with suspected retinal detachment may complain of a painless change in vision. Ask patients if they have experienced "floaters" or black spots, flashing lights (photopsia), or the sensation of a curtain being pulled over the field of vision. Some patients report feeling as if they are looking through a veil or through cobwebs.

PHYSICAL EXAMINATION. The most common symptoms are **photopsia, floaters,** and **visual loss**. A thorough visual examination is done to detect changes in vision and evaluate the visual fields. Conduct an examination to determine if external eye trauma has occurred and check the pupil reaction. Inspect the retina with an ophthalmoscope to determine the extent of the tear. Generally, a specialized clinician will check the intraocular pressure and perform a dilated fundus examination with ophthalmoscopy. Assess the patient's ability to ambulate safely and to perform the normal activities of daily living.

PSYCHOSOCIAL. If the patient is employed, determine the effect of visual impairment on the patient's ability to perform the job. Determine the effects of visual changes on leisure activities. Assess the patient's support system, access to healthcare, and financial resources.

Diagnostic Highlights

Test	Normal Result	Abnormality With Condition	Explanation
Ophthalmoscopic examination	Normal retina	Gray bulge or fold in retina; may be able to see jagged or irregularly shaped tear	Allows examiner to view the internal and external structures of the eye

Other Tests: Ultrasound, electroretinogram, fluorescein angiography, optical coherence tomography

PRIMARY NURSING DIAGNOSIS

DIAGNOSIS. Risk for injury as evidenced by visual alterations and/or visual loss

OUTCOMES. Vision compensation behavior; Fall prevention behavior; Risk control; Neurological status: Cranial sensory/motor function; Knowledge: Medication

INTERVENTIONS. Eye care; Vision screening; Fall prevention; Medication management; Teaching: Procedure/treatment

PLANNING AND IMPLEMENTATION
Collaborative

If a retinal tear is suspected, the patient should be kept at rest, immobile, and NPO until treatment decision can be made. If possible, protect the involved eye with a metal eye shield. Avoid any pressure on the eye. The main objective in treating a tear or hole is to prevent a retinal detachment. Photocoagulation, cryotherapy, and diathermy are used to produce an inflammatory response that creates an adhesion or scar, which seals the edges of the tear. These therapies differ in the mechanism used to cause the scarring effect. Photocoagulation uses light beams; cryotherapy uses cold to freeze the tissues; and diathermy uses energy from a high-frequency current. All three result in sealing of the hole to prevent the vitreous from spilling between the layers. Vitrectomy in the past was reserved for complicated retinal detachments but is now used to treat primary uncomplicated retinal detachments as well.

If the retina is detached, surgical repair is required. The objective of the surgical procedure is to force the retina into contact with the choroid. The scleral buckling procedure places the retina back into position.

Preoperatively, the patient is on bedrest and has activity restrictions depending on the size and location of detachment. Total eye rest may be needed. The patient may not read, watch television, or participate in any activity that causes rapid eye movements. An eye patch may be prescribed. It is important to position the patient either to keep the retinal tear lowermost within the eye or in the dependent position to allow the retina to fall back against the epithelium, which prevents further detachment.

To obtain direct access to the damaged retina, a retina specialist performs a vitrectomy, removes the vitreous humor gel, and repairs the retina. A gas bubble is injected to wall off the repaired retina to allow it to heal. When gas is used, the physician asks the patient to remain in a position that keeps the bubble against the repaired area of the retina. The head is usually kept parallel to the floor and turned to the side with the unaffected eye down. It may take 4 to 8 days for the bubble to absorb. The patient cannot fly or travel to high altitudes until the gas bubble is gone because a rapid increase in altitude can increase the intraocular pressure and result in a redetachment of the retina. Reading, writing, close work, watching television, shampooing, shaving, and combing the hair may be restricted.

Pharmacologic Highlights

Medication or Drug Class	Dosage	Description	Rationale
Cyclopentolate hydro-chloride (Cyclogyl)	Drops as prescribed	Cycloplegic agent	Causes dilation of the pupil and rest of the muscles of accommodation
Antibiotics	Drops as prescribed	Gentamicin; prednisolone acetate	Prevent eye infections

Other Drugs: Antiemetics and analgesics are ordered to manage nausea, vomiting, and pain.

Independent

Assure the patient that it is normal for vision to continue to be distorted after surgery because of postoperative inflammation and cycloplegic eyedrops. Inform the patient that vision will return to normal over several weeks. During hospitalization, keep the bed in a low position, and the call light within the patient's reach. Provide a safe environment and identify potential safety hazards.

The patient needs to assume the position that was ordered by the physician for postoperative management. Assist the patient to use an over-the-bed table if necessary or place pillows to support the arms and lower back. Place a sign at the head of the bed, giving each practitioner instructions on the position to be maintained. Observe the eye patch for drainage and notify the physician for drainage other then serous. Once the initial eye patch has been removed, place cool compresses over the closed eyelid for relief of discomfort. The eye may be swollen, reddened, and ecchymotic for several days, and the conjunctiva may persist for weeks. If the patient experiences postoperative nausea and vomiting, maintain an odor-free environment and apply cool compresses to the forehead.

Evidence-Based Practice and Health Policy

Xu, D., Uhr, J., Patel, S., Pandit, R., Jenkins, T., Khan, M., & Ho, A. (2021). Sociodemographic factors influencing rhegmatogenous retinal detachment presentation and outcome. *Ophthalmology Retina, 5,* 337–341.

- The authors aimed to analyze the impact of sociodemographic factors on the presenting symptoms and outcomes for people with rhegmatogenous retinal detachment (RRD) in the United States. Factors included age, gender, race, and mean household income as well as visual acuity at baseline and after repair and whether the fovea was attached or not (fovea on or off). The investigators analyzed data from a single health sciences center (N = 4,061) in the United States.
- Older age, male sex, non-White race, and lower household income were independent risk factors for fovea-off presentation of RRD. The 12-month postoperative visual acuity was worse in patients who were fovea-off, older, male, and non-White, but household income was not related. The authors concluded that socioeconomic disparities can negatively impact the prognosis of patients with RRD.

DOCUMENTATION GUIDELINES

- Visual acuity
- Reaction to activity restrictions; ability of patient to participate in activities of daily living independently
- Complications such as bleeding, infection, pain or discomfort, decreased visual acuity, falls
- Response to medications and ability of the patient to instill eyedrops
- Understanding of eye care at home

DISCHARGE AND HOME HEALTHCARE GUIDELINES

Have the patient or significant others demonstrate the correct technique for instilling eyedrops. Instruct the patient to wash the hands before and after removing the dressing; using a clean washcloth, cleanse the lid and lashes with warm tap water; tilt the head backward and inclined slightly to the side so the solution runs away from the tear duct and other eye to prevent contamination; depress the lower lid with the finger of one hand. Tell the patient to look up when the solution is dropped on the averted lower lid; do not place drop directly on the cornea.

Do not touch any part of the eye with the dropper; close the eye after instillation, and wipe off the excess fluid from the lids and cheeks. Close the eye gently so the solution stays in the eye longer.

Teach the patient to use warm or cold compresses for comfort several times a day. Note that the patient should wear either an eye shield or glasses during the day, during naps, and at night. Teach the patient to avoid vigorous activities and heavy lifting for the immediate postoperative period. The discharge instructions may be detailed, and careful explanations are essential. Teach the patient the symptoms of retinal detachment and the action to take if it occurs again. Instruct the patient about the importance of follow-up appointments, which may be every few days for the first several weeks after surgery.

Rheumatic Fever, Acute

DRG Category:	315	
Mean LOS:	3.6 days	
Description:	MEDICAL: Other Circulatory System Diagnosis With Complication or Comorbidity	
DRG Category:	546	
Mean LOS:	4.4 days	
Description:	MEDICAL: Connective Tissue Disorders With Complication or Comorbidity	

Rheumatic fever is an autoimmune disorder that follows an upper respiratory infection with group A beta-hemolytic streptococci (GABHS) and causes an inflammatory response. Only 3% of people who have a pharyngeal streptococcal infection develop rheumatic fever, but when it occurs, a variety of organs and tissues are affected. Rheumatic fever affects the heart, central nervous system, skin, and musculoskeletal system, and many people experience recurrences after the initial illness.

Acute rheumatic fever is most destructive to the heart. Rheumatic heart disease (RHD) occurs in up to 60% of patients with acute rheumatic fever and may affect any of the layers of the heart during the acute phase. Endocarditis leads to leaflet swelling of the valves, leaflet erosion, and deposits of blood and fibrin, known as vegetation, on the valves. Myocarditis causes cellular swelling, damage to collagen, and formation of fibrosis and scarring. Pericarditis can occur as well, which can lead to pericardial effusion. In addition to valvular disease, acute rheumatic fever can lead to severe carditis and life-threatening heart failure. Complications lead to a 20% death rate within the first 10 years after the initial illness. In addition to valve and myocardial muscle complications, the patient may experience cardiac dysrhythmias and heart failure.

CAUSES

Acute rheumatic fever is caused by a prior streptococcal infection and is often associated with nasopharyngitis or upper respiratory infections. The GABHS infection, which may have been mild and even unnoticed and untreated, usually occurs 2 to 6 weeks before the development of symptoms of acute rheumatic fever. Experts suspect that rheumatic fever is an autoimmune response triggered by antibodies that are produced in response to the streptococcal infection. The antibodies react with the body's cells and produce characteristic lesions in the target organs. Risk factors include family history, skin infections, and environmental factors such as overcrowding and poor sanitation. Children who have untreated streptococcal throat infections are at high risk.

GENETIC CONSIDERATIONS

Increased susceptibility to rheumatic fever is known to occur in families and has a strong genetic component (heritability of ~ 60%). Variants in the *MASP2* gene, which encodes a protein of the complement system, have been associated with rheumatic fever. About 50% of cases also have damage to heart valves, which greatly increases the risk of developing RHD. The human leukocyte antigen type DR7DR53 has been associated with the development of valve lesions in patients with severe RHD. Other genetic variants that increase risk have been suggested but need further research to fully define.

SEX AND LIFE SPAN CONSIDERATIONS

Although acute rheumatic fever primarily targets the school-age population, it also occurs in adults. It is particularly common in children ages 5 to 20 years, with a median age of 10 years, and with hospitalizations significantly more common among children ages 6 to 11 years. It rarely occurs in people over age 30 years. Valvular heart disease is most likely to damage the mitral valve in females and the aortic valve in males. In both genders, tricuspid and pulmonic valve damage occurs rarely. While rheumatic fever occurs in equal numbers in women and men, women's complications are more frequent and severe.

HEALTH DISPARITIES AND SEXUAL/GENDER MINORITY HEALTH

Asian and Pacific Islander persons are overrepresented in hospital admissions for rheumatic fever. The proportion of rheumatic fever hospitalizations is greater in the northeastern United States and lower in the southern United States (Bradely-Hewitt et al., 2019). Children from disadvantaged backgrounds are at risk for rheumatic fever; as median income decreases, the frequency of the disease increases. Crowded living conditions increase transmission because children and adults with untreated infection are contagious for weeks after resolution of the pharyngitis (sore throat). Sexual and gender minority status has no known effect on the risk for rheumatic fever.

GLOBAL HEALTH CONSIDERATIONS

Around the world, 95% of cases occur in tropical countries, those with limited resources, and those with underrepresented Indigenous groups. Particular regions of risk for children are Africa, the Middle East, South America, and India. The World Health Organization reports that approximately 15 million people have RHD, approximately 300,000 new cases of rheumatic fever occur each year, and 33,000 deaths occur each year. In developing countries, acute rheumatic fever is the most common acquired heart disease from childhood to young adulthood and is the cause of up to half of all intensive care admissions.

ASSESSMENT

HISTORY. Establish the timeline of symptoms with the patient. Usually, the patient has a sore throat and a fever of at least 100.4°F (38°C) for a few days to several weeks before the onset. This latent period between the acute infection of streptococcal pharyngitis and acute rheumatic fever averages 18 days. The patient may not have been treated with antibiotics or may not have completed a full course of treatment. Determine if the patient has experienced migratory joint tenderness (polyarthritis), chest pain, fever, and fatigue. Some patients describe unexplained nosebleeds as well. Patients with pericarditis may describe sharp pain over the shoulder that radiates to the neck, back, and arms. The pain may increase with inspiration and decrease when the patient leans forward from a sitting position. Patients with heart failure may describe shortness of breath, cough, and right upper quadrant abdominal pain. In addition, the patient may describe fatigue or activity intolerance, along with periorbital, abdominal, or pedal edema.

PHYSICAL EXAMINATION. The patient may have a **distinctive red rash**, referred to as *erythema marginatum*, **fever**, and **joint and muscle pain**. This nonpruritic rash appears primarily on the trunk of the body, the buttocks, and the extremities; it appears on the face in only rare instances. In addition, subcutaneous nodules of less than 1 cm in diameter form on the skin. Painless and movable, they usually appear over bony prominences: the hands, wrists, elbows, knuckles, feet, and vertebrae. If the patient has heart failure, there may be peripheral edema.

The patient may also demonstrate chorea (previously referred to as *St. Vitus dance*). Mild chorea produces hyperirritability, problems concentrating, and illegible handwriting. Severe chorea causes purposeless, uncontrollable, jerky movements and muscle spasms, speech disturbances, muscle fatigue, and incoordination. Transient chorea may not appear until several months after the initial streptococcal infection.

When the joints are palpated, the patient may have migratory polyarticular arthritis (more than four joints are progressively involved). The most frequently involved joints include the knees, elbows, hips, shoulders, and wrists. These joints are extremely warm and tender to the touch, and even a light palpation can cause pain. The pain usually subsides after the patient becomes afebrile.

Heart murmurs serve as an indicator that carditis has occurred. The aortic and mitral valves are particularly involved as a result of the Aschoff bodies (small nodules of cells and leukocytes) that form on the tissues of the heart. Audible heart murmurs are more likely auscultated at the third intercostal space right of the sternum for the aortic valve and at the apex of the heart if the mitral valve is involved. When palpating peripheral pulses, you may note a rapid heart rate.

PSYCHOSOCIAL. The disease is likely to occur at an age when children are active and industrious. Those who require extended bedrest may have trouble coping with the limitations placed on them.

Diagnostic Highlights

According to the modified Jones criteria (American Heart Association major and minor criteria), to make the diagnosis of acute rheumatic fever, there needs to be evidence of a previous streptococcal infection and two major Jones criteria or one major plus two minor Jones criteria. For recurrent acute rheumatic fever, there needs to be two major Jones criteria and two minor criteria, or three minor criteria.

Criteria	Description	Explanation
Major manifestations	Carditis	Cardiomegaly, new murmur, congestive heart failure, pericarditis
	Polyarthritis	Polyarticular, involves the large joints
	Subcutaneous nodules (Aschoff bodies)	Firm, painless fibrous nodules on the extensor surfaces of the wrists, elbows, and knees
	Erythema marginatum	Long-lasting rash
	Chorea (St. Vitus dance)	Movement disorder, rapid and purposeful movements of face and arms; generally, movements cease during sleep
Minor manifestations	Clinical findings	Polyarthralgia, fever ≥ 101.3°F (38.5°C), erythrocyte sedimentation rate ≥ 60 mm in the first hour and/or C-reactive protein ≥ 3.0 mg/dL, prolonged PR interval on electrocardiogram

Laboratory Findings

Test	Normal Results	Abnormality With Condition	Explanation
Throat cultures	Negative culture	Positive for GABHS	Identifies causative organism in the acute phase of pharyngeal infection; positive culture found in 25% of patients
Antistreptolysin O (ASO) titer	< 166 Todd units	< 250 Todd units for an inactive infection; 500–5,000 Todd units for an active infection	Antibody to the streptolysin O enzyme produced by GABHS; titers rise about 7 days after infection and gradually return to baseline after 12 mo

(highlight box continues on page 1060)

Diagnostic Highlights (continued)

Other Tests: Complete blood count, blood cultures, rapid antigen test, C-reactive protein, erythrocyte sedimentation rate, chest x-ray, echocardiogram, chest computed tomography scan, chest magnetic resonance imaging

PRIMARY NURSING DIAGNOSIS

DIAGNOSIS. Acute pain related to joint and muscle inflammation as evidenced by self-reports of pain, facial grimacing, and/or protective behavior

OUTCOMES. Pain level; Pain control; Symptom severity; Symptom control; Knowledge: Pain management

INTERVENTIONS. Pain management: Acute; Analgesic administration; Medication administration; Teaching: Prescribed medication

PLANNING AND IMPLEMENTATION
Collaborative

The goal of management is to end the infection, relieve the symptoms, and prevent recurrence. Complete eradication of the streptococcal infection is necessary so that the heart and kidneys are not damaged. The physician may prescribe intramuscular benzathine penicillin G, if the patient has no known history of allergy to penicillin. Reinforce the need for the patient to complete all medications and to watch for potential side effects, such as rash, hives, wheezing, or anaphylaxis. Activity restrictions are required to ensure full recovery. In patients with active carditis, strict bedrest may be needed for approximately 5 weeks. The physician then prescribes a progressive increase in activity. If valvular dysfunction leads to persistent heart failure, the patient may need surgery to correct the deficit in heart function.

Pharmacologic Highlights

Medication or Drug Class	Dosage	Description	Rationale
Benzathine penicillin G or procaine penicillin G	2.4 million units IM	Antibiotic	Eradicates the infection; injections may be given in the hospital or by a home health nurse; oral penicillin may be given, with erythromycin as an alternative in those allergic to penicillin
Aspirin	650 mg PO as needed	NSAID	Treats the arthralgia (muscle achiness); monitor for side effects such as tinnitus, gastric upset, and petechiae

Other Drugs: Erythromycin; penicillin VK; sulfadiazine, azithromycin; naproxen; prednisone (to treat the carditis); furosemide (for patients with congestive heart failure). After the acute phase of the disease, the physician usually prescribes monthly injections of benzathine penicillin G or daily oral antibiotics. Preventive treatment with antibiotics may last at least for 5 years. Anticonvulsants such as valproic acid or carbamazepine may be recommended for severe involuntary movements associated with chorea.

Independent

Explain to the child and the family the need to take all antibiotics until they are completed. This information needs to be conveyed to promote compliance, not to communicate guilt.

Remind the parents that failure to seek treatment for a streptococcal infection is common because the symptoms are so mild. The patient is likely to remain on oral antibiotics indefinitely through life. Because symptoms from heart damage may not present for several years after the infection, it is important for the patient and family to report symptoms when they occur and include them in their medical history. Regular heart examinations may be required for long-term follow-up.

Managing activity restrictions is a challenging goal in working with a young person of school age who is on bedrest. As the chorea decreases, the child needs to participate in therapeutic play activities that promote a sense of industry and minimize any feelings of inferiority—activities such as reading, board games, and video game play. Encourage the parents to obtain a tutor so the patient can keep up with schoolwork during convalescence. To protect the patient who develops chorea and has an unsteady gait, make sure that all obstructions are cleared out of the way during ambulation to reduce the risk of injury.

Evidence-Based Practice and Health Policy
Beaton, A., Kamalembo, F., Dale, J., Kado, J., Karthikeyan, G., Kazi, D., Longenecker, C., Mwangi, J., Okello, E., Ribiero, A., Taubert, K., Watkins, D., Wyber, R., Zimmerman, M., & Carapetis, J. (2020). The American Heart Association's call to action for reducing the global burden of rheumatic heart disease. *Circulation, 142*, 3358–3368.

- RHD remains a condition of health disparities in the United States in underserved areas. RHD mortality parallels other cardiovascular disease disparity, with hot spots along the Mississippi River Valley, southern states, and western states. Available data suggest an urgent need to improve epidemiological surveillance in these areas and among other high-risk groups such as Native Americans, Alaskan Native, Hawaiian Natives, and those living in Puerto Rico or one of the U.S. Pacific territories, notably among Samoan youths.
- The American Heart Association (AHA) recommends four interventions: development and maintenance of a rheumatic fever/RHD registry, health worker training, access to benzathine penicillin G (BPG), and access to cardiac ultrasound. The organization advocates for disseminating the best science on real and perceived risks of BPG administration and support research to better quantify adverse reactions. AHA also argues for updating scientific statements to include BPG best practices, including minimization of pain with administration, considerations in advanced RHD, and improved management of adverse drug reactions.

DOCUMENTATION GUIDELINES
- The extent of the skin lesions for the erythema marginatum rash and subcutaneous nodules
- The extent of chest pain and cardiac involvement
- The extent of the chorea and joint involvement
- Reaction to bedrest and activity restriction

DISCHARGE AND HOME HEALTHCARE GUIDELINES
Teach the patient or parents to prevent any further streptococcal infections by good hand washing and avoiding people with sore throats. Encourage the patient or parents to contact the primary healthcare provider if a sore throat occurs. Explain all medications, including dosage, action, route, and side effects. Encourage the patient to resume activity gradually and to use an elevator, if one is available, at school. Teach the patient to return to physical education classes or extracurricular sports gradually, with the guidance of the physician. Encourage the patient to take frequent naps and rest periods.

Rheumatoid Arthritis

DRG Category: 546
Mean LOS: 4.4 days
Description: MEDICAL: Connective Tissue Disorders With Complication or Comorbidity

Rheumatoid arthritis (RA) is a chronic, progressive, systemic disease characterized by recurrent inflammation of connective tissue, primarily diarthrodial joints (hinged joints that contain a cavity within the capsule that separates the bony elements to allow freedom of movement) and their related structures. RA affects approximately 2% of all adults, and in the United States, approximately 1.5 million people have RA.

The disease generally begins with inflammation of the synovial membrane, which becomes thickened and edematous. The thickened synovium, or pannus, erodes the articular cartilage and underlying bone, causing joint destruction. The small peripheral joints of the hand and wrist and the joints of the knees, ankles, elbows, and shoulders are usually affected symmetrically. The cervical spine may also be affected. Extra-articular involvement of the disease includes inflammation of the tendon sheaths; the bursae; and the connective tissue of the heart, lungs, pleurae, and arteries.

If the disease is left untreated, the inflammatory process of RA moves through four stages. In the first stage, synovitis is caused by congestion and edema of the synovial membrane and joint capsule. In the second stage, the formation of pannus, thickened layers of granulation tissue that cover and invade cartilage begins, and this leads to eventual destruction of the joint capsule and bone. In the third stage, fibrous ankylosis is noted in the inflammatory process; this is the fibrous invasion of the pannus and scar formation that occludes joint space. In the fourth and final stage, the fibrous tissue calcifies, causing ankylosis and total immobility.

Complications caused by RA include temporomandibular joint disease, which impairs the patient's chewing and causes headaches. Infection, osteoporosis, myositis, myocardial infarction, inflammatory pulmonary disease, carpal tunnel syndrome, lymphadenopathy, and peripheral neuritis may also occur.

CAUSES

Although the specific cause of RA is unknown, there is speculation about multiple causation, which includes infection, autoimmunity, and genetic factors and also environmental and hormonal factors. Heredity seems to account for up to 50% of the risk for RA. The strongest evidence of an autoimmune cause is supported by the findings of rheumatoid factor (RF) in the serum of more than 80% of affected individuals. Risk factors include family history, imbalance of intestinal microbes, cigarette smoking and nicotine exposure, diet with high sugar content, obesity, hormone imbalances, infection with Epstein-Barr virus, and environmental exposure.

GENETIC CONSIDERATIONS

Familial recurrence risk in RA is small compared with that of other autoimmune diseases, with heritability estimated at 20% to 50%. The strongest susceptibility risk factor that has been demonstrated is the HLA DRB1*0404 allele, with two other genetic risk factors mapping within the HLA complex locus. This finding seems consistent across many studied populations. Polymorphisms in the *SLC22A4*, *STAT4*, *PTPN8*, *MHC2TA*, *IRF5*, and *NFKBIL1* genes also appear to be associated with RA susceptibility. Various tumor necrosis factor (TNF) alleles have also been linked with RA. Finally, there are also polymorphisms in the interleukin 6 gene (*IL6*) and the macrophage migration inhibitory factor gene (*MIF*) that are associated with juvenile-onset RA.

SEX AND LIFE SPAN CONSIDERATIONS

RA is two to three times more common in women than in men. The disease can occur at any age, although the onset peaks between ages 35 and 50 years. A higher RA risk may occur among women with a history of preeclampsia, hyperemesis, or hypertension during pregnancy. These conditions may indicate a reduced immune adaptability to pregnancy and a predisposition to RA. The first 5 years after a pregnancy seem to offer some protection from RA.

HEALTH DISPARITIES AND SEXUAL/GENDER MINORITY HEALTH

RA seems to be more common in Native American persons and less common in Black persons from the Caribbean region as compared to other groups. Experts suggest that gender and sexual minority persons have higher levels of chronic health conditions such as asthma, diabetes, obesity, and rheumatoid arthritis than other groups. They are also more likely to delay testing and screening for chronic health conditions because of stigma, lack of healthcare providers' awareness, or insensitivity to the unique needs of this community. If care is delayed and they are left untreated, the conditions may become severe (Downing & Przedworski, 2018).

GLOBAL HEALTH CONSIDERATIONS

RA occurs in all countries and in all peoples. Approximately 3 people per 10,000 develop RA each year, with an overall prevalence of 1% in the world's population.

ASSESSMENT

HISTORY. Ask if the patient has experienced paresthesia (tingling) of the hands and feet or joint pain with swelling and warmth in the joint. Note that RA symptoms most commonly occur in the hands and feet but may occur in any joint lined by a synovial membrane. Determine if the patient has experienced fatigue, malaise, low-grade fever, weight loss, anemia, or anorexia, which are all common early symptoms of RA. Ask about stiffness: Does it occur before or after physical activity, and does the patient need to "limber up" after inactivity, such as sleeping? Determine whether the patient is taking medication for pain and, if so, ask about the dosage and frequency. Ask if the patient has had involvement of organs such as the skin, heart, lungs, and eyes. Ask if the patient has had carpal tunnel syndrome.

PHYSICAL EXAMINATION. Common symptoms include **morning joint stiffness, symmetrical joint pain and tenderness in the small joints of the hands and feet**, and **joint swelling**. Many patients experience systemic effects such as fever, weakness, fatigue, and malaise before joint swelling actually occurs. As the disease progresses, patients may experience deformity, limited range of motion, and rheumatoid nodules. The most common joints involved are the metacarpophalangeal (MCP, knuckles of the hand) joints, the wrist, the proximal interphalangeal joints, the knee, the metatarsophalangeal (MTP, feet) joints, the shoulder, and the ankle. Observe the patient initially for pallor and signs of fatigue and immobility. Assess all joints carefully, looking for deformities, contractures, immobility, and inability to perform the activities of daily living. Inspect the patient's fingers for edema or congestion in the joints. Inspect the elbows for rheumatoid nodules, which are subcutaneous, rounded, nontender masses. Note skin lesions or leg ulcers caused by vasculitis. Check for a positive Babinski sign, which is caused by spinal cord compression if the vertebrae are involved. If the patient is able to participate, assess the MCP joints by having the patient dorsiflex, extend, and flex the fingers. Assess the patient's ability to perform radial and ulnar deviation. Also ask the patient to straighten the fingers, then abduct and adduct them. Test the muscle strength of the patient's hand by having the patient squeeze your hands simultaneously. Ask the patient to make a fist and resist your attempt to pry it open.

To assess the patient's elbow and shoulder range of motion, ask the patient to flex and extend the arms and to abduct and adduct each extended arm. Test the trapezius muscles by placing your hands on the patient's shoulders and asking the patient to shrug the shoulders as you press down on them. Look for subcutaneous nodules around the elbows.

Observe the range of motion of the hips, knees, and ankles by asking the patient to walk about and to sit down in a chair. If the patient is in pain, you can defer the examination, relying instead on observations of the patient as you observe the patient in the setting.

PSYCHOSOCIAL. Initially, assess patients' understanding of what the disease means and what they believe life holds in the future. Identify the patients' support systems and how available support persons are. If the patients had RA for some time, assess their current level of functioning. Determine if the disease affected relationships, work, or leisure activities.

Diagnostic Highlights

Test	Normal Result	Abnormality With Condition	Explanation
Anticyclic citrullinated peptide (anti-CCP) antibodies, IgG, serum	< 20 units	20–39.9 units (weak positive); 40–59.9 units (positive); ≥ 60 units (strong positive)	Differentiates RA from other connective tissue diseases that might mimic the signs of arthritis
Rheumatoid factor	Negative: < 20 International Unit/mL	20–80 International Unit/mL (weakly positive); greater than 80 International Unit/mL (positive)	Identifies unusual immunoglobulin G and M antibodies that develop against connective tissue disease
Antinuclear antibody	Negative	< 1:80	Identifies antibodies to the body's own DNA and nuclear material

Other Tests: Complete blood count, C-reactive protein, erythrocyte sedimentation rate, serum protein electrophoresis, serum complement, serum protein electrophoresis, synovial fluid analysis, immunoglobulin analysis, bone x-rays, computed tomography scan, magnetic resonance imaging

PRIMARY NURSING DIAGNOSIS

DIAGNOSIS. Chronic pain related to joint swelling and deformity as evidenced by changes in hand strength, decreased fine motor movement of the hands, self-reports of pain, facial grimacing, and/or protective behavior

OUTCOMES. Comfort status; Pain control; Pain level; Symptom severity; Symptom control; Knowledge: Pain management; Knowledge: Medication; Knowledge: Disease process

INTERVENTIONS. Pain management: Chronic; Analgesic administration; Teaching: Prescribed medication; Teaching: Disease process; Exercise promotion: Strength training

▓ PLANNING AND IMPLEMENTATION
Collaborative

The goals of treatment are to relieve pain, inhibit the inflammatory response, preserve joint function, and prevent deformity. Initial medical treatment consists of pharmacologic measures. An appropriate ongoing exercise program is prescribed by the physical therapist; this includes teaching proper body mechanics. Therapy may also include the use of moist heat, but ice may be prescribed in some cases. Splints are provided for painful joints. The physical therapist teaches the patient to use a walker and cane if indicated.

Some patients may undergo surgery to restore joint function. One type of procedure, a synovectomy, involves removal of the inflamed synovium early in the disease process. Patients who are in relatively good physical and mental condition may be candidates for joint reconstructive surgery (arthroplasty). The effectiveness of hip and joint replacement is considered quite good, although replacement surgery associated with other joints is less efficacious. Osteotomy involves cutting the bone to realign the joint and to shift the pressure points to a less denuded area of the joint; this shift relieves pain. Tendon transfers may prevent deformities or relieve contractures.

Pharmacologic Highlights

Medication or Drug Class	Dosage	Description	Rationale
NSAIDs	Varies by drug	Ibuprofen, piroxicam, phenylbutazone, indomethacin, propoxyphene, nabumetone, celecoxib, or naproxen	Relieve pain; may be given with misoprostol (Cytotec) to minimize gastrointestinal symptoms
Methotrexate (considered first-line therapy)	7.5–20 mg PO or sc once a week	Nonbiologic disease-modifying antirheumatic drugs (DMARDs)	Retards or prevents progression of RA, joint destruction, loss of function; note increased susceptibility to infection; blocks several enzymes involved in the immune response
Other nonbiologic DMARDs	Varies by drug	Hydroxychloroquine (HCQ), azathioprine (AZA), sulfasalazine (SSZ), leflunomide	Retards or prevents progression of RA, joint destruction, loss of function; note increased susceptibility to infection
Biologic DMARDs	Varies by drug	Etanercept, infliximab, adalimumab, certolizumab, golimumab, rituximab, anakinra, abatacept, tocilizumab	Retards or prevents progression of RA, joint destruction, loss of function; note increased susceptibility to infection
Prednisone	5–60 mg PO daily	Corticosteroid	Reduces inflammation; used as a bridge to treatment with DMARDs or as rescue therapy when symptoms occur

Other Drugs: Opioids for pain relief

Independent

Teach the patient assistive techniques to manage joint pain, such as meditation, biofeedback, and distraction. Advise the patient to take warm to hot showers or baths in the morning or evening to help relieve the pain. During acute stages of the disease, encourage the patient to avoid exercising the inflamed joints; help the patient understand the need to rest; however, patients do need to maintain mobility and movement of joints that are not involved. Provide necessary assistance with the activities of daily living and prevent flexion contractures by having the patient lie prone with the feet hanging between the mattress and the footboard several times a day. Keep the patient warm and provide meticulous skin care.

During subacute and chronic stages of RA, the patient needs to return to as much independence as possible. When mobility improves, encourage the patient to assume more responsibility for self-care. Promote adequate rest, especially after activity, and plan rest periods during the day. Assist the patient with nutrition to prevent anorexia, which contributes to anemia, causing further weakness and activity intolerance. Determine whether the patient has a firm mattress and straight-back chairs with arm rests at home to support proper positioning. Show the patient how to avoid flexion contractures of the large muscle groups while sleeping and sitting.

Teach the patient to avoid putting pillows under the legs while sitting and sleeping and to avoid sitting in soft, low chairs. When the acute inflammatory stage subsides and the patient is ready for discharge from the hospital, teach the patient to take medications as prescribed, stressing the need to maintain therapeutic blood levels of the drug. Suggest that the patient use dressing aids such as a long-handled shoehorn, elastic shoelaces, a zipper pull, and a buttonhook. Recommend the use of handheld shower nozzles, grab bars, and hand rails. As RA progresses and deformity becomes pronounced, patients may suffer with body image disturbances and inability to engage in sexual activity. Assist the patient and partner to cope with these problems.

Evidence-Based Practice and Health Policy

Navarro-Millan, I., Rajan, M., Lui, G., Kern, L., Pinheiro, L., Safford, M., Sattui, S., & Curtis, J. (2020). Racial and ethnic differences in medication use among beneficiaries of social security disability insurance with rheumatoid arthritis. *Seminars in Arthritis and Rheumatism, 50,* 988–995.

• The aim of the study was to determine racial and ethnic differences in the use of conventional synthetic or biologic DMARDS and long-term glucocorticoid use among people on Social Security Insurance with RA. The authors used the Centers for Medicare and Medicaid Services claims data to study people younger than age 65 years with RA and no longer working because they were disabled.

• Conventional DMARDS included methrotrexate, leflunomide, hydroxychloroquine, sulfasalazine, and azathioprine. Biologic DMARDS included drugs such as adalimumab, etanercept, and abatacept. The use of conventional DMARDS without biologic DMARDS was higher in Black patients compared to White patients, and the use of biologic DMARDS was lower in Black patients compared to White patients. The use of biologic DMARDS was higher in Hispanic as compared to White patients. The authors suggested these differences may be due to physician prescribing behaviors or patient preferences.

DOCUMENTATION GUIDELINES

• Physical findings: Deformed joints, swollen nodes, range of motion, strength and dexterity of extremities
• Response to medication and treatments, level of pain, degree of pain relief, understanding of RA medications
• Ability to perform self-care and tolerance to activity

DISCHARGE AND HOME HEALTHCARE GUIDELINES

The medications used to treat RA can be complicated. Make sure the patient understands the medication regime and how often to have laboratory tests drawn to monitor their side effects. Ensure that the patient understands the appropriate methods for pain relief and the need to notify a home-care agency or physician if the regimen is ineffective. Be sure the patient understands any pain medication prescribed, including dosage, route, action, and side effects. Ensure that the patient understands the rest-activity cycle, use of assistive devices, exercise routine, and proper body mechanics. Determine whether a home-care agency needs to evaluate the home for safety equipment such as rails and grab bars and whether ongoing supervision is required. The Arthritis Foundation, which publishes information about arthritis, is engaged in a national education program about living with the condition. Help the patient get in touch with this organization.

Rocky Mountain Spotted Fever

DRG Category: 868
Mean LOS: 4.6 days
Description: MEDICAL: Other Infectious and Parasitic Diseases Diagnoses With Complication or Comorbidity

Rocky Mountain spotted fever (RMSF) is a tick-borne disease that is found in all 48 contiguous states in the United States; approximately 5,000 cases occur each year. A concentration of cases occurs in the southwestern, southern, and southeastern United States along with Cape Cod and Long Island in the Northeast. Highest rates of disease occur in North Carolina, Missouri, and Tennessee. The illness occurs as a small, intracellular parasite, *Rickettsia rickettsii*, is released from the salivary glands of some adult ticks. The primary result is small-vessel vasculitis, which results in vascular lesions throughout the body that lead to symptoms such as severe headache, myalgias, and rash. After exposure, the incubation period is usually about a week, but in cases of severe infection, it can be as short as 2 days.

The patient outcome is directly related to accurate, early diagnosis and appropriate treatment. Without treatment, the disease has a mortality rate of up to 40%. With treatment, the mortality rate declines to less than 10%. Complications, although uncommon, include meningitis, pneumonia, pneumonitis, middle-ear infections, and parotitis. If the infection is left untreated, the associated rash may lead to peeling skin and even gangrene of the elbows, fingers, and toes. Life-threatening complications—such as disseminated intravascular coagulation, shock, respiratory failure, liver failure, and acute renal failure—occur rarely.

CAUSES

R rickettsii is implicated as the cause of RMSF and is spread by exposure from two types of ticks. The mountain wood tick is found mainly in the west and is called *Dermacentor andersoni*. The dog tick, *D variabilis*, is more commonly found in the east. The ticks attach themselves to exposed body areas such as the neck, hair, and ankles. The tick then not only engorges itself on the blood of the host but also infects the host during a prolonged bite of 4 to 6 hours. Risk factors include being out of doors in high-risk areas without protective clothing and not checking for ticks after being out of doors in a high-risk area.

GENETIC CONSIDERATIONS

Heritable immune responses could be protective or could increase susceptibility.

SEX AND LIFE SPAN CONSIDERATIONS

Most reports indicate that those infected are mostly male (60%) and under age 20 years (50%), although another peak in incidence occurs in men ages 60 to 69 years. The clinical symptoms of RMSF vary with age. Patients older than 15 years fit the most common clinical description of the disease (fever up to 104°F [40°C], headache, joint and muscle pain, rash), with the mortality rate the highest in patients over 30 years. Patients younger than 15 years (and their parents) often wait longer to seek medical treatment, have a later onset of rash, and manifest more severe disease. These younger patients experience cardiac dysrhythmias and pneumonia more often than do mature patients.

HEALTH DISPARITIES AND SEXUAL/GENDER MINORITY HEALTH

Native American persons have a higher risk and poorer outcomes than other groups. White persons have twice the incidence of Black persons. However, the clinical course is more difficult and mortality is higher in persons with dark skin, possibly because of slowed diagnosis due to the practitioner's difficulty visualizing a rash. Sexual and gender minority status has no known effect on the risk for RMSF.

GLOBAL HEALTH CONSIDERATIONS

The entire western hemisphere is the primary location for exposure for RMSF. In Brazil, the disease is more common from October to February and in North America during the warmer months (April to September), but in countries located in the tropics, there is little seasonal variation.

ASSESSMENT

HISTORY. At least 50% of patients presenting with RMSF display the classic triad of symptoms: fever, rash, and history of exposure to ticks. Ask about the dates of recent outdoor activities and known tick exposure. Note that only about 75% of patients actually recall tick exposure when they are diagnosed with RMSF. Determine if the patient has pets because dogs are another source of the infection. Ask about common symptoms such as fever; severe headache; pain of the joints, muscles, and bones; malaise; and lethargy. Gastrointestinal symptoms are also common, including nausea, vomiting, diarrhea, constipation, anorexia, and abdominal pain. RMSF should be considered in any patients with an unexplained fever if they have traveled to a location where tick-borne disease is endemic.

PHYSICAL EXAMINATION. The most common symptoms are **fever, rash**, and a **history of exposure to ticks**. The hallmark hemorrhagic rash associated with this disease appears 1 to 15 days after the onset of illness, most commonly around the third day, and therefore may not be present on the initial examination. The associated rash occurs in 80% to 90% of patients but is a major diagnostic sign. It is a maculopapular eruption on the wrists and ankles with pink 2- to 5-mm macules that blanch with pressure. Three days after the rash appears, it becomes fixed and darker red with a petechial appearance. The rash then extends to the trunk and extremities and ultimately to the palms and soles of the feet. The patient appears acutely ill, with skin that is warm to the touch. Fevers from 102°F to 104°F (38.9°C–40°C) are almost a universal symptom.

The patient may develop a rapid respiratory rate, shallow breathing, and a bronchial cough. Changes in mental status, such as confusion, agitation, and restlessness, may indicate a worsening condition. Fever and dehydration can lead to a rapid and thready peripheral pulse, hypotension, delayed capillary blanching, respiratory failure, and shock. Late signs of complications include hepatomegaly and splenomegaly on palpation and pitting peripheral edema.

PSYCHOSOCIAL. Assess the patient's social support network and consider the effect the illness has on the patient's family. Expect them to be anxious and fearful about a sudden, unexpected serious illness. The patient may have to take time off from high school, college, or work and may worry about unmet financial, family, or educational obligations. Note the patient's developmental stage and recognize the age-related concerns that a sudden illness creates.

Diagnostic Highlights

Most often the diagnosis of RMSF is made as a result of clinical findings because diagnostic titers of antibodies are only detectable 10 days after the onset of illness. Other tests may include complement fixation titer, indirect hemagglutination titer, indirect immunofluorescence titer, and latex agglutination. Complete blood count may show thrombocytopenia and anemia (30% of patients). Electrolytes may show hyponatremia (30% of patients).

PRIMARY NURSING DIAGNOSIS

DIAGNOSIS. Risk for infection as evidenced by fever, rash, myalgia, tachypnea, and tachycardia.

OUTCOMES. Infection severity; Immune status; Risk control: Infectious process; Symptom severity; Symptom control; Knowledge: Infection management; Knowledge: Disease process; Knowledge: Medication

INTERVENTIONS. Infection protection; Medication administration; Temperature regulation; Teaching: Prescribed medication; Teaching: Disease process

▓ PLANNING AND IMPLEMENTATION

Collaborative

If the patient needs to have a tick removed, wear gloves and place gentle traction on the tick with either tweezers or the fingers. Do not crush the tick because inhaling the bacteria may lead to disease exposure. Do not apply noxious chemicals onto the tick. Because the patient may be further injured if a match is used on the tick, do not apply a match to the skin to remove the tick. Patients who have severe cases of RMSF are admitted to the hospital, possibly to the intensive care unit. Central parenteral administration of fluids and antibiotics is often necessary, and the patient may also be monitored with a pulmonary artery catheter if hemodynamically unstable. Oxygen therapy and electrolyte replacement may be necessary.

Pharmacologic Highlights

Medication or Drug Class	Dosage	Description	Rationale
Doxycycline	100 mg every 12 hr IV or PO for 7–14 days or 3 days after becoming afebrile is the treatment of choice for adults; dose for children is 2.2 mg/kg body weight every 12 hr	Broad-spectrum tetracycline class antibiotic	Kill the microorganism and fight infection

Other Drugs: For symptom management, antipyretics are usually necessary for temperature control, and analgesia is used to control discomfort. Usually, the physician avoids prescribing aspirin because of the added risk of platelet dysfunction.

Independent

Nursing care focuses on increasing comfort, monitoring for complications, and educating the patient. Implement nonpharmacologic strategies to manage discomfort, such as tepid sponge baths for fever, frequent linen changes for excessive diaphoresis, and age-appropriate diversions for discomfort. Teach the patient guided imagery, deep-breathing techniques, and music therapy to manage pain and boredom. Provide age-appropriate activities for young adults, such as television, radio, videos, and music, to help them pass the time and to take their minds off discomfort. To conserve the patient's energy during a time of increased metabolic demand, assist with activities of daily living and space all caregiving activities with periods of rest to decrease the patient's oxygen expenditure.

Monitor the patient's skin rash for signs of infection, such as sloughing, redness, warmth, and purulent drainage. Help the patient move in bed to positions of comfort every hour or two and pad the elbows and heels to prevent skin breakdown. Provide mouth care every 4 hours and offer the patient mentholated lotions to decrease the itching associated with the rash. If possible, maintain a cool room temperature to help the patient control the itching. When the patient's condition has stabilized, discuss methods to avoid tick bites in the future. Encourage the patient to avoid tick-infested areas. If the patient chooses to be out of doors in such an area, teach the patient to wear protective clothing (long pants, tucked-in shirt, laced boots), to use tick repellent, and to inspect the entire body every 4 hours for ticks. If a tick bite occurs, explain that the tick should be removed with a tweezers by steady traction and then discarded immediately without crushing. Encourage homeowners to spray their yards for ticks.

Evidence-Based Practice and Health Policy

Omodior, O. (2021). A space-time permutation scan statistic for evaluating county-level tick-borne disease clusters in Indiana, 2009–2016. *Health Security*, *19*, 108–115.

- The authors aimed to identify age group, sex, rural-urban differences, and spatiotemporal clusters of tick-borne disease diagnoses in Indiana. They analyzed retrospective surveillance data for Lyme disease, ehrlichiosis, RMSF, typhus/rickettsial diseases, and tularemia.
- Approximately 60% of people infected were male. They found more Lyme disease diagnoses among Indiana residents younger than 45 years of age as compared to older adults. Conversely, more ehrlichiosis, RMSF, and tularemia were reported in Indiana residents aged 45 years and older. An analysis of summated tick-borne disease by county showed significantly higher diagnoses reported in urban counties, compared with rural and rural-mixed counties.

DOCUMENTATION GUIDELINES

- Patient history: Recent trips and outdoor activities specific to possible tick exposure, exposure to pets, and early physical signs
- Physical findings: Pink macular rash, trend of vital signs, fluid intake and output, respiratory assessment, and level of oxygenation (measured by pulse oximetry)
- Patient's response to antibiotic treatment, antipyretics, other measures to control temperature, analgesics, and discussion of tick prevention

DISCHARGE AND HOME HEALTHCARE GUIDELINES

To prevent RMSF, teach patients to avoid tick exposure if possible. Encourage them to wear dark, hooded clothing that is tight around the ankles and wrists when walking in wooded areas and tall grasses. Boots that lace provide additional protection. Explain that after spending time in infested areas, patients should examine their skin and especially hair for the presence of ticks. Remind patients to use a tick repellent spray on their clothing. Teach patients to avoid spraying tick repellents directly on the skin and check the labels before using them on children.

Be sure the patient understands the importance of continuing to take antibiotics for the entire course. The most commonly prescribed antibiotic for adults is doxycycline. Antibiotics are prescribed for up to 2 weeks after the fever is gone. Teach the patient to report increasing shortness of breath, inability to take oral food and fluids, or a rash that appears infected. Encourage patients to report a fever that does not respond to the doses of acetaminophen given every 4 hours.

Salmonella Infection (Salmonellosis)

DRG Category:	868
Mean LOS:	4.6 days
Description:	MEDICAL: Other Infectious and Parasitic Diseases Diagnoses With Complication or Comorbidity

Salmonellosis is a bacterial infection caused by gram-negative bacilli of the genus *Salmonella*. Sometimes classified as food poisoning because it is frequently acquired by ingesting food that has been contaminated with the *Salmonella* bacterium, salmonella syndromes can be divided into five categories: gastroenteritis, enteric fever, bacteremia, localized infection, and a chronic carrier state (see Table 1). The most severe form of salmonellosis is typhoid, which can cause perforation or hemorrhage of the intestines, pneumonia, toxemia, acute circulatory failure, and cerebral thrombosis. Only about 3% of *Salmonella* infections are confirmed by laboratory testing, but an estimated 1.4 million people are infected each year in the United States.

Experts suggest that a large dose of the organism is needed to survive acid in the stomach. Once the *Salmonella* bacterium is ingested, it multiplies rapidly in the mucosal layers of the stomach and small intestine. The greater the number of organisms ingested, the shorter is the incubation period; typically, incubation is 8 to 48 hours after ingestion of contaminated food or liquid, and symptoms usually last for 3 to 5 days. An inflammatory response in the tissues produces gastroenteritis. The infection may stop there, or the salmonella organisms may travel via the lymph and vascular system throughout the body. The dissemination of organisms produces lesions in other organs or, possibly, sepsis. Systemic lesions may result in appendicitis, peritonitis, otitis media, pneumonia, osteomyelitis, or endocarditis. Symptoms of intermittent fever, chills, anorexia, and weight loss indicate sepsis. Other complications include intestinal perforation, hemorrhage, cholecystitis, arteritis, or abscess formation. Patients diagnosed with severe salmonellosis have increased risk for developing cancer of the ascending/transverse colon.

• TABLE 1 Types of *Salmonella* Infections

TYPE	INCIDENCE AND INCUBATION	DESCRIPTION
Gastroenteritis	Most common in May through October; incubation is 8–48 hr	Acute onset of fever and chills for 72 hr, nausea and vomiting, cramping, diarrhea for 3–7 days; diarrhea is usually not bloody
Enteric (typhoid fever)	Transmission from contaminated water or animal by-products; incubation 5–21 days	First 10 days: Headache, cough, anorexia, fatigue, weakness, sore throat, gastrointestinal complaints such as abdominal pain or changes in bowel habits; relative bradycardia during period of fever; after 10 days, abdominal distention, abdominal pain, bradycardia, rash (rose spots), confusion may occur; condition either resolves after 4 wk or complications such as intestinal perforation or endocarditis occur
Bacteremia	Occurs in people who are immunosuppressed	Fever, infection
Local infection	Occurs in 5% of infected people	Infections of heart, brain, lungs, bones, kidneys, muscles
Carrier	Stool or urine for more than 1 yr	< 1% in nontyphoid *Salmonella* and 4% with untreated *Salmonella*

CAUSES

Salmonellosis is caused by any of more than 2,000 serotypes of *Salmonella* bacteria. *Salmonellae* can be nontyphoidal or typhoidal depending on the organism type. Typhoid fever is caused by *Salmonella* Typhi bacterium transmitted through ingestion of water that has been contaminated with the feces of infected persons. Salmonellosis may also be contracted by eating infected raw eggs or egg products or uncooked meat or poultry, ingesting raw milk, or handling infected animals. *Salmonella* can survive for an extended period of time in water, sewage, ice, and food. Although cooking food thoroughly can reduce the risk of salmonellosis, it cannot eliminate it.

GENETIC CONSIDERATIONS

Heritable immune responses could be protective or increase susceptibility. Mutations in the interleukin-12 receptor (*IL12RB1*) appear to increase susceptibility to mycobacteria and salmonella infections.

SEX AND LIFE SPAN CONSIDERATIONS

All people are susceptible. Although the disease is rarely fatal, severity may be pronounced in infants and persons with neoplastic, immunosuppressive, or other debilitating conditions. Enterocolitis and bacteremia are more common among infants. People in hospitals and nursing homes have a higher prevalence of this disease than the general population. Women over age 50 years are the most common carriers of typhoid. Patients infected with *Salmonella* tend to be most commonly either younger than 20 years of age or older than 70 years.

HEALTH DISPARITIES AND SEXUAL/GENDER MINORITY HEALTH

People with HIV disease are susceptible to recurrent bacteremia caused by salmonellae. Black and Hispanic people bear a disproportionate burden of HIV disease compared with other populations. The Centers for Disease Control and Prevention reported in 2018 that 69% of new HIV diagnoses in the United States were in gay and bisexual men. In young people ages 13 to 24 years, young gay and bisexual men account for 83% of all new HIV diagnoses.

GLOBAL HEALTH CONSIDERATIONS

Developed countries have frequencies of salmonella infections resulting in gastroenteritis similar to that of the United States. Estimates of global *Salmonella* gastritis range widely, from 200 million to 1.4 billion cases each year. Experts estimate that at least 3 million people die annually from infections. In countries where people acquire typhoid fever, most cases occur in children between the ages of 5 and 19 years. The areas where typhoid fever is endemic include southern and southeastern Asia and southern Africa, as well as some parts of Latin America.

ASSESSMENT

HISTORY. Establish a history of fever (often 102°F [38.9°C] and higher), nausea, abdominal pain and cramping, vomiting, anorexia, and diarrhea that has persisted for at least 4 days. Ask about headache or constipation, which are symptoms of typhoid. The first symptoms generally appear between 8 and 48 hours after ingesting the bacteria; ask the patient about possible sources of the infection. Ask if the patient has had recent contact with an infected person or animal. Determine if the patient has ingested uncooked egg or meat products. If so, ask the patient whether the potentially contaminated food was prepared at home or at another location, such as a restaurant or public gathering. Elicit a history of recent travel to other countries that have endemic typhoid.

PHYSICAL EXAMINATION. The patient appears to be weak and pale because of **fever, nausea, headache, vomiting, abdominal pain**, and **diarrhea**. Young children and debilitated patients may show signs of dehydration. Fevers range from 101°F to 105°F (38.3°C–40.6°C). Rose spots (pink, blanchable, raised macules) may appear on the trunk, and joints may be painful. Palpation of the abdomen may be difficult because of tenderness. Stools are usually greenish-brown, watery, and foul smelling. They contain mucus, pus, or blood. A sudden worsening abdominal pain may indicate perforation of the bowel.

PSYCHOSOCIAL. Patients with salmonellosis feel ill and may be apprehensive about the diagnosis. Patients feel guilty if they inadvertently exposed others to the disease through food preparation or angry if they have been exposed to the illness at a restaurant or other public gathering. Parents of young children are apt to be anxious and afraid for their child's life.

Diagnostic Highlights

Test	Normal Result	Abnormality With Condition	Explanation
Cultures of feces, urine, vomitus, pus, or blood	Negative for pathogens	Presence of *Salmonella*	Determines presence of *Salmonella* in various samples; stool culture is the definitive diagnostic tool for salmonellosis; stool culture should be fresh

Other Tests: Complete blood count to determine the response to infection, liver function tests, serum electrolytes, blood urea nitrogen, creatinine, bone marrow aspirate and culture (highly sensitive for enteric fever but rarely done)

PRIMARY NURSING DIAGNOSIS

DIAGNOSIS. Risk for infection as evidenced by fever, nausea, vomiting, headache, abdominal pain, and/or diarrhea

OUTCOMES. Infection severity; Immune status; Knowledge: Infection management; Risk control; Risk detection; Knowledge: Medication

INTERVENTIONS. Infection control; Infection protection; Medication management; Environmental management: Home preparation; Teaching: Disease process

PLANNING AND IMPLEMENTATION

Collaborative

Patients with systemic infections are placed on the antibiotic that is most appropriate for their condition. Symptom management is accomplished by fluid and electrolyte replacement and control of fever. Because antidiarrheal and antispasmodic agents slow intestinal mobility, some experts do not recommend their use because they retard the intestinal transit of the infecting organisms.

The patient with salmonellosis is placed on bedrest during the acute phase and should be on enteric precautions until the diarrhea stops. Observe the patient's stools for consistency and blood. Bleeding or abdominal pain may indicate the complication of bowel perforation; check for a sudden fall in temperature or blood pressure and a rising pulse rate. Many patients with *Salmonella* infection are not hospitalized but recover at home. Report *Salmonella* infection to the local health authority, particularly if the patient is employed in a food-handling occupation.

Pharmacologic Highlights

Medication or Drug Class	Dosage	Description	Rationale
Antibiotics are reserved for patients with severe disease or who are at a high risk of invasive disease (infants, older patients, or immunocompromised)	Varies with drug	Ciprofloxacin (Cipro), ampicillin, azithromycin (Zithromax), ceftriaxone (Rocephin), chloramphenicol, trimethoprim, and sulfamethoxazole (Bactrim DS, Septra)	Kill bacteria and halt infection; treatment with antibiotics for gastroenteritis is controversial; experts suggest that antibiotics do not shorten the disease but prolong the time that the patient is a carrier
Nonsystemic antidiarrheals	Varies with drug	Kaolin/pectin (Kaopectate), loperamide	Coat the intestinal mucosa, decrease intestinal secretions, and reduce discomfort; use sparingly because may prolong the infection

Independent

Encourage the patient to drink fluids so as not to become dehydrated. During the acute phase, encourage adults to drink water and suck on ice chips. Children should drink oral rehydration solutions. Provide regular skin and mouth care, and turn the patient often. While the patient is infected, allow the patient as much rest as possible between activities. Provide a restful atmosphere. To help reduce the patient's temperature, apply tepid wet towels to the patient's groin and axillae. Use universal precautions. Employ scrupulous hand-washing techniques before and after working with the patient who has salmonellosis. Wear gloves when you dispose of feces or any objects that have been contaminated by the patient's feces.

Explain to the patient the need to report salmonella infections to the local health authority. To prevent future infections, instruct the patient and family to wash their hands thoroughly after defecation and before handling food. Also, instruct the patient to avoid raw eggs or foods prepared with raw eggs, to cook meat and poultry thoroughly, to refrigerate food below 46°F (7.5°C), and to wash hands after handling animals.

Evidence-Based Practice and Health Policy

Mughini-Gras, L., Pijnacker, R., Duijster, J., Heck, M., Wit, B., Veldman, K., & Franz, E. (2020). Changing epidemiology of invasive non-typhoid *Salmonella* infection: A nationwide population-based registry study. *Clinical Microbiology and Infection, 26*, 941.e9–941.e14.

* The authors examined the epidemiology of invasive nontyphoid *Salmonella* (iNTS) to determine trends, risk factors, serotype distribution, antimicrobial resistance (AMR), and sources of iNTS infection in a high-income setting. They used national surveillance registries in the Netherlands to obtain 22,837 records of culture-confirmed human salmonellosis cases and 10,008 serotyped *Salmonella* isolates from five putative animal reservoirs (pigs, cattle, broilers, layers, reptiles) for the years 2005 to 2018.
* Increased iNTS infection risk was associated with wintertime, male sex, older age, and living in rural areas. Cattle were a larger source of iNTS than non-iNTS infections.

DOCUMENTATION GUIDELINES

* Physical findings: Vital signs; dehydration; intake of food and fluids; tolerance of food, including instances of vomiting; output; and diarrhea or constipation with description of stool
* Notification of the local health authority
* Response to treatment: Changes in symptoms, increased comfort, and decrease in body temperature

DISCHARGE AND HOME HEALTHCARE GUIDELINES

Instruct the patient and family about the cause, transmission, and symptoms of the disease and preventive measures. Teach the family how to care for the patient at home. Treat mild fever with antipyretics and maintain a good fluid intake. Ice pops and soda may increase fluid intake for young children. Avoid the use of laxatives. Gradually increase the patient's activity level as tolerated. Explain the need to report complications of bleeding, dehydration, or the return of symptoms to the physician at once. Be sure the patient understands any medications prescribed, including dosage, route, action, and side effects. Stress the importance of completing the antibiotic regimen even after symptoms diminish.

When the diarrhea subsides, surfaces should be cleaned with soap and then a bleach solution of 250 parts per million free chlorine. Clean all surfaces, utensils, and the bathroom. Vinegar and water is an adequate cleaner for day-to-day kitchen use after meal preparation to prevent *Salmonella* infections.

Sarcoidosis

DRG Category: 196
Mean LOS: 6.2 days
Description: MEDICAL: Interstitial
Lung Disease With Major
Complication or Comorbidity

S arcoidosis, formerly called *Boeck sarcoid*, is a noncontagious multisystem disorder characterized by epithelioid granular tumors (granulomas) that most frequently affect the lung; more
than 90% of cases involve lung or intrathoracic lymph nodes. Pulmonary sarcoidosis is usually
a chronic disorder associated with an intense cellular immune response in the alveolar structures of the lungs. A series of interactions between lymphocytes (primarily responsible for the
granuloma formation), macrophages/monocytes (primarily responsible for interstitial fibrosis),
epithelioid cells, and giant cells lead to the formation of noncaseating granulomas. The granulomas can lead to fibrosis, which affects the lung's ability to exchange gases. Other recurrent sites
include the liver, lymph nodes, bone marrow, skin, and eyes. Sarcoidosis is detected occasionally in the spleen, joints, heart, skeletal muscle, phalangeal bones, parotid glands, and central
nervous system (CNS).

About 65% to 70% of the cases of sarcoidosis usually resolve spontaneously within 2 years.
Without treatment, however, sarcoidosis can lead to chronic progressive sarcoidosis, which is
associated with complications such as pulmonary fibrosis, scarring, and progressive pulmonary
disease. In such cases, when the heart can no longer pump against the noncompliant fibrotic
lungs, cor pulmonale can develop. Other potentially lethal complications are superinfections
by organisms such as *Aspergillus*. The overall mortality is less than 5% for patients who do not
receive treatment.

CAUSES

Sarcoidosis is a complex and mysterious disease of unknown origin, although 80% of patients
with sarcoidosis have high titers of the Epstein-Barr virus. It is not a malignant disease, and it
is not an autoimmune disease. There is increasing evidence that a triggering agent strikes and
stimulates an enhanced cell-mediated immune process at the site of involvement. The triggering
agent may be a fungus, an atypical mycobacterium, pine pollen, or a toxic chemical such as
zirconium or beryllium, which can lead to illnesses resembling sarcoidosis. Because there is a
slightly higher incidence of sarcoidosis in the same family, the triggering agent may be genetic.
The primary risk factor seems to be a family history, but environmental exposure to toxins and
chemicals may contribute. The risk seems to be enhanced in people working in jobs related to
agriculture, water, construction, metal work, education, and health. Smoking is also a risk factor.

GENETIC CONSIDERATIONS

Allelic variation in human leukocyte antigen (HLA)-DRB1 increases susceptibility for sarcoidosis. A mutation near the *HLA-DRB1* gene, in the *BTNL2* gene, also independently affects
susceptibility to sarcoidosis, while mutations in the *NOD2* gene cause an early-onset form of
sarcoidosis. Polymorphisms in the *ANXA11* gene are also associated with sarcoidosis, a result
that is consistent across ethnic groups. Confusingly, familial clustering of this disease may also
be due to a shared environment. The much greater frequency of Black people with sarcoidosis
as compared to other groups in the United States suggests a genetic contribution to etiology.
A genome-wide association study conducted in Black individuals demonstrated an SNP in the
NOTCH4 gene as well as the *XAF1* gene. Familial transmission patterns do not always follow
simple Mendelian rules, making complex transmission combining both genetic and environmental factors most likely.

SEX AND LIFE SPAN CONSIDERATIONS

Disease onset is usually between ages 20 and 30 years or between 45 and 65 years. It is more frequent among women than men, and women have poorer outcomes.

HEALTH DISPARITIES AND SEXUAL/GENDER MINORITY HEALTH

Frequency of sarcoidosis is 10 times higher in Black persons as compared to White persons, and Black women of childbearing age develop sarcoidosis twice as frequently as Black men. Black patients experience more severe pulmonary disease, more multi-organ involvement, higher rates of hospitalization, and a worse prognosis than other groups. The financial strain of the condition is highest among women and Black persons (Ogundipe et al., 2019 [see Evidence-Based Practice and Health Policy]). Sexual and gender minority status has no known effect on the risk for sarcoidosis.

GLOBAL HEALTH CONSIDERATIONS

The overall global prevalence of sarcoidosis is similar to that in the United States. The highest reported prevalence is in Sweden, and the lowest is in Poland. People of Scandinavian ancestry have higher rates of the disease than their other European counterparts. In developing countries without experience with the disease or without diagnostic capabilities, it may be misdiagnosed as tuberculosis.

ASSESSMENT

HISTORY. Sarcoidosis is known as the great masquerader because it presents in a variety of guises from lymphadenopathy to erythema nodosum (red and painful nodules on the legs, associated with rheumatism). Establish a history of arthralgia in the wrists, ankles, and elbows, which is an initial symptom of sarcoidosis. Ask if the patient has experienced fatigue, malaise, weakness, anorexia, fever, or weight loss. Elicit a history of respiratory difficulties, such as breathlessness, cough (generally nonproductive but may be blood tinged [hemoptysis]), or substernal chest pain. Ask if the patient has had any visual deficits or any eye pain, night sweats, seizures, or cranial or peripheral nerve palsies, which are signs of CNS involvement. Determine if a family history of sarcoidosis exists. Ask if the patient has been exposed to a viral or bacterial infection or to chemicals such as beryllium or zirconium.

PHYSICAL EXAMINATION. Common symptoms are organ specific but may include **fever**, **fatigue**, **anorexia**, **muscle pain**, **dyspnea**, **cough**, and **chest pain**. Examine the patient's skin for lesions, plaques, papules, and subcutaneous nodules on the face, neck, and extremities. A common skin lesion, erythema nodosum, is seen in 10% of cases; other lesions, such as lupus pernio (hard, blue-purple, swollen, shiny lesions of the nose, cheeks, lips, ears, fingers, and knees), are seen in 15% of patients. When granulomas affect the face, they tend to occur around the nose and may cause nasal destruction and disfigurement. Note the patient's skin tone for signs of jaundice.

Up to 60% of patients develop intraocular symptoms. Examine the patient's eyes for signs of enlarged tear glands, conjunctival infections, and granulomatous uveitis; if the patient has noted visual difficulties, perform a vision examination. Bilateral granulomatous uveitis occurs in 15% of cases and can lead to loss of vision because of secondary glaucoma. Other ocular symptoms may include retinal periphlebitis, lacrimal gland enlargement, and conjunctival infiltration, which can result in blurred vision, ocular pain, conjunctival infections, and iritis.

Inspect the patient's legs and arms for muscle wasting and enlarged or reddened joints. Ask the patient to move the joints in full range of motion to determine if pain or tenderness occurs. Palpate the salivary and parotid glands to determine if nontender enlargement is present. Palpate the lymph nodes to assess for lymphadenopathy and the abdomen for an enlarged liver and spleen. Auscultate the patient's chest to determine if diminished breath sounds indicate pulmonary fibrosis, infiltration, or restrictive disease. If breath sounds are not audible in one lung, suspect a pneumothorax. If you hear adventitious breath sounds or lung consolidation, suspect pulmonary infection. Auscultate the patient's heart and note any irregularities that might indicate bundle-branch block or ventricular ectopy.

PSYCHOSOCIAL. Sarcoidosis is associated with fatigue and can be linked with depression, bipolar disorder, panic disorder, or anxiety disorder. As with any chronic disease, the patient and family need continual support and caring from healthcare professionals. Assess the patient's and family's ability to cope with a chronic disease and the change in roles that a chronic disease demands. The patient may also be distressed over changes in appearance that have been caused by lesions on the face in particular.

Diagnostic Highlights

General Comments: Sarcoidosis is primarily diagnosed by exclusion or by finding characteristic noncaseating granulomas in the affected organs.

Test	Normal Result	Abnormality With Condition	Explanation
Tuberculin skin test, fungal serologies, and sputum cultures for mycobacteria and fungi	Negative	Used to make a differential diagnosis; positive results indicate diagnosis other than sarcoidosis	Rule out tuberculosis
Tissue biopsy	Negative	Used to make a differential diagnosis; positive results indicate diagnosis other than sarcoidosis	Rule out other conditions
High-resolution computed tomography	Clear lung fields with no lymphadenopathy	Active alveolitis or fibrosis	Demonstrates extent of air trapping

Other Tests: Tests include complete blood count, serum electrolytes with calcium, gallium-67 scanning, electrocardiogram, bronchoalveolar lavage, pulmonary function tests, antinuclear antibodies, rheumatoid factor levels, and hypergammaglobulinemia. Other tests may include serum amyloid A (SAA), soluble interleukin-2 receptor (sIL-2R), alkaline phosphatase, lysozyme, angiotensin-converting enzyme (ACE), and glycoprotein KL-6.

PRIMARY NURSING DIAGNOSIS

DIAGNOSIS. Impaired gas exchange related to altered alveolar-capillary membrane changes and decreased oxygen-carrying ability as evidenced by fatigue, dyspnea, diminished breath sounds, and/or cough

OUTCOMES. Respiratory status: Gas exchange; Respiratory status: Ventilation; Symptom severity; Symptom management; Knowledge: Disease process

INTERVENTIONS. Airway management; Oxygen therapy; Respiratory management; Respiratory monitoring; Ventilation assistance; Teaching: Disease process

PLANNING AND IMPLEMENTATION
Collaborative

Asymptomatic sarcoidosis requires no treatment, although ongoing assessment is called for. Sarcoidosis with ocular, respiratory, CNS, cardiac, or systemic symptoms requires treatment with systemic or topical corticosteroids. Other treatment includes a low-calcium, high-calorie nutritional diet with an increase in fluids to prevent malnutrition, hypercalcemia, and dehydration. A low-sodium diet may be indicated if sodium retention occurs because of prednisone. Ongoing monitoring of the patient's physical condition by physical examination and diagnostic tests indicates the patient's response to treatment and the appearance of complications.

Pharmacologic Highlights

Medication or Drug Class	Dosage	Description	Rationale
Prednisone	May range from 30–60 mg/day PO, tapering over 4–8 wk to a maintenance dose of 10–15 mg for 6 mo every other day	Corticosteroids remain the mainstay of therapy for the first 1–2 yr, but some patients may require life-long steroid therapy	Relieves symptoms and reverses fibrosis of pulmonary tissue

Other Drugs: Optic agents such as methylcellulose eyedrops and other ophthalmic ointments are used to treat ocular manifestations. Antidysrhythmic agents are used to treat ventricular ectopy. Salicylates and other NSAIDs are used for the treatment of arthritis manifestations. Cytotoxic agents such as methotrexate may be used to inhibit T-cell production. Other medications used to treat cutaneous sarcoidosis include hydroxychloroquine, azathioprine, cyclosporine, chlorambucil, allopurinol, doxycycline, and infliximab.

Independent

Because many patients have pulmonary granulomas that have the potential to affect airway, breathing, and gas exchange, the primary nursing focus is to ensure that these essential functions are preserved. Maintain an oral airway and endotracheal intubation equipment near the patient at all times in case they are needed to clear airway obstruction. Support the patient's breathing by positioning the patient for comfort (often with the head of the bed elevated and the arms raised slightly on pillows). Adjust the patient's activity to reduce oxygen demands. Space all activities with adequate periods of rest. Provide uninterrupted periods of sleep at night and at least one 2-hour rest period during the day. Schedule diagnostic tests to provide adequate rest and work with the family and other visitors to conserve the patient's energy.

Changes in vision place the patient at risk for injury. Teach the patient to scan the area for obstructions before beginning to walk. Remove any obstructions or rugs in the path between the patient's bed and the bathroom. Encourage the patient to wear well-fitting shoes or slippers when ambulating. The patient's impaired vision, intolerance to activity, and any lesions on the face may lead to a disturbance in self-concept or body image. From the patient, elicit priorities for a "good" appearance and support those activities that the patient finds beneficial. Those activities may include extra hair care, using makeup, wearing clothing from home, maintaining a beard or moustache, or other similar grooming strategies. Help the patient maintain the highest level of activity that the disease allows. As with any chronic, debilitating disease with no cure, the patient is expected to have times of depression and anxiety. Use a supportive, nonjudgmental approach and active listening. Answer the patient's questions honestly and provide information about the long-range prognosis of the condition. If the patient or family demonstrates ineffective coping, refer the patient or significant others for counseling or to a support group.

Evidence-Based Practice and Health Policy

Ogundipe, F., Mehari, A., & Gillum, R. (2019). Disparities in sarcoidosis mortality by region, urbanization, and race in the United States: A multiple cause of death analysis. *American Journal of Medicine, 132*, 1062–1068. https://doi.org/10.1016/j.rmed.2017.11.008

- The goal of this study was to assess if the disparity of the sarcoidosis-related mortality rates varies by sex, race/ethnicity, region, and urbanization. U.S. data for multiple causes of death for 1999 to 2016 were used to determine numbers of deaths (N = 28,923) and age-adjusted rates for sarcoidosis as a cause of death. In the years 2008 to 2016, 9,112 deaths had sarcoidosis as the underlying cause (56%) compared with 16,129 with sarcoidosis listed as any cause.
- Age-adjusted annual death rates were higher for females than males and lower for Hispanics than for non-Hispanics. Rates in non-Hispanic Blacks were eight times those in non-Hispanic Whites. Among females, the highest rate was in non-Hispanic Blacks in the East-Central division. Sarcoidosis-related multiple cause of death mortality rates were highest in females and in non-Hispanic Blacks, and they varied geographically.

DOCUMENTATION GUIDELINES

- Physical findings: Breath sounds, respiratory rate and depth, heart sounds, cardiac rhythm, visual changes, ability to ambulate safely, appearance of skin lesions, tolerance to activities, and extent of fatigue
- Pain: Degree of joint and muscle pain; location, duration, and type of pain; response to analgesics; degree of mobility or immobility
- Response to corticosteroid therapy, changes in activity tolerance, ability to perform self-care

DISCHARGE AND HOME HEALTHCARE GUIDELINES

Teach the patient the purpose, dosage, schedule, precautions, potential side effects, interactions, and adverse reactions of all prescribed medications. Stress the need for compliance with prescribed steroid therapy. Stress the importance of regular follow-up and treatment. If appropriate, refer the patient with failing vision to community support and resources such as the American Foundation for the Blind (https://www.afb.org).

Teach the patient the signs and symptoms of possible complications, such as dizziness, anorexia, and peripheral edema (cor pulmonale); diminished vision and massive urine output (diabetes insipidus); flank pain (kidney stones); headache and fever (meningitis); and fever and productive cough (infection), that need to be reported to the primary healthcare provider.

Septic Shock

DRG Category:	292
Mean LOS:	3.9 days
Description:	MEDICAL: Heart Failure and Shock With Complication or Comorbidity

Septic shock is a clinical syndrome associated with severe systemic infection. It is a severe critical illness with healthcare costs exceeding $62 billion a year in the United States. Sepsis, a life-threatening organ dysfunction due to an abnormal response to infection, leads to multiple organ dysfunction; it is accompanied by circulatory and metabolic abnormalities associated with an increased risk for death. Septic shock is a sepsis-induced shock with hypotension (mean arterial pressure < 65 mm Hg) requiring vasopressors to maintain blood pressure, despite adequate fluid replacement, and with a serum lactate level greater than 2 mmol/L. Patients have perfusion abnormalities, including lactic acidosis, oliguria (urine output < 400 mL/day), or an acute alteration in mental status. Often septic shock is characterized by decreased organ perfusion, hypotension, and organ dysfunction. Septic shock is the major cause of death in intensive care units; the mortality rate is as high as 20% to 40% depending on the patient population. The incidence has increased during the past 50 years in the United States, probably owing to an increased number of patients who are immunocompromised, the increased use of invasive devices, and a longer life span for older adults.

While the physiology of septic shock is not completely understood, most experts note that it occurs because of a complex interaction between an infecting agent and the patient's immune system. The syndrome usually begins with the development of a local infectious process, but in septic shock, the response is not local but rather systemic. Bacteria from the local infection enter the systemic circulation and release toxins into the bloodstream. Gram-negative bacteria release endotoxins from their cell membrane as they lyse and die, whereas gram-positive bacteria release exotoxins throughout their life span. These toxins trigger the release of cytokines (proteins released by cells to signal other cells) and other mediators such as the interleukins, tumor necrosis factor, interferon, nitric oxide, complement, and platelet-activating factor. They also activate phagocytic cells such as the macrophages. The complex chemical reactions lead to multiple system effects such as disruption to the vascular endothelium, increased vascular permeability, vasodilation, and thrombosis at the organ level. Endothelial damage leads to further inflammatory responsiveness, coagulation, and further organ damage. As the syndrome progresses, blood flow becomes more sluggish, tissues become hypoxemic, and acidosis develops. Ultimately, if the infection is not reversed, the major organ systems (such as the lungs, kidneys, liver, and blood coagulation) fail, which leads to multiple organ dysfunction syndrome and death.

CAUSES

Respiratory tract, abdominal, urinary tract, and soft tissue infections are the most frequent causes of sepsis. Although any microorganism may cause septic shock, it is most often associated with gram-negative bacteria such as *Escherichia coli*, *Klebsiella pneumoniae*, and *Pseudomonas*. Gram-positive bacteria such as *Staphylococcus aureus* and *Streptococcus pneumoniae* can also cause septic shock. A fungal infection causes septic shock in less than 3% of the cases. Lower respiratory infections cause 35% to 50% of the cases of septic shock, urinary tract infections cause 25%, and soft tissue infections cause 15% of the cases.

Common factors or conditions associated with septic shock include diabetes mellitus, chronic kidney disease, malnutrition, alcohol abuse, chronic liver disease, respiratory infections, hemorrhage, cancer, and surgery. People with traumatic injuries with either peritoneal contamination, burns, prolonged IV cannulation, abscesses, or multiple blood transfusions are at particular risk as well. People at greatest risk have an impaired immune system, advanced age, infection with a resistant organism, and poor functional status at baseline.

GENETIC CONSIDERATIONS

Studies of genetic epidemiology have indicated that there is a strong genetic component involved in individual responses and outcomes of sepsis. The contributions of candidate inflammatory response genes are being investigated. These include tumor necrosis factor alpha (*TNF*) and tumor necrosis factor beta (*LTA*) genes. Additional candidate genes include FOXP3, interleukin 1 receptor associated kinase 3 (*IRAK3*), *IL6*, *IL10*, *IL12* receptor, *CD14*, toll-like receptor 4 (*TLR4*) and *TLR2*.

SEX AND LIFE SPAN CONSIDERATIONS

Septic shock occurs at all ages. Adults over 60 years of age are at high risk because of the immunocompromise associated with the aging process and make up the largest proportion of patients with septic shock. More males than females develop septic shock, and males have a slightly higher mortality rate. In neonates, the most common cause of septic shock is an immature immune system. Clinical manifestations may differ in the adult and pediatric populations. For instance, poor feeding and decreased activity levels may be early indicators of septic shock in infants. Pediatric patients may also maintain vital signs within normal limits for longer periods of time before circulatory failure occurs. Older individuals may never have an increased temperature and may remain hypothermic throughout the course of the disease.

HEALTH DISPARITIES AND SEXUAL/GENDER MINORITY HEALTH

Some epidemiological studies indicate that Black, Hispanic, and Native American persons have a higher prevalence of septic shock, possibly because of decreased access to healthcare and increased prevalence of multiple comorbidities. Epidemiological studies show that the highest risk for sepsis is found in Black men. Experts suggest that gender and sexual minority persons have higher levels of chronic health conditions such as asthma, diabetes, obesity, and rheumatoid arthritis than other groups. They also have higher rates of health behaviors such as tobacco use and heavy drinking. Gender and sexual minority persons are also more likely to delay testing and screening for chronic health conditions because of stigma, lack of healthcare providers' awareness, or insensitivity to the unique needs of this community (Caceres et al., 2019; Downing & Przedworski, 2018). These factors place them at risk for septic shock.

GLOBAL HEALTH CONSIDERATIONS

While septic shock occurs around the globe, there are no data on global prevalence.

ASSESSMENT

HISTORY. Patients with sepsis have nonspecific symptoms such as fever, chills, anxiety, confusion, dyspnea, nausea, vomiting, and fatigue. Patients may also have organ-based symptoms depending on the location of the infection, such as respiratory distress. Because of the severity of patients' condition, you may not be able to interview them for a complete history. You may obtain a great deal of information from the family and from other healthcare providers when the patient is transferred to your care. Because patients with septic shock are among the most critical of all patients treated in a hospital, they are admitted to a critical care unit for management.

Patients often have a history of either an infection or a critical event, such as a traumatic injury, recent major surgery, perforated bowel, or acute hemorrhage. Some patients may also have a longstanding IV catheter or a Foley catheter. Determine the cause for the patient's admission to the hospital and any history of a chronic disease such as cancer, diabetes mellitus, or pneumonia. Note any brief periods of decreased tissue perfusion such as hemorrhage, severe hypotension, or cardiac arrest that may demand emergency management before the development of septic shock. Take a thorough medication history, with particular attention to recent antibiotic administration, immunosuppressive medications, or total parenteral nutrition. Ask if the patient has been exposed to any treatment—such as organ transplantation, radiation therapy, or chemotherapy—that would lead to immunosuppression.

PHYSICAL EXAMINATION. Common symptoms are **fever, tachycardia, fatigue, chills, confusion, agitation**, and **dyspnea**. Three stages have been identified, but all patients do not progress with the same pattern of symptoms. In early septic shock (early hyperdynamic, compensated stage), some patients are tachycardic, with warm and flushed extremities and a normal blood pressure. As shock progresses, the diastolic blood pressure drops, the pulse pressure widens, and the peripheral pulses are bounding. The patient's temperature may be within normal limits, elevated, or below normal, and the patient may be confused or agitated. Often, the patient has a rapid respiratory rate, and peripheral edema may develop. In the second stage (late hyperdynamic, uncompensated stage), widespread organ dysfunction begins to occur. Blood pressure falls, and the patient becomes hypotensive. Increased peripheral edema becomes apparent. Respirations become more rapid and labored; you can hear rales when you auscultate the lungs; and the patient's sputum may become copious, pink, and frothy. In late septic shock, the blood pressure falls below 90 mm Hg for adults, the patient's extremities become cold, and signs of multiple organ failure (decreased urinary output, abdominal distention, absence of bowel sounds, bleeding from invasive lines, petechiae, cardiac dysrhythmias, hypoxemia, and hypercapnia) develop.

PSYCHOSOCIAL. As the syndrome progresses, patients may develop symptoms that change their behavior and appearance and experience situations that increase their anxiety and that of their family members. Ultimately, the family may be faced with the death of a loved one. Continuously assess the coping mechanisms and anxiety levels in both patients and families.

Diagnostic Highlights

Test	Normal Result	Abnormality With Condition	Explanation
Cultures and sensitivities	Negative for pathological bacterial flora or fungi	Positive for pathological bacterial flora or fungi	Identifies infecting organism in blood, urine, sputum, or wounds; note that in less than 50% of patients who develop septic shock, no bacterium is ever identified in cultures
Serum lactate level	0.5–2 mmol/L	> 2 mmol/L	Elevated under conditions of anaerobic metabolism due to hypoxemia or decreased perfusion

Other Tests: Tests include complete blood count, serum electrolytes, creatine, blood urea nitrogen, arterial blood gases, serum glucose, liver function tests, albumin level, prothrombin, and partial thromboplastin levels. In the later stages of septic shock, as complications develop, serial chest x-rays are essential to follow the progression of conditions such as pulmonary congestion and adult respiratory distress syndrome (ARDS), abdominal ultrasound, and echocardiography.

PRIMARY NURSING DIAGNOSIS

DIAGNOSIS. Risk for infection as evidenced by increased or decreased temperature, chills, confusion, agitation, hypotension, fatigue, and/or dyspnea

OUTCOMES. Immune status; Infection severity; Knowledge: Infection management; Risk control; Risk detection; Symptom severity; Symptom control; Fluid balance

INTERVENTIONS. Infection control; Medication management; Oxygen therapy; Respiratory monitoring; Medication administration; Fluid/Electrolyte management; Vital signs monitoring; Teaching: Disease process

PLANNING AND IMPLEMENTATION
Collaborative

The primary goals of treatment in septic shock are to identify and treat the infection, maintain oxygen delivery to the tissues, and restore the vascular volume, blood pressure, and cardiac output. IV fluids are administered to increase the volume within the vascular bed; crystalloids (normal saline solution or lactated Ringer's injection) are usually the fluids of choice. Vasopressors, such as dopamine, norepinephrine (Levophed), phenylephrine, or vasopressin may also be required to maintain an adequate blood pressure. The patient is also placed on broad-spectrum IV antibiotics. If the patient's hemoglobin and hematocrit are insufficient to manage oxygen delivery, the patient may need blood transfusions. A pulmonary artery catheter or central venous catheter may be inserted to monitor fluid, circulatory, and gas exchange status.

If complications such as ARDS develop, more aggressive treatment is instituted. Intubation, mechanical ventilation with low tidal volumes, and oxygenation are required for severe respiratory distress or failure. Patients often need ventilator adjuncts, such as positive end-expiratory pressure, pressure-control ventilation, or inverse inspiration-to-expiration ratio ventilation. Airway stabilization and management are essential to allow for ventilator management. An aggressive search for the source of sepsis is an essential part of the treatment. Any indwelling catheters, whether they are urinary, intravascular, intracerebral, or intra-arterial, are discontinued if possible or moved to another location. A surgical consultation may be performed to search for undrained abscesses or to débride wounds.

Total parenteral feeding or enteral feedings may be instituted for patients who are unable to consume adequate calories. Monitor the success of nutritional therapy with daily weights. During supportive care, the entire healthcare team needs to monitor the patient's condition carefully with serial cardiopulmonary assessments, including vital signs, physical assessment, and continuous hemodynamic monitoring. Patients should be attached to a pulse oximeter for continuous assessment of the arterial oxygen saturation. The patient's level of consciousness is important. In children, monitor the child's activity level and the response to parents or significant others.

Pharmacologic Highlights

Medication or Drug Class	Dosage	Description	Rationale
Vasopressors	Varies by drug	First line of care: Dopamine, norepinephrine; second line of care: dobutamine, phenylephrine, vasopressin, synthetic human angiotensin II	Maintain an adequate blood pressure
Broad-spectrum antibiotics	Varies by drug	Examples: Vancomycin, gentamicin, cefotaxime (Claforan), ceftriaxone, cefuroxime (Zinacef), piperacillin and tazobactam (Zosyn), ticarcillin and clavulanate, imipenem and cilastatin (Primaxin), clindamycin, meropenem (Merrem), metronidazole (Flagyl), ciprofloxacin (Cipro), levofloxacin, cefepime	Eradicate bacteria

Other Drugs: Administration of corticosteroid in septic shock remains controversial but is often performed if hypotension is poorly responsive to fluid resuscitation and vasopressor therapy; generally corticosteroids need to be started within 8 hours of onset of severe septic shock.

Independent

Priorities of nursing care for the patient with septic shock include maintaining airway, breathing, and circulation; preventing the spread of infection; increasing the patient's comfort; preventing injury; and supporting the patient and family. Monitor the patient continuously for airway compromise, and prepare for intubation when necessary. Maintain strict aseptic technique when you manipulate invasive lines and tubes. Use universal precautions at all times. Unless the patient is endotracheally intubated, place patients with a decreased level of consciousness in a side-lying position, and turn them every 2 hours to protect them from aspiration. To increase the intubated patient's comfort, provide oral care at least every 2 hours.

Maintain skin integrity by placing the patient on an every-2-hour turning schedule. Post the schedule at the head of the bed to increase the visibility of the routine. Implement active and passive range of motion as appropriate to the patient's condition. Provide the family with information about diagnosis, prognosis, and treatment. Expect the patient and family to have high levels of anxiety and fear given the grave nature of septic shock. Support effective coping strategies and provide adequate time for the expression of feelings.

Evidence-Based Practice and Health Policy

Chinai, B., Gaughan, J., & Schorr, C. (2020). Implementation of the Affordable Care Act: A comparison of outcomes in patients with severe sepsis and septic shock using the National Inpatient Sample. *Critical Care Medicine, 48*, 783–789.

• The authors note that sepsis is the most common and costly diagnosis in U.S. hospitals and yet accounts for more than 50% of hospital deaths. The aim of the study was to evaluate changes in insurance coverage and outcomes in patients with severe sepsis and septic shock as a result of the Affordable Care Act. They used a national data set and examined patients ages 18 to 64 years ($N = 361,323$) before the Affordable Care Act and after it was implemented.

• They found that there was a 5% increase in Medicaid coverage and a 2% decrease in the uninsured in patients with severe sepsis and septic shock. Overall in-hospital mortality decreased from 23% to 19%, and patients with Medicaid had the greatest reduction in mortality. The authors concluded that there was an increase in insured patients post Affordable Care Act initiation, and the improvement in outcomes was likely because of advances in management, earlier presentation, earlier treatment, and patients being less severely ill.

DOCUMENTATION GUIDELINES

• Cardiovascular response: Heart rate and rhythm; presence and character of peripheral pulses; capillary refill time; pulmonary artery pressure, central venous pressure, left atrial pressure, and right atrial pressure; cardiac output and index; oxygen delivery and oxygen consumption
• Respiratory response: Rate and rhythm; lung expansion; breath sounds; oxygen saturation; color of oral mucosa and skin; type, location, and patency of an artificial airway
• Neurological response: Level of consciousness, orientation, strength and movement of extremities, activity level, response to the parents or significant others
• Signs of infection: Response to antibiotics

DISCHARGE AND HOME HEALTHCARE GUIDELINES

Instruct patients who have been identified as high risk to call the healthcare provider at the first signs of infection. Discuss signs and symptoms of complications that may occur. Teach high-risk individuals to avoid exposure to communicable diseases and to use good hand-washing technique. Reinforce the need for immunizations against infectious diseases such as influenza. Encourage patients to consume a healthy diet, get adequate rest, and limit their alcohol intake. Instruct patients and families about the purpose, dosage, route, desired effects, and side effects of all medications. Explain that it is particularly important that the patient take the entire antibiotic prescription until it is finished.

Sickle Cell Disease

DRG Category:	812
Mean LOS:	3.4 days
Description:	MEDICAL: Red Blood Cell Disorders Without Major Complication or Comorbidity

Sickle cell disease (SCD) is a genetic autosomal recessive disorder that results in abnormalities of the globin genes of the hemoglobin (Hg) molecule of the red blood cells (RBCs), called hemoglobin S (HbS). It is more common in Black people than in other groups in the United States. SCD is the most common inherited blood disorder in the United States; approximately 100,000 people have the disease in the United States; and 8% of Black Americans have the sickle cell gene. Sickle cell anemia, the severest of the sickle cell disorders, is homozygous and has no known cure. Sickle cell trait occurs when a child inherits normal adult Hg (also called HgA) from one parent and HgS from the other; people with the sickle cell trait are carriers only and rarely manifest the clinical signs of the disorder. Individuals who have SCD have some protective advantage against malaria, which is likely the reason people with SCD are concentrated in malaria-endemic areas in Africa and the Mediterranean, or have ancestors from the area.

RBCs that contain more HgS than HgA are prone to sickling when they are exposed to decreased oxygen tension in the blood. The cells become more elongated, thus the term *sickle*, and form a gel-like substance. Once sickled, RBCs are more rigid, fragile, and rapidly destroyed. The RBCs therefore have a short survival time (30–40 days, as compared with a normal 120-day survival rate), a decreased oxygen-carrying capacity, and low Hg content. They cannot flow easily through tiny capillary beds and may become clumped and cause obstructions. The obstructions can lead to ischemia and necrosis, which produce the major clinical manifestations of pain. In people with SCD, approximately 50% do not survive beyond age 20 years, and most people do not live past age 50 years. Complications include stroke, chronic obstructive pulmonary disease, congestive heart failure, and infarction of organs such as the spleen, retina, and kidneys.

CAUSES

SCD is caused by a genetic mutation that produces Hb changes in solubility and molecular stability in different situations. The abnormal properties of Hb are responsible for the clinical expression of sickling, during which the Hb decreases its solubility, increases blood viscosity, and forms polymers. Two factors have been identified as producing sickling. The first is hypoxemia, which is caused by low oxygen tension in the blood from high altitudes, strenuous exercise, or low oxygen concentration during anesthesia. The second is a change in the condition of the blood, such as decreased plasma volume, decreased blood pH, or increased plasma osmolality as a result of dehydration. The primary risk is heredity.

GENETIC CONSIDERATIONS

Sickle cell anemia is the result of mutant beta globin (*HBB* gene) in which a mutation causes aggregation of hemoglobin and sickling of RBCs. Sickle cell anemia (also known as homozygous sickle cell disease and Hb SS disease) accounts for 60% to 70% of sickle cell disease in the United States. Sickle cell anemia is an autosomal recessive disease, and prevalence is much higher in people of African descent. Heterozygous carriers have a reduced risk of infection by the parasite that causes malaria. SCD may also result from co-inheritance of the HbS mutation with another abnormal hemoglobin variant. The C allele of the gene *BCL11A* is associated with reduced severity of sickle cell anemia, likely because of increased production of fetal hemoglobin.

SEX AND LIFE SPAN CONSIDERATIONS

Clinical symptoms rarely appear before the child is 6 months old and occur in both boys and girls, but once they occur, the disease lasts the child's entire life. Males and females have SCD in equal measure, but males are more likely to have sickle cell nephropathy, which occurs in approximately one-third of children with SCD. The average time for renal failure to occur in SCD is 23 years of age, and when that occurs, life expectancy is 4 years in spite of dialysis treatments.

HEALTH DISPARITIES AND SEXUAL/GENDER MINORITY HEALTH

Sickle cell occurs most frequently in Black persons but also occurs in African, Mediterranean, Caribbean, Middle Eastern, and Central American populations. Approximately 1 of 12 Black persons has sickle cell trait, and the sickle gene is present in approximately 8% of Black persons. Approximately 2 million people in the United States have sickle cell trait. Sexual and gender minority status has no known effect on the risk for sickle cell disease.

GLOBAL HEALTH CONSIDERATIONS

SCD is most commonly found in people with ancestry in sub-Saharan Africa, where in some sections of the continent the prevalence of sickle cell trait is 30%. It is also found in the

Mediterranean region (Sicily, Greece, Turkey), the Middle East, and India. Experts suspect that this geographic concentration is related to the survival advantage during malaria epidemics.

ASSESSMENT

HISTORY. Most infants do not develop symptoms during the first 6 months because fetal Hg has a protective effect. The parents or the child may describe a history of lung infections or cardiomegaly (hypertrophy of the heart). Children with the disease may have a history of chronic fatigue, dyspnea, joint pain and swelling, and chest pain. Determine when the symptoms occurred, whether or not the child has had a vaso-occlusive crisis (microcirculation is obstructed by sickled RBCs leading to ischemic injury), how often, and the type and nature of the resulting pain. Determine how long the pain lasts and the location of the pain. Note that some children have six or more crises each year, and others have rare episodes or none at all. Determine if the parent knows the patient's triggers, such as dehydration or changes in body temperature. Determine the child's growth history, height, and weight. Ask about the child's nutritional, sleep, and exercise patterns; how the child is doing in school; and the child's social interactions.

PHYSICAL EXAMINATION. The most common symptoms are a result of a vaso-occlusive crisis: **sudden pain in the abdomen, soft tissues, bones, and joints** and **swelling of the hands and feet**. The extent of the symptoms depends on the amount of HgS that is present. The general signs are similar to the other types of hemolytic anemia (anemia as a result of destruction of RBCs): malaise, fatigue, pallor, jaundice, and irritability. Children begin to fall below the growth curve in height and weight at around 7 years, and puberty is usually delayed. They are often small for their age and may have narrow shoulders and hips, long extremities, and a curved spine. You may note jaundice and pale skin. Often, the children have heart rates that are faster than normal and heart murmurs; you may find a large liver and spleen. Eventually, all body systems, including the heart, lungs, central nervous system, kidneys, liver, bones and joints, skin, and eyes, are affected. The most severe problem is sickle cell crisis (Table 1).

• TABLE 1 Sickle Cell Crisis

TYPE/DESCRIPTION	SYMPTOMS
Vaso-occlusive crisis: Most common type; usually appears after age 5 yr; the result of sickling in the microcirculation that leads to vasospasm, thrombosis, and local infection	Severe pain: Joint, abdominal, muscle, and thoracic; jaundice; dark urine; fever; elevated white blood cell (WBC) count; lethargy; fatigue; sleepiness
Sequestration crisis: Occurs in infants between 8 and 24 mo; massive pooling of RBCs in the liver and spleen	Lethargy, pale skin, hypovolemia, tachycardia, cool extremities, dropping urinary output, delayed capillary refill
Aplastic crisis: Results from bone marrow depression and is associated with viral infections; leads to compensatory increase in RBCs and RBC lysis	Lethargy, pale skin, shortness of breath, altered mental status, sleepiness
Hyperhemolytic crisis: Rare; result of certain medications or infections	Abdominal distension, jaundice, dark urine

Sickle cell crisis may be preceded by a recent infection or a stressor such as dehydration, fever, changes in environmental temperature, strenuous activity, or high altitude leading to hypoxemia. Other assessment findings include changes in mental status, such as sleepiness, listlessness, and irritability. Fever; severe pain; bloody urine; and pallor of the lips, tongue, palms, and nails may also occur.

PSYCHOSOCIAL. Children with SCD have a chronic, potentially fatal genetic disorder. Frequent hospitalizations and delayed growth and development put them at risk for low self-esteem and body image problems. In addition, because of the genetic nature of the disease, parents may experience guilt feelings. Families need extensive genetic and psychological counseling to avoid problems. Assess the child and the family for coping skills and knowledge deficits about the cause and prevention of sickle cell crisis.

Diagnostic Highlights

Test	Normal Result	Abnormality With Condition	Explanation
Genetic testing	Negative	Mutant gene	Identifies expressed mutations in single genes; prenatal diagnosis is available through chorionic villus sampling at 8–12 wk of gestation
Peripheral blood smear	Normal RBCs	Classic distorted, sickle-shaped RBCs	RBCs have a characteristic sickle shape caused by structurally abnormal Hg molecules
Hg electrophoresis	No HgS	Presence of HgS	Identifies SCD by identifying HgS; a stained blood smear can show sickling cells
Complete blood count	RBCs: 3.6–5.8 million/mcL; hemoglobin: 11.7–17.3 g/dL; hematocrit: 36%–52%; white blood cells: 4,500–11,100/mcL; platelets: 150,000–450,000/mcL	RBCs: Decreased, generally 5–10 g/dL; WBCs: Chronic neutrophilia with leukocytosis; platelets often increased	Short RBC survival time because of genetic mutation and sickling; elevation of WBC with left shift indicates infection; elevated platelets may indicate reduced spleen function leading to reduction in platelet destruction
Transcranial Doppler	Normal cerebral blood flow velocity	Abnormal high cerebral blood flow velocity in large arteries of circle of Willis	Identifies children at risk for stroke

PRIMARY NURSING DIAGNOSIS

DIAGNOSIS. Risk for delayed child development as evidenced by delayed growth, delayed puberty, fatigue, and/or malaise

OUTCOMES. Child development: Middle childhood; Child development: Adolescence; Physical maturation: Male/female; Caregiver-patient relationship; Parenting performance; Nutritional status; Knowledge: Disease process

INTERVENTIONS. Nutritional monitoring; Nutrition therapy; Teaching: Disease process; Developmental enhancement: Child; Developmental enhancement: Adolescent; Parenting promotion

PLANNING AND IMPLEMENTATION
Collaborative

Although SCD cannot be cured, there are many treatment alternatives to prevent exacerbations, limit complications, and manage sickle cell crises. Medical management centers on the treatment of vaso-occlusive crisis, management of pain, management of anemia, prevention of infections, management of complications, prevention of stroke, and detection of pulmonary hypertension. Sequestration and aplastic crises are treated with analgesia, oxygen if they are hypoxemic, IV fluids, transfusions of packed RBCs to support the Hg, and bronchodilators if needed. A vaso-occlusive crisis is treated with analgesia, oxygen, and increased hydration. Pain levels should be assessed frequently and corrected quickly. Current pain guidelines indicate that a patient with acute, painful crisis should receive analgesia within 30 minutes of arrival at the hospital. Avoid using aspirin, which may increase acidosis. Children may not express the need for pain medication because of fear of the route of administration. Patient-controlled analgesia, therefore, may be used, with morphine sulfate as the drug of choice. Iron supplements may be used if folic acid levels are lower than normal. Infections are treated with appropriate antibiotics. The patient and family may consider a bone marrow transplant or cord blood stem cell transplantation.

Counsel families to avoid the causes of crisis (dehydration, infection, hypoxia, high altitudes, vigorous exercise, and stress). To prevent aplastic crisis, prophylactic daily doses of penicillin are given to infants beginning when they are about 4 months old. Periodic transfusions should be considered when Hg levels drop, and children benefit from physical therapy and nutritional consultation. Hydroxyurea is used to inhibit sickling and to provide relief from frequent and severe pain in adults and some children. Newer therapies include phosphodiesterase type 5 inhibitors and endothelin receptor antagonists for pulmonary hypertension. Management to prevent crises include P-selectin inhibitors and hemoglobin oxygen-affinity modulators.

Pharmacologic Highlights

Medication or Drug Class	Dosage	Description	Rationale
Hydroxyurea (Hydrea)	• Initial: 10 mg/kg • After 6 wk: 15 mg/kg • Goal: Maximally tolerated dose up to 35 mg/kg without signs of toxicity	Antimetabolite	Inhibits production of HgF, which inhibits sickling; provides relief from frequent and severe pain
Analgesia	Varies by drug	Oxycodone and aspirin, methadone, morphine sulfate, oxycodone and acetaminophen, fentanyl, ketorolac	Relieves pain

Independent

Counsel children and families on the importance of maintaining hydration even when the child is ill and during hot weather. Encourage oral fluid intake in addition to IV fluids when children are in the hospital. Increase fluid intake to 1.5 times the normal maintenance volume if the child's cardiac function is adequate.

In cases of acute crisis, pain is the overriding problem. In addition to prescription medicines, employ other pain-reducing interventions, such as diversion, imagery, and general comfort measures. Keep the pain level within tolerable limits for the individual. Encourage families to maintain a normal life for the child with SCD. Arrange for genetic counseling so that families can make informed decisions. When appropriate, and depending on the age, include siblings in the care.

Evidence-Based Practice and Health Policy

Cisnero, G., & Thein, S. (2020). Recent advances in the treatment of sickle cell disease. *Frontiers in Physiology*. Advance online publication. https://doi.org/10.3389/fphys.2020.00435

• The authors intended to focus on the most important advances in the last decade in understanding and treating SCD. The authors reviewed recent advances in therapy: modifying the patient's genotype, targeting hemoglobin S (HbS) polymerization, targeting vaso-occlusion, and targeting inflammation. They note that in the last 30 years, SCD, because of its genetic simplicity, has been at the forefront of numerous scientific discoveries.

• Progress has been made in understanding its pathophysiology and pathobiological complexities, but developing treatments has been slow and elusive. The future holds the possibility for translating insights into better therapeutic options—pharmacologic and genetic—particularly for those most in need in Africa, where patients have less access to resources, medical treatment, and facilities, and the consequences of the disease are devastating.

DOCUMENTATION GUIDELINES

• Response to pain medication and other pain-reduction methods
• Physical findings of pain: Location and duration
• Response to hydration methods, ability to identify and respond to triggers
• Presence of complications: Unresolved pain, stroke, kidney impairment

DISCHARGE AND HOME HEALTHCARE GUIDELINES

Teach the patient and family the causes, signs, and symptoms of crisis and ways to avoid future crisis. Emphasize good nutrition and the avoidance of caffeine and smoking. Patients and families need to be taught the signs and symptoms of complications, such as stroke, embolism, thrombophlebitis, cardiopulmonary dysfunction, increased intracranial pressure, and renal impairment. The patient and family need to be taught the importance of taking daily antibiotics and the side effects, dosage, and route of medication. If the patient is on pain medications, care should be taken to ensure that the medication is not abused but is taken when the patient is in need. Patients and families need to understand the need for genetic counseling, the potential long-term effects of SCD, and the possible complications. Older children and parents need to deal with the delayed sexual maturity that occurs. Long-term, follow-up care is essential for patients with SCD. Refer patients to the Web site for the Sickle Cell Disease Association of America (https://www.sicklecelldisease.org) for patient and family information.

Sjögren Syndrome

DRG Category:	546
Mean LOS:	4.4 days
Description:	MEDICAL: Connective Tissue Disorders With Complication or Comorbidity

Sjögren syndrome (SS) is the most common autoimmune rheumatic disorder after rheumatoid arthritis (RA). It is a chronic, progressive disease that occurs 50% of the time as a primary disorder in the absence of other conditions. It may also be associated with connective tissue disorders, such as RA, scleroderma, systemic lupus erythematosus (SLE), and primary biliary cirrhosis.

SS is characterized by failure of exocrine glands and by diminished tearing and salivary secretion leading to dry eyes and dry mouth. Manifestations of SS are referred to as sicca symptoms, taken from the Latin word, siccus, or "dry." It results from chronic exocrine gland dysfunction, although the disorder may also involve other organs such as the skin, lung, and kidney. Tissue damage results either from infiltration by lymphocyte or the deposition of immune complexes. The diagnosis is made if patients have at least four of the following criteria, including at least one of the final two criteria (see Table 1). The overall prognosis for patients with SS is good, although the disease is associated with pulmonary disease, gastrointestinal disease, anemia, leukopenia, lymphadenopathy, neuropathy, vasculitis, and lymphoma.

• TABLE 1

1. Ocular symptoms	Dry eyes for more than 3 mo, foreign body sensation, use of tear substitutes more than three times a day
2. Oral symptoms	Feeling of dry mouth, recurrent swollen salivary glands, frequent use of liquids to aid swallowing
3. Ocular signs	Schirmer test performed without anesthesia (< 5 mm in 5 min), positive vital dye staining results (determines if tear ducts produce adequate tears)
4. Oral signs	Abnormal salivary scintigraphy findings, abnormal parotid sialography findings, abnormal sialometry findings (contrast media infected into salivary glands with x-rays or gamma scanning)
5. Salivary gland	Positive minor salivary gland biopsy findings
6. Antibody results	Positive SSA/Ro or SSB/La antibody results (see Diagnostic Highlights)

CAUSES

The direct cause of SS is not well understood. It seems likely that both environmental and genetic factors (see Genetic Considerations) contribute to its development. Environmental or internal antigens may trigger an inflammatory response in the exocrine glands. In a genetically susceptible individual, either bacterial or viral infection or exposure to pollen may be the catalyst for SS. The primary risk factor is rheumatic diseases.

GENETIC CONSIDERATIONS

SS is believed to be a complex disorder with a genetic susceptibility and an environmental trigger. Associations with the human leukocyte antigen variants DRB1, DRB1*03, and DQB1*02 as well as the lymphotoxin and tumor necrosis factor genes have been described. Other immunology-related genes that have also been associated with SS by genome-wide association study include *STAT4, IRF5, CXCR4, IL12A*, and *BLK*.

SEX AND LIFE SPAN CONSIDERATIONS

SS occurs mainly in women: 9 out of 10 patients are female. The mean age of occurrence is 50 years, although it has been reported in children who develop parotid gland enlargement. A small percentage of women who develop SS may have accompanying nonlymphoma and lymphoid malignancies.

HEALTH DISPARITIES AND SEXUAL/GENDER MINORITY HEALTH

Ethnicity, race, and sexual/gender minority status have no known effect on the risk for SS.

GLOBAL HEALTH CONSIDERATIONS

SS occurs around the globe with similar prevalence to that found in the United States.

ASSESSMENT

HISTORY. Establish a history of either autoimmune or lymphoproliferative disorders. Rule out other causes of oral and ocular dryness; ask about any history of sarcoidosis, endocrine disorders, anxiety or depression, and radiation therapy to the head and neck. Many commonly used medications produce dry mouth as a side effect (antidepressants, anticholinergics, beta blockers, diuretics, antihistamines), so take a thorough history of medications. In patients with salivary gland enlargement and severe lymphoid infiltration, rule out malignancy. Approximately 50% of patients with SS have confirmed RA. When you ask about symptoms, the patient may report gritty or sandy sensations in the eye or a film across the visual field. Patients may also report dryness of the mouth, burning oral discomfort, difficulty in chewing and swallowing dry foods, increased thirst, and reduced taste. The patient may also report the incidence of many dental caries, chronic middle ear infections, and nasal dryness or bleeding. Patients may describe dry skin and pruritus. Dryness of the vagina and vulva leads to reports of painful urination, itching, and painful or difficult sexual intercourse.

PHYSICAL EXAMINATION. The most common symptoms are **dry eyes** and **dry mouth**. Patients are usually referred to an ophthalmologist for a thorough eye examination. Patients have a decreased tear pool in the lower conjunctiva. They may have dilated vessels in the conjunctiva and corneal lesions as well as inflamed eyelids. The patient's tongue is often red and dry with atrophic taste buds, and the saliva pool under the tongue is usually small. Unilateral or bilateral parotid and salivary glands may be hardened and nontender. Dental caries are a common finding. The dryness may make talking difficult. Patients may have a dry, chronic cough and an increased incidence of upper and lower respiratory tract infections, which resulted in a chronic vocal hoarseness. Nasal mucosa may be dry and reddened, and the patient may have nose bleeding. Gastrointestinal tract involvement may lead to gastritis, esophageal mucosal atrophy, and difficulty in swallowing. Genitalia may appear dry and possibly ulcerated. Involvement of the exocrine glands leads to dry, tough, scaly skin; decreased sweat; and chronic itching.

PSYCHOSOCIAL. The patient with SS has complaints that may have been attributed to multiple causes, possibly over years. Because SS is closely related to SLE and RA, the patient may have been misdiagnosed, causing considerable emotional distress. Because SS affects senses, such as sight and taste, and also sexuality, assess the patient's ability to cope with the presenting symptoms and other common complaints.

Diagnostic Highlights

Test	Normal Result	Abnormality With Condition	Explanation
Salivary gland biopsy	Normal salivary gland cells	Presence of inflammatory cells and immune complexes	Identifies abnormal cells in secretory glands and ducts
Enzyme-linked immunosorbent assay (ELISA) for anti-SSA/Ro and anti-SSB/La antibodies	Negative	Positive antibody titers; antibodies against SSA/Ro are found in 50% and antibodies against SSB/La are present in 40%–50% of patients with SS	Immune response to triggers of SS leads to antibody production
Slit-lamp examination	Normal examination	Detection of dryness of conjunctiva and reduced tearing	Identifies reduced tear film and dryness of eyes

Other Tests: Complete blood count, antinuclear antibodies, rheumatoid factor, anti-alpha-fodrin antibody, erythrocyte sedimentation rate, tear osmolarity, fluorescence clearance test, parotid flow rate, radionuclide scan, Schirmer test (test strip of number 41 Whatman filter paper placed near the lower conjunctival sac to measure tear formation; healthy persons wet 15 mm or more after 5 min), sialography, scintigraphy

PRIMARY NURSING DIAGNOSIS

DIAGNOSIS. Risk for dry eye as evidenced by decreased tear pool, inflamed eyelid, and corneal lesions.

OUTCOMES. Dry eye severity; Tissue integrity: Skin and mucous membranes; Symptom severity; Symptom control; Knowledge: Disease process; Knowledge: Treatment regimen

INTERVENTIONS. Dry eye prevention; Medication management; Medication administration; Teaching: Disease process; Teaching: Prescribed treatment

PLANNING AND IMPLEMENTATION

Collaborative

Care of the patient with SS is designed to treat symptoms. Instill artificial tears as often as every 30 minutes to prevent corneal ulcerations or opacifications that may be caused by insufficient lacrimal secretions. Medications that contribute to the symptoms of SS need to be evaluated collaboratively by the physician and patient to determine if they can be avoided.

Patients who also have RA may benefit from a combined program of medical, rehabilitative, and surgical treatments. The management is anchored by administration of biologic and nonbiologic disease-modifying antirheumatic drugs (DMARDs). The primary goals are suppression of further joint and tissue inflammation, maintenance of joint and tissue function, repair of joint damage, and relief of pain.

Pharmacologic Highlights

Medication or Drug Class	Dosage	Description	Rationale
Cyclosporine ophthalmic eyedrops	Apply 1% or 2% solution bid	Immunosuppressant	Suppresses T-cell formation and has been used to increase lacrimal gland function in SS
Rituximab	1,000 mg IV infusion and repeat after 2 wk	Monoclonal antibody	Directed against antigen on B lymphocytes to reduce immune response

Other Drugs: Corticosteroids; eye lubricants; omega-3 fish oil; sustained-release cellulose capsules (hydroxypropyl cellulose) may be used. Topical (diquafosol) and systematic (pilocarpine, cevimeline) stimulators of tear secretion may be used. If eye infection develops, the patient receives antibiotics; topical steroids are avoided. Biologic therapies: rituximab; immunosuppressives: cyclophosphamide.

Independent

Suggest the use of sunglasses to protect the patient's eyes from strong light, wind, and dust. To reduce the risk of infection caused by dry eyes, advise the patient to keep the face clean and to avoid rubbing the eyes. Encourage the patient to use warm soaks over the eyes for 10 minutes, once a day, to improve eye lubrication. Mouth dryness can be relieved by using a swab or spray and by drinking plenty of fluids, especially at mealtime. Sugarless throat lozenges can also relieve mouth dryness without promoting tooth decay. Meticulous oral hygiene should include regular brushing, flossing, and fluoride treatment at home, along with frequent dental checkups. Teach the patient to avoid medications that decrease saliva production, such as atropine derivatives, antihistamines, anticholinergics, and antidepressants. Suggest high-protein, high-calorie liquid supplements to patients with painful mouth lesions. Soft foods may be easier for patients to swallow. Parotid gland enlargement can be treated with local heat and analgesia.

Respiratory dryness can be reduced by using a humidifier at home and at work. Nasal dryness can be relieved by the use of normal saline solution drops. Moisturizing lotions can ease skin dryness, as can avoiding lengthy hot showers or baths. Patients should avoid sunburn and any lengthy exposure to the sun; recommend using a sunscreen when outdoors. Water-soluble lubricating jelly is an effective lubricant during sexual intercourse.

Evidence-Based Practice and Health Policy
Chu, L., Cui, K., & Pope, J. (2020). Meta-analysis of treatment for primary Sjögren's syndrome. *Arthritis Care & Research, 72*, 1011–1021.

- The authors present a review to assess the efficacy and safety of immunomodulation on primary SS from randomized clinical trials. The authors consulted five electronic databases and chose primary outcome measures of ocular dryness, oral dryness, tear production, and salivary function. They also assessed serious adverse events (AEs) and withdrawals due to AEs. The search yielded 32 trials evaluating 19 different medications.
- The average duration of diagnosis was up to 9.2 years. Twenty-two trials examined ocular and oral dryness, but only two and four trials showed statistically significant improvements, respectively. No studies found a benefit for tear production; few studies found improvements for unstimulated salivary flow and stimulated salivary flow. The authors concluded that reducing inflammation potentially improves salivary gland function and that no individual immunomodulatory drugs demonstrated a consistent benefit in dry mouth and dry eye symptoms.

DOCUMENTATION GUIDELINES
- Physical findings of dysphagia (difficulty swallowing)
- Physical findings of presence of red, irritated, or ulcerated mucosal membranes
- Reaction to remoisturizing eyes, mouth, and other affected areas

DISCHARGE AND HOME HEALTHCARE GUIDELINES
Instruct the patient to avoid sugar; tobacco; alcohol; and spicy, salty, and highly acidic foods. Recommend high-calorie, protein-rich liquid supplements to patients with painful mouth lesions. Teach the patient how to instill eyedrops, ointments, or sustained-release capsules. Advise the patient to avoid over-the-counter medications that include saliva-decreasing compounds, such as antihistamines, antidepressants, anticholinergics, and atropine derivatives.

Skin Cancer

DRG Category:	577
Mean LOS:	6.6 days
Description:	SURGICAL: Skin Graft Except for Skin Ulcer or Cellulitis With Complication or Comorbidity
DRG Category:	592
Mean LOS:	7.4 days
Description:	MEDICAL: Skin Ulcers With Major Complication or Comorbidity
DRG Category:	606
Mean LOS:	5.9 days
Description:	MEDICAL: Minor Skin Disorders With Major Complication or Comorbidity

Skin cancer is the most common malignancy in the United States, accounting for over 50% of all diagnosed cancers. The majority of skin cancers (more than 90%) are classified as nonmelanoma skin cancers (NMSCs) of which there are two types: basal cell carcinoma (BCC) and squamous cell carcinoma (SCC). Approximately 80% of skin cancers are BCC; SCC is the next most common skin cancer, followed in frequency by melanoma. According to the American Cancer

Society (ACS), about 5.4 million SCC and BCC are diagnosed each year in about 3.3 million Americans. Other, less frequently occurring skin cancers include skin adnexal tumors, Kaposi sarcoma, various other types of sarcomas, Merkel cell carcinoma, and cutaneous lymphoma, all of which together account for fewer than 1% of NMSCs. BCC and SCC are very treatable conditions.

BCC is a slow-growing, nonmetastasizing neoplasm of the nonkeratinizing cells of the basal layer of the epidermis, which extends wide and deep if left untreated. BCC is the least likely cancer to metastasize, but if distant metastasis does occur to the bone, brain, lung, and liver, the prognosis is grave. BCC is most frequently found on the head, on the neck, and on skin that has hair. There are two types of BCC. The nodular ulcerative BCC is a nodulocystic structure that begins as a small, flesh-colored, smooth nodule that enlarges over time. A central depression forms that progresses to an ulcer surrounded by a waxy border. The superficial BCC is often seen on the chest or back and begins as a flat, nonpalpable, erythematous plaque that enlarges and becomes red and scaly with nodular borders. Although BCC can be treated effectively, it is not uncommon for it to return after treatment. Of people diagnosed with one BCC, 35% to 50% will develop a new skin cancer within 5 years of the first diagnosis.

SCC leads to an invasive tumor that can metastasize to the lymph nodes and visceral organs. SCC, which constitutes 20% of all skin cancers, is characterized by lesions on the squamous epithelium of the skin and mucous membranes. SCC appears as a red, scaling, keratotic, slightly elevated lesion with an irregular border, usually with a shallow chronic ulcer. The risk of metastasis is associated with the size and penetration of the tumor, the tumor morphology, and the causative factors. Complications of NMSCs include disfigurement of facial structures and metastasis to other tissues and organs.

The ACS estimates that 2,000 people die each year from NMSC, but most are older people who have not sought treatment for skin cancer and have experienced metastatic disease. The 5-year survival rate for patients with BCC is greater than 99%; although BCCs rarely spread to lymph nodes or other organs, those patients who do have metastasized BCC have a 5-year survival rate of only 10%. The overall 5-year survival rate for patients with SCC is more than 90%; for patients with spread of SCC to lymph nodes or other organs, the 5-year survival rate is 25% to 45%. Complications, which are rare, are scarring, disfigurement, metastasis, and death.

CAUSES

The cause of NMSCs may be environmental (ultraviolet [UVA, long wave, black light] radiation or UVB [medium wave, absorbed by the ozone] exposure), occupational (arsenic, mineral oils, or ionizing radiation exposure), viral (HIV or human papillomavirus [HPV]), related to medical conditions (immunosuppression or scars from removed SCC or BCC), or related to heredity (xeroderma pigmentosum, albinism). More than 90% of NMSCs are attributed to the primary risk factor, exposure to UV radiation from the sun. Indoor tanning beds are also an avoidable risk factor for NMSC.

GENETIC CONSIDERATIONS

NMSC has a significant genetic component (heritability of ~40%), although it is less than melanoma. Polymorphisms in several genes (*TNFR2*, *IL10*, *IL4R*) have been proposed to increase risk, especially after UV exposure. There are also several heritable syndromes that increase susceptibility to NMSC. These include xeroderma pigmentosum (*XPA* and *POLH* genes), nevoid basal cell carcinoma syndrome, albinism, and epidermodysplasia verruciformis (*TMC6* and *TMC8*), which produces multiple warts on the hands and feet and is linked to susceptibility to HPV.

SEX AND LIFE SPAN CONSIDERATIONS

BCC has the highest incidence in people 50 to 80 years of age. Mean age at diagnosis is 67 years. Approximately 15% of cases of BCC occurs in patients 20 to 40 years of age.

Average age for SCC is 70 years. However, younger people are now more likely to develop skin cancer, perhaps because of greater exposure to the sun. Children rarely have the disease, although the incidence increases with each decade of life. Men are more likely than women to develop BCC (2:1 ratio) and SCC (3:1 ratio). People with fair skin and freckles are at especially high risk.

HEALTH DISPARITIES AND SEXUAL/GENDER MINORITY HEALTH

The ratio of White to Black persons who develop skin cancer is 20:1. However, skin cancer assessment in Black individuals is critical because they have a higher mortality rate possibly due to delayed diagnosis. Skin cancer is uncommon in people of Asian ancestry. People with low incomes also have an increased risk of all-cause mortality from skin cancer as compared to people with high incomes. Experts note that people living in rural areas have more sun exposure than in urban areas, and skin cancer prevention efforts should address this health disparity. Sexual minority men have higher rates of indoor tanning bed use and skin cancer than heterosexual men. Sexual minority women use tanning beds less frequently than heterosexual women and do not have an elevated risk of skin cancer. Gender-nonconforming individuals have a higher lifetime prevalence of any skin cancer compared to cisgender men (cisgender is a term used to describe persons whose gender identity and gender expression are aligned with their assigned sex listed on their birth certificate) (Singer et al., 2020).

GLOBAL HEALTH CONSIDERATIONS

Rates are increasing worldwide. People who live close to the equator tend to present with skin cancer at a younger age than people who live more distant to it. The highest rates are thought to be in Australia, where there is a high concentration of people with fair skin and heavy sun exposure. In general, countries with large numbers of people with European ancestries have the highest rates of skin cancer.

ASSESSMENT

HISTORY. Assess the patient for a personal or family history of skin cancer. Ask if the patient has an exposure to risk factors, including environmental or occupational exposure, at-risk medical conditions, or exposure to viruses. Take a history of the amount of sunbathing the patient engages in, and take a sunburn history. Note that outdoor recreation or employment and living in a sunny, warm climate such as the southeastern (Florida) or southwestern (New Mexico, Arizona, California) United States, Australia, or New Zealand place the patient at risk. Question the patient about any bleeding lesions or changes in skin color. Explore the history of non-healing wounds or lesions that have been present for weeks or even several years without any change and bleed when traumatized. Question the patient about the presence of atypical moles, an unusual number of moles, or any noticeable change in a mole.

PHYSICAL EXAMINATION. The most common symptoms are the **appearance of a new skin lesion** or a **change in a mole or skin growth**. Inspect the patient for additional risk factors, such as light skin and hair (red, blond, light brown), freckling, and light eye color (blue or green). Examine the patient's skin for the presence of lesions. Use a bright white light and magnification during the skin examination. Stretch the skin throughout the examination to note any nodules or translucent lesions. Examine folds or wrinkles in the skin. Assess the skin for ulcerations, sites of poor healing, old scars, drainage, pain, and bleeding. Because more than 70% of NMSCs occur on the face, head, and neck, closely examine these areas. Complete the skin assessment, considering that in order of frequency, the remainder of NMSCs occurs on the trunk, upper extremities, lower extremities, and lastly, the genitals. Determine if the patient has precursor lesions of SCC, such as actinic keratoses (a hornlike projection on the skin from excessive sun exposure) and/or Bowen disease (intraepidermal carcinoma). No assessment of precursor lesions for BCC is necessary because no equivalent lesions exist.

Assess for the characteristic lesions of BCC, which tend to be asymptomatic, grow slowly, are 0.5 to 1 cm in size, and have overlying telangiectasis (vascular lesions formed by dilated blood vessels). BCCs are classified as nodular (the most common type), superficial, pigmented, morpheaform, and keratotic. Nodular BCC appears as a translucent, nodular growth. Superficial BCC, frequently appearing on the trunk, presents as a scaly lesion with a distinct, raised, pearly margin. Pigmented BCC has a characteristic dark or bluish color with a raised and pearly border. The morpheaform BCC lesion is poorly demarcated, is light in color, and has a plaquelike appearance. Keratotic BCC lesions appear similar to ulcerating nodular BCC.

Assess for the characteristic lesions of SCC, which are usually found on sun-damaged skin. The lesions tend to be scaly, 0.5 to 1.5 cm in size, and likely to metastasize; they also grow rapidly. SCC lesions are usually covered by a warty scale surrounded by erythema that bleeds easily with minimal trauma. The tumor appears nodular, plaquelike, and without a distinct margin. When SCC is invasive, the lesion appears firm, dome-shaped, erythematous, and with an ulcerating core.

PSYCHOSOCIAL. Determine the patient's willingness to follow primary prevention strategies and to institute changes that decrease the risk of skin cancer or its recurrence. Of particular concern are patients who are adolescents and young adults who place a high premium on physical appearance. If the patient has metastatic disease, assess the ability to cope with highly stressful situations. Determine if the patient has support systems and the ability to cope with major lifestyle changes.

Diagnostic Highlights

General Comments: The initial diagnosis of skin cancer is made by clinical observation and is confirmed by histological studies through biopsy.

Test	Normal Result	Abnormality With Condition	Explanation
Shave biopsy	No cancer cells present	Presence of cancer cells	Scraping off the top layers of skin; may not be thick enough to determine the degree of cancer invasion
Punch biopsy	No cancer cells present	Presence of cancer cells	Deep sample of skin is removed after numbing the site; cuts through all layers of skin
Incisional and excisional biopsy	No cancer cells present	Presence of cancer cells	Surgical knife is used to cut through full thickness of skin, and a wedge of skin is removed; incisional biopsy removes only a portion; excisional biopsy removes entire tumor
Fine-needle aspiration biopsy	No cancer cells present	Presence of cancer cells	Thin needle is used to remove very small tissue fragment; may be used to biopsy a lymph node near a melanoma to determine extent of disease

PRIMARY NURSING DIAGNOSIS

DIAGNOSIS. Impaired skin integrity related to cutaneous lesions as evidenced by changes in moles and/or development of skin growths

OUTCOMES. Tissue integrity: Skin and mucous membranes; Wound healing: Primary intention; Knowledge: Treatment regimen; Knowledge: Disease process

INTERVENTIONS. Incision site care; Wound care; Skin surveillance; Medication administration; Infection control

▒ PLANNING AND IMPLEMENTATION

Collaborative

Treatment depends on the patient's characteristics; whether the lesion is a primary or recurrent tumor; and its size, location, and histology. The goal of treatment is to eliminate the tumor while preserving function and physical appearance. For some primary SCCs and BCCs, therapies may include electrosurgery, surgical excision, cryosurgery, photodynamic therapy, and radiation therapy, which all have comparable cure rates of greater than 90%. Tumors best suited to such methods are generally small, superficial, well defined, and slow growing. Treatment is done on an outpatient basis unless the tumor involves deep anatomic sites and surgery cannot be performed under local anesthesia. Mohs micrographic surgery is the preferred procedure for invasive SCCs, incomplete excisions, and recurrences. The procedure is also preferred for BCCs that are greater than 2 cm, are located in high-risk areas, have aggressive morphology, or have ill-defined borders. This time-consuming procedure involves removing a layer of skin, immediately checking the removed tissue for cancer cells, and continuing this process until the removed skin samples are cancer free. Reconstructive surgery may be necessary after Mohs surgery or extensive excision. For BCC, chemotherapeutic agents for metastatic tumors include vismodegib and sonidegib.

Topical fluorouracil may be used to manage some SCC and BCC skin lesions. During treatment, the patient's skin is more sensitive than usual to the sun. Healing generally occurs in 1 to 2 months. With metastatic SCC, radiation, chemotherapy, and surgery may be combined. The chemotherapeutic agent commonly used is cisplatin or carboplatin, but other antineoplastic medications may also be used in combination therapy. Monoclonal antibodies cemiplimab and pembrolizumab may be used in patients who are not candidates for curative surgery or curative radiation. External beam radiation therapy may be used in cases where a tumor is difficult to remove surgically because of its size or location and in situations in which the patient's health precludes surgery. As an adjuvant therapy after surgery, radiation can be used to kill small deposits of cancer cells that were not visible during surgery. Radiation may also be used when NMSC has spread to other organs or to lymph nodes. If the patient undergoes radiation therapy, prepare the patient for common side effects such as nausea, vomiting, diarrhea, hair loss, and malaise.

Pharmacologic Highlights

Medication or Drug Class	Dosage	Description	Rationale
Chemotherapeutic agents	Topical application	Fluorouracil (5-FU)	Manage premalignant conditions such as actinic keratosis
Biological response modifier	Topical application	Imiquimod	Causes the body to react and destroy the lesion
Cetuximab	400 mg/m² IV with subsequent doses of 250 mg/m² every wk	Epidermal growth factor receptor inhibitors	Adjuvant therapy for highest-risk cases of SCC and BCC

Independent

Nursing care focuses on wound management, threats to body image and self-esteem, and prevention. Teach the patient how to care for the wound aseptically. Coordinate a consistent, standard plan so that the patient can begin to assume care for the wound. If the wound is large and infected, keep it dry and clean. If it has an odor, control the odor with odor-masking substances such as oil of cloves or balsam of Peru in the room.

Patients are often upset about the changes in their appearance. Listen to the patients' fears and anxieties and accept the patients' perception of their appearance. Assist patients and significant others to have realistic expectations. Help patients present a pleasant appearance by assisting with hair care and clothing. Some patients experience increased self-esteem when they wear their own clothing rather than hospital-issued clothing, if hospitalization is needed. If hair loss occurs during radiation, encourage patients to wear any type of head covering that improves body image, such as baseball caps, wigs, scarves, or bandanas. If appropriate, arrange for patients to interact with others who have a similar problem. If the patient has end-stage disease, listen to the patient's and significant others' fears and concerns. Identify the needs of the family, and investigate mechanisms for support from the chaplain, the ACS, or a local hospice.

If patients cannot continue with their present occupation, arrange for job counseling to evaluate possible occupational alternatives. Encourage patients to avoid excessive sun exposure by using sunscreen and wearing protective clothing. Explain the necessity of examining the skin weekly or monthly for precancerous lesions and to obtain healthcare when any unusual skin changes occur.

Evidence-Based Practice and Health Policy
Sommers, M., Fargo, J., Regueira, Y., Brown, K., Beachman, B., Perfetti, A., Everett, J., & Margolis, D. (2019). Are the Fitzpatrick skin phototypes valid for cancer risk assessment in a racially and ethnically diverse sample of women? *Ethnicity & Disease, 29*, 505–512.

- The authors aimed to determine the criterion-related validity of self-reported Fitzpatrick skin phototype (FSP) when compared with skin color and sunburn history, controlling for age, race/ethnicity, and geography. The FSP is an instrument used to classify skin color and the skin's response to ultraviolet light. They used data from a study of skin injury that enrolled 466 women of diverse ancestries to answer the study aims. The sample was 45% White or White Hispanic, 40% Black or Black Hispanic, and 15% other backgrounds.
- Skin color, sunburn history, and race/ethnicity explained 72% of the variance in FSP for the entire sample. However, in the Black and Black Hispanic sample, only 5% of the variance in FSP was explained. The authors note that the FSP does not perform well for skin color and sunburn history in Black and Black Hispanic people and may result in inaccurate clinical data for skin cancer risk assessment.

DOCUMENTATION GUIDELINES
- Physical findings related to skin cancer: Location and description of lesions, degree of healing, appearance and healing of surgical wound
- Patient's history related to skin cancer and associated risk factors
- Psychological response: Psychosocial state related to diagnosis of skin cancer, self-esteem, body image, level of anxiety and fear about prognosis, coping ability
- Response to diagnostic and treatment interventions: Surgery, chemotherapy, radiation

DISCHARGE AND HOME HEALTHCARE GUIDELINES
Teach the patient primary prevention strategies:

- Perform skin self-assessments, including the use of a buddy or a mirror during the self-assessment.
- Use sunscreens and lip balms with a sun protection factor of 15; to apply sunscreens 15 to 30 minutes before every exposure to the sun; and to follow the reapplication guidelines.
- Use wraparound sunglasses with 99% to 100% UV absorption to protect the eyes and the skin area around the eyes.
- Avoid sun exposure, particularly between 10 a.m. and 3 p.m.

- Use available shade, avoid artificial tanning, and wear protective clothing.
- Be aware of photosensitivity because certain medications and cosmetics can enhance UV ray exposure.
- Encourage members of the family to follow all prevention strategies.

Spinal Cord Injury

DRG Category: 53
Mean LOS: 3.5 days
Description: MEDICAL: Spinal Disorders and Injuries Without Complication or Comorbidity or Major Complication or Comorbidity

Spinal cord injury (SCI), trauma to the spinal cord, results in a temporary or permanent change in motor, sensory, or autonomic functioning. It affects approximately 18,000 Americans every year; approximately 300,000 people in the United States live with spinal cord injuries. Half of the injuries produce paraplegia and half tetraplegia, formerly known as quadriplegia. According to the International Standards for Neurological and Functional Classification of Spinal Cord Injury (ISNCSCI), paraplegia is injury in the spinal cord in the thoracic, lumbar, or sacral segments, including the cauda equina and conus medullaris. T12 and L1 are the most common levels of injury in paraplegia. Tetraplegia, which most often occurs in C5, is injury to the spinal cord in the cervical region, with associated loss of muscle strength in all four extremities. The ISNCSCI classifies impairment from Class A through Class E. Class A is loss of motor functions and sensation. Class B is sensory impairment. Class C is some sensory and motor function preserved. Class D indicates useful motor function is retained. Class E is normal function.

SCI is a dynamic process that triggers a physiological cascade of events and leads to neuronal damage and neurological deficits. The injury to the spinal cord occurs initially from direct trauma, followed by cord compression from bone fragments, hematoma, or material from the disks. Finally, ischemia occurs because of lack of perfusion from the spinal arteries. The initial injury causes a release of glutamate, which causes cellular damage and petechial hemorrhages at the injury site. Calcium influx into the neuron is caused by thrombus formation. This alteration in calcium triggers the arachidonic acid cascade to be initiated, leading to free radical formation, lactic acidosis, and lipid peroxidation. This final series of events hastens ischemia of the white matter and microvasculature destruction, with resultant neuronal damage and permanent neurological deficit. With aggressive medical interventions and nursing management, approximately 90% of patients with acute SCI survive, but many have permanent disability.

Several complications may occur after SCI. Neurogenic shock occurs with hypotension, bradycardia, and peripheral vasodilation, often accompanied by hypothermia. It occurs because of severe autonomic nervous system dysfunction and loss of sympathetic nervous system control. Spinal shock after SCI is defined as a temporary (hours to several days) but complete loss of sensorimotor function below the level of injury. Other complications include cardiac dysrhythmias, hypotension, hypertension, ileus, loss of bowel and bladder function, sexual dysfunction, spastic or flaccid paralysis, depression, and skin pressure injuries.

SCI can be classified by a variety of methods: complete and incomplete cord injury, mechanism of injury, and the level of injury. In a complete SCI, the patient loses all function below the neurological injury level (the lowest neurological segment with intact motor and sensory function). In an incomplete SCI, some motor or sensory function below the neurological injury level remains intact (Table 1).

• TABLE 1 Types of Incomplete Spinal Cord Injury

INJURY	MECHANISM	DESCRIPTION	FUNCTIONS PRESERVED	FUNCTIONS IMPAIRED
Brown-Séquard syndrome	Penetrating trauma	One side of the cord is affected	Opposite-side pain and temperature sensation; same-side movement, proprioception, light touch	Opposite-side movement, proprioception, light touch; same-side pain and temperature sensation
Posterior cord syndrome	Extension	Loss of posterior column sensory function; motor paralysis	Pain sensation; temperature sensation	Vibratory sensation; proprioception
Anterior cord syndrome	Flexion	Hypalgesia; hypesthesia, motor paralysis, posterior column sensory function preserved	Light touch, proprioception, vibratory sensation	Pain sensation, motor function, temperature sensation, touch
Central cord syndrome	Flexion or extension	Injury to central gray matter	Motor functions of lower extremities but possible loss of sensation below the site of injury	Motor functions of upper extremities

CAUSES

Leading causes of SCI include motor vehicle crashes (MVCs; 56%), falls (14%), acts of violence/firearm injuries (9%), and sporting injuries (7%). SCIs caused by violence have increased dramatically in the last decade. The mechanism of injury influences the type of SCI and the degree of neurological deficit. Associated factors are risk taking (e.g., speeding), ignoring seat belts in vehicles, violent or aggressive behaviors, bone and joint disorders, alcohol misuse and abuse, and substance abuse.

GENETIC CONSIDERATIONS

No clear genetic contributions to susceptibility have been defined.

SEX AND LIFE SPAN CONSIDERATIONS

Acute SCIs occur in both children and adults, although the majority occur between the ages of 16 and 30 years. The vast majority, approximately 80%, involve males. The financial impact of acute SCIs is tremendous for the patient and society, and it is related to the age of most patients and the degree of disability. Older adults have greater functional and mental status decline after an SCI as compared to their younger counterparts.

HEALTH DISPARITIES AND SEXUAL/GENDER MINORITY HEALTH

Ethnicity, race, and sexual/gender minority status have no known effect on the risk of SCI. However, Black, Hispanic, and Native American persons as well as sexual and gender minority persons and persons with low incomes are known to experience discrimination, stigma, and insensitivity to their unique needs when interacting with the healthcare system. In the setting of SCI, these issues may interfere with referral, rehabilitation, and recovery and lead to significant health disparities.

GLOBAL HEALTH CONSIDERATIONS

The World Health Organization estimates that each year, there are approximately 250,000 to 500,000 traumatic SCIs from injuries and violence. Road traffic injuries are decreasing in developed regions but increasing in developing regions due to the growing number of vehicles on the road, poor infrastructure, and difficulty enforcing laws. Males between the ages of 20 to 30 years are most at risk, but traumatic SCIs from falls among older adults is increasing in developed and developing regions; falls are common from trees, roofs, and balconies and at construction sites.

ASSESSMENT

HISTORY. The initial triage is done according to ABCDE principles of the primary survey: airway maintenance with stabilization of the cervical spine, breathing and ventilation, circulation with control of hemorrhage, disability assessment and neurological examination, and exposure along with environmental control. The secondary survey is a complete head-to-toe assessment that occurs later as part of the physical assessment. Sometime during the first 48 hours, a tertiary survey is performed to discover any subtle injuries that may have been missed during the initial assessment.

Determine the mechanism of injury in addition to taking a detailed report from the first responders about the patient with an acute SCI. Question the first responders, significant others, or witnesses about the situation surrounding the injury. If the patient was involved in a traffic injury, determine the speed and type of the vehicle, whether the patient was restrained, the patient's position in the vehicle, whether the patient was thrown from the vehicle on impact, or if the patient was a pedestrian. If the patient fell, the distance of the fall is important to know during the initial assessment and evaluation phase. If it was a sports-related injury, determine the sport and the patient's activities at the time of the injury. Determine if the patient has ingested alcohol or other drugs of abuse. A key component of the history in the patient with a suspected acute SCI is information about the patient's motor and sensory function at the scene as well as the severity of the injury. Determine if the patient also experienced a loss of consciousness. Determine any other organ dysfunction such as chronic heart, lung, or kidney conditions.

PHYSICAL EXAMINATION. Common symptoms include **pain, changes in strength and motion of the extremities, changes in sensation**, and **changes in bowel and bladder function**. Changes may be an autonomic response (urinary retention, constipation, paralytic ileus, hypotension, hypothermia, and bradycardia), a motor response (hemiplegia or hemiparesis, paraplegia or paraparesis, tetraplegia or tetraparesis), or sensory changes at a particular cord level. Assess the patient as soon as possible after the primary injury and again each hour during the acute period. Neurological assessments usually include the Glasgow Coma Scale and pupil reflexes. Assess the patient's injury level. Test the patient's ability to distinguish a pinprick from dull pain at each level of the dermatomes. Rectal examination helps determine if the sphincter tone is normal and if the SCI is complete or incomplete. Normal sphincter tone and anal winking indicate an incomplete SCI. Evaluate the patient's motor strength to help determine the injury level. Test the patient's motor movement. Patients may demonstrate agitation, anxiety, and restlessness. All patients with SCI should also be assessed for head injury.

Examine the patient for signs of neurogenic shock, which usually occurs within 30 to 60 minutes after the SCI when sympathetic nerves have lost their normal connections to the central nervous system (CNS). Signs to look for include decreased heart rate and pronounced hypotension (systolic pressure below 90 mm Hg). Assess the patient's respiratory status, paying particular attention to the rate and depth of respirations, chest wall expansion, and breath sounds.

PSYCHOSOCIAL. Acute SCI is catastrophic and alters not only the lives of patients but also the lives of their families, partners, friends, and the community they live in. Single people are more likely to have an SCI than married people, and the marriage rate after SCI is 60% lower than their noninjured counterparts. Divorce rates for married people with SCI are 2.5 times that of the general population after an SCI. Physiological alterations are significant in patients with acute SCIs, as are the psychosocial adjustments. The likelihood of employment after injury is higher for people with formal education and people who were employed at the time of injury. Ongoing assessment of patients' and families' coping skills is critical in planning meaningful support and interventions to assist patients in reaching their functional potential.

Diagnostic Highlights

Test	Normal Result	Abnormality With Condition	Explanation
Spine x-rays	Normal body structures	May show spine fractures or injury such as dislocation or subluxation	Determines the integrity of bony structures of spine
Computed tomography scan	Normal body structures	Determines degree and extent of injury; may show spine fractures or injury such as dislocation or subluxation	Determines the integrity of bony structures of spine; highly sensitive to detect spinal fractures
Magnetic resonance imaging	Normal body structures	Determines degree and extent of injury; may show spine fractures or injury such as dislocation or subluxation	Determines the integrity of bony structures of spine; identifies cord lesions, ligamentous injuries, and soft tissue injuries

Other Tests: Electromyography, somatosensory-evoked potentials, motor-evoked potentials, complete blood count, urinalysis, arterial blood gases, serum lactate levels

PRIMARY NURSING DIAGNOSIS

DIAGNOSIS. Ineffective airway clearance related to hypoventilation or airway obstruction as evidenced by cough, stridor, wheezing, decreased chest excursion, dyspnea, air hunger, anxiety, and/or restlessness

OUTCOMES. Respiratory status: Airway patency; Respiratory status: Gas exchange; Respiratory status: Ventilation; Symptom severity; Symptom control; Neurological status

INTERVENTIONS. Airway insertion; Airway management; Airway suctioning; Oxygen therapy; Respiratory monitoring; Mechanical ventilation: Invasive; Oral health promotion; Neurologic monitoring

PLANNING AND IMPLEMENTATION
Collaborative

Maintenance of ABCs is the highest priority in patients with SCI. The patient with a cervical or high thoracic injury is at risk for developing pulmonary insufficiency, problems with airway clearance, and ineffective breathing patterns. They may have a pneumothorax or hemothorax due to the traumatic impact. The patient may require endotracheal intubation or tracheostomy with mechanical ventilation. Assess tidal volume and vital capacity every 2 hours in the patient who is not endotracheally intubated. The patient likely needs a nasogastric tube to manage an ileus and to prevent aspiration of stomach contents. Hydration may be provided by IV crystalloid fluids or by dextran, a plasma expander that may be used to increase capillary blood flow. The systolic blood pressure should be maintained above 90 to 100 mm Hg. Neurogenic shock needs to be differentiated from hypovolemic shock by assessment of vital signs, laboratory testing, and hemodynamic monitoring, if necessary. The most common sources of a hidden hemorrhage after SCI are injuries to the chest, abdomen, retroperitoneum, and bone fractures. Hypothermia often accompanies both neurogenic shock and fluid resuscitation. The patient's temperature needs continuous monitoring, and interventions must be initiated to warm the patient if needed.

The benefits of early spinal stabilization are decreased morbidity and decreased length of hospital stay, but the neurological benefits are controversial. Although this is a temporary intervention, external stabilization may be accomplished by Gardner-Wells tongs, which can be applied until surgical stabilization can be performed. A halo apparatus can be applied either as a primary intervention or to protect a surgical repair. This device immobilizes the cervical spine but allows the patient increased mobility. Patients with stable thoracolumbar spine fractures require only support with a rigid external brace for several months. Timing for surgical (internal) stabilization of cervical spine injuries is controversial. Some suggest that early surgical stabilization enhances neurological recovery and decreases morbidity, but others believe that early stabilization may increase biochemical alterations and vascular instability.

Patients with unstable thoracolumbar spine fractures are managed with metal rods and surgical decompression. Neurological outcome may be improved by postponing surgery until spinal cord edema is decreased.

Postoperative patients may require a rigid cervical collar or rigid external brace to protect the surgical repair. Patients with acute SCI from penetrating trauma may require surgical intervention for débridement and closure of the dura if cerebrospinal fluid leakage persists. If x-ray films demonstrate that a bullet or other foreign body is within the spinal cord, surgical removal may be recommended to decrease the likelihood of chronic radicular pain.

Current thinking about corticosteroid administration after complete or incomplete spinal cord injuries is that it is associated with significant improvement in motor and sensory function if initiated within 8 hours after injury.

Pharmacologic Highlights

Medication or Drug Class	Dosage	Description	Rationale
Methylprednisolone	30 mg/kg IV as a loading dose, followed by a 48-hr IV infusion of 5.4 mg/kg per hr	Corticosteroid; dexamethasone may also be used	Reduces inflammation and improves motor and sensory function
Inotropic agents	Varies by drug	Dopamine, norepinephrine	Improve systemic vascular resistance and blood pressure
Atropine	1 mg IV as needed	Anticholinergic	Manages symptomatic bradycardia

Other Drugs: Prophylactic anticoagulants may prevent the formation of deep vein thrombosis when the patient is no longer at risk for hemorrhage. Histamine-receptor antagonists decrease gastric acid secretion by inhibiting the receptor sites in the parietal cells and reducing the risk of stress ulcers. Pregabalin may be administered for neuropathic pain. Antacids may be administered to neutralize gastric acid.

Independent

The most critical nursing intervention for the patient with an acute SCI is to maintain airway, breathing, and circulation. Maintain cervical alignment and immobilization. An abdominal binder may be beneficial in patients with SCIs to provide additional support of the abdominal musculature, a major contributor to respiratory excursion. A potentially life-threatening complication associated with acute SCI is autonomic dysreflexia. This dysfunction may occur after the acute phase and is characterized by a hypersympathetic response to some noxious stimuli; this response is commonly found in patients with SCIs above the T8 level (Box 1). Deep vein thrombosis may also occur. Apply sequential compression devices or foot pumps as prescribed.

• BOX 1 Autonomic Dysreflexia

PRECIPITATING FACTORS	CLINICAL MANIFESTATIONS
• Bladder distension or urinary tract infection	• Paroxysmal hypertension
• Bowel distention	• Pounding headache
• Pressure ulcers	• Blurred vision
• Thrombophlebitis	• Bradycardia
• Gastric ulcers, gastritis	• Diaphoresis above the level of injury
• Pulmonary emboli	• Piloerection
• Menstruation	• Nasal congestion
• Constrictive clothing	• Nausea
• Pain	• Pupillary dilation
• Sexual activity; ejaculation	
• Manipulation of bowel or bladder	
• Spasticity	
• Exposure to hot or cold stimuli	

Check bony prominences and areas under the brace or jacket for skin breakdown. Aggressive physical and occupational therapy early in the acute phase may be beneficial to the patient's overall rehabilitation. Joint range-of-motion exercises prevent contractures and severe muscle wasting. Some patients may require splints for the upper and lower extremities to prevent flexion contractures and footdrop.

Prevent urinary tract infections by instituting an intermittent catheterization protocol early. Protocols vary, but most begin with catheterizing every 4 hours. Monitor the residual urine volume; when it is less than 400 mL, catheterization can be done every 6 hours. Record the amount of urine voided and the postvoid residuals. As the amount of residual volume decreases, increase the time intervals between catheterizations. Before catheterization, assist the patient in emptying the bladder by Crede method or by gently tapping or percussing the bladder. Establish bowel continence early in the acute phase.

When the patient is eating by mouth or is being tube fed, administer stool softeners as ordered. If the patient has not had a bowel movement, administer bisacodyl (Dulcolax) suppository. If the patient is NPO (nothing by mouth), administer bisacodyl every other night. Digital stimulation is used in conjunction with the bowel program. Adequate fluid volume status is important for a successful bowel and bladder program.

Provide diversionary activities to help pass the time. Arrange for the patient or family to consult with a clinical nurse specialist, chaplain, or social worker to assist in coping with anxiety and stress if it is deemed necessary. The disruption in the patient's life is extraordinary, and supporting the patient's psychological health is critical. If the patient has little hope for recovery, consider speaking with the family about donating the patient's organs if appropriate.

If the patient is scheduled for discharge, teach the patient and family about the recommended activity level and rehabilitative exercises. Explain how to recognize the signs and symptoms of infection or a deteriorating level of consciousness. Instruct the patient and family in the name, dosage, action, and potential adverse effects of all prescribed medications. Show them the proper care for wounds and lacerations. Make sure the patient and family are aware of the schedule for follow-up medical care.

Evidence-Based Practice and Health Policy

Burkhart, L., Skemp, L., Siddiqui, S., & Bates-Jensen, B. (2021). Developing a decision support tool to prevent community-acquired pressure injuries in spinal cord injury in ambulatory care: A nurse-led protocol for mix methods research. *Nursing Outlook, 69,* 127–135.

• The authors described a plan to create and test a decision support tool to prevent community-acquired pressure injuries (CAPrIs) in people with SCI. They identified mental models of

CAPrI prevention from the perspectives of Veterans and Veterans Health Administration SCI providers through a mix of photovoice, guided tours, and interviews.
- They used triangulation to compare the two mental models that led to the development of a decision support tool and used Delphi approaches for validation strategies. Their research protocol provides a systematic map to explore, address, and translate research on SCI into evidence-based practice.

DOCUMENTATION GUIDELINES

- Physical findings: Vital signs, hemodynamic parameters, urinary output, tidal volumes, vital capacity, level of consciousness
- Presence of complications: Pulmonary infections, urinary tract infection, deep vein thrombosis, alterations in skin integrity, autonomic dysreflexia
- Presence of bowel and bladder continence
- Psychological findings, mood, coping, family dynamics, need for alcohol or substance abuse assessment or counseling

DISCHARGE AND HOME HEALTHCARE GUIDELINES

Encourage the patient to participate in therapies. Instruct the patient to communicate any abnormalities that are recognized. Explain the use of compression stockings as prescribed, with correct application. Teach the patient to maintain the bowel and bladder program. Verify that the patient and family understand the causes and symptoms of autonomic dysreflexia. Be sure the patient understands any medication prescribed. Verify that the patient and family have demonstrated safe use of all assistive devices: wheelchair, transfers, adaptive feeding equipment, and toileting practices. Review with the patient and family all follow-up appointments that are arranged. Verify that all at-home arrangements have been completed. If appropriate, refer the family to the Christopher & Dana Reeve Foundation (https://www.christopherreeve.org) for information on living with paralysis.

Stroke

DRG Category:	70
Mean LOS:	6.2 days
Description:	MEDICAL: Nonspecific Cerebrovascular Disorders With Major Complication or Comorbidity
DRG Category:	84
Mean LOS:	2.6 days
Description:	MEDICAL: Traumatic Stupor and Coma, Coma > 1 Hour Without Complication or Comorbidity or Major Complication or Comorbidity
DRG Category:	955
Mean LOS:	11.0 days
Description:	SURGICAL: Craniotomy for Multiple Significant Trauma

Stroke, formerly known as *cerebrovascular accident* (CVA), is the interruption of normal blood flow in one or more of the blood vessels that supply the brain. The tissues become ischemic, leading to hypoxia or anoxia with destruction or necrosis of the neurons, glia, and vasculature. According to the American Heart Association (AHA), stroke is the fifth leading cause of death in the United States and affects close to 800,000 Americans annually with approximately 130,000 deaths per year. The incidence of first-time strokes is approximately 610,000 per year, but as the population ages, the incidence will increase to 1 million per year by 2050. The AHA reports that stroke is the leading cause of serious long-term disability in the United States.

Stroke is an acute neurological injury that occurs because of changes in the blood vessels of the brain with a corresponding loss of neurological function. Blood vessel changes can be intrinsic to the vessel (atherosclerosis, inflammation, arterial dissection, dilation of the vessel, weakening of the vessel, obstruction of the vessel) or extrinsic, such as when an embolism travels from the heart. Although reduced blood flow interferes with brain function, the brain can remain viable with decreased blood flow for long periods of time. However, total cessation of blood flow produces irreversible brain infarction within 3 minutes. Once the blood flow stops, toxins released by damaged neurons, cerebral edema, and alterations in local blood flow contribute to neuron dysfunction and death. Complications of stroke include unstable blood pressure, pneumonia, contractures, pulmonary emboli, pain, sensory and motor impairment, speech impairment, memory loss, cognitive loss, labile emotions, infection (encephalitis), cerebral edema, coma, and death.

CAUSES

Thrombosis, embolism, and hemorrhage are the primary causes of ischemic stroke, characterized by the sudden loss of blood circulation to an area of the brain. Experts estimate that 87% of strokes in the United States are ischemic, 10% are secondary to intracerebral hemorrhage, and 3% are due to subarachnoid hemorrhage. In cerebral thrombosis, the most common cause of stroke, a blood clot obstructs a cerebral vessel. The most common vessels involved are the carotid arteries of the neck and the arteries in the vertebrobasilar system at the base of the brain near the circle of Willis. Cerebral thrombosis also contributes to transient ischemic attacks (TIAs), which are temporary episodes (10–30 min) of poor cerebral perfusion caused by partial occlusion of the arterial lumen. A thrombotic stroke that causes a slow evolution of symptoms over several hours is called a *stroke in evolution*. When the condition stabilizes, it is called a *completed stroke*.

In an embolic stroke, a clot is carried into the cerebral circulation, usually by the carotid arteries. Blockage of an intracerebral artery results in a localized cerebral infarction. Hemorrhagic stroke results from hypertension, rupture of an aneurysm, arteriovenous malformations, or bleeding disorder. Risk factors thought to cause blood vessel changes that cause vessel walls to be more susceptible to rupture and hemorrhage include elevated low-density lipoprotein and lowered high-density lipoprotein levels, cigarette smoking, and a sedentary lifestyle. Other risk factors for stroke include hypertension, cigarette smoking, exposure to secondary smoke, diabetes mellitus, obstructive sleep apnea, heart failure, myocarditis, endocarditis, cardiac dysrhythmias, and family history.

GENETIC CONSIDERATIONS

Stroke is considered a complex disease with both genetic and environmental risk factors (heritability is estimated to be ~38%). Several susceptibility loci have been reported. Variants in the genes phosphodiesterase 4D (*PDE4D*), *SELP*, *IL4*, *F5*, prothrombin (*F2*), *MTHFR*, *ACE*, *ALOX5AP*, *EPHX2*, and *PRKCH* have been shown to increase the risk of ischemic stroke. Other risk factors include atrial fibrillation (*PITX2*), coronary artery disease (*ABO*, *HDAC9*, *ALDH2*), high blood pressure, and smooth muscle cell development (*FOXF2*). For hemorrhagic stroke, *APOE* and *PMF1*.

There are also several single-gene disorders for which stroke is a common feature, although the exact genetic mechanism is unknown. These include cerebral autosomal dominant arteriopathy with subcortical infarcts and leukoencephalopathy (CADASIL; an autosomal dominant stroke syndrome affecting small cerebral vessels), Marfan syndrome, Ehlers-Danlos syndrome, and sickle cell anemia.

SEX AND LIFE SPAN CONSIDERATIONS

Five percent of the population in North America over age 65 years is affected by stroke. Stroke affects men slightly more often than women and is more common after 50 years, although drug use is causing an increase in strokes in younger people. Approximately 35% of people hospitalized with stroke are less than 65 years of age. Experts note that women are more disabled than men after surviving a stroke, with more problems with mobility, self-care, usual activity, pain/discomfort, and anxiety/depression. They experience more limitation of activity, worse quality of life, and greater levels of poststroke depression than men. Women's symptoms at presentation also differ from men's. They are more likely to experience incontinence, difficulty swallowing, and loss of consciousness, whereas both men and women experience traditional symptoms such as limb weakness, facial weakness, dysarthria, paresthesia, and dysphagia.

HEALTH DISPARITIES AND SEXUAL/GENDER MINORITY HEALTH

Black persons have a 2.5 times higher rate of stroke than White persons because of the former's higher incidence of hypertension. Black persons also suffer greater physical impairment and are nearly twice as likely as White persons to die from stroke. Hispanic persons have a lower overall incidence of stroke than other groups. Health disparities exist for rural dwellers who have stroke. Rural patients, as compared to their urban counterparts, are less likely to receive IV thrombolysis or endovascular therapy and have higher in-hospital mortality.

Sexual and gender minority persons have higher odds for multiple chronic conditions and poor quality of life and are more apt to have disabilities than cisgender males and females. (Cisgender is a term used to describe persons whose gender identity and gender expression are aligned with their assigned sex listed on their birth certificate.) Gender-affirming hormone therapy is the use of hormone therapy for gender transition or gender affirmation and can be masculinizing or feminizing. It may also affect cardiovascular health in transgender females. In a large sample, researchers have found that transgender men and women are more likely to be overweight than cisgender women. Compared to cisgender women, transgender women reported higher rates of diabetes, ischemic stroke, angina/coronary disease, and myocardial infarction. Gender-nonconforming men and women reported higher odds of myocardial infarction than cisgender women. Transgender women also had higher rates of any cardiovascular disease than cisgender men (Cacerese, Jackman, et al., 2020; Connelly et al., 2019). While large-scale studies are not available, these factors likely place sexual and gender minority persons at risk for stroke.

GLOBAL HEALTH CONSIDERATIONS

The World Health Organization and the AHA report that 25.7 million people experience stroke globally each year, with 10.3 million people having a first stroke. It is the second leading cause of death, after ischemic heart disease, in the world. Stroke is also a leading cause of serious disability in the world.

▓ ASSESSMENT

HISTORY. Determine if the patient is on any medications or abuses IV drugs. Determine if the patient has any of the following conditions: hypertension, diabetes mellitus, tobacco use, elevated cholesterol, heart disease, heart failure, or atrial fibrillation. Ask about cocaine use, recent trauma, migraine headaches, and oral contraceptive use. Elicit a history of neurological deficits (Table 1). Determine if the patient has experienced a loss of consciousness, an inability to recognize familiar objects or persons through sensory stimuli (agnosia) or any memory loss (amnesia). Elicit a history of speech difficulties such as an inability to understand language or express language (aphasia), poorly articulated speech (dysarthria), or any other form of speech impairment (dysphasia). Note if urinary incontinence occurred. Determine if the patient has lost the ability to comprehend written words (alexia), read written words (dyslexia), or write (agraphia). Establish a history of visual difficulties such as double vision (diplopia), defective vision, or blindness in the right or left halves of the visual fields of both eyes (homonymous hemianopia), lack of depth perception, color blindness, blindness, blurring on the affected side, or drooping eyelids (ptosis).

• TABLE 1 Stroke Sites and Neurological Deficits

STROKE SITE	SIGNS AND SYMPTOMS
Posterior cerebral artery	Visual field deficits, sensory impairments; reading difficulty (dyslexia); coma; cortical blindness resulting from ischemia in the occipital area; paralysis (rarely)
Vertebral or basilar artery	Numbness around the lips and mouth; dizziness; weakness on the affected side; vision deficits (color blindness; lack of depth perception; double vision [diplopia]); poor coordination; difficulty swallowing (dysphagia); slurred speech; amnesia; staggering gait (ataxia)
Internal carotid artery	Headache; weakness; paralysis; numbness; sensory changes; vision disturbances (blurring on the affected side or blindness); altered level of consciousness; bruits over the carotid artery; defective language function (aphasia); speech impairment (dysphasia); eyelid drooping (ptosis)
Middle cerebral artery	Defective language function (aphasia); speech impairment (dysphasia); reading difficulty (dyslexia); visual field deficits; hemiparesis on the affected side (more severe in the face and arm than in the leg)

Elicit a history of motor difficulties such as the inability to move the muscles (akinesia), inability to perform purposeful acts or manipulate objects (apraxia), poor coordination, impairment of voluntary movement (dyskinesia), muscular weakness or partial paralysis affecting one side of the body (hemiparesis), or paralysis of one side of the body (hemiplegia). Ask if the patient has experienced numbness, and ascertain the specific location. Determine if the patient has experienced headaches. Establish a history of personality changes such as flat affect or distractibility.

PHYSICAL EXAMINATION. Symptoms vary based on the location of the stroke. Common symptoms include **altered consciousness, visual defects, speech and language impairment, motor impairment, sensory impairment, paralysis, eyelid or mouth drooping,** and **numbness.** If the patient appears unconscious, quickly determine the patient's airway status and level of consciousness. If the patient is conscious, the patient may be experiencing a TIA or a stroke in evolution. Determine the level of orientation; ability to respond to questions of intellectual functioning; and speech, hearing, and vision ability. Lightly touch the patient's skin on various parts of the body and ask the patient to identify the location. Apply firm pressure to various parts of the body and observe the patient's responses. Be sure to test skin sensations sensed in both hemispheres of the body and compare the responses.

Begin your assessment by determining the patient's understanding of your commands and the appropriateness of the patient's verbal and nonverbal responses. In left-hemisphere stroke, there is likely to be loss of language ability, although memory may be intact. In right-hemisphere stroke, patients are often confused and disoriented, but the ability to speak remains. Determine the presence of hemiplegia or hemiparesis and the patient's muscle strength, gait, and balance. Assess the patient's cranial nerves (V, VII, IX, X, and XII) to determine tongue movement and ability to chew and swallow, as well as the presence of a gag reflex. Assess the patient for the presence of hemianopia by observing whether the patient sees objects on either side of the mid-visual field. If the patient is disoriented or has lost the ability to understand language (receptive aphasia), assessing hemianopia is difficult. Try handing the patient a fork on the affected side and ask the patient to tell you what it is you are holding or ask the patient to pick up the fork.

PSYCHOSOCIAL. During the early stages of their condition, many patients with stroke experience great despair and frustration trying to communicate their needs. The inability to communicate causes profound depression. Although patients may laugh or cry or display outbursts of anger and frustration at unusual times, it is impossible to know with any certainty if these responses are inappropriate for the patient.

Diagnostic Highlights

Test	Normal Result	Abnormality With Condition	Explanation
Computed tomography (CT)	Intact cerebral anatomy	Identification of size and location of site of hemorrhage or infarction	Shows anterior to posterior slices of the brain to highlight abnormalities

Other Tests: Magnetic resonance imaging is more sensitive than CT if the stroke is small and/or in the brainstem. Carotid duplex scanning is used in patients with acute ischemic stroke when carotid artery stenosis or occlusion is suspected. Transcranial Doppler ultrasound is used to evaluate the middle cerebral, intracranial carotid, and vertebrobasilar arteries. Echocardiography is used for patients with acute ischemic stroke when cardiogenic embolism is suspected. Continuous oximetry and electrocardiographic monitoring provide surveillance. Laboratory tests include complete blood count with differential, platelet count, prothrombin time, activated partial thromboplastin time, electrolytes, creatinine, and glucose. Other diagnostic tests that help evaluate cerebral blood flow, identify abnormalities, or locate the stroke include positron emission tomography, cerebral blood flow studies, and transthoracic two-dimensional echocardiography to identify intracardiac sites for thrombi.

PRIMARY NURSING DIAGNOSIS

DIAGNOSIS. Risk for ineffective cerebral tissue perfusion as evidenced by motor impairment, sensory impairment, speech and/or language impairment, confusion, and/or visual defects

OUTCOMES. Cognitive orientation; Tissue perfusion: Cerebral; Neurological status: Cranial sensory/motor function; Knowledge: Stroke management; Self-management: Stroke

INTERVENTIONS. Cerebral perfusion promotion; Cerebral edema management; Vital signs monitoring; Oxygen therapy; Neurological monitoring; Self-care assistance; Teaching: Disease process

PLANNING AND IMPLEMENTATION
Collaborative

MEDICAL. The primary goal for treatment is to preserve tissue, which might be ischemic but not infarcted. Likely this can be achieved by restoring blood flow to the area of ischemia and supporting collateral circulation. The treatment needs to be initiated rapidly (within 6 hr of the onset of symptoms) to preserve as much brain tissue as possible. Medical management for patients with strokes typically includes support of vital functions and ongoing surveillance to identify early neurological changes as the patient's condition evolves. Although the hallmark of stroke is the abrupt onset of neurological symptoms and deficits due to the interruption of the vascular supply to a specific brain region, therapeutic intervention may save tissue that is at risk for infarction. Recombinant tissue-plasminogen activator (rt-PA) can improve outcome for some patients with acute nonhemorrhagic ischemic stroke if it is given within 3 hours of the onset of symptoms. Medication management centers on these four areas: anticoagulation, reperfusion, antiplatelet function, and neuroprotective function.

SURGICAL. When a stroke has occurred, the treatment consists of maintaining life, reducing intracranial pressure (ICP), limiting the extension of the stroke, and preventing complications. For patients who cannot maintain airway, breathing, and circulation independently, assist with endotracheal intubation, ventilation, and oxygenation as prescribed. In hemorrhagic stroke, surgery may be required to evacuate a hematoma or to stop bleeding. A ventricular shunt may be placed to drain cerebrospinal fluid.

Physical therapy is begun as soon as the patient's condition stabilizes. Flaccid muscles soon become spastic and subject to contractures. Use passive range-of-motion exercises on the affected side. Strengthening the unaffected side assists the patient in compensating for the losses of the opposite hemisphere. The physical therapist teaches the patient to transfer with the use of assistive devices, and the physical or occupational therapist teaches the patient how to perform self-care activity.

Pharmacologic Highlights

Medication or Drug Class	Dosage	Description	Rationale
Recombinant tissue-plasminogen activator (rt-PA) (alteplase, recombinant)	0.9 mg/kg up to a maximum of 90 mg with the first 10% given IV over 1 min and the remainder given by infusion pump over 1 hr	Thrombolytic; activates the fibrinolytic system by directly cleaving the bond in plasminogen-producing plasmin; increases perfusion to ischemic areas	Increases perfusion to at-risk tissue; note that aspirin, heparin, and warfarin are not given during the first 24 hr; can be given up to 4.5 hr after symptom onset
Antiplatelet agents	Varies by drug	Block prostaglandin synthetase action, which then inhibits prostaglandin synthesis and prevents formation of platelet-aggregating thromboxane A2; aspirin, dipyridamole, clopidogrel	Decrease blood clotting and prevent embolic stroke

Pharmacologic Comments: Contraindications to rt-PA: Duration of stroke for more than 4.5 hours, recent surgery, head injury or gastrointestinal/urinary hemorrhage, seizure at stroke onset, bleeding disorder, hypertension. Some patients receive anticonvulsant agents to reduce the risk of seizures (diazepam, lorazepam), stool softeners to decrease straining, corticosteroids to decrease cerebral edema, and analgesics to reduce headache. Cerebral edema may be reduced through dehydrating measures and the use of steroids and osmotics. For thromboembolic strokes, pharmacologic agents such as warfarin, apixaban, and dabigatran are used to limit the extension of the stroke.

Independent

Position the patient to maintain a patent airway by elevating the head of the bed 30 degrees to promote pulmonary drainage and limit upper airway obstruction. Suction the patient's mouth and, if needed, the nasopharynx and trachea. Before suctioning, oxygenate the patient well; to minimize ICP increases, limit suctioning to 20 to 30 seconds at a time.

The patient with a stroke is at extremely high risk for complications caused by immobility. If appropriate, use compression boots to promote venous return and help prevent phlebitis. To reduce the risk of pulmonary infection, promote skin integrity, and prevent contractures, turn and reposition the patient every 2 hours. Keep the patient's joints in a functional position and keep the affected hand elevated slightly on a pillow. Use a trochanter roll to prevent external rotation of the hip. Keep the patient safe by putting the bed in a low position and keeping the side rails up.

Prevent aspiration pneumonia by first determining the patient's ability to handle solids and liquids. Keep a suction machine nearby while feeding the patient. Some patients have difficulty with liquids, so thicken fluids with soft foods like cooked cereal, applesauce, soup, or mashed potatoes.

Make sure the patient has a bowel movement each morning after breakfast to stimulate normal peristalsis and prevent constipation. A catheter may be in place immediately after the stroke, but the goal is to have the patient gain control through a bladder training program. If the patient has expressive aphasia (inability to transform sounds into speech), give the patient ample time to respond to questions and be supportive if the patient becomes frustrated during speech. Be sure to accept any method of self-expression the patient uses, such as pointing, gesturing, or writing. Some patients find it easier to point to a picture that describes a word rather than trying to say the word.

Remember that the patient's family undergoes a struggle to deal with the patient's illness and needs support. If the patient or family seems to be coping poorly, arrange for a referral to a clinical nurse specialist, chaplain, or social worker. A magazine, *Stroke Connection*, can be subscribed to by writing AHA Stroke Connection, 7272 Greenville Avenue, Dallas, TX 75231 or http://strokeconnection.strokeassociation.org.

Evidence-Based Practice and Health Policy

Kim, Y., Twardzik, E., Judd, S., & Colabianchi, N. (2021). Neighborhood socioeconomic status and stroke incidence: A systematic review. *Neurology*. Advance online publication. https://doi .org/10.1212/WNL.0000000000011892

- The authors aimed to summarize the impact of neighborhood socioeconomic status on stroke incidence using a systematic review of existing literature. The authors reviewed four electronic databases and contacted corresponding authors to locate additional studies.
- They found that higher neighborhood disadvantage was associated with higher stroke risk in some studies but not all. The relationship between neighborhood socioeconomic status and stroke risk within different racial and ethnic groups in the United States was inconclusive, possibly because of individual-level characteristics and neighborhood-level racial composition.

DOCUMENTATION GUIDELINES

- Physical findings: Neurological deficits, level of orientation, Glasgow Coma Scale, pupil responses, gait, range of motion, gag reflex, visual deficits
- Ability to communicate verbally and nonverbally
- Ability to perform self-care; bowel and bladder control
- Presence of complications, infections, contractures, skin breakdown
- Emotional response: Ability to cope, presence of depression, ability to socialize with others, anxiety and frustration over speech difficulties

DISCHARGE AND HOME HEALTHCARE GUIDELINES

Teach the family to check for skin breakdown and the development of contractures and to take appropriate preventative measures. Be sure the family performs frequent range-of-motion activities, as taught in the rehabilitation unit. Advise the family whom to call in an emergency. Be sure the patient and family understand the importance of maintaining the mobility and self-care routine developed in the rehabilitation unit. Be sure the social worker or rehabilitation personnel have provided the family with a list of resources for in-home care. Determine whether a home-care agency will be providing in-home supervision and ongoing physical therapy support. Advise the family how to seek ongoing support for home maintenance.

ONLINE SUPPORT GROUPS.

American Stroke Association: https://www.strokeassociation.org/STROKEORG
National Institute of Neurological Disorders and Stroke: https://www.ninds.nih.gov

Subarachnoid Hemorrhage

DRG Category:	26
Mean LOS:	5.5 days
Description:	SURGICAL: Craniotomy and Endovascular Intracranial Procedures With Complication or Comorbidity
DRG Category:	70
Mean LOS:	6.2 days
Description:	MEDICAL: Nonspecific Cerebrovascular Disorders With Major Complication or Comorbidity

Subarachnoid hemorrhage (SAH) is the direct hemorrhage of arterial blood into the subarachnoid between the pia mater and arachnoid mater. SAH and intracerebral hemorrhage are the two forms of hemorrhagic stroke. SAH usually occurs from a ruptured cerebral aneurysm or an arteriovenous malformation (AVM). Immediately after the extravasation of blood, intracranial pressure (ICP) rises, resulting in a fall in cerebral perfusion pressure (CPP = mean arterial pressure − ICP). The expanding hematoma acts as a space-occupying lesion as it compresses or displaces brain tissue. Blood in the subarachnoid space may impede the flow and reabsorption of cerebrospinal fluid (CSF), resulting in hydrocephalus. The bleeding ceases with the formation of a fibrin-platelet plug at the point of the rupture and by tissue compression. As the clot, which forms initially to seal the rupture site, undergoes normal lysis or dissolution, the risk of rebleeding increases. More than 30,000 people in the United States have a ruptured intracranial aneurysm each year, although the annual incidence is probably underestimated because death is attributed to other reasons.

Cerebral vasospasm, or narrowing of the vessel lumen, is a common complication of SAH; it occurs in 35% to 49% of individuals with SAH. The pathophysiology of vasospasms is not clearly understood, but it is believed that they are precipitated by certain vasoactive substances (e.g., prostaglandins, serotonin, and catecholamines), which are released by the blood into the subarachnoid space. When vasospasm develops, it may last for several days or even several weeks. By decreasing cerebral blood flow, a vasospasm produces complications such as neurological deterioration, cerebral ischemia, and cerebral infarction. Other short-term complications of SAH are hydrocephalus and rebleeding. Long-term complications include speech and language deficits, weakness or paralysis of the extremities, visual derangements, seizures, headaches, problems with attention or concentration, memory loss, and personality changes.

CAUSES

Both genetic and environmental factors are related to SAH. SAH typically results from cerebral aneurysm rupture (70%), which occurs when the blood vessel wall becomes so thin that it can no longer withstand the surrounding arterial pressure. Stress occurs on the arterial walls, particularly where the arteries branch where the blood is most turbulent. Some types of aneurysms form because the adventitia is very thin in intracranial arteries, which makes them prone to aneurysm formation. Because aneurysm-forming vessels usually lie in the space between the arachnoid and the brain, hemorrhage from an aneurysm usually occurs in the subarachnoid space. Another less common cause of SAH is AVM, an abnormal tangle of vessels that diverts blood from the arteries to the veins without oxygenating tissue. Risks of SAH include smoking, cocaine use, oral contraception use, hypertension, cerebral atherosclerosis, persistent headache, pregnancy, family history of stroke, and long-term analgesic use.

GENETIC CONSIDERATIONS

SAH appears to cluster in families independent of environmental factors, as does the propensity to have vasospasm following surgery. First-degree relatives have a three- to sevenfold higher risk of SAH, and 10% of all cases have a family history. There are six known risk-associated loci, although no genes have been definitively identified. Patients with the apolipoprotein E (ApoE)-e4 allele have demonstrated poorer outcomes after aneurysmal SAH than those with other variants of this gene even though an association between ApoE and incidence of SAH has not been well documented. Autosomal dominant polycystic kidney disease has also been associated with an increased incidence of SAH. There are multiple other syndromes that manifest with vascular abnormalities or aneurysms, which greatly increase the risk of intracranial bleeding and SAH. These include Loeys-Dietz syndrome (*TGFBR1*, *TGFBR2*, or *TGFB2* mutations), Marfan syndrome (*FBN1* mutations), vascular Ehlers-Danlos syndrome (*COL3A1* mutations), neurofibromatosis type 1 (NF1), and tuberous sclerosis complex (*TSC1* or *TSC2* mutations).

SEX AND LIFE SPAN CONSIDERATIONS

The peak incidence of aneurysm rupture is between ages 40 and 65 years. In persons under age 40 years, SAH occurs more commonly in men, but after age 50 years, it is more common in women. Few aneurysms rupture in persons younger than 20 years of age. Pregnancy creates a significant risk of SAH, which is higher in the third trimester of pregnancy and a leading cause of parental mortality. The peak incidence of SAH from arteriovenous malformation is between ages 30 and 40 years.

HEALTH DISPARITIES AND SEXUAL/GENDER MINORITY HEALTH

In the United States, Black persons have a greater risk for SAH than White persons. In urban, safety net hospitals that primarily take care of uninsured persons, patients have longer time between SAH and intervention and poorer outcomes than patients cared for in university hospitals or major medical centers. These differences create significant health disparities, which also exist among rural versus urban patients. Prompt diagnosis and treatment is important in SAH. Patients residing in rural locations have almost a threefold increase in time to neurosurgical admission when compared to patients who live near major medical centers within cities (Nichols et al., 2020 [see Evidence-Based Practice and Health Policy]), potentially leading to delays in the management of SAH.

Risk factors such as smoking, hypertension, and atherosclerosis place persons at risk for SAH. Sexual and gender minority persons have higher rates of smoking than the general population (Centers for Disease Control and Prevention, 2021), which may place them at risk for SAH. Transgender is a term used to describe persons whose gender identity is different from their sex assigned at birth. Approximately 1% of the U.S. population identify themselves as transgender. Cisgender is a term used to describe persons who have gender identity and gender expression aligned with their assigned sex listed on their birth certificate. Compared to cisgender women, transgender women reported higher rates of diabetes, ischemic stroke, angina/coronary disease, and myocardial infarction. Gender-nonconforming men and women reported higher odds of myocardial infarction than cisgender women. Transgender women also had higher rates of any cardiovascular disease than cisgender men (Cacerese, Jackman, et al., 2020; Connelly et al., 2019). While large-scale studies are not available, these factors may place some sexual and gender minority persons at risk for SAH.

GLOBAL HEALTH CONSIDERATIONS

SAH occurs around the world, with reported rates varying widely between 5 and 30 cases per 100,000 individuals. The Middle East, China, and India have low reported rates, which may partly be due to the low rates of cardiovascular disease for people living in these regions. High rates occur in the United States, Finland, Japan, and Australia.

☀ ASSESSMENT

HISTORY. Ask if the patient has had a sudden brief loss of consciousness followed by a severe headache; this sign has been reported by 45% of patients who survive SAH and may occur because of sentinel, or warning, leaks. Sentinel leaks often occur approximately 2 weeks before an aneurysm rupture. Many also report a severe headache associated with exertion but no loss of consciousness. Patients often describe the headache as "the worst headache of my life." Establish any recent history of dizziness, vomiting, stiff neck, orbital pain, ptosis (drooping eyelid), seizures, or partial paralysis. Ask the patient if any visual changes occurred, such as photophobia, double vision, or vision loss. Establish any history of personal or family cerebral aneurysms.

PHYSICAL EXAMINATION. The most common symptoms are **severe headache, diplopia and visual loss, loss of consciousness, neck pain and stiffness,** and **limited neck flexion.** The physical examination, however, may be normal. Approximately 50% of patients have mild or moderate hypertension. Observe the patient for signs and symptoms of cranial nerve deficits, especially cranial nerves III, IV, and VI. Meningeal irritation may lead to nausea, vomiting, stiff neck, pain in the neck and back, and possible blurred vision or photophobia. Examine for symptoms of stroke syndrome, such as hemiparesis, hemiplegia, aphasia, and cognitive deficits. Cerebral edema, increased ICP, and seizures may also occur. Assess the vital signs for bradycardia, hypertension, and a widened pulse pressure. Other symptoms may result from pituitary dysfunction, caused by irritation or edema, leading to diabetes insipidus (excessive urinary output, hypernatremia) or hyponatremia. Several days after the event, the patient may become febrile because the meninges are irritated from the hemorrhaged blood.

SAHs are graded as follows (Hunt and Hess grading system):

- Grade 0: Unruptured aneurysm
- Grade I: Asymptomatic or mild headache and slight nuchal rigidity
- Grade II: Cranial nerve palsy, moderate to severe headache, nuchal rigidity
- Grade III: Mild focal deficit, lethargy, or confusion
- Grade IV: Stupor, moderate to severe hemiparesis, early decerebrate rigidity
- Grade V: Deep coma, decerebrate rigidity, moribund appearance

PSYCHOSOCIAL. Provide emotional support for the patient and family. Encourage the patient to verbalize fears of death, disability, dependency, and becoming a burden. Answer the patient's and family's questions and involve both the patient and the family or the significant others in all aspects of planning care. SAH is a life-threatening condition that may change the patient's quality of life permanently. Be sensitive to the fact that the event is life-changing for the patient and family, and expect stresses and strains on their coping ability. If necessary, make home health referrals before the patient's discharge.

Diagnostic Highlights

Test	Normal Result	Abnormality With Condition	Explanation
Computed tomography (CT) scan without contract (urgent)	Normal brain and supporting structures	Blood collection in subarachnoid space often in the cisterns or sylvian fissure	Identifies areas of bleeding

Diagnostic Highlights (continued)

Other Tests: Lumbar puncture, complete blood count, coagulation studies, cerebral angiogram, arterial blood gases, serum electrolytes, digital subtraction cerebral angiography, multidetector CT angiography, electrocardiogram, magnetic resonance imaging if no lesion is found on angiogram

PRIMARY NURSING DIAGNOSIS

DIAGNOSIS. Risk for ineffective cerebral tissue perfusion as evidenced by headache, neck pain, neck stiffness, changes in level of consciousness, and/or changes in vision

OUTCOMES. Cognitive orientation; Neurological status; Tissue perfusion: Cerebral; Cranial sensory/motor function; Communication: Expressive; Communication: Receptive

INTERVENTIONS. Cerebral perfusion promotion; Cerebral edema management; ICP monitoring; Neurological monitoring; Peripheral sensation management; Hypovolemia management; Vital signs monitoring; Emergency care; Medication management

PLANNING AND IMPLEMENTATION

Collaborative

Surgery is the treatment of choice for a cerebral aneurysm that has ruptured into the subarachnoid space. Repair of the ruptured aneurysm may be accomplished by surgical clipping or coiling. The timing of surgery is controversial, but most experts recommend that surgery should take place within 72 hours. Until a decision about surgery is made, however, the management of the patient is focused on preventing secondary injury and relieving symptoms.

Endotracheal intubation and mechanical ventilation should be performed for patients who are unresponsive and cannot maintain their own airway. Experts recommend that the mean arterial blood pressure be kept below 130 mm Hg with the use of IV beta blockers that can be adjusted minute by minute. Beta blockers are also used to control hypertension to prevent rebleeding, which occurs most often within the first 24 hours after rupture. The overall mortality rate of rebleeding is as high as 78%, so measures such as sedation and analgesia are important to reduce the risk. Hypotension must be avoided at all costs because it worsens ischemic deficits and can lead to cerebral ischemia. Monitoring ICP to detect brain swelling and hydrocephalus is essential. In patients with elevated ICP, mechanical ventilation is titrated to achieve a $Paco_2$ of 30 to 35 mm Hg. The intravascular volume status is assessed with either a central venous access monitor or pulmonary artery catheter, depending on the patient's condition. Fluid volume is maintained within a normal range because dehydration increases hemoconcentration, which may increase the incidence of vasospasm. If cerebral edema is present, a moderate fluid restriction is employed. The administration of corticosteroids (dexamethasone, methylprednisolone) to manage ICP remains controversial. Vasospasm is managed with calcium channel blockers such as nimodipine, although transluminal balloon angioplasty may be used if other therapy fails.

Complications during the immediate postoperative period include brain swelling, bleeding at the operative site, fluid and electrolyte disturbances, hydrocephalus, and the onset of cerebral vasospasm. If an intracranial monitoring system is in place, generally ICP rises over 15 mm Hg are reported to the neurosurgeons, and CPP is maintained at more than 50 mm Hg. Goals of medication management include control of blood pressure, prevention of seizures, treatment of symptoms (pain, nausea), maintenance of cerebral perfusion, and prevention of elevated ICP and vasospasm.

Pharmacologic Highlights

Medication or Drug Class	Dosage	Description	Rationale
Nimodipine	60 mg PO every 4 hr beginning within 96 hr of event	Calcium channel blocker	Reduces vasospasm and cerebral ischemia
Labetalol	20 mg IV over 2 min, then 40–80 mg IV every 10 min not to exceed 300 mg; may also be given by infusion 1–2 mg/min not to exceed 300 mg	Beta blocker	Lower blood pressure to maintain a range that allows for sufficient cerebral perfusion
Fentanyl	50–100 mcg IV	Opioid analgesic	Ensures comfort and relieves pain, has sedating properties that allow for rest; can be reversed rapidly; has a short half-life

Other Drugs: Mannitol (osmotic diuretic) may be ordered to decrease cerebral edema, stool softeners, sedatives and opioids may be used to induce rest, anticonvulsants (phenytoin, phenobarbital, fosphenytoin), analgesics (acetaminophen or codeine) to control headache, antiemetics, anticonvulsants, loop diuretics

Independent

Accurate, detailed, and serial assessments are essential. Frequently, the first signs of rebleeding and vasospasm are evidenced through subtle changes in the neurological examination. At any time during the course of SAH, maintenance of airway, breathing, and circulation is the top priority. In the postoperative period, unless otherwise indicated, maintain the bed at an elevation of 30 to 40 degrees. Prevent flexion of the head and maintain proper alignment of the head and neck with towel rolls or sandbags. Avoid hip flexion greater than 90 degrees. Suction the patient as needed to keep the airway open. If deep endotracheal suctioning is indicated, hyperventilate and hyperoxygenate the patient before suctioning and limit suctioning to less than 30 seconds.

To prevent complications from postoperative immobility, turn the patient often and provide skin care. Perform active or passive range-of-motion exercises and encourage deep-breathing exercises when the patient is able. Space all nursing care activities to maintain ICP less than 15 mm Hg. Allow ICP to drop between all activities. Encourage other departments to space x-rays, therapies, and interviews to allow adequate rest and to avoid ICP elevations. Avoid conversations at the bedside that might be disturbing to the patient. Explain all procedures even if the patient does not appear to respond. Use soft restraints only when absolutely necessary; fighting restraints raises ICPs and thereby impedes venous outflow from the brain.

After surgery, monitor the dressing for bleeding or CSF leakage. If either occurs, notify the physician and reinforce the dressing. Inspect the surgical site with all dressing changes for redness, drainage, poor wound healing, and swelling.

Evidence-Based Practice and Health Policy

Nichols, L., Stirling, C., Stankovich, J., & Gall, S. (2020). Time to treatment following an aneurysmal subarachnoid hemorrhage, rural place of residence and inter-hospital transfer. *Australasian Emergency Care, 23,* 225–232.

- The authors aimed to examine the effect of geographical location, socioeconomic status, and interhospital transfer on time to treatment following an aneurysmal subarachnoid hemorrhage. They initiated a retrospective cohort study using medical records and calculated time intervals from time of the hemorrhage event to treatment.

- The median time to the intervention was 13.78 hours. Socioeconomic disadvantage was associated with a 1.5-fold increase in time to arrival at the hospital and a 1.76-fold increase in time to neurosurgical admission. Residing in an outer regional location was associated with a 2.27-fold increase in time to neurosurgical admission, and interhospital transfer led to a 6.26-fold increase in time to neurosurgical admission. The authors concluded that time to treatment was negatively influenced by socioeconomic disadvantage, geographical distance from hospitals, and interhospital transfer.

DOCUMENTATION GUIDELINES

- Neurological findings: Level of consciousness; pupillary size, shape, and reaction to light; motor function of extremities; other cranial nerve deficits (blurred vision, extraocular movement deficits, drooping eyelids, facial weakness); speech loss; headache and facial pain; photophobia; and stiff or painful neck; deterioration of neurological status; vital signs and ICP
- Coping: Patient comfort, family anxiety, response to explanations of the patient's condition
- Cardiopulmonary response: Blood pressure control, airway patency, ventilatory management, adequacy of oxygenation

DISCHARGE AND HOME HEALTHCARE GUIDELINES

Prepare the patient and family for the possible need for rehabilitation after the acute care phase of hospitalization. Instruct the patient to report any deterioration in neurological status to the physician. Teach the patient signs and symptoms of deterioration in neurological status. Stress the importance of follow-up visits with the physician. If the patient has had surgery, teach the patient or caregiver to notify the physician for any signs of wound infection or poor incisional healing. Be sure the patient understands all medications, including dosage, route, action, adverse effects, and the need for routine laboratory monitoring for anticonvulsants.

Subdural Hematoma

DRG Category:	70
Mean LOS:	6.2 days
Description:	MEDICAL: Nonspecific Cerebrovascular Disorders With Major Complication or Comorbidity
DRG Category:	955
Mean LOS:	11.0 days
Description:	SURGICAL: Craniotomy for Multiple Significant Trauma

Subdural hematoma (SDH) is an accumulating mass of blood, usually clotted, or a swelling that is confined to the space between the dura mater and the subarachnoid membrane. SDHs are space-occupying lesions and thus categorized as focal brain injuries, thereby concentrated in one part of the brain rather than a diffuse injury. They have a mortality as high as 80% because of associated underlying brain injuries, with younger people having lower mortality and older people having higher mortality. Sometimes an SDH is referred to as a *mass lesion* because it occupies critical space in the cranial vault. It is the most common type of traumatic intracranial mass lesion. Deaths from SDH usually occur because the expanding mass lesion leads to excessive brain swelling and herniation, causing brainstem ischemia and hemorrhage.

SDHs are classified as either acute or chronic on the basis of when symptoms appear. Clinical findings in acute SDHs are evident within 24 to 72 hours after the traumatic event. A subacute

SDH produces symptoms within 2 to 10 days; symptoms appear in chronic SDH within weeks or months (Table 1). Generally, head trauma involves both a primary injury and a secondary injury. The primary injury results from the initial impact, which causes immediate neurological damage and dysfunction. The secondary injury follows the initial trauma and probably stems from cerebral hypoxia and ischemia that then lead to cerebral edema, increased intracranial pressure (ICP), and brain herniation. A consequence of increased ICP, brain herniation is a life-threatening condition in which brain structures protrude through an opening in the brain cavity. Complications of SDH include headaches, difficulty problem-solving, memory difficulty, attention deficits, mood swings, brain herniation, coma, and death.

• **TABLE 1** Types of Subdural Hematomas

TYPE	DESCRIPTION	ONSET OF SYMPTOMS	SYMPTOMS
Acute	Usually results from brain laceration with injury to the small pial veins bridging the subdural space	24–72 hr	Decreased level of consciousness, hemiparesis, unilateral pupil dilation, extraocular eye movement, paralysis, cranial nerve dysfunction
Subacute chronic	Similar to acute	3–21 days	Similar to acute
Chronic	Usually occurs in older adults or in problem drinkers who experience atrophy of the brain; often associated with falls but up to 50% have no history of head trauma	3 wk or more	Interval when patient appears to recover and then progressive deterioration occurs; confusion, drowsiness, inattention, personality changes, headache; progresses to hemiparesis, pupil changes, decreased mental status, problems with gait or balance

CAUSES

The mechanisms of injury associated with the development of SDH are a strong, direct-force, high-speed impact to the head or an acceleration-deceleration force. When the brain accelerates and then decelerates, it hits fixed brain structures and can tear blood vessels. The torn vessel may be a vein connecting the surface of the brain to the dural sinus, leading to bleeding in the subdural space. SDH can occur from motor vehicle crashes, auto-pedestrian crashes, falls, and assaults. Child abuse, including shaken baby syndrome, is also a cause of SDH in children. Chronic SDH is most commonly associated with falls in older adults, particularly those on anti-coagulants, and in problem drinkers. Risks for SDH include aging, alcohol and substance abuse, anticoagulation, cigarette smoking, extreme exertion, contact sports such as football, seizure disorders, atherosclerosis, diabetes mellitus, and hypertension.

GENETIC CONSIDERATIONS

Intracerebral hematoma owing to aneurysm rupture has been associated with autosomal dominantly inherited polycystic kidney disease. Hereditary coagulation defects can also increase risk of hematoma.

SEX AND LIFE SPAN CONSIDERATIONS

SDH can occur at any time in life—no one is exempt. Most head injuries are associated with traffic injuries, which are more common in males than females by a 3:1 ratio. Serious industrial accidents are also more common in men. The average age of a patient with trauma and an SDH is approximately 40 years. Experts note that as people age and the brain atrophies, the veins are more fragile after impact leading to bleeding, which is why patients are older than the average trauma patient. Men have different patterns of injury than women, and a higher injury severity. Analyses of trauma outcomes indicate that, following traumatic injury, males have higher rates of multiple organ failure, pneumonia, and sepsis than females, creating health disparities for men (Marcolini et al., 2019). Trauma is the third leading cause of death in people 45 to 65 years of age and the seventh leading cause of death in people older than age 65 years. Older women in particular are at risk for SDH from falls. The very old population and chronic abusers of alcohol have cortical atrophy, which places them at risk for chronic SDH, which occurs most often in the 50- to 79-year-old age group. Men have a higher incidence of chronic SDH than women.

HEALTH DISPARITIES AND SEXUAL/GENDER MINORITY HEALTH

Traffic injuries are one of the leading causes of subdural hematoma. In recent years, Black persons have been killed in traffic crashes at a rate almost 25% higher than White persons (National Highway Traffic Safety Administration [NHTSA], 2021). Native American persons have the highest rate of traffic crash injury in the United States, more than twice the rate of Black persons (NHTSA, 2021). Experts have noted that Black and Native American communities tend to be crisscrossed by more dangerous roads than other locations, placing people from those communities at risk for injury. Healthy People 2020 reports that non-Hispanic Black persons have the highest injury death rate in the United States (79.9 injury deaths per 100,000 people), followed by non-Hispanic White people (79.2), Native American people (78.2), Hispanic people (45.5), and Asian/Pacific Islander people (25.6).

Recent work has shown evidence that rural populations have injury mortality rates that are more than twice as high as urban rates. Many factors contribute to these health disparities, including the risk of traffic injury in narrow rural roads, the lack of graded curves and lighted traffic signals on rural highways, and the distance from major trauma centers. Many of the most dangerous occupations, such as mining and agriculture, are found in rural areas and can result in injury, disability, and death. Sexual and gender minority persons have high risk for dating and interpersonal violence, violence related to bullying, and intentional and unintentional injury (Healthy People 2020).

GLOBAL HEALTH CONSIDERATIONS

Falls and traffic crashes occur around the world and may lead to SDH. Internationally, falls from heights of less than 5 meters are the leading cause of injury overall, and traffic crashes are the next most frequent cause. More men than women globally have SDH.

▓ ASSESSMENT

HISTORY. Question the prehospital care provider, significant others, or witnesses about the situation when the injury occurred, which is usually a traffic crash, fall, or violent event. If the patient was in a traffic crash, determine the speed and type of vehicle, whether the patient was restrained, the patient's position in the vehicle, and whether the patient was thrown from the vehicle on impact. If the injury occurred in a motorcycle crash, ask if the patient was wearing a helmet. If the patient fell, determine the point of impact, distance of the fall, and type of landing surface. If the patient was assaulted, determine the context and if a weapon was used. Ask if the patient experienced momentary loss of reflexes or momentary arrest of respiration, followed by loss of consciousness. If the patient was unconscious at any time, find out for how long. Determine if the patient experienced a headache, nausea, vomiting, dizziness, convulsions, decreased respiratory rate, or progressive insensitivity to pain (obtundity). Ask about the patient's alcohol and substance use, and if the patient was involved in the injury. If you suspect that a patient has a chronic SDH, establish if the patient had symptoms such as decreased levels of consciousness, headache, memory loss, unstable gait, balance problems, personality changes, motor deficits, or aphasia.

PHYSICAL EXAMINATION. The most common symptoms are **headache, decreased level of consciousness, drowsiness, inattention, hemiparesis,** and **unilateral pupil dilation**. The headache is usually accompanied by nausea and vomiting and is worsened by coughing, straining, or exercise. The initial evaluation or primary survey of the patient with a head injury is centered on assessing the airway, breathing, circulation, and disability (neurological status). Exposure (undressing the patient completely) is incorporated as part of the primary survey. The secondary survey, a head-to-toe assessment including vital signs, is then completed.

The initial neurological assessment of the patient with SDH includes monitoring the vital signs, assessing the level of consciousness, examining pupil size and level of reactivity, and assessing on the Glasgow Coma Scale, which evaluates eye opening, best verbal response, and best motor response. Determine if the patient had a seizure, which sometimes accompanies SDH. Clinical findings may include a rapidly changing level of consciousness from confusion to coma, ipsilateral pupil dilation, hemiparesis, and abnormal posturing, including flexion and extension. A neurological assessment is repeated at least hourly during the first 24 hours after the injury.

Examine the entire scalp and head for lacerations, abrasions, contusions, and bony abnormalities. Take care to maintain cervical spine immobilization during the examination. Patients with SDH may have associated cervical spine injuries or thoracic, abdominal, or extremity trauma. Examine the patient for signs of basilar skull fractures, such as periorbital ecchymosis (raccoon eyes), subscleral hemorrhage, retroauricular ecchymosis (Battle sign), hemotympanum (blood behind the eardrum), and leakage of cerebrospinal fluid (CSF) from the ears (otorrhea) or nose (rhinorrhea). Gently palpate the facial bones, including the mandible and maxilla, for bony deformities and step-offs. Examine the oral pharynx for lacerations, and check for any loose or fractured teeth.

PSYCHOSOCIAL. The patient may be anxious about their condition during intervals of lucidity. Assess the patient's ability to cope with a sudden illness and the change in roles that a sudden illness demands. Explain to the patient's family that personality changes and mood swings sometimes occur with SDH. Determine the significant others' responses to the injury. Expect parents of children who are injured to feel anxious, fearful, and sometimes guilty. Note if the injury was related to alcohol consumption (approximately 40% to 60% of head injuries occur when the patient has been drinking), and elicit a drinking history from the patient or significant others. Assess the patient for signs of alcohol withdrawal 1 to 14 days after admission. Depending on the patient's prognosis, initiate a discussion about end-of-life care and the need for hospice. Determine the patient's and family's desires about resuscitation.

Diagnostic Highlights

Test	Normal Result	Abnormality With Condition	Explanation
Computed tomography scan	Normal brain and supporting structures	Blood collection on brain surface	Identified mass lesion

Other Tests: Magnetic resonance imaging, cervical spine x-rays to rule out cervical spine injury; transcranial Doppler ultrasound; skull x-rays; complete blood count; arterial blood gases; serum electrolytes, blood urea nitrogen, creatinine, serum glucose

PRIMARY NURSING DIAGNOSIS

DIAGNOSIS. Ineffective airway clearance related to hypoventilation or airway obstruction as evidenced by wheezing, stridor, decreased chest excursion, dyspnea, and/or apnea

OUTCOMES. Respiratory status: Airway patency; Respiratory status: Gas exchange; Respiratory status: Ventilation; Symptom severity; Symptom control; Knowledge: Disease process

INTERVENTIONS. Airway management; Airway insertion and stabilization; Oxygen therapy; Airway suctioning; Mechanical ventilation management; Respiratory monitoring

▩ PLANNING AND IMPLEMENTATION
Collaborative
MEDICAL. Endotracheal intubation and mechanical ventilation are critical to ensure oxygenation and ventilation and to decrease the risk of pulmonary aspiration. A Pao_2 greater than 100 mm Hg and a $Paco_2$ between 30 and 35 mm Hg may decrease cerebral blood flow and intracranial swelling. The routine use of hyperventilation is controversial, and some physicians are using $Sjvo_2$ (saturation of jugular venous bulb) monitoring to assess the response to changes in Pao_2 and $Paco_2$. Generally, the $Paco_2$ is maintained at 35 to 40 mm Hg if cerebral swelling is not a risk.

SURGICAL. Prompt surgical evacuation of the hematoma is generally the first-line therapy for patients, but if the underlying brain injury is severe and the patient has a poor prognosis, the surgical team and the family will need to consult about the best outcome for the patient. Surgical management is evacuation of the clot, control of the hemorrhage, and resection of nonviable brain tissue. Rapid surgical intervention is essential. If surgical evacuation is delayed for more than 4 hours, these lesions produce a higher mortality rate. The surgeon exposes the area involved, the clot is evacuated, bleeding from surface vascular structures is controlled with bipolar coagulation, and bridging veins are controlled with Gelfoam or muscle tissue. The surgical site may be drained postoperatively by using a Jackson-Pratt drain for 24 to 48 hours. Possible postoperative complications include intracranial hypertension, reaccumulation of the clot, intracerebral hemorrhage, and development of seizures.

Patients with critical head injuries who have a high probability of developing intracranial hypertension may require invasive ICP monitoring with an intraventricular catheter. Some physicians use a Glasgow Coma Scale score of less than 7 as an indicator for monitoring ICP. The goal is to maintain the ICP at less than 10 mm Hg and the cerebral perfusion pressure (CPP) greater than 80 mm Hg. Management of intracranial hypertension may also be done by draining CSF through a ventriculostomy, either intermittently or continuously according to a predetermined ICP measurement. IV mannitol is given if the patient manifests signs of impending brain herniation.

Patients with chronic SDH without symptoms may be observed over time. In some patients, the hematoma may remain stable or even resolve. Patients who are on anticoagulants and antiplatelet therapy usually have those therapies halted for approximately 2 to 4 weeks after injury depending on clinical indication.

Pharmacologic Highlights

Medication or Drug Class	Dosage	Description	Rationale
Diuretics	Varies by drug	Furosemide, mannitol	Assist in managing intracranial hypertension (although their use remains controversial)
Sedatives	Varies by drug	Short-acting sedatives: Midazolam, propofol (Diprivan), fentanyl	Control intermittent increases in ICP with a resultant decrease in CPP; short action of drugs allows for temporarily stopping infusion so that neurological assessment can be performed

(highlight box continues on page 1122)

Pharmacologic Highlights (continued)

Medication or Drug Class	Dosage	Description	Rationale
Chemical paralysis	Varies by drug	Mivacurium, atracurium (short-acting agents that have few hypotensive effects)	Improves oxygenation and ventilation for some patients with severe head injuries
Anticonvulsants	Prophylactically	Phenytoin (Dilantin)	Controversial in the routine management of subdural hematoma; overall effectiveness has yet to be determined

Other Drugs: Other drugs include antibiotics and barbiturates (persistently elevated ICP despite routine interventions may be managed with the induction of a barbiturate coma, which reduces the metabolic rate of brain tissue). Mannitol for impending brain herniation and uncontrolled increased intracranial pressure.

Independent

The highest priority in managing patients with SDH is to maintain a patent airway, appropriate ventilation and oxygenation, and adequate circulation. Make sure the patient's endotracheal tube is anchored well. If the patient is at risk for self-extubation, maintain the patient in soft restraints. Note the lip level of the endotracheal tube to determine if tube movement occurs. Notify the physician if the patient's Pao_2 drops below 80 mm Hg, $Paco_2$ exceeds 40 mm Hg, or if severe hypocapnia ($Paco_2 < 25$ mm Hg) occurs.

Help control the patient's ICP. Maintain normothermia by avoiding body temperature elevations. Elevate the patient's bed to 30 degrees and avoid flexing, extending, or rotating the patient's neck because these maneuvers limit venous drainage of the brain and thus raise ICP. Avoid hip flexion, which limits venous drainage, by maintaining the patient in a normal body alignment. Maintain a quiet, restful environment with minimal stimulation; limit visitors as appropriate. Time nursing care activities carefully to limit prolonged ICP elevations. Use caution when suctioning the patient: Hyperventilate the patient beforehand, and suction only as long as necessary. When turning the patient, prevent Valsalva maneuver by using a draw sheet to pull the patient up in bed. Instruct the patient not to hold on to the side rails.

Strategies to maximize the coping mechanisms of the patient and family are directed toward providing support and encouragement. Provide simple educational tools about head injuries. Teach the patient and family appropriate rehabilitative exercises, as necessary. Help the patient cope with long stretches of immobility by providing diversionary activities appropriate to the patient's mental and physical abilities. Head injury support groups may be helpful. Referrals to clinical nurse specialists, pastoral care staff, and social workers are helpful in developing strategies for support and education.

Evidence-Based Practice and Health Policy

Rauhala, M., Helén, P., Huhtala, H., Heikkila, P., Iverson, G., Niskakangas, T., Öhman, J., & Luoto, T. (2020). Chronic subdural hematoma—Incidence, complications, and financial impact. *Acta Neurochirurgica, 162*, 2033–2043.

- The authors had two goals: to examine the population-based incidence, complications, and total, direct hospital costs of chronic subdural hematoma (CSDH) treatment in a neurosurgical clinic during a 26-year period and to estimate the necessity of planned postoperative follow-up computed tomography. The authors used medical records to create a retrospective cohort of adult patients with CSDH in Finland ($N = 1,148$). They calculated direct hospital costs and all costs from hospital admission to the last neurosurgical follow-up visit, following all patients until death or the end of 2017.

• The sample was 65% male with a median age of 76 years. Eighty-five percent underwent surgery. Patients undergoing re-operations experienced more seizures, empyema, and pneumonia compared with patients with no surgery. The treatment cost for recurrent CSDHs was 132% higher than the treatment cost of nonrecurrent CSDHs, most likely because of longer hospital stay for readmissions and more frequent outpatient follow-up with CT. The authors noted that CT was only necessary for symptomatic patients.

DOCUMENTATION GUIDELINES

• Trauma history, description of the event, time elapsed since the event, whether or not the patient had a loss of consciousness and, if so, for how long
• Adequacy of airway, breathing, and circulation; serial vital signs
• Appearance, bruising or lacerations, drainage from the nose or ears
• Physical findings related to the site of head injury: Neurological assessment, presence of accompanying symptoms, presence of complications (decreased level of consciousness, unequal pupils, loss of strength and movement, confusion or agitation, nausea and vomiting), CPP, ICP
• Signs of complications: Seizure activity, infection (fever, purulent discharge from any wounds), aspiration pneumonia (shortness of breath, pulmonary congestion, fever, productive cough), increased ICP
• Response to surgery and clot evacuation: Mental status changes, incisional healing, presence of complications (infection, hemorrhage), response to analgesia and sedation

DISCHARGE AND HOME HEALTHCARE GUIDELINES

Review proper care techniques for wounds and lacerations. Discuss the recommended activity level and explain rehabilitative exercises as appropriate. Teach the patient and family to recognize symptoms of infection or a deteriorating level of consciousness. Stress the need to contact the physician on the appearance of such signs or symptoms. Teach the patient the purpose, dosage, schedule, precautions, potential side effects, interactions, and adverse reactions of all prescribed medications. Review with the patient and family all follow-up appointments that have been arranged. If the patient drinks above the recommended alcohol limits, refer the patient to a counselor or for evaluation for outpatient treatment.

Sudden Infant Death Syndrome

DRG Category:	92
Mean LOS:	3.9 days
Description:	MEDICAL: Other Disorders of Nervous System With Complication or Comorbidity

Sudden infant death syndrome (SIDS) is the sudden, unexplained death of an infant under age 1 year for reasons that remain unexplained even after autopsy. A typical scenario is when a seemingly healthy infant of 2 to 3 months of age is put to bed without concern over illness but is later found dead. SIDS occurs worldwide with an incidence of 0.2 to 3 per 1,000 live births. SIDS is the most common cause of death in infants under 6 months of age. To make the diagnosis, a case investigation is necessary to rule out metabolic disorders, hyperthermia, hypothermia, child abuse or neglect, or suffocation. Without thorough investigation, deaths are considered sudden unexpected infant deaths (SUIDs), which include SID, unknown causes, and accidental suffocation and strangulation in bed. The most recent statistics were published in 2019, indicating that approximately 1,250 SIDS-related; 1,200 unknown; and 1,000 accidental suffocation deaths occur in the United States per year (Centers for Disease Control and Prevention [CDC], 2021).

Recent statistics have shown that the prevalence of SIDS has decreased by approximately 50% following public health campaigns, such as Safe to Sleep, which is focused on placing infants supine (face upward) for sleep. This recommendation was based on studies that demonstrated that the risk of SIDS was highest for prone-sleeping (face down) infants. Although there is great uncertainty in the scientific community about risk factors for SIDS, several genetic, environmental, and social factors have been linked with SIDS. Approximately 20% of SIDS occurs in childcare facilities. Many of these deaths occur within the first week of child care, thereby suggesting a disruption in sleep patterns. More SIDS deaths occur between the hours of midnight and 9 a.m., and more occur in colder rather than warmer months.

CAUSES

A wide variety of findings have been reported in infants who have died of SIDS. Some of these findings include retarded postnatal growth, low Apgar scores at birth, increased pulmonary arterial smooth muscle, increased right ventricular muscle mass, and a variety of cardiopulmonary and neurological cellular abnormalities. The cellular findings suggest that SIDS may be caused by exposure to chronic hypoxia and respiratory failure. However, the direct evidence is controversial and has led to multiple theories. Several theories suggest that SIDS may be caused by sleep apnea, congenital central nervous system (CNS) anomaly, decreased serotonergic receptor binding in the brainstem, neuromuscular infantile botulism, accidental suffocation, abnormal upper airway dysfunction, cardiac abnormalities, or inborn errors of metabolism. Risk factors include premature births (particularly associated with apnea or bronchopulmonary dysplasia); low birth weight; overbundling; bed-sharing; young, unmarried birthing parents; lack of prenatal care; prenatal and postnatal parental smoking or anemia; birthing parent substance use; cold weather; and low-income housing. Protective factors include room-sharing, breastfeeding, and dummy pacifier use.

GENETIC CONSIDERATIONS

Mutations in several genes have been associated with SIDS. The metabolic disease MCAD deficiency (*ACADM* mutations) is the most common fatty acid oxidation defect and has been associated with SIDS. The ion channel genes that cause long QT syndrome (*SCN5A, CACNA1C, CAV3, KCNE1/KCNE2*, and *KCNQ1*) have been shown to cause some cases of SIDS, and the mitochondrial genes *MT-TL1* and *MT-ND1* may play a role in other cases. There is also evidence for an association between SIDS and mutation in the 5-hydroxytryptamine transporter gene (5-HT).

SEX AND LIFE SPAN CONSIDERATIONS

Boys are affected more than girls. The incidence is highest during the second and third months of life; few cases occur in the first 2 weeks of life or after 6 months of age.

HEALTH DISPARITIES AND SEXUAL/GENDER MINORITY HEALTH

Although racial and ethnic differences are unexplained, Black and Native American babies have a higher incidence of SIDS than Hispanic and White babies. Poverty is associated with SUID, which is more than two times higher in counties in the United States with high as compared to counties with low poverty. Sexual and gender minority status has no known effect on the risk for SID.

GLOBAL HEALTH CONSIDERATIONS

The lowest rates of SIDS are found in developed countries in Western Europe and in some Asian countries such as Japan.

ASSESSMENT

HISTORY. If you suspect that an infant is at risk for SIDS, elicit a history of risk factors. Determine if the infant has a history of brief resolved unexplained events (BRUE), formerly known as apparent life-threatening events (ALTEs). In BRUE, three observations have occurred: cyanosis, breathing difficulties, and/or abnormal limb movements. The infant may have ceased breathing, developed pallor, had a marked change in muscle tone, choked or gagged, or become unresponsive, and yet the child recovered or was successfully resuscitated. This "near miss" is thought to be a warning sign for future SIDS. Determine details surrounding the situation, the activities that occurred prior to the event (sleeping, sleeping position, feeding), any illness in the weeks prior to the event, the period of apnea, a description of color changes and any changes in muscle tone, the duration of the event, and any treatment that was administered. If parents have lost a child to SIDS, the history of the event needs to be elicited carefully and with compassion because of the loss and grief patients are experiencing.

PHYSICAL EXAMINATION. Common symptoms of a life-threatening event include **cyanosis, breathing irregularities or difficulties**, and **abnormal limb movements related to changes in muscle tone**. Infants with BRUE who are brought to the emergency department after an event often have a normal physical examination. Approximately 25% have fever and 25% have an infection. Symptoms that may occur in infants at risk for BRUE or SIDS may show increased incidence of periodic breathing during sleep with pauses of up to 10 seconds and possibly increased respiratory rates. Some infants have faster heart rates than normal, less heart rate variability, and shorter Q-T intervals.

PSYCHOSOCIAL. If an infant has had a BRUE, parents are likely to be anxious and afraid. Provide a referral to a support group and consider providing them with counseling to deal with their anxiety. For a family who has lost a child to SIDS, management is directed to assisting the family to cope with loss of an infant. Sadness and feelings of despair or hopelessness may evolve; patients and families should be encouraged to discuss these openly. Parents, grandparents, and siblings will likely experience feelings of guilt or anger and will need opportunities to express these feelings.

Diagnostic Highlights

No test is diagnostic for BRUEs or SIDS. In suspected cases of BRUEs, a full diagnostic investigation should include complete blood count, blood chemistries, blood urea nitrogen, blood gas analysis, chest x-ray with magnification of the upper airways, upper gastrointestinal barium study, electrocardiogram, 24-hour monitoring electrocardiogram, a variety of respiratory studies, electroencephalogram, esophageal pH, and sleep studies.

PRIMARY NURSING DIAGNOSIS

DIAGNOSIS. Risk for maladaptive grieving as evidenced by alterations in sleep or activity patterns, anger, blaming, despair, detachment, distress, and/or finding meaning in a loss

OUTCOMES. Coping; Grief resolution; Psychosocial adjustment: Life change; Self-esteem; Mood equilibrium

INTERVENTIONS. Counseling; Family support; Active listening; Coping enhancement; Crisis intervention; Emotional support; Grief work facilitation: Perinatal death

PLANNING AND IMPLEMENTATION
Collaborative

A full work-up for infants following a BRUE should include a search for infectious diseases, metabolic abnormalities, environmental factors, and structural problems such as congenital heart, respiratory, and CNS lesions. Following a BRUE or with infants at risk for SIDS, a number of preventive measures can occur. Positioning is one measure that appears to aid in the prevention of SIDS. Encourage all parents to place infants on their backs to sleep until at least 1 year of age. Because of publicity on the link between sleep position and SIDS, the use of prone and side-lying sleeping positions for infants has decreased in the United States from 75% to as low as 11.3%. The Centers for Disease Control and Prevention reported that the SIDS rate has fallen by 58% in the United States with the Safe to Sleep campaign.

Encourage parents to use a firm mattress for their infants. Explain that they should not use soft bedding or have stuffed animals in the bed with the infant, and infants should not sleep on a waterbed or with parents (bed sharing). Discuss that head coverings or bedding that is covering the infant's head may be related to SIDS. Parents should avoid overheating the infant's room (temperature should be in the range of 68°F to 72°F [20°C to 22°C]), and a fan may be useful. Explain that the use of a pacifier may be beneficial, and experts suggest that breastfeeding may serve as protection for SIDS. Co-sleeping in the same room, but not the same bed, is recommended for at least the first 6 months. Recommend that birthing parents avoid alcohol and drug use during pregnancy and breastfeeding; explain that parents should not allow passive inhalation of cigarette smoke by the infant.

Home monitoring may be recommended for infants with BRUEs or for siblings of infants who have died from SIDS. However, the rate of SIDS in succeeding children is difficult to determine. Because monitoring cannot prevent the occurrence of SIDS, some controversy exists about home monitoring for succeeding infants. Monitors exist to measure heart rate, heart rate variability, and respiratory rate. Apnea monitors, however, may not detect complete airway obstruction as infants continue to make respiratory efforts even when the airway is obstructed. There is little information available to determine whether home monitoring is necessary, and the decision is generally made by the physician or nurse practitioner and the parents. If monitoring is initiated, the abilities of members of the household to handle and interpret monitors become important so that true and false alarms may be handled appropriately. In addition, parents should receive appropriate training in infant cardiopulmonary resuscitation and proper use of monitoring equipment.

Pharmacologic Highlights

No pharmacologic management is known to prevent SIDS and BRUEs.

Independent

The following information is helpful to parents to prevent SIDS: (1) Place babies supine for sleep, (2) pacifier use may reduce risk for SIDS, (3) avoid overbundling babies, (4) avoid excessively soft or padded sleep mattresses, (5) remove all blankets and toys from the crib, (6) breastfeeding may be protective, (7) co-sleeping in the same room but not the same bed is recommended for the first 6 to 12 months, and (8) avoid secondhand cigarette smoke exposure and create a smoke-free zone. Management after the death of an infant from SIDS is focused on helping the family cope with loss of the infant. Parents often react with disbelief, anger, or shock. Confusing the situation with child abuse, which will compound the family's emotional trauma, should be avoided.

A thorough investigation of the incident is important, but questions need to be asked carefully and with compassion. Obtain a thorough history from the caretaker about the situation, but be careful not to accuse the family of mistakes in caregiving. Obtain the information within a few hours of the event so as to obtain a thorough history. Reassure the family and caretaker that SIDS was not their fault and was unpreventable. Offer support and counseling and provide a referral as appropriate. Many online support groups and informational sources exist for families of children with SIDS, including Compassionate Friends (https://www.compassionatefriends .org), First Candle (https://www.firstcandle.org), The SUDC Foundation (Sudden Unexplained Death in Childhood, https://sudc.org), and Share (https://nationalshare.org).

Remember to assist the surviving siblings, who may need referrals for counseling to understand their feelings of guilt, loss, or vulnerability. Help parents deal with their other children and with their own need for extra attention and concern.

Evidence-Based Practice and Health Policy

Anderson, T., Ferres, J., Ren, S., Moon, R., Goldstein, R., Ramirez, J., & Mithcell, E. (2019). Maternal smoking before and during pregnancy and the risk of sudden unexpected infant death. *Pediatrics*, *143*, 1–8.

- The authors investigated the effects of maternal prepregnancy smoking, reduction during pregnancy, and smoking during pregnancy on SUID. They analyzed data from the Centers for Disease Control and Prevention with over 20 million births and 19,127 babies with SUID. They defined SUID as death prior to 1 year of age.
- They found that SUID risk more than doubled with any maternal smoking during pregnancy. For mothers who smoked 1 to 20 cigarettes per day, the probability of SUID increased linearly with each additional cigarette smoked per day. They noted that if causality is assumed, 22% of SUIDs in the United States can be directly attributed to maternal smoking during pregnancy.

DOCUMENTATION GUIDELINES

- Description of the SIDS event: Precipitating factors, risk factors, situation, timing, sleep and wake patterns of infant, position during sleep, type of mattress
- Health history of infant: Previous illnesses, birth weight and length of gestation, history of BRUEs
- Health history of birthing parent: Tobacco and substance use, parity, nutrition, socioeconomic status

DISCHARGE AND HOME HEALTHCARE GUIDELINES

Make sure the caregiver and family have contact information for support services. Encourage the family to receive grief counseling and let them know that grieving takes many months or even more time. Arrange for a visit with the primary care provider at the end of a year to evaluate family functioning. If home monitoring is instituted for succeeding children, make sure the caregiver understands the monitors and can make decisions about true and false alarms. Teach the caregiver infant cardiopulmonary resuscitation if it is deemed appropriate.

Syndrome of Inappropriate Antidiuretic Hormone

DRG Category:	644
Mean LOS:	4.3 days
Description:	MEDICAL: Endocrine Disorders With Complication or Comorbidity

Syndrome of inappropriate antidiuretic hormone (SIADH), a disorder of the posterior pituitary gland, is a condition of excessive release of antidiuretic hormone (ADH) that results in excessive water retention and hyponatremia. Hyponatremia is the most common electrolyte imbalance that occurs while patients are in the hospital, and SIADH is a common cause. SIADH occurs when ADH secretion is activated by factors other than hyperosmolarity (increased concentration of solutes in the blood) or hypovolemia (decreased blood volume), which usually controls ADH secretion. The excess ADH secretion increases renal tubular permeability and reabsorption of water into the circulation, resulting in excess extracellular fluid volume, reduced plasma osmolality, decreased serum sodium levels, and increased glomerular filtration rates.

The hyponatremia in this syndrome is not related to sodium loss but rather to water excess and the movement of water into the brain. In the process, brain cells lose potassium and amino acids. Without treatment, SIADH can lead to life-threatening complications. Water intoxication accompanied by sodium deficit and cerebral edema lead to complications such as seizures, coma, and death.

CAUSES

Several conditions contribute to SIADH. Central nervous system (CNS) responses to fear, pain, psychoses, and acute distress are known to increase the rate of ADH secretion by the posterior pituitary gland. Physiological conditions that increase intracranial pressure, such as acute CNS infections, brain trauma, anoxic brain death, stroke, and brain surgery, may lead to SIADH. Other conditions associated with SIADH include peripheral neuropathy, delirium tremens, and Addison disease. Certain medications, such as analgesics, anesthetics, thiazide diuretics, opiates, chlorpropramide, carbamezapine, vincristine, and nicotine, are also associated with SIADH. Some tumors have been associated with ADH production, such as cancer of the lungs, pancreas, and prostate as well as Hodgkin disease. Risk factors include head trauma, stroke, cardiopulmonary arrest, cancer of the lung, pneumonia, positive pressure ventilation, meningitis, alcohol withdrawal, low body weight, and certain medications (as listed previously).

GENETIC CONSIDERATIONS

No clear genetic contributions to susceptibility have been defined.

SEX AND LIFE SPAN CONSIDERATIONS

Both children and adults are at risk, but being a hospitalized patient over age 30 years is a risk factor, as is low body weight, which may result in more women than men being affected. Women are also are more affected by drug-induced and exercise-induced hyponatremia than men, who are more prone to develop mild hyponatremia. Typical childhood conditions that can lead to SIADH include pneumonia, meningitis, head trauma, and subarachnoid bleeding. In adults, the condition is most commonly associated with CNS disorders. The very old and very young develop symptoms with smaller decreases in serum sodium levels than adults.

HEALTH DISPARITIES AND SEXUAL/GENDER MINORITY HEALTH

Ethnicity, race, and sexual/gender minority status have no known effect on the risk for SIADH.

GLOBAL HEALTH CONSIDERATIONS

While SIADH and hyponatremia occur around the world, no prevalence data are available.

✺ ASSESSMENT

HISTORY. Because SIADH is usually hospital acquired, the condition is noted because of hyponatremia found in laboratory testing. Given the serious nature of the related causes, often the patient will have urinary output monitored hourly. Ask if the patient has experienced alterations in urinary patterns. Question the patient about recent weight gain. Signs of sodium deficit generally occur slowly. Ask if the patient has experienced recent signs of hyponatremia such as fatigue, weakness, nausea, anorexia, or headaches.

PHYSICAL EXAMINATION. The most common sign of SIADH is a **dropping serum sodium level**. Often no clinical signs are obvious, and the severity of symptoms does not always correlate with the degree of hyponatremia. Late signs include nausea, vomiting, muscle weakness, decreased reaction time, irritability, decreased level of consciousness, seizures, and even coma. Note that the most severe, life-threatening signs of SIADH are not fluid overload and pulmonary congestion but rather the CNS effects from acute sodium deficiency. Perform a neurological assessment to determine if the patient has experienced changes in the level of consciousness, which can range from confusion to seizure activity. Life-threatening symptoms such as seizures may indicate acute water excess, whereas nausea, muscle twitching, headache, and weight gain are more indicative of chronic water accumulation.

PSYCHOSOCIAL. The family and significant others may be fearful if the patient has experienced CNS changes that alter behavior and alertness. If the patient has had seizures, note that family members may have many questions. The patient's and family's responses to SIADH are often a reflection of their responses to these other conditions, which are important to consider in any evaluation of patient and family coping.

Diagnostic Highlights

Test	Normal Result	Abnormality With Condition	Explanation
Urine osmolality (osmolality refers to a solution's concentration of solute particles per kilogram of solvent)	200–1,200 mOsm/L	> 100 mOsm/L	Excretion of inappropriately concentrated urine and hyponatremia caused by overproduction of ADH
Blood osmolality	275–295 mOsm/L	< 275 mOsm/L	Sodium loss in urine and water intoxication lead to hemodilution
Serum sodium	135–145 mEq/L	< 120 mEq/L	Sodium loss in the urine leads to hyponatremia and hemodilution
Urine sodium	< 20 mEq/L	> 40 mEq/L	Sodium loss in the urine

Other Tests: Blood urea nitrogen, urine specific gravity, serum electrolytes, plasma cortisol, computed tomography of head, radioimmunoassay of ADH

PRIMARY NURSING DIAGNOSIS

DIAGNOSIS. Excess fluid volume related to retention of free water as evidenced by fatigue, weakness, nausea, anorexia, and/or headache

OUTCOMES. Fluid balance; Hydration; Electrolyte balance; Circulation status; Cardiac pump effectiveness; Knowledge: Disease process; Knowledge: Medication

INTERVENTIONS. Fluid monitoring; Fluid management; Electrolyte management: Hyponatremia; IV therapy; Circulatory care; Vital signs monitoring; Medication management

PLANNING AND IMPLEMENTATION
Collaborative

Restoration of normal electrolyte and fluid balance and normal body fluid concentration are the treatment goals. Treatment involves correction of the underlying cause and correction of hyponatremia. If the patient's life is not in danger from airway compromise or severe hyponatremia, the physician often restricts fluids initially to 600 to 800 mL or less per 24 hours. With fluid restriction, the hormone aldosterone is released by the adrenal gland and the patient begins to conserve sodium in the kidneys. As serum sodium increases, SIADH gradually corrects itself. The patient needs assistance to plan fluid intake, and a dietary consultation is also required for consistency in fluid management.

If fluid restriction is unsuccessful, the physician may prescribe an IV infusion of a 3% to 4.5% saline solution. Correction of hyponatremia is done carefully, because fluid could move rapidly from the brain into the circulation by osmosis, causing damage to the brain. In complicated cases, consultation with a neurologist may be important because of the risk of neurological deficits if correction is not done carefully. Use caution in administering these hypertonic solutions and always place them on an infusion control device to regulate the infusion rate precisely. Correction of the serum sodium levels by 6 mEq/L in 24 hours is recommended by many experts, or if in an emergency, 6 mEq/L in 6 hours and then cease correction for the rest of the day. Monitor the patient carefully because sodium and water retention may also result, leading to pulmonary congestion and shortness of breath.

Diuretics to remove excess fluid volume may be used in patients with cardiac symptoms if they are symptomatic.

Pharmacologic Highlights

Medication or Drug Class	Dosage	Description	Rationale
Vasopressin receptor antagonists	Varies with drug	Conivaptan; tolvaptan	Block vasopressin receptors; used for hypervolemic and euvolemic (normal volume) hyponatremia when serum sodium level < 125 mEq/L, when hyponatremia is symptomatic, and when there has been inadequate response to fluid restriction
Diuretics	Varies with drug	Thiazide diuretics; loop diuretics (furosemide)	Remove excess fluid volume (may be used in patients with cardiac symptoms)

Other Drugs: Osmotic diuretics mannitol and urea; tetracycline derivative demeclocycine is no longer recommended because of its delayed mechanism of action and nephrotoxic side effects.

Independent

If the patient is at risk for airway compromise because of low serum sodium levels or seizure activity, maintaining a patent airway is the primary nursing concern. Insert an oral or nasal airway if the patient is able to maintain breathing or prepare the patient for endotracheal intubation if it is needed. If the patient is able to maintain airway and breathing, consider positioning the patient so that the head of the bed is either flat or elevated no more than 10 degrees. This position enhances venous return and increases left atria filling pressure, which, in turn, reduce the release of ADH.

Explore with the patient methods to maintain the fluid restriction. If thirst and a dry mouth cause discomfort, try alternatives such as hard candy (if the patient is awake and alert) or chewing gum. Allocate some of the restricted fluids for ice chips to be used throughout the day at the patient's discretion. Work with the patient to determine the amount of fluid to be sent on each tray so that fluid intake is spread equitably throughout the day. If the patient is receiving fluids in IV piggyback medications, consider those volumes as part of the 24-hour intake. Work with the pharmacy to concentrate all medications in the lowest volume that is safe for the patient.

Promote range-of-motion exercises for patients who are bedridden, and turn and reposition them every 2 hours to limit the complications of immobility. Initiate seizure precautions to ensure the patient's safety.

Evidence-Based Practice and Health Policy

Mentrasti, G., Scortichini, L., Torniai, M., Giamperi, R., Morgese, F., Rinaldi, S., & Berardi, R. (2020). Syndrome of inappropriate antidiuretic hormone secretion (SIADH): Optimal management. *Therapeutics and Clinical Risk Management, 16,* 663–672.

- The authors note that while hyponatremia (sodium concentration < 135 mEq/L) is the most common electrolyte balance disorder in clinical practice, SIADH is the most relevant in hospitalized patients. The author describes the pathophysiology and clinical aspects and biochemical tests related to SIADH.
- Management strategies include fluid restriction of 500 to 800 cc per day, infusion of hypertonic saline (3%) with a bolus of 100 to 150 mL over 10 minutes, and the administration of tolvaptan, an arginine vasopressin (AVP) antagonistic agent. The authors note that the decrease of serum sodium levels lowers quality of life and leads to poorer survival in some critical medical conditions, such as congestive heart failure, hepatic cirrhosis, and renal disease, especially in older patients in treatment.

DOCUMENTATION GUIDELINES

- Physical findings: Status of airway, assessment of CNS, fluid volume status (presence of edema, skin turgor, intake and output), serum sodium level
- Response to fluid restriction, ability to maintain fluid restriction, response to diuretics and other medications, electrolyte levels
- Presence of complications: Changes in lung or cardiac sounds; changes in level of consciousness; seizures

DISCHARGE AND HOME HEALTHCARE GUIDELINES

Be sure the patient and significant others understand the medication regimen, including the dosage, route, action, adverse effects, and need for follow-up laboratory tests (ADH level, serum sodium and potassium, blood urea nitrogen and creatinine, urine and serum osmolality). Instruct the patient to report changes in voiding patterns, level of consciousness, presence of edema, symptoms of hyponatremia, reduced neurological functioning, nausea and vomiting, and muscle cramping. If the patient is going home on fluid restriction, be sure to discuss methods of limiting fluid intake and encourage the patient to obtain weight daily to monitor for fluid retention.

Syphilis

DRG Category:	868
Mean LOS:	4.6 days
Description:	MEDICAL: Other Infectious and Parasitic Diseases Diagnoses With Complication or Comorbidity

Syphilis is a chronic, infectious, systemic, sexually transmitted vascular infection characterized by five stages: incubation, primary, secondary, latency, and late. The incubation stage begins with the penetration of the infecting organism, the spirochete *Treponema pallidum*, into the skin or mucosa of the body. Within 10 to 90 days after the initial infection, the primary stage begins with the appearance of a firm, painless lesion called a chancre at the site of entry. In women, the chancre often forms in the vagina or on the cervix and therefore goes unnoticed. If it is left untreated, the chancre heals spontaneously in 1 to 5 weeks. As this primary stage resolves, systemic symptoms appear, signaling the start of the secondary stage. Secondary stage symptoms include malaise, headache, nausea, fever, loss of appetite, sore throat, stomatitis, alopecia, condylomata lata (reddish-brown lesions that ulcerate and have a foul discharge), local or generalized rash, and silver-gray eroded patches on the mucous membranes. These symptoms subside in 1 week to 6 months, and the infected person enters a latent stage, which may last from 1 to 40 years. During latency, periodic symptoms of secondary syphilis may recur.

Approximately one-third of patients with untreated syphilis eventually progress to the late or tertiary stage of syphilis; the complications are often disabling and life-threatening. In this stage, destructive lesions called *gummas* develop in the skin, bone, viscera, central nervous system, or cardiovascular system. Three subtypes of late syphilis are late benign syphilis, cardiovascular syphilis, and neurosyphilis. Late benign syphilis can result in destruction of the bones and body organs, which leads to death. Cardiovascular syphilis develops in approximately 10% of untreated patients and can cause aortitis, aortic regurgitation, aortic valve insufficiency, and aneurysm. Neurosyphilis develops in approximately 8% of untreated patients and can cause meningitis and paresis.

CAUSES

Syphilis is a communicable disease caused by the organism *T pallidum*. Transmission usually occurs through direct contact with open lesions, body fluids, or the secretions of infected persons during sexual contact. Blood transfusions; placental transfer; and, in rare cases, contact with contaminated articles are also modes of transmission. Susceptibility to syphilis is universal, but only 10% of exposures lead to active infection. Risk behaviors that may lead to syphilis include engaging in unprotected sexual intercourse, having sex with multiple partners, and using alcohol and other drugs of abuse. Men who have sex with men and people who have HIV disease are at risk.

GENETIC CONSIDERATIONS

Heritable immune responses could be protective or could increase susceptibility.

SEX AND LIFE SPAN CONSIDERATIONS

Syphilis is most reported in the 15- to 30-year-old age group. It occurs more frequently in men, but the incidence in women is steadily rising. Prenatal transmission from an infected birthing parent to the fetus is possible and occurs in at least 50% to 80% of exposed neonates. In the past, one-third of fetal demises were caused by parental syphilis, but this number has decreased significantly with fewer incidences in pregnant people today.

HEALTH DISPARITIES AND SEXUAL/GENDER MINORITY HEALTH

The incidence of syphilis varies depending on sexual practices, numbers of partners, drug use, and cultural norms. The highest rates of syphilis are reported in Black and Hispanic men who have sex with men, among urban populations, and among impoverished groups (Sullivan et al., 2018). In 2000, the incidence in the United States reached an all-time low, but rates have been gradually increasing since then, with the increase occurring most notably in men who have sex with men and people who live in the southern and western states.

GLOBAL HEALTH CONSIDERATIONS

According to the World Health Organization (WHO), more than 12 million people around the world have syphilis, with the highest proportion of infected people in sub-Saharan Africa, South and Southeast Asia, and Central/South America. They estimate that an average of 12% of men who have sex with men and an average of 11% of sex workers globally have syphilis. The WHO estimates that 1% to 10% of pregnant persons making an antenatal visit across the globe will test positive for syphilis. They note that syphilis is the second leading cause of stillbirth globally and also results in prematurity, low birth weight, neonatal death, and infections in newborns (WHO, 2021).

ASSESSMENT

HISTORY. Establish a sexual history, including the number of sexual partners, the types of sexual behaviors in which the patient engages, and whether the patient was protected by a condom during intercourse. Determine if any of the patient's partners were infected with a sexually transmitted infection (STI). Question the patient about IV drug use, alcohol use, and previous STIs. With an infant, establish the sexual history of the birthing parent. Ask when the patient's last menstrual period occurred.

Elicit a history of chancres. Ask the patient to describe the appearance, location, and duration of any chancres, particularly if they are no longer present. Establish a history of fever, headaches, nausea, anorexia, weight loss, sore throat, mild fever, hair loss, or rashes, symptoms of the primary and secondary stages. Determine if the patient has experienced paresis, seizures, arm and leg weakness, alterations in judgment, or personality changes, all of which are symptoms of late-stage syphilis.

PHYSICAL EXAMINATION. Common symptoms include **lesions on the sex organs, fingers, mouths, and tongue.** Carefully inspect the patient's genitalia, anus, mouth, breasts, eyelids, tonsils, or hands for a primary lesion. With female patients, be sure to determine if chancres have developed on internal structures such as the cervix or the vaginal wall. Chancres vary in appearance and location, depending on which stage the disease has entered, so record a detailed description of any lesions (Table 1).

• **TABLE 1** Syphilitic Lesions	
STAGE OF DISEASE	**DESCRIPTION OF LESION**
Primary	Chancres that start as painless papules and then erode; have indurated, raised edges and clear bases. Found on genitals, lips, tongue, nipples, tonsils, anus, fingers, and eyelids
Secondary	Macular, papular, pustular, or nodular rash. Lesions are uniform in size, well defined, generalized. Lesions may enlarge and erode, producing highly contagious pink or grayish-white lesions (condylomata lata). Found on palms, arms, soles, face, scalp, perineum, scrotum, vulva, and between rolls of body fat
Latent late	Absence of lesions. Gummas: Chronic, superficial nodules or deep, granulomatous lesions. Solitary, asymmetric, painless, indurated. Found on bones and in organs

If a chancre exists, palpate the surrounding lymph nodes for hard, painless nodules. Also inspect the scalp, skin, and mucous membranes for hair loss, rashes, or mucoid lesions, which are characteristic of the secondary stage. Inspect the fingernails for signs of pitting.

If late syphilis is suspected, assess the patient for the characteristic complications. Observe for joint deformities or disfiguring lesions on the palate. Note areas of numbness or paralysis and hyperactive reflexes. Assess the pupils for size and reaction to light. Assess the patient for pulmonary congestion. Auscultate for heart sounds to determine irregularities, which may indicate valvular degeneration.

PSYCHOSOCIAL. Use sensitivity taking a sexual history. Be accepting of the sexual behaviors the patient describes. The patient with syphilis may be embarrassed by the infection and may be reluctant to seek out and continue treatment. Be nonjudgmental. Assure the patient that privacy and confidentiality will be maintained during examination, diagnosis, and treatment, although all sexual partners need to be notified so that they can be examined and treated as needed. Let the patient know that depending on the regulations of states, STIs are reportable to the public health department and partner notification will occur.

Diagnostic Highlights

General Comments: Diagnostic tests for syphilis include nontreponemal serology tests. *T pallidum* cannot be cultured; diagnostic tests are based on the detection of specific and nonspecific antibodies that are produced.

Test	Normal Result	Abnormality With Condition	Explanation
Venereal Disease Research Laboratory (VDRL)	Negative or nonreactive	Positive, returns to negative eventually after treatment	Detects *Treponema* antibodies; becomes positive 2 wk after inoculation
Rapid plasma reagin (RPR)	Negative or nonreactive	Positive, returns to negative eventually after treatment	A sensitive test that detects a nontreponemal antibody called reagin
Fluorescent treponemal antibody absorption test (FTA-ABS)	Negative	Positive, remains positive for life	Done if VDRL or RPR is positive; sensitive test that confirms the diagnosis of syphilis 4–6 wk after inoculation; used as confirmatory test
T pallidum particle agglutination (TP-PA)	Negative	Positive, remains positive for life	Done if VDRL or RPR is positive; sensitive test that confirms the diagnosis of syphilis 4–6 wk after inoculation; used as confirmatory test (Marshall, 2020 [see Evidence-Based Practice and Health Policy])

PRIMARY NURSING DIAGNOSIS

DIAGNOSIS. Risk for infection as evidenced by skin lesions on the sex organs, mouth, fingers, and/or tongue

OUTCOMES. Infection severity; Immune status; Risk control: Sexually transmitted diseases; Symptom severity; Symptom control; Knowledge: Infection management

INTERVENTIONS. Infection protection; Medication administration; Medication management; Teaching: Safe sex; Teaching: Prescribed medication

PLANNING AND IMPLEMENTATION
Collaborative

Medical treatment for syphilis infection at any stage consists of antibiotic therapy to destroy the infecting bacteria. After treatment, patients are instructed to refrain from sexual contact for at least 2 weeks or until lesions heal and to return for serology testing in 1 month and then every 3 months for 1 year.

Carefully question patients about penicillin sensitivity before treatment. They should also be warned about the Jarisch-Herxheimer reaction, which is believed to be caused by toxins that are released from dying spirochetes. The reaction develops 6 to 12 hours after the initial penicillin dose and causes fever, headache, nausea, tachycardia, and hypotension. Instruct the patient to rest, drink fluids, and take antipyretics.

Tell the patient that the disease must be reported to the local health authority and that confidentiality will be maintained. Identifying and treating sexual partners of the infected patient is an important intervention. If the patient is treated in the primary or secondary stage, attempt to contact all sexual partners from the past 3 months. If the patient is in the later stages of the disease, contacts from the previous year should be screened. Handle the "contact discovery" interview carefully, and if possible, have a public health professional conduct the interview.

Pharmacologic Highlights

Medication or Drug Class	Dosage	Description	Rationale
Benzathine penicillin G; for people with penicillin allergies, doxycycline is the best alternative	2.4 million units IM, single dose (some recommend a second dose 1 wk later)	Antibiotic, penicillin	Effective for primary, secondary, and latent syphilis of less than 1-yr duration
Benzathine penicillin G; for people with penicillin allergies, doxycycline is the best alternative	2.4 million units, IM, weekly, for three doses	Antibiotic, penicillin	Effective treatment for latent syphilis of more than 1-yr duration or cardiovascular or late benign syphilis
Aqueous crystalline penicillin G	2–4 million units IV every 4 hr for 10–14 days	Antibiotic, penicillin	Recommended to treat neurosyphilis

Other Drugs: Other antibiotics include doxycycline, azithromycin, and ceftriaxone.

Independent

Provide care for the patient's lesions. Keep them clean and dry. Properly dispose of contaminated materials from draining lesions. Use universal precautions when you come in direct contact with the patient, when collecting specimens, and when caring for the lesions.

Focus on prevention. Educate patients about the course of the disease and the need to return for follow-up treatment or blood tests. Patients need to understand that although their lesions may heal, the infection may not be gone. Approximately 10% of patients do not respond to the first round of antibiotics, so additional treatment may be necessary.

Teach patients how to reduce risk factors to prevent future infections by limiting the number of sexual partners and practicing safer sex. Using condoms with spermicide and inspecting partners for any rashes or lesions may reduce exposure to the disease. Patients need ongoing emotional support to make lifestyle changes. Explain the need for regular laboratory testing (VDRL) every 3 months for 2 years to detect a relapse. Urge patients in the latent or late stages to have blood tests every 6 months for 2 years. Explain the relationship between HIV and syphilis and perform HIV testing if the patient wishes.

Evidence-Based Practice and Health Policy

Marshall, A. (2020). Update on syphilis for women's health. *AWHONN Journal, 24*, 128–133.

- The author discussed the rising rate of syphilis and the lack of adequate screening and treatment. Untreated syphilis can have major health consequences for pregnant women and newborns. The author recommended that nurses take a thorough sexual history at the first prenatal visit or any women's health visit while establishing rapport and limiting judgmental comments.
- She noted to never assume a woman is heterosexual whether she is pregnant or not, and to avoid biased language, avoid assuming she has had only male partners, or assuming that she

is in a monogamous relationship. She recommended to look for risk factors for syphilis such as age under 30 years, excessive alcohol use, depression, low self-esteem, and sexual fluidity.

DOCUMENTATION GUIDELINES
- Description of lesions; rashes; and any neurological, visual, or cardiac abnormalities
- Reactions to medications, including the site and dosage of intramuscular (IM) injections
- Information for follow-up, including report of disease incidence to the local health authority and names of patient contacts (to maintain confidentiality, this information may not be kept in the patient's treatment record)

DISCHARGE AND HOME HEALTHCARE GUIDELINES
PREVENTION. Instruct the patient to avoid sexual contact for at least 2 weeks or as prescribed by the practitioner. Tell the patient to contact the practitioner if any new lesions or rashes are noted. Teach the patient how to prevent infection from STIs through safer sex practices. Empower the patient to take steps for self-protection by insisting on condom use during sexual activity. Inform the patient that most state public health regulations require STIs to be reported to the public health department. To prevent the spread of the STI and to provide treatment, partner notification will occur.

MEDICATIONS. Teach the patient the purpose, dosage, schedule, precautions, potential side effects, interactions, and adverse reactions of all prescribed medications. Recommend that patients treated as outpatients wait in the clinic or office for at least 30 minutes after administration of penicillin IM or IV to make sure there is no allergic reaction. Instruct patients given oral tetracycline to take the medication 1 hour before or 2 hours after meals and to avoid dairy products, antacids, iron, and sunlight while taking the drug.

PATIENT TEACHING. Teach the patient the importance of follow-up care and make sure the patient knows the dates and times for follow-up appointments. Teach the patient the cause, symptoms, and mode of transmission for syphilis. Emphasize the importance of testing and treating all of the patient's sexual partners; urge the patient to provide the names of sexual partners.

Tendinitis

DRG Category:	509
Mean LOS:	4.7 days
Description:	SURGICAL: Arthroscopy
DRG Category:	558
Mean LOS:	3.8 days
Description:	MEDICAL: Tendinitis, Myositis, and Bursitis Without Major Complication or Comorbidity

Tendinitis is a painful inflammation or tearing of tendons, tendon-muscle attachments, or tendon sheaths. Commonly affected joints include the shoulder (rotator cuff), elbow, knee, heel (Achilles tendinitis), and hamstring. The disorder is characterized by restricted joint movement and pain in the joint area. Fluid accumulation causes swelling early in the course of the disorder, but calcium deposits can increase swelling and cause further joint immobility or acute calcific bursitis.

Tendons transmit forces of the muscles to the skeleton and thus are exposed to repeated mechanical loads during activity. Microscopic findings include inflammation, mucoid degeneration, fibrosis, microtearing, and necrosis. It can be difficult to differentiate tendinitis from bursitis in the initial stages of both conditions, particularly in the shoulder. Bursitis is an inflammation of one or more bursae, the padlike sacs that contain synovial fluid; these sacs reduce the friction between tendons, ligaments, and bones. Bursitis therefore can be distinguished from tendinitis by fluid in the bursa. Untreated tendinitis can result in bursitis, which can cause joint immobilization. Other complications include ruptured tendon, tenosynovitis, contractures, scarring/adhesions, muscle wasting, and disability.

CAUSES

The most common cause of tendinitis is overuse. Tendinitis may result from a traumatic injury, strenuous exercise, or repetitive movement at a rapid pace. It can also be caused by postural misalignment, defective body development, or complications from another disease process such as any of the rheumatic diseases.

Work-related causes include intense, repeated, and sustained exertion; cold temperatures; extreme postures; and vibration. It is associated with risks such as repetitive work, a high workload, and pressure to complete work. Other risks include playing the following sports: baseball, basketball, bowling, golf, running, swimming, and tennis.

GENETIC CONSIDERATIONS

Heritable inflammatory responses could be protective or increase susceptibility.

SEX AND LIFE SPAN CONSIDERATIONS

Tendinitis can occur in any age group in anyone who performs an activity that stresses or overloads a joint on a repetitive basis. Middle-aged adults are more susceptible to tendinitis than other groups because, as they begin to age, they attempt to perform activities that they were accustomed to at a younger age. Women are more prone to tendinitis in their middle and older years. Older men also develop the disorder as their joints and soft tissues undergo the changes that occur with aging.

HEALTH DISPARITIES AND SEXUAL/GENDER MINORITY HEALTH

Ethnicity, race, and sexual/gender minority status have no known effect on the risk for tendinitis.

GLOBAL HEALTH CONSIDERATIONS

While no prevalence data exist, tendinitis occurs around the globe.

ASSESSMENT

HISTORY. Ask the patient to describe normal and unusual exercise and activity patterns. Determine if the patient has had localized joint swelling, pain, and restricted movement and which joints have been affected. Ask if the pain has affected sleeping patterns. Establish a history of repetitive joint stress or trauma. Ask the patient to describe any medications taken for pain relief. Determine if the patient has either a congenital musculoskeletal condition that might have caused the tendinitis or a history of rheumatic disease. Determine if the patient has allergies to specific corticosteroids or local anesthetics, which are sometimes prescribed for tendinitis.

PHYSICAL EXAMINATION. The affected joint may be **red, warm, painful, swollen, and tender to touch**. Note to what degree mobility is restricted, the type of pain that occurs when the joint is moved, and the number and location of joints that are involved.

PSYCHOSOCIAL. Patients may be concerned about permanent long-term immobility or restricted movement and how it will affect their occupation, leisure activities, family responsibilities, and lives. Assess their coping abilities.

Diagnostic Highlights

Test	Normal Result	Abnormality With Condition	Explanation
X-rays, ultra-sound, magnetic resonance imaging (MRI)	Normal bone and soft tissue structure and alignment	Detect bony abnormalities and arthritic changes	Exclude bony abnormalities and arthritis; tendons are generally not visible on x-rays; ultrasonography may offer the best view of tendons, and MRI assesses pathology of the tendon
Arthrogram	Intact soft tissue structures of the joint; absence of lesions or tears	Detects damage to tendons	Fluoroscopic and radiographic examination of a joint after injection of air and/or radiographic dye

Other Tests: Arthrocentesis, magnetic resonance imaging to assess cartilage injuries, bony abnormalities, injury to ligaments

PRIMARY NURSING DIAGNOSIS

DIAGNOSIS. Acute pain related to inflammation and swelling of the tendon as evidenced by gait changes, decreased range of motion of limbs, self-reports of pain, facial grimacing, and/or protective behavior

OUTCOMES. Comfort status; Pain control; Pain level; Symptom severity; Symptom control; Knowledge: Pain management

INTERVENTIONS. Pain management: Acute; Analgesic administration; Teaching: Prescribed medication; Heat/cold application; Teaching: Disease process

PLANNING AND IMPLEMENTATION
Collaborative

The goal of treatment is to reduce pain and regain function. In addition to rest, first-line therapy is often pharmacologic. Applications of heat, cold, and ice (for the first 24–48 hours) may be indicated to promote relief of pain and inflammation. The physician may also prescribe immobilization using a sling, splint, or cast. Strengthening and stretching exercises may be recommended once the pain has subsided. Fluid removal by aspiration and physical therapy to prevent "frozen" joints and preserve motion constitute supplementary treatment. In rare situations, arthroscopic or open surgery may be necessary to loosen calcification.

Pharmacologic Highlights

Medication or Drug Class	Dosage	Description	Rationale
NSAIDs	Varies with drug	Ibuprofen, naproxen	Relieve pain and reduce inflammation
Analgesics	Varies with drug	Aspirin, 650 mg PO every 4 hr as needed; acetaminophen with 15 or 30 mg of codeine PO every 4–6 hr	Relieve pain and reduce inflammation

Other Drugs: Corticosteroids, local injection with corticosteroids or lidocaine for immediate pain relief

Independent

Focus on symptom relief. Encourage the patient to elevate the affected joint as often as possible to promote venous drainage and decrease the swelling. After the patient has received an intra-articular injection, apply ice for about 4 hours to help control the pain. Teach the patient how to apply ice and heat properly to prevent burning or chilling.

Explain to patients the need to rest and reduce stress on the affected joints by modifying their lifestyle or activities until the condition has improved. If a sling is prescribed, teach patients how to wear it properly. Instruct patients to wear a splint during sleep to protect an affected shoulder. When the patients' joint pain has diminished, assist with range-of-motion and strengthening exercises. To limit the risk of re-injury, encourage patients to use proper shoes for exercise and to lose weight if needed.

Explain the importance of anti-inflammatory medications and teach the patient to take them with milk to minimize gastrointestinal (GI) distress. Also caution the patient to report distress, GI upset, nausea, and vomiting. Explain the seriousness of vomiting coffee ground–like material and the need to seek medical help immediately. Encourage the patient to take medications with food to minimize gastric distress.

Evidence-Based Practice and Health Policy

Louwerens, J., Sierevelt, I., Kramer, E., Boonstra, R., van den Bekerom, M., van Royen, B., Eygendaal, D., & van Noort, A. (2020). Comparing ultrasound-guided needling combined with a subacromial corticosteroid injection versus high-energy extracorporeal shockwave therapy for calcific tendinitis of the rotator cuff: A randomized controlled trial. *Arthroscopy, 36,* 1823–1833.

- The authors compared clinical and radiographic outcomes after treatment with standardized high-energy extracorporeal shock wave therapy (ESWT) and ultrasound-guided needling (UGN) in patients with symptomatic calcific tendinitis of the rotator cuff who were nonre-sponsive to conservative treatment. They employed a randomized controlled trial with the ESWT group receiving four sessions with 1-week intervals and the UGN group receiving needling with corticosteroid ultrasound-guided subacromial bursa injection. Shoulder function was assessed at 6 weeks and 3, 6, and 12 months.
- Eighty-two patients were treated (56 female, 65%; mean age 52.1). At 1-year follow-up, the UGN group showed similar results as the ESWT group with regard to the change from baseline. The mean calcification size showed a greater decrease in the UGN group and twice as many in the ESWT group received additional treatment because of persistent symptoms. The authors concluded that UGN is more effective in eliminating the calcific deposit, and the amount of additional treatments was greater in the ESWT group.

DOCUMENTATION GUIDELINES

- Physical findings: Joint mobility, tenderness, color, warmth
- Response to analgesic and anti-inflammatory medications, change in symptoms, and presence of side effects
- Tolerance of immobility and exercise regimen

DISCHARGE AND HOME HEALTHCARE GUIDELINES

Help the patient find alternatives to repetitive or stressful joint movement. Be sure the patient understands any medications prescribed, including dosage, route, action, and side effects. Caution the patient not to take aspirin with other NSAIDs. Encourage the patient to use heat or cold therapy as prescribed. Teach the patient to use a barrier between the skin and heat or to use cold therapy to prevent burning or frostbite. Remind the patient to keep follow-up appointments with the physician.

Testicular Cancer

DRG Category:	712
Mean LOS:	3.1 days
Description:	SURGICAL: Testes Procedures Without Complication or Comorbidity or Major Complication or Comorbidity
DRG Category:	715
Mean LOS:	6.6 days
Description:	MEDICAL: Other Male Reproductive System Operating Room Procedures for Malignancy With Complication or Comorbidity or Major Complication or Comorbidity

Testicular cancer is a rare tumor that arises from the germinal cells (cells that produce sperm) of the embryonal tissues and causes less than 1% of all cancer deaths in men. The American Cancer Society estimates that in 2021, there will be 9,470 new cases of testicular cancer diagnosed and that 440 people will die from this disease. The cure rate exceeds 90%, and the 5-year survival rate is 73% to 99% depending on the stage at diagnosis. The risk of developing this cancer is 1 in 250.

Testicular tumors are classified as seminomas or nonseminomas. Seminomas are composed of uniform, undifferentiated cells that resemble primitive gonadal cells. This type of tumor represents 40% of all testicular cancer and is usually confined to the testes and retroperitoneal nodes. There are two types of seminomas: classical seminomas (occur between the late 30s and early 50s) and spermatocytic seminomas (occur around age 55 years, grow slowly, and do not metastasize). Nonseminomas show varying degrees of cell differentiation and include embryonal carcinoma (occurs most often between ages 20 and 30 years, grows rapidly, and metastasizes), teratoma (can occur in children and adults), choriocarcinoma (rare and highly malignant), and yolk cell carcinoma derivatives (most common in children up to age 3 years and have a very good prognosis). Sometimes, testicular tumors are "mixed," containing elements distinctive to both groups. Complications of testicular cancer include infertility, organ toxicity (lung, kidney, heart), hearing loss from chemotherapy, leukemia, and malignancy.

CAUSES

Although specific causative factors for testicular cancer are unknown, research findings suggest a connection between the incidence of cryptorchidism (failure of testicles to descend) and testicular cancer. If an undescended testis is noted in a child, orchiopexy (surgical descent of the testes into its normal position within the scrotum) is recommended as soon as possible after birth. Although orchiopexy does not completely eliminate the risk of testicular cancer, it is believed that the sooner after birth orchiopexy is performed, the less chance there is of developing testicular cancer later in life. An increased incidence of testicular cancer has been found in men infected with HIV (seminomas) and men with testicular disorders such as Klinefelter syndrome.

Exogenous estrogen has also been linked to testicular cancer. Offspring of mothers who took diethylstilbestrol during their pregnancy have an increased risk of developing testicular cancer. In addition, patients who have had mumps, orchitis, or a childhood inguinal hernia are also considered to be at higher risk for developing testicular cancer. Infertility is considered a risk factor. Nonseminomatous testicular germ cell tumors have been linked to exposure to marijuana smoking and cigarette smoking. Other risk factors include maternal infection with Epstein-Barr virus and cytomegalovirus, placing offspring at risk for testicular cancer.

GENETIC CONSIDERATIONS

Approximately 1% to 3% of patients with testicular cancer report a family history of the disease. Overall heritability is estimated at 30%. In patients with a family history, brothers of an affected patient are 8 to 10 times more likely to develop the disease, and when a father is affected, his son is four times as likely to develop testicular cancer as sons of unaffected fathers. Recent genetic studies have identified 15 loci that confer susceptibility to testicular cancer. These include genes in the KIT-KITL signaling pathway, microtubule assembly (*TEX14*, *CENPE*, *WDR73*, and *PMF1*) and telomerase regulation (*TERT*, *ATF7IP*, and *PITX1*). Recent genome-wide association studies have also implicated genes involved in germ cell specification-sex determination, including *PRDM14*, *DMRT1*, and *SALL4*.

SEX AND LIFE SPAN CONSIDERATIONS

Testicular cancer most commonly occurs in men ages 15 to 40 years, but it can affect males from infancy to old age. Approximately 6% of cases occur in children and teens. Approximately 50% of the cases occur in men 20 to 34 years of age, and the most common age for a diagnosis of testicular cancer is 33 years. A second group of cases occur at approximately 50 to 60 years of age.

HEALTH DISPARITIES AND SEXUAL/GENDER MINORITY HEALTH

Testicular cancer incidence in White men is fivefold higher than in Black men. Hispanic and Native American men have a lower incidence than White men and a higher incidence than Black men. In the past 10 years, Asian and Pacific Islander men have experienced the greatest increase in testicular cancer compared to other groups. Significant health disparities exist for Black men, however, because they tend to present with higher-grade disease, receive treatment later, and have a poorer prognosis than White men. Men living in rural areas have a 3% increase in testicular cancer as compared to urban-dwelling men. Transgender is a term used to describe persons whose gender identity is different from their sex assigned at birth. Approximately 1% of the U.S. population identify themselves as transgender. Sexual and gender minority persons have higher odds for multiple chronic conditions, cancer, and poor quality of life, and are more apt to have disabilities than cisgender males and females. (Cisgender is a term used to describe persons whose gender identity and gender expression are aligned with their assigned sex listed on their birth certificate.) Gender-affirming hormone therapy is the use of hormone therapy for gender transition or gender affirmation and can be masculinizing or feminizing. The incidence of testicular cancer in transgender women is relatively understudied. In one cohort study of 3,026 transgender women using feminizing hormone treatment, the authors found a testicular cancer risk similar to the risk in cisgender men (de Nie et al., 2022). The risks may be complicated by a reluctance of transgender women to examine their testes for lumps because of anatomical dysphoria (a person's anatomy does not match their inner sense of self and gender identity).

GLOBAL HEALTH CONSIDERATIONS

The global incidence of testicular cancer is 1.6 per 100,000 males per year. The incidence is three times higher in developed than in developing countries. The highest incidence of testicular cancer occurs in northern and eastern Europe, and experts are monitoring the reasons for increasing rates in these locations.

ASSESSMENT

HISTORY. Obtain a thorough health history, particularly about the occurrence of risk factors. Any patients born between 1940 and 1971 should be asked if their mother took any drugs to maintain her pregnancy. The earliest sign of testicular cancer is a small, hard, painless lump that cannot be separated from the testicle; it is occasionally accompanied by low back pain. Patients often describe a feeling of "heaviness" or "dragging" in the testicles. These symptoms are often mistaken for epididymitis or muscle strain. Tenderness in the breast may also be present. Inquire about back pain, vague abdominal pain, nausea and vomiting, anorexia, and weight loss, which are all findings that suggest metastasis. Only 25% of patients experience symptoms related to metastasis prior to diagnosis.

PHYSICAL EXAMINATION. The testes may be enlarged and swollen. A hydrocele or hematocele may be present. A testicular tumor can be distinguished from a hydrocele by transillumination (inspection of the testes by passing a light through its walls): A tumor does not transilluminate, whereas a hydrocele appears red and a normal testicle illuminates clearly. Because the tumor produces estrogen, inspect the patient for gynecomastia.

A testicular examination is accomplished by placing the index and middle finger on one side of the testicle with the thumb on the other side. Digital separation of the anterior testes from the posterior elements, including the epididymis and cord, is performed with care so that the intrascrotal contents can be palpated. A gentle rolling motion enables the examiner to palpate each testicle completely. A normal testicle is egg-shaped and feels smooth and firm but not hard. One testicle may naturally be larger than the other. A change in size or the presence of a lump is considered to be an abnormal finding. With testicular cancer, the lump is generally painless. Also, palpate the surrounding area for the presence of enlarged lymph nodes. Lymphadenopathy, especially in the abdominal and supraclavicular regions, is also found in more advanced disease.

PSYCHOSOCIAL. The diagnosis of cancer at any time is a lifestyle-altering event, but it is particularly disrupting to the young population. Interruption of school or work schedules, financial coverage for medical expenses, transportation to and from scheduled therapies, and childcare issues are a few of the concerns expressed by patients. Testicular cancer raises serious concerns for patients and their partners, not only about long-term well-being but also about sexual function, impotence, intimacy, and fertility.

Diagnostic Highlights

General Comments: Most testicular tumors are found in routine checkups or by self-examination; they often cause no symptoms.

Test	Normal Result	Abnormality With Condition	Explanation
Scrotal ultrasound, computed tomography (CT)	Normal size, shape, and configuration of the testicles	Solid, malignant mass is identified	Noninvasive visualization of the testicles
Radical orchiectomy, followed by a biopsy	NA	Solid mass is removed, 100% prove to be malignant	Needle biopsy would lead to open spread of the cancer cells, thus the biopsy is done after the testicle is removed

Other Tests: Serum laboratory analysis of beta-subunit human chorionic gonadotropin and α-fetoprotein, lactic hydrogenase, complete blood count, chest x-ray or CT for lung metastasis, abdominal and pelvic CT or magnetic resonance imaging to check for retroperitoneal lymph node metastasis, IV pyelography to check for urinary tract involvement

PRIMARY NURSING DIAGNOSIS

DIAGNOSIS. Acute pain related to inflammation, tissue damage, tissue compression, or nerve irritation from tumor metastasis in the perineum, groin, or abdomen as evidenced by self-reports of pain, facial grimacing, and/or protective behavior

OUTCOMES. Comfort status; Pain control; Pain level; Symptom severity; Symptom control; Knowledge: Pain management; Knowledge: Disease process

INTERVENTIONS. Analgesic administration; Pain management: Acute; Teaching: Prescribed medication; Teaching: Disease Process

PLANNING AND IMPLEMENTATION
Collaborative
SURGICAL. The initial treatment for testicular cancer is surgical resection of the involved testicle (orchiectomy). A testicular prosthesis can be placed if the patient so desires. If a bilateral orchiectomy is performed, the patient may need hormonal replacement. It is controversial whether or not the retroperitoneal nodes should be resected or treated with chemotherapy. Surgical resection carries with it the likelihood of impotence. To preserve fertility, nerve-sparing retroperitoneal lymph node surgery protects the nerves and allows for normal ejaculation.

Postoperatively, edema and intrascrotal hemorrhage are the two most common problems. Monitor the patient closely for swelling and bleeding. Elevate the scrotum on a rolled towel and apply ice to assist with discomfort and decrease swelling. Observe for signs of infection. Encourage the patient to wear an athletic supporter during ambulation to minimize discomfort. Usually, the patient is encouraged to do so within 12 hours of surgery.

RADIATION AND CHEMOTHERAPY. Depending on staging of the disease, radiation or chemotherapy may also be used. Tumors classified as seminomas are especially radiosensitive. External beam radiation is usually given after surgery if the peritoneal lymph system is disease-positive or if the pelvis and mediastinal and supraclavicular lymph nodes are involved. Inform the patient that although the unaffected testicle is shielded during radiation, it does receive some radiation that is scattered, which may decrease spermatogenesis. Nonseminomatous tumors are not radiosensitive, and chemotherapy is the preferred treatment. Most patients can produce viable sperm after chemotherapy, but experts recommend waiting for 3 months after completion of chemotherapy before attempting to conceive a child.

Pharmacologic Highlights

Medication or Drug Class	Dosage	Description	Rationale
Antineoplastic agents	Varies by drug	Carboplatin, bleomycin, etoposide, cisplatin	Inhibition of cell growth and tumor proliferation; drugs are often used in combination
Acetaminophen/ NSAIDs; opioids; combination opioids/ NSAIDs	Depends on the drug	Analgesic	Analgesics used are determined by the severity of pain; pain may be postoperative or caused by metastasis

Independent
Nurses can play a role in the early detection of testicular cancer. Patients should be taught how to do a testicular self-examination and should be encouraged to perform the examination monthly. Provide private time for the patient and the patient's partner to ask questions, express concerns, and clarify information. Offer the patient an opportunity for sexuality and fertility counseling after discussing the impact of the surgery on anatomy and function. Make sure the patient understands the need to perform coughing and deep-breathing exercises to limit pulmonary complications. Before surgery, instruct the patient on the use of an incentive spirometer.

Because stomatitis is a common occurrence, check the mouth regularly for open irritated areas and encourage the patient to use warm mouthwashes. If the patient becomes nauseated, offer small, frequent feedings and eliminate any noxious stimuli such as bad odors. In addition, have the patient drink at least 3 L of fluid per day to ensure adequate hydration. If the patient is receiving radiation, monitor for side effects. Avoid rubbing the skin near the site of radiation to prevent discomfort and skin breakdown.

Ask about pain regularly and assess pain systematically. Believe the patient and family in their reports of pain. Inform the patient and family of options for pain relief as proposed by the National Cancer Institute (pharmacologic, physical, psychosocial, and cognitive behavioral interventions), and involve the patient and family in determining pain relief measures. To manage the discomfort of chemotherapy in addition to medications, consider the use of biofeedback or other alternative relaxation techniques.

The diagnosis of testicular cancer is a devastating one to most patients. Discuss the patient's concerns, and assess the partner's responses as well. Explain the role of hormonal replacement in maintaining secondary sex characteristics. If the patient is at risk for sterility, explain sperm banking procedures before treatment if infertility and impotence may result from surgery. Refer the patient to a support group or ask that another patient who has experienced a similar diagnosis and treatment share experiences to provide support. If the patient or partner is struggling to cope with the diagnosis, arrange for a counselor.

Evidence-Based Practice and Health Policy

Li, Y., Lu, Q., Wang, Y., & Ma, S. (2020). Racial differences in testicular cancer in the United States: Descriptive epidemiology. *BMC Cancer*. https://doi.org/10.1186/s12885-020-06789-2

- The authors aimed to discern whether there may be important racial differences in recent trends in testicular cancer, which is the most common malignancy in young adult men. The authors analyzed data from a large, national data set for patients from the following groups: non-Hispanic White, Hispanic White, Black, and Asian/Pacific Islander persons. Patient characteristics, age-adjusted incidence rates, and survival were compared across racial groups, and the authors evaluated factors including marital status, age group, histologic type, treatment, stage, and tumor location.
- Non-Hispanic White persons had the highest incidence rates of testicular cancer, followed by Black, Hispanic, and Asian/Pacific Islander persons. Highest survival rates were in non-Hispanic White persons and lowest survival rates were in Black persons. Black persons experience health disparities in testicular cancer, and further work needs to be done to determine the causes.

DOCUMENTATION GUIDELINES

- Physical findings: Operative incisions, patency of IV lines, healing of incisions, vital signs, testicular assessment findings
- Response to treatments: Side effects from medications or radiation therapy; management and control of symptoms, concern about health and long-term well-being, concern about fertility and sexual function
- Presence of complications: Infection, bleeding, respiratory distress, unrelieved pain or nausea

DISCHARGE AND HOME HEALTHCARE GUIDELINES

MEDICATIONS. If hormonal replacement is ordered, be sure the patient understands the dosage, schedule, actions, and side effects of the medication.

PREVENTION. Have the patient demonstrate a testicular self-examination before leaving the hospital. The patient should understand that testicular cancer can recur in the remaining testes and that early detection is a critical factor in the outcome.

SEXUALITY. Inform the patient that if a unilateral orchiectomy was performed, the patient is still fertile and should not experience impotence. Make sure the patient has an understanding of the option of undergoing reconstructive surgery and placement of a testicular prosthesis. Refer the patient to the American Cancer Society to assist with obtaining information and support. Consider referring the patient to a support group to manage issues of sexuality, intimacy, and infertility.

HOME CARE. Teach the patient to do the following:

• Avoid prolonged standing because this can increase scrotal edema.
• Wear an athletic supporter or snug-fitting undershorts until the area is completely healed.
• Avoid heavy lifting for 4 to 6 weeks.
• Take a 20-minute tub bath three times a day for 1 week after discharge.

Tetanus

DRG Category:	868
Mean LOS:	4.6 days
Description:	MEDICAL: Other Infectious and Parasitic Diseases Diagnoses With Complication or Comorbidity

Tetanus, or lockjaw, is a preventable but often fatal disorder caused by the bacterium *Clostridium tetani*, a spore-forming anaerobe. The bacterium exists in spore form in an aerobic environment until it is exposed to an anaerobic environment. The organism then changes to the vegetative form, multiplies, and produces neurotoxins. Less than 50 cases of tetanus occur each year in the United States, and in recent years, approximately half occurred in people with injected drug use.

When the tetanus bacteria enter an open wound, they multiply and produce a potent neurotoxin called tetanospasmin, which enters the bloodstream and acts on the spinal ganglia and central nervous system by interfering with the function of the postsynaptic inhibitory potentials. The anterior horn cells become overstimulated, resulting in excessive muscle contraction. Toxins may also act directly on skeletal muscle and cause muscle contraction. Complications include lung disorders such as pneumonia, pulmonary emboli, atelectasis, cardiac dysrhythmias, gastric ulcers, and flexion contractures. Tetanus results in approximately five deaths per year in the United States; death usually results from complications such as autonomic dysfunction leading to extremes in blood pressure, cardiac dysrhythmia, or cardiac arrest.

CAUSES

Because *C tetani* is commonly found in soil, tetanus is more common in agricultural regions. Any break in the skin or mucous membrane can result in a tetanus infection, but wounds that are contaminated with soil or those that produce a relatively anaerobic environment are at greater risk. Wounds that produce an anaerobic environment include those with purulent or necrotic tissue, puncture wounds, burns, gunshot wounds, animal bites, and complex fractures. Drug abusers who engage in "skin popping," or subcutaneous injections, are also at risk for a tetanus infection. Bacterially contaminated quinine may be used to dilute heroin and expose the user to *C tetani*. Risk factors include failure to receive vaccination, history of puncture wounds or trauma, IV drug abuse, foot ulcers, and history of surgical procedures.

GENETIC CONSIDERATIONS

Heritable immune responses could be protective or could increase susceptibility.

SEX AND LIFE SPAN CONSIDERATIONS

People of all ages and genders are at risk for tetanus if they have not been vaccinated. In the United States, approximately 60% of cases and 75% of deaths occur in people age 60 years or older. Older adults are at risk even when they are immunized because of the waning effects of past immunizations. Only 28% of people over 70 years of age are immune to tetanus; the rest lack a booster dose or have never been vaccinated.

HEALTH DISPARITIES AND SEXUAL/GENDER MINORITY HEALTH

The incidence of tetanus in the United States is highest among Hispanics and White persons as compared to Black persons. Sexual and gender minority status has no known effect on the risk for tetanus.

GLOBAL HEALTH CONSIDERATIONS

Tetanus is generally an infection of developing regions located in warm, damp climates, and in Africa in particular. Infants, children, and young adults are particularly at risk in developing regions. In developing countries, tetanus is a common cause of neonatal death when infants are delivered in unsterile conditions. The World Health Organization has targeted vaccination programs focused on developing regions of the world to reduce the incidence of tetanus. Developed regions have incidences of tetanus similar to those in the United States.

ASSESSMENT

HISTORY. Classically, patients have a dirty (often soil-contaminated) puncture wound or laceration and describe pain or paresthesia at the puncture site. Frequently, the wound may be unnoticed. Patients may report a history of IV drug abuse, dental infection, umbilical stump infection (infants), or penetrating eye infection and inadequate tetanus immunization. The average incubation period is 7 days, but incubation ranges from 4 to 14 days. If the wound has been left untreated, early symptoms include difficulty chewing or swallowing and a sore throat. The patient may have a mild fever or painful muscle contractions or spasms in the affected region. Infants may be unable to suck.

PHYSICAL EXAMINATION. The most common symptoms are **pain or paresthesia at the puncture site of the wound, sore throat,** and **dysphagia.** Because most cases of tetanus result in a systemic reaction, inspect the patient for neuromuscular changes. Spasms begin in the facial and jaw muscles and progress to muscles of the neck, extremities, and respiratory/pharyngeal regions. Muscles ultimately become rigid, with painful spasms in response to any external stimuli. You may note seizures, posturing, and muscle rigidity; during seizure activity, the patient is awake and in severe pain. Autonomic disturbances include diaphoresis, increased heart rate, cardiac dysrhythmias, and blood pressure fluctuations. Spasms of respiratory and pharyngeal muscles may make it difficult to maintain a patent airway. Patients may exhibit increased respiratory rate, increased inspiratory effort, poor lung expansion, and decreased airflow. Late findings include risus sardonicus (a grotesque, grinning expression), trismus (lockjaw), and opisthotonos (rigid somatic muscles that lead to an arched-back posture). With supportive care, signs and symptoms reverse after the toxin has been metabolized in about 6 weeks.

The "spatula test" may be performed. The test involves touching the oropharynx with a tongue blade, which elicits a gag reflex in uninfected people. Patients with tetanus have a reflex spasm of the masseters and bite the spatula in a positive test result.

PSYCHOSOCIAL. The family may feel guilty if the patient has not been vaccinated. Assess the patient's and family's levels of anxiety and their ability to cope. The length of hospitalization and the seriousness of the diagnosis place the patient and family at risk for alterations in growth and development. Assess levels of growth and development using age-appropriate milestones and developmental tasks as guidelines.

Diagnostic Highlights

General Comments: There are no definitive tests for tetanus.

Test	Normal Result	Abnormality With Condition	Explanation
Lumbar (not necessary for diagnosis but may be used to differentiate tetanus from other conditions if symptoms are not clear)	Normal opening pressures and clear and sterile cerebrospinal fluid (CSF)	Normal opening pressures and clear and sterile CSF	Procedure is used to differentiate between meningitis (positive CSF cultures) and tetanus (negative CSF cultures)

PRIMARY NURSING DIAGNOSIS

DIAGNOSIS. Ineffective airway clearance related to muscle spasms and trismus as evidenced by dyspnea, stridor, air hunger, decreased chest excursion, and/or tachypnea

OUTCOMES. Respiratory status: Airway patency; Respiratory status: Gas exchange; Respiratory status: Ventilation; Symptom severity; Symptom control; Knowledge: Treatment regime

INTERVENTIONS. Airway insertion and stabilization; Airway management; Airway suctioning; Oxygen therapy; Respiratory monitoring; Teaching: Disease process

PLANNING AND IMPLEMENTATION
Collaborative

To prevent tetanus, within 3 days of a puncture wound, patients with no previous tetanus immunization require immediate passive immunization with tetanus immunoglobulin for temporary protection. Active immunization with tetanus toxoid is also provided. If the patient had a previous immunization more than 5 years before the injury, a booster injection of tetanus toxoid is warranted at the time of injury. Goals of treatment include neutralizing the toxin, preventing complications, and eliminating the source of the toxin. One-half of the dose is administered by infiltrating the wound, and the remaining half is administered intramuscularly. Active immunity is given by administering tetanus toxoid at a site remote from the globulin injections. The affected wound is thoroughly débrided after the antitoxin has been administered. Cultures of the wound may be obtained at that time. Parenteral antibiotics (metronidazole in particular) are administered for 10 days.

Patients are generally admitted to an intensive care unit to manage airway, breathing, circulation, and the neurological manifestations of the illness. Respiratory distress may necessitate intubation or tracheostomy and mechanical ventilation with supplemental oxygen. Nasogastric tubes are inserted to prevent gastric distension. Patients with difficulty swallowing may require nutritional support with total parenteral nutrition or enteral feeding by a nasogastric or nasointestinal tube.

Pharmacologic Highlights

Medication or Drug Class	Dosage	Description	Rationale
Human tetanus immunoglobulin	One-half dose is administered by infiltrating the wound; remaining half is administered intramuscularly; total dose is 3,000–6,000 units	Immunoglobulin	Provides passive immunization; administered immediately

(highlight box continues on page 1148)

Pharmacologic Highlights (continued)

Medication or Drug Class	Dosage	Description	Rationale
Tetanus toxoid	Series of three 0.5-mL doses provide protection in 90% of patients; administered at a site remote from globulin injections	Toxoid	Provides active immunization against tetanus; affected wound is débrided after antitoxin has been administered; patient will need two follow-up vaccinations at 1–2 mo and then 6–12 mo
Antimicrobials	Metronidazole (Flagyl): Current drug of choice; 0.5 g PO every 6 hr for 7–10 days; alternatively, 1 g IV every 12 hr for 7–10 days; other antibiotics: penicillin G, clindamycin, erythromycin, tetracycline, vancomycin, doxycycline,	Antibiotic	Prevent or combat infection

Other Drugs: Others drugs include neuromuscular blocking agents; antipyretics; analgesics; and anticoagulants; sedatives, antianxiety agents, and muscle relaxants such as diazepam are administered to decrease muscle spasms. Neuromuscular blocking agents may be required to paralyze the patient if other agents cannot control the spasms or seizures. Antidysrhythmic drugs are given if cardiac rhythm disturbances arise, antipyretics are administered for fever, and analgesics are provided for pain relief. Prophylactic anticoagulation therapy may be instituted to prevent thrombus formation.

Independent

Nursing care focuses on maintaining a patent airway, regular breathing, and adequate circulation and on providing comfort management, protection from injury, and psychosocial support of the patient and family. If muscle spasms or seizure activity places the patient at risk for airway compromise, use the chin lift or jaw thrust to maintain an open airway if possible. Insert an oral or nasal airway before seizures, but if the patient has lockjaw, do not attempt to force an airway in place because you may injure the patient and worsen the airway patency. Have intubation and suction equipment immediately available at the bedside should the patient require it. Anchor the endotracheal tube firmly, and document the lip level of the endotracheal tube in the progress notes for continuity.

Institute seizure precautions as soon as the patient is admitted to the unit. Pad the side rails of the bed and provide immediate access to oxygen, suction, intubation equipment, artificial airways, and a resuscitation bag. Place the patient in a quiet, dark room to reduce environmental stimuli. Position the patient who is unconscious or paralyzed from pharmacologic agents in a side-lying position and turn the patient every 2 hours.

Provide clarification of information about the patient's diagnosis, prognosis, and treatment to the patient and family. Make sure that the family has adequate time for expression of their feelings each day. Support effective coping mechanisms and provide appropriate referrals to the chaplain, clinical nurse specialist, or counselor if the patient or family demonstrates ineffective coping behaviors.

Evidence-Based Practice and Health Policy

Kriss, J., Albert, A., Carter, V., Jiles, A., Liang, J., Mullen, J., Rodriguez, L., Howards, P., Orenstein, W., Omer, S., & Fisher, A. (2019). Disparities in Tdap vaccination and vaccine information needs among pregnant women in the United States. *Maternal and Child Health Journal, 23*, 201–211.

- The authors aimed to evaluate disparities in Tdap vaccination among pregnant women in the United States and to assess if race and ethnicity were associated with factors that inform pregnant women's decisions about vaccination. They conducted a national, Web-based survey of pregnant women with the primary outcome of self-reported vaccination status during pregnancy. Secondary outcomes included factors that influenced the decision about vaccination.
- Of the women surveyed, 41% reported that they received Tdap during the current pregnancy, and of women in the third trimester, 52% had received it. Hispanic women had the highest rate of vaccination (53%) as compared to White (38%) and Black (36%) women. Higher income and residing in the western United States were associated with vaccination. Twenty-six percent of surveyed women who had not yet been vaccinated intended to receive it during pregnancy. The most common reason for not receiving the vaccine was concern about its safety.

DOCUMENTATION GUIDELINES

- Respiratory response: Rate and rhythm; lung expansion, respiratory effort, presence of retractions or nasal flaring (infants); presence of adventitious breath sounds; oxygen saturation; placement and patency of an artificial airway; character and amount of respiratory secretions; color of mucous membranes
- Presence, location, duration, and description of muscle spasms or seizures
- Physical responses: Condition of skin; bowel and urinary elimination patterns; description of stool and urine; pain and comfort level; condition of wound and dressings; weight; response to feedings; response to IV infusions, analgesics, muscle relaxants, and antipyretics
- Growth and development level, growth and development activities, response

DISCHARGE AND HOME HEALTHCARE GUIDELINES

Teach the patient and family that tetanus is a preventable disease. Inform them of the appropriate immunization and booster schedule and encourage them to follow it. If the patient was not vaccinated prior to admission, remind the patient and family that two more booster doses are needed at 1 to 2 months and 6 to 12 months. Note that the patient may experience pain, tenderness, redness, and muscle stiffness in the limb in which the tetanus injection(s) is (are) given. Explain that the convalescent period following tetanus may be prolonged. The patient may need multidisciplinary rehabilitation and home nursing.

Thoracic Aortic Aneurysm

DRG Category:	270
Mean LOS:	9.4 days
Description:	SURGICAL: Other Major Cardiovascular Procedures With Major Complication or Comorbidity
DRG Category:	299
Mean LOS:	5.1 days
Description:	MEDICAL: Peripheral Vascular Disorders With Major Complication or Comorbidity

A thoracic aortic aneurysm is an abnormal widening of the aorta between the aortic valve and the diaphragm. An aneurysm is defined as dilation of the aorta that is more than 150% of its normal diameter for a given segment. The diameter of the thoracic aorta is approximately

3.0 cm. If the diameter exceeds 3.5 cm, it is considered a dilated thoracic aorta, and if the diameter is greater than 4.5 cm (150% increase), the patient would meet the criteria for a thoracic aneurysm.

Thoracic aneurysms account for approximately 25% of all aneurysms, and approximately 25% of people with thoracic aneurysms also have abdominal aneurysms. Although aneurysms may be located on the ascending, transverse (aortic arch), or descending part of the aorta or may involve the entire thoracic aorta, they commonly develop between the origin of the left subclavian artery and the diaphragm.

Aneurysm formation is caused by a weakening of the medial layer of the aorta, which stretches outward, causing an outpouching of the aortic wall. Thoracic aortic aneurysms take four forms: fusiform, saccular, dissecting, and false aneurysms (Table 1). Dissection of the aorta can occur with or without an aneurysm but is most often associated with the presence of a preexisting aneurysm. Thoracic aortic aneurysms may lead to serious or fatal complications if they are left untreated. For example, a thoracic dissecting aneurysm may rupture into the pericardium, resulting in cardiac tamponade, hemorrhagic shock, and cardiac arrest.

• TABLE 1 Forms of Thoracic Aortic Aneurysm

TYPE	DESCRIPTION
Fusiform	Spindle-shaped bulge that encompasses the entire circumference of the aorta
Saccular	Unilateral pouchlike bulge with a narrow neck, most frequently at a bifurcation that involves only a portion of the vessel circumference
Dissecting	Hemorrhagic separation of the medial and intimal layers, creating a false lumen
False	Pulsating hematoma that results from a rupture of the aorta, secondary to trauma

CAUSES

The single most important cause is atherosclerosis. The atherosclerotic process damages the arterial wall by weakening the medial muscle layer and distending the lumen. Destruction of the medial layer allows the artery to increase in size circumferentially (a fusiform shape), or the artery develops a saccular outpouching at the weakened area. Tobacco use is also related to aneurysm formation, but the underlying explanation for this relationship is unknown. Other factors that contribute include Marfan syndrome (hereditary musculoskeletal disorder), Ehlers-Danlos syndrome (an inherited disorder of elastic connective tissue), coarctation of the aorta, fungal infections (mycotic aneurysms) of the aortic arch, a bicuspid aortic valve, aortitis, and trauma (external, blunt trauma or iatrogenic trauma that occurs during invasive diagnostic procedures).

GENETIC CONSIDERATIONS

Thoracic aortic aneurysm has a genetic component, as numerous susceptibility loci have been identified. These include mutations in genes involved in vascular smooth muscle contraction and extracellular matrix adhesion such as *TGFB1*, *ACTA2*, *MYH11*, *MYLK*, *PRKG1*, *MFAP5*, *LOX*, and *FOXE3*. Thoracic aortic aneurysms and dissections are mainly associated with medial necrosis in which there is degeneration of elastic fibers, a loss of smooth muscle cells, and an accumulation of basophilic ground substance. Medial necrosis and thoracic aortic aneurysm/dissection are known to occur in certain heritable connective tissue diseases such as Marfan syndrome (*FBN1*) and vascular (type IV) Ehlers-Danlos syndrome (*COL3A1*). Medial necrosis has also been seen to cluster in families in the absence of a clearly identifiable syndrome.

SEX AND LIFE SPAN CONSIDERATIONS

The most common thoracic aortic aneurysm is an ascending aortic aneurysm, which is usually seen in hypertensive men under age 60 years. A descending aortic aneurysm is most common in older hypertensive men or younger patients with a history of traumatic chest injury. Some experts report that at least 3% to 4% of people older than age 65 years have aortic aneurysms. The incidence of thoracic aortic aneurysm is higher in men than in women by a ratio of 3:1.

HEALTH DISPARITIES AND SEXUAL/GENDER MINORITY HEALTH

The incidence of thoracic aortic aneurysm is more common in White persons than in other populations. Black patients are younger and have more comorbidities prior to surgery than White patients (Yin et al., 2021 [see Evidence-Based Practice and Health Policy]), but Black and White patients have similar outcomes. Transgender is a term used to describe persons whose gender identity is different from their sex assigned at birth. Approximately 1% of the U.S. population identify themselves as transgender. Sexual and gender minority persons have higher odds for multiple chronic conditions, cancer, and poor quality of life and are more apt to have disabilities than cisgender males and females. (Cisgender is a term used to describe persons whose gender identity and gender expression are aligned with their assigned sex listed on their birth certificate.) Gender-affirming hormone therapy is the use of hormone therapy for gender transition or gender affirmation and can be masculinizing or feminizing. It may also affect cardiovascular health in transgender females. In a large sample, researchers have found that transgender men and women are more likely to be overweight than cisgender women and more likely to smoke cigarettes. Compared to cisgender women, transgender women reported higher rates of diabetes, angina/coronary disease, and myocardial infarction. These factors, particularly smoking and atherosclerosis, place transgender women at risk for thoracic aortic aneurysm (Caceres, Jackman, et al., 2020).

GLOBAL HEALTH CONSIDERATIONS

The global incidence of thoracic aortic aneurysm is similar to that in the United States, where the incidence is approximately six cases per 100,000 individuals.

ASSESSMENT

HISTORY. Many patients are asymptomatic when they are diagnosed with a thoracic aortic aneurysm, which often is found at the time of a chest x-ray. Establish a history of atherosclerosis, hypertension, hypercholesteremia, smoking, obesity, diabetes, and familial tendencies. Elicit a history of pain, including a description and location (Table 2). Establish a history of pulmonary symptoms, such as wheezing, coughing, hemoptysis, dyspnea, or stridor, which may be caused by a descending thoracic aortic aneurysm that compresses the tracheobronchial tree. Ask if the patient has had difficulties swallowing, hoarseness, dyspnea, or dry cough, all of which may be caused by a transverse arch thoracic aortic aneurysm.

• **TABLE 2** Characteristic Signs and Symptoms of Thoracic Aortic Aneurysms

LOCATION OF ANEURYSM	LOCATION OF PAIN	TYPE OF PAIN
Ascending aorta	Substernal chest pain (reminiscent of angina), extending to the neck, shoulders, lower back, or abdomen but not generally to the jaw or arms; more severe on right side	Severe, boring, ripping; patient may also have signs of heart failure
Transverse arch of aorta	Neck pain radiating to the shoulders	Sudden, sharp tearing
Descending aorta	Back and shoulder pain radiating to the chest	Sharp, tearing

PHYSICAL EXAMINATION. The most common symptom is **severe chest, neck, and/or back pain.** The physical examination of a patient with a thoracic aortic aneurysm usually does not reveal the presence of the aneurysm. Certain physical findings, however, should raise your level of suspicion. Complete a neurological examination to determine the adequacy of tissue perfusion. Take the patient's blood pressure in both arms because an ascending thoracic aortic aneurysm may cause a contralateral (opposite side) difference. Take both the patient's right carotid and left radial pulses and note any differences. Auscultate for pericardial friction rub and aortic valve insufficiency murmur, indicating the extension of an ascending aortic aneurysm proximally into the aortic valve. Note any signs of bradycardia.

PSYCHOSOCIAL. Assess the patient's and significant others' understanding of the implications of the condition. Assess the ability of the patient and significant others to cope with a sudden life-threatening illness, a prolonged hospitalization, and the role changes that a sudden illness requires. Assess the patient's level of anxiety about the illness, potential surgery, and complications.

Diagnostic Highlights

General Comments: Because this condition often causes no symptoms, it is often diagnosed through routine physical examinations or chest x-rays.

Test	Normal Result	Abnormality With Condition	Explanation
Computed tomography (CT) scan, magnetic resonance imaging (MRI)	Negative study; normal aorta and aortic valve	Locates outpouching within the aortic wall	Assesses size and location of aneurysm
Transesophageal echocardiography (TEE)	Negative study; normal aorta and aortic valve	Location and size of aneurysm	Assesses size and location of aneurysm; high sensitivity and specificity for diagnosing aortic aneurysm
Chest x-ray	Negative study; normal aorta	May show widened mediastinum or enlarged calcified aortic shadow; traumatic aneurysm may be associated with skeletal fractures	Assesses size and location of aneurysm

Other Tests: Electrocardiogram, TEE with Doppler color flow mapping, aortic angiography

PRIMARY NURSING DIAGNOSIS

DIAGNOSIS. Risk for decreased cardiac and ineffective cerebral tissue perfusion as evidenced by tachycardia, hypotension, apnea, and/or loss of consciousness

OUTCOMES. Cardiac pump effectiveness; Cardiopulmonary status; Tissue perfusion: Cerebral, Peripheral, Cardiac, Pulmonary; Respiratory status; Neurological status; Vital sign status; Fluid balance; Electrolyte balance

INTERVENTIONS. Cardiac care; Airway management; Fluid/electrolyte management; Medication management; Medication administration; IV insertion; IV therapy; Neurologic monitoring; Oxygen therapy; Emergency care; Laboratory data interpretation

☀ PLANNING AND IMPLEMENTATION

Collaborative

A thoracic aortic aneurysm that is 4 to 5 cm in size or less may be treated with oral antihypertensives or a beta-blocking agent to control hypertension. Frequent diagnostic testing (every 6 months) is necessary to determine the size of the aneurysm. A thoracic aortic aneurysm that is 5.5 cm (ascending) or 6.5 cm (descending) or greater in diameter is usually treated surgically. Other indications for surgical intervention include dissection, intractable pain, and an unstable aneurysm (one that is changing size). Surgical procedures vary, depending on the location of the aneurysm. An ascending arch aneurysm may be replaced with an interposition graft, a composite valved conduit, or a supracoronary graft with separate aortic valve replacement. A transverse arch aneurysm is usually repaired with anastomoses and reconstructions. A graft is used to repair descending thoracic and thoracoabdominal aneurysms. Open repairs of thoracic aortic aneurysms are technically challenging and have a high risk for complications. In contrast, endovascular aneurysm repair (EVAR) is a minimally invasive method that involves the placement of an expandable stent graft within the aorta through a small incision in the groin. EVAR is associated with lower perioperative and long-term mortality than is open surgical repair, as well as with more graft-related complications, higher cost, and generally a shorter hospital stay.

The primary complication for thoracic aortic aneurysms is dissection. Monitor the patient for any changes in the quality of peripheral pulses; changes in vital signs; changes in the level of consciousness; and onset of sudden, severe, ripping, or tearing pain in the chest, neck, back, or shoulders. A ruptured thoracic aortic aneurysm requires immediate emergency resuscitation and immediate surgical intervention. Preoperatively, assess the patient's peripheral pulses, taking care to compare one side with the other. Take the patient's blood pressure measurement in both arms and auscultate for an aortic insufficiency murmur to establish a baseline for postoperative comparison. Also, administer large volumes of IV fluids and blood products to maintain circulation until surgery is performed. Postoperatively, monitor cardiopulmonary states, especially for patients with heart failure, because beta-blocking agents may worsen it. If the patient has hypercholesteremia that cannot be controlled with diet, a cholesterol-lowering agent may be prescribed by the physician.

Pharmacologic Highlights

Medication or Drug Class	Dosage	Description	Rationale
Antihypertensives	Varies by drug	Beta blockers: Esmolol, labetalol, metoprolol, propranolol	Reduce blood pressure so that hypertension does not stress graft suture lines
Nitroprusside	0.5–10 mcg/kg/min, titrated to reduce blood pressure IV	Antihypertensive	Reduces blood pressure in acute or critical situations
Morphine	1–10 mg IV	Opioid analgesic	Relieves surgical pain
Fentanyl	50–100 mcg IV	Opioid analgesic	Relieves surgical pain

Other Drugs: Diuretics

Independent

Focus on maintaining adequate circulation, preventing complications, and implementing patient education. For the nonsurgical patient, patient teaching includes information about low-fat, low-cholesterol diets to prevent progression of the atherosclerotic process and to treat hypercholesteremia. Urge the patient to stop smoking cigarettes and provide information about smoking cessation.

For the surgical patient, focus on maintaining adequate circulation preoperatively and postoperatively, preventing complications, and patient teaching. Preoperative care of the elective surgical patient is the same as for any patient who undergoes general anesthesia. Postoperatively, care is similar to that of a patient who undergoes any chest surgery. Provide aggressive pulmonary hygiene every 1 to 2 hours to prevent pulmonary complications. Assist with range-of-motion exercises to limit the effects of immobility. Provide emotional support for the patient and significant others.

Evidence-Based Practice and Health Policy

Yin, K., AlHajri, N., Rizwan, M., Locham, S., Dakour-Aridi, H., & Malas, M. (2021). Black patients have a higher burden of comorbidities but a lower risk of 30-day and 1-year mortality after thoracic endovascular aortic repair. *Journal of Vascular Surgery*, *73*, 2071–2080.

* The authors aimed to examine the clinical characteristics, perioperative outcomes, and 1-year survival of Black and White patients who underwent less invasive thoracic endovascular aortic repair. They used a national vascular surgery database with data from 9 years to analyze data from 2,669 patients, 24.3% of whom were Black.
* Black patients were younger and had more comorbidities, were more likely to be symptomatic, present with acute dissection, and undergo emergency surgery. There was no significant difference in 30-day mortality risk between Black and White patients, and Black patients had better 1-year survival than White patients. The authors concluded that although Black patients had a higher burden of comorbidities preoperatively, racial disparities did not persist postoperatively.

DOCUMENTATION GUIDELINES

* Physical findings: Vital signs, pain (location, onset, severity), heart sounds, urine output, healing of incision
* Assessment of circulation: Blood pressure in both arms, quality of peripheral pulses in all extremities, capillary blanch test
* Response to acute, life-threatening illness: Anxiety, fear, coping
* Response to surgery: Incision, wound healing, wound drainage, signs of complications

DISCHARGE AND HOME HEALTHCARE GUIDELINES

The nonsurgical patient is discharged to the home setting. The surgical patient is usually discharged to the home setting if a support system can be identified. An extended-care facility may be required for a short time if a support system is not in place for the patient at the time of discharge. Be sure the patient understands all medications prescribed, including dosage, route, action, and side effects. Provide patients and their families with information about a low-fat, low-cholesterol diet (reduced calorie if obese). Be sure the patient understands the importance of controlling blood pressure and blood cholesterol levels in the prevention of progression of the atherosclerotic process.

Provide patients who smoke and their families with information about how to stop smoking. Be sure the patient understands that smoking is a risk factor for hypertension and atherosclerosis. Make sure the nonsurgical patient with a thoracic aortic aneurysm understands the necessity for follow-up examinations at regular intervals to determine the size of the aneurysm and the rate of enlargement. The surgical patient is restricted from activity for 6 to 12 weeks postoperatively. Teach the patient to restrict activities by avoiding heavy lifting, pushing or pulling strenuously, and straining. Give the surgical patient specific instructions for wound care. Teach the patient to examine the incision site for signs of infection and to report any to the physician.

Thrombophlebitis

DRG Category:	253
Mean LOS:	5.4 days
Description:	SURGICAL: Other Vascular Procedures With Complication or Comorbidity
DRG Category:	299
Mean LOS:	5.1 days
Description:	MEDICAL: Peripheral Vascular Disorders With Major Complication or Comorbidity

Thrombophlebitis, inflammation of a vein with an associated blood clot (thrombus), typically occurs in the veins of the lower extremities when fibrin and platelets accumulate at areas of stasis or turbulence near venous valves. Deep vein thrombophlebitis (deep vein thrombosis [DVT]) occurs more than 90% of the time in small veins, such as the lesser saphenous, or in large veins, such as the femoral and popliteal. DVT and its possible consequence, pulmonary embolism, are the leading causes of preventable mortality in hospitalized patients in the United States. DVT occurs in approximately 1 in every 20 individuals over their lifetime, but in hospitalized patients, the incidence of DVT ranges from 20% to 70%.

DVT is potentially more serious than superficial vein thrombosis (SVT) because the deep veins carry approximately 90% of the blood flow as it leaves the lower extremities. Once a thrombus begins to move, it becomes an embolus (a detached intravascular mass carried by the blood). If it reaches the lungs, a pulmonary embolus, it is potentially fatal. Another complication is postphlebitic syndrome, which leads to lasting and disabling pain, swelling, and heaviness in the affected leg.

CAUSES

Venous stasis, hypercoagulability, and vascular injury are major causes of thrombophlebitis. Venous stasis results from prolonged immobility, pregnancy, obesity, chronic heart disease such as congestive heart failure or myocardial infarction, recovery from major surgery (surgical procedures lasting more than 30 minutes), cerebrovascular accidents, and advanced age. Hypercoagulability is associated with pregnancy, cigarette smoking, dehydration, deficiencies of substances involved in clot breakdown, tamoxifen use, long airplane flights, disseminated intravascular coagulation, estrogen supplements and oral contraceptives, malignancy, and sepsis. Vascular injury can occur with lower extremity fractures, surgery, burns, multiple trauma, childbirth, infections, irritating IV solutions, venipuncture, and venulitis. Other diseases that may lead to thrombus formation are cancer of the lung, gastrointestinal tract, and genitourinary tract and also atrial fibrillation; individuals older than 55 years are also particularly susceptible to thrombophlebitis.

GENETIC CONSIDERATIONS

Coagulopathies such as factor V Leiden, a thrombophilia that predisposes to thrombophlebitis, is due to a very poor response to activated protein C. This is caused by mutations in factor V (F5) that render it resistant to cleavage. Factor V Leiden increases clot formation in heterozygote carriers, but homozygotes are most severely affected. Testing for factor V Leiden should be considered when a person has a thrombophlebitis meeting any of the following criteria: onset before age 50 years, idiopathic venous thromboembolism at any age, recurrent thromboembolism, and venous thrombosis at unusual sites (e.g., cerebral, mesenteric, portal, and hepatic veins). Testing has also been recommended when thrombophlebitis occurs during pregnancy, in the postpartum period, or in association with oral contraceptive use or hormone replacement therapy. Anyone with a strong family history should also be tested for factor V Leiden. The prothrombin 20210G-A variant also increases the risk of thrombophilia, especially in combination with the factor V Leiden mutation.

SEX AND LIFE SPAN CONSIDERATIONS

Young women and older adults are more likely to develop thrombophlebitis than adult men because young adult women may have many risk factors (pregnancy, oral contraceptives, smoking, obesity). Women over age 30 years who smoke and use oral contraceptives are at particular risk. The older person's increased tendency for immobility, platelet aggregation, and elevated fibrinogen levels increases their risk.

HEALTH DISPARITIES AND SEXUAL/GENDER MINORITY HEALTH

Ethnicity, race, and sexual/gender minority status have no known effect on the risk for thrombophlebitis.

GLOBAL HEALTH CONSIDERATIONS

Global incidence is likely similar to that of the United States and Western Europe. Little is known about the incidence in developing countries, and definitive diagnosis is often difficult or even impossible in low-resourced areas.

ASSESSMENT

HISTORY. Although almost half of the patients with DVT and SVT are asymptomatic, patients with DVT may have complaints of swelling, pain, and warm erythema over the site of the thrombosis. Take a thorough medical and family history, and determine any recent (past 3 months) infections, surgeries, trauma, or stroke. Ask about any previous thrombosis or pulmonary emboli, when they occurred, and how they were managed. Obtain an obstetric history, including whether patients are pregnant, have had any recurrent spontaneous abortions (may indicate a factor deficiency), or use birth control pills and the date of their last menstrual period. Determine if patients have any signs of malignancy, such as fever, bone pain, weight loss, or bruising. Ask patients if they have had any recent travel involving being in a car, train, bus, or airplane for more than 4 hours.

PHYSICAL EXAMINATION. While patients may have no symptoms, common complaints may be **calf muscle or groin tenderness** and a **firm, tender, erythematous cord** in the area of a vein in the leg. Other signs include pain, fever (rarely above 101°F [38.4°C]), chills, general weakness, and lethargy. Observe both legs, noting alterations in symmetry, color, and temperature of one leg compared with the other. In DVT, the affected limb may reveal redness, warmth, swelling, and discoloration when compared with the contralateral limb. In addition, superficial veins over the area may be distended. Note the presence of calf pain with dorsiflexion of the foot of the affected extremity, which is a positive Homans sign. This positive finding occurs in 33% of patients with DVT and is considered an inconsistent and unreliable physical sign.

SVT may be asymptomatic or may lead to pain, redness, induration, and swelling in the local area of the thrombus. Note the presence of local redness and nodules on the skin or extremity edema, which is rare. Palpate over the suspected vein involved. It may feel like a cord or thickness that extends upward along the entire length of the vein.

PSYCHOSOCIAL. The patient has not only an unexpected, sudden illness, but also an increased risk for life-threatening complications such as pulmonary embolism. Assess the patient's ability to cope. In addition, assess the patient's degree of anxiety about the illness and potential complications.

Diagnostic Highlights

Test	Normal Result	Abnormality With Condition	Explanation
D-dimer, measured by latex agglutination or by an enzyme-linked immunosorbent assay test	< 400 ng/mL	> 500 ng/mL	D-dimer fragments are present in a fresh fibrin clot and levels are elevated for 7 days when clots form
Doppler ultrasound; duplex Doppler venous scanning	Normal blood flow velocity	Diminished flow caused by phlebitis	Records sound waves reflected from moving red blood cells in arteries and veins
Partial thromboplastin time (activated; APTT)	Varies by laboratory; generally 25–35 sec	Prolonged when on anticoagulation; on heparin maintain APTT 60–85 sec	Indicates how long it takes for recalcified, citrated plasma to clot after partial thromboplastin is added
Prothrombin time (PT)	Varies by laboratory; generally 10–13 sec	Prolonged when on anticoagulation	Prothrombin is a vitamin K–dependent glycoprotein necessary for firm clot formation; converts to thrombin in clotting cascade; see INR
International normalized ratio (INR)	< 2	2–3 for patient receiving treatment for thrombophlebitis	Laboratories convert PT values to an international norm for accuracy

Other Tests: Magnetic resonance venography, compression ultrasonography, I-125–labeled fibrinogen leg scan, radio-opaque venographyvenous thrombosis, complete blood count, platelet count, inherited hypercoagulability factors

PRIMARY NURSING DIAGNOSIS

DIAGNOSIS. Risk for ineffective peripheral tissue perfusion as evidenced by swelling, pain, and/or warmth of the extremity

OUTCOMES. Tissue perfusion: Peripheral; Tissue integrity: Skin and mucous membranes; Circulation status; Knowledge: Thrombus threat reduction; Knowledge: Disease process; Vital signs

INTERVENTIONS. Embolus precautions; Embolus care: Peripheral; Vital signs monitoring; Teaching: Disease process

PLANNING AND IMPLEMENTATION
Collaborative

To prevent thrombus formation, most physicians prescribe compression of the legs by graduated compression stockings to reduce venous stasis in low-risk general surgical patients. In higher-risk patients, intermittent pneumatic compression boots prevent venous stasis and increase the normal breakdown of fibrin in the body with increased fibrinolytic activity.

The location of the thrombus dictates the treatment. If a DVT is suspected, anticoagulation is used to prevent pulmonary emboli. For patients with SVT, low molecular weight heparin (LMWH) is the treatment of choice. Most patients who develop thrombophlebitis are placed on bedrest with extremity elevation to avoid dislodging the thrombus. Local heat with warm soaks may also be used to reduce venospasm and decrease inflammation, but data are not clear whether or not this therapy improves outcomes. Generally, the patient is given analgesics for pain control along with the anticoagulant therapy to prevent further clot formation. From 1 to 3 days later, warfarin therapy is started. LMWH is usually discontinued 48 hours after the patient's PT reaches a therapeutic value. (Box 1).

• BOX 1 Caring for the Patient on Anticoagulants

ASSESSMENT

Monitor coagulation profile (PT, partial thromboplastin time, INR) daily and report values below and above the therapeutic range to the physician.

Monitor for overt bleeding such as bruising, tarry stools, coffee ground or bloody vomitus, oozing gums, hematuria, vaginal bleeding, and heavy menstruation.

Monitor for occult bleeding demonstrated by flank pain or abdominal pain and for changes in mental status.

MANAGEMENT CONSIDERATIONS

Have the antidote for heparin (protamine sulfate) and warfarin (vitamin K) available for emergency use in case of hemorrhage.

Avoid administering aspirin to patients on anticoagulants because the synergistic effect may induce bleeding.

Avoid the following procedures if possible because of the risk of increased bleeding: intramuscular injections, central line insertions, arterial cannulation, lumbar puncture, and surgical procedures.

Note that the following conditions are relative contraindications to anticoagulant therapy: active bleeding, cerebrovascular accident, severe hypertension, pericarditis and endocarditis, pregnancy (particularly warfarin therapy), and chronic alcoholism.

Note that the following medications may interact with warfarin:

• Increased activity: Allopurinol, cimetidine, indomethacin, metronidazole, oral hypoglycemic agents, phenothiazines, quinidine, tricyclic antidepressants

• Decreased activity: Barbiturates, oral contraceptives, rifampin. Apply pressure on all punctures for 5 minutes or as long as needed to stop bleeding.

Some patients may continue heparin subcutaneously for several weeks before changing to warfarin. Because prothrombin assays are performed in various ways, PT results are now also reported as an INR. The target INR for oral anticoagulation is at least 2; current recommendations are to stop heparin therapy after 5 to 7 days of joint therapy when the INR is 2 to 3 with the patient off heparin. For patients with massive DVT in proximal veins, thrombolytic therapy may be considered. Before initiating therapy, the risk that the clot presents to the patient is compared with the risk of bleeding from thrombolytic agents.

SURGICAL. Other treatments that may be used for severe, obstructive DVT are thrombectomy (surgical clot removal) and surgical prophylaxis against pulmonary embolism with implantation of an umbrella filter in the inferior vena cava.

Pharmacologic Highlights

Medication or Drug Class	Dosage	Description	Rationale
Fibrinolytic agents	Varies with drug	Reteplase (r-PA, Retavase), Alteplase (t-PA, Activase)	Breakdown of the blood clot for extensive DVT but usually not SVT
Anticoagulants	Varies with drug and patient weight	LMWH: Enoxaparin (Lovenox), dalteparin (Fragmin), and tinzaparin (Innohep); warfarin	Standard treatment is to initiate IV heparin to reduce further formation of clots; leads to early discharge for some patients

Pharmacologic Highlights (continued)

Medication or Drug Class	Dosage	Description	Rationale
NSAIDs	Varies with drug	Ibuprofen, naproxen	Resolve symptoms and prevent extension of thromboembolism

Other Drugs: Analgesics; antibiotics if infection is suspected

Independent

The most important nursing interventions focus on prevention. Decrease the risk of venous stasis in a bedridden patient by performing early ambulation and active or passive range-of-motion exercises several times a day. Avoid using the knee bed adjustment because of the risk of popliteal pressure and venous stasis with the knees bent; encourage patients not to cross their legs, especially when sitting. If pillows are needed to elevate extremities, position them along the entire length of the extremity to prevent additional pressure on veins and to allow for adequate venous drainage. If the patient is immobile and not on fluid restriction, encourage the patient to drink at least 3 L of fluid a day to prevent dehydration and venous stasis.

To prevent injury to vessel walls, monitor IV cannulas to prevent infiltration. If IV medications are irritating to the vein, IV cannulas should be changed and rotated to new sites more often than the standard procedure.

Discuss activity restrictions with the patient and family. The patient usually feels confined and may become resentful because of the need for absolute bedrest. To increase mobility in bed, install an orthoframe and trapeze system to the bed. A sheepskin, air mattress, foam pad, foot cradle, or heel pads can reduce the risk of skin breakdown while the person is on bedrest. Provide diversional activities to reduce anxiety.

Evidence-Based Practice and Health Policy

Marone, E., Bonalumi, G., Curci, R., Arzini, A., Chierico, S., Marazzi, G., Diaco, D., Rossini, R., Boschini, S., & Rinaldi, L. (2020). Characteristics of venous thromboembolism in COVID-19 patients: A multicenter experience from Northern Italy. *Annals of Vascular Surgery, 68*, 83–87.

- The authors aimed to determine the characteristics of DVT and pulmonary embolism in COVID-19 patients based on four high-volume hospitals in Italy. They reviewed all cases of patients undergoing duplex ultrasound for clinically suspected DVT
- Of 101 ultrasounds performed, 42 were positive for DVT, 7 for SVT, and 24 for pulmonary emboli. Most patients had moderate (44%) or mild (17%) pneumonia. Diagnosis of thrombophlebitis and pulmonary embolism was generally during the first 2 weeks of hospitalization. Two-thirds of the pulmonary emboli occurred in the absence of a recognizable DVT.

DOCUMENTATION GUIDELINES

- Physical findings of affected extremity: Presence of redness, tenderness, swelling
- Response to pain medications, heat application, elevation, rest
- Reaction to immobility and bedrest
- Presence of complications: Bleeding tendencies, respiratory distress, unrelieved discomfort

DISCHARGE AND HOME HEALTHCARE GUIDELINES

Teach the patient preventive strategies. Demonstrate how to apply compression stockings correctly if they have been prescribed. Be sure the patient understands all medications, including the dosage, route, action, adverse effects, and need for routine laboratory monitoring for anticoagulants. If the patient is being discharged on subcutaneous heparin, the patient or family needs to demonstrate the injection technique. The patient also needs to know to avoid over-the-counter medications, particularly those that contain aspirin. Explain the need to avoid activities that could cause bumping or injury and predispose the patient to excessive bleeding. Instruct the patient to notify the physician if abdominal or flank pain, heavy bleeding during menstruation, and bloody urine or stool occur.

Recommend using a soft toothbrush and an electric razor to limit injury. Remind the patient to notify the physician or dentist of anticoagulant use before any invasive procedure. Instruct the patient to report leg pain or swelling, skin discoloration, or decreases in peripheral skin temperature to the physician. In addition, if the patient experiences signs of possible pulmonary embolism (anxiety, shortness of breath, pleuritic pain, hemoptysis), the patient should go to the emergency department immediately.

Thyroid Cancer

DRG Category:	626
Mean LOS:	3.5 days
Description:	SURGICAL: Thyroid, Parathyroid, and Thyroglossal Procedures With Complication or Comorbidity
DRG Category:	644
Mean LOS:	4.3 days
Description:	MEDICAL: Endocrine Disorders With Complication or Comorbidity

Thyroid cancer is the most common endocrine cancer in the United States. The American Cancer Society (ACS, 2021) estimates that in 2021, there will be 44,280 new cases of thyroid cancer diagnosed and approximately 2,200 deaths in the United States. Most thyroid nodules or tumors develop from thyroid follicular cells; 95% of these nodules and tumors are benign. The remaining 5% of thyroid nodules or tumors are cancerous, and there are several forms of thyroid cancer. Papillary carcinoma is the most common form of primary thyroid cancer. It is also the slowest-growing thyroid cancer and is usually multifocal and bilateral in distribution. Papillary carcinoma metastasizes slowly into the cervical lymph nodes and the nodes of the mediastinum and lungs. Follicular cancer is the next most common form. It is more likely to recur than other forms; it generally metastasizes to the regional lymph nodes and is spread by the blood to distant areas such as the bones, liver, and lungs. More than 90% of patients treated for either papillary or follicular carcinoma will live for 15 years or longer after their diagnosis.

Anaplastic carcinoma of the thyroid is a less common form of thyroid cancer and is resistant to both surgical resection and radiation; the 5-year survival rate is 7%. Anaplastic cells metastasize quickly, invade the trachea and surrounding tissues, and compress vital structures. Medullary cancer is even less common (3% to 4% of thyroid cancers); it originates in the parafollicular cells of the thyroid. Metastasis occurs to the bones, liver, and kidneys if the disease is not treated. In addition to metastases, other life-threatening complications include compression of surrounding structures (particularly in the neck), leading to difficulty swallowing and breathing. Surgery can cure medullary thyroid cancer; depending on stage, the 5-year survival rate ranges from nearly 38% to nearly 100%. The primary complications for thyroid cancer are metastasis and recurrence.

CAUSES

The cause of thyroid cancer is unclear, but like many cancers, it is related to both genetic and environmental factors. It occurs when thyroid cancer cells mutate, leading thyroid cells to proliferate rapidly and abnormally. People who have been exposed to radiation therapy to the neck are particularly susceptible to thyroid cancer, including those exposed to low-dose radiation as children and others exposed to high-dose radiation for malignancies. About 25% of individuals who had radiation in the 1950s to shrink an enlarged thymus gland, tonsils, or adenoids develop thyroid nodules; approximately 25% of those with nodules actually develop thyroid cancer (6% of those exposed to neck radiation in the first place). Other factors related to thyroid cancer include prolonged secretion of thyroid-stimulating hormone (TSH) because of radiation and chronic goiter. Risk factors include exposure to high levels of radiation, family history of thyroid disease, female sex, and Asian ethnicity.

GENETIC CONSIDERATIONS

Most cases of thyroid cancer are sporadic (75% in a Swedish study and 60% in a French national registry). Rearrangements of the *RET* or *NTRK1* gene to form chimeric oncogenes are observed in about 50% of cases. Familial cases are usually due to the presence of multiple endocrine neoplasia type II (MEN II), a group of autosomal dominantly inherited disorders caused by mutations in the *RET* oncogene. Mutations in *NKX2-1* cause nonmedullary thyroid cancer with autosomal dominant inheritance. To date, 14 genes have been associated with familial susceptibility: *DICER1, FOXE1, PTCSC2, PTCSC3, MYH9, SRGAP1, HABP2, BRCA1, CHEK2, ATM, RASAL1, SRRM2, XRCC1,* and *NKX2-1.*

SEX AND LIFE SPAN CONSIDERATIONS

Although benign thyroid nodules and thyroid cancers can occur in people of all ages, those between ages 30 and 50 years are most likely to develop papillary and follicular thyroid cancer. Women are three times as likely as men to have thyroid cancer, but there does not seem to be a difference in mortality between women and men. Solitary thyroid nodules are more likely to be malignant in people older than 60 and younger than 30 years of age.

HEALTH DISPARITIES AND SEXUAL/GENDER MINORITY HEALTH

Ethnicity and race have no known effects on the risk for thyroid cancer, except for people with Asian ancestry, who are more at risk for the disease (Patel et al., 2020 [see Evidence-Based Practice and Health Policy]). Health disparities occur in thyroid cancer for persons living in rural areas, which tend to be at a distance from cancer centers. Five- and 10-year survival rates are significantly lower in rural areas of the United States as compared to urban areas, possibly because of healthcare disparities or differences in therapies (McDow et al., 2020). Sexual and gender minority status have no known effect on the risk for thyroid cancer, but gender and sexual minority persons experience fear of discrimination, have low rates of health insurance, and have negative experiences with healthcare providers (ACS, 2021). These factors may create barriers to obtaining healthcare.

GLOBAL HEALTH CONSIDERATIONS

Globally, thyroid cancer is more common in females than in males. The incidence of thyroid cancer is approximately 3 per 100,000 females, as compared to 1 per 100,000 males. People in developed countries have two to three times the incidence of thyroid cancer as compared to people in developing countries.

ASSESSMENT

HISTORY. Most patients present with an asymptomatic neck mass. Note that malignant thyroid nodules are usually painless, and rapid growth of a nodule is of great concern. Less commonly, patients may also have complaints of neck discomfort, hoarseness, dysphagia (difficulty swallowing), feeling as if they are "breathing through a straw," and rapid nodule growth. Elicit a family history, particularly of chronic goiter, because some forms of thyroid cancer are inherited. Ask if patients have had exposure to low- or high-dose radiation because of diagnostic testing, treatment for other cancers, in an occupational setting, or through an environmental disaster. If the thyroid has been completely destroyed by cancer cells, the patient may report a history of sensitivity to cold, weight gain, and apathy from hypothyroidism. If the thyroid has become overstimulated, the patient may describe signs of hyperthyroidism: sensitivity to heat, nervousness, weight loss, and hyperactivity. Changes in thyroid function may also lead to gastrointestinal changes such as diarrhea and anorexia.

PHYSICAL EXAMINATION. The most common symptoms are a **palpable thyroid nodule, hoarseness, difficulty swallowing,** and **neck discomfort.** Observe the patient's neck, noting any mass or enlargement. Patients with anaplastic thyroid cancer may have a rapidly growing tumor that distorts the neck and surrounding structures. Palpate the thyroid gland for size, shape, configuration, consistency, tenderness, and presence of any nodules. Single nodules can vary from soft to hard in consistency. Describe the number of nodules present and whether the nodule is smooth or irregular, soft or hard, or fixed to underlying tissue. Note the presence of enlarged cervical lymph nodes, which occurs in 25% of patients with the disease. Auscultation may reveal bruits if the thyroid enlargement results from an increase in TSH, which increases thyroid circulation and vascularity.

PSYCHOSOCIAL. Assess the patient's ability to cope with the sudden illness and the diagnosis of cancer. Determine what a diagnosis of cancer means to the patient. Consider the type of cancer (and the speed of cancer growth) when assessing the patient's and family's response to the disease.

Diagnostic Highlights

Test	Normal Result	Abnormality With Condition	Explanation
Fine-needle aspiration (FNA) biopsy; usually the first intervention and most important diagnostic tool	Microscopic viewing reveals no cancerous cells	Microscopic viewing reveals cancer cells	A thin needle guided by ultrasound is placed directly into the nodule several times to sample different areas; 5% of FNA biopsies reveal cancer, while 60% to 80% clearly show that the nodule is benign
Ultrasound of the thyroid and/or computed tomography	Normal structures	Identifies primary tumor and associated cervical lymph nodes	Provides information on tumor location, size, echogenicity, hypervascularity, architecture, calcification, tumor invasion
Thyroid scan	Homogenous uptake of radioactive tracer; normal size and shape of thyroid	Abnormal areas of the thyroid may contain less radioactivity (cold nodules with decreased uptake) or more radioactivity (hot nodules with increased uptake)	A small quantity of radioactive iodine is taken orally or intravenously; after the chemicals concentrate in the thyroid, a special camera measures the amount of radiation in the thyroid gland
Thyroid-stimulating hormone (TSH; thyrotropin)	< 4 mIU/L	Normal or elevated	Used to determine if radioactive iodine will work as therapy
Serum calcitonin	< 40 pg/mL	Increased in medullary cancer of thyroid; levels 500 to 2,000 pg/mL are often associated with cancer	Thyroid gland polypeptide hormone produced by thyroid even when no mass is palpable

Diagnostic Highlights (continued)

Other Tests: Magnetic resonance imaging, octreotide scan used for determining cancer staging and spread, lymph node biopsy, serum calcium

PRIMARY NURSING DIAGNOSIS

DIAGNOSIS. Ineffective airway clearance related to swelling and obstruction as evidenced by stridor, wheezing, dyspnea, and/or decreased chest excursion

OUTCOMES. Respiratory status: Airway patency; Respiratory status: Gas exchange; Respiratory status: Ventilation; Symptom severity; Knowledge: Disease process; Vital signs; Knowledge: Cancer management

INTERVENTIONS. Airway management; Airway insertion and stabilization; Anxiety reduction; Oxygen therapy; Airway suctioning; Respiratory monitoring

PLANNING AND IMPLEMENTATION
Collaborative

Most physicians prescribe surgical treatment of thyroid cancer, with the definitive treatment depending on the size of the nodule. Surgical interventions range from a thyroid lobectomy for cancers smaller than 1 cm that show no signs of metastasis to a total thyroidectomy and, possibly, a modified neck dissection if lymph nodes need to be removed. To prevent complications after the thyroidectomy, careful monitoring for airway obstruction and stridor is essential. A tracheostomy tray should be kept near the patient at all times during the immediate recovery period. In addition, monitor for signs of thyrotoxicosis (tachycardia, diaphoresis, increased blood pressure, anxiety) and hypocalcemia (tingling of the fingers and toes, carpopedal spasms, and convulsions). The surgical dressing and incision also need to be assessed for excessive drainage or bleeding during the postoperative period. If the patient complains that the dressing feels tight, the surgeon needs to be alerted immediately.

Generally, after surgery is completed, the patient is started on synthetic levothyroxine therapy to suppress TSH levels and establish a euthyroid (normal) state. Most patients do not have chemotherapy or radiotherapy because these modalities are usually ineffective with rapidly growing thyroid cancers. Chemotherapy is usually reserved as an adjuvant measure to halt the spread of metastasis; the chemotherapeutic drugs include doxorubicin and CHOP (cyclophosphamide, hydroxydaunomycin, oncovin [vincristine], and prednisone). Radiation may be used for people with differentiated thyroid cancer.

Radioactive iodine (^{131}I) may be used to destroy any remaining thyroid tissue not removed by surgery and to treat affected lymph nodes. For radioiodine therapy to be most effective, patients need to have high serum TSH levels; thus, an intentional hypothyroid condition is induced by stopping thyroid medications for 1 to 2 weeks. This temporary condition causes the pituitary gland to release more TSH.

Pharmacologic Highlights

Medication or Drug Class	Dosage	Description	Rationale
Levothyroxine (Synthroid)	2.6 mcg/kg per day for 7–10 days or for life, if the thyroid was completely removed	Synthetic T4 hormone	Suppresses TSH levels and establishes a euthyroid state postoperatively

Independent

Nursing interventions focus on teaching and prevention of complications. When you prepare patients before surgery, discuss not only the procedure and aftercare, but also the methods for postoperative communication such as a magic slate or a point board. Explain that the patient will be able to speak only rarely, will need to rest the voice for several days, and should expect to be hoarse. Answer all questions before surgery. After the procedure, monitor the patient's ability to speak with each measurement of vital signs. Assess the patient's voice tone and quality and compare it with the preoperative voice.

Maintaining a patent airway is the most important intervention. Maintain the bed in a high-Fowler position to decrease edema and swelling of the neck. To avoid pressure on the suture line, encourage the patient to avoid neck flexion and extension. Support the head and neck with pillows or sandbags; if the patient needs to be transferred from stretcher to bed, support the head and neck in good body alignment. Be prepared to initiate emergency care if the patient's airway is compromised if an emergency tracheostomy is needed. If the patient had a total thyroidectomy, hypocalcemia may occur if the parathyroid glands were damaged. Monitor for hypocalcemia (paresthesias, muscle spasms) and supplement calcium as prescribed.

Before discharge, make sure the patient has a follow-up appointment for a postdischarge assessment. Make sure the patient has the financial resources to obtain all needed medications; some patients require thyroid supplements for the rest of their lives. Refer the patient or family to the American Cancer Society for additional information.

Evidence-Based Practice and Health Policy

Patel, S., Pappoppula, L., Guddati, A., & Annamaraju, P. (2020). Analysis of race and gender disparities in incidence-based mortality in patients diagnosed with thyroid cancer from 2000 to 2016. *International Journal of General Medicine, 13*, 1589–1594.

- The authors aimed to analyze the rates of mortality for anaplastic thyroid cancer with respect to gender and race: White, Black, American Indian, and Asian/Pacific Islander. They used a national cancer database and grouped the sample by race.
- The incidence-based mortality for men and women were the same. Anaplastic thyroid cancer had a higher mortality rate in White and Asian women compared to men, and Asian women had a higher mortality rate compared to all White and Black patients. The authors noted that additional resources should be devoted to decreasing the disparity in mortality for women.

DOCUMENTATION GUIDELINES

- Physical findings: Patency of airway, breathing patterns, voice
- Physical findings of incision: Wound edges, hematoma formation, bleeding, infection
- Presence of complications: Thyrotoxicosis, hypocalcemia, hypothyroidism
- Reaction to diagnosis of thyroid cancer
- Understanding of and interest in cancer support groups

DISCHARGE AND HOME HEALTHCARE GUIDELINES

To maintain a euthyroid state, teach the patient and family the symptoms of hypothyroidism for early detection of problems: weakness, fatigue, cold intolerance, weight gain, facial puffiness, periorbital edema, bradycardia, and hypothermia. Be sure the patient understands all medications, including the dosage, route, action, and adverse effects. Explain that the patient needs routine follow-up laboratory tests to check TSH and thyroxine (T4) levels. Be sure the patient knows when the first postoperative physician's visit is scheduled. Explain any wound care and that the patient should expect to be hoarse for a week or so after the surgical procedure.

Tonsillitis

DRG Category:	145
Mean LOS:	2.4 days
Description:	SURGICAL: Other Ear, Nose, Mouth Throat Operating Room Procedures Without Complication or Comorbidity or Major Complication or Comorbidity

Tonsils are the masses of lymphatic tissue located in the depressions of the mucous membranes of the fauces (constricted opening leading from the mouth to the oral pharynx) and pharynx. The tonsils act as a filter to protect the body from bacterial invasion via the oral cavity and also to produce white blood cells. Tonsillitis is generally referred to as an inflammation of a tonsil, particularly a faucial tonsil. Acute tonsillitis is considered acute pharyngitis. When tonsillar involvement is severe, the term tonsillopharyngitis or tonsillitis is used; when the involvement is minor, the term nasopharyngitis is used. Nearly all children have at least one episode of tonsillitis during their childhood. Complications include difficulty or disrupted breathing, abscesses, and sepsis, and if caused by group A beta-hemolytic streptococci (GABHS), rheumatic fever, scarlet fever, septic arthritis, and poststreptococcal glomerulonephritis.

CAUSES

Viral infection is the leading cause of nasopharyngitis. Adenovirus is the most common infecting agent, but other viruses include enteroviruses, herpes virus, and Epstein-Barr virus. A nonviral cause is *Mycoplasma pneumoniae*. Bacterial causes include GABHS, *Neisseria gonorrheae*, and *Corynebacterium diphtheriae*. Risk factors include childhood and frequent exposure to infectious agents such as often found at a school or day-care center.

GENETIC CONSIDERATIONS

Heritable immune responses could be protective or could increase susceptibility.

SEX AND LIFE SPAN CONSIDERATIONS

Viral tonsillitis is unusual in infants under age 2 years and is most common in children of both sexes ages 4 to 5 years. Bacterial infections are most common in children ages 5 to 11 years.

HEALTH DISPARITIES AND SEXUAL/GENDER MINORITY HEALTH

Ethnicity, race, and sexual/gender minority status have no known effect on the risk for tonsillitis. Sore throat and swollen lymph nodes (adenopathy) are early signs of HIV infection as well as tonsillitis. The Centers for Disease Control and Prevention (2020) reported in 2018 that 69% of new HIV diagnoses in the United States were in gay and bisexual men. In young people ages 13 to 24 years, young gay and bisexual men account for 83% of all new HIV diagnoses. If persons are at risk for HIV and have signs of tonsillitis, they should have HIV testing.

GLOBAL HEALTH CONSIDERATIONS

Children develop tonsillitis in all regions of the world. Recurrent tonsillitis has a prevalence of 10% to 12% in many developed regions; no data are available in developing regions.

☀ ASSESSMENT

HISTORY. Usually, the symptoms of viral tonsillitis have a gradual onset. Elicit a description of the history and progression of the signs and symptoms. Expect that the predominant symptom is rhinorrhea (a runny nose), which is the key symptom. Ask parents if the child also demonstrates other common symptoms: sore throat, dysphagia, mild cough, hoarseness, and a low-grade fever. Ask if any members of the household have had a cold or upper respiratory infection. Bacterial infections have an abrupt onset without rhinorrhea, and viral infections are associated with adenopathy (enlarged lymph nodes). Generally, parents will describe fever, weakness, sore throat, dysphagia, nausea, abdominal discomfort, and vomiting. Symptoms usually resolve in several days but may last longer than a week in some children.

PHYSICAL EXAMINATION. Children with viral and bacterial infections will have symptoms that reflect the infecting organism (Table 1). Common symptoms include **sore throat; foul breath; swollen, painful cervical nodes**; and **difficult, painful swallowing**.

• TABLE 1 Symptoms of Tonsillitis Based on Causative Agent

MICROORGANISM	TONSIL APPEARANCE	OTHER FINDINGS
Epstein-Barr virus	Exudate on tonsils, petechiae on soft palate	Diffuse adenopathy, consider mononucleosis
Adenovirus	Exudate on tonsils	Cervical adenopathy
Enterovirus	Vesicles and sores on tonsils	Vomiting, diarrhea, rhinorrhea
Herpes simplex virus	Tonsil ulcers	Diffuse adenopathy
Bacteria (GABHS is most common)	Red tonsils and uvula, exudates on tonsils, petechiae on soft palate	Anterior cervical adenopathy, rash

PSYCHOSOCIAL. The parents and child will be apprehensive. Assess the parents' ability to cope with the acute situation and intervene as appropriate. Note that many children are treated at home rather than in the hospital; your teaching plan may need to consider home rather than hospital management.

Diagnostic Highlights

General Comments: Diagnostic testing involves identifying the causative organism, determining oxygenation status, and ruling out masses as a cause of obstruction.

Test	Normal Result	Abnormality With Condition	Explanation
Throat culture	Negative for bacteria	Positive for bacteria	To differentiate between viral and bacterial infections (particularly viral from group A beta-hemolytic streptococcus)
Rapid antigen detection test (RADT)	Negative	Positive	Detects the presence of GABHS cell wall carbohydrate; less sensitive than throat culture

Other Tests: Complete blood count, heterophil antibody test to rule out mononucleosis, sleep study to detect sleep apnea or sleep disturbances.

PRIMARY NURSING DIAGNOSIS

DIAGNOSIS. Risk for infection as evidenced by difficulty swallowing, fever, cough, hoarseness, adenopathy, refusal to eat, irritability, sleeplessness, or foul breath.

OUTCOMES. Infection severity; Immune status; Risk control: Infectious process; Symptom control; Symptom severity; Knowledge: Infection management; Knowledge: Medication

INTERVENTIONS. Infection protection; Medication administration; Temperature regulation; Teaching: Prescribed medication

PLANNING AND IMPLEMENTATION
Collaborative

The aim of treatment for a viral infection is to provide supportive care. Usually, fever and sore throat pain can be managed with over-the-counter analgesia. Antibiotic therapy is appropriate for bacterial infections. Allow the child to get rest and provide adequate fluid intake. If the child continues to have symptoms in spite of appropriate antibiotic therapy after cultures and sensitivities, the child may represent a "treatment failure" and may need a different antibiotic. If a relapse occurs, a second course of antibiotics may be needed, and a family member may be a carrier.

Chronic tonsillitis occurs in children with recurrent throat infections (seven in the past year or five in each of the past 2 years). Tonsillectomy and adenoidectomy decrease the incidence of these problems during childhood, although those who do not have surgery also have a decreased incidence of infection. Current recommendations generally encourage physicians to avoid surgery in most cases. Watchful waiting, as compared to tonsillectomy, has been shown to have similar outcomes with quality of life. A Cochrane review shows that tonsillectomy and adenoidectomy are most effective with children who are most severely affected with pharyngitis and that some children will get better without surgery. The decision to remove the tonsils relates directly to hypertrophy, obstruction, chronic infection, and parent/child choice.

Pharmacologic Highlights

Medication or Drug Class	Dosage	Description	Rationale
Non-narcotic analgesia and antipyretics	Varies with drug	Acetaminophen, ibuprofen	Relieve aches and pains and reduce fever
Antibiotics	Varies with drug	Benzathine penicillin G, potassium penicillin V, erythromycin, first-generation cephalosporin, amoxicillin, dicloxacillin, cefdinir, cefuroxime	Halt replication of the bacteria in bacterial infections
Corticosteroids	Varies with drug	Dexamethasone, predni-sone, prednisolone	Reduces inflammation to allow for adequate airway, breathing, and swallowing

Independent

Children should be allowed to rest as much as possible to conserve their energy; organize interventions to limit disturbances. Provide age-appropriate activities. Crying increases the child's difficulty in breathing and should be limited if possible by comfort measures and the presence of the parents; parents should be allowed to hold and comfort the child as much as possible. Provide adequate hydration to liquefy secretions and to replace fluid loss from increased sensible loss (increased respirations and fever). The child might also have a decreased fluid intake during the illness. Apply lubricant or ointment around the child's mouth and lips to decrease the irritation from secretions and mouth breathing. Instruct parents to provide soft foods for swallowing difficulties. Using saltwater gargles, warm liquids, or cold foods may help with throat soreness.

Evidence-Based Practice and Health Policy

Abdel-Naby Awad, O. (2020). Echinacea can help with Azithromycin in prevention of recurrent tonsillitis in children. *American Journal of Otolaryngology*. Advance online publication. https://doi.org/10.1016/j.amjoto.2019.102344

- The authors employed a prospective randomized clinical trial design to evaluate children in the Ear, Nose, Throat Clinic with recurrent tonsillitis who were scheduled for a tonsillectomy. Children were divided into three groups: those who did not receive any prophylactic antibiotics, those who received azithromycin daily for 6 days every month for 6 months, and the last group who received the same antibiotic treatment but also added echinacea to their treatment plan three times daily for 10 days every month for 6 months.
- The first group showed no statistically significant difference between number of tonsillitis episodes compared to the pre-study duration. In the group receiving just the antibiotic treatment, there were a smaller number of tonsillitis episodes reported in comparison to the pre-study duration. The group receiving both the antibiotics and supplemental echinacea reported a significantly less number of attacks during the study than those in the second group. The author concluded that the combined use of azithromycin and echinacea produced more favorable outcome than azithromycin alone in patients with recurrent tonsillitis.

DOCUMENTATION GUIDELINES

- Pain and sore throat: Type, location, severity, response to medications
- Respiratory status: Rate, quality, depth, ease, breath sounds
- Child's response to illness, feeding, rest, and activity; dietary patterns, ability to swallow, fluid intake
- Parent's emotional response

DISCHARGE AND HOME HEALTHCARE GUIDELINES

Most children will be managed at home. Caregivers need to understand the rationale for all medications. If the child has a viral infection, explain to the parents why an antibiotic is not indicated. If the child has a bacterial infection, make sure the parents understand the importance of taking the entire prescription and to report new onset of symptoms if they occur. Reassure parents that frequent infections are not unusual, but if the infections persist, they need to report them to a healthcare provider. The home should be a smoke-free environment to decrease irritation to the child's respiratory tract.

Toxoplasmosis

DRG Category:	868
Mean LOS:	4.6 days
Description:	MEDICAL: Other Infectious and Parasitic Diseases Diagnoses With Complication or Comorbidity

Toxoplasmosis, a parasitic infection that is widespread throughout the world, is caused by *Toxoplasma gondii*, an intracellular protozoan parasite. In the United States, approximately 225,000 cases of toxoplasmosis are reported annually, resulting in 750 deaths. Toxoplasmosis refers to clinical or pathological manifestations of a *T gondii* infection, which occurs when the protozoa invade the cells but does not usually cause symptoms in patients with normal immune systems. Conversion of chronic *T gondii* infection into active toxoplasmosis occurs primarily in severely immunocompromised hosts.

There are three forms of *T gondii*: oocysts, tissue cysts, and tachyzoites. Oocysts are oval shaped and have been found only in cats; this form of *T gondii* can live outside of the host in a warm, moist environment for over a year and therefore may play a major role in transmission of *T gondii* infection. Tissue cysts can contain up to 3,000 organisms. Tachyzoites are the crescent-shaped invasive form of *T gondii*. This form is seen in acute *T gondii* infection and invades all mammalian cells except non-nucleated red blood cells.

Toxoplasmosis is the most common cause of intraocular inflammation. When the organism reaches the eye via the circulation, an infection may begin in the retina, particularly in immunocompromised individuals. Ultimately, a cyst forms, and because the cyst is resistant to the host's defenses, a chronic infection develops. When the person's immune function declines, the cyst wall ruptures and organisms are released into the retina. Other organs can be infected by the organism as well. These organs include the gray and white matter of the brain, the alveolar lining of the lungs, the heart, and the skeletal muscles. HIV-associated toxoplasma encephalitis can result from reactivation of a chronic infection, and congenital toxoplasmosis may be associated with many fetal anomalies such as microcephaly, microphthalmia, hydranencephaly, and hydrocephalus. Complications include encephalitis and seizures. In pregnancy, it can cause stillbirths and miscarriages, and in infants, it can cause seizures, liver and spleen enlargement, jaundice, and eye infections. In children, toxoplasmosis can lead to hearing loss, mental disability, epilepsy, spasticity, palsies, and impaired vision.

CAUSES

The prevalence of a *T gondii* infection seems to be highest in warm, humid climates at lower altitudes; it occurs less frequently in areas at the extremes of temperatures and at high altitudes. The two major routes of *T gondii* transmission to humans are oral and congenital. Tissue cysts are found in a large percentage of meat used for human consumption, especially in lamb and pork. Vegetables and other food products contain a large number of oocysts. Exposure to cat feces also plays a major role in transmission of infection. Risk factors include immunosuppression, HIV disease, pregnancy, and taking immunosuppressive medications such as chemotherapy drugs and corticosteroids.

GENETIC CONSIDERATIONS

Heritable immune responses could be protective or could increase susceptibility.

SEX AND LIFE SPAN CONSIDERATIONS

Toxoplasmosis can occur in at-risk patients of any age and gender. Neonatal toxoplasmosis may occur as a result of acute infection of the pregnant person during pregnancy. Congenitally infected infants who are symptomatic at birth have an 80% chance of developing severe disabilities. As individuals age, most develop antitoxoplasma antibodies. Adults with multiple organ involvement are at high risk for mortality or permanent organ failure. It is more common in the southern United States, in Florida especially, than in other regions, as well as in regions that are underresourced and with people on low incomes.

HEALTH DISPARITIES AND SEXUAL/GENDER MINORITY HEALTH

Ethnicity and race have no known effect on the risk for toxoplasmosis. However, toxoplasmosis can occur in people with immunosuppression caused by HIV disease. Black and Hispanic persons bear a disproportionate burden of HIV disease in the United States compared with other populations. The Centers for Disease Control and Prevention reported in 2018 that 69% of new HIV diagnoses in the United States were in gay and bisexual men. In young people ages 13 to 24 years, young gay and bisexual men account for 83% of all new HIV diagnoses. Therefore, gay and bisexual men, as well as men who have sex with men, are at risk for toxoplasmosis.

GLOBAL HEALTH CONSIDERATIONS

The proportion of people who are seropositive varies by global region. Experts report that in El Salvador and France, up to 75% of people are seropositive in their 30s, whereas in other parts of Western Europe, Africa, and Central/South America, 50% of people are infected. Prevalence is low in China. In South and Central America and Africa, experts estimate that 50% of pregnant people are seropositive for toxoplasmosis.

ASSESSMENT

HISTORY. Most patients are asymptomatic. Ask the patient or significant others if fever or changes in mental state have occurred. Explore the presence of conditions that cause an immunocompromised state, such as HIV disease, organ transplantation accompanied by immunosuppressive therapy, cancer chemotherapy, and hematological malignancies. The term acquired toxoplasmosis is reserved for immunocompetent individuals who have developed clinical manifestations in response to acute infection. Ask about enlarged lymph nodes; a rash; or problems with the heart, liver, lungs, brain, or muscles. Ask patients if they have experienced blurred vision, pain, photophobia, and visual impairment.

Question parents of infants about potential exposure or manifestations of *T gondii* infection that may have occurred during pregnancy. If you suspect congenital toxoplasmosis, which is transmitted in utero from birthing parent to fetus, ask the parent(s) to describe any central nervous system (CNS) or ocular dysfunction. The baby's clinical manifestations may include microcephalus, hydrocephalus, strabismus, cataracts, glaucoma, deafness, or psychomotor retardation.

PHYSICAL EXAMINATION. Signs of low-grade *T gondii* infection include **fever of unknown origin, asymptomatic lymph node enlargement, malaise, headache, sore throat, rash**, and **muscle soreness**. The most common finding is asymptomatic lymphadenopathy, either confined to a single area or region or generalized. Usually, the lymph nodes normalize within a few weeks, but the problem may recur over several months. You may be able to see a rash and palpate an enlarged liver and spleen. Some patients also have signs of dysfunction of the organ or tissue involved (heart, liver, lungs, brain, or muscle). In infants with congenital toxoplasmosis, you may note changes in the shape of the head denoting microcephalus or hydrocephalus, or you may find jaundice and a rash. When you palpate the infant's abdomen, you may feel an enlarged liver or spleen. There may also be signs of myocarditis, pneumonitis, and lymphadenopathy (enlarged lymph nodes).

Ocular toxoplasmosis, which occurs in both acquired and congenital toxoplasmosis, typically causes a lesion on the retina that leads to inflammation of the retina and choroid (retinochoroiditis). An ophthalmoscopic examination reveals patches of yellow-white, cottonlike lesions on the retina. The area around the lesions is usually engorged with blood. Acute toxoplasmosis in the immunocompromised patient is associated with a unique set of clinical manifestations. The patient may have any of the signs and symptoms seen in patients with normal immunity but is more likely to have serious organ involvement as well. More than 50% of these patients have manifestations of CNS involvement, such as altered consciousness, motor impairment, neurological deficits, and seizures. These findings indicate a large *T gondii* brain abscess, or meningoencephalitis. Severe myocarditis and pneumonitis are also common findings in immunocompromised patients with toxoplasmosis.

PSYCHOSOCIAL. Death is a real possibility in toxoplasmosis patients with immune dysfunction. Fear of death and feelings of despair or hopelessness may evolve; patients and families should be encouraged to discuss these openly. Birthing parents of infants with congenital toxoplasmosis may experience feelings of guilt because of their transmission of the infection.

Diagnostic Highlights

Test	Normal Result	Abnormality With Condition	Explanation
Enzyme-linked immunosorbent assay	Negative	Pinpoints specific toxoplasmosis antibody (immunoglobin G [IgG] and M [IgM])	Identify presence of antibodies to parasitic infection

Diagnostic Highlights (continued)

Test	Normal Result	Abnormality With Condition	Explanation
Serum toxoplasmosis antibody assay	IgM titer < 1:64	IgM titer increased	Identify presence of antibodies to parasitic infection
Immunofluorescence	IgG titer < 1:1024	IgG titer increased	Identify presence of antibodies to parasitic infection
Tissue and fluid cultures; fluids are cerebrospinal fluid, lymph node aspirate	Negative for *T gondii*	Positive for *T gondii*	Identify presence of parasitic infection

Other Tests: Serum globulin (increased), complete blood count, lymph node biopsy, brain biopsy, computed tomography scan of the brain, magnetic resonance imaging of the brain, tests for hemagglutination (Sabin-Feldman dye test; generally done only as a reference test in special laboratories because it requires live organisms), brain biopsy, lymph node biopsy, lumbar puncture

PRIMARY NURSING DIAGNOSIS

DIAGNOSIS. Risk for injury as evidenced by visual changes, gait changes, neurological deficits, and/or motor dysfunction

OUTCOMES. Cognitive orientation; Neurological status: Consciousness; Neurological status: Central motor control; Gait; Sensory function: Vision

INTERVENTIONS. Surveillance; Fall prevention; Neurological monitoring; Vision screening; Environmental management: Safety

PLANNING AND IMPLEMENTATION
Collaborative

The challenge in treating toxoplasmosis is that *T gondii* protozoa are resistant to many antimicrobial agents, and they typically invade tissue that is difficult for many drugs to reach. The ideal duration for pharmacotherapy has not been established. Acute acquired toxoplasmosis should be treated only if the patient is extremely symptomatic or severely immunodeficient. The duration of treatment for immunosuppressed patients depends largely on the duration of the immunocompromised state. Patients with permanent immunocompromised states, such as patients with HIV disease with very low CD4 counts, need prophylactic antitoxoplasmosis therapy for the rest of their lives. Because the immune-inflammatory response is thought to be responsible for the pathological processes in ocular toxoplasmosis, glucocorticoid steroids may be ordered in some situations. Steroids have been shown to decrease retinochoroiditis and improve vision but cause further decreased immune function in the immunocompromised patient.

Pharmacologic Highlights

General Comments: The combination of pyrimethamine and sulfadiazine is the treatment of choice for patients with HIV disease who have toxoplasma encephalitis. Trimethoprim sulfamethoxazole is effective in preventing toxoplasma encephalitis in patients with HIV disease who are at risk.

(highlight box continues on page 1172)

Pharmacologic Highlights (continued)

Medication or Drug Class	Dosage	Description	Rationale
Pyrimethamine	75 mg PO loading dose; then 25 mg PO daily	Antiprotozoal	Eradicates the protozoa; given together with sulfonamides or clindamycin; folinic acid (leucovorin) is given to reduce bone marrow toxicity
Sulfonamides and antimicrobials	Varies with drug	Sulfadiazine, tri-methoprim and sulfa-methoxazole, dapsone, trisulfapyrimidines	Eradicates the protozoa; given together with sulfonamides; folinic acid is given to reduce bone marrow toxicity

Other Drugs: Clindamycin, azithromycin, atovaquone; spiramycin is used for pregnant person or fetal toxoplasmosis

Independent

Patients with toxoplasmosis do not require any special precautions to prevent the spread of infection; universal precautions are sufficient. There is no evidence that toxoplasmosis can be spread from person to person. The sensory and neurological deficits associated with acute disseminated toxoplasmosis present the greatest nursing challenges. During the management of patients with acute neurological changes, assess the neurological status at least hourly. Include assessments of orientation, memory, and thought processes; the strength and motion of the extremities; sensory alterations; pupil response; and the patient's speech, emotional response, and behaviors. Provide adequate safety measures as indicated: bed location where the patient can be closely monitored, padding of side rails, and assistance with ambulation or activities of daily living. Reorient the patient as often as necessary, provide opportunities for undisturbed sleep, and ensure appropriate amounts of sensory stimulation. Have the patient talk about topics of interest and importance, such as hobbies, family, occupation, or current sports and news. Encourage family members to bring pictures and other items from home that help the patient focus on pleasant memories. Institute active or passive range-of-motion exercises to maintain neuromuscular function and prevent contractures. Initiate seizure precautions for patients with suspected brain involvement.

Because toxoplasmosis can affect virtually every tissue in the body, the patient often experiences pain and nausea. Choice of analgesic and antinausea agents requires close consultation with the physician, taking into consideration actual or potential neurological alterations. Nonpharmacologic pain relief methods can be instituted to augment the effect of analgesics, such as relaxation techniques, frequent repositioning to level of comfort, soothing music, and massage therapy. If vision is impaired, the patient needs assistance with activities of daily living. Everyone entering the room should identify themselves by name. Referral to social work services or community organizations for the blind may be indicated if ocular involvement is severe.

Evidence-Based Practice and Health Policy

Fernandes, S., Dias, A., & Miranda-Scippa, A. (2020). Association between exposure to toxoplasmosis and major psychiatric disorders: A systematic review. *Brazilian Journal of Psychiatry*, *43*, 438–445.

- The authors wanted to assess the association between exposure to toxoplasmosis and major psychiatric disorders through a systematic review of the literature. They used multiple electronic databases and evaluated the quality of 31 studies.
- The majority of the articles reported an association between exposure to toxoplasmosis and schizophrenia (58%) or bipolar disorder (55%), but not major depressive disorder. The authors

noted that the results indicate an association with both bipolar disorder and schizophrenia, despite their heterogeneity. They suggested that further studies should be performed with more specific variables so that the nature of these relationships can be understood further.

DOCUMENTATION GUIDELINES

- Neurological status: Memory, orientation, thought processes, behaviors, emotions, motor function, sensory function, speech, pupil response
- Patient's or family members' mood and emotional response to the diagnosis of toxoplasmosis and the associated poor prognosis
- Physical responses: Status of lymph nodes (enlargement, any changes from baseline), presence of fever, response to interventions
- Abnormal assessment findings from organs commonly affected by acute toxoplasmosis: Heart, liver, lungs, eyes (visual disturbances)

DISCHARGE AND HOME HEALTHCARE GUIDELINES

Teach the patient and family about the medications. Pyrimethamine can cause folic acid deficiency. The patient should report bleeding, bruising, visual changes, and feelings of fatigue. Folic acid supplements may be recommended by the physician. Pyrimethamine should be taken just before or after meals to minimize gastric distress. Sulfadiazine can cause decreased white blood cell count, cause fever and rash, and lead to crystals in the urine; it should be taken with a full glass of water, and daily fluid intake should be at least 2,000 mL. Sulfadiazine causes increased sensitivity to the sun; the patient should avoid prolonged sun exposure and wear sunscreen when going outdoors.

If the patient has HIV disease or some other condition that causes a permanent immunocompromised state, emphasize that these drugs probably are needed throughout the patient's lifetime. If the patient has neuromuscular defects, teach family members the exercises needed to maintain muscle strength and joint range of motion. If the patient has neurological involvement and is not on antiseizure medications, teach the patient and significant others how to recognize a seizure and what to do if it occurs. Discuss the long-term prognosis for acquired toxoplasmosis; assist the patient and family in drawing up an appropriate plan of action.

Tuberculosis

DRG Category: 177
Mean LOS: 6.9 days
Description: MEDICAL: Respiratory Infections and Inflammations With Major Complication or Comorbidity

Tuberculosis (TB) is an infectious disease caused by *Mycobacterium tuberculosis*, an aerobic acid-fast bacillus and the most common cause of infectious disease mortality in the world. Although it is most frequently a pulmonary disease, more than 15% of patients experience extrapulmonary TB that can infect the meninges, kidneys, bones, or other tissues. Pulmonary TB can range from a small infection of bronchopneumonia to diffuse, intense inflammation, necrosis, pleural effusion, and extensive fibrosis.

Although TB at one time was thought to be preventable and treatable, the number of cases increased steadily in the 1980s in the United States until approximately 1993. The increase was thought to be due to a high infection rate in patients with HIV disease and patients who were exposed to others hospitalized with TB, as well as a new strain of the disease that is resistant to traditional drugs such as isoniazid (isonicotinylhydrazide [INH]) and rifampin (RIF). Since 1993, the incidence of TB decreased by 61% in the United States due to intensive public health efforts to prevent and control the disease, and it is now at the lowest levels in history. In 2020, 7,163 cases of TB were reported to the Centers for Disease Control and Prevention (CDC, 2021). Complications include pulmonary hemorrhage, joint damage, meningitis, liver and kidney dysfunction, and pericarditis.

CAUSES

TB is transmitted by respiratory droplets through sneezing or coughing by an infected person. Most infected persons have had a sustained exposure to the active agent rather than a single one. The *M tuberculosis* bacilli are inspired into the respiratory tract and usually lodge in the lower part of the upper lobe or the upper part of the lower lobe. The TB bacilli need high levels of oxygen to survive. When they reach the lungs, they multiply rapidly.

Mycobacteria that are not destroyed lie dormant until there is a decrease in the host's resistance. Of individuals who inhale mycobacteria, 5% develop clinical TB at that time, and 95% have been infected and have no clinical symptoms but enter a latent phase and are at risk to develop TB later. People who are immunocompromised, such as those with HIV disease, are at risk for developing TB as well as people who travel from an area where TB is endemic; people who are malnourished; and people who live in underresourced, crowded housing.

GENETIC CONSIDERATIONS

Mutations in several genes have been associated with increasing susceptibility to TB. These include variants in human leukocyte antigen DQB1 (*HLA-DQB1*), *SLC11A1*, the vitamin D receptor, the mannose-binding protein (*MBL2*), *CD209*, and *MCP1*. These gene variants have been studied in populations where TB was endemic.

SEX AND LIFE SPAN CONSIDERATIONS

TB can occur at any age but is most common in the older population, in men as compared to women, and in those who are immunosuppressed. Since 1980, the largest increase in TB has been in men ages 25 to 44 years and in children under age 15 years.

HEALTH DISPARITIES AND SEXUAL/GENDER MINORITY HEALTH

In the United States, approximately 70% of TB cases occur among underrepresented and vulnerable groups. The states with the highest numbers of cases are California, New York, Texas, and Florida, and Alaska has the highest incidence. Foreign-born individuals, particularly people born in Asia (India, Vietnam, China, Philippines) and Mexico, are more likely to have TB than people born in the United States (CDC, 2021). Other high-risk groups are hospital employees, urban dwellers, drug and alcohol abusers, people who are homeless, nursing home residents, and people who are incarcerated. In Black, Hispanic, and Asian persons, the median age of onset of the infection is 39 years, whereas in White persons, the median age of onset is 62 years. TB can occur in people with immunosuppression caused by HIV disease. Black and Hispanic people bear a disproportionate burden of HIV disease in the United States compared with other populations. The CDC reported in 2018 that 69% of new HIV diagnoses in the United States were in gay and bisexual men. In young people ages 13 to 24 years, young gay and bisexual men account for 83% of all new HIV diagnoses. Therefore, gay and bisexual men, as well as men who have sex with men, are a group that is at risk for TB.

GLOBAL HEALTH CONSIDERATIONS

TB is a disease of poverty, economic distress, vulnerability, stigma, and discrimination, but it is also curable (World Health Organization [WHO], 2020). TB is one of the leading causes of death internationally, and approximately 95% of all TB cases occur in the poorest countries where resources are limited and HIV disease is common. Approximately 10 million cases occur yearly, and annual mortality worldwide is estimated at more than 1.2 million people without HIV disease and approximately 250,000 with HIV disease. Sub-Saharan regions in Africa have the highest incidence rates of multidrug-resistant (MDR) TB, while Southeast Asia (India and China in particular) has the largest number of infected people overall (WHO, 2020).

ASSESSMENT

HISTORY. Ask patients about a previous history of TB or Hodgkin disease, diabetes mellitus, leukemia, gastrectomy, silicosis (a disease resulting from inhalation of quartz dust), and immunosuppressive disorders such as HIV infection. A history of corticosteroid or immunosuppressive drug therapy can also increase the likelihood of TB infection. Other risk factors include a history of multiple sexual partners; abuse of drugs or alcohol; foreign travel to endemic areas; or being homeless, housed in a shelter, or incarcerated. Determine if the patient has had recent contact with a newly diagnosed TB patient or has resided in any type of long-term facility. Take an occupational history as well to determine if the patient is a healthcare worker and therefore at risk.

Ask the patient to describe any symptoms. The patient often reports generalized weakness and fatigue, activity intolerance, and shortness of breath on exertion. Anorexia and weight loss occur because of altered taste and indigestion. The patient may also describe difficulty sleeping, chills or night sweats (or both), chest pain, and either a productive or a nonproductive cough.

PHYSICAL EXAMINATION. Common symptoms are **cough, hemoptysis, night sweats, fever, chest pain, weight loss, anorexia, muscle wasting, malaise,** and **fatigue.** The patient looks acutely ill on inspection, with muscle wasting, poor muscle tone, loss of subcutaneous fat, poor skin turgor, and dry flaky skin. When you auscultate the chest, you may hear a rapid heart rate, rapid and difficult breathing, and stridor. Diminished or absent breath sounds may be present bilaterally or unilaterally from pleural effusion or pneumothorax. Tubular breath sounds or whispered pectoriloquia may be heard over large lesions, as may crackles over the apex of the lungs during quick inspiration after a short cough. Other findings include fever and lymphadenopathy. Some patients have confusion, coma, and neurological deficits if they have central nervous system involvement.

The sputum appears green, purulent, yellowish, mucoid, or blood tinged. The patient may have pain, stiffness, and guarding of the affected painful area. Accumulation of secretions can decrease oxygenation of vital organs and tissues. You may note cyanosis or a change in skin color, mucous membranes, or nailbeds and changes in mental status, such as distraction, restlessness, inattention, or marked irritability.

PSYCHOSOCIAL. Patients dependent on alcohol or drugs, those who are economically disadvantaged, and those who live in crowded conditions are at risk. The living environment needs careful assessment. Ask about living conditions, including the number of people in the household. Patients may have recent or longstanding stress factors, adjustment to recent immigration, financial concerns, and feelings of helplessness or hopelessness. They may experience feelings of alienation or rejection because they have a communicable disease and are in isolation. They may have changes in patterns of responsibility, physical strength, and capacity to resume roles because of TB. Assess the patient's ability to cope. Assess the degree of anxiety or depression about the illness, the change in health status, and the change in roles.

Diagnostic Highlights

Test	Normal Result	Abnormality With Condition	Explanation
Fluorochrome or acid-fast bacilli sputum	Negative	Positive; three samples are often obtained	Mycobacterium tuberculosis is a bacterium that resists decolorizing chemicals after staining
Chest x-ray, Computed tomography	Normal lung structures	Identification of active TB or old lesions	Radiographic assessment of the lungs

(highlight box continues on page 1176)

Diagnostic Highlights (continued)

Other Tests: Histology or tissue analysis, needle biopsy, purified protein derivative (Mantoux test), blood cultures, urine cultures, HIV testing, enzyme-linked immunospot (ELISpot) and enzyme-linked immunosorbent assay (ELISA) to detect TB antigens

PRIMARY NURSING DIAGNOSIS

DIAGNOSIS. Risk for infection as evidenced by fever, hemoptysis, night sweats, chest pain, and/or weight loss

OUTCOMES. Infection severity; Immune status; Symptom severity; Symptom control; Knowledge: Infection management; Risk control: Infectious process

INTERVENTIONS. Infection protection; Medication management; Medication administration; Teaching: Prescribed medication; Teaching: Disease process

▒ PLANNING AND IMPLEMENTATION
Collaborative

Because TB typically becomes resistant to any single-drug therapy, patients generally receive a combination of drugs. The most common combination of drugs prescribed in the United States is INH, RIF, pyrazinamide (PZA), and either ethambutol (ETB) or streptomycin. Some experts recommend up to 9 months of drug therapy, whereas patients with drug-resistant strains of TB may require as much as 24 months of treatment. IV fluids, total parenteral nutrition, and food supplements may be needed for those with nutritional compromise. Humidity and oxygen are administered to correct hypoxia and to decrease the thickness of secretions. Emergency intubation and mechanical ventilation may be needed in extreme cases.

Teach the patient how and when to take medication and to complete the course of drug therapy because one of the primary reasons for the development of drug-resistant TB strains is the failure of patients to complete medication regimens. If you suspect that the patient may not adhere to the medication regimen, a home health referral is important after the patient is discharged.

Pharmacologic Highlights

The WHO has initiated a directly observed treatment short course (DOTS) of medications, which consists of five medications in a short-course chemotherapy regimen (INH, RIF, PZA, and ETB and/or streptomycin). DOTS involves people directly observing patients taking their anti-TB medications. This strategy is considered a cost-effective intervention and has been adopted by more than 100 countries. Multiple resistances to medications remain a significant problem. MDR-TB is resistant to either INH and/or RIF, whereas extensive drug-resistant (XDR) TB is resistant to at least INH and RIF, resistant to fluoroquinolone, and resistant to at least one of the following: amikacin, capreomycin, or kanamycin. Note that combinations of the drugs below are titrated to obtain the optimal response. One protocol suggested by the Centers for Disease Control and Prevention is as follows for daily therapy: initially for 2 months by mouth, INH 300 mg daily, RIF 600 mg daily, PZA 2 g daily, and ETB 2 g daily. For the final 4 months following negative smear and improvement in symptoms, INH 300 mg daily and RIF 600 mg daily.

Medication or Drug Class	Dosage	Description	Rationale
INH	5 mg/kg per day PO once a day	Antitubercular	Inhibits synthesis of bacterial cell wall and hinders cell division

Pharmacologic Highlights (continued)

Medication or Drug Class	Dosage	Description	Rationale
RIF	10 mg/kg per day PO once a day	Antitubercular	Interferes with RNA synthesis; able to kill slower-growing organisms that reside in granuloma in lungs or other organs
PZA	15–30 mg/kg PO once a day	Antitubercular	Bacteriostatic or bacteriocidal
ETB	15 mg/kg PO once a day	Antitubercular	Interferes with cell metabolism and multiplication by inhibiting bacterial metabolites
Streptomycin	1,000 mg IM or IV daily	Aminoglycoside antibiotic	Transported across cell membrane, binds to receptor proteins, and prevents cell reproduction

Other Drugs: Second-line medications include cycloserine, ethionamide, and capreomycin sulfate. Mucolytics are used to thin secretions and facilitate expectoration. Increased fluid intake decreases secretions. Bronchodilators increase the lumen size of the bronchial tree and decrease resistance to airflow. Corticosteroids are used in extreme cases when inflammation causes life-threatening hypoxia. Newer drugs include rifapentine, ofloxacin, levofloxacin, gatifloxacin, and immune amplifiers.

Independent

Nursing priorities are to maintain and achieve adequate ventilation and oxygenation; prevent the spread of infection; support behaviors to maintain health; promote effective coping strategies; and provide information about the disease process, prognosis, and treatment needs. Arrange for identification and prophylactic treatment of all family members and household and community contacts.

Use respiratory isolation precautions (masks only) for all patients with pulmonary TB who require hospitalization. Whenever they leave their rooms or receive treatment from the hospital staff, patients should wear masks to help prevent transmission of TB. The masks need to fit tightly and not gap. Teach the patient to cover the mouth when coughing and to dispose of all tissues. For patients with excessive secretions or those who are unable to cooperate with respiratory isolation, gowns and gloves may be necessary for hospital staff. The nurse should always remember to wash hands before and after patient contact.

Position the patient in a Fowler or semi-Fowler position and assist with coughing and deep-breathing exercises. Demonstrate and encourage pursed-lip breathing on expiration, especially for patients with fibrosis or parenchymal destruction. Promote bedrest and activity restrictions and assist with self-care activities as needed.

Teach the patient and family how to use proper protection methods to prevent infection or reinfection. In the case of treatment at home, the family has probably already been exposed to the patient before diagnosis, so wearing masks is not necessary. Advise the family members that they need regular TB testing to ensure that they have not contracted TB. Teach the patient about complications of TB, such as recurrence and hemorrhage, and the need for proper nutrition.

Evidence-Based Practice and Health Policy

Leung, C., Huang, H., Rahman, M., Nomura, S., Abe, S., Saito, E., & Shibuya, K. (2020). Cancer incidence attributable to tuberculosis in 2015: Global, regional, and national estimates. *BMC Cancer, 20,* 412.

• Because TB is associated with increased risk of cancer, the authors wanted to assess the impact of TB on global cancer burden, which is currently unknown. The authors conducted meta-analyses of studies reporting the association between TB and cancer risks by searching electronic databases through June 1, 2019. Population attributable fractions (PAFs) of cancer

incidence attributable to TB were calculated using relative risks by age, sex, and country. The authors included 49 studies of 52,480 cancer cases.
• TB was associated with head and neck cancer, hepatobiliary cancer, Hodgkin lymphoma, lung cancer, gastrointestinal cancer, non-Hodgkin lymphoma, pancreatic cancer, leukemia, kidney and bladder cancer, and ovarian cancer. The authors estimated that 2.33% of global cancer incidences in 2015 were attributable to TB. Attribution varied by sociodemographics ranging from 1.28% in the high-income countries to 3.51% in the middle-income countries. Individually, China and India accounted for 47% of all TB-related cancer cases. TB is associated with increased risk of cancer at 10 locations in the body. The burden of TB-attributable cancer skewed toward lower-resource countries.

DOCUMENTATION GUIDELINES
• Physical changes: Breath sounds, quality and quantity of sputum, vital signs, mental status
• Tolerance to activity and level of fatigue
• Complications and changes in oxygen exchange or airway clearance
• Response to medications

DISCHARGE AND HOME HEALTHCARE GUIDELINES
Advise the patient to quit smoking, avoid excess alcohol intake, maintain adequate nutrition, and avoid exposure to crowds and others with upper respiratory infections. Teach appropriate preventive measures. Be sure the patient understands all medications, including the dosage, route, action, and adverse effects. Instruct the patient to abstain from alcohol while on INH and refer for eye examination after starting and then every month while taking ethambutol. Teach the patient to recognize symptoms such as fever, difficulty breathing, hearing loss, and chest pain that should be reported to healthcare personnel. Discuss the patient's living condition and the number of people in the household. Give the patient a list of referrals if the patient is homeless or economically at risk.

Ulcerative Colitis

DRG Category:	394
Mean LOS:	3.8 days
Description:	MEDICAL: Other Digestive System Diagnoses With Complication or Comorbidity
DRG Category:	329
Mean LOS:	13.1 days
Description:	SURGICAL: Major Small and Large Bowel Procedures With Major Complication or Comorbidity

Ulcerative colitis is a chronic inflammatory disease of the colon, and 20% of the cases occur before the individual reaches age 20 years. Approximately 1 million people have ulcerative colitis in the United States. Usually, the disease begins in the rectum and sigmoid colon and gradually spreads up the colon in a continuous distribution pattern. The inflammatory process involves the mucosa and submucosa of the colon.

Gradually, multiple ulcerations and abscesses form at the inflamed areas. As the disease progresses, the colon mucosa becomes edematous and thickened with scar tissue formation, which results in altered absorptive capabilities of the colon. The severity of the disease ranges from a mild form that is localized in specific areas of the bowel to a critical syndrome with life-threatening complications. The most common complications are nutritional deficiencies; other complications include sepsis, fistulae, abscesses, and hemorrhage. For unknown reasons, patients with ulcerative colitis also have a high risk for arthritis and cancer, but all those conditions have immune dysregulation in common.

CAUSES

Research has not established a specific cause for ulcerative colitis. Several theories are being pursued, including infectious agents such as a virus or bacteria, immune factors, environmental factors such as geographic location, and genetic factors. Current thinking holds that psychosomatic factors such as emotional stress are a result of the chronic and severe symptoms of ulcerative colitis rather than a cause, as was once thought. Risk factors include smoking, consumption of milk products, use of NSAIDs, psychological stress, and family history.

GENETIC CONSIDERATIONS

Ulcerative colitis, a form of inflammatory bowel disease (IBD) is caused by the action of multiple genes working together (polygenic). There have been 163 risk loci identified for IBD, with most variants occurring in patients with both ulcerative colitis and Crohn disease. There has been an association between ulcerative colitis and rare variations in intestinal mucin-3 gene (*MUC3A*). Mutations in several immune-modulating genes certainly appear to be modulators of IBD risk, including the *IL6R*. Heritable immune responses could be protective or increase susceptibility. In addition, recent evidence indicates that the *GLI1* gene, which has not been previously associated with immune modulation, appears to be important for an appropriate inflammatory response in both humans and mice. Studies are ongoing.

SEX AND LIFE SPAN CONSIDERATIONS

The peak incidence occurs during the early adolescent and young adult years, often between ages 15 and 25 years, thus hampering normal growth and development. Girls are affected more often than boys. There is also evidence of a second peak incidence among those ages 55 to 65 years. Two factors that may predispose the older population to ulcerative colitis are their increased vulnerability to infection and their susceptibility to inadequate blood supply to the bowel.

HEALTH DISPARITIES AND SEXUAL/GENDER MINORITY HEALTH

Some studies show that ulcerative colitis occurs more frequently in White persons than Black, Hispanic, and Asian persons. However, Black persons are more likely than White persons to receive their diagnosis at a later age and present with more complications and with more advanced disease. Delays in diagnosis for Black patients may occur because of limited access to specialists or provider bias. White patients are also more likely to receive biologic agents and immunotherapy compared to all other patients, demonstrating health disparities for non-White groups (Barnes et al., 2021). While people who are sexual and gender minorities have no known specific risk for ulcerative colitis, they are at risk for multiple chronic conditions, experience fear of discrimination, have low rates of health insurance, and have negative experiences with healthcare providers (ACS, 2021). These factors may create barriers to obtaining healthcare and may lead to risk.

GLOBAL HEALTH CONSIDERATIONS

Ulcerative colitis exists around the world, but prevalence varies. The prevalence rate is 35 to 100 cases per 100,000 individuals in North America and Western Europe, and prevalence rates are lower in South America, Asia, and Africa.

ASSESSMENT

HISTORY. A patient with acute ulcerative colitis typically reports rectal bleeding with numerous episodes of bloody diarrhea and mucus discharge from the rectum. The number of stools may range from 4 to 5 to 10 to 25 per day during severe episodes, often causing sleepless nights. In addition, the patient may describe abdominal pain and cramping that is relieved with defecation.

Ask the patient about accompanying symptoms such as fatigue, abdominal distention, anorexia, nausea, and weight loss. Some patients will have a history of low-grade fevers. Take a medical history to determine if other inflammatory conditions exist, such as pleuritis, uveitis (inflammation of the uvea of the eye), ankylosing spondylitis (spinal arthritis), and other joint swelling.

PHYSICAL EXAMINATION. The most common symptoms are **abdominal pain and cramping that is relieved with defecation of bloody stools.** Other symptoms may include **fatigue, diminished appetite with weight loss, low-grade fever,** and **nausea with vomiting.** Because ulcerative colitis is a chronic disease, which may cause periods of anorexia, diarrhea, and intestinal malabsorption, inspect for the signs of malnutrition and dehydration: dry mucous membranes, poor skin turgor, muscle weakness, and lethargy. Palpate the patient's abdomen for tenderness and pain. Typically, pain is noted in the left lower quadrant of the abdomen. Auscultate the patient's abdomen; bowel sounds are often hyperactive during the inflammatory process.

Assess the patient for infection. During the acute inflammatory process, monitor the patient's vital signs every 4 hours or more frequently if the patient's condition is unstable. Watch for temperature elevations and rapid heart rate, which often indicate an infectious process.

PSYCHOSOCIAL. The effects of chronic illness and debilitating symptoms often result in psychological problems for the patient with this disease. Note the patient's current psychological status because depression is common for those with ulcerative colitis. Because emotional stress increases bowel activity and plays a critical role in the exacerbation of the disease, it is also important to assess the patient's current life stressors. In addition, determine the need for instruction on stress reduction techniques.

Diagnostic Highlights

Test	Normal Result	Abnormality With Condition	Explanation
Colonoscopy; sigmoidoscopy	Normal bowel mucosa	Edematous, friable bowel mucosa with loss of vascular pattern and frequent ulcerations	Direct visualization of mucosa by endoscopic examination
Barium enema with air contrast	Normal bowel	Identifies distribution and depth of disease involvement	Fluoroscopic and radiographic examination of large intestine after rectal instillation of barium sulfate to identify structural abnormalities (use with caution in severe cases)

Other Tests: Complete blood count, transabdominal bowel sonography, computed tomography, abdominal x-ray, plasma electrolytes, stool culture and sensitivity, biopsy, serology markers such as antineutrophil cytoplasmic antibodies

PRIMARY NURSING DIAGNOSIS

DIAGNOSIS. Imbalanced nutrition: less than body requirements related to anorexia, diarrhea, and/or decreased absorption from the intestines as evidenced by diminished appetite and/or weight loss

OUTCOMES. Nutritional status: Food and fluid intake; Nutritional status: Nutrient intake; Bowel elimination; Fluid balance; Electrolyte balance

INTERVENTIONS. Nutrition management; Nutrition therapy; Nutritional counseling; Nutrition monitoring; Fluid/electrolyte management; Enteral tube feeding; IV therapy; Total parenteral nutrition administration

✳ PLANNING AND IMPLEMENTATION
Collaborative
MEDICAL. Treatment depends on the stage, extent, and severity of the disease. Drug therapy is the typical method used to control the inflammatory process. Mesalazine suppository and budesonide foam are the primary drugs used to achieve remission for mild disease. After remission is established, dosages are generally reduced, and patients continue on this agent for at least 1 year after an acute attack. Oral mesalazine or sulfasalazine may also be given.

To maintain fluid and electrolyte balance during acute attacks, IV fluids are generally prescribed, and electrolytes may be added to the solutions as needed. Blood transfusions may also be prescribed if the patient is anemic because of numerous bloody diarrheal stools. To achieve bowel "rest," the patient is usually given nothing by mouth. During this time, nutritional deficits may be managed through the use of total parenteral nutrition with vitamin supplements. Helping patients maintain an adequate nutritional status, fluid balance, and electrolyte balance is a priority nursing measure. Record intake and output accurately every shift. Note the number of stools and stool characteristics.

Gradually, as the acute attack subsides and inflammation clears, the patient is placed on a low-residue, low-fat, high-calorie, high-protein, and lactose-free diet.

SURGICAL. Surgery may be performed when patients fail to respond to conservative treatment, if acute episodes are frequent, or when a complication such as bleeding or perforation occurs. The standard surgical procedure, when performed, is a total proctocolectomy with ileostomy. This procedure is considered a permanent cure for ulcerative colitis. To prepare the patient for surgery, administer bowel preparations such as laxatives and enemas.

Pharmacologic Highlights

Medication or Drug Class	Dosage	Description	Rationale
Mesalamine (Asacol, Pentasa), sulfasalazine, balsalazide	Varies by drug	Anti-inflammatory agents	Treatment of choice to induce and maintain remission
Tumor necrosis factor inhibitors	Varies with drug	Infliximab, golimumab, adalimumab	Prevents endogenous cytokines from binding to receptors
Corticosteroids	Varies with drug	Methylprednisolone, prednisone, hydrocortisone, budesonide	Used in acute exacerbations to reduce the inflammatory response; agents are administered until clinical symptoms subside, at which time steroidal agents are tapered off

Other Drugs: Other drugs include immunosuppressant agents (cyclosporine, azathioprine). Antidiarrheal agents alleviate symptoms of abdominal cramping and diarrhea in patients with mild symptoms or postresection diarrhea. Metronidazole (Flagyl) is effective in colon disease; it treats infections with fistulae and perianal skin breakdown and is beneficial in patients who have not responded to other agents. Some patients suffering with severe abdominal pain may require narcotic analgesics such as meperidine (Demerol). Also, patients who develop deficiencies because of problems of malabsorption may require vitamin B_{12} injections monthly or iron replacement therapy. Other nutritional supplements include calcium, magnesium, folate, and other micronutrients.

Independent
Promote patient physical and emotional comfort. Encourage the patient to assume the position of comfort. Instruct in distraction techniques as needed. Promote mental comfort by encouraging

the patient to share thoughts and feelings and provide supportive, empathetic care. Discuss measures to decrease life stressors. Teach the patient about the disease process and the typical treatment regimen. Areas to include in the teaching plan are the signs of disease complications, the importance of rest and stress reduction, and any dietary adjustments.

If the patient requires surgery, several nursing interventions are important in the preoperative phase. First, conduct preoperative teaching sessions on deep-breathing techniques and leg exercises. Also, discuss the operative procedure and the typical postoperative course. When appropriate, discuss with the patient information on stoma placement and stoma care. After surgery, ensure a healthy respiratory status for the patient by encouraging the patient to cough and deep-breathe every 1 to 2 hours. Manage patient pain and discomfort with prescribed analgesics and proper positioning techniques. Monitor for adequate wound healing by checking the color and approximation of the wound and noting any wound drainage or odor. Note the stoma size and color during every shift, and immediately report any duskiness noted at the stoma site. Note the condition of the skin around the stoma; protect the skin with appropriate barrier products because ileostomy drainage is extremely caustic to skin tissues. Finally, encourage the patient's participation in ostomy care. Assess whether a community resource person from the United Ostomy Associations of America is needed to offer the patient additional support.

Evidence-Based Practice and Health Policy

Barnes, E., Jiang, Y., Kappelman, M., Long, M., Sandler, R., Kinlaw, A., & Herfarth, H. (2020). Decreasing colectomy rate for ulcerative colitis in the United States between 2007 and 2016: A time trend analysis. *Inflammatory Bowel Diseases, 26*, 1225–1231.

* The authors aimed to estimate the quarterly rates for colectomy before and after the emergence of newly available biologic therapies in 2014. They used a retrospective cohort design analyzing 93,930 patients, 2.4% of whom underwent colectomy, in a database of commercially insured patients in the United States.
* Rates of biologic use increased significantly from 2007 to 2016, from 131 per 1,000 to 589 per 1,000. Colectomy rates decreased significantly to 7.8 per 1,000 (2007) to 4.2 per 1,000 (2016). The authors concluded that as biologic use rates increased, colectomy rates deceased, suggesting that new therapies may have contributed to decreased colectomy rates.

DOCUMENTATION GUIDELINES

* Evidence of stability of vital signs, hydration status, bowel sounds, and electrolytes
* Response to medications, tolerance of foods, and ability to eat and select a well-balanced diet
* Location, intensity, frequency of pain, and factors that relieve pain
* Number of diarrheal episodes and stool characteristics
* Description of discharge and follow-up instructions given to the patient
* Presence of complications: Hemorrhage, bowel strictures, bowel perforation, infection
* Patient participation in care of stoma and periostomal skin

DISCHARGE AND HOME HEALTHCARE GUIDELINES

The patient must understand all prescribed medications, including actions, side effects, dosages, and routes. Emphasize ways to prevent future episodes of inflammation (rest, relaxation, stress reduction, well-balanced diet). Review the symptoms of inflammation. Teach the patient to seek medical attention if such symptoms occur. Be certain the patient understands symptoms of complications, such as hemorrhage, bowel strictures and perforation, and infection. The patient must know to seek medical attention if these complications should occur. Ensure that the patient understands the importance of close follow-up because of the high incidence of colon and rectal cancer in patients with ulcerative colitis.

Urinary Tract Infection

DRG Category:	689
Mean LOS:	4.2 days
Description:	MEDICAL: Kidney and Urinary Tract Infections With Major Complication or Comorbidity

Urinary tract infections (UTIs) are common and usually occur because of the entry of bacteria into the urinary tract at the urethra. Approximately 20% to 40% of women have a UTI sometime during their lifetime, and acute UTIs account for approximately 7 million healthcare visits per year. About 20% of women who develop a UTI experience recurrences. Women are more prone to UTIs than men because of natural anatomical variations. The female urethra is only about 1 to 2 inches in length, whereas the male urethra is 7 to 8 inches long. The female urethra is also closer to the anus than the male urethra, increasing women's risk for fecal contamination. The motion during sexual intercourse also increases the female's risk for infection.

Urinary reflux is one reason that bacteria spread in the urinary tract. Vesicourethral reflux occurs when pressure increases in the bladder from coughing or sneezing and pushes urine into the urethra. When pressure returns to normal, the urine moves back into the bladder, taking with it bacteria from the urethra. In vesicoureteral reflux, urine flows backward from the bladder into one or both of the ureters, carrying bacteria from the bladder to the ureters and widening the infection. If they are left untreated, UTIs can lead to chronic infections, pyelonephritis, and even systemic sepsis and septic shock. If infection reaches the kidneys, permanent renal damage can occur, which leads to acute and chronic renal failure.

CAUSES

The pathogen that accounts for about 90% of UTIs is *Escherichia coli*. Other organisms that are commonly found in the gastrointestinal tract and may contaminate the genitourinary tract include *Enterobacter, Pseudomonas*, group B beta-hemolytic streptococci, *Proteus mirabilis, Klebsiella* and *Proteus* species, and *Serratia*. Two growing causes of UTIs in the United States are *Staphylococcus saprophyticus* and *Candida albicans*.

Risk factors are urethral damage from childbirth, catheterization, or surgery; decreased frequency of urination; other medical conditions such as diabetes mellitus; and in women, frequent sexual activity and some forms of contraceptives (poorly fitting diaphragms, use of spermicides).

GENETIC CONSIDERATIONS

Increased susceptibility to UTIs has been observed in women and female children who have no anatomical predisposing factors, making genetic contributions suspect. Incidence of UTIs among first-degree female relatives has been reported to be 50% higher than in nonrelatives. In some families, the predisposition has suggested a dominantly inherited trait determined by a single gene, while in others, recessive or polygenic inheritance seems more likely.

SEX AND LIFE SPAN CONSIDERATIONS

UTIs are uncommon in children. The largest group of individuals with UTI is adult women, and the incidence increases with age. Once young and adult women become sexually active, the incidence of UTI increases dramatically. UTIs are common during pregnancy and are caused by the hormonal changes and urinary stasis that result from ureteral dilation. Men secrete prostatic fluid that serves as an antibacterial defense, particularly during their teen and early adulthood years. As men age past 50 years, however, the prostate gland enlarges, which increases the risk for urinary retention and infection. As women age, vaginal flora and lubrication change; decreased lubrication increases the risk of urethral irritation in women during intercourse. By age 70 years, prevalence is similar for men and women.

HEALTH DISPARITIES AND SEXUAL/GENDER MINORITY HEALTH

Ethnicity, race, and sexual/gender minority status have no known effect on the risk for UTI.

GLOBAL HEALTH CONSIDERATIONS

In men living in developed countries, the incidence is comparable to that in the United States. In developing countries with a shorter life expectancy, rates are lower for men than in the United States, possibly because of the reduced incidence of prostatic hypertrophy in younger men. UTIs in both developed and developing countries are extremely common in women.

ASSESSMENT

HISTORY. The patient with a UTI has a variety of symptoms that range from mild to severe. The typical complaint is of one or more of the following: frequency, burning, urgency, nocturia, blood or pus in the urine, and suprapubic fullness. If the infection has progressed to the kidney, there may be flank pain (referred to as costovertebral tenderness) and low-grade fever.

Question the patient about risk factors, including recent catheterization of the urinary tract, pregnancy or recent childbirth, neurological problems, volume depletion, frequent sexual activity, and presence of a sexually transmitted infection (STI). Ask the patient to describe current sexual and birth control practices because poorly fitting diaphragms, the use of spermicides, and certain sexual practices such as anal intercourse place the patient at risk for a UTI.

PHYSICAL EXAMINATION. The most common symptoms are **frequency, burning, urgency**, and **hematuria**. Physical examination is often unremarkable in the patient with a UTI, although some patients have costovertebral angle tenderness in cases of pyelonephritis. On occasion, the patient has fever, chills, and signs of a systemic infection. Inspect the urine to determine its color, clarity, odor, and character. Surveillance for STIs is recommended as part of the examination. If vaginal discharge is present, a pelvic examination is needed to determine if vaginitis, cervicitis, or pelvic inflammatory disease is causing the dysuria.

PSYCHOSOCIAL. UTIs rarely result in disruption of the patient's normal activities. The infection is generally acute and responds rapidly to antibiotic therapy. The general guidelines to increase fluid intake and concomitant frequent urination may be problematic for some patients in restrictive work environments. The accompanying discomfort may result in temporary restriction of sexual activity, especially if an STI is diagnosed.

Diagnostic Highlights

General Comments: Guidelines from the American College of Obstetricians and Gynecologists indicate that a urine culture is not necessary for the initial treatment of lower UTI. Follow-up testing demonstrates the effectiveness of treatment.

Test	Normal Result	Abnormality With Condition	Explanation
Leukocyte esterase dip test	Negative	Positive (purple shade)	Presence of leukocyte esterase indicates UTI; 90% accurate in detecting white blood cells (WBCs) in the urine
Urine culture and sensitivity	< 10,000 colony forming units (cfu)/mL	> 10,000 cfu/mL or > 1,000 cfu in acutely symptomatic patients in some situations	Identifies causative organism; determines appropriate antibiotic

Diagnostic Highlights (continued)

Test	Normal Result	Abnormality With Condition	Explanation
Urinalysis	WBCs: < 5/hpf; red blood cells (RBCs): < 5/hpf; nitrites: none; pH: 4.6–8; no crystals; clear, aromatic	Increased WBCs, RBCs, pH, nitrites, crystals; cloudy, odor present	Presence of bacteria in the urine is indicated by several changes noted in a urinalysis

Other Tests: Voiding cystoureterography may detect congenital anomalies that predispose patients to recurrent UTI; dynamic computed tomography; complete blood count; high-power field (hpf)

PRIMARY NURSING DIAGNOSIS

DIAGNOSIS. Impaired urinary elimination related to swelling and inflammation as evidenced by frequency, burning, and/or urgency

OUTCOMES. Urinary elimination; Self-management: Infection; Knowledge: Infection management; Knowledge: Medication, Symptom severity; Symptom control

INTERVENTIONS. Medication prescribing; Medication administration; Teaching: Prescribed medication; Teaching: Disease process; Urinary elimination management

PLANNING AND IMPLEMENTATION

Collaborative

The treatment for a UTI is primarily pharmacologic, with a focus on prevention because of the frequency of recurrences. An acid-ash diet may be encouraged. A diet of meats, eggs, cheese, prunes, cranberries, plums, and whole grains can increase the acidity of the urine. Foods not allowed on this diet include carbonated beverages, anything containing baking soda or powder, fruits other than those previously stated, all vegetables except corn and lentils, and milk and milk products. Because the action of some UTI medications is diminished by acidic urine (nitrofurantoin), review all prescriptions before instructing patients to follow this diet.

UTIs are treated with antibiotics specific to the invading organism, although there is a growing interest in offering a 48-hour delayed prescription to be used at the patient's discretion. By waiting to see if a patient's symptoms subside without antibiotics, that process may reduce antibiotic resistance. Without treatment, 20% to 40% of women with uncomplicated cystitis will resolve without antibiotics. Often, a 3-day course of antibiotics is prescribed, but single-dose regimens (fosfomycin) are also used. Older patients may need a longer course of therapy. Women being treated with antibiotics may contract a vaginal yeast infection during therapy; review the signs and symptoms (cheesy discharge and perineal itching and swelling) and encourage the woman to purchase an over-the-counter antifungal or to contact her primary healthcare provider if treatment is indicated.

Pharmacologic Highlights

Medication or Drug Class	Dosage	Description	Rationale
Trimethoprim-sulfamethoxazone (Bactrim, Septra)	1 tablet (160 mg/800 mg) PO twice a day for 3 days	Sulfonamide	Interferes with folic acid, which is essential for bacterial development

(highlight box continues on page 1186)

Pharmacologic Highlights (continued)

Medication or Drug Class	Dosage	Description	Rationale
Antibiotics	Varies by drug	Nitrofurantoin monohydrate, nitrofurantoin macrocrystals, fosfomycin, trimethoprim, ciprofloxacin, ofloxacin, levofloxacin, ampicillin, amoxicillin/clavulanate, cefaclor, cefuroxime	Bacteriocidal

Other Drugs: Depending on the organism, many antibiotics are available. Acetaminophen may be given for discomfort.

Independent

Encourage patients with infections to increase fluid intake to promote frequent urination, which minimizes stasis and mechanically flushes the lower urinary tract. Strategies to limit recurrence include increasing vitamin C intake, drinking cranberry juice, wiping from front to back after a bowel movement (women), regular emptying of the bladder, avoiding tub and bubble baths, wearing cotton underwear, and avoiding tight clothing such as jeans. These strategies have been beneficial for some patients, although there is little research that supports the efficacy of such practices.

Encourage the patient to take over-the-counter analgesics unless contraindicated for mild discomfort but to continue to take all antibiotics until the full course of treatment has been completed. If the patient experiences perineal discomfort, sitz baths or warm compresses to the perineum may increase comfort.

Evidence-Based Practice and Health Policy

Hoffmann, T., Peiris, R., Del Mar, C., Cleo, G., & Glasziou, P. (2020). Natural history of uncomplicated urinary tract infection without antibiotics: A systematic review. *British Journal of General Practice, 10,* e714–e722.

- Uncomplicated UTI is commonly treated with antibiotics. However, the duration of symptoms without antibiotics is not established, which would inform decision making about antibiotic use. The authors aimed to determine the natural history of uncomplicated UTI in adults by performing a review of electronic databases to locate studies that involved adults with UTIs in a placebo group of randomized trials that did not use antibiotics and measured symptom duration.
- Over the first 9 days, the percentage of participants who were symptom free or reported improved symptoms was reported as rising to 42%. At 6 weeks, the percentage of such participants was 36%; up to 39% of participants failed to improve by 6 weeks. The rate of adverse effects was low. The authors concluded that some women appear to improve or become symptom free spontaneously, and most improvement occurs in the first 9 days.

DOCUMENTATION GUIDELINES

- Physical response: Pain, burning on urination, urinary frequency; vital signs; nocturia; color and odor of urine; patient history that may place the patient at risk
- Location, duration, frequency, and severity of pain; response to medications
- Absence of complications such as pyelonephritis

DISCHARGE AND HOME HEALTHCARE GUIDELINES

Treatment of a UTI occurs in the outpatient setting. Teach the patient an understanding of the proposed therapy, including the medication name, dosage, route, and side effects. Explain the signs and symptoms of complications such as pyelonephritis and the need for follow-up before leaving the setting.

Explain the importance of completing the entire course of antibiotics even if symptoms decrease or disappear. If the patient experiences gastrointestinal discomfort, encourage the patient to continue taking the medications but to take them with a meal or milk unless contraindicated. Warn the patient that drugs with phenazopyridine turn the urine orange.

Urinary Tract Trauma

DRG Category:	659
Mean LOS:	8.1 days
Description:	SURGICAL: Kidney and Ureter Procedures for Non-Neoplasm With Major Complication or Comorbidity
DRG Category:	663
Mean LOS:	4.9 days
Description:	SURGICAL: Minor Bladder Procedures With Complication or Comorbidity
DRG Category:	699
Mean LOS:	4.2 days
Description:	MEDICAL: Other Kidney and Urinary Tract Diagnoses With Complication or Comorbidity

U rinary tract trauma includes injury to the kidneys, ureters, urinary bladder, and urethra. These injuries occur in approximately 3% to 10% of patients admitted to the hospital for abdominal trauma, and the damage can threaten life and lead to lifelong impaired urinary dysfunction. Most urinary tract trauma affects the kidneys. Blunt renal injury is classified as minor, major, and critical trauma. Minor renal trauma occurs when organ tissue is bruised or when superficial lacerations of the renal cortex occur without disruption of the renal capsule. Major renal trauma occurs with major lacerations that extend through the renal cortex, medulla, and renal capsule. Critical renal trauma occurs when the kidney is shattered or when the renal pedicle (stem that contains the renal artery and vein) is injured.

Bladder injury occurs in up to 40% of urinary tract trauma, usually involves bladder rupture, and can be either intraperitoneal or extraperitoneal. Intraperitoneal bladder rupture occurs with blunt trauma to the lower portion of the abdomen, usually when the bladder is full. The bladder ruptures at the dome (the point of least resistance), and blood and urine collect in the peritoneal cavity. Extraperitoneal bladder rupture usually occurs in conjunction with a pelvic fracture when a sharp bone fragment perforates the bladder at its base. Blood and urine then collect in the space surrounding the bladder base. Urethral injury occurs in 8% to 10% of cases of urinary tract trauma and is also associated with a pelvic fracture, whereas ureteral trauma is rarer.

Although renal trauma is unusual, it is associated with a 6% to 12% mortality rate, possibly because of the kidneys' high vascularity. Complications of urinary tract trauma include hemorrhage and exsanguination, hypovolemic shock, peritonitis, septic shock, acute renal failure, urinary incontinence, pyelonephritis, dyspareunia, and impotence.

CAUSES

Urinary tract trauma is caused by either blunt or penetrating trauma. Traffic crashes are the most common cause of blunt trauma. Other causes include falls, assaults, occupational (crush) injuries, bicycle injuries, and sports injuries. The energy of the trauma is dissipated throughout the cavity, which frequently causes rupturing of the bladder or kidney or tearing of the urethra. Pelvic fractures are often associated with urinary tract trauma, as are direct kicks to the groin and straddling injuries associated with bicycling. Penetrating trauma to the urinary tract is frequently the result of a gunshot wound or a stabbing injury. The degree and severity of the damage from a gunshot wound depend on the velocity and trajectory of the bullet. The result is usually localized tissue damage and potential hemorrhage in the highly vascular kidney or the distended bladder. A small proportion of people have urinary tract trauma from medical procedures such as laparoscopic hysterectomy and laparoscopically assisted vaginal hysterectomy. Risk factors include alcohol and substance use that may lead to falls or traffic crashes, aggressive behaviors that lead to fights and assaults, and undergoing urinary procedures such as laparoscopy.

GENETIC CONSIDERATIONS

No clear genetic contributions to susceptibility have been defined.

SEX AND LIFE SPAN CONSIDERATIONS

Traumatic injuries, which are usually preventable, are the leading cause of death in the first four decades of life. Most blunt abdominal and urinary tract trauma is associated with traffic crashes, which are two to three times more common in males than in females in the 15- to 24-year-old age group. Penetrating injuries from gunshot wounds and stab wounds, which are on the increase in preteens, teens, and young adults in the United States, are more common in males than females. Men have different patterns of injury than women, and a higher injury severity. Analyses of trauma outcomes indicate that, following traumatic injury, males have higher rates of multiple organ failure, pneumonia, and sepsis than females, creating health disparities for men (Marcolini et al., 2019). Trauma is the third leading cause of death in people ages 45 to 65 years and the seventh leading cause of death in people older than age 65 years. The other group at risk are women undergoing laparoscopic hysterectomies.

HEALTH DISPARITIES AND SEXUAL/GENDER MINORITY HEALTH

In recent years, Black persons have been killed in traffic crashes at a rate almost 25% higher than White persons (National Highway Traffic Safety Administration [NHTSA], 2021). Native American persons have the highest rate of traffic injury in the United States, more than twice the rate of Black persons (NHTSA, 2021). Experts have noted that Black and Native American communities tend to be crisscrossed by more dangerous roads than other locations, placing people from those communities at risk for injury. Recent work has shown evidence that rural populations have injury mortality rates that are more than twice as high as urban rates. Many factors contribute to these health disparities, including the risk of traffic injury in narrow rural roads, the lack of graded curves and lighted traffic signals on rural highways, and the distance from major trauma centers. Many of the most dangerous occupations, such as mining and agriculture, are found in rural areas and can result in injury, disability, and death. Sexual and gender minority persons have high risk for dating and interpersonal violence, violence related to bullying, and intentional and unintentional injury (Healthy People 2020). All of these factors and situations put people at risk for urinary tract trauma.

GLOBAL HEALTH CONSIDERATIONS

Falls and traffic crashes occur around the world and may lead to urinary tract trauma. Internationally, falls from heights of less than 5 meters are the leading cause of injury overall, and traffic crashes are the next most frequent cause. Regions of the world with war or civil unrest may have increased incidence of penetrating injury because of penetrating injuries from guns and knives. When rape is used as a weapon of war, urinary tract trauma may occur.

ASSESSMENT

HISTORY. Obtain a relevant history from the patient or significant others. If the patient is critically injured, note that the history, assessment, and early management merge in the primary survey. Determine as much as you can from witnesses to the trauma or the life squad. Determine the patient's position in the vehicle if a crash has occurred, or the size of the stabbing weapon or the caliber of the gun.

If the patient's condition is stable enough to warrant a separate history, ask questions about allergies, current medications, preexisting medical conditions, recent medical procedures, and factors surrounding the injury. Take a sexual history to rule out rape. Note that patients with preexisting renal diseases such as polycystic kidney disease and pyelonephritis are at higher risk for renal injury than those with normal kidneys. If you suspect a lower urinary tract injury, ask if the patient has experienced suprapubic tenderness, the inability to void spontaneously, or bloody urine. If you suspect kidney injury, ask if the patient is experiencing flank pain, pain at the costovertebral angle, back tenderness, colicky pain with the passage of blood clots, or bloody urine. Note that if the patient has a positive blood alcohol level, the patient may not be sensitive to painful stimuli even if the patient has experienced a severe injury.

PHYSICAL EXAMINATION. Common symptoms include **urethral bleeding, bruising along the flank, urinary retention or inability to void, lower abdominal distention and pain**, and **swelling and edema of the genitalia**. If the patient is stable enough for you to perform a complete head-to-toe assessment, determine if there are any physical signs indicating kidney injury. Note, however, that physical signs may be masked because of the protection of the kidneys by the abdominal organs, muscles of the back, and bony structures. Inspect the area over the 11th and 12th ribs and flank area for obvious hematomas, wounds, contusions, or abrasions. Inspect the lower back and flank for Grey Turner sign or bruising because of a retroperitoneal hemorrhage. Note any abdominal distention. To identify lower urinary tract trauma, inspect the urinary meatus to determine the presence of blood. Note any bruising, edema, or discoloration of the genitalia or tracking of urine into the tissues of the thigh or abdominal wall. Signs of penile trauma include loss of skin, swelling, and angulation, and of scrotal trauma include loss of skin, swelling, discoloration, and pain.

Auscultate for the presence of bowel sounds in all quadrants. Although the absence of bowel sounds does not indicate urinary tract injury for certain, increase your index of suspicion when bowel sounds are absent because abdominal injury often accompanies urinary tract injury. If you note a bruit near the renal artery, notify the physician at once because an intimal tear may have occurred in the renal artery. Percussion may reveal excessive dullness in the lower abdomen or flank. When you palpate the flank, upper abdomen, lumbar vertebrae, and lower rib cage, the patient may experience pain. Other signs of urinary tract trauma include crepitus and a flank mass. Bladder rupture leads to severe pain in the hypogastrium on palpation or swelling from extravasation of blood and urine in the suprapubic area. Signs of peritoneal irritation (abdominal rigidity, rebound tenderness, and voluntary guarding) may also be present because of extravasation of blood or urine into the peritoneal cavity.

PSYCHOSOCIAL. The patient with urinary tract trauma requires immediate emotional support because of the nature of any sudden traumatic injury. The sudden alteration in comfort, potential body image changes, and possible impaired functioning of vital organ systems can often be overwhelming and can lead to maladaptive coping. Determine the patient's and family's level of anxiety and their ability to cope with stressors.

Diagnostic Highlights

Test	Normal Result	Abnormality With Condition	Explanation
Retrograde urethrogram, retrograde cystogram	Normal structure of urethra, normal structure of bladder	Transected or torn urethra; extravasation indicates ruptured bladder	Contrast indicates location and extent of injury
Kidney-ureter-bladder x-ray and radionuclide imaging, computed tomography	Normal structures of urinary tract	Location and extent of injury	Contrast media and radiography used to identify areas of injury
Renal and lower urinary tract computed tomography	Normal structures of urinary tract	Location and extent of injury	Identifies radiographic slices with or without contrast

Other Tests: Complete blood count, urinalysis, renal ultrasound, excretory urogram (IV pyelogram), cystography, cystoscopy, ultrasound

PRIMARY NURSING DIAGNOSIS

DIAGNOSIS. Acute pain related to tissue damage and swelling as evidenced by self-reports of pain, facial grimacing, and/or protective behavior

OUTCOMES. Comfort status; Pain control; Pain level; Symptom severity; Symptom control; Knowledge: Pain management

INTERVENTIONS. Pain management: Acute; Analgesic administration; Heat/cold application; Teaching: Disease process; Medication management; Teaching: Prescribed medication

PLANNING AND IMPLEMENTATION
Collaborative

MEDICAL. The initial care of the patient with urinary tract trauma involves airway, breathing, and circulation. Measures to ensure adequate oxygenation and tissue perfusion include establishing an effective airway and supplemental oxygen source, supporting breathing, controlling the source of blood loss, and replacing intravascular volume. As with any traumatic injury, treatment and stabilization of any life-threatening injuries are completed immediately.

SURGICAL. Patients with renal trauma may need urinary diversion with a nephrostomy tube, depending on the location of injury or in situations in which pancreatic and duodenal injury coexist with renal trauma. If the patient is unable to void, the trauma team considers urinary catheterization. If the patient has blood at the urinary meatus or if there is any resistance to catheter insertion, a retrograde urethrogram is performed to evaluate the integrity of the urethra. In the presence of urethral injury, an improperly placed catheter can cause long-term complications, such as incontinence, impotence, and urethral strictures. A suprapubic catheter may be used to manage severe urethral lacerations and urethral disruption. Extraperitoneal bladder rupture is usually managed not with surgery but with urethral or suprapubic catheter drainage. Ongoing monitoring of the amount, character, and color of the patient's urine is important during treatment and recovery. In a patient without renal impairment, the physician usually maintains the urine output at 1 mL/kg per hour. Note any blood clots in the urine and report an obstructed urinary drainage system immediately.

The indications for surgery depend on the severity of injury. Patients with major renal trauma who are hemodynamically unstable and patients with critical trauma need surgical exploration. Patients with urethral disruption and severe lacerations may have surgery delayed for several weeks or even months, or the surgeon may choose to perform surgical reconstruction immediately. A growing number of surgeons are performing endoscopic realignment with fluoroscopy for urethral injuries. Patients with an intraperitoneal bladder rupture have the bladder surgically repaired, with the extravasated blood and urine evacuated during the procedure. Usually, suprapubic drainage is used during recovery. Laceration of the ureter is immediately repaired surgically or the patient risks loss of a kidney.

Minor renal trauma is usually managed with bedrest and observation. Minor extraperitoneal bladder tears can be managed with insertion of a Foley catheter for drainage, along with antibiotic therapy. Many urethral tears can be managed with insertion of a suprapubic catheter and delayed surgical repair or plasty, provided that bleeding can be controlled. The patient needs to be monitored for complications throughout the hospital stay, such as infection (dysuria, low back pain, suprapubic pain, and foul or cloudy urine), impaired wound healing (seepage of urine from repair sites, flank or abdominal mass from pockets of urine, and crepitus from urine seepage into tissues), and impaired renal function (nausea, irritability, edema, hypertension, oliguria, and anuria).

Pharmacologic Highlights

Medication or Drug Class	Dosage	Description	Rationale
Antibiotics	Varies by drug	Ampicillin and sulbactam, cefotetan	To prevent infection of the urinary tract

Other Drugs: Analgesics such as fentanyl, morphine sulfate; antispasmodics may be needed for bladder spasm.

Independent

The most important priority is to ensure the maintenance of an adequate airway, oxygen supply, breathing patterns, and circulatory status. If the patient is stable, apply ice to the perineal area, the scrotum, or the penis to help relieve pain and swelling. Use care to avoid cold burns from ice packs that are in contact with the skin for a prolonged period of time. For severe scrotal swelling, some experts recommend a scrotal support to reduce pain. Use either a commercially available support or a handmade support using an elastic wrap as a sling.

Patients may or may not have residual problems with urinary incontinence or sexual functioning. Loss of urinary continence leads to self-esteem and body image disturbances. Provide the patient with information on reconstructive techniques and methods to manage incontinence. Listen to the patient and offer support and understanding. Patients often view injury to the urinary tract system as a threat to their sexuality. Reassure patients who are not at risk for sexual dysfunction that their sexuality is not impaired. Sexual concerns should not be ignored during the acute phase of recovery. Be alert to questions about sexuality, which may be phrased in terms that are familiar in the patient's culture. Answer questions honestly and listen to the patient's questions and responses carefully to understand the full meaning.

Note that the inability to function sexually is an enormous loss to patients of both sexes. It may occur with posterior urethral injury in men when nerve damage occurs in the area. Urinary tract injury in men is often associated with injury to the penis and testes as well. Sexual dysfunction may also occur in women if the ovaries, uterus, vagina, or external genitalia are damaged along with urinary tract structures or the pelvis. Provide specific answers to the patient's questions, such as alternative techniques to intercourse (oral sex, use of a vibrator, massage, or masturbation). Give the patient information about the feasibility and safety of resuming sexual activity and include the partner in all discussions.

Emotional support of the patient and family is also a key intervention. Patients and their families are often frightened and anxious. If the patient is awake as you implement strategies to manage the airway, breathing, and circulation, provide a running explanation of the procedures to reassure the patient. Explain to the family the treatment alternatives and keep them updated as to the patient's response to therapy.

Evidence-Based Practice and Health Policy

Luchristt, D., Brown, O., Geynisman-Tan, J., Mueller, M., Kenton, K., & Bretschneider, E. (2020). Timing of diagnosis of complex lower urinary tract injury in the 30-day postoperative period following benign hysterectomy. *American Journal of Obstetrics and Gynecology, 224,* e1–e12.

- The authors described the time to diagnosis of complex lower urinary tract injury among women undergoing hysterectomy and to identify the intraoperative risk factors in the 30-day postoperative period. They used a retrospective analysis of a national data set using all benign hysterectomy cases ($N = 100,823$). Sociodemographic factors, health status, surgeon type, and other operative characteristics were included. A complex lower urinary tract injury was defined as ureteral obstruction, ureteral fistula, or bladder fistula.
- Median time to diagnosis was 10 days and varied significantly based on type of injury with ureteral obstruction recognized first. Approximately 99% of complex lower urinary tract injuries were diagnosed on the day of surgery. Total laparoscopic hysterectomy had the lowest rate of complex lower urinary tract injury, and abdominal hysterectomy and vaginal hysterectomy had greater odds of ureteral obstruction. The authors note that intraoperative risk factors should be considered when assessing for complex lower urinary tract injury in the 30-day postoperative period.

DOCUMENTATION GUIDELINES

- Urinary tract assessment: Urinary drainage system (patency, color of urine, presence of bloody urine or clots, amount of urine, appearance of catheter insertion site); fluid balance (intake and output, patency of IV catheters, speed of fluid resuscitation); wound healing (wound drainage, extravasation of urine from wound, tracts of urine extending beneath the skin)
- Assessment of level of anxiety, degree of understanding, adjustment, family or partner's response, and coping skills
- Concern over sexual dysfunction, content of conversations, and content taught

DISCHARGE AND HOME HEALTHCARE GUIDELINES

Provide a complete explanation of all emergency treatments and answer the patient's and family's questions. Explain the possibility of complications to recovery, such as poor wound healing, infection, and anemia. As needed, provide information about any follow-up laboratory procedures that might be required after discharge from the hospital. Provide the dates and times that the patient is to receive follow-up care with the primary healthcare provider or the trauma clinic. Give the patient a phone number to call with questions or concerns. Provide information on how to manage urinary drainage systems if the patient is discharged with them in place. Demonstrate catheter care, emptying the bag, and the need for frequent hand washing. Explain when the patient can resume sexual activity. If the patient has sexual dysfunction, provide the patient with information about alternatives to intercourse; refer the patient to a support group if interested.

Uterine Cancer

DRG Category:	740
Mean LOS:	3.9 days
Description:	SURGICAL: Uterine and Adnexa Procedures for Non-Ovarian and Non-Adnexal Malignancy With Complication or Comorbidity
DRG Category:	755
Mean LOS:	4.1 days
Description:	MEDICAL: Malignancy, Female Reproductive System With Complication or Comorbidity

Uterine cancer most commonly occurs in the endometrium, the mucous membrane that lines the inner surface of the uterus. Endometrial cancer, specifically adenocarcinoma (involving the glands), accounts for more than 95% of the diagnosed cases of uterine cancer. In 2021, the American Cancer Society predicts that 66,570 new cases of uterine cancer will occur in the United States and 12,940 deaths will occur from the disease. Women have a lifetime risk of 3.1% for uterine cancer. There has been an increase in the number of women with endometrial cancer, partly owing to women living longer and more accurate reporting. Endometrial cancer is the third most common cause of cancer in women, ranking behind breast and lung cancer. It is the most common neoplasm of the pelvic region and reproductive system of the female, and it occurs in 1 in 100 women in the United States. Other uterine tumors include adenocarcinoma with squamous metaplasia (previously referred to as *adenoacanthoma*), endometrial stromal sarcomas, and leiomyosarcomas.

Endometrial cancer can infiltrate the myometrium, resulting in an increased thickness of the uterine wall, and it can eventually infiltrate the serosa and move into the pelvic cavity and lymph nodes. It can also spread by direct extension along the endometrium into the cervical canal; pass through the fallopian tubes to the ovaries, broad ligaments, and peritoneal cavity; or move via the bloodstream and lymphatics to other areas of the body. It is a slow-growing cancer, taking 5 or more years to develop from hyperplasia to adenocarcinoma. Endometrial cancer is very responsive to treatment, provided it is detected early. Prognosis depends on the stage, uterine signs, and lymph node involvement, with 5-year survival rates in localized disease as 95%, and 5-year survival rates in distant disease as 17%. Complications of uterine cancer include abnormal bleeding, anemia, uterine perforation, and metastasis.

CAUSES

The exact cause of uterine cancer is not known, although it is considered to be dependent on excess endogenous (internal) or exogenous (external) hormonal levels for growth. Risk factors associated with the development of uterine adenocarcinoma include age, genetic and familial factors, early menarche (before age 12 years), late menopause (after 52 years), hypertension, nulliparity, unopposed estrogen hormonal replacement therapy, pelvic irradiation, polycystic ovarian disease, obesity, tamoxifen use, and diabetes mellitus. Women who have used oral fertility medications, specifically clomiphene, may have an increased risk of uterine cancer. Smoking may decrease the risk of endometrial cancer by decreasing estrogen levels and leading to an earlier menopause.

GENETIC CONSIDERATIONS

Uterine cancer has a smaller genetic component than some other cancers, with heritability of ~27%. However, there are some familial cases, as an estimated 1 in 10 women with uterine cancer may have a genetic predisposition. Genetic risk is higher if uterine cancer occurs before age 50 years; occurs along with another cancer, such as colon, ovarian, stomach, or bile duct; occurs when there is a history of colon polyps before age 40 years; or occurs when the patient has family members with other gastrointestinal cancers or polyps. Women with hereditary non-polyposis colorectal cancer (HNPCC) have a risk of uterine cancer that is 50% higher than that of the general population. Uterine cancer is so common in this population that some families with HNPCC gene variants will have only cases of uterine cancer and no colon cancer. Mutations in *TP53*, which causes Li-Fraumeni syndrome, also increase the incidence of uterine cancer. Other gene mutations associated with uterine and breast cancer include *MSH6*, *CHEK2*, *BRCA1*, *BRCA2*, *ATM*, *PMS2*, *PALB2*, *MSH2*, and *PTEN*.

SEX AND LIFE SPAN CONSIDERATIONS

Uterine cancer occurs primarily in middle-aged and older women who are postmenopausal, with a mean age of diagnosis at 60 years. Only 10% of the cases occur in women under age 50 years, and it is rare in women under age 30 years.

HEALTH DISPARITIES AND SEXUAL/GENDER MINORITY HEALTH

The incidence of uterine cancer is highest among White and Black women as compared to other groups (Centers for Disease Control and Prevention [CDC], 2018). With endometrial cancer, mortality is higher in Black as compared to White women, with a mortality rate of nine deaths per 100,000 individuals in Black women and four to five deaths per 100,000 individuals in White women. Differences in mortality are thought to be related to late diagnosis for Black women due to problems with access to care.

Transgender is a term used to describe persons whose gender identity is different from their sex assigned at birth. Approximately 1% of the U.S. population identify themselves as transgender. Sexual and gender minority persons have higher odds for multiple chronic conditions, cancer, and poor quality of life and are more apt to have disabilities than cisgender males and females. (Cisgender is a term used to describe persons whose gender identity and gender expression are aligned with their assigned sex listed on their birth certificate.) Gender-affirming hormone therapy is the use of hormone therapy for gender transition or gender affirmation and can be masculinizing or feminizing. Transgender men are at risk for gynecological malignancies but are an underserved group who experience discrimination and marginalization that contribute to health disparities. The risks may be complicated by a reluctance of transgender men to have routine gynecologic examinations because of anatomical dysphoria (a person's anatomy does not match their inner sense of self and gender identity). There is no evidence that hormone use leads to an increased risk of gynecological cancers in transgender men, but there are limited data available (Stenzel et al., 2020). Lesbian and bisexual women may have an increased risk for gynecological cancers due to a higher prevalence of obesity and lower pregnancy rates than heterosexual women (Panganiban & O'Neil, 2021).

GLOBAL HEALTH CONSIDERATIONS

The global incidence of uterine cancer is 6.5 per 100,000 females per year. The incidence is 10 times higher in developed than in developing countries, in part because of higher rates of obesity and lower parity in developed countries.

ASSESSMENT

HISTORY. Establish a history of risk factors. The major presenting symptom is abnormal vaginal bleeding. The patient may also describe pelvic pressure. A mucoid and watery discharge may be noted several weeks to months before bleeding begins. Postmenopausal patients may report bleeding that began a year or more after menses stopped. A mucosanguineous, odorous vaginal discharge is noted if metastases to the vagina has occurred. Younger patients may have spotting and prolonged, heavy menses.

Inquire about pain, fever, weight loss, anorexia, and bowel/bladder dysfunction, which are late symptoms of uterine cancer. Assess the use and effectiveness of any analgesics for pain relief and also the location, onset, duration, and intensity of the pain.

PHYSICAL EXAMINATION. The major initial symptom of endometrial cancer occurring in 85% of women is **abnormal, painless vaginal bleeding, either menometrorrhagia (prolonged, excessive uterine bleeding and more frequent than normal) or postmenopausal bleeding.** Conduct a general physical and gynecological examination. The patient should be directed to not douche or bathe for 24 hours before the examination so that tissue is not washed away. Inspection of any bleeding or vaginal discharge is imperative. The characteristics and amount of bleeding should be noted. Upon palpation, the uterus will feel enlarged and may reveal masses.

PSYCHOSOCIAL. Patients with the disease often exhibit depression and anger, especially if they are a nulligravida and desired a pregnancy. Therefore, a thorough assessment of the patient's perception of the disease process and coping mechanisms is required. The family or partner should also be included in the assessment to examine the extent of support they can provide for the patient. Family anger, ineffective coping, and role disturbances may interfere with family functioning and need careful monitoring.

Diagnostic Highlights

General Comments: Several diagnostic tests may be done to confirm the diagnosis and to check for metastases.

Test	Normal Result	Abnormality With Condition	Explanation
Endometrial biopsy; fractional dilation and curettage of the uterus	No malignant cells found	Malignant cells found	Obtain specimen of endometrium and endocervix for pathological examination
Transvaginal ultrasound	Normal endometrial thickness	Detection of endometrial carcinoma or atypical endometrial hyperplasia with a thickness > 5.0 mm	Allows for calculation of endometrial thickness
Papanicolaou examination (Pap smear)	No abnormality or atypical cells noted	High-class/grade cytological results	Initial screening; can detect approximately 50% of cases of uterine cancer

Other Tests: CA-125 blood test is used for surveillance for advanced uterine cancer. Other tests include sonography, sonohysterography, hysteroscopy, chest x-ray, IV pyelography, cystoscopy, proctoscopy, computed tomography scan, and magnetic resonance imaging.

PRIMARY NURSING DIAGNOSIS

DIAGNOSIS. Deficient knowledge related to treatment procedures, treatment regimens, medications, and disease process as evidenced by inaccurate follow-through of instruction, insufficient knowledge to manage care, and/or anxiety over lack of knowledge

OUTCOMES. Knowledge: Treatment procedure; Knowledge: Treatment regimens; Knowledge: Medications; Knowledge: Disease process

INTERVENTIONS. Teaching: Disease process; Teaching: Prescribed medication; Teaching: Procedure/treatment; Teaching: Preoperative

PLANNING AND IMPLEMENTATION
Collaborative

SURGICAL. If uterine cancer is detected early, the treatment of choice is surgery. A total abdominal hysterectomy (TAH) with removal of the fallopian tubes and ovaries, bilateral salpingo-oophorectomy (BSO), is generally performed. Common complications after a hysterectomy are hemorrhage, infection, and thromboembolic disease. Premenopausal patients who have a BSO become sterile and experience menopause. Hormone replacement therapy may be warranted and is appropriate. Laparoscopic or robot-assisted staging is becoming more common, resulting in loss operative blood loss, less complications, shorter hospital stay, and faster recovery. In a total pelvic exenteration (evisceration or removal of the contents of a cavity), the surgeon removes all pelvic organs, including the bladder, rectum, and vagina. This procedure is performed if the disease is contained in the areas without metastasis. If the lymph nodes are involved, this procedure is usually not curative.

RADIATION AND CHEMOTHERAPY. A growing trend is to use more chemotherapy as compared to radiation therapy for extrauterine metastasis (see Pharmacologic Highlights). Radiation may provide local tumor control for patients who are not candidates for surgery but has not improved survival rates with metastatic disease. Radiation therapy may be given in combination with the surgery (before or after), or it may be used alone depending on the staging of the disease, whether the tumor is not well differentiated, or whether the carcinoma is extensive. Radiation may be used for the very older patient with an advanced stage of endometrial cancer for whom surgery would not improve quality of life. With radiation, the possible complications are hemorrhage, cystitis, urethral stricture, rectal ulceration, or proctitis.

Intracavity radiation (brachytherapy) or external radiation therapy may be used for some people with extensive extrauterine pelvic disease. An internal radiation device may be implanted during surgery (preloaded) or at the patient's bedside (afterloaded). If the device is inserted during the surgical procedure, the postoperative management needs to include radiation precautions. Provide a private room for the patient and follow the key principle to protect against radiation exposure: distance, time, and shielding. The greater the distance from the radiation source, the less exposure to ionizing rays. Brachytherapy may also be given in three sessions that each last 10 minutes by inserting a tampon-like device into the vagina. Outside of the procedure itself, the patient does not emit radiation and can receive treatments as an outpatient.

Pharmacologic Highlights

Medication or Drug Class	Dosage	Description	Rationale
Doxorubicin; cisplatin; carboplatin; ifosfamide; gemcitabine	Given in combination	Antineoplastic	Response rate of 4%–30%
Paclitaxel (Taxol)	Depends on patient tolerance and condition	Antineoplastic	Response rate of 35%; premedicate with corticosteroids, diphenhydramine, and H_2 antagonists
Acetaminophen; NSAIDs; opioids; combination	Depends on the drug and patient condition and tolerance	Analgesics	Analgesics used are determined by the severity of pain

Other Drugs: Tamoxifen (Nolvadex), progestin, or antiestrogen therapy (medroxyprogesterone acetate, megestrol) may be used.

Independent

The major emphasis is prevention, either primary by reduction of risk factors or secondary by early detection. Encourage patients to seek regular medical checkups, which should include gynecological examination. Discuss risk factors associated with the development of endometrial cancer, particularly as they apply or do not apply to the particular patient. Encourage the older menopausal patient to continue with regular examinations. If the patient is bleeding heavily, monitor closely for signs of dehydration and shock (dry mucous membranes, rapid and thready pulses, delayed capillary refill, restlessness, and mental status changes). Encourage the patient to drink liberal amounts of fluids and have the equipment available for IV hydration if necessary. A balanced diet promotes wound healing and maintains good skin integrity.

Patients require careful instruction before chemotherapy, radiation therapy, or surgery. Explain the procedures carefully and notify the patient what to expect after the procedure. For surgical candidates, teach coughing and deep-breathing exercises. Fit the patient with antiembolism stockings. If the patient is premenopausal, explain that removal of the ovaries induces menopause. Unless the patient undergoes a total pelvic exenteration, the vagina is intact and sexual intercourse remains possible. During external radiation therapy, the patient needs to know the expected side effects (diarrhea, skin irritation) and the importance of adequate rest and nutrition. Explain that the patient should not remove ink markings on the skin because they direct the location for radiation. If a preloaded radiation implant is used, the patient has a preoperative hospital stay that includes bowel preparation, douches, an indwelling urinary catheter, and diet restrictions the day before surgery.

If the patient has pain from either the surgical procedure or the disease process, teach the patient pain-relief techniques such as imagery and deep breathing. Encourage the patient to express anger and feelings without fear of being judged. Note that surgery and radiation may profoundly affect the patient's and partner's sexuality. Answer any questions honestly, provide information on alternatives to traditional sexual intercourse if appropriate, and encourage the couple to seek counseling if needed. If the patient's support systems and coping mechanisms are insufficient to meet the patient's needs, help the patient find others. Provide a list of support groups that may be helpful.

Evidence-Based Practice and Health Policy

Li, P., Sung, F., Yan, Y., Chen, W., Wang, J., Lin, S., & Ding, D. (2020). Aspirin associated with a decreased incidence of uterine cancer: A retrospective population-based cohort study. *Medicine.* Advance online publication. https://doi.org/10.1097/MD.0000000000021446

- Because clinical studies on the preventive effects of aspirin (ASA) on uterine cancer are inconsistent, the authors aimed to conduct a population-based, retrospective cohort study to evaluate uterine cancer in ASA users. They used insurance claims data to identify women who received ASA treatment and a comparison group of the same sample size.
- The incidence of uterine cancer in the ASA cohort was 10% of that in the comparison group. Hormone therapy was associated with the increase of uterine cancer risk in both cohorts but less in ASA users than the comparison group. The authors concluded that ASA use is associated with a decreased risk of uterine cancer and advised further prospective work in the area.

DOCUMENTATION GUIDELINES

- Physiological response: Amount and characteristics of any vaginal bleeding or discharge, vital signs, intake and output if appropriate, weight loss or gain, sleep patterns, response to all therapies
- Emotional response: Signs of stress, ability to cope, degree of depression, relationship with partner and significant others
- Comfort: Location, onset, duration, and intensity of pain; effectiveness of analgesics and pain-reducing techniques

DISCHARGE AND HOME HEALTHCARE GUIDELINES

PREVENTION. Teach the need for regular gynecological examinations even though the patient has had a hysterectomy. Teach the patient to report any abnormal vaginal bleeding to the healthcare provider. The patient who has had a TAH with BSO is at risk for developing osteoporosis. Recommend a daily intake of up to 1,500 mg of calcium through diet and supplements. Recommend vitamin D supplements to enable the body to use the calcium. Stress the need for regular exercise, particularly weight-bearing exercise. Discuss the exercise schedule and type with the patient in light of the treatment and expected recovery time.

MEDICATIONS. Ensure that the patient understands the dosage, route, action, and side effects of any medication that is to be taken at home. Note that to monitor the patient's response, some of the medications require the patient to have routine laboratory tests following discharge from the hospital.

POSTOPERATIVE. Discuss any incisional care. Encourage the patient to notify the surgeon of any unexpected wound discharge, bleeding, poor healing, or odor. Teach the patient to avoid heavy lifting, sexual intercourse, and driving until the surgeon recommends resumption.

RADIATION. To decrease bulk, teach the patient to maintain a diet high in protein and carbohydrates and low in residue. If diarrhea remains a problem, instruct the patient to notify the physician or clinic because antidiarrheal agents can be prescribed. Encourage the patient to limit exposure to others with colds because radiation tends to decrease the ability to fight infections. To decrease skin irritation, encourage the patient to wear loose-fitting clothing and avoid using heating pads, rubbing alcohol, and irritating skin preparations.

FOLLOW-UP CARE. Teach the patient appropriate self-care for the specific treatment. Teach the patient to be able to identify where assistance can be obtained should postoperative or post-treatment complications occur. Make sure the significant others are aware of the expectations of a normal convalescence and whom to call should concerns arise.

Vaginal Cancer

DRG Category:	734
Mean LOS:	4.9 days
Description:	SURGICAL: Pelvic Evisceration, Radical Hysterectomy, and Radical Vulvectomy With Complication or Comorbidity or Major Complication or Comorbidity
DRG Category:	755
Mean LOS:	4.1 days
Description:	MEDICAL: Malignancy, Female Reproductive System With Complication or Comorbidity

Vaginal cancer (VC) is a neoplastic disease of cells within the vaginal canal. The American Cancer Society estimates that approximately 5,000 new cases of VC will be diagnosed in 2021, and 1,200 women will die from the disease. Because primary cancer of the vagina is rare (it accounts for only 3% of all gynecological malignancies), VC is usually secondary as a result of metastasis from choriocarcinoma (cancer of the cervix or adjacent organs). VC often extends to the bladder and rectum, which makes treatment difficult. Approximately 85% to 90% of vaginal cancers are squamous cell carcinomas, which begin in the epithelial lining in the upper areas of the vagina near the cervix. Less common are adenocarcinomas, which develop in women over age 50 years who were exposed to diethylstilbestrol (DES) in utero; melanomas, which tend to affect the lower or outer portion of the vagina; or sarcomas that form in the deep wall of the vagina.

The vagina has a thin wall and extensive lymphatic drainage; the severity of the cancer, therefore, varies depending on its location in relation to the lymphatic system and the thickness of the neoplastic involvement. Localized VC (limited to the vaginal wall) has a 5-year survival rate of 66%, whereas distant VC (cancer has spread to distant organs such as lungs or liver) has a 5-year survival rate of 21%.

Low survival rates are caused by the advanced stage of the disease at the time of diagnosis, difficulty in treatment resulting from the proximity of important structures, and the rarity of the disease that makes it difficult to determine the best treatment. Complications from VC include recto-vaginal fistulae, metastases, recurrence, or depression. Complications from treatment include dyspareunia, early menopause, and/or bladder or bowel dysfunction.

CAUSES

The cause of VC is not known, although ingestion of DES, a drug given to women at one time (1940–1970) to prevent pregnancy loss in the first trimester, has been identified as one possible cause. Evidence is growing that human papillomavirus (HPV) types 16 and 18 may interfere with tumor suppressor gene production, which helps to suppress tumor growth. Therefore, the presence of HPV in the vagina may increase the likelihood of tumors. There may be some association with VC and late menarche. Many cases of VC are believed to start out as precancerous changes in the cells of the vagina, called *vaginal intraepithelial neoplasia*. Risk factors include a previous malignancy of the vagina, vulva, or cervix and advancing age. Women who have had cervical cancer previously should be examined on a regular basis to assess for vaginal lesions. Other risk factors include exposure to DES in utero, the improper use of pessaries (infrequent cleaning, infrequent examination to ensure proper fit), exposure to radiation therapy, trauma, exposure to chemical carcinogens found in some sprays and douches, a history of HPV, alcohol misuse and abuse, and smoking.

GENETIC CONSIDERATIONS

No clear genetic contributions to susceptibility have been defined.

SEX AND LIFE SPAN CONSIDERATIONS

VC occurs in menopausal and postmenopausal women, typically over age 50 years. The average age at the time of diagnosis is 67 years.

HEALTH DISPARITIES AND SEXUAL/GENDER MINORITY HEALTH

VC is rare in Black and Jewish women. Women living in rural areas of the United States have significantly higher rates of gynecological cancers, including VC, that are related to HPV as compared to women living in urban areas. Experts suggest this difference is related to high rates of HPV in rural males, lower vaccination rates, poor geographic access, and patient-provider miscommunication (Zahnd et al., 2018).

Transgender is a term used to describe persons whose gender identity is different from their sex assigned at birth. Approximately 1% of the U.S. population identify themselves as transgender. Sexual and gender minority persons have higher odds for multiple chronic conditions, cancer, and poor quality of life and are more apt to have disabilities than cisgender males and females. (Cisgender is a term used to describe persons whose gender identity and gender expression are aligned with their assigned sex listed on their birth certificate.) Gender-affirming hormone therapy is the use of hormone therapy for gender transition or gender affirmation and can be masculinizing or feminizing. Transgender men are at risk for gynecological malignancies but are an underserved group who experience discrimination and marginalization that contribute to health disparities. The risks may be complicated by a reluctance of transgender men to have routine gynecologic examinations because of anatomical dysphoria (a person's anatomy does not match their inner sense of self and gender identity). There is no evidence that hormone use leads to an increased risk of gynecological cancers in transgender men, but there are limited data available (Stenzel et al., 2020). Lesbian and bisexual women may have an increased risk for VC due to a higher prevalence of cigarette smoking and alcohol use than heterosexual women (Panganiban & O'Neil, 2021).

GLOBAL HEALTH CONSIDERATIONS

While VC occurs globally, no prevalence data are available.

ASSESSMENT

HISTORY. A complete reproductive history of the patient and the patient's mother is important. Because the average time between the start of symptoms and diagnosis is 6 to 12 months, take a reproductive history of the previous 12 months. Evaluate the patient for any risk factors. Ask if the patient's mother was taking DES when pregnant with the patient. Establish if the patient has uterine prolapse and has used a pessary. Determine a thorough history of the patient's physical symptoms, and note that up to 25% of patients are asymptomatic. One of the symptoms of VC is spontaneous vaginal bleeding after either intercourse or a pelvic examination. Vaginal discharge of a watery nature may also be present. Other symptoms include pain, urinary or rectal symptoms, pruritus, dyspareunia (pain during sexual intercourse), and groin masses.

Question the patient about any pain. Assess the use and effectiveness of any analgesics for pain. Document the location, onset, duration, and intensity of the pain. The patient may also describe urinary retention or urinary frequency if the lesion is near the bladder neck.

PHYSICAL EXAMINATION. Painless vaginal bleeding is the most common symptom, and some women have pelvic pain. Inspection of any bleeding or vaginal discharge, with particular attention to the characteristics and amount of bleeding, is imperative. Palpate the groin area to detect any masses. A pelvic examination may reveal an ulcerated vaginal lesion or vaginal prolapse. During the internal vaginal examination, all walls of the vagina need to be inspected and palpated to check for raised or hardened areas.

PSYCHOSOCIAL. A thorough assessment of each patient's perception of the disease process and the patient's coping mechanisms is required. Changes in sexual patterns and body image present stressors to patients. The family of the patient should also be included in the assessment to examine the extent of support they can provide. The patient's partner may experience anxiety over the potential loss of their partner or fear about altered patterns of sexuality.

Diagnostic Highlights

General Comments: VC is often well advanced before diagnosis is made.

Test	Normal Result	Abnormality With Condition	Explanation
Lugol solution applied to vaginal areas	Normal tissue stains	Areas that do not stain indicate suspect areas	Identifies areas to be biopsied; malignant cells lack glycogen and do not stain brown
Colposcopy	Normal structures visualized	Lesions noted	A magnifying lens is used to view the walls of the vagina to identify areas that should be biopsied
Biopsy	Benign	Malignant	Confirms the diagnosis

Diagnostic Highlights (continued)

Other Tests: CA-125 blood test may be elevated with some cancer types. Other tests include Papanicolaou (Pap) test, barium enema, computed tomography, and endoscopic tests to check for metastasis.

PRIMARY NURSING DIAGNOSIS

DIAGNOSIS. Ineffective sexuality pattern related to tissue damage, pain, and change in body structures as evidenced by dyspareunia, difficulty with sexual activity, change in sexual role, and/or alteration in sexual behavior

OUTCOMES. Sexual functioning; Knowledge: Sexual functioning; Anxiety level; Quality of life

INTERVENTIONS. Sexual counseling; Coping enhancement; Teaching: Sexuality; Anxiety reduction

PLANNING AND IMPLEMENTATION

Collaborative

Because the number of women with VC is small, large-scale clinical trials have not been established to determine the best treatment plan. Most often, the treatment of choice for VC is chemoradiation, a combination of chemotherapy with cisplatin concurrently with radiation therapy, delivered either by external beam or internally (brachytherapy). Treatment decisions are based on the extent of the lesion and the age and condition of the patient. Patients with early-stage disease are treated so that the malignant area is removed but the vagina is preserved. Laser surgery is often used during stages 0 and 1. Patients in the later stages of disease are treated with surgery or radiation. The type of surgery or radiation depends on the extent of the disease, the patient's desire to preserve a functional vagina, and the location of the lesion. A radical hysterectomy may be done with removal of the upper vagina and dissection of the pelvic nodes. Most patients receive total external pelvic radiation therapy to shrink the tumor before surgery or before internal intracavity radiation. Internal radiation with radium or cesium into the vagina can be provided for 2 to 3 days.

Collaborative postoperative management includes analgesics for pain relief and careful assessment for signs of postoperative infection or poor wound healing. Before discharge, discuss with the physician the patient's timetable for resumption of physical and sexual activity and be certain that the patient understands any limitations.

Pharmacologic Highlights

Medication or Drug Class	Dosage	Description	Rationale
Antineoplastic alkylating agents	Varies by drug	Cisplatin, carboplatin, fluorouracil, paclitaxel, docetaxel	May be given concurrently with radiation or for metastatic disease to kill cancer cells
Acetaminophen, NSAIDs, opioids, combinations of opioids and NSAIDs	Depends on the drug and patient condition and tolerance	Analgesics	Choice of drug depends on the severity of pain

Independent

The nursing management of patients with VC is challenging because of the interaction between the patient's physical and emotional needs. Provide information to the patient and family about what to expect from the treatment of choice, whether it is radiation, chemotherapy, surgery, or a combination of any of those options. If the patient has pain from either the surgical procedure or the disease process, explore pain-control methods such as imagery and breathing techniques to manage discomfort. The patient may be depressed and angry. Allow the patient to express anger and concerns without fear of being judged or discouraged. Provide a private place for the patient to discuss concerns with the nurse or significant others. Provide a list of support groups for the patient and partner.

Teach all female patients to be alert for signs of VC, particularly any unusual discharge or bleeding. Encourage all women over age 18 years to seek annual checkups, including gynecological examination. Women should also be taught to perform a genital self-examination at the same time they perform breast self-examination. Teach them to use a mirror to inspect for any changes in the female anatomy and to report any lesions, sores, lumps, or the presence of a persistent itch.

Evidence-Based Practice and Health Policy

Messelt, A., Thomaier, L., Jewett, P., Lee, H., Teoh, D., Everson-Rose, S., Blaes, A., & Vogel, R. (2021). Comparisons of emotional health by diagnosis among women with early stage gynecological cancers. *Gynecologic Oncology, 160*, 805–810.

- The authors set out to assess self-reported emotional health in a cohort of women with early-stage gynecological cancers and to explore differences based on primary cancer type. The authors analyzed survey data ($N = 242$) from a study of gynecological cancer patients treated at a cancer center. Variables included cancer-related quality of life, distress, depression, anxiety, posttraumatic stress disorder (PTSD), and posttraumatic growth. Potential confounders included age, stage, education, income, partner status, treatment status, and race.
- Patients with cervical and vaginal/vulvar cancers reported greater cancer-related distress, anxiety, and PTSD symptoms, and patients with endometrial cancer reported the lowest posttraumatic growth scores. No significant differences in cancer-related quality of life were observed based on primary care site. Women with early-stage gynecological cancer have different patterns of mental health disorders based on cancer location.

DOCUMENTATION GUIDELINES

- Physical response: Amount and characteristics of any vaginal bleeding or discharge, vital signs, pain (location, onset, duration, intensity, response to interventions)
- Emotional response: Support system, ability to deal with terminal diagnosis, emotional well-being; ability to cope with sexuality issues
- Patient's appetite, general appearance, and sleep patterns

DISCHARGE AND HOME HEALTHCARE GUIDELINES

TEACHING. Explain any procedures such as wound care or skin care that need to be continued at home. If the patient has had internal radiation therapy, teach the patient to use a stent or dilator to prevent vaginal stenosis; sexual intercourse also prevents vaginal stenosis. Teach the patient any limitations on the resumption of sexual activity or activity such as lifting or driving. Emphasize the importance of follow-up visits, which may include procedures such as x-rays, computed tomography scans, ultrasound, or magnetic resonance imaging. If the patient had vaginal reconstruction, teach the patient about the need for using a lubricant during sexual intercourse. Also inform the patient that, owing to neural pathways, the patient may feel as if the thigh is being stroked during intercourse.

COMPLICATIONS. Teach the patient with VC to report any further vaginal bleeding or signs of infection (fever, poor wound healing, fatigue, drainage with an odor).

COPING. Discuss helpful coping patterns with the patient if this was not done previously. Encourage the patient to be open about concerns and needs with family and friends. Provide the patient with a referral to the American Cancer Society if appropriate.

PREVENTION. Teach patients who have been exposed to DES to have examinations at least once annually regardless of the absence of symptoms of VC. Practicing safe sex will reduce the likelihood of contracting HPV, which is a contributing factor to the development of VC.

Vaginitis

DRG Category:	761
Mean LOS:	2.2 days
Description:	MEDICAL: Menstrual and Other Female Reproductive System Disorders Without Complication or Comorbidity or Major Complication or Comorbidity

Vaginitis is an inflammation of the vagina that includes three infections: candidiasis, trichomoniasis, and bacterial vaginosis. Approximately 7 million new cases of bacterial vaginosis occur each year in the United States. Generally, it occurs with a hormonal imbalance and an infection with a microorganism. Vaginitis is associated with changes in normal flora, alkaline pH, insertion of foreign bodies such as tampons and condoms, chemical irritations from douches and sprays, and medications such as broad-spectrum antibiotics. As women age, they also may develop genitourinary syndrome of menopause, which is atrophic vaginitis, or vulvovaginal atrophy, which affects approximately half of all postmenopausal women. Complications of vaginitis include pelvic inflammatory disease, increased susceptibility to HIV infection, endometritis, vaginal cellulitis, and in pregnancy, premature rupture of the membranes, preterm labor, low birth weight infants, and preterm delivery.

CAUSES

Trichomoniasis is an infection caused by *Trichomonas vaginalis*, a single-celled, anaerobic, protozoan parasite that is shaped like a turnip and has three or four anterior flagella. This parasite feeds on the vaginal mucosa and ingests bacteria and leukocytes. Among sexually active adolescents, approximately 2% to 3% have *T vaginalis*.

Vulvovaginal candidiasis is caused by *Candida albicans* (most often), *C glabrata*, or *C tropicalis*. These organisms are normally present in approximately 50% of women and cause no symptoms until the vaginal environment is altered. Contributing factors to altering the vaginal environment and causing an overgrowth of *Candida* are taking broad-spectrum antibiotics, which alter the protective bacterial flora; higher hormone levels from birth control pills and pregnancy, which increase glycogen stores that facilitate yeast growth; and diabetes mellitus or HIV infection, which alters the immune system. Repeated candida infections may be an indicator of unrecognized HIV infections.

Bacterial vaginosis (nonspecific vaginitis) is characterized by an imbalance in the vaginal flora (absence of the normal *Lactobacillus* species) and an overgrowth of *Gardnerella* and *Mycoplasma* species, and anaerobic bacteria. The anaerobe raises the vaginal pH, producing favorable conditions for bacterial growth. Cervicitis and urethritis are frequent manifestations of gonococcal or chlamydial infections and result from infection by *Neisseria gonorrhoeae* or *Chlamydia trachomatis*, but other agents may also cause vaginitis. Group B streptococcus is a cause of vaginitis, and patients culturing positive have vaginal mucosa with small, macular blotches of erythema. Group A streptococcus is rarely a concern in adults but is the causative factor in 21% of vulvovaginitis in prepubescent girls. Atrophic vaginitis may result from estrogen deficiency. As women age, a decrease in estrogen leads to the genitourinary syndrome of menopause, which is also called *atrophic vaginitis*. Risk factors for vaginitis include hormonal changes associated with pregnancy, birth control pills, or menopause; sexual activity; multiple partners; having a sexually transmitted infection (STI); antibiotics and corticosteroid; use of spermicides for birth control; and diabetes mellitus.

GENETIC CONSIDERATIONS

Heritable immune or inflammatory responses could be protective or could increase susceptibility.

SEX AND LIFE SPAN CONSIDERATIONS

Most women have some form of vaginitis at least once in their lifetime. Yeast infection is rare in the pediatric population but more common in adolescents. Vaginitis usually occurs in young, sexually active women after puberty and during pregnancy or when taking oral contraceptives.

HEALTH DISPARITIES AND SEXUAL/GENDER MINORITY HEALTH

Vaginitis is more common in female diabetics than in the general population. Females with multiple sex partners or who have impaired immune systems or HIV disease are also more susceptible. Incidence rates are higher in Black women and lower in Asian women. Little is known about the extent of STIs and bacterial vaginosis transmission in women who have sex with women, but bacterial vaginosis is more common than STIs in this group.

GLOBAL HEALTH CONSIDERATIONS

Vaginitis occurs in women around the world. No prevalence data are available.

⬛ ASSESSMENT

HISTORY. Elicit a history of the onset and description of symptoms, paying particular attention to the nature and amount of vaginal discharge (quantity, duration, color, consistency, and odor). Establish a history of external inflammation, pain, and pruritus. Patients may describe exertional dysuria, dyspareunia, and vulvular inflammation. Determine the medications that the patient is taking, paying particular attention to antibiotics, hormone replacement therapy, and contraceptives. Take a menstrual history and a medical history. Ask about the patient's rest, sleep, nutrition, exercise, and hygiene practices. Ask if the patient is pregnant or a diabetic, both of which place the patient at risk for vaginitis. Take a sexual history to determine the number of partners, the frequency of intercourse, the types of sexual practices, and the type of birth control that was used. Note that sexual history taking is sensitive and should be done by an experienced practitioner with great sensitivity. Notify the patient that some STIs are mandated to be reported to the state public health department, as are the names of the patient's sexual partner(s).

PHYSICAL EXAMINATION. The most common symptom is a **vaginal discharge, which may be frothy, thick, or malodorous.** The patient is likely to have external swelling of the vulva, internal inflammation, pain, and itching. Vaginal examination should take place under the following conditions: not during menses, no douching or vaginal sprays for 24 hours prior to examination, and no sexual intercourse without a condom for 24 hours prior to the examination. Physical examination generally reveals some type of discharge, such as frothy, malodorous, greenish-yellow, purulent vaginal discharge (trichomoniasis); thick, cottage cheese–like discharge (candidiasis); or malodorous, thin, grayish-white, foul, fishy odor discharge (bacterial). The external and internal genitalia are often reddened, inflamed, and painful on examination. Patients with candidiasis often have patches on their vaginal walls and cervix and signs of inflammation. Patients with trichomoniasis have a strawberry spot on the vaginal surface and cervix. Note that bacterial vaginitis may be asymptomatic with a normal vaginal mucosa. Palpate the patient's abdomen for tenderness or pain, which may indicate pelvic inflammatory disease.

PSYCHOSOCIAL. Psychosocial assessment should include evaluation of the patient's home situation and a sexual history. Ask patients about the type of contraception they and their partner use. Provide a private environment to allow patients to answer questions without being embarrassed.

Diagnostic Highlights

Test	Normal Result	Abnormality With Condition	Explanation
Saline wet mount (wet prep)	Negative for organism (not visualized under microscope)	Positive for organism (visualized under microscope); clue cells seen for bacterial vaginosis	Identifies the organism
Potassium hydroxide preparation (KOH) ("whiff test")	Negative for fungus/bacteria	Positive for fungus/bacteria; fishy, amine odor present for bacteria	Identifies candidiasis (Candida species) and bacteria
Vaginal pH	3.8–4.5	Candida: pH < 4.5; trichomonas: pH 5.0–7.0; bacterial vaginosis: pH 5.0–6.0	Identifies the type of infection

PRIMARY NURSING DIAGNOSIS

DIAGNOSIS. Risk for infection as evidenced by vaginal discharge, pain, and/or itching

OUTCOMES. Infection severity; Immune status; Knowledge: Infection management; Risk control: Infectious process; Symptom severity; Symptom control; Knowledge: Medication; Risk control: Sexually transmitted disease

INTERVENTIONS. Infection protection; Medication administration; Medication management; Perineal care; Teaching: Sexuality; Teaching: Safe sex; Teaching: Prescribed medication

PLANNING AND IMPLEMENTATION
Collaborative

Once vaginitis is diagnosed, the primary treatment is pharmacologic. Patients are told to stop using any douches and feminine hygiene sprays, to observe good nutrition, and to maintain healthy exercise patterns. Sexual intercourse may increase the severity. Many patients with candidiasis use over-the-counter treatment, which may or may not be effective.

Pharmacologic Highlights

Medication or Drug Class	Dosage	Description	Rationale
Antifungals	Varies with drug; given as a vaginal cream or suppository or PO	Miconazole nitrate, clotrimazole, nystatin, terconazole, butoconazole, fluconazole	Treat vaginal candidiasis
Metronidazole	Single 2-g dose PO for patient and sexual partner; 500 mg bid for 7 days for bacterial vaginosis	Antibacterial	Disrupts susceptible microorganisms and acts as a bactericidal drug; used to treat trichomoniasis or bacterial vaginosis

(highlight box continues on page 1206)

Pharmacologic Highlights (continued)

> Other Drugs: Bacterial vaginosis may also be treated with metronidazole vaginal gel, oral clindamycin, and clindamycin vaginal cream.

Independent

Encourage the patient to get adequate rest and nutrition. Encourage the patient to use appropriate hygiene techniques by wiping from front to back after urinating or defecating. Teach the patient to avoid wearing tight-fitting clothing (pantyhose, tight pants, or jeans) and to wear cotton underwear rather than synthetics. Teach the patient that douching is not recommended because it can flush out normal healthy microbes from the vagina, change the pH of the vagina, and make the patient more susceptible to vaginal infections. Explain to the patient that the risk of getting vaginal infections increases if one has sex with more than one person. Teach the patient to abstain from sexual intercourse until the infection is resolved. If the patient has *Trichomonas*, the partner needs treatment as well. Teach the patient that the inflammation caused by the *Trichomonas* increases susceptibility to HIV disease. Male circumcision may decrease the incidence of vaginitis in partners.

The pain and itching from vaginitis may be quite intense until the medication is effective. Some patients find that by applying wet compresses and then using a hair dryer on a cool setting several times a day provides some relief of itching. Other women find that a cool sitz bath provides comfort. For yeast infections, tepid sodium bicarbonate baths and applying cornstarch to dry the area may increase comfort during treatment. Be informed about which sexually transmitted diseases need to be reported to the local health department.

Evidence-Based Practice and Health Policy

Felix, T., Borges de Araujo, L., Von Dolinger de Brito Roder, D., & dos Santos Pedroso, R. (2020). Evaluation of vulvovaginitis and hygiene habits of women attended in primary health care units of the family. *International Journal of Women's Health, 12*, 49–56.

- The authors investigated the occurrence of vulvovaginal infections related to genital hygiene habits in women ($N = 100$). Data were obtained through medical records and also from in-person interviews.
- Women without vulvovaginal infections cleaned their genital areas three or more times a day after urination and defecation, whereas women with vulvovaginal infections cleaned their genital area twice a day. Women without vulvovaginal infections cleaned their genital area after a bowel movement in the front to back method, whereas women with vulvovaginal infections tended to use the opposite method. More than half the women who had vulvovaginitis wore cotton underwear (70%) and tight pants (83%) that allowed no ventilation.

DOCUMENTATION GUIDELINES

- Discomfort: Character, location, duration, precipitating factors
- Discharge: Odor, amount, color
- Medication management: Understanding of drug therapy, response to medications
- Response to teaching: Safe sex behaviors, response to lifestyle recommendations

DISCHARGE AND HOME HEALTHCARE GUIDELINES

Teach the patient how to maintain lifestyle changes regarding rest, nutrition, and medication management. Make sure the patient understands all aspects of the treatment regimen with particular attention to taking the full course of medication therapy. Make sure the patient understands the necessity of any follow-up visits.

Varicose Veins

DRG Category:	263
Mean LOS:	6.2 days
Description:	SURGICAL: Vein Ligation and Stripping
DRG Category:	299
Mean LOS:	5.1 days
Description:	MEDICAL: Peripheral Vascular Disorders With Major Complication or Comorbidity

Varicose veins (varicosities) are the visible manifestations of abnormally dilated, tortuous veins that have an underlying problem of reversed blood flow. Varicose veins occur most often in the lower extremities but can appear anywhere in the body. Primary varicosities are caused by incompetent valves in the superficial saphenous veins, whereas secondary varicosities are the result of impaired blood flow in the deep veins. Primary varicosities tend to occur in both legs, whereas secondary varicosities usually occur in only one leg. Normally, in a ladderlike fashion, perforator veins connect the deep vein and the superficial vein systems, promoting drainage of the lower extremities. Blood can be shunted from one system to the other in the event of either system being compressed. Incompetence in one system can lead to varicosities. The underlying problem of varicose veins is reverse venous flow, which is also known as *venous insufficiency syndrome*. Venous blood flow deviates from a normal flow path, flows in a retrograde or reversed direction, and causes congestion. The blood that is circulated by retrograde flow has already been circulated once, is poorly oxygenated, and contains lactate. It does not provide body tissues with helpful nutrients, and it contributes to congestion. Fluid accumulates in the extremity, causing swelling, inflammatory dermatitis, and skin breakdown.

Varicose veins are considered a chronic disease and, along with valvular incompetence, can progress to chronic venous insufficiency (CVI). Other complications include infection, cellulitis, discoloration, ulceration, thrombophlebitis, and loss of limbs.

CAUSES

The development of varicose veins is caused by a combination of heredity and environment. Primary varicose veins occur because of incompetent venous valves that result in venous hypertension. They occur most commonly at the saphenofemoral junction. Some people have an inherited tendency for elevated superficial venous pressures, and others have weakness of vein walls in the absence of elevated venous pressure. Several behavioral and environmental factors cause increased venous pressure and venous stasis that result in dilation and stretching of the vessel wall. Increased venous pressure results from being erect, which shifts the full weight of the venous column of blood to the legs. Prolonged standing increases venous pressure because leg muscle use is less; therefore, blood return to the heart is decreased. Secondary varicose veins result from deep venous thrombosis and its sequelae or congenital anatomical abnormalities.

Heavy lifting, genetic factors, obesity, thrombophlebitis, pregnancy, trauma, abdominal tumors, congenital or acquired arteriovenous fistulae, trauma to the legs, and congenital venous malformations are among the risk factors for varicose veins. Chronic liver diseases such as cirrhosis can cause varicosities in the rectum, abdomen, and esophagus.

GENETIC CONSIDERATIONS

Genetic transmission of varicose veins has been reported since the 1950s with various modes of transmission suggested. Several loci have been identified through linkage analysis (*FOXC2,*

LIPH), and candidate genes are being further investigated. Disruption of production of the gene coding for vascular endothelial growth factor (*VEGFA*) is one implicated mechanism. Family history accounts for an estimated 50% of the risk of disease. A recent study also implicated several other genes (*EBF1, STIM2, GATA2, NFATC2*, and *SOX9*) as candidates for further research as potential drug targets.

SEX AND LIFE SPAN CONSIDERATIONS

About 20% to 25% of all adults in the United States have varicose veins. Prevalence increases with age, peaking in the 50s and 60s and decreasing dramatically after age 70 years. In the population over age 30 years, four times as many women as men are affected. Varicose veins are more common in women because veins become more distensible under the effects of progesterone during the menstrual cycle and pregnancy. In the third trimester, the enlarged uterus compresses the vena cava, which leads to venous congestion, venous hypertension in the lower extremities, and pregnancy-related varicose veins, which may or may not resolve after pregnancy.

HEALTH DISPARITIES AND SEXUAL/GENDER MINORITY HEALTH

Ethnicity, race, and sexual/gender minority status have no known effect on the risk for varicose veins.

GLOBAL HEALTH CONSIDERATIONS

Varicose veins affect an estimated one in five persons in the world. The prevalence of venous disease and varicose veins is higher in developed than in developing countries, likely due to alterations in lifestyle, nutrition, body mass index, and physical activity. Prevalence statistics are not available from the developing world.

ASSESSMENT

HISTORY. Elicit a history of symptoms, paying particular attention to pain and discomfort, changes in appearance of vessels and skin, and complaints of a sensation of fullness or tingling of the lower extremities. Determine if the patient has experienced any bleeding from the varicose veins, as well as leg edema and dermatitis, pruritus, exercise intolerance, tenderness along the course of the vein, burning sensations, or cramping. Ask the patient to describe the amount of time each day spent standing. Take an occupational history with particular attention to those jobs that require long hours of walking or standing. Question the patient about lifetime weight changes, such as changes during pregnancy and sustained periods of being overweight. Ask the patient if there is a personal or family history of heart disease, obesity, thrombophlebitis or other vascular diseases, or varicose veins.

PHYSICAL EXAMINATION. Superficial veins can be inspected for **distension and prominence** as well as accompanying symptoms such as **ulceration, swelling, blanching**, and a **sense of fullness of the legs**. The number, severity, and type of varicosities determine the symptoms experienced by the individual. With the patient standing, examine the legs from the groin to the foot in good lighting. Inspect the ankles, measure the calves for differences, and assess for edema and discoloration. Time of examination is a factor because secondary varicosities are more symptomatic earlier in the day. Palpate both legs for dilated, bulbous, or corkscrew vessels. Patients may complain of heaviness, aching, edema, muscle cramps, increased fatigue of lower leg muscles, and itching. Determine if the patient has discoloration, ulcerations, translucent or shiny skin, and swelling of the legs. Severity of discomfort may be difficult to assess and is unrelated to the size of the varicosity.

PSYCHOSOCIAL. The patient with varicose veins has usually been dealing with a progressively worsening condition. Assess the patient for any problems with body image because of the changed appearance of skin surface that is caused by varicose veins. Question the patient to determine possible lifestyle adjustments to decrease symptoms. The patient may need job counseling or occupational retraining.

Diagnostic Highlights

General Comments: Incompetency of the deep and superficial veins can be diagnosed by several tests.

Test	Normal Result	Abnormality With Condition	Explanation
Duplex ultrasound (most commonly used diagnostic tool)	Normal Doppler venous signal with spontaneous respirations; no evidence of occlusion	Reversal of blood flow is noted as a result of incompetent valves in varicose veins	Detects moving red blood cells, thus demonstrating venous patency
Trendelenburg test	Veins fill from below in about 30 sec after the tourniquet is in place and the client stands; no further blood fills the veins from above after the tourniquet is released	Additional blood flows into the vein from above, indicating a valve is incompetent and has allowed a backflow of blood	Detects abnormal filling time and incompetent valves; veins normally fill from below; if the vein fills from above, the incompetent valve is allowing blood to flow backward
Magnetic resonance venography and magnetic resonance imaging	Normal blood flow without evidence of occlusion	Reversal of blood flow noted	Examines blood flow in extremities
Venography (in many centers, duplex ultrasonography has replaced this test but may be used in confusing cases)	No evidence of obstruction	Abnormal venous flow seen	X-ray study designed to locate thrombi in lower extremities

Other Tests: Contrast venography and color-flow duplex ultrasonography

PRIMARY NURSING DIAGNOSIS

DIAGNOSIS. Risk for ineffective peripheral tissue perfusion as evidenced by leg ulceration, swelling, blanching, and/or feelings of fullness in the legs

OUTCOMES. Tissue perfusion: Peripheral; Tissue integrity: Skin and mucous membranes; Wound healing: Primary intention; Knowledge: Wound management

INTERVENTIONS. Circulatory care: Venous insufficiency; Pain management: Chronic; Skin surveillance; Wound care; Exercise promotion

PLANNING AND IMPLEMENTATION
Collaborative

MEDICAL. The primary goal of treatment is the ablation of the pathways that have retrograde flow, thereby improving venous circulation, reducing injury, and reducing venous pressure. Pharmacologic treatment is not indicated for varicose veins. To give support and promote venous return, physicians recommend wearing graded elastic compression stockings. When obesity is a factor, a weight loss program is helpful in relieving symptoms. Experts also recommend that the patient stop smoking to prevent vasoconstriction of the vessels.

A nonsurgical treatment is the use of sclerotherapy for varicose and spider veins (telangiectasia, dilated or broken vessels near the skin's surface) to prevent retrograde blood flow. Sclerotherapy is palliative, not curative, and is often done for cosmetic reasons after surgical intervention. A sclerosing agent, such as sodium tetradecyl sulfate (Sotradecol) or polidocanol, is injected into the vein, followed by a compression bandage for a period of time. The expert application of this therapy is important because some of the underlying problems may be in deeper, subsurface veins. Newer techniques, such as radiofrequency ablation and endovenous laser therapy, are also available with expert consultation.

SURGICAL. A surgical approach to varicose veins is vein ligation (tying off) or stripping (removal) of the incompetent veins. Removal of the vein is performed through multiple short incisions from the ankle to the groin. A compression dressing is applied after surgery and is maintained for 3 to 5 days. Patients are encouraged to walk immediately postoperatively. Elevate the foot of the bed 6 to 9 inches to keep the leg above the heart when the postoperative client is in bed.

Pharmacologic Highlights

> No medications are generally used to treat varicose veins, except for analgesics following surgery.

Independent

Nursing interventions are aimed at educating the patient to decrease venous stasis, promote venous return, and prevent tissue injury. To prevent vein distention by compression of superficial veins, teach the patient to apply elastic support stockings before standing and to avoid long periods of standing. The patient should be encouraged to engage in an exercise program of walking to strengthen leg muscles. Teach the patient to avoid crossing the legs when sitting and to elevate the legs when sitting or lying down. The patient should be taught to observe the skin when removing graded elastic compression stockings to check for signs of irritation, edema, decreased nerve sensation, and discoloration. Preventive measures are similar to those for a patient with thrombophlebitis.

For patients who have had sclerotherapy, teaching should focus on activity restrictions. The patient should learn to avoid heavy lifting. Teach the patient to wait 24 to 48 hours after the procedure before showering and to avoid tub baths. Prepare patients by advising them to expect ecchymosis and some scarring, which will fade in several weeks. Caution patients that some residual brown staining may remain at the injection sites. Inform patients that the sclerotherapy may need to be repeated in other areas.

Evidence-Based Practice and Health Policy

Gong, J., Du, J., Han, D., Wang, X., & Qi, S. (2020). Reasons for patient non-compliance with compression stockings as a treatment for varicose veins in the lower limbs: A qualitative study. *PLoS ONE.* Advance online publication. https://doi.org/10.1371/journal.pone.0231218

• The authors wanted to explore the reasons for patients' nonadherence with graded elastic compression stockings (GECS) for treatment of lower limb varicose veins. The authors applied phenomenological analysis to understand the meaning and essence of participants' experiences in this specific situation—GECS treatment for varicose veins. Patients diagnosed with lower limb varicose veins and undergoing elective surgery who had low adherence to GECS therapy were invited to have semi-structured, in-depth, face-to-face interviews.

• Colaizzi method was employed to analyze the data to illuminate emerging themes associated with the reasons for patients' low adherence. Four themes emerged from the data: (1) gaps in the knowledge of GECS therapy as a treatment for lower limb varicose veins, (2) few recommendations from the doctors and nurses with the therapy not described in detail, (3) disadvantages of GECS such as the effort to put them on and the discomfort of wearing them, and (4) sociopsychological factors such as their price and appearance. The authors noted that practitioners and policy makers should share in the responsibility with patients to ensure that adherence occurs.

DOCUMENTATION GUIDELINES

• Physical assessment of both extremities: Presence of edema, pain, discoloration
• Reaction to the medications used for sclerotherapy and pain management
• Tolerance to activity and exercise

DISCHARGE AND HOME HEALTHCARE GUIDELINES

PREVENTION. To prevent worsening of varicosities, teach the patient to avoid prolonged standing in one place, to avoid sitting with the legs crossed, to elevate the legs frequently during the day, to wear compression stockings as ordered, and to drink 2 to 3 L of fluid daily. The patient should wear shoes that fit comfortably and are not too tight. Weight loss and smoking cessation need to be supported.

MEDICATIONS. Teach the patient the purpose, dosage, route, and side effects of any medications ordered.

COMPLICATIONS. Teach the patient to recognize and observe daily for signs of thrombophlebitis, which include redness, local swelling, warmth, discoloration (not related to surgery area), and back pain on bending. Teach the patient which signs to report to the physician.

POSTOPERATIVE COMPLICATIONS. Teach the patient to report any signs of infection, such as redness at incision sites or injection sites, severe pain, purulent drainage, fever, or swelling.

Ventricular Dysrhythmias

DRG Category:	309
Mean LOS:	2.9 days
Description:	MEDICAL: Cardiac Arrhythmia and Conduction Disorders With Complication or Comorbidity

A ventricular dysrhythmia is a disturbance in the normal rhythm of the electrical activity of the heart that arises in the ventricles (Fig. 1). Experts estimate that sudden cardiac death occurs in approximately 300,000 cases each year in the United States, and up to one-third are attributable to ventricular fibrillation (VF) (Fig. 3). People who have survived a major cardiac event, such as myocardial infarction or cardiac arrest, are at increased risk for VF up to 2 years after the event. Types of ventricular dysrhythmias include premature ventricular contractions (PVCs), which can have one focus or can arise from multiple foci; ventricular tachycardia (VT) (Fig. 2), which can lead to VF or sudden cardiac death; VF, which results in death if not treated immediately; and ventricular asystole (cardiac standstill) (Fig. 4), in which no cardiac output occurs and full cardiopulmonary arrest results (Table 1).

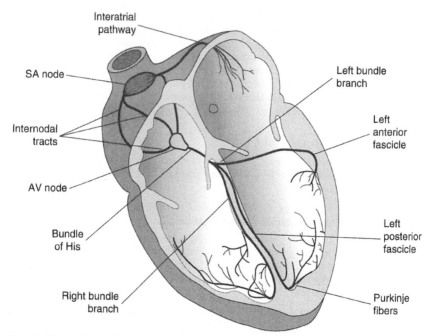

Figure 1 Electrical Conduction System of the Heart

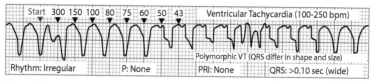

Figure 2 Ventricular Tachycardia

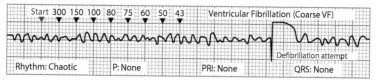

Figure 3 Ventricular Fibrillation

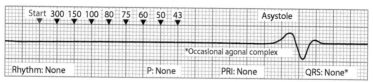

Figure 4 Asystole

• TABLE 1 Types of Ventricular Dysrhythmias

TYPE	DESCRIPTION	CAUSE
PVC	Early ectopic beats that arise from the ventricles Atrial rate: Regular Ventricular rate: Irregular QRS complex: Wide and distorted, usually longer than 0.14 sec Occurrence: Singly, in pairs, or alternating with regular sinus beats	Heart failure Myocardial infarction Cardiac trauma Myocardial irritation from pacemaker or pulmonary artery catheter insertion Hypercapnia, hypokalemia, or hypocalcemia Medication toxicity (digitalis, aminophylline, tricyclic antidepressants, beta-adrenergic stimulants) Caffeine, tobacco, or alcohol use; physiological and psychological stress
VT	Three or more premature ventricular contractions in a row dissociated from the atrial contraction P waves: In sustained VT, none are identifiable; usually buried within aberrant, bizarre ventricular contractions Ventricular rate: Usually 100–220 beats per min Ventricular rhythm: May start and stop suddenly	Myocardial ischemia Myocardial infarction Rheumatic heart disease Mitral valve prolapse Heart failure Cardiomyopathy Electrolyte imbalances such as hypokalemia, hypomagnesemia, and hypercalcemia or hypocalcemia Medication toxicities: Digitalis, procainamide, epinephrine, or quinidine
VF	Disorganized, ineffective contraction of the ventricle P waves: None QRS complex: None Ventricular rhythm: Chaotic rhythm with a wavy baseline	Coronary heart disease, myocardial infarction, myocardial ischemia, cardiomyopathy, heart failure, low ejection fraction Medication toxicities: Digitalis, procainamide, epinephrine, or quinidine
Ventricular asystole (cardiac standstill)	Atrial rhythm: None P, QRS, T waves: None Ventricular rhythm: None	Myocardial ischemia Myocardial infarction Valvular disease Severe heart failure pH and electrolyte imbalances (severe acidosis, hypokalemia, or hyperkalemia in particular) Electric shock Pulmonary embolism Cardiac rupture Cardiac tamponade Cocaine overdose

Most sudden deaths are caused by either VT or VF. Many patients have nonfatal VT, and it is often associated with chronic heart failure, cardiomyopathy, and ischemic heart disease. VF causes approximately 50% of deaths that occur from coronary heart disease (CHD). The highest incidence of VF occurs in people with chronic heart failure with low ejection fractions, and people who are recovering after a cardiac arrest or a myocardial infarction. Typically, VF occurs in the first 24 months after these events. Complications include syncope, brain injury, seizures, myocardial infarction, acute renal insufficiency, or sudden death.

CAUSES

Conditions associated with cardiac dysrhythmias include myocardial ischemia, myocardial infarction, structural heart disease such as cardiomyopathy, inherited conduction disturbances, electrolyte imbalances (hypokalemia, hypocalcemia, hypomagnesemia), drug toxicity, and degeneration of the conduction system by necrosis. A dysrhythmia can be the result of a disturbance in the ability of the myocardial cell to conduct an impulse (conductivity), a disturbance in the ability to initiate and maintain an inherent rhythm spontaneously (automaticity), or a combination of both. Risk factors include CHD, use of recreational drugs such as cocaine, smoking, electrolyte abnormalities, family history of rhythm disorders, and toxicities from medications such as digitalis, procainamide, epinephrine, aminophylline, tricyclic antidepressants, beta-adrenergic stimulants, or quinidine.

GENETIC CONSIDERATIONS

Mutations in a variety of genes have been associated with the production of familial ventricular dysrhythmias (*LQT1, LMNA, MVP*). The long QT syndrome (caused by mutations in potassium, sodium channels, and an anchoring protein) can result in a polymorphic VT called torsades de pointes. Long QT can be passed as an autosomal dominant (Romano-Ward) or recessive (Jervell and Lange-Nielsen) trait. Brugada syndrome is caused by a sodium channel mutation (*SCN5A*) and results in episodes of VF and sudden cardiac death. Catecholaminergic polymorphic VT results from defects in calcium or potassium channel genes.

SEX AND LIFE SPAN CONSIDERATIONS

Although these rhythms can occur at any point in the life span and in both sexes, they are more common in older adults because of the increased incidence of cardiac diseases, atherosclerosis, and degenerative hypertrophy of the left ventricle. Intrinsic degeneration of the conduction system and a higher propensity toward drug toxicity because of altered metabolism and excretion are contributing factors as patients age. In addition, many of the medications that aging people take to manage heart failure (digitalis and diuretics in particular) place them at risk for drug toxicities and electrolyte imbalances. Men are three times more likely than women to have VF, and slightly more men than women have VT. VT and VF are unusual in children. Women are less likely to receive placement of resynchronization therapy devices with defibrillator as compared to men, creating health disparities for women.

HEALTH DISPARITIES AND SEXUAL/GENDER MINORITY HEALTH

The Centers for Disease Control and Prevention report that 11.5% of White persons, 9.5% of Black persons, 7.4% of Hispanic persons, and 6.0% of Asian persons have heart disease. Black persons have higher morbidity and mortality rates of CHD and sudden cardiac death; the burden for Black persons is higher than for White persons because of the prevalence of hypertension, obesity, metabolic syndrome, and Black, Indigenous, and other people of color are known to receive care less often guided by standard cardiac care guidelines than White persons. Unless patients have health insurance, White patients are more likely to receive coronary angiograms and other coronary interventions than Black and Hispanic patients. Black and Hispanic persons are also less likely to be referred to cardiologists and cardiac surgeons than White persons

(Batchelor et al., 2019). In the United States, Asian Indian persons have a higher prevalence of CHD than White persons.

Transgender is a term used to describe persons whose gender identity is different from their sex assigned at birth. Approximately 1% of the U.S. population identify themselves as transgender. Sexual and gender minority persons have higher odds for multiple chronic conditions, cancer, and poor quality of life and are more apt to have disabilities than cisgender males and females. (Cisgender is a term used to describe persons whose gender identity and gender expression are aligned with their assigned sex listed on their birth certificate.) Gender-affirming hormone therapy is the use of hormone therapy for gender transition or gender affirmation and can be masculinizing or feminizing. It may also affect cardiovascular health in transgender females. Several case reports suggest that feminizing hormone therapy may place transgender women at risk for dysrhythmias. In a large sample, researchers have found that transgender men and women are more likely to be overweight than cisgender women. Compared to cisgender women, transgender women reported higher rates of diabetes, ischemic stroke, angina/coronary disease, and myocardial infarction. Gender-nonconforming men and women reported higher odds of myocardial infarction than cisgender women. Transgender women also had higher rates of any cardiovascular disease than cisgender men (Cacerese, Jackman, et al., 2020; Connelly et al., 2019). While large-scale studies are not available, these factors may place some sexual and gender minority persons at risk for ventricular dysrhythmias.

GLOBAL HEALTH CONSIDERATIONS

While people around the world have ventricular dysrhythmias, no data are available on prevalence. VT and VF are common throughout most of the developed world but are less common in developing countries. VF is prevalent worldwide, and the largest number of people with VF live in the northern hemisphere; this prevalence is likely due to nutritional, occupational, and lifestyle factors as well as heredity.

ASSESSMENT

HISTORY. If the patient is unable to provide a history of the life-threatening event, obtain it from a witness. Many patients with suspected cardiac dysrhythmias describe a history of symptoms indicating periods of decreased cardiac output. They may report dizziness, syncope, fatigue, dyspnea, palpitations, diaphoresis, chest pain, and activity intolerance. Question patients to determine if they have seen a medical provider recently; many patients who experience VT or VF have seen their physician recently for vague complaints such as fatigue, palpitations, or shortness of breath. In particular, question the patient or family about the onset, duration, and characteristics of the symptoms and the events that precipitated them. Determine if the patient has experienced a previous myocardial infarction, syncope, cardiomyopathy, or valvular disease. Obtain a complete history of all illnesses, dietary and fluid restrictions, activity restrictions, and a current medication history.

PHYSICAL EXAMINATION. Patients with VT may be awake and symptomatic. Common symptoms are **dizziness, fatigue, activity intolerance, a "fluttering" in their chest, shortness of breath**, and **chest pain**. They may have syncope from decreased perfusion to the brain, pallor, diaphoresis, hypotension, and dyspnea from diminished perfusion to the lungs. Changes in cerebral perfusion may be manifested by anxiety, agitation, lethargy, or coma. Lethal dysrhythmias such as VF and ventricular asystole usually lead to a **full cardiopulmonary arrest**. If the patient does not have adequate airway, breathing, or circulation (ABCs), initiate cardiopulmonary resuscitation (CPR) as needed. If the patient is stable, complete a general head-to-toe physical examination. Pay particular attention to the cardiovascular system by inspecting the skin for changes in color, presence of peripheral pulses, or presence of edema. Auscultate the heart rate and rhythm and note the first and second heart sounds and also any adventitious sounds. Auscultate the blood pressure. Perform a full respiratory assessment and note any adventitious breath sounds or labored breathing. Perform a neurological examination to determine level of responsiveness and presence of reflexes.

PSYCHOSOCIAL. Ventricular dysrhythmias may cause a life-threatening event and a great deal of anxiety and fear because of the potential alterations to current lifestyle and functioning. Assess the ability of the patient and significant others to cope. If the dysrhythmia requires a pacemaker insertion or an automatic implantable cardioverter defibrillator (ICD), determine the patient's response.

Diagnostic Highlights

Test	Normal Result	Abnormality With Condition	Explanation
12-lead electro-cardiogram (ECG)	Regular sinus rhythm	Varies with dysrhyth-mias (Table 1)	Detects specific conduction defects; monitors the patient's cardiac response to electrolyte imbalances, drug effects, and toxicities

Other Tests: Resting and exercise ECG, Holter monitoring, serum electrolytes, serum calcium, ionized calcium, serum magnesium, cardiac enzymes, creatine kinase, complete blood count, arterial blood gases, toxic screen, thyroid-stimulating hormone, B-type natriuretic peptide, electrophysiological studies, echocardiogram, chest x-ray, nuclear imaging to assess myocardial damage

PRIMARY NURSING DIAGNOSIS

DIAGNOSIS. Risk for decreased cardiac and ineffective cerebral tissue perfusion as evidenced by dizziness, decreased level of consciousness, chest pain, shortness of breath, pulselessness, apnea, shock, and/or cardiopulmonary arrest

OUTCOMES. Respiratory status; Circulation status; Cardiac pump effectiveness; Cardiopulmonary status; Tissue perfusion: Cardiac, Pulmonary, Cerebral, Peripheral; Vital signs, Neurological status

INTERVENTIONS. Airway management; Dysrhythmia management; Emergency care; Vital signs monitoring; Cardiac care; Oxygen therapy; Fluid/electrolyte management; Fluid monitoring; Shock management: Cardiac; Medication administration; Resuscitation

PLANNING AND IMPLEMENTATION
Collaborative

It is important to follow the most current Advanced Cardiac Life Support algorithms, which are updated regularly based on scientific evidence and best practices. In out-of-hospital resuscitations, the American Heart Association recommends chest-compression-only CPR, also known as *cardiocerebral resuscitation*. If the patient is in full arrest, use current CPR guidelines. CPR for patients in the hospital is performed with a compression-to-ventilation ratio of 30:2 until the defibrillator arrives. If the patient is not in full arrest, the first step of treatment is to maintain ABCs. Low-flow oxygen by nasal cannula or mask may decrease the rate of PVCs. Higher flow rates are usually needed for the patient with VT, and if pulseless VT or VF occurs, the patient needs immediate endotracheal intubation, and support of breathing with a manual resuscitator bag. The most important intervention for a patient with pulseless VT or VF is rapid defibrillation (electrical countershock). If a defibrillator is not available, and the arrest was witnessed, begin chest compressions and, as soon as possible, give a sharp blow to the precordium (precordial thump or thumpversion) to try to convert VT or VF into a regular sinus rhythm. Maintain CPR between all other interventions for patients without adequate breathing and circulation.

The drugs of choice to manage PVCs or VT with a pulse depend on the morphology of the ventricular beats and include amiodarone, lidocaine, or depending on the morphology of the electrocardiogram, magnesium sulfate. If the patient has pulseless VT or VF, the treatment of choice is to defibrillate the patient as discussed previously, intubate the patient, administer epinephrine, and then administer amiodarone or lidocaine. If the patient has electrolyte imbalances, or they are suspected, supplemental potassium, calcium, and/or magnesium is administered IV. Procainamide may be given to treat sustained ventricular tachycardia or recurrent VF if other interventions have not been successful. Long-term management may be done by ICDs.

The patient with ventricular asystole is managed with CPR. Initiate CPR, intubate the patient immediately, provide oxygenated breathing with a manual resuscitator bag, and obtain IV access. Confirm the ventricular asystole in a second lead to make sure the patient is not experiencing VF, which would indicate the need to defibrillate. If the rhythm still appears as ventricular asystole, administer epinephrine every 3 to 5 minutes in an attempt to have the patient regain an effective cardiac rhythm. Depending on setting and expertise, practitioners may consider a transcutaneous or transvenous pacemaker, but if efforts do not convert the cardiac rhythm, the physician may terminate resuscitation efforts.

Pharmacologic Highlights

Medication or Drug Class	Dosage	Description	Rationale
Epinephrine	1 mg IV or intraosseous (IO) 1:10,000 solution; repeat every 3–5 min	Catecholamine	Cardiac stimulant
Amiodarone	VF and pulseless VT: 300 mg IV or IO after dose of epinephrine if no initial response to defibrillation; repeat 150 mg IV in 3–5 min; Wide complex QRS: 150 mg IV with calcium chloride 1 gm IV	Antidysrhythmic agent	For VF and pulseless VT; prolongs action potential and repolarization
Lidocaine	1–1.5 mg/kg of body weight IV	Antidysrhythmic agent	Manages PVCs or VT with a pulse; inhibits conduction of nerve impulses

Other Drugs: Vasopressors/sympathomimetics (epinephrine, vasopressin, dopamine, norepinephrine), atropine, procainamide, sodium bicarbonate, propranolol, electrolytes (magnesium sulfate, calcium chloride)

Independent

As with all potentially serious conditions, the first priority is to maintain the patient's ABCs. If the patient is not having a cardiopulmonary arrest, maximize the amount of oxygen available to the heart muscle. During periods of abnormal ventricular conduction, encourage the patient to rest in bed until the symptoms are treated and subside. Remain with the patient to ensure rest and to allay anxiety.

For some patients with asymptomatic short runs of PVCs, strategies to reduce stress help limit the incidence of the dysrhythmia. A referral to a support group or counselor skilled at stress reduction techniques is sometimes helpful. Teach the patient to reduce the amount of caffeine intake in the diet. Explain the need to read the ingredients of over-the-counter medications to limit caffeine intake. If appropriate, encourage the patient to become involved in an exercise program or a smoking-cessation group.

Patients who experience dysrhythmias are often facing alterations in their lifestyle and job functions. Provide information about the dysrhythmia, the precipitating factors, and mechanisms to limit the dysrhythmia. If the patient is placed on medications, teach the patient and significant others the dosage, route, action, and side effects. If the patient is at risk for electrolyte imbalance, teach the patient any dietary considerations to prevent electrolyte depletion of vital substances.

The most devastating outcome of a ventricular dysrhythmia is sudden cardiac death. If the patient survives the episode, provide an honest accounting of the incident and support the patient's emotional response to the event. If the patient does not survive, remain with the family and significant others, support their expression of grief without being judgmental if it varies from your own ways to express grief, and notify a chaplain or clinical nurse specialist if appropriate to provide additional support.

Evidence-Based Practice and Health Policy

Long, B., Brady, W., Bridwell, R., Ramzy, M., Montrief, T., Singh, M., & Gottlieb, M. (2021). Electrocardiographic manifestations of COVID-19. *American Journal of Emergency Medicine*, *41*, 96–103.

- The authors note that although COVID-19 is a lower respiratory condition, the disease can also impact the cardiovascular system and lead to abnormal electrocardiographic findings. Up to 90% of patients who are critically ill with COVID-19 have cardiac dysrhythmias. There are a number of causes, such as cytokine storm, hypoxic injury, electrolyte imbalances, microthrombi, or direct endothelial injury.
- Although sinus tachycardia is the most common dysrhythmia during COVID-19, ventricular dysrhythmias such as ventricular tachycardia and fibrillation often occur. Rhythm presentations that are associated with poor outcomes include atrial fibrillation, ST segment and T wave changes, ventricular tachycardia, and ventricular fibrillation.

DOCUMENTATION GUIDELINES

- Cardiopulmonary assessment: Heart and lung sounds, cardiac rate and rhythm on the cardiac monitor, blood pressure, quality of the peripheral pulses, capillary refill, respiratory rate and rhythm
- Activity tolerance and ability to perform self-care
- Complications: Dizziness, syncope, hypotension, electrolyte imbalance, loss of consciousness, uncorrected cardiac dysrhythmias, ineffective patient or family coping

DISCHARGE AND HOME HEALTHCARE GUIDELINES

Explain to the patient the importance of taking all medications. If the patient needs periodic laboratory work to monitor the effects of the medications (e.g., serum electrolytes or drug levels), discuss with the patient the frequency of these laboratory visits and where to have the tests drawn. Explain the actions, the route, the side effects., the dosage, and the frequency of the medication. Discuss methods for the patient to remember to take the medications, such as numbered medication boxes or linking the medications with other activities such as meals or sleep. Teach the patient how to take the pulse and recognize an irregular rhythm. Explain that the patient needs to notify the healthcare provider when symptoms such as irregular pulse, chest pain, shortness of breath, and dizziness occur.

Stress the importance of stress reduction and smoking cessation. If the patient has a pacemaker or an ICD, provide teaching about the settings, signs of pacemaker failure (dizziness, syncope, palpitations, fast or slow pulse rate), and when to notify the physician. Explain any environmental hazards based on the manufacturer's recommendations, such as heavy machinery and airport security checkpoints. Make sure the patient understands the schedule for the next physician's checkup. If the patient has an ICD, encourage the patient to keep a diary of the number of times the device discharges. Most physicians want to be notified the first time the ICD discharges after implantation.

Volvulus

DRG Category:	329
Mean LOS:	13.1 days
Description:	SURGICAL: Major Small and Large Bowel Procedures With Major Complication or Comorbidity
DRG Category:	389
Mean LOS:	4.0 days
Description:	MEDICAL: Gastrointestinal Obstruction With Complication or Comorbidity

Volvulus, from the Latin for "to twist," is a mechanical obstruction of the bowel that occurs when the intestine twists at least 180 degrees on itself and is one of the leading causes of large bowel obstruction in the United States. The most common anatomical sites for volvulus are the sigmoid colon (80%), the cecum (15%), the transverse colon (3%), and the splenic flexure (2%). Volvulus is a disease associated with immobility and institutionalization. Experts estimate that approximately 50% of people with volvulus are admitted to the hospital from psychiatric and long-term care institutions.

Although volvulus can occur in either the large or the small bowel, the most common areas in adults are the sigmoid and ileocecal areas. Compression of the blood vessels occurs, and an obstruction both proximal and distal to the volvulus also occurs. The direction of the chyme flow is obstructed, but the secretions of bile, pancreatic juices, and gastric juices continue. The internal pressure of the bowel rises when fluids and gases accumulate, causing a temporary stimulation of peristalsis that increases the distention of the bowel and causes colicky pain. The bowel wall becomes edematous and capillary permeability increases, causing fluid and electrolytes to enter the peritoneal cavity.

These changes place the patient at risk for severe electrolyte imbalance, decreased circulating blood volume, and development of peritonitis. When the volvulus is near or within the ileum, regurgitation and vomiting increase fluid, electrolyte, and acid-base imbalances. Blockage within the cecum or large intestine leads to bowel distention and eventual perforation. Reflux can occur if the ileocecal valve is incompetent. Other complications include perforation of the bowel, which releases bacteria and endotoxins into the peritoneal cavity, endotoxic shock, and death.

CAUSES

In some patients, the cause of volvulus is never discovered. In most cases, however, the condition occurs at the site of an anomaly, tumor, diverticulum, foreign body (dietary fiber, fruit pits), or surgical adhesion. Volvulus can occur in people with chronic constipation who have sigmoid elongation, resulting in extra looping and lengthening of the colon or can be caused by a birth defect during fetal development that causes a malrotation leading to symptoms early in life. Drugs that contribute to decreased motility include excessive use of laxatives and psychotropic drugs. Risk factors include laxative misuse, high-fiber diets that overload the sigmoid colon, immobility, prolonged bedrest, nursing home admission, Parkinson disease, and spinal cord injury.

GENETIC CONSIDERATIONS

There have been several cases of intestinal volvulus occurring in several members of the same family, so it appears that in at least a few cases, it may be familial. No gene mutations have yet been identified.

SEX AND LIFE SPAN CONSIDERATIONS

Intestinal obstructions may occur at any age. More male infants than female have volvulus in the first week of life. Volvulus can occur in infants with cystic fibrosis because of a meconium ileus. In children, the most common site is the small bowel. Older people are at risk because of the increased incidence of constipation and diverticula in that age group. Cecal volvulus is most common in adults, particularly women in their 50s, whereas sigmoid volvulus is more common in older adults and children.

HEALTH DISPARITIES AND SEXUAL/GENDER MINORITY HEALTH

Ethnicity, race, and sexual/gender minority status have no known effect on the risk for volvulus.

GLOBAL HEALTH CONSIDERATIONS

Volvulus in adults has a much higher frequency in Africa, Asia, and Middle Eastern, Eastern European, and South American countries as compared to those in North America and Western Europe because of very high-fiber diets in those geographic regions. More male children than female children in these regions have sigmoid colon volvulus. Chagas disease in Brazil causes a significant number of cases in people of all ages.

▓ ASSESSMENT

HISTORY. Many patients admitted with volvulus are debilitated and older adults, making history-taking a challenge. If possible, take a complete history of the patient's eating patterns, bowel patterns, onset of symptoms, and distention. Elicit a gastrointestinal history from the patient, paying particular attention to those with a history of constipation and Meckel diverticulum (a blind pouch found in the lower portion of the ileum). Elicit information about the patient's medications. Ask if the patient has had abdominal surgery because adhesions make the patient at risk for volvulus. Ask the patient to describe any symptoms, which may include abdominal distention, thirst, and abdominal pain. Patients may also report anorexia and food intolerance, with vomiting after eating. Late signs include colicky abdominal pain of sudden onset and vomiting with sediment and a fecal odor. The patient may also describe chronic constipation with no passage of gas or feces, or when a stool is passed, there may be blood in it.

PHYSICAL EXAMINATION. The patient usually appears in **acute distress from abdominal pain and pressure.** The patient's abdomen appears distended, and the patient may show signs of dehydration such as poor skin turgor and dry mucous membranes. Measure the abdominal girth to identify the amount of distension. When you auscultate the abdomen, you may hear no bowel sounds at all, indicating a paralytic ileus, or you may hear high-pitched peristaltic rushes with high metallic tinkling sounds, indicating intestinal obstruction. You may be able to palpate an abdominal mass, although the patient experiences pain and guarding on palpation.

PSYCHOSOCIAL. The patient may have lived with constipation for a long time and may be embarrassed to discuss the issue of bowel movements or may hold certain beliefs about the frequency and consistency of bowel movements. Assess the patient's self-image and the patient's ability to cope with possible body disfigurement from surgical correction. If the patient is an adult, determine the patient's ability to provide self-care.

Diagnostic Highlights

Test	Normal Result	Abnormality With Condition	Explanation
Abdominal x-rays	Normal abdominal structures	Distended loops of bowel; may be normal x-ray	Identifies blockage of lumen of bowel with distal passage of fluid and air (partial) or complete obstruction

Diagnostic Highlights (continued)

Test	Normal Result	Abnormality With Condition	Explanation
Computed tomography scan	Normal abdominal structures	Location of the site of the torsion and evidence of resulting ischemia; upward displacement of the appendix with large bowel obstruction is a definitive sign of cecal volvulus	Locates the site of the twisted bowel
Barium enema	Normal abdominal structures	Partial or complete blockage of lumen of bowel	Identifies site of volvulus; should not be used if there are signs of peritonitis

Other Tests: Complete blood count, colonoscopy, sigmoidoscopy, stool heme test

PRIMARY NURSING DIAGNOSIS

DIAGNOSIS. Acute pain related to inflammation as evidenced by self-reports of pain, facial grimacing, and/or protective behavior

OUTCOMES. Comfort status; Pain control; Pain level; Symptom severity; Symptom control; Knowledge: Pain management

INTERVENTIONS. Pain management: Acute; Analgesic administration; Medication management; Patient-controlled analgesia assistance; Teaching: Prescribed medication

PLANNING AND IMPLEMENTATION
Collaborative

If the patient does not have peritonitis, sigmoidoscopy or colonoscopy and rectal tube placement can successfully decompress the bowel. The objective of treatment is to relieve the obstruction and ensure circulation to the bowel. Often the patient is then prepped for surgery in case it is necessary. Emergency surgery occurs for adult patients with sigmoid volvulus who have evidence of ischemic bowel or peritonitis. In cases where the cause is not apparent, it may be discovered only during surgery. Vascular and mechanical obstructions are relieved by the surgeon, who excises the affected bowel. Depending on the location and extent of the bowel resection, a colostomy or bypass procedure may be performed.

The collaborative postoperative management often includes IV analgesia with narcotic agents or patient-controlled analgesia, antibiotic therapy, nasogastric drainage to low continuous or intermittent suction, and IV fluids. Monitor the patient for complications such as wound infection (fever, wound drainage, poor wound healing), pneumonia (lung congestion, shallow breathing, fever, productive cough), and bleeding at the surgical site.

Pharmacologic Highlights

Medication or Drug Class	Dosage	Description	Rationale
Antibiotics	Varies with drug	Broad spectrum	Prevent peritonitis or postoperative infection

Other Drugs: Patient-controlled anesthesia in adults

Independent

When the patient is first admitted to the hospital, the patient is in acute discomfort. Usually, strategies are initiated immediately to correct the underlying condition rather than provide analgesia to minimize the discomfort. Explain to the patient that large doses of analgesics mask the symptoms of volvulus and may place the patient at risk for perforation. Remain with the patient as much as possible until the decision is made to use surgical or nonsurgical treatment to correct volvulus. Provide a brief explanation of all procedures and what the patient can expect postoperatively. Have the patient practice coughing and deep breathing, and reassure the patient that postoperative analgesia will be available to manage pain. When the patient returns from surgery, use pillows to splint the abdomen during coughing and deep-breathing exercises. Get the patient out of bed for chair rest and ambulation as soon as the patient can tolerate activity. Notify the physician when bowel sounds resume, and gradually advance the patient from a clear liquid diet to solid food. If the patient experiences any food intolerance at all (nausea, vomiting, pain), notify the surgeon immediately.

If a colostomy or other surgical diversion is needed, work with the patient to accept the change in body image and body function. Allow the patient to verbalize feelings about the ostomy and begin a gradual program to assist the patient to assume self-care. Be honest and explain whether the ostomy is temporary or permanent. If the patient or significant other is going to care for the ostomy at home and is having problems coping, contact the enterostomal therapist or clinical nurse specialist to consult with the patient. Provide teaching about strategies to limit constipation, such as diet, adequate fluid intake, and appropriate exercise.

Evidence-Based Practice and Health Policy

Chung, J., Kim, W., & Kim, S. (2021). Comparison of total midgut volvulus and segmental volvulus in neonates. *Journal of Pediatric Surgery, 56,* 1375–1377.

- This retrospective study divided infants after surgery for small bowel volvulus a month after birth into the following groups: total midgut volvulus ($n = 27$) and segmental volvulus ($n = 17$). Clinical characteristics, diagnosis, management, and outcomes were compared between the two groups. There was no significant difference between groups with regard to gender and gestational age. All cases of total midgut volvulus were associated with malrotation, while those with segmental volvulus were not.
- There was a significant difference for patients diagnosed with total midgut volvulus presenting with bilious vomiting, while those in the small bowel volvulus group presented with abdominal distention. The presentation of symptoms began in the total midgut volvulus at 4 days after birth, while the small bowel volvulus group showed symptoms on day of birth. When evaluating for coexisting congenital anomalies, cardiac anomalies were mainly seen in the small bowel volvulus group while nonexistent in the total midgut volvulus patients. Although this study was small, bilious vomiting was a classic sign of malrotation in this cohort, and it should be suspected until ruled out.

DOCUMENTATION GUIDELINES

- Physical response: Abdominal assessment (return of bowel sounds, relief of distention, and elimination patterns), vital signs, intake and output, pertinent laboratory findings
- Comfort: Location, type, and degree of pain; response to analgesia and other interventions
- Nutrition: Presence of nausea and vomiting, food tolerance, daily weights
- Postoperative recovery: Status of incisions and dressings, presence of complications (infection, lung collapse, hemorrhage), intractable pain

DISCHARGE AND HOME HEALTHCARE GUIDELINES

Teach the patient about strategies to maintain healthy bowel function, such as diet, exercise, drinking fluids, and avoiding laxatives. Provide phone numbers for agencies that can be supportive, such as colostomy and ileostomy groups. Encourage the patient to report any recurrence of symptoms immediately. Encourage patients who have had surgery to avoid strenuous activity for up to 6 weeks.

Index

Note: Page numbers followed by *f* refer to figures, *t* refer to tables, and *b* refer to boxes.